Interpretation of Diagnostic Tests

EIGHTH EDITION

Interpretation of Diagnostic Tests

EIGHTH EDITION

Jacques Wallach, M.D.

Clinical Professor of Pathology
State University of New York
Health Science Center at Brooklyn
Emeritus Attending Pathologist
Kings County Hospital Center
Brooklyn, New York

 Wolters Kluwer | Lippincott Williams & Wilkins
Health
Philadelphia · Baltimore · New York · London
Buenos Aires · Hong Kong · Sydney · Tokyo

Acquisitions Editor: Sonya Seigafuse
Managing Editor: Nancy Winter
Developmental Editor: Dvora Konstant
Marketing Manager: Kimberly Schonberger
Project Manager: Nicole Walz
Manufacturing Coordinator: Kathy Brown
Design Coordinator: Stephen Druding
Cover Designer: Joseph DePinho
Production Services: TechBooks, Inc.
Printer: R. R. Donnelley, Crawfordsville

Printed in the United States of America

Library of Congress Cataloging-in-Publication Data

Wallach, Jacques B. (Jacques Burton), 1926-
    Interpretation of diagnostic tests / Jacques Wallach.—8th ed.
        p. ; cm.
    Includes bibliographical references and index.
    ISBN-13: 978-0-7817-3055-6
    ISBN-10: 0-7817-3055-4
        1. Diagnosis, Laboratory—Handbooks, manuals, etc.   I. Title.
    [DNLM: 1. Laboratory Techniques and Procedures.   2. Diagnostic
    Techniques and Procedures.   QY 25 W195i 2007]
    RB38.2.W35 2007
    616.07'56—dc22   2006033587

Care has been taken to confirm the accuracy or the information presented and to describe
generally accepted practices. However, the authors, editors, and publisher are not responsible
for errors or omissions or for any consequences from application of the information in this
book and make no warranty, expressed or implied, with respect to the currency,
completeness, or accuracy of the contents of the publication. Application of this information
in a particular situation remains the professional responsibility of the practitioner.
    The author, editors, and publisher have exerted every effort to ensure that drug selection
and dosage set forth in this text are in accordance with current recommendations and
practice at the time of publication. However, in view of ongoing research, changes in
government regulations, and the constant flow of information relating to drug therapy and
drug reactions, the reader is urged to check the package insert for each drug for any change
in indications and dosage and for added warnings and precautions. This is particularly
important when the recommended agent is a new or infrequently employed drug.
    Some drugs and medical devices presented in this publication have Food and Drug
Administration (FDA) clearance for limited use in restricted research settings. It is the
responsibility of the health care provider to ascertain the FDA status of each drug or device
planned for use in their clinical practice.
    To purchase additional copies of this book, call our customer service department at
(800) 638-3030 or fax orders to (301) 824-7390. International customers should call
(301) 223-2300.
    Visit Lippincott Williams & Wilkins on the Internet: http://www.LWW.com.
Lippincott Williams & Wilkins customer service representatives are available from
8:30 am to 6:00 pm, EST.

10 9 8 7 6 5 4 3 2 1

To Doris
and
To Kim, Lisa, and Tracy
and
To Gabriel, Jonah, Zachary, Ariel
and
To Anthony

CONTENTS

The history is important in the selection of appropriate diagnostic tests and for an estimate of prior prevalence for interpreting the test sensitivity and specificity. Laboratory tests have greater specificity and sensitivity than the physical examination for many disorders.

Test selection depends largely on the clinical purpose for testing (e.g., screening, case finding, monitoring the course of disease, following the effects of therapy, determining drug levels or drug effects) and on the patient population being evaluated. Whereas formerly it was common to order a multiphasic panel of blood chemistry and hematology tests, this practice is now discouraged to decrease costs and to avoid the "Ulysses syndrome."

Appropriate diseases for screening should be sufficiently prevalent, life threatening, disabling, or financially burdensome; detectable by tests of sufficient sensitivity and specificity with high predictive value; and susceptible to available therapy that can prevent, ameliorate, or delay the onset of disease or prolong useful life. Common examples of conditions for screening and case finding in asymptomatic persons include cytology for cervical cancer, testing for HIV and other transmissible diseases in blood donors, and for phenylketonuria (PKU) and hypothyroidism in newborns.

Laboratory tests are an increasing part of most patient-physician relationships and contribute greatly to the selection of additional diagnostic procedures and, ultimately to diagnosis and treatment. They often precede the history and physical examination. The use of physician office laboratories and increased consolidation of distant reference laboratories diminishes the opportunity for clinicians to consult with local laboratory directors even as there are greater economic constraints and criticisms regarding inappropriate utilization of health resources.

Many remarkable advances have occurred in laboratory medicine since the first edition of *Interpretation of Diagnostic Tests* was published in 1970. A wealth of new laboratory tests has become essential to the modern practice of medicine, and each edition has paralleled these changes by including more recently described disorders and newer tests, which accounts for the increased size of each edition. The number, cost, complexity, sophistication, variety, utility, and availability of laboratory tests continues to grow along with clinicians' dependence on them.

Many diagnoses can only be established, or etiologies confirmed or appropriate therapy selected, by such tests. The size of this medical knowledge database defies and challenges the ability of any individual to use it to its greatest advantage.

I have attempted to address these issues in the following ways:

1. The result is that *Interpretation of Diagnostic Tests, Eighth Edition* has transformed itself from a pocket manual into a reference text but still maintains the original characteristic format, style, ease of use, nominal cost, thoroughness, and practical utility combined with improved organization.
2. Making significant improvements through extensive editing, remodeling, cross referencing, and book design (e.g., edge tabs) to make the data more readable and more accessible.
3. With the increasing complexity of diseases and volume of test procedures, I have added brief definitions to many topics which will make the book more useful.
4. Information about tests and diseases has been extensively updated, including newer technologies such as monoclonal antibodies, DNA probes, polymerase chain reaction, specific hormone assays, immunochemical and cytochemical staining, flow cytometry, HPLC, cytogenics, and chromosomal studies that have markedly improved our accuracy and diagnostic ability. Outmoded or rarely used tests have been deleted.
5. Additional algorithms and tables should clarify and expedite the patient's workup.
6. More data on test sensitivity, specificity, and positive and negative predictive values is included to aid in selecting tests.

7. Current references have replaced older ones in keeping with more up-to-date information.
8. Reorganization includes improved organization of the laboratory tests immediately preceding diseases of that organ system within each chapter. This has allowed deleting redundancies and repetitions that may have crept in during previous years. An extensive index that characterized previous editions is provided; the reader can find answers quickly and expeditiously.
9. I have continued to use symbols to mark tests that are diagnostic for a disease (♦), and a different icon (○) is used for those tests that are suggestive or supportive or should arouse suspicion of, but are not diagnostic for, that disease, thus encouraging more cost effective and immediate diagnosis; these have met with very positive feedback. Unmarked tests simply let the reader know that such test results may occur and are nonspecific, although they may occasionally provide useful collateral information in the differential diagnosis of an individual problem.
10. The effect of drugs on laboratory tests that appeared in a separate chapter in previous editions has been included with the tests themselves, diminishing the need for the reader to cross check between chapters and possible redundancy.
11. On-line versions are available for easier pursuit of information and cross referencing and ultimately for integration with computerized laboratory test reporting.
12. A more concise pocket version (Handbook of Interpretation of Diagnostic Tests) may be a possibility for those who may need less detail and more portability.
13. This edition continues to mostly use conventional rather than Système International (SI) units because many journals do so and especially because most physicians are more familiar with them; a table for converting units is included in Appendix B.
14. Computerized consolidation of laboratory results brings clinicians closer to the goal of integrating these results and clinical findings with their interpretation and constitutes an increasing unique opportunity in medicine.

These modifications should permit this book to continue to meet the needs of seasoned pathologists, laboratorians, clinicians, as well as house officers, students in medicine, dentistry, nursing, laboratory technology, and veterinary medicine, as well as a wide range of health care providers. Its success is indicated in the use of many hundreds of thousands of copies of earlier editions in various languages and countries for more than 35 years, the many favorable comments received, and the number of authors who have tried to emulate it. Readers are encouraged to continue their suggestions and criticisms.

The author's perspective as a practicing pathologist, laboratory director, clinician, and teacher who personally needs current, concise, and practical diagnostic data without the distraction of other material, such as methodology, technology, and Medicare code numbers, has informed the preparation of this edition and continues to distinguish it from other laboratory books.

J.W.

Results of laboratory tests may aid in
  Discovering occult disease
  Preventing irreparable damage (e.g., phenylketonuria)
  Early diagnosis after onset of signs or symptoms
  Differential diagnosis of various possible diseases
  Determining the stage of the disease
  Estimating the activity of the disease
  Detecting the recurrence of disease
  Monitoring the effect of therapy
  Genetic counseling in familial conditions
  Medicolegal problems, such as paternity suits
This book is written to help the physician achieve these purposes the least amount of
  Duplication of tests
  Waste of patient's money
  Overtaxing of laboratory facilities and personnel
  Loss of physician's time
  Confusion caused by the increasing number, variety, and complexity of tests cur-
    rently available. Some of these tests may be unrequested but performed as part
    of routine surveys or hospital admission multitest screening.
In order to provide quick reference and maximum availability and usefulness, this
  handy-sized book features
  Tabular and graphic style of concise presentation
  Emphasis on serial time changes in laboratory findings in various stages of disease
  Omission of rarely performed, irrelevant, esoteric, and outmoded laboratory tests
  Exclusion of discussion of physiologic mechanisms, metabolic pathways, clinical
    features, and nonlaboratory aspects of disease
  Discussion of only the more important diseases that the physician encounters
    and should be able to diagnose
This book is not
  An encyclopedic compendium of clinical pathology
  A technical manual
  A substitute for good clinical judgment and basic knowledge of medicine
Deliberately omitted are
  Technical procedures and directions
  Photographs and illustrations of anatomic changes (e.g., blood cells, karyo-types, iso-
    tope scans)
  Discussions of quality control
  Selection of a referral laboratory
  Performance of laboratory tests in the clinician's own office
  Bibliographic references, except for the most general reference texts in medicine,
    hematology, and clinical pathology and for some recent references to specific
    conditions
The usefulness and need for a book of this style, organization, and contents have been
  increased by such current trends as
  The frequent lack of personal assistance, advice, and consultation in large commer-
    cial laboratories and hospital departments of clinical pathology, which are often
    specialized and fragmented as well as impersonal
  Greater demand for the physician's time

The development of many new tests
Faculty and administrators still assume that this essential area of medicine can be
learned "intuitively" as it was 20 years ago and that it therefore requires little for-
mal training. This attitude ignores changes in the number and variety of tests now
available as well as their increased sophistication and basic value in establishing a
diagnosis.

The contents of this book are organized to answer the questions most often posed by
physicians when they require assistance from the pathologist. There is no other single
adequate source of information presented in this fashion. It appears from numerous
comments I have received that this book has succeeded in meeting the needs not only
of practicing physicians and medical students but also of pathologists, technologists,
and other medical personnel. It has been adopted by many schools of nursing and of
medical technology, physicians assistant training programs, and medical schools. Such
widespread acceptance confirms my original premise in writing this book and is most
gratifying.

A perusal of the table of contents and index will quickly show the general organization of the material by type of laboratory test or organ system or certain other categories. In order to maintain a concise format, separate chapters have not been organized for such categories as newborn, pediatric, and geriatric periods or for primary
psychiatric or dermatologic diseases. A complete index provides maximum access to
this information.

Obviously these data are not original but have been adapted from many sources over
the years. Only the selection, organization, manner of presentation, and emphasis are
original. I have formulated this point of view during 40 years as a clinician and pathologist, viewing with pride the important and growing role of the laboratory but deeply
regretting its inappropriate utilization.

This book was written to improve laboratory utilization by making it simpler for the
physician to select and interpret the most useful laboratory tests for his clinical problems.

J.W.

ACKNOWLEDGMENTS

I thank colleagues in various parts of the world who continue to share their clinical and laboratory problems with me and have encouraged the continuation of this book. The universal need to convert an ever expanding mass of raw laboratory data into accessible, cost effective, clinically usable information continues to be a matter of increasing significance throughout the medical community and a chief concern of mine in producing this book and in other teaching and research efforts. The need for expeditious, unencumbered information has been repeatedly confirmed during teaching of medical students and house officers, in the daily practice of pathology, by discussions with physicians in many countries that I have visited or in which I have worked or taught, and by the translation of this volume into various other languages. I am rewarded by numerous instances of friendship, criticism, kindness, and help and by learning far more than I could include in this small volume. I continue to be gratified and stimulated beyond expectation.

My thanks to Managing Editor Nancy Winter for her diligent and tireless work on this project, and to the other people behind the scenes at Lippincott Williams & Wilkins who were so helpful; to Max Leckrone, the project manager, and his associates at Techbooks — The Content Transformation Company, for their meticulous and careful proofreading.

My special thanks to Dr. Anthony Auteri for his suggestions on Gastrointestinal and Hepatobiliary diseases, to Bennett J. Daidone, Chief of Virology Section for checking the virology portion of the manuscript, and to Dr. Martin J. Salwen, Distinguished Service Professor at SUNY Downstate for his advice on Endocrine Diseases.

The friendship, love, care, and generosity of my wife, Doris, can never be sufficiently acknowledged.

Normal Values

1 Introduction to Normal Values (Reference Ranges)

General Principles

The purpose of all testing (laboratory, radiologic, ECG, etc.) is to reduce clinical uncertainty. The degree of reduction varies with the test characteristics and clinical situation. Modern medicine has superseded Voltaire's dictum that "the art of medicine consists of amusing the patient while nature cures the disease."

Many clinicians are still largely unaware of the reasoning process that they pursue in seeking a diagnosis. They tend to follow an empirical path that was previously successful or was learned during early training periods by observing their mentors during clinical rounds without appreciating the rationale for selecting, ordering, and interpreting laboratory tests. This is often absorbed in a subliminal, informal, or rote fashion. The need to control health care costs and many recent studies on laboratory test use have emphasized the need for a selective approach.

Some important principles in using laboratory (and all other) tests are as follows:

1. Under the best of circumstances, no test is perfect (e.g., 100% sensitivity, specificity, predictive value). In any specific case, the results may be misleading. The most sensitive tests are best used to rule out a suspected disease so that the number of false-negative tests is minimal; thus a negative test tends to exclude the disease. The most specific tests are best used to confirm or exclude a suspected disease and minimize the number of false-positive results. Sensitivity and specificity may be markedly altered by the coexistence of other disorders or complications or sequelae of the primary disease. (See Table 1-1.)

2. Choice of tests should be based on the prior probability of the diagnosis being sought, which affects the predictive value of the test. This prior probability is determined by the history, physical examination, and prevalence of the suspected disorder (in that community at that time), which is why history and physical examination should precede ordering tests. The clinician need not know the exact prior probability of the disease. It is usually sufficient to estimate this as high, intermediate, or low. Moderate errors in estimating prior probability have only relatively limited effects on interpretation of the tests. If the prior prevalence is high, a positive result tends to confirm the presence of the disease but an unexpected negative result is not very useful in ruling out the disease. Conversely, when the prior prevalence is low, a normal result tends to rule out the disease but an unexpected positive result is not very useful in confirming the disease. If the prior probability

3

Table 1-1.	Definition of Terms	
Test Result	Disease Present	Disease Absent
Positive	A (true-positive)	B (false-positive)
Negative	C (false-negative)	D (true-negative)
Total		

Sensitivity = A/(A + C).
Specificity = D/(B + D).
Positive predictive value (PPV) = A/(A + B).
Negative predictive value (NPV) = D/(C + D).

Table 1-2.	Assuming a Low Prior Probability (10%) (in 1,000 Tests, Disease is Present in 100 and Absent in 900)	

Prevalence = (90 + 10)/(90 + 180 + 10 + 720) or (100/1,000) = 10%

Test Result	Disease Present	Disease Absent
Positive	90 (true-positive)	180 (false-positive)
Negative	10 (false-negative)	720 (true-negative)
Total	100	900

With a test of high sensitivity (e.g., 90%), the positive predictive value (probability that those with a positive test have the disease) is only 33% [90/(90 + 180)]. In contrast, the negative predictive value (% of those with a negative test who do not have the disease) [720/(10 + 720)] = 99%. Thus a negative test indicates 99% probability of no disease. The specificity = 720/(180 + 720) = 80%.

Table 1-3.	Assuming a High (90%) Prior Probability (in 1,000 Tests, Disease is Present in 900 and Absent in 100)	

Prevalence = (810 + 90)/(810 + 20 + 90 + 80) or (90/1,000) = 90%

Test Result	Disease Present	Disease Absent
Positive	810 (true-positive) (A)	20 (false-positive) (B)
Negative	90 (false-negative) (C)	80 (true-negative) (D)
Total	900	100

With a test of high sensitivity (e.g., 90%), the positive predictive value (probability that those with a positive test have the disease) is 98% [810/(810 + 20)], indicating near certainty that disease is present. In contrast, the negative predictive value (% of those with a negative test who do not have the disease) is 47% [80/(90 + 80)]. Thus a negative test (probability of no disease) indicates that the patient still has a fairly high possibility of having the disease (47%). The specificity = 80/(20 + 80) = 80%.

of a disease is high, only a negative test on a very sensitive test can lower the probability sufficiently to rule out that disease. (See Tables 1-2 and 1-3.)
3. In most laboratory measurements, the combination of short-term physiologic variation and analytic error is sufficient to render the interpretation of single determinations difficult when the concentrations are in the borderline range. For example, the individual's coefficient of variation (CV) for cortisone over 7 days is 21% and for C-reactive protein (CRP) for 1 to 6 months is 57%, whereas the CV for sodium is 0.6% and for calcium is 1.8%. Any particular laboratory result may be incorrect for many reasons regardless of the high quality of the laboratory; all unexpected or suspicious results should be rechecked. If indicated, a new specimen sample should be submitted with careful confirmation of patient identification,

prompt delivery to the laboratory, and immediate processing. In some circumstances, confirmation of test results at another laboratory may be appropriate.

4. Strive to avoid random analytic error in an analytic method including changes in temperature, volume of reagent or sample, and so on.[1] Imprecision is measured by calculating the mean, standard deviation (SD), and CV. Imprecision does not include preanalytic variables (e.g., specimen collection, transport, and receipt in laboratory as well as diet; time of eating; menstrual, circadian, and seasonal rhythms; posture, exercise, and mobilization; recent transfusion; environmental temperature, altitude, and geography, etc.) or postanalytic variables (e.g., transcription and telephone reports, absent reference ranges, etc.). Preanalytic errors constitute 31% to 75% of all laboratory errors, postanalytic errors constitute 9% to 30% of all laboratory errors, and analytic errors (e.g., subjective interpretation, contamination, interferences, cross-reactions, methodology) constitute 13% to 31% of all laboratory errors.[2]

It should be remembered that imprecision depends on the concentration of the analyte.

The following illustrations may be useful:

Serum cholesterol has decreased from 250 mg/dL to 220 mg/dL during 6 months. Assuming a zero analytic bias and CV of 3% and a 95% confidence interval, at a 250 mg/dL concentration, the cholesterol concentration is between 235 and 265 mg/dL. At the concentration of 220 mg/dL, the 95% confidence interval is 207 to 233 mg/dL. Since the confidence intervals do not overlap, this is a true analytic change. However, the physiologic variation is approximately 6%. Using the formula,[3] the 95% confidence interval for these values of 250 mg/dL (216–284) and 220 mg/dL (186–254) results in overlapping values that are not significantly different.

A test with high sensitivity (i.e., few false-negatives) is used when there are significant consequences to missing the diagnosis. A test with high specificity is used (i.e., few false-positives) to avoid labeling a patient who does not have the disease. Sensitivity and specificity can be calculated at different cutoff points to generate a receiver-operating-characteristic (ROC) curve. Ideally, a test will be highly sensitive through the whole range of specificity. The most useful tests show the largest area under the ROC curve.

The likelihood ratio (LR) is independent of the prevalence (unlike the predictive value) and helps to assess the diagnostic benefit of a positive or negative test. It is a ratio of the probability that the test result is positive in a patient who has the disease compared with the probability that the test result is positive in a person who does not have the disease. LR = 1 indicates equal likelihood of disease presence or absence; higher values mean disease is that many times more likely to be present than absent, and lower values mean the opposite.

LR shows the magnitude and direction of a change from pretest to posttest probability for which a nomogram or formula[4] can be used:

$$\text{Posttest probability} = \text{pretest probability} \times LR/[1 + \text{pretest probability} \times (LR - 1)]$$

A change of 1 to 2 from pretest to posttest probability makes little difference, but a change in LR of <0.1 or >10 from pretest to posttest probability may be diagnostic.

5. Based on the statistical definition of "normal" as 95% range of values, 5% of independent tests will be outside this normal range in the absence of disease. If 12 tests are performed, at least one abnormal result will occur in 46% of normal persons; for 20 tests, 64% of normal persons will have at least one abnormal result. The

[1]Grenache DG. Imprecision and physiological variation. Impact on uncertainty of clinical laboratory results. *Clin Lab News* March 2004:12.
[2]Matlow AG, Berte LM. Sources of error in laboratory medicine. *Lab Med* 2004;35:331.
[3]Standard error of the mean estimate: $N = (1.96 \times [CV_A^2 + CV_1^2]^{0.5} \text{ divided by } D^2)$ where:
    1.96 is the 95% probability level
    CV_A = analytic imprecision at homeostatic set point
    CV_1 = individual's biologic variation
    D = % deviation from the "acceptable" homeostatic set point
[4]http://bmj.com/cgi/eletters/324/7341/824#21308

greater the degree of abnormality of the test result, the more likely that a confirmed abnormality is significant or represents a real disorder. Most slightly abnormal results are due to preanalytic factors.

6. Tables of reference values represent statistical data for 95% of the population; values outside these ranges do not necessarily represent disease. Results may still be within the reference range but be elevated above the patient's baseline, which is why serial testing is important in a number of conditions. For example, in acute myocardial infarction, the increase in serum total creatine kinase (CK) may be abnormal for that patient although the value may be within "normal" range.

7. An individual's test values when performed in a good laboratory tend to remain fairly constant over a period of years when performed with comparable technology; comparison of results with previous values obtained when the patient was not ill (if available) are often a better reference value than "normal" ranges.

8. Multiple test abnormalities are more likely to be significant than single test abnormalities. When two or more tests for the same disorder are positive, the results reinforce the diagnosis; however, when only one test is positive and the other is not positive, the strength of the interpretation is diluted. Similarly, ratios of various analytes are often useful (e.g., BUN:creatinine, albumin:globulin, chloride:phosphate, liver function tests), and the clinician may find useful clues in these.

9. The degree of abnormality (signal strength) is useful. Thus a value increased ten times the upper reference range is much more likely to be clinically significant than one that is only slightly increased.

10. Characteristic laboratory test profiles that are described in the literature and in this book represent the full-blown picture of the well-developed or far advanced case, but all abnormal tests may be present simultaneously in only a small fraction (e.g., one-third) of patients with that condition. Even when a test profile (combination of tests) is characteristic of a particular disorder, other disorders or groups of conditions may produce exactly the same combination of laboratory test changes.

11. Excessive repetition of tests is wasteful, and the excess burden increases the possibility of laboratory errors. Appropriate intervals between tests should be dictated by the patient's clinical condition.

12. Tests should be performed only if they will alter the patient's diagnosis, prognosis, treatment, or management. Incorrect test values or isolated individual variation in results may cause Ulysses syndrome and result in loss of time, money, and peace of mind.

13. Clerical errors are far more likely to cause incorrect results than are technical errors. Greatest care should be taken to completely and properly label and identify every specimen, which should *always* be accompanied by a test requisition form. Busy hospital laboratories receive inordinate numbers of unlabeled, unidentified specimens each day, which are useless, burdensome, and sometimes dangerous.

14. Reference ranges vary from one laboratory to another; the user should know what these ranges are for each laboratory used and should also be aware of variations due to age, sex, race, size, physiologic status (e.g., pregnancy, lactation, diet, diurnal variation) that may apply to the particular patient. These "normal" ranges represent collected statistical data rather than classification of patients as having disease or being healthy. This is best illustrated in the use of *multitest* chemical profiles for screening persons known to be free of disease. The probability of any given test being abnormal is about 2% to 5%, and the probability of disease if a screening test is abnormal is generally low (0% to 15%). The frequency of abnormal single tests is 1.5% (albumin) to 5.9% (glucose) and up to 16.6% for sodium. Based on statistical expectations, when a panel of eight tests is performed in a multiphasic health program, 25% of the patients have one or more abnormal results; when the panel includes 20 tests, 55% have one or more test abnormalities.[5]

15. The effect of drugs on laboratory test values must never be overlooked. The clinician should always be aware of what drugs the patient has been taking, including over-the-counter medications, vitamins, iron, and so on. These effects may produce false-negative as well as false-positive results; for example, vitamin C may produce a false-negative test for occult blood in the stool. Complementary and alternative medicines may cause increased serum bilirubin and liver enzymes (e.g., kava-kava,

[5]Friedman GD, Goldberg M, Ahuja JN, et al. Biochemical screening tests: effect of panel size on medical care. *Arch Int Med* 1972;129:91.

Table 1-4. Reference Ranges for Complete Blood Cell Count at Various Ages

Age	RBC ($\times 10^6$/cu mm)	Hb (g/dL)	Hct (%)	MCV (fL)	MCH (pg)	RDW (%)
Newborn	4.1–6.7	15.0–24.0	44–70	102–115	33–39	13.0–18.0
1–23 mos	3.8–5.4	10.5–14.0	32–42	72–88	24–30	11.5–16.0
2–9 yrs	4.0–5.3	11.5–14.5	33–43	76–90	25–31	11.5–15.0
10–17 yrs						
Males	4.2–5.6	12.5–16.1	36–47	78–95	26–32	11.5–14.0
Females	4.1–5.3	12.0–15.0	35–45	78–95	26–32	11.5–14.0
>18 yrs						
Males	4.7–6.0	13.5–18.0	42–52	78–100	27–31	11.5–14.0
Females	4.2–5.4	12.5–16.0	37–47	78–100	27–31	11.5–14.0

Mean platelet volume = 6.0–9.5 fL for all age groups. Platelets = 150,000–450,000/cu mm for all age groups. Mean corpuscular hemoglobin concentration = 32–36 gm/dL for all age groups.
Source: Clinical Laboratories of Children's Hospital of Buffalo.

chaparral, comfrey, germander). Unexpected high digoxin levels may be due to interference by Chan Su, Dan Shen, or ginseng. Reduced cyclosporine levels are reported due to use of St. John's wort. Contamination by heavy metals (e.g., arsenic, lead, mercury) in many Chinese medicines may cause toxicity.

16. The reader must be aware of the effect of artifacts causing spurious values and of factitious disorders *especially in the face of discrepant laboratory results*.
17. Negative laboratory values (or any other type of tests) do not necessarily rule out a clinical diagnosis.

Typical Reference Values

These are typical references values. Readers are referred to these and other sources and especially their own laboratories for more detailed data.[6,7,8]

Hematology Reference Values

Complete blood count (CBC)	See Tables 1-4, 1-5, 1-6, and 1-7
Carboxyhemoglobin (WB)	
Smoker	2.1%–4.2%
Nonsmoker	<2.3%
Erythrocyte sedimentation rate (ESR) (WB)	
Westergren	
Males	0–15 mm/1 hr
Females	0–25 mm/1 hr
Wintrobe	
Males	0–10 mm/1 hr
Females	0–15 mm/1 hr
Neonate/child	3–13 mm/1 hr
Newborn	0–4 mm/1 hr
Erythropoietin (S)	3–20 mIU/L
Ferritin (S)	
Newborns	25–200 ng/mL
1 month	200–600 ng/mL

[6]Greer JP, et al., eds. *Wintrobe's Clinical Hematology*. 11th ed. Philadelphia: Lippincott Williams & Wilkins; 2004.
[7]McMillan JA, et al., eds. *Oski's Pediatrics*. 4th ed. Philadelphia: Lippincott Williams & Wilkins; 2006.
[8]*Quest Diagnostics*. Chantilly, VA: Nichols Institute Directory of Services; 2003.

Table 1-5. Reference Ranges for White Blood Cell Count (WBC) at Various Ages (Differential Count in Absolute Numbers)

Age	WBC (×1,000/cu mm)	Total Neutrophils*	Segs	Bands	Lymphs	Monos	Eos	Baso
Newborn	9.1–34.0	6.0–23.5	6.0–20.0	<3.5	2.5–10.5	<3.5	<2.0	<0.4
1–23 mos	6.0–14.0	1.1–6.6	1.0–6.0	<1.0	1.8–9.0	<1.0	<0.7	<0.1
2–9 yrs	4.0–12.0	1.4–6.6	1.2–6.0	<1.0	1.0–5.5	<1.0	<0.7	<0.1
10–17 yrs	4.0–10.5	1.5–6.6	1.3–6.0	<1.0	1.0–3.5	<1.0	<0.7	<0.1
>18 yrs	4.0–10.5	1.5–6.6	1.3–6.0	<1.0	1.5–3.5	<1.0	<0.7	<0.1

Segs = segmented neutrophils; Bands = band neutrophils; Lymphs = lymphocytes; Monos = monocytes; Eos = eosinophils; Baso = basophils.
*Total Neutrophils = Segs + Bands.
Source: Clinical Laboratories of Children's Hospital of Buffalo.

Table 1-6. Reference Ranges for Blood Cell Count at Various Fetal Ages

	Age (wks)			
	18–20	21–22	23–25	25–30
RBC ($\times 10^6$/cu mm)	2.35–2.95	2.70–3.22	2.80–3.32	3.20–3.84
Hb (gm/dL)	10.7–12.3	11.4–13.2	12.1–12.7	12.2–14.5
Hct (%)	33–39	35–41	36–41	38–45
MCV (fL)	125–142	123–136	119–132	112–124
WBC ($\times 1,000$/cu mm)	3.6–5.0	3.4–5.0	3.3–4.6	3.5–5.2
Platelets ($\times 1,000$/cu mm)	208–277	203–312	217–301	216–290

RBC = red blood cell count; Hb = hemoglobin; Hct = hematocrit; MCV = mean corpuscular volume; WBC = white blood cell count.
Source: Daffos F. Fetal blood sampling. In: Harrison WR, Globus MS, Filly RA, eds. *The unborn patient*, 2nd ed. Philadelphia: WB Saunders, 1991:79.

2–5 months	50–200 ng/mL
6 months–15 years	7–140 ng/mL
Adult males	30–300 ng/mL
Adult females	10–200 ng/mL
Borderline (males or females)	10–20 ng/mL
Iron excess	>400 ng/mL
Folate (RBCs)	>280 ng/mL
Folate (S)	3–25 ng/mL
Free erythrocyte protoporphyrin (FEP)	16–36 μg/dL packed RBCs
Glucose-6-phosphate dehydrogenase (RBCs)	6.1–9.3 IU/g Hb
Haptoglobins (S)	Genetic absence in 1% of population
Newborns	Absent in 90%; 10 mg/dL in 10%
Age 1–6 months	Gradual increase to 30 mg/dL
6 months–17 years	40–180 mg/dL
Adults	16–199 mg/dL
Hematocrit (WB)	41%–53%
Hemoglobin (P)	<1–5 mg/dL
Hemoglobin (WB)	13.5–17.5 g/dL
Hemoglobin electrophoresis (WB)	
HbA ($\alpha_2\beta_2$)	
0–30 days	10%–40%
6 months to adult	95%–98%
HbA$_2$ ($\alpha_2\delta_2$)	
<1 year	<2%
1 year to adult	1.5%–3.5%
HbF ($\alpha_2\gamma_2$)	<2%
Other Hb variants	None
Iron (liver tissue)	530–900 μg/g dry weight
Iron (S)	
Newborn	100–250 μg/dL
Infant	40–100 μg/dL
Child	50–120 μg/dL
Adults	
Male	65–175 μg/dL
Female	50–170 μg/dL
Iron-binding capacity (IBC)	224–428 μg/dL
% saturation	15%–50%
Leukocyte alkaline phosphatase (LAP) score	40–100
Lysozyme (muramidase) (S)	7.0–15.0 μg/mL
Marrow sideroblasts	≥30% of normoblasts

Table 1-7. Pediatric Reference Ranges for Lymphocyte Counts

Lymphocytes	Age (mos)						
	0–6	6–12	12–18	18–24	24–30	30–36	>36
Total %	62–72	60–69	56–63	52–29	45–57	38–53	22–69
Total absolute	5,395–7,211	5,284–6,714	4,943–5,943	4,431–5,508	3,855–5,248	3,315–5,058	1,622–5,370
CD4 %	5,057	4,955	4,651	4,248	3,846	3,344	2,757
CD4 absolute	2,780–3,908	2,630–3,499	2,307–2,864	1,919–2,472	1,538–2,213	1,216–2,009	562–2,692
CD8 %				8–31			14–34
CD8 absolute				351–2,479			331–1,445
CD2 %				55–88			65–84
CD2 absolute	3,929–5,275	3,806–4,881	3,516–3,868	3,101–3,868	2,640–3,639	2,236–3,463	1,230–4,074
CD3 %				55–82			55–82
CD3 absolute	3,505–5,009	3,409–4,575	3,156–3,899	2,766–3,508	2,324–3,295	1,923–3,141	1,072–3,890
CD19 %				11–45			9–29
CD19 absolute				4,32–3,345			200–1,259
Helper-suppressor ratio				1.2–6.2			0.98–3.24

Source: Riley Hospital for Children, Indiana University Medical Center, 1992.

Methemoglobin (WB)   <1% of total Hb
Osmotic fragility of RBCs   Increased if hemolysis occurs in >0.5% NaCl
                                                  Decreased if incomplete in 0.30% NaCl
Pyruvate kinase (RBCs)   13–17 IU/g Hb
RBC survival time (^{51}Cr)   Half-life: 25–35 days
Reticulocyte count (WB)   0.5–2.5% of RBCs
Reticulocyte hemoglobin content,   See Chapter 11
   reticulocyte index, mean volume,
   parameter, hemoglobin.
   Immature reticulocyte fraction.
Ringed sideroblasts   None
Transferrin (S)   240–480 mg/dL
Transferrin receptor (S)   0.57–2.8 μg/L
Transferrin saturation   **Males**   **Females**
                                                  14.2%–58.4%   15.2%–49.3%
TfR-F index (sTfR:log serum   **Males**   **Females**
   ferritin)   0.45–1.88   0.46–13.29
Unsaturated vitamin B$_{12}$-binding   870–1,800 pg/mL
   capacity
Vitamin B$_{12}$ (S)   190–900 ng/L
Volume (mL/kg body weight)   **Males**   **Females**
   Blood   75   67
   RBC   30   24
   Plasma   44   43

RBCs, red blood cells; S, serum; WB, white blood.

Blood Coagulation Tests—Reference Values

Activated clotting time (WB)   70–180 sec
Activated protein C resistance   Ratio >2.1
   (factor V Leiden) (P)
Alpha$_2$-antiplasmin (P)   80%–130%
Antiphospholipid-antibody panel
   Partial thromboplastin time—   Negative
      lupus anticoagulant screen (P)
   Dilute Russell viper venom time   Negative
      (dRVVT) (P)
   Platelet-neutralization (P)   Negative
   Anticardiolipin antibody IgG or   0–15 U
      IgM (S)
Antithrombin III (P)
   Immunologic   22–39 mg/dL
   Functional   80%–130%
Anti-Xa assay (heparin) (P)
   Unfractionated   0.3–0.7 IU/mL
   Low-molecular-weight   0.5–1.0 IU/mL
   Danaparoid   0.5–0.8 IU/mL
Bleeding time (Simplate)   2–9.5 minutes
Clot retraction, qualitative (WB)   Begins in 1/2–1 hr;
                                                  50%–100% in 2 hr
Cryofibrinogen (P)   Negative
D-dimer (P)   <0.5 μ/mL

Coagulation factor assay (P)	Activity	Plasma levels
I (fibrinogen)		150–400 mg/dL
II (prothrombin)	60%–140%*	100 μg/mL
V	60%–140%*†	10 μg/mL
VII	60%–140%*†	0.5 μg/mL
VIII (AHG)	50%–200%*	0.1 μg/mL
IX	60%–140%*†	5 μg/mL
X	60%–140%*†	10 μg/mL
XI	60%–140%*	5 μg/mL

XII	60%–140%* 　　　30 μg/mL
XIII screen	No deficiency detected
Fibrin and fibrinogen degradation products (P)	<2.5 μ/mL
Partial thromboplastin time, activated (aPTT) (P)	25–38 sec
Plasminogen (P)	
Antigenic	8–14 mg/dL
Functional	80%–130%
Platelet aggregation	>65% aggregation in response to ADP, epinephrine, collagen, ristocetin, arachidonic acid
Platelet count	150,000–350,000/μL
Protein C, total antigen or functional (P)	70%–140%
Protein S, total or free antigen or functional (P)	70%–140%
Prothrombin-gene mutation G20210A	Absent
Prothrombin time (P)	11–13 sec
Reptilase time (P)	16–24 sec
Thrombin time (P)	16–24 sec
Ristocetin cofactor (functional vWF) (P)	
Blood Group O	75% mean of normal
Blood Group A	105% mean of normal
Blood Group B	115% mean of normal
Blood Group AB	125% mean of normal
von Willebrand factor (factor VIII:R) antigen (P)	
Blood Group O	75% mean of normal
Blood Group A	105% mean of normal
Blood Group B	115% mean of normal
Blood Group AB	125% mean of normal
von Willebrand factor multimers (P)	Normal distribution
Coagulation time (Lee-White)	6–17 minutes (glass tubes) 19–60 minutes (siliconized tubes)
Euglobulin lysis	No lysis in 2 hours
Fibrinogen split products	Negative at >1:4 dilution Positive at >1:8 dilution
Fibrinolysins (WB)	No clot lysis in 24 hours
Platelet antibody (S)	Negative

P, plasma; S, serum; WB, whole blood.
*Infants may not reach adult level until age 6 months.
†Increases with age in elderly.

Blood Chemistries—Reference Values

These values will vary, depending on the individual laboratory as well as the methods, reagents, and instruments used. Each clinician should compare the applicability of these data to his or her own situation.

Acetoacetate (P)	<1 mg/dL
Acetone (S, P)	0.3–2.0 mg/dL
Aldolase (S)	
Neonate	<32 U/L
Child	<16 U/L
Adults	1.0–8.0 U/L
Alkaline phosphatase (S)	30–120 U/L
Alpha$_1$ antitrypsin (S)	85–213 mg/dL
Alpha-fetoprotein (S)	<15 ng/mL
Ammonia (P)	19–60 μg/dL

Newborn at term or premature	<50 U/L	
Amylase, total (S)	+	
Angiotensin-converting enzyme (ACE) (S)	<40 U/L	
Anion gap (calculated)	8–16 or 10–20 mEq/L (See Chapter 12)	
Apolipoprotein A-1 (S)	120–240 mg/dL	
Apolipoprotein B (S)	50–160 mg/dL	
Apolipoprotein B/apolipoprotein A1 ratio	0.35–98	
Base, excess		
Newborns	−10 to −2 mEq/L	
Infant	−7 to −1 mEq/L	
Child	−4 to +2 mEq/L	
Adult	−3 to +3 mEq/L	
Beta-hydroxybutyrate (P)	<3 mg/dL	
Bicarbonate (arterial WB)		
<2 years	20–25 mEq/L	
Adult	22–28 mEq/L	
Bilirubin[9] (S)		
Total	**Term**	**Preterm**
Cord	<2.0 mg/dL	<2.0 mg/dL
<1 day	<6.0 mg/dL	<8.0 mg/dL
1–2 days	<8.0 mg/dL	<12.0 mg/dL
3–5 days	<12.0 mg/dL	<16.0 mg/dL
>1 month	<1.0 mg/dL	<2.0 mg/dL
Adult	≤1.0 mg/dL	
Direct 1 month to adult	0.1–0.3 mg/dL	
Brain-type natriuretic peptide (BNP) (S)	BNP = 80–100 pg/mL. NT-proBNP = 125 pg/mL for age <75 years; 450 pg/mL for age >75 years	
Calcium, total (S)		
<1 week	7.0–12.0 mg/dL	
Child	8.0–11.0 mg/dL	
Adult	9.0–10.5 mg/dL	
Calcium, ionized (WB)	3.0–4.5 mg/dL	
Carbon dioxide		
CO_2 content (P)	21–30 mEq/L	
pCO_2 (partial pressure) (arterial WB)	35–45 mm Hg	
Carbon monoxide (WB)	See Chapter 17	
Ceruloplasmin (S)	27–37 mg/dL	
Chloride (S)	98–106 (mEq/L)	
Cholesterol (P)		
Total cholesterol (adult)		
Desirable	<200 mg/dL	
Borderline high	200–239 mg/dL	
High	≥240 mg/dL	
Total cholesterol (<19 years old)		
Desirable	<170 mg/dL	
Borderline high	170–199 mg/dL	
High	≥200 mg/dL	
High-density lipoprotein (HDL) cholesterol		
High	≥60 mg/dL	
Low	<40 mg/dL	
Low-density lipoprotein (LDL) cholesterol		
Optimal	<100 mg/dL	
Near normal	100–129 mg/dL	

[9]Bock BJ, et al. The data warehouse as a foundation population-based reference intervals. *Am J Clin Pathol* 2003;120:662.

Borderline high	130–159 mg/dL
High	160–189 mg/dL
Very high	≥190 mg/dL
Cholinesterase (S)	5–12. U/mL (See Chapter 17)
Complement (S)	
Total complement, CH_{50}	75–160 U/mL
C3 <3 months	53–131 mg/dL
C3, 3 months–1 year	62–180 mg/dL
C3, 1–10 years	77–195 mg/dL
C3, adult	83–177 mg/dL
Factor B (C3 proactivator)	17–42 mg/dL
C4 cord blood	6.6–23 mg/dL
C4 <3 months	7–28 mg/dL
C4 3 months–1 year	7–42 mg/dL
C4 1–10 years	9.2–40 mg/dL
C4 adult	15–45 mg/dL
Copper (S)	70–140 µg/dL
Copper (U)	3–35 µg/dL
Creatine kinase (CK), total (S)	
Males	60–400 U/L
Females	40–150 U/L

Creatine kinase isoenzyme (S) (See Chapter 5)	CK-MB (<5% of total) or <5 ng/mL	CK-BB (trace)	CK-MM (94%–96% of total)
Male	24–195 IU/L		
Female	24–170 IU/L		
MB index (CK-MB/total CK) (calculated)	<2.5		

Creatinine (S)	
Newborn	0.3–1.0 mg/dL
Infant	0.2–0.4 mg/dL
Child	0.3–0.7 mg/dL
Adolescent	0.5–1.0 mg/dL
Adult	<1.5 mg/dL
Cryoglobulins (P)	Negative
Gamma-glutamyl transferase (GGT) (S)	6–19 U/L
Glucose (fasting)	60–100 mg/dL (depends on method) (See Chapter 13)
Homocysteine, total (P)	4–12 µmol/L
Isocitrate dehydrogenase (ICD) (S)	3–85 U/L
Lactate (venous P)	5–15 mg/dL
Lactate dehydrogenase (LDH) (S)	
Newborn	160–1,500 U/L
Infant	150–360 U/L
Child	150–300 U/L
Adult	100–190 U/L
Lactate dehydrogenase isoenzymes (S) (See Chapter 3)	
LD-1	14%–26%
LD-2	29%–39%
LD-3	20%–26%
LD-4	8%–16%
LD-5	6%–16%
Lead (S) (See Chapter 17)	
Adults	<10 µg/dL
≤15 years	<9 µg/dL
Leptin (<15% body fat in men, <25% in women)	1–16 µg/L
Leucine aminopeptidase (LAP) (S)	1.1–3.4 U/mL
Lipase (S)	0–160 U/L

Magnesium (S)	1.8–3.0 mg/dL
Myoglobin (S)	
Male	19–92 μg/L
Female	12–76 μg/L
5′-Nucleotidase (S)	0–11 U/L
Osmolality (P)	285–295 mOsm/kg
Osmolality (U)	300–900 mOsm/kg
Oxygen (WB)	
Saturation, arterial	96%–100%
Saturation, venous	60%–85%
Partial pressure (pO$_2$)	80–100 mm Hg
Oxygen dissociation, P^{50} (RBCs)	26–30 mm Hg
pH (WB)	7.38–7.44
Phenylalanine (S, P)	
<1 month	38–137 μmol/L
1–24 months	31–75 μmol/L
2–18 years	26–91 μmol/L
>18 years	35–85 μmol/L
Phosphatase, acid (PAP)	0–5.5 U/L
Phosphatase, alkaline (ALP) (S)[10]	
1–3 years	145–320 U/L
4–6 years	150–380 U/L
7–9 years	175–420 U/L

	Males	**Females**
10–11 years	135–530 U/L	130–560 U/L
12–13 years	200–495 U/L	105–420 U/L
14–15 years	130–525 U/L	70–230 U/L
16–19 years	48–261 U/L	40–136 U/L
Adult	30–120 U/L	

Phosphorus, inorganic (S)	
1–5 days	4.8–8.2 mg/dL
1–3 years	3.8–6.5 mg/dL
4–11 years	3.7–5.6 mg/dL
12–15 years	2.9–5.4 mg/dL
16–19 years	2.7–4.7 mg/dL
Adult	3.0–4.5 mg/dL
Phospholipids (S)	150–264 mg/dL
Potassium (S)	3.5–5.0 mEq/L
Prealbumin (transthyretin)	
<6 weeks	4–36 mg/dL
≥16 years	13–27 mg/dL
Adult	19.5–35.8 mg/dL
Prostate-specific antigen (PSA)	
(S) Males	
Values higher in black men than in white men. Increases with age.	
Normal	<4.0 ng/mL
Borderline	4–10 ng/mL
40–49 years	1.5 ng/mL
50–59 years	2.5 ng/mL
60–69 years	4.5 ng/mL
70–79 years	7.5 ng/mL
PSA, free, males (S)	>25% associated with BPH
PSA (S) females	<0.5 ng/dL

Proteins (S)	**Total (g/dL)**	**Albumin (g/dL)**
Term	4.6–7.4	2.5–3.4
7–19 years	6.3–8.6	3.7–5.6
Adult	5.5–8.0	3.5–5.5

[10]Bock BJ, et al. The data warehouse as a foundation for population-based reference intervals. *Am J Clin Pathol* 2003;120:662.

	Globulin (g/dL)
<1 year	0.4–3.7
1–3 years	1.6–3.5
4–9 years	1.9–3.4
Adult	2.0–3.5
Electrophoresis (S)	
Albumin	3.5–5.5 g/dL (50%–60%)
Globulin	
Alpha$_1$	0.2–0.4 g/dL (4.2%–7.2%)
Alpha$_2$	0.5–0.9 g/dL (6.8%–12%)
Beta	0.6–1.1 g/dL (9.3%–15%)
Gamma	0.7–1.7 g/dL (13%–23%)

Immunoglobulins (95% confidence interval [CI]) (S)

	IgG (mg/dL)	**IgM (mg/dL)**	**IgA (mg/dL)**
Cord blood	636–1,606	6.3–25	1.4–3.6
1 month	251–906	20–87	1.3–53
2 months	206–601	17–105	2.8–47
3 months	176–581	24–89	4.6–46
4 months	196–588	27–101	4.4–73
5 months	172–814	33–108	8.1–84
6 months	215–704	35–102	8.1–68
7–9 months	217–904	34–126	11–90
10–12 months	294–1,069	41–149	16–84
1 years	345–1,213	43–173	14–106
2 years	424–1,051	48–168	14–123
3 years	441–1,135	47–200	22–159
4–5 years	463–1,236	43–196	25–154
6–8 years	633–1,280	48–207	33–202
9–10 years	608–1,572	52–242	45–236
Adult	639–1,349	56–152	70–312

Immunoglobulins G subclasses (95% CI) (S)

	IgG$_1$ (mg/dL)	**IgG$_2$ (mg/dL)**	**IgG$_3$ (mg/dL)**	**IgG$_4$ (mg/dL)**
0–1 year	190–620	30–140	9–62	6–63
1–2 years	230–710	30–170	11–98	4–43
2–3 years	280–830	40–240	6–130	3–120
3–4 years	350–790	50–260	9–98	5–180
4–6 years	360–810	60–310	9–160	9–160
6–8 years	280–1,120	30–630	40–250	11–620
8–10 years	280–1,740	80–550	22–320	10–170
10–13 years	270–1,290	110–550	13–250	7–530
13 years–adult	280–1,020	60–790	14–240	11–330
IgD (S)	0–14 mg/dL			

IgE (95% CI) (S)

0 days	0.04–1.28 IU/mL
6 weeks	0.08–6.12 IU/mL
3 months	0.18–3.76 IU/mL
6 months	0.44–16.3 IU/mL
9 months	0.76–7.31 IU/mL
1 years	0.80–15.2 IU/mL
2 years	0.31–29.5 IU/mL
3 years	0.19–16.9 IU/mL
4 years	1.07–68.9 IU/mL
7 years	1.03–161.3 IU/mL
10 years	0.98–570.6 IU/mL
14 years	2.06–195.2 IU/mL
17–85 years	1.53–114.0 IU/mL
Bence Jones protein (S)	0

Qualitative (U)	0 in 50× concentrated specimen
Quantitative (U)	
Kappa (κ)	<2.5 mg/dL
Lambda (λ)	<5.0 mg/dL
Beta$_2$-microglobulin (S)	<0.27 mg/dL
Beta$_2$-microglobulin (U)	<120 μg/day

Sodium — 135–145 mEq/L

Transaminases
  Aspartate aminotransferase
    (AST; serum glutamic oxaloacetic
    transaminase [SGOT])[11]

1–3 years	20–60 U/L
4–6 years	15–50 U/L
7–9 years	15–40 U/L
10–11 years	10–60 U/L
>16 years	0–35 U/L

	Males	**Females**
12–15 years	15–40 U/L	10–30 U/L
>16 years	0–35 U/L	

Alanine aminotransferase (ALT;
  serum glutamic pyruvic
  transaminase [SGPT])[11]

1–3 years	May be slightly higher in young children
10 years–adult	0–35 U/L
Triglyceride (S)	25–175 mg/dL
Troponin I (S)	<1.6 ng/mL
Troponin T (S)	<0.1 ng/mL
Urea nitrogen (BUN) (S)	10–20 mg/dL

Uric acid (S)	**Males**	**Females**
	2.5–8.0 mg/dL	1.3–6.0 mg/dL

Urobilinogen (U)	1–3.5 mg/24 hr
Viscosity (correlates with fibrinogen, HDL-cholesterol) (S, P)	1.6–2.0 relative units
Vitamin A (S)	20–100 μg/dL
Vitamin B$_1$ (thiamine) (S)	0–2 μg/dL
Vitamin B$_2$ (riboflavin) (S)	4–24 μg/dL
Vitamin B$_6$ (S)	5–30 ng/dL
Vitamin C (ascorbic acid) (S)	0.4–1.0 mg/dL
Vitamin D3 (1,25-dihydroxy-vitamin D) (S)	25–45 pg/mL
Vitamin D3 (25-dihydroxy-vitamin D) (S)	10–68 ng/mL
Vitamin E (S)	5–18 μg/dL
Vitamin K (S)	0.13–1.19 ng/mL

P, plasma; S, serum; U, urine; WB, whole blood.

Blood and Urine Hormone—Reference Values

Adrenocorticotropic hormone
  (ACTH) (P)

0800 hours	25–100 pg/mL
1800 hours	<60 pg/mL

Aldosterone (S)

Normal sodium diet (supine)	1–16 ng/dL
Normal sodium diet (standing)	4–31 ng/dL
Low sodium diet (supine)	2–5× supine value

[11]Bock BJ, et al. The data warehouse as a foundation for population-based reference intervals. *Am J Clin Pathol* 2003;120:662.

Table 1-8.	Comparison of Umbilical Artery and Vein Analytes*	
Analyte	Umbilical Artery	Umbilical Vein
pH	7.33 ± 0.07	7.38 ± 0.06
CO_2 pressure (mm Hg)	45 ± 10	38 ± 8
Bicarbonate (mEq/L)	23 ± 5	23 ± 5
O_2 content		
O_2 pressure (mm Hg)	35 ± 15	41 ± 20
Hb (g/dL)	13	13

*Henderson Z, Ecker JL. Fetal scalp blood sampling—limited role in contemporary obstetric practice: part 1. *Lab Med*. 2003;34:548.

Aldosterone (U)
  Normal sodium diet — 6.0–25 μg/24 hr
  Low sodium diet — 17.0–44.0 μg/24 hr
  High sodium diet — 0.0–6.0 μg/24 hr
Androstenedione (S)
  Child — 5–50 ng/dL
  Adult — 50–250 ng/dL
Angiotensin-converting enzyme (ACE) (S) — <40.0 U/L
Calcitonin (P)
  Basal
  Calcium infusion (2.4 mg calcium/kg)
  Pentagastrin infusion (0.5 μg/kg)

Males, <19 pg/mL; females, <14 pg/mL. Normal increase is <0.2 ng/mL above basal level. See Chapter 13.

Catecholamine fractionation (free) (P)

	Supine (at least 30 min.)	Standing
Norepinephrine	100–400 pg/mL	300–900 pg/mL
Epinephrine	≤70 pg/mL	≤110 pg/mL
Dopamine	<30 pg/mL (any posture)	

Catecholamine fractionation (U)
Norepinephrine
  <1 year — 0–10 μg/24 hr
  1–2 years — 1–17 μg/24 hr
  2–3 years — 4–29 μg/24 hr
  5–7 years — 8–45 μg/24 hr
  8–10 years — 13–65 μg/24 hr
  >11 years — 15–100 μg/24 hr

Epinephrine
  <1 year — <2.5 μg/24 hr
  2 years — <3.5 μg/24 hr
  3–4 years — <6.0 μg/24 hr
  5–7 years — <10 μg/24 hr
  >8 years — <20 μg/24 hr

Dopamine
  <1 year — <85 μg/24 hr
  2 years — 10–140 μg/24 hr
  3–4 years — 40–260 μg/24 hr
  >5 years — 60–400 μg/24 hr

Catecholamine metabolites fractionation (U)

Homovanillic acid (HVA) (random)
  <1 year — <32.6 μg/mg creatinine
  2–4 year — <22 μg/mg creatinine
  5–9 years — <15.1 μg/mg creatinine
  10–19 years — <12.8 μg/mg creatinine

>20 years	<7.6 µg/mg creatinine
24-Hour urine	<8 mg/24 hr
Metanephrines (U)	<1.3 mg/24 hr
Metanephrines (S)	<0.50 nmol/L
Nounatanephrines (S)	<0.50 nmol/L
Vanillylmandelic acid (VMA)	
Random	4–11.8 µg/mg creatinine
24-Hour urine	2.6–7.7 mg/24 hr
Chorionic gonadotropins, beta-subunit (S)	
Females, nonpregnant	<5 IU/L
Postmenopausal females	<9 IU/L
Males	<2.5 IU/L
Cerebrospinal fluid (CSF)	≤1.5 IU/L
Cortisol (for general screening) (S)	8 AM–noon: 5–25 µg/dL
	Noon–8 PM: 5–15 µg/dL
	8 PM –8 AM: 0–10 µg/dL
Cortisol, free (U)	20–70 µg/24 hr
Deoxycorticosteroids	AM: 0–5 µg/dL
(for metyrapone test), plasma	PM: 0–3 µg/dL

Dehydroepiandrosterone (DHEA) (S)

	Males	Females
<6 years	26–72 ng/dL	19–42 ng/dL
6–8 years	29–66 ng/dL	73–165 ng/dL
8–10 years	53–135 ng/dL	74–180 ng/dL
10–12 years	183–383 ng/dL	234–539 ng/dL
12–14 years	240–520 ng/dL	224–611 ng/dL
Adult	180–1,250 ng/dL	130–980 ng/dL

Dehydroepiandrosterone sulfate (DHEA-S) (S)

	Males	Females
1–5 years	<10 µg/mL	
6–11 years	10–150 µg/mL	
12–17 years	30–550 µg/mL	
Adult	10–619 µg/mL	12–535 µg/mL premenopausal; 30–160 µg/mL postmenopausal

Estradiol (S, P)	
Adult males	<20 pg/mL
Premenopausal females	
Follicular phase	≤145 pg/mL
Midcycle peak	112–443 pg/mL
Luteal phase	≤241 pg/mL
Postmenopausal females	<59 pg/mL
Estrone (S, P)	
Female	
Follicular phase of menstrual cycle	1.5–15.0 pg/mL
Luteal phase of menstrual cycle	1.5–20 0 pg/mL
Postmenopausal	1.5–5.5 pg/mL
Male	1.5–6.5 pg/mL
Estrogen and progesterone receptor assays (tissue)	
Negative	<3 fmol/mg cytosol protein
Borderline	3–9 fmol/mg cytosol protein
Positive	≥10 fmol/mg cytosol protein
Follicle-stimulating hormone (FSH) (S/P)	
Adult male	1–12 mIU/L
Adult female, menstruating	
Follicular	3.0–20.0 mIU/L
Ovulatory	9.0–26.0 mIU/L
Luteal	1.0–12.0 mIU/L
Postmenopausal	18–153 mIU/L

Fructosamine (S)	1.61–2.68 mmol/L
Gastrin, serum (S)	<100 pg/mL
Glucagon (P)	20–100 pg/mL
Growth hormone (S)	0.5–17 ng/mL
5-Hydroxyindolaeacetic acid (5-HIAA) (U)	<6 mg/24 hr
17-Hydroyxprogesterone (U)	
Males	5.0–250 ng/dL
Prepubertal	0–80 ng/dL
Females	
Follicular phase	20–100 ng/dL
Luteal phase	100–500 ng/dL
Postmenopausal	≤70 ng/dL
Prepubertal	0–90 ng/dL
Insulin (S, P)	2–20 μU/mL
17-Ketogenic steroids (total adrenal corticosteroids) (U)	
Adults, males	5–23 mg/24 hr
Females	3–15 mg/24 hr
Children, <1 year	<1 mg/24 hr
1–10 years	2.3–3.8 mg/24 hr
17-Ketosteroids (U)	
Adults, males	8–20 mg/24 hr
Females	6–15 mg/24 hr
Children, <1 year	<1 mg/24 hr
1–4 years	<2 mg/24 hr
5–8 years	<3 mg/24 hr
9–12 years	3–10 mg/24 hr
13–16 years	5–12 mg/24 hr
17-Ketosteroids, fractionation (U)	See Table 1-9
Luteinizing hormone (LH) (S)	
Prepuberty	<5.0 mIU/L
Adult males	2.0–12 mIU/L
Adult females, follicular	2.0–15 mIU/L
Adult females, midcycle	22.0–105.0 mIU/L
Adult females, luteal	0.6–19.0 mIU/L
Postmenopausal females	16.0–64.0 mIU/L
Parathyroid hormone (PTH) (S)	10–60 pg/mL

Pregnanetriol (U)	**Males**	**Females**
0–5 years	<0.1 mg/24 hr	<0.1 mg/24 hr
6–9 years	<0.3 mg/24 hr	<0.3 mg/24 hr
10–15 years	0.2–0.6 mg/24 hr	0.1–0.6 mg/24 hr
>16 years	0.2–2.0 mg/24 hr	0.0–1.4 mg/24 hr
Pregnenolone (S)	10–200 ng/dL	10–230 ng/dL

Progesterone (S)	
Males	≤1.4 ng/mL
Females	
Follicular phase	<0.2 ng/mL
Midluteal phase	3.0–20.0 ng/mL
Prolactin (S)	
Males	0–15 ng/mL
Females	0–20 ng/mL
Pregnancy	9–200 ng/dL
Renin activity (peripheral vein) (PRA) (sodium-replete, upright) (P)	0.00–364 ng/mL/hour
Sex hormone binding globulin (SHBG) (S)	
Adult males	13–71 nmol/L
Adult nonpregnant females	18–114 nmol/L
Somatomedin-C (insulinlike growth factor; IGF-I) (S, P)	

Table 1-9. 17-Ketosteroids (F=actionation), Urine (mg/24 hrs)

	Adult Females	Adult Males	Males 10–15 yrs	Females 10–15 yrs	6–9 yrs	3–5 yrs	1–2 yrs	0–1 yr
Pregnanediol	0–4.5	0–1.9	0.1–1.2	0.1–0.7	<0.5	<0.3	<0.1	<0.1
Androsterone	0–3.1	0.9–6.1	0.2–2.0	0.5–2.5	0.1–1.0	<0.3	<0.3	<0.1
Etiocholanolone	0.1–3.5	0.9–5.2	0.1–1.6	0.7–3.1	0.3–1.0	<0.7	<0.4	<0.1
Dehydroepiandrosterone	0–1.5	0–3.1	<0.4	<0.4	<0.2	<0.1	<0.1	<0.1
Pregnanetriol	0–1.4	0.2–2.0	0.2–0.6	0.1–0.6	<0.3	<0.1	<0.1	<0.1
Δ5-Pregnanetriol	0–0.4	0–0.4	<0.3	<0.3	<0.2	<0.2	<0.1	<0.1
11-Ketoandrosterone	0–0.3	0–0.5	<0.1	<0.1	<0.1	<0.1	<0.1	<0.1
11-Ketoetiocholanolone	0–1.0	0–1.6	<0.3	0.1–0.5	0.1–0.5	<0.4	<0.1	<0.1
11-Hydroxyandrosterone	0–1.1	0.2–1.6	0.1–1.1	0.2–1.0	0.4–1.0	<0.4	<0.3	<0.3
11-Hydroxyetiocholanolone	0.1–0.8	0.1–0.9	<0.3	0.1–0.5	0.1–0.5	<0.4	<0.1	<0.1
11-Ketopregnanetriol	0–0.5	0–0.5	<0.3	<0.2	<0.2	<0.2	<0.2	<0.2

Source: Leavelle DE, ed. *Mayo Medical Laboratories Handbook*. Rochester, MN: Mayo Medical Laboratories, 1995.

Table 1-10.   Thyroid Function Tests by Age (Serum Concentrations)

Age	Thyroid-stimulating Hormone (TSH) Reference Range (mU/L)	Thyroxine, Free (fT_4) Reference Range (ng/dL; pmol/L)
Midgestation fetus	0.7–11	0.15–0.34 (2–4)
Term infant	1.3–19	0.8–1.9 (10–22)
3 days	1.1–17	1.8–4.1 (22–49)
10 weeks	0.6–10	0.8–1.7 (9–21)
14 months	0.4–7.0	0.6–1.4 (8–17)
5 years	0.4–6.0	0.8–1.7 (9–20)
14 years	0.3–5.0	0.6–1.4 (8–17)
Adult	0.3–4.0	0.8–1.8 (9–22)
Pregnancy		
First trimester	0.3–4.5	0.7–2.0 (9–26)
Second trimester	0.5–4.6	0.5–1.6 (6.5–21)
Third trimester	0.8–5.2	0.5–1.6 (6.5–21)

*National health and nutrition examination survey. *J Clin Endocrinol Metab*. 2002;87:489.

Age	Males	Females
2 mo–5 years	17–248 ng/mL	17–248 ng/mL
6–8 years	88–474 ng/mL	88–474 ng/mL
9–11 years	110–565 ng/mL	117–771 ng/mL
12–15 years	202–597 ng/mL	261–1,096 ng/mL
Adult		
16–24 years	182–780 ng/mL	
25–39 years	114–492 ng/mL	
40–54 years	90–360 ng/mL	
>55 years	71–290 ng/mL	

	Total	Free
Testosterone (S)		
Males	270–1,070 ng/dL	12–40 ng/dL
Females	6–86 ng/dL	0.2–3.1 ng/dL
Thyroxine, total (T_4) (S)	4.5–10.9 µg/dL	
Triiodothyronine, total (T_3) (S)	60–181 ng/dL	
Triiodothyronine, free (fT_3) (S)	1.4–4.4 pg/dL	
Reverse T_3 (rT_3) (S)	0.09–0.35 ng/mL	
Thyroglobulin (S)	0–60 ng/mL	
Thyroid-binding globulin (S)	16–24 µg/mL	
Thyroid microsomal (S)	<1:100	
Thyroglobulin antibodies (S)	<2.0 IU/mL	
Thyroid peroxidase antibodies (S)	<2.0 IU/mL	
Thyrotropin	0.4–6.0 IU/mL	
Vasoactive intestinal polypeptide (VIP) (P)	<75 µg/mL	

P, plasma; S, serum; U, urine.

Blood Antibody—Reference Values

Acetylcholine (Ach) (S)	
Receptor-binding antibodies	≤0.02 nmol/L
Receptor-blocking antibodies	<25% blockade of ACh receptors
Receptor-modulating antibodies	<20% loss of ACh receptors
Antiadrenal antibody (S)	Negative at 1:10 dilution
Antiglomerular basement membrane antibody (S)	
Qualitative	Negative
Quantitative	<5 U/mL

Antinuclear antibodies (ANA) (S)	Negative at 1:40 dilution
Antimitochondrial antibodies (S)	Negative
Antibodies to Scl 70 antigen (S)	Negative
Antibodies to Jo 1 antigen (S)	Negative
Anti-La antibody (S)	Negative
Anti-ds-DNA (double-stranded) (native) antibodies (S)	Negative at 1:10 dilution
Antiextractable nuclear antigens (anti-RNP, anti-Sm, anti-SSB, anti-SSA) (S)	Negative
Antineutrophil cytoplasmic autoantibody, cytoplasmic (c-ANCA) (S)	
Qualitative	Negative
Quantitative	<2.8 U/mL
Antineutrophil cytoplasmic autoantibody, perinuclear (p-ANCA) (S)	
Qualitative	Negative
Quantitative	<1.4 U/mL
Antigranulocyte antibodies (S)	Negative

HLA-B27 present in: (S)

Whites:	Blacks:	Asians:
6%–8%	3%–4%	1%

Intrinsic factor blocking antibody (S)	Negative
Parietal cell antibodies (S)	Negative at 1:20 dilution
Antiplatelet antibodies (S)	Negative
Rheumatoid factor (S, JF)	<30 IU/mL
Anti–smooth muscle antibodies (S)	Negative at 1:20 dilution
Anti–striated muscle antibodies (S)	Negative at <1:60
Antithyroglobulin antibodies (S)	Negative
Antithyroid antibodies (S)	<0.3 IU/mL

S, serum.

Blood Levels for Metabolic Diseases—Reference Values

Acid mucopolysaccharides (U)		
<14 years		Age dependent
>14 years		<3.4 mg/mmol creatinine
Alpha$_1$ antitrypsin (S)		85–213 mg/dL
Alpha-fucosidase	(F)	Compare with controls
	(L)	0.49–1.76 U/g cellular protein
Alpha-galactosidase (Fabry disease)	(S)	0.016–0.2 U/L
	(F)	0.24–1.10 U/g cellular protein
	(L)	0.60–3.63 U/10^{10} cells
Alpha-glucosidase	(F)	0.13–1.84 U/g protein
Alpha-L-iduronidase (Hurler, Scheie syndrome)	(F)	0.44–1.04 U/g cellular protein
	(L)	0.17–0.54 U/10^{10} cells
Alpha-mannosidase (mannosidosis)	(F)	0.71–5.92 U/g cellular protein
	(L)	1.50–3.33 U/10^{10} cells
Alpha-N-acetylglucosaminidase (Sanfilippo type B)	(S)	0.09–0.58 U/L
	(F)	0.076–0.291 U/g cellular protein
Arylsulfatase A (mucolipidosis, Type II and III)	(F)	2.28–15.74 U/g cellular protein
	(L)	≥2.5 U/10^{10} cells
	(U)	>1 U/L
Arylsulfatase B	(F)	1.6–14.9 U/g cellular protein
Beta-galactosidase (Gm$_1$, gangliosidosis, Morquio syndrome)	(F)	4.7–19.1 U/g cellular protein
	(L)	1.01–6.52 U/10^{10} cells
Beta-glucosidase (Gaucher disease)	(F)	3.80–8.70 U/g cellular protein
	(L)	0.08–0.35 U/10^{10} cells
Beta-glucuronidase (MPS VII)	(F)	0.34–1.24 U/g cellular protein

NORMAL

Carbohydrate (U)	Negative
Cystine (U)	
<1 month	64–451 μmol/g creatine
1–5 months	66–375 μmol/g creatine
6–11 months	70–316 μmol/g creatine
1–2 years	53–244 μmol/g creatine
3–15 years	11–53 μmol/g creatine
≥16 years	28–115 μmol/g creatine
Linoleate	≥25% of fatty acids in serum lipids
Arachidonate	≥6% of fatty acids in serum lipids
Palmitate	18%–26% of fatty acids in serum lipids
Phytanate	≤0.3% of fatty acids in serum lipids (>0.5% suggests Refsum disease 0.3%–0.5% borderline)
Free fatty acids (S)	239–843 μEq/L
Galactose (U)	Not detectable
Galactose 1-phosphate (RBC)	
Nongalactosemic	5–49 μg/g Hb
Galactosemic (galactose-restricted diet)	80–125 μg/g Hb
Galactosemic (unrestricted diet)	>125 μg/g Hb
Galactose-1-phosphate uridylyl-transferase (galactosemia) (WB)	18.5–28.5 U/g Hb
<2 years old	20–80 mU/g Hb
≥2 years old	12–40 mU/g Hb
Galactosylceramide-beta-galactosidase (F)	10.3–89.7 mU/g cellular protein
(Krabbe's disease, globoid cell leukodystrophy) (L)	>21.5 mU/g cellular protein
Glucose-6-phosphate dehydrogenase (G-6-PD) (WB)	4.6–13.5 U/g Hb
Glucose phosphate isomerase (B)	49–81 U/g Hb
Hexosaminidase (≥5 years old) (Tay-Sachs, GM_2 gangliosidosis)	
Total (S)	10.4–23.8 U/L
Hexosaminidase A	
Noncarrier	>55% of total
Indeterminate	51%–54% of total
Carrier	≤55% of total
Total (L)	16.4–36.2 U/g cellular protein
Hexosaminidase A	63%–75% of total
Total (F)	92–184.5 U/g cellular protein
Hexosaminidase A	41%–65% of total
Homogentisic acid (U)	Negative
Hydroxyproline, free (U)	<1.3 mg/24 hr
Hydroxyproline, total (U)	
<5 years old	100–400 μg/mg creatinine
5–12 years	100–150 μg/mg creatinine
Females ≥19 years	0.4–2.9 mg/2 hr specimen
Males ≥19 years	0.4–5.0 mg/2 hr specimen
^{35}S Mucopolysaccharide (MPS I, II, III, VI, VII) (F)	Normal or abnormal turnover
≤1 week of age	0.69–2.0 mg/dL (42–124 μmol/L)
<16 years old	0.43–1.4 mg/dL (26–86 μmol/L)
>16 years old	0.68–1.1 mg/dL (41–68 μmol/L)
Phytanate (phytanic acid) (S)	<0.3% normal 0.3%–0.5% borderline >0.5% suggests Refsum disease
Porphyrins, Qualitative (U)	None
Porphyrins, Qualitative (St)	None
Porphyrins, total (RBC)	16–60 μg/dL packed cells
Uro (octacarboxylic)	≤2 μg/dL
Hepatocarboxylic	≤1 μg/dL

Hexacarboxylic	≤1 μg/dL
Pentacarboxylic	≤1 μg/dL
Copro (tetracarboxylic)	≤2 μg/dL
Porphyrins, Total (P)	≤1 μg/dL
Fractionation	≤1 μg/dL for any fraction
Porphyrins (St)	
Coproporphyrin	≤200 μg/24 hr
Protoporphyrin	≤1,500 μg/24 hr
Uroporphyrin	≤1,000 μg/24 hr
Porphyrins, fractionation (U)	
Uroporphyrins	<45 μg/24 hr
Hepatocarboxylic	<13 μg/24 hr
Hexacarboxyl porphyrin	<6 μg/24 hr
Pentacarboxylporphyrin	<5 μg/24 hr
Coproporphyrin	<110 μg/24 hr
Porphobilinogen	<2.0 mg/24 hr
Protoporphyrins, zinc (WB)	
<15 years	<35 μg/dL
>15 years	<50 μg/dL
Sphingomyelinase (Niemann-Pick disease) (F)	1.53–7.18 U/g cellular protein
Tyrosine (P)	
<1 month	55–147 μmol/L
1–24 months	22–108 μmol/L
2–18 years	24–115 μmol/L
>18 years	34–112 μmol/L
Uroporphyrinogen-1-synthase (WB)	9.2–19.1 nmol/sec/L RBC

F, skin fibroblasts; JF, joint fluid; L, leukocytes; P, plasma; RBC, erythrocytes; S, serum; St, stool; U, urine; WB, whole blood.

Critical values may indicate the need for prompt clinical intervention. Any *sudden changes* may also be critical. These values are also called *action values* or *automatic call back values*.

Values will vary according to the laboratory performing the tests as well as patient age and other factors.[1,2]

Amniotic Fluid

Abnormality	
Bilirubin	Increased in hemolytic disease of newborn
Lecithin/sphingomyelin ratio	<2.0 (see Chapter 14)
Color	Yellow, red, green, brown (see Chapter 14)
Abnormal metabolites	See Chapter 12
Chromosomal abnormalities	See Chapter 12

Blood Chemistry

	Low	High
Ammonia	None	>40 μmol/L
Amylase	None	>200 U/L
Arterial pCO_2	<20 mm Hg	>75 mm Hg
Arterial pH	<7.10 units	>7.59 units
Arterial pO_2 (adult)	<40 mm Hg	None
Arterial pO_2 (newborn)	<37 mm Hg (SD = 7)	92 mm Hg (SD = 12)
Bicarbonate	<10 mEq/L	>40 mEq/L
Bilirubin, total (<3 mo of age)	None	>20 mg/dL
Calcium	<6.5 mg/dL	>14.0 mg/dL
Carbon dioxide	<11 mEq/L	>40 mEq/L

[1]Some data from: Emmancipator K. Critical values. ASCP practice parameter. *Am J Clin Path.* 1997;108:247.
[2]Dighe AS, et al. Analysis of laboratory critical value reporting at a large academic medical center. *Am J Clin Path* 2006;125:758.

Cardiac troponin		
cTnT	None	>0.1 μg/L
cTnI	None	>1.6 μg/L
Chloride	<80 mEq/L	>115 mEq/L
Creatine kinase (CK)	None	>3–5× ULN
CK-MB	None	>5% or ≥10 μg/L
Creatinine (except dialysis patients)	None	>5.0 mg/dL
Glucose	<45 mg/dL	>500 mg/dL
Glucose (newborns)	<30 mg/dL	>300 mg/dL
Magnesium	<1.0 mg/dL	>4.7 mg/dL
Osmolality	<250 mOsmol/kg	>600 mOsmol/kg
Phosphorus	<1.1 mg/dL	None
Potassium	<2.8 mEq/L	>6.2 mEq/L
Potassium (newborns)	<2.5 mEq/L	>8.0 mEq/L
Sodium	<120 mEq/L	>160 mEq/L
Urea nitrogen (BUN) (except dialysis patients)	2 mg/dL	>80 mg/dL

Cerebrospinal Fluid (CSF)

	Low	High
Glucose	<80% of blood level	
Protein, total	None	>45 mg/dL
White blood cells (WBCs) in CSF	None	>10/μL
Positive bacterial stain (e.g., Gram, acid-fast), antigen detection, culture or India ink preparation		
Presence of malignant cells or blasts or any other body fluid		

Hematology

	Low	High
Hematocrit (packed cell volume)	<20 vol%	>60 vol%
Hemoglobin	<7 g/dL	>20 g/dL
Platelet count (adult)	<50,000/μL	>1,000,000/μL
Platelet count (pediatric)	<20,000/μL	>1,000,000/μL
Activated partial thromboplastin time	None	>100 seconds
Prothrombin time	None	>30 seconds or >3× control level
Positive test for fibrin split products, protamine sulfate, high heparin level		
Fibrinogen	<100 mg/dL	>700 mg/dL
White blood cells (WBC)	<2,000/μL	>30,000/μL

Presence of blast cells, sickle cells
New diagnosis of leukemia, sickle cell anemia, aplastic crisis
Presence of tumor cells in bone marrow

Inherited or Metabolic Disorders

See Chapter 12.
Any chromosomal abnormalities
Any abnormal prenatal screen (e.g., maternal serum α-fetoproteins [AFP], unconjugated estriol, human chorionic gonadotropin [hCG,] maternal serum Inhibin A, p-aminopropiophenone-A [PAPP-A], free β-hCG)
Any abnormal newborn spot test confirmed by MS/MS

Microbiology

Positive blood culture

Positive Gram stain or culture from any body fluid (e.g., pleural, peritoneal, joint)

Positive bacterial stain (e.g., Gram, acid-fast), antigen detection, culture or India ink preparation from CSF

Positive acid-fast stain or culture from any site

Positive culture or isolate for *Corynebacterium diphtheriae, Cryptococcus neoformans, Bordetella pertussis, Neisseria gonorrhoeae,* dimorphic fungi (e.g., *Histoplasma, Coccidioides, Blastomyces brasiliensis, Paracoccidioides*)

Presence of organisms in peripheral blood smear or bone marrow (e.g., malaria, *Babesia,* microfilaria), heart valve, or other tissue (e.g., *Heliobacter pylori*)

Positive antigen detection (e.g., *Cryptococcus,* group B streptococci, *Haemophilus influenzae* B, *Neisseria meningitidis, Streptococcus pneumoniae*)

Respiratory culture showing heavy growth of pathogens

Pneumocystis, fungi, or viral cytopathic changes in bronchial washings, brushings, or BAL

Any invasive organism in surgical pathology specimens

Stool culture positive for *Salmonella, Shigella, Campylobacter, Vibrio,* or *Yersinia*

Serology

Incompatible cross-match

Positive direct and indirect antiglobulin (Coombs) test on routine specimens

Positive direct antiglobulin (Coombs) test on cord blood

Titers of significant red blood cell (RBC) alloantibodies during pregnancy

Transfusion reaction workup showing incompatible unit of transfused blood

Failure to call within 72 hours for RhIg following possible or known exposure to Rh-positive RBCs

Confirmed positive test for hepatitis, syphilis, AIDS

Increased blood antibody levels for infectious agents (See Chapter 15)

Therapeutic Drugs

	Blood Levels
Acetaminophen	>150 µg/mL
Carbamazepine	>20 µg/mL
Chloramphenicol	>50 µg/mL (peak)
Digoxin	>2.5 ng/mL
Digitoxin	>35 ng/mL
Ethosuximide	>200 µg/mL
Gentamicin	>12 µg/mL
Imipramine	>400 ng/mL
Lidocaine	>9 µg/mL
Lithium	>2 mEq/L
Phenobarbital	>60 µg/mL
Phenytoin	>40 µg/mL
Primidone	>24 µg/mL
Quinidine	>10 µg/mL
Salicylate	>700 µg/mL
Tobramycin	>12 µg/mL (peak)
Theophylline	>25 µg/mL

See Chapter 18 for toxic levels of various therapeutic drugs and toxic substances.

In addition, the physician is promptly notified of any of the following:

Serum glucose, fasting	>130 mg/dL
Serum glucose, random	>250 mg/dL
Serum cholesterol	>300 mg/dL
Serum total protein	>9.0 mg/dL

Blood lead	>10 μg/dL or increased free erythrocyte protoporphyrin (FEP). FEP ≥190 μg/dL is almost always due to lead intoxication. See Chapter 17.
Respiratory culture	Heavy growth of pathogens
Peripheral blood smear	Atypical lymphocytes, plasma cells, organisms

Urinalysis

Strongly positive test for glucose and ketone
Reducing sugars in infants
Presence of pathologic crystals (urate, cysteine, leucine, tyrosine)
Presence of pus, blood, or protein ≥2+
Urine colony count/culture with >50,000 colonies/mL of a single organism

CRIT. VALUES

II

Specific Laboratory Examinations

Acid Phosphatase

Acid phosphatase is a hydrolytic enzyme secreted by various cells; it has five isoenzymes. The greatest amount is found in semen (prostate); it is also detectable in bone, liver, spleen, kidney, red blood cells (RBCs), and platelets.

Use

Formerly used for diagnosis of prostate cancer; increased serum level indicates extension of prostatic cancer beyond the capsule. Now replaced by prostate-specific antigen (PSA).

Occasionally useful to monitor postsurgical treatment, especially if PSA is not useful because of androgen deprivation treatment, which has no effect on acid phosphatase. It should become undetectable with complete tumor resection.

Detection in vaginal fluid indicates sexual intercourse (e.g., rape), with peak in first 12 hours, and remains increased for ≤4 days.

Alkaline Phosphatase[1]

Alkaline phosphatase (ALP) catalyzes hydrolysis of organic phosphate esters at alkaline pH. There are at least five isoenzymes derived from liver (sinusoidal and bile canalicular surface of hepatocytes), bone, intestine (brush border of mucosal

---

[1]Dufour DR, Lott JA, Nolte FS, et al. Diagnosis and monitoring of hepatic injury. I. Performance characteristics of laboratory tests. *Clin Chem* 2000;46:2027–2049.

cells), placenta, and tumor-associated tissues separated by electrophoresis. Placenta and tumor-associated ALP are the most heat resistant to inactivation. More than 95% of total ALP activity comes from bone and liver (~1:1 ratio). The half-life of ALP is 7 to 10 days.

See Chapter 8.

Use

Diagnosis of causes and monitoring of course of cholestasis (e.g., neoplasm, drugs)

Diagnosis of various bone disorders (e.g., Paget disease, osteogenic sarcoma)

Interferences

Intravenous injection of albumin; sometimes marked increase (e.g., 10× normal level) lasting for several days (placental origin); total parenteral nutrition

Decreased by collection of blood in ethylenediaminetetraacetic acid (EDTA), fluoride, or oxalate anticoagulant

Increased (up to 30%) by standing at room or refrigerator temperature

Increased In

Bone origin—increased deposition of calcium.

- Hyperparathyroidism.
- Paget disease (osteitis deformans) (highest reported values 10× to 20× normal). *Marked elevation in absence of liver disease is most suggestive of Paget disease of bone or metastatic carcinoma from prostate.*
- *Increase in cases of metastases to bone is marked only in prostate carcinoma.*
- Osteoblastic bone tumors (osteogenic sarcoma, metastatic carcinoma).
- Osteogenesis imperfecta (due to healing fractures).
- Familial osteoectasia.
- Osteomalacia, rickets.
- Polyostotic fibrous dysplasia.
- Osteomyelitis.
- Late pregnancy; reverts to normal level by 20th day postpartum.
- Children <10 years of age and again during prepubertal growth spurt may have 3× to 4× adult values; adult values by age 20.
- Administration of ergosterol.
- Hyperthyroidism.
- Transient hyperphosphatasemia of infancy.
- Hodgkin disease.
- Healing of extensive fractures (slightly).

Liver disease (see Chapter 8): Any obstruction of biliary system (e.g., stone, carcinoma, primary biliary cirrhosis); is a sensitive indicator of intrahepatic or extrahepatic cholestasis. Whenever the alkaline phosphatase (ALP) is elevated, a simultaneous elevation of 5'-nucleotidase (5'-N) establishes biliary disease as the cause of the elevated ALP. If the 5'-N is not increased, the cause of the elevated ALP must be found elsewhere (e.g., bone disease).

- Liver infiltrates (e.g., amyloid, or leukemia)
- Cholangiolar obstruction in hepatitis (e.g., infectious, toxic)
- Hepatic congestion due to heart disease
- Adverse reaction to therapeutic drug (e.g., chlorpropamide) (progressive elevation of serum ALP may be first indication that drug therapy should be halted); may be 2× to 20× normal
- Increased synthesis of ALP in liver
    Diabetes mellitus—44% of diabetic patients have 40% increase of ALP
    Parenteral hyperalimentation of glucose
- Liver diseases with increased ALP
    <3× to 4× increase lacks specificity and may be present in all forms of liver disease.
    2× increase: acute hepatitis (viral, toxic, alcoholic), acute fatty liver, cirrhosis.
    2× to 10× increase: nodules in liver (metastatic or primary tumor, abscess, cyst, parasite, tuberculosis [TB], sarcoid); is a sensitive indicator of a hepatic infiltrate.
    Increase >2× upper limits of normal in patients with primary breast or lung tumor with osteolytic metastases is more likely caused by liver than bone metastases.

5× increase: infectious mononucleosis, postnecrotic cirrhosis.

10× increase: carcinoma of head of pancreas, choledocholithiasis, drug cholestatic hepatitis.

15 to 20× increase: primary biliary cirrhosis, primary or metastatic carcinoma. Gamma-glutamyltransferase (GGT)/ALP ratio >2.5 is highly suggestive of alcohol abuse.

Chronic therapeutic use of anticonvulsant drugs (e.g., phenobarbital, phenytoin).

Placental origin—appears 16th to 20th week of normal pregnancy, increases progressively to 2× normal up to onset of labor, disappears 3 to 6 days after delivery of placenta. May be increased during complications of pregnancy (e.g., hypertension, preeclampsia, eclampsia, threatened abortion) but difficult to interpret without serial determinations. Lower in diabetic than nondiabetic pregnancy.

Intestinal origin—is a component in ~25% of normal sera; increases 2 hours after eating in persons with blood type B or O who are secretors of H-blood group. Has been reported to be increased in cirrhosis, various ulcerative diseases of the gastrointestinal (GI) tract, severe malabsorption, chronic hemodialysis, acute infarction of intestine.

Benign familial hyperphosphatasemia.

Ectopic production by neoplasm (Regan isoenzyme) without involvement of liver or bone (e.g., Hodgkin disease; cancer of lung, breast, colon, or pancreas; highest incidence in ovary and cervical cancer).

Vascular endothelium origin—some patients with myocardial, pulmonary, renal (one third of cases), or splenic infarction, usually after 7 days during phase of organization.

Hyperphosphatasia (liver and bone isoenzymes).

Hyperthyroidism (liver and bone isoenzymes). Increased ALP alone in a chemical profile, especially with a decreased serum cholesterol and lymphocytosis should suggest excess thyroid medication or hyperthyroidism.

Primary hypophosphatemia (often increased).

ALP isoenzyme determinations are not widely used clinically; heat inactivation may be more useful to distinguish bone from liver source of increased ALP (extremely 90% heat-labile: bone, vascular endothelium, reticuloendothelial system; extremely 90% heat-stable: placenta, neoplasms; intermediate 60%–80% heat-stable: liver, intestine). Also differentiate by chemical inhibition (e.g., L-phenylalanine) or use serum GGT, leucine aminopeptidase (LAP).

Children—mostly bone; little or no liver or intestine.

Adults—liver with little or no bone or intestine; after age 50, increasing amounts of bone.

Normal In

Inherited metabolic diseases (Dubin-Johnson, Rotor, Gilbert, Crigler-Najjar syndromes; types I to V glycogenoses, mucopolysaccharidoses; increased in Wilson disease and hemochromatosis related to hepatic fibrosis).

Consumption of alcohol by healthy persons (in contrast to GGT); may be normal even in alcoholic hepatitis.

In acute icteric viral hepatitis, increase is <2× normal in 90% of cases, but when ALP is high and serum bilirubin is normal, infectious mononucleosis should be ruled out as cause of hepatitis.

Decreased In

Excess vitamin D ingestion

Milk-alkali (Burnett) syndrome

Congenital hypophosphatasia (enzymopathy of liver, bone, kidney isoenzymes)

Achondroplasia

Hypothyroidism, cretinism

Pernicious anemia (one third of patients)

Celiac disease

Malnutrition

Scurvy

Zinc deficiency

Magnesium deficiency

Postmenopausal women with osteoporosis taking estrogen replacement therapy

Therapeutic agents (e.g., corticosteroids, trifluoperazine, antilipemic agents, some hyperalimentation)

Cardiac surgery with cardiopulmonary bypass pump

Ammonia

Ammonia is derived mostly from amino acid metabolism in the liver via the urea cycle.

Use

Should be measured in cases of unexplained lethargy and vomiting, encephalopathy, or any neonate with unexplained neurologic deterioration

Not useful to assess degree of dysfunction (e.g., in Reye syndrome, hepatic function improves and the ammonia level falls, even in patients who finally die of these disorders)

Increased In

Certain inborn errors of metabolism (e.g., defects in urea cycle, organic acid defects) (see Chapter 12).

Transient hyperammonemia in newborn; unknown etiology; may be life-threatening in first 48 hours.

May occur in any patient with severe liver disease (e.g., acute hepatic necrosis, terminal cirrhosis, and after portacaval anastomosis). Increased in most cases of hepatic coma but correlates poorly with degree of encephalopathy. Not useful in known liver disease but may be useful in encephalopathy of unknown cause.

Moribund children. Moderate increases ($\leq$300 μmol/L) without being diagnostic of a specific disease.

Genitourinary (GU) tract infection with distention and stasis.

Ureterosigmoidostomy.

Some hematologic disorders, including acute leukemia and after bone marrow transplant.

Total parenteral nutrition.

Smoking, exercise, valproic acid therapy.

Decreased In

Hyperornithinemia (deficiency of ornithine aminotransaminase activity) with gyrate atrophy of choroid and retina

Antistreptococcal Antibody Titers

Use

Serial determinations are most desirable; a 4× increase in titer confirms an immunologic response to streptococcal organisms when cultures are no longer positive. A high or rising titer is indicative only of current or recent streptococcal infection.

* Direct diagnostic value in
    Scarlet fever
    Erysipelas
    Streptococcal pharyngitis and tonsillitis
* Indirect diagnostic value in
    Rheumatic fever
    Glomerulonephritis (GN)
    Detection of subclinical streptococcal infection
    Differential diagnosis of joint pains of rheumatic fever and rheumatoid arthritis (RA)

Interferences

Early use of penicillin prevents rise of titers.

False-positive results are associated with TB, liver disease (e.g., active viral hepatitis), bacterial contamination.

Latex agglutination method may give a false-positive result in markedly lipemic or contaminated specimens.

Interpretation

♦ Increased serologic titer of antistreptococcal antibodies. One titer is elevated in 95% of patients with acute rheumatic fever (RF); if all are normal, a diagnosis of RF is less likely. This is its primary use.

* Antistreptolysin O titer (ASOT) increase indicates recent Group A streptococcus pharyngitis within the last 2 months (Table 3-1). Increased titer develops 7 to 14 days after infection, rises rapidly to a peak in 4 to 6 weeks, and declines rapidly over the next 4 to 6 months. Increasing titer is more significant than a single determination. Titer is usually >250 IU; it is more significant if above 400 to 500 IU. A normal

BLOOD ANALYT

Table 3-1. Factors Affecting Various Enzymes Other Than Liver Injury

	AST	ALT	ALP	GGT	Bilirubin	NH$_3$
Time of day		H in PM, L at night[a]				
Daily	5%–10%[b]	45%[b]	5%–10%[a,b]	10%–15%	15%–30%	
Race/gender	15% H in black men		15% H in black men; 10% H in black women	2× H in blacks	33% L in black men; 15% in black women	
BMI	≤50% H with H BMI[c]		≤25% H with H BMI	25% H in mild; 50% if BMI >30		
Eating	0	0	I ≤30 U/L[d]	D after meals	≤2× I with fasting up to 48 hours	
Strenuous exercise	3 × H[e]	20% L or if do not exercise[e]	Not significant	Not significant	30% H in men	≤3× I
Pregnancy			2×–3× H in third trimester due to placental isoenzyme	25% L in early pregnancy	D 33% by second trimester	
Drugs			20% L with oral contraceptives	I by various drugs[f]	15% L with oral contraceptives	
Smoking			10% H	1 pack/d: 10% H; ~2× if heavier		I 10 μmol/L after 1 cigarette
Alcohol				Direct relationship to intake		

Storage	Serum stable at room temp for 3 days; refrigerate for 3 weeks; ~10% D	Serum stable ≤7 days in refrigerator	Serum stable at room temp for ≤7 days	I 20% in 1 hour; 100% by 2 hours
Hemolysis	Significant I	Inhibited by hemoglobin		I indirect bilirubin
Muscle injury	Significant I	Mod I	Mod I	
Other	Macroenzymes	H in bone disease, certain tumors; L in hypophosphatasia, severe enteritis in children		≤50% after 1 hour light exposure

0 = no effect; BMI = body mass index; D = decrease; daily = daily variation; H = higher/highest; I = increase; L = lower/lowest; mod = moderate; PM = afternoon.

[a] Similar in liver disease and health.
[b] Similar in elderly and young.
[c] Direct relationship to weight.
[d] Remains I ≤12 hours in persons with blood groups B and O due to intestinal isoenzyme.
[e] Exercise effect mostly in men.
[f] Oral contraceptives, phenytoin, valproic acid, phenobarbital, furosemide, heparin, others.

Adapted from: Dufour DR, Lott JA, Nolte FS, et al. Diagnosis and monitoring of hepatic injury. I. Performance characteristics of laboratory tests. *Clin Chem* 2000;46:2027–2049.

titer helps to rule out clinically doubtful RF. Sometimes ASOT is not increased, even when other titers are increased. Even in severe streptococcal infection, ASOT will be increased in only 70% to 80% of patients. The height of the titer is not related to severity, and the rate of fall is not related to the course of the disease. ASOT is increased in only 30% to 40% of patients with streptococcal pyoderma, 50% of patients with poststreptococcal GN, and ,20% of cases of membranoproliferative GN.

- Anti-DNAse-B assay should also be performed (normal <170 IU/mL varies with age and season) (significant titer >10 in other units) since >15% of patients with acute RF will not have an increased ASOT. This test is superior to ASOT to detect antibodies after group A streptococcal skin infections and is less prone to false-positive reactions; its longer period of reactivity (detectable for several months) is helpful in patients with isolated chorea or carditis, who may have a long latent period before manifesting RF by which time ASOT may have returned to normal. DNAse antibodies are the most sensitive indicators of these conditions.
- Antihyaluronidase titer of 1,000 to 1,500 follows recent streptococcus A disease and ≤4,000 (significant titer >128 different units) with RF. Average titer is higher in early RF than in subsiding or inactive RF or nonrheumatic streptococcal disease or nonstreptococcal infections; is increased as often as ASOT and antifibrinolysin titer.
- Antifibrinolysin (antistreptokinase) titer is increased in RF and in recent hemolytic streptococcus infections.

Conditions	Usual ASOT (Todd Units)
Normal persons	12–166
Active rheumatic fever	500–5,000
Inactive rheumatic fever	12–250
Rheumatoid arthritis	12–250
Acute poststreptococcal glomerulonephritis	500–5,000
Streptococcal upper respiratory tract infection	100–333
Collagen diseases	12–250

Autohemagglutination, Cold

Use
Aid in diagnosis of primary atypical (*Mycoplasma*) pneumonia (found in 30%–90% of patients by early in second week); titer ≥1:14 to 1:224. Not ruled out by negative titer.

Increased In
Atypical hemolytic anemia
Paroxysmal hemoglobinuria
Raynaud disease
Cirrhosis of the liver
Trypanosomiasis
Malaria
Infectious mononucleosis
Adenovirus infections
Influenza
Psittacosis
Mumps
Measles
Scarlet fever
Rheumatic fever
Some cases of lymphoma

Bilirubin[2,3]

Bilirubin is a tetrapyrrole pigment. About 70% to 80% of it is derived from breakdown of senescent RBC hemoglobin (Hb) (≤300 mg/day); 20% to 30% is derived

---

[2]Dufour DR, Lott JA, Nolte FS, et al. Diagnosis and monitoring of hepatic injury. I. Performance characteristics of laboratory tests. *Clin Chem* 2000;46:2027–2049.
[3]Stevenson DK, Wong RJ, Vreman HJ. Reduction in hospital readmission rates for hyperbilirubinemia is associated with use of transcutaneous bilirubin measurements [Editorial]. *Clin Chem* 2005;51481–5482.

from prematurely destroyed marrow erythroid cells and hemoproteins elsewhere (chiefly the liver). Breakdown of RBCs in reticutoendothilial (RE) cells forms bilirubin, which is bound to albumin for transport to the liver, where it is conjugated to glucuronic acid (glucuronides, now called "direct-acting"), which are transported to the bile canaliculi, then to the duodenum. In the bowel, bilirubin is hydrolyzed to unconjugated bilirubin by bacteria (now called urobilinogens); 80% to 90% is excreted in the feces unchanged or oxidized (urobilins); 10% to 20% is reabsorbed, returned to the liver, and re-excreted. Less than 3 mg/dL filters through the glomeruli to the urine as urobilinogen.

See Chapter 8.

Use

Differential diagnosis of diseases of hepatobiliary system and pancreas and other causes of jaundice. Jaundice becomes apparent clinically at >2.5 mg/dL.

Transcutaneous bilirubin measurement has been used as a surrogate in neonatal hyperbilirubinemia.

Interferences

Exposure to either white or ultraviolet light decreases total and indirect bilirubin by 2% to >20%.

Fasting for 48 hours produces a mean increase of 240% in normal persons and 194% in those with hepatic dysfunction.

Increased Conjugated (Direct) Bilirubin In

Hereditary disorders (e.g., Dubin-Johnson syndrome, Rotor syndrome).

Hepatic cellular damage (e.g., viral, toxic, alcohol, drugs). *Increased conjugated bilirubin may be associated with normal total bilirubin in up to one third of patients with liver diseases.*

Methodologic interference:

- Evelyn-Malloy (dextran, novobiocin)
- Diazo reaction (ethoxazene, histidine, indican, phenazopyridine, rifampin, theophylline, tyrosine)
- Sequential Multiple Analysis 12/60 (aminophenol, ascorbic acid, epinephrine, isoproterenol, levodopa, methyldopa, phenelzine)
- Spectrophotometric methods (drugs that cause lipemia)

Other effects (e.g., toxic, cholestasis).

Biliary duct obstruction (extrahepatic or intrahepatic).

Infiltrations, space-occupying lesions (e.g., metastases, abscess, granulomas, amyloidosis).

Direct bilirubin:

- 20% to 40% of total: more suggestive of hepatic than posthepatic jaundice
- 40% to 60% of 1: occurs in either hepatic or posthepatic jaundice
- >50% of total: more suggestive of posthepatic than hepatic jaundice

Total serum bilirubin >40 mg/dL indicates hepatocellular rather than extrahepatic obstruction.

Increased Unconjugated (Indirect) Bilirubin In
(Conjugated, 20% of Total)

Increased bilirubin production

    Hemolytic diseases (e.g., hemoglobinopathies, RBC enzyme deficiencies, disseminated intravascular coagulation [DIC], autoimmune hemolysis)

    Ineffective erythropoiesis (e.g., pernicious anemia)

    Blood transfusions

    Hematomas

Hereditary disorders (e.g., Gilbert disease, Crigler-Najjar syndrome)

Drugs (e.g., causing hemolysis)

Decreased In

Drugs (e.g., barbiturates)

Interferences

Presence of hemoglobin

Exposure to sunlight of fluorescent light

Note: Increased total serum bilirubin (0.58 mg/dL or 10 μmol/L) is related to a lower risk of cardiovascular events (e.g., coronary artery disease [CAD], acute coronary syndrome, AMI) in men for unknown reasons. (See Chapter 5).

BLOOD ANALYT

Calcium

Ninety-nine percent of the body's calcium is in bone. Of the remainder (of 1%) in blood about 5% is ionized (free), about 10% is bound to anions (e.g., phosphate, bicarbonate), about 40% (of 1%) in blood, is bound to plasma proteins, (80% of 40%) of that to albumin.

Total Calcium

See Figure 13-8 and Table 13-7; see also "Parathyroid Hormone," Chapter 13.

Use

Diagnosis of parathyroid dysfunction and hypercalcemia of malignancy. *Ninety percent of cases of hypercalcemia are caused by hyperparathyroidism, neoplasms, or granulomatous diseases. Hypercalcemia of sarcoidosis, adrenal insufficiency, and hyperthyroidism tend to be found in clinically evident disease.*

Blood calcium should be monitored in renal failure, as an effect of various drugs, in acute pancreatitis, and following thyroidectomy and parathyroidectomy.

Interferences

Increased by

• Hyperalbuminemia (e.g., multiple myeloma, Waldenström macroglobulinemia)
• Dehydration
• Venous stasis during blood collection by prolonged application of tourniquet
• Use of cork-stoppered test tubes
• Hyponatremia (<120 mEq/L), which increases the protein-bound fraction of calcium, thereby slightly increasing the total calcium (opposite effect in hypernatremia)

Decreased by

• Hypomagnesemia (e.g., due to cisplatin chemotherapy)
• Hyperphosphatemia (e.g., laxatives, phosphate enemas, chemotherapy of leukemia or lymphoma, rhabdomyolysis)
• Hypoalbuminemia
• Hemodilution

Total serum protein and albumin should always be measured simultaneously for proper interpretation of serum calcium levels, since 0.8 mg of calcium is bound to 1.0 g of albumin in serum; to correct, add 0.8 mg/dL for every 1.0 g/dL that serum albumin falls below 4.0 g/dL; binding to globulin only affects total calcium if globulin >6 g/dL.

Increased In

Hyperparathyroidism

• Primary
• Secondary

Acute and chronic renal failure
Following renal transplant
Osteomalacia with malabsorption
Aluminum-associated osteomalacia
Malignant tumors (especially breast, lung, kidney; 2% of patients with Hodgkin or non-Hodgkin lymphoma)

• Direct bone metastases (up to 30% of these patients) (e.g., breast cancer, Hodgkin and non-Hodgkin lymphoma, leukemia, pancreatic cancer, lung cancer)
• Osteoclastic activating factor (e.g., multiple myeloma, Burkitt lymphoma; may be markedly increased in human T-cell leukemia virus-I–associated lymphoma [see Chapter 11])
• Humoral hypercalcemia of malignancy (parathyroid hormone–related peptide [PTH])
• Ectopic production of 1,25-dihydroxy-vitamin D_3 (e.g., Hodgkin and non-Hodgkin lymphoma)

Granulomatous disease (e.g., uncommon in sarcoidosis, TB, leprosy; more uncommon in mycoses, berylliosis, silicone granulomas, Crohn disease, eosinophilic granuloma, cat scratch fever)

Effect of drugs

- Vitamin D and A intoxication
- Milk-alkali (Burnett) syndrome (rare)
- Diuretics (e.g., thiazides)
- Others (estrogens, androgens, progestins, tamoxifen, lithium, thyroid hormone, parenteral nutrition)

Renal failure, acute or chronic
Other endocrine conditions

- Thyrotoxicosis (in 20%–40% of patients; usually <14 mg/dL)
- More uncommon: Some patients with hypothyroidism, Cushing syndrome, adrenal insufficiency, acromegaly, pheochromocytoma (rare), VIPoma syndrome
- Multiple endocrine neoplasia

Acute osteoporosis (e.g., immobilization of young patients or in Paget disease)
Miscellaneous

- Familial hypocalciuric hypercalcemia
- Rhabdomyolysis causing acute renal failure
- Porphyria
- Dehydration with hyperproteinemia
- Hypophosphatasia
- Idiopathic hypercalcemia of infancy

Concomitant hypokalemia is not infrequent in hypercalcemia. Concomitant dehydration is almost always present because hypercalcemia causes nephrogenic diabetes insipidus.

Decreased In
Hypoparathyroidism

- Surgical
- Idiopathic
- Infiltration of parathyroids (e.g., sarcoid, amyloid, hemochromatosis, tumor)
- Hereditary (e.g., DiGeorge syndrome)

Pseudohypoparathyroidism
Chronic renal disease with uremia and phosphate retention, Fanconi syndromes, renal tubular acidosis
Malabsorption of calcium and vitamin D, obstructive jaundice
Insufficient calcium, phosphorus, and vitamin D ingestion

- Bone disease (osteomalacia, rickets)
- Starvation
- Late pregnancy

Altered bound calcium citrate

- Multiple citrated blood transfusions
- Dialysis with citrate anticoagulation

Hyperphosphatemia (e.g., phosphate enema/infusion)
Rhabdomyolysis
Tumor lysis syndrome
Acute severe illness (e.g., pancreatitis with extensive fat necrosis, sepsis, burns)
Respiratory alkalosis
Certain drugs

- Cancer chemotherapy drugs (e.g., cisplatin, mithramycin, cytosine arabinoside)
- Fluoride intoxication
- Antibiotics (e.g., gentamicin, pentamidine, ketoconazole)
- Chronic therapeutic use of anticonvulsant drugs (e.g., phenobarbital, phenytoin)
- Loop-active diuretics
- Calcitonin

Osteoblastic tumor metastases
Neonates born of complicated pregnancies

- Hyperbilirubinemia
- Respiratory distress, asphyxia

- Cerebral injuries
- Infants of diabetic mothers
- Prematurity
- Maternal hypoparathyroidism

Hypermagnesemia (e.g., magnesium [Mg] for treatment of toxemia of pregnancy)
Magnesium deficiency
Toxic shock syndrome
Temporary hypocalcemia after subtotal thyroidectomy in >40% of patients; >20% are symptomatic

Hypocalcemic Disorders	Serum PO$_4$	PTH	25(OH)D	1,25(OH)$_2$D
Hypoparathyroidism	I	D	N	D
Pseudohypoparathyroidism	I	I	N	D
Vitamin D deficiency	D	I	D	Low N
1α-Hydroxylase deficiency	D	I	N	D
1,25(OH)$_2$D resistance	D	I	N	I

PO$_4$, phosphate; N, normal; I, increased; D, decreased.

Hypocalcemia Associated With	Increased	Decreased
Serum PTH	Pseudohypoparathyroidism	Hypoparathyroidism
	Renal failure, acute/chronic	Acute pancreatitis
	Malabsorption	Magnesium deficiency
	Vitamin D deficiency	
	Phosphate administration	
Serum phosphorus	Hypoparathyroidism	Vitamin D deficiency
	Pseudohypoparathyroidism	Acute pancreatitis
	Renal failure, acute (oliguric phase)/chronic	Renal failure, acute (diuretic phase)
	Phosphate administration	Malabsorption
Serum bicarbonate and pH	Hypoparathyroidism	
Serum Mg	Renal failure, acute/chronic	Magnesium deficiency
		Acute pancreatitis
		Renal failure, acute (diuretic phase)
Urine calcium	Hypoparathyroidism	Other causes of hypocalcemia
Urine phosphate	Renal failure, chronic	Hypoparathyroidism
	Vitamin D deficiency	Pseudohypoparathyroidism
	Malabsorption	Magnesium deficiency
	Phosphate administration	
Urine cAMP	Renal failure, chronic	Hypoparathyroidism
	Vitamin D deficiency	Pseudohypoparathyroidism
	Malabsorption	

cAMP, cyclic adenosine monophosphate.

Calcium, Ionized

Ionized calcium is the physiologically active form of calcium. Ionized calcium homeostasis is regulated by the parathyroid glands, bone, kidney, and intestine.

Use

In patients with hypocalcemia or hypercalcemia with borderline serum calcium and altered serum proteins.

~50% of calcium is ionized; 40% to 45% is bound to albumin; 5% to 10% is bound to other anions (e.g., sulfate, phosphate, lactate, citrate); only the ionized fraction is physiologically active. Total calcium values may be deceiving, since they may be unchanged even if ionized calcium values are changed; (e.g., increased blood pH increases protein-bound calcium and decreases ionized calcium and PTH has the opposite effect) (*blood pH should always be performed with ionized calcium* which is increased in acidosis and decreased in alkalosis). However, in critically ill patients, elevated total serum calcium usually indicates ionized hypercalcemia, and a normal total serum calcium is evidence against ionized hypocalcemia.

Ionized calcium is the preferred measurement rather than total calcium, because it is physiologically active and can be rapidly measured, which may be essential in certain situations (e.g., liver transplantation and rapid or large transfusion of citrated blood make interpretation of total calcium nearly impossible).

Life-threatening complications are frequent when serum ionized calcium <2 mg/dL.

With multiple blood transfusions, ionized calcium <3 mg/dL may be an indication to administer calcium.

Reference ranges for ionized calcium vary with methodology and should be determined by each laboratory.

Interferences

Hypomagnesemia or hypermagnesemia; patients respond to serum Mg that becomes normal but not to calcium therapy. *Serum Mg should always be measured in any patient with hypocalcemia.*

Increase of ions to which calcium is bound:

* Phosphate (e.g., phosphorus administration in treatment of diabetic ketoacidosis, chemotherapy causing tumor lysis syndrome, rhabdomyolysis).
* Bicarbonate.
* Citrate (e.g., during blood transfusion).
* Radiographic contrast media containing calcium chelators (edetate, citrate).

Increased In

Normal total serum calcium associated with hypoalbuminemia may indicate ionized hypercalcemia.

About 25% of patients with hyperparathyroidism have normal total but increased ionized calcium levels.

Acidosis.

Decreased In

Alkalosis, (e.g., hyperventilation, to control increased intracranial pressure) (total serum calcium may be normal), administration of bicarbonate to control metabolic acidosis

Increased serum free fatty acids (increased calcium binding to albumin) due to:

* Certain drugs (e.g., heparin, intravenous lipids, epinephrine, norepinephrine, isoproterenol, alcohol)
* Severe stress (e.g., acute pancreatitis, diabetic ketoacidosis, sepsis, AMI)
* Hemodialysis

Hypoparathyroidism (primary, secondary)

Vitamin D deficiency

Toxic shock syndrome

Fat embolism

Hypokalemia protects patient from hypocalcemic tetany; correction of hypokalemia without correction of hypocalcemia may provoke tetany

Chloride

Chloride is the major extracellular anion; it is not actively regulated normally. It reflects changes in sodium; if it changes independent of sodium, this is usually due to an acid-base disorder.

See Chapter 12.

Use

With sodium, potassium, and CO_2 to assess electrolyte, acid-base, and water balance. Chloride usually changes in the same direction as sodium except in metabolic acidosis with bicarbonate depletion and metabolic alkalosis with bicarbonate excess, when serum sodium levels may be normal.

Interferences

Hyperlipidemia (artifactual change)

Increased In

Metabolic acidosis associated with prolonged diarrhea with loss of sodium bicarbonate ($NaHCO_3$)

Renal tubular diseases with decreased excretion of H^+ and decreased reabsorption of HCO_3^- ("hyperchloremic metabolic acidosis")

Respiratory alkalosis (e.g., hyperventilation, severe central nervous system [CNS] damage)

Drugs

Excessive administration of certain drugs (e.g., ammonium chloride [NH_4Cl], intravenous [IV] saline, salicylate intoxication, acetazolamide therapy)

False (methodologic) increase due to bromides or other halogens

Retention of salt and water (e.g., corticosteroids, guanethidine, phenylbutazone)

Some cases of hyperparathyroidism

Diabetes insipidus, dehydration

Sodium loss > chloride loss (e.g., diarrhea, intestinal fistulas)

Ureterosigmoidostomy

Decreased In

Prolonged vomiting or suction (loss of hydrochloric acid)

Metabolic acidosis with accumulation of organic anions

Chronic respiratory acidosis

Salt-losing renal diseases

Adrenocortical insufficiency

Primary aldosteronism

Expansion of extracellular fluid (e.g., syndrome of inappropriate secretion of antidiuretic hormone [SIADH], hyponatremia, water intoxication, congestive heart failure)

Burns

Drugs

Alkalosis (e.g., bicarbonates, aldosterone, corticosteroids)

Diuretic effect (e.g., ethacrynic acid, furosemide, thiazides)

Other loss (e.g., chronic laxative abuse)

Creatine

Creatine is synthesized in the liver, taken up by muscle for stored energy as creatine phosphate, and broken down to creatinine; it then enters the circulation and is excreted by the kidneys.

Use

Rarely used clinically

Increased In

High dietary intake (meat)

Destruction of muscle

Hyperthyroidism (this diagnosis is almost excluded by normal serum creatine)

Active RA

Testosterone therapy

Decreased In

Not clinically significant

Drugs (e.g., trimethoprim-sulfamethoxazole, cimetidine, cefoxitin)

Interferences

Artifactual decrease in diabetic ketoacidosis

Creatine Kinase Total

Creatine kinase (CK) is an enzyme that catalyzes the interconversion of adenosine triphosphate and creatine phosphate, controlling energy flow within cells, principally muscle.

Use

Marker for injury or diseases of cardiac muscle with good specificity

Measurement of choice for striated muscle disorders (see Chapter 10)

Increased In

Necrosis or inflammation of cardiac muscle (see Chapter 5)

• Disorders listed under CK–myocardial band [MB] (CK index usually >2.5%)

Necrosis, inflammation, or acute atrophy of striated muscle (see Chapter 10)

* Disorders listed under CK-MB (CK index usually <2.5%)
* Muscular dystrophy
* Myotonic dystrophy
* Amyotrophic lateral sclerosis (>40% of cases)
* Polymyositis (70% of cases; average 20× upper limit of normal [ULN])
* Thermal and electrical burns (values usually higher than in AMI)
* Rhabdomyolysis (especially with trauma and severe exertion); marked increase may be 1,000× ULN
* Severe or prolonged exercise as in marathon running (begins 3 hours after start of exercise; peaks after 8–16 hours; usually normal by 48 hours); smaller increases in well-conditioned athletes
* Status epilepticus
* Parturition and frequently the last few weeks of pregnancy
* Malignant hyperthermia
* Hypothermia
* Familial hypokalemic periodic paralysis
* McArdle disease (see Chapter 12)

Drugs and chemicals

* Cocaine
* Alcohol
* Emetine (ipecac)—(e.g., bulimia)
* Chemical toxicity; benzene ring compounds (e.g., xylene) depolarize the surface membrane and leach out low-molecular-weight enzymes, producing very high levels of total CK (100% fraction muscle [MM]) with increased lactate dehydrogenase (LD) (three to five times normal)

Half of patients with extensive brain infarction. Maximum levels are reached in 3 days; the increase may not appear before 2 days; levels are usually lower than in AMI and remain increased for a longer time; levels return to normal within 14 days; high mortality is associated with levels >300 IU. Elevated serum CK in brain infarction may obscure diagnosis of concomitant AMI.

Some persons with large muscle mass (≤2× normal) (e.g., football players)

Slight Increase (Occasionally) In

Intramuscular (IM) injections. Variable increase after IM injection to two to six times normal level. Returns to normal 48 hours after cessation of injections. Rarely affects CK-MB, LD-1, aspartate aminotransferase (AST).

Muscle spasms or convulsions in children

Moderate hemolysis

Normal In

Pulmonary infarction

Renal infarction

Liver disease

Biliary obstruction

Some muscle disorders

* Thyrotoxicosis myopathy
* Steroid myopathy
* Muscle atrophy of neurologic origin (e.g., old poliomyelitis, polyneuritis)

Pernicious anemia

Most malignancies

Scleroderma

Acrosclerosis

Discoid lupus erythematosus

Decreased In

Decreased muscle mass (e.g., elderly, malnutrition, alcoholism)

Rheumatoid arthritis (about two thirds of patients)

Untreated hyperthyroidism

Cushing disease

Connective tissue disease not associated with decreased physical activity

Pregnancy level (8th to 12th week) is said to be ~75% of nonpregnant level

BLOOD ANALYT

Various drugs (e.g., phenothiazine, prednisone, estrogens, tamoxifen, ethanol), toxins, and insecticides (e.g., aldrin, dieldrin)
Metastatic tumor in liver
Multiple organ failure
Intensive care patients with severe infection or septicemia

Creatine Kinase isoenzymes

CK-MB Isoenzyme

Use
CK-MB is a widely used early marker for myocardial injury.

CK-MB Increased In
Necrosis or inflammation of cardiac muscle (*CK index >2.5%; in all other causes, CK index usually <2.5%*):

- AMI.
- Cardiac contusion.
- After thoracic/open heart surgery, values return to baseline in 24 to 48 hours. AMI is difficult to diagnose in the first 24 postoperative hours.
- Resuscitation for cardiac arrest may increase CK and CK-MB in ~50% of patients, with peak at 24 hours, due to defibrillation (>400 J) and chest compression, but CK-MB/CK total ratio may not be increased, even with AMI.
- Percutaneous transluminal coronary angioplasty.
- Myocarditis.
- Prolonged supraventricular tachycardia.
- Cardiomyopathies (e.g., hypothyroid, alcohol).
- Collagen diseases involving the myocardium.
- Coronary angiography (transient).

Necrosis, inflammation, or acute atrophy of striated muscle (see Chapter 10):

- Exercise myopathy; slight to significant increases in 14% to 100% of persons after extreme exercise (e.g., marathons); smaller increases in well-conditioned athletes
- Skeletal muscle trauma with rhabdomyolysis, myoglobinuria
- Skeletal muscle diseases (e.g., myositis, muscular dystrophies, polymyositis, collagen vascular diseases [especially systemic lupus erythematosus (SLE)])
- Familial hypokalemic periodic paralysis
- Electrical and thermal burns and trauma (~50% of patients; but not supported by LD-1 > LD-2)
- Drugs (e.g., alcohol, cocaine, halothane [malignant hyperthermia], ipecac)

Endocrine disorders (e.g., hypoparathyroid, acromegaly, diabetic ketoacidosis; hypothyroidism—total CK four to eight times ULN in 60% to 80% of cases; becomes normal within 6 weeks of replacement therapy)
Some infections:

- Viral (e.g., HIV, Epstein-Barr, influenza, picornaviruses, Coxsackievirus, echovirus, adenoviruses)
- Bacterial (e.g., *Staphylococcus, Streptococcus, Clostridium, Borrelia*)
- Rocky Mountain spotted fever
- Fungal
- Parasitic (e.g., trichinosis, toxoplasmosis, schistosomiasis, cysticercosis)

Others:

- Malignant hyperthermia; hypothermia
- Reye syndrome
- Peripartum period for first day beginning within 30 minutes
- Acute cholecystitis
- Hyperthyroidism and chronic renal failure, which may cause persistent increase although the proportion of CK-MB remains low
- Acute exacerbation of obstructive lung disease

- Drugs (e.g., aspirin, tranquilizers)
- Carbon monoxide poisoning

Some neoplasms:

- For example, prostate, breast
- 90% of patients following cryotherapy for prostate carcinoma with peak at 16 hours to about five times ULN; similar increase in total CK

% Activity Distribution of CK Isoenzymes in Tissue

	CK-MM	CK-MB	CK-BB
Skeletal muscle	99	1	0
Myocardium	77	22	1
Brain	4	0	96

A CK-MB above 15% to 20% should raise the possibility of an atypical macro CK-MB.

CK-MB Not Increased In

Increase in angina pectoris, coronary insufficiency, exercise testing for CAD, or pericarditis implies some necrosis of cardiac muscle, even if a discrete infarct is not identified.

Following cardiopulmonary bypass, cardiac catheterization (including Swan-Ganz), cardiac pacemaker and coronary arteriography, unless the myocardium has been injured by a catheter

IM injections (total CK may be slightly increased)

Seizures (total CK may be markedly increased)

Brain infarction or injury (total CK may be increased)

CK-BB Isoenzyme

Use

Rarely encountered clinically

CK-BB May Be Increased In

Malignant hyperthermia, uremia, brain infarction or anoxia, Reyes syndrome, necrosis of intestine, various metastatic neoplasms (especially prostate), biliary atresia

Atypical Macro Isoenzyme

This isoenzyme is a high-molecular-mass complex of a CK isoenzyme and immunoglobulin, most often CK-BB and monoclonal IgG and a kappa light chain.

It may cause falsely high or low CK-MB results (depending on type of assay), resulting in an incorrect diagnosis of myocardial infarction or delayed recognition of a real myocardial infarction.

The atypical macro isoenzyme is discovered in <2% of all CK isoenzyme electrophoresis studies.

	Type 1	Type 2
Electrophoretic location	Between CK-MM and CK-MB	Cathode side of CK-MM
Prevalence (%)	0.43	1.30
Associated disorders	Myositis Autoimmune disease	Malignancy

Creatinine

Creatinine is formed by the hydrolysis of creatine and phosphocreatine in muscle and by ingestion of meat. It is freely filtered at the glomerulus, secreted at the proximal tubule; some is resorbed.

Use

Serum creatinine levels can be used to diagnose renal insufficiency. *Serum creatinine is a more specific and sensitive indicator of renal disease than BUN. Use of simultaneous BUN and creatinine determinations provides more information in conditions.*

Serum creatinine and blood urea nitrogen (BUN) are not useful in discovering early renal insufficiency, because they do not become abnormal until 50% of renal function has been lost. Serum creatinine shows poor sensitivity but very good specificity.

An increase in serum creatinine occurs in 10% to 20% of patients taking aminoglycosides and ≤20% of patients taking penicillins (especially methicillin).

Serum creatinine levels are a proxy for reduced skeletal muscle mass.

Creatinine clearance is used to measure the glomerular filtration rate (GFR).

Increased In
Diet: Ingestion of creatinine (roast meat)

Muscle disease: gigantism, acromegaly

Prerenal azotemia (see section on BUN)

Postrenal azotemia (see section on BUN)

Impaired kidney function; 50% loss of renal function is needed to increase serum creatinine from 1.0 to 2.0 mg/dL; therefore the test is not sensitive for mild to moderate renal injury

Decreased In
Pregnancy—normal value is 0.4 to 0.6 mg/dL. *A value higher than 0.8 mg/dL is abnormal and should alert the clinician to further diagnostic evaluation.*

Creatinine secretion is inhibited by certain drugs (e.g., cimetidine, trimethoprim).

Proxy for reduced skeletal muscle mass.

Interferences
(Depending on methodology; can be avoided by measuring *rate* of color development)

Artifactual decrease by

* Marked increase of serum bilirubin
* Enzymatic reaction (glucose >100 mg/dL)

Artifactual increase due to

* Reduction of alkaline picrate (e.g., glucose, ascorbate, uric acid). *Ketoacidosis may substantially increase serum creatinine results with alkaline picrate reaction.*
* Formation of colored complexes (e.g., acetoacetate, pyruvate, other ketoacids, certain cephalosporins).
* Enzymatic reaction: 5-fluorocytosine may increase serum creatinine ≤0.6 mg/dL.
* Other methodologic interference (e.g., ascorbic acid, PSP, L-Dopa, phenolsulfonphthalein)

5'-Nucleotidase

5'-nucleotidase is widely distributed in the body, mostly attached to cell membranes; it is primarily derived from the liver, in the canaliculi and sinusoidal membranes.

Use
Is rarely used

May aid in differential diagnosis of hepatobiliary disease occurring during pregnancy

See also Chapter 8.

Increased Only In
Obstructive types of hepatobiliary disease

May be an early indication of liver metastases in the cancer patient, especially if jaundice is absent

Normal In
Pregnancy and postpartum period (in contrast to serum leucine aminopeptidase [LAP] and alkaline phosphatase [ALP])

Gamma-Glutamyl Transferase[4]

Gamma-glutamyl transferase (GGT) is a membrane-bound enzyme that is present (in decreasing order of abundance) in the liver (in cells lining the bile ductules

[4]Dufour DR, Lott JA, Nolte FS, et al. Diagnosis and monitoring of hepatic injury. I. Performance characteristics of laboratory tests. *Clin Chem* 2000;46:2027–2049.

and canaliculi), the proximal renal tubules, the brain, the prostate, and the pancreas (ductules and acinar cells). GGT is responsible for the extracellular metabolism of glutathione, the main antioxidant in cells. Its half-life is 7 to 10 days.

See also Chapter 8.

Use

In liver disease, GGT levels generally parallel changes in serum ALP.

GGT is a sensitive indicator of occult alcoholism; the half-life increases $\geq$28 days.

GGT aids in diagnosis of liver disease in the presence of bone disease, pregnancy, or childhood, which increase serum ALP and LAP but not GGT.

Increased In

Liver disease—generally parallels changes in serum ALP, LAP, and 5'-nucleotidase but is more sensitive.

- Acute hepatitis. Elevation is less marked than that of other liver enzymes, but it is the last to return to normal and therefore is useful to indicate recovery.
- Chronic active hepatitis. Increased (average >7× ULN) more than in acute hepatitis. More elevated than AST and alanine aminotransferase (ALT). In dormant stage, may be the only enzyme elevated.
- Alcoholic hepatitis, average increase >3.5× ULN.
- Alcohol abuse; a GGT/ALP ratio >2.5 is highly suggestive.
- Cirrhosis. In inactive cases, average values are lower (4× ULN) than in chronic hepatitis. Increases of more than 10 to 20 times normal in cirrhotic patients suggest superimposed primary carcinoma of the liver (average increase >21× ULN).
- Primary biliary cirrhosis. Elevation is marked: average >13× ULN.
- Fatty liver. Elevation parallels that of AST and ALT but is greater.
- Obstructive jaundice. Increase is faster and greater than that of serum ALP and LAP. Average increase >5× ULN.
- Liver metastases. Parallels ALP; elevation precedes positive liver scans. Average increase >14× ULN.
- Cholestasis. In mechanical and viral cholestasis, GGT and LAP are increased about equally, but in drug-induced cholestasis, GGT is much more increased than LAP. Average increase >6× ULN.
- Children. Much more increased in biliary atresia than in neonatal hepatitis (300 IU/L is useful differentiating level). Children with α_1-antitrypsin deficiency have higher levels than other patients with biliary atresia.

Pancreatitis. The GGT level is always elevated in acute pancreatitis. In chronic pancreatitis, it is increased when there is involvement of the biliary tract or active inflammation.

AMI. Increased in 50% of patients. Elevation begins on the fourth to the fifth day, reaching a maximum at 8 to 12 days. With shock or acute right heart failure, an early peak may appear within 48 hours, with a rapid decline followed by a later rise.

Is increased risk factor for myocardial infarction and cardiac death.

Heavy use of alcohol: *Is the most sensitive indicator and a good screening test for alcoholism*, since elevation exceeds that of other commonly assayed liver enzymes.

Various drugs (e.g., barbiturates, phenytoin (Dilantin), tricyclic antidepressants, acetaminophen).

Some cases of carcinoma of prostate.

Neoplasms, even in absence of liver metastases; especially malignant melanoma, carcinoma of breast and lung; highest levels seen in hypernephroma.

Others (e.g., gross obesity [slight increase], renal disease, cardiac disease, postoperative state).

Normal In

Pregnancy (in contrast to serum ALP, LAP) and children over 3 months of age; therefore may aid in differential diagnosis of hepatobiliary disease occurring during pregnancy and childhood

Bone disease or patients with increased bone growth (children and adolescents); therefore useful in distinguishing bone disease from liver disease as a cause of increased serum ALP

Renal failure

Strenuous exercise

BLOOD ANALYT

Glucose

Use

Diagnosis of diabetes mellitus (defined by World Health Organization as an unequivocal increase of fasting serum [or plasma] glucose $\geq$126 mg/dL on more than one occasion or any glucose $\geq$200 mg/dL)

Control of diabetes mellitus

Diagnosis of hypoglycemia

May Be Increased In

Diabetes mellitus, including

- Hemochromatosis
- Cushing syndrome (with insulin-resistant diabetes)
- Acromegaly and gigantism (with insulin-resistant diabetes in early stages; hypopituitarism later)

Increased circulating epinephrine

- Adrenalin injection
- Pheochromocytoma
- Stress (e.g., emotion, burns, shock, anesthesia)

Acute pancreatitis

Chronic pancreatitis (some patients)

Wernicke encephalopathy (vitamin B_1 deficiency)

Some CNS lesions (subarachnoid hemorrhage, convulsive states)

Effect of drugs (e.g., corticosteroids, estrogens, alcohol, phenytoin, thiazides, propranolol, chronic hypervitaminosis A)

May Be Decreased In

Pancreatic disorders

- Islet cell tumor, hyperplasia
- Pancreatitis
- Glucagon deficiency

Extrapancreatic tumors

- Carcinoma of adrenal gland
- Carcinoma of stomach
- Fibrosarcoma
- Other

Hepatic disease

- Diffuse severe disease (e.g., poisoning, hepatitis, cirrhosis, primary or metastatic tumor)

Endocrine disorders

- Hypopituitarism*
- Addison disease
- Hypothyroidism
- Adrenal medulla unresponsiveness
- Early diabetes mellitus

Functional disturbances

- Postgastrectomy
- Gastroenterostomy
- Autonomic nervous system disorders

Pediatric anomalies

- Prematurity*
- Infant of diabetic mother*
- Ketotic hypoglycemia
- Zetterstrom syndrome
- Idiopathic leucine sensitivity
- Spontaneous hypoglycemia in infants

*May cause neonatal hypoglycemia.

Enzyme diseases

* von Gierke disease*
* Galactosemia*
* Fructose intolerance*
* Amino acid and organic acid defects*
    Methylmalonic acidemia*
    Glutaric acidemia, Type II*
    Maple syrup urine disease*
    3-hydroxy, 3-methyl glutaric acidemia*
* Fatty acid metabolism defects*
    Acyl CoA dehydrogenase defects*
    Carnitine deficiencies*
    Other
* Exogenous insulin (factitious)
* Oral hypoglycemic medications (factitious)
* Leucine sensitivity
* Malnutrition
* Hypothalamic lesions
* Alcoholism

*May cause neonatal hypoglycemia.

Interferences

Blood samples in which serum is not separated from blood cells will show glucose values decreasing at rate of 3% to 5% per hour at room temperature.

Most glucose strips and meters quantify whole blood glucose, whereas most laboratories use plasma or serum, which reads 10% to 15% higher.

Postprandial capillary glucose is ≤36 mg/dL higher than venous glucose at peak of 1 hour postprandial; usually returns to negligible fasting difference within 4 hours but in ~15% of patients, there may still be >20 mg/dL difference.

There is considerable imprecision between glucose meters from the same manufacturer and between different types of meters.

Only fresh capillary blood should be used with some reflectance meters; low oxygen content (e.g., venous blood, high altitudes >3,000 meters) gives falsely increased values.

Reflectance meter value on capillary blood of ~160 mg/dL corresponds to venous plasma level of ~135 mg/dL in most cases.

Immunologic Tests

See Table 3-2.

Inflammatory Reactants, Acute

Acute-phase reactants in serum are not used for this purpose (except C-reactive protein [CRP]), but it is important to recognize this cause of increase when they are used in testing for other conditions (e.g., ferritin, ceruloplasmin):

* Fibrinogen usually increases by 200% to 400%; this is reflected in the erythrocyte sedimentation rate (ESR)
* Alpha$_1$-antitrypsin increases by 200% to 400%
* Alpha$_2$-macroglobulin
* Haptoglobin increases by 200% to 400%
* Ferritin usually increases by 50%
* Ceruloplasmin
* Alpha$_1$-acid glycoprotein
* Serum amyloid A

Acute phase reactants in serum that are useful include:

* CRP, which can increase up to 1,000% in severe tissue injury
* Serum complement, which usually increases by 50%
* Total white blood cell (WBC) count, neutrophils, and bands
* ESR

BLOOD ANALYT

Table 3-2.	Immunologic Tests
Antibody Test	**Interpretation**
Anti–acetylcholine receptor	Result <1 IU makes the diagnosis of myasthenia gravis. May be negative in ocular myasthenia, Eaton-Lambert syndrome, and treated or inactive generalized myasthenia gravis.
Antistriational	Found in >80% of cases of myasthenia gravis with thymoma; ≤25% of cases of thymoma without myasthenia gravis; 30% of patients with myasthenia gravis alone; in 25% of drug reactions caused by penicillamine.
Antiadrenal	High titers are characteristic of autoimmune hypoadrenalism (70%); rarely found in Addison disease caused by tuberculosis.
Anti–glomerular basement membrane	See Rapidly Progressive Nonstreptococcal GN, Chapter 14.
Anti-intrinsic factor	Antibodies indicate overt or latent pernicious anemia; present in ~75% of cases.
Parietal cell antibodies	See Chapter 11.
Antimitochondrial	Strongly positive in >90% of patients with primary biliary cirrhosis but almost never in extrahepatic biliary obstruction; therefore useful in differentiating these two conditions. May also be found in 5% of chronic hepatitis cases.
Anti-IgA endomysial, Anti-IgA Ttg, Antigliadin IgA antibodies	See Chapter 7
Anti-skin, interepithelial	Positive test confirms diagnosis of pemphigus and is helpful in evaluating bullous disease. Positive in >90% of pemphigus cases; absence largely excludes that diagnosis. Rise and fall of titer may indicate impending relapse or effective control of disease. High sensitivity; lower specificity.
Anti-skin, dermal-epidermal	Positive in >80% of bullous pemphigus cases. Absence does not exclude that diagnosis. Some correlation of titer and severity. Low sensitivity; high specificity.
Anti–smooth muscle (antiactin)	Titer ≥1:160 in 95% of patients with autoimmune chronic active hepatitis. Less often in other liver and viral diseases.
Antithyroglobulin and antithyroid microsome antibodies	Absence of both antibodies is strong evidence against autoimmune thyroiditis (see Chapter 13).
Thyroid-stimulating immunoglobulin (TSI)	Elevated TSI occurs only in Graves disease. Failure of TSI to fall after antithyroid therapy predicts relapse. Elevated TSI in a patient who is HLA-DR3 positive predicts poor response to antithyroid therapy and suggests need for alternate mode of treatment.
Rheumatoid factor	See Rheumatoid Arthritis, Chapter 10, and Table 10-7.
Neutrophil antibodies	
Cytoplasmic (e-ANCA)	Wegener granulomatosis.
Perinuclear (p-ANCA)	Vasculitis, Churg-Strauss syndrome, microscopic polyarteritis nodosa, ulcerative colitis.

ANCA, antineutrophil cytoplasmic antibodies.
Source: Peter JP. *The Use and Interpretation of Tests in Clinical Immunology,* 8th ed. Santa Monica, CA: Clinical Immunology Laboratories, 1991.

C-Reactive Protein, High Sensitivity

High-sensitivity CRP (hsCRP) is an acute-phase reactant produced by hepatocytes, induced by the release of interleukin 1 and 6, that reflects activation of systemic inflammation.

Use/Increased In

Disorders due to acute inflammation or infections. Values ≥1 mg/L may also represent subclinical infection/inflammation and should be repeated in 3 to 4 weeks.

♦ Significant independent risk factor for CAD, stroke, and peripheral vascular disease in apparently healthy persons and adds to predictive value of total cholesterol/HDL-C for future events. Risk increases progressively by amount: Low risk: <1.0 mg/L; average risk = 1.0 to 3.0 mg/L; high risk ≥3.0 mg/L. Risk increases incrementally as well for peripheral vascular disease and stroke.

May be a criterion for metabolic syndrome.

♦ Inflammatory disorders:

Monitoring course and effect of therapy:

- In any acute inflammatory change, CRP shows an earlier (begins in 4 to 6 hours) more intense increase rise than ESR; with recovery, disappearance of CRP precedes the return to normal of ESR. CRP disappears when inflammatory process is suppressed by steroids or salicylates. Generally parallels ESR but is not influenced by anemia and other disorders that affect ESR.
- Indicator of activity in rheumatic disease (e.g., RA, rheumatic fever), seronegative arthritides (e.g., Reiter syndrome), vasculitis syndromes (e.g., hypersensitivity vasculitis).
- Inflammatory bowel disease: significantly higher in Crohn disease than in ulcerative colitis and corresponds to relapse, remission, and response to therapy in Crohn disease.
- Chronic inflammatory diseases: usually <10.0 mg/L; if >10.0 mg/L, superimposed infection should be ruled out.
- Acute inflammation: 40 to 200 mg/L; mild inflammation: 10 to 40 mg/L.

♦ Tissue injury or necrosis:

- AMI.
- Has been reported as a risk factor for the development of hypertension.[5]
- Ischemia or infarction of other tissues.
- Level of 150 mg/L distinguishes mild from severe acute pancreatitis.
- Rejection of kidney or marrow transplant but not of heart transplant.
- Malignant (but not benign) tumors, especially breast, lung, GI tract; >10 mg/L in one third of cases. May be a useful tumor marker, since a high CRP is often present when carcinoembryonic antigen and other tumor markers are not increased.
- Following surgery: CRP increases within 4 to 6 hours and peaks at 48 to 72 hours (usually at 25 to 35 mg/L). It begins to decrease after third postoperative day and returns to normal by fifth to seventh day; failure to fall is a more sensitive indicator of complications (e.g., infection, pulmonary infarction) than WBC count, ESR, temperature, pulse rate. A baseline preoperative value should be obtained; the serial pattern is different with complicating infection or tissue necrosis.
- Burns, trauma (≤1,000 mg/L).

♦ Infection.

- Indicates presence of infection (30 to 35 mg/L in 80% to 85% of acute bacterial infections and <20 mg/L in viral infections, but it is not useful to differentiate bacterial from viral infections).
- Exclusion of infection (with a normal value).
- Monitoring of recovery from infection (spontaneous or due to therapy).
- Diagnosis of postoperative and intercurrent infection: After surgery, CRP begins to increase in 4 to 6 hours, peaks by 48 to 72 hours (usually 25 to 35 mg/L), and begins to decrease after the third day to normal by the fifth to seventh day. A

[5]Sesso HD, Buring JE, Rifai N, et al. C-reactive protein and the risk of developing hypertension. *JAMA* 2003;290:2945–2951.

BLOOD ANALYT

baseline preoperative value should be obtained; the serial pattern is different with complicating infection or tissue necrosis.
- Highest levels are found in acute bacterial infections (>30 mg/dL; usually <20 mg/dL in most acute viral infections), but may be very high in both.
- Infections in various sites, (e.g., neonatal, GU, GI and biliary tracts, pelvic inflammatory disease, CNS) or due to other organisms (e.g., parasites, fungi).
    In premature rupture of membranes, CRP >12.5 mg/L in cord blood strongly suggests chorioamnionitis.
    Increased CRP in a seriously ill neonate is indication for immediate vigorous antibiotic therapy.
    In children under 6 years old with meningitis, CRP >20 mg/L after 12 hours (50 mg/L in older patients) suggests bacterial rather than viral cause. CRP in the cerebrospinal fluid has been reported as specific to differentiate bacterial from viral meningitis.

Leukemia: Fever, blast crisis, or cytotoxic drugs cause only modest elevation of CRP, but intercurrent infection stimulates significantly higher CRP levels and is particularly useful to monitor response to antibiotic therapy. Not useful to differentiate graft-versus-host disease from infection after marrow transplant.

Not Increased
Autoimmune diseases (e.g., SLE, mixed connective tissue disease, dermatomyositis, scleroderma): little or no increase unless infection is present
Pregnancy
Strenuous exercise
Angina
Cerebrovascular accident other than atherosclerosis
Seizures
Asthma
Common cold
Rejection of heart transplant

Complement Components

These are circulating glycoproteins that promote inflammation. They identify and destroy foreign cells and microorganisms by lysis, opsonization, or by attracting phagocytes. The three major activation pathways are classical (antibody-sensitized cells), *alternative* (early defense against microorganisms), and *mannan-binding Lectin* (MBLectin) (recognizes microorganisms).

Use
Evaluation of role of complement in immune disorders
To determine whether a deficiency is acquired or genetic

Normal In
Renal diseases

- IgG-IgA nephropathy (Berger disease)
- Idiopathic rapidly progressive GN
- Antiglomerular basement membrane disease
- Immune complex disease
- Negative immunofluorescence findings

Systemic diseases

- Polyarteritis nodosa
- Hypersensitivity vasculitis
- Wegener granulomatosis
- Schönlein-Henoch purpura
- Goodpasture syndrome
- Visceral abscess

Decreased In (Acquired)
*Common Diseases Associated with **Arthritis***

- Active SLE, particularly associated with renal disease
- Prodromal HBV hepatitis
- Essential mixed cryoglobulinemia

- Sjögren syndrome
- Serum sickness
- Short bowel syndrome

Common Diseases Associated with *Vasculitis*

- Rheumatoid vasculitis
- Essential mixed cryoglobulinemia
- Sjögren syndrome
- Hypocomplementemic vasculitis
- Wegener granulomatosis

Common Diseases Associated with *Nephritis*

	% of Cases in Which Occurs
Acute poststreptococcal GN	Transient (3–8 week) decline in C3
Membranoproliferative GN	
Type I ("classic" MPGN)	50%–80%
Type II ("dense deposit disease")	80%–90%; C3 often remains depressed
SLE	
Focal	75%
Diffuse	90%
Subacute bacterial endocarditis	90%
Cryoglobulinemia	85%
"Shunt" nephritis	90%
Serum sickness	—
Atheromatous emboli	—

Decreased In (Inherited)	Deficient Complement
SLE	C1qINH, C1q, C1r, C1s, C2, C4, C5, C8
Hereditary angioedema	C1qINH
Familial Mediterranean fever	C5aINH
Urticarial vasculitis	C3
GN	C1r, C2
Severe combined immunodeficiency	C1q
X-linked hypogammaglobulinemia	C1q
Recurrent infections	C3, C3bINH
Recurrent neisserial infections	C5, C6, C7, C8

Increased In

Inflammatory conditions that increase acute-phase reactants

Use of Individual Complement Levels

CH50 detects activation of classical pathway; measures functional activity of C1 through C9; is useful for screening since a normal result indicates classic complement pathway is functionally intact. Decrease indicates that 50% to 80% of normal amounts have been depleted. Detects all inborn and most acquired complement deficiencies.

AH50 measures only activity of alternative pathway.

C3 is useful for screening for classic and activation of alternate complement pathway. May be increased in subacute inflammation, biliary obstruction, nephrotic syndrome, and corticosteroid therapy. May be decreased in immune complex disease (especially lupus nephritis), acute poststreptococcal GN, hypercatabolism (especially C3b inactivator deficiency), massive necrosis and tissue injury, sepsis, viremia, hereditary deficiency, infancy.

C3 or CH50 may be useful for monitoring disease activity in SLE, but usefulness may vary from case to case.

C4 may be decreased in immune complex disease (especially lupus nephritis), hereditary angioneurotic edema, hereditary deficiency, acute GN, infancy, or when classic pathway is activated.

Decreased C3 and C4 indicates initiation of classic activation pathway and activation of functional unit (e.g., active viral hepatitis, immune complex formation).

Normal C3 with decreased C4 suggests a C4 deficiency (e.g., hereditary angioedema, malaria, some SLE patients).

BLOOD ANALYT

Normal C4 with decreased C3 suggests congenital C3 deficiency, deficiency of the C3b inactivator, or activation of functional unit by alternate pathway (e.g., Gram-negative toxemia).

Normal C3 and C4 with decreased C50 indicates isolated deficiency of another complement component, and further testing is indicated.

C2 may be decreased in immune complex disease (especially lupus nephritis), hereditary angioedema, hereditary deficiency, infancy.

C1 esterase inhibitor deficiency is characteristic of hereditary angioedema. In heterozygotes, C1 inhibitor is substantially decreased. Patients have low CH100, C4, and C2 during attacks.

C1q can be very low in acquired angioedema, severe combined immunodeficiency, and X-linked hypogammaglobulinemia; it may be decreased in SLE and infancy.

An absence of or marked decrease in any of the components of complement will cause an absence of or marked decrease in the total hemolytic complement assay, but mild to moderate decrease of an individual component of complement may not alter this total.

Deficiency of early classic pathway components (C1q, C1r, C1s, C2, C4):

- Serum shows absence of hemolytic complement activity.
- The affected component is absent or decreased on immunochemical testing.
- Opsonic activity and generation of chemotactic activity are defective.
- Infections are not a problem (due to alternative pathway being intact).
- Symptoms due to collagen vascular disorders (e.g., nephritis, arthritis).

Hereditary deficiency of C2 results in severe invasive and often repeated infections (especially septicemia, meningitis) due to *Streptococcus pneumoniae.*[6]

Deficiency of C3 and C5:

- Serum shows absence of hemolytic complement activity.
- C3 or C5 is absent or decreased in serum.
- Defective opsonic capacity and chemotactic activity are present.
- Severe recurrent infections (e.g., pneumonia, sepsis, otitis media, chronic diarrhea) are present.
- These often respond to fresh plasma.

Deficiency of late classic pathway components (C6, C7, C8):

- Serum shows absence of hemolytic complement activity.
- Normal opsonization and generation of chemotactic factor are present.
- There is a total absence of the individual component.
- Recurrent systemic infections take place due to *Neisseria gonorrhoeae* or *Neisseria meningitides.*

Erythrocyte Sedimentation Rate

See Table 3-3.

Use

○ *Indicates presence and intensity of an inflammatory process; never diagnostic of a specific disease. Changes are more significant than a single abnormal occurrence.*

To detect occult disease (e.g., screening program), but a normal ESR does not exclude malignancy or other serious disease.

♦ To confirm or exclude a diagnosis (a normal ESR virtually excludes diagnosis of temporal arteritis or polymyalgia rheumatica; >50 mm/hr in 90% of these patients).

To monitor the course or response to treatment of certain diseases (e.g., temporal arteritis, polymyalgia rheumatica, acute rheumatic fever, RA, SLE, Hodgkin disease, TB, bacterial endocarditis). *ESR is normal in 5% of patients with RA or SLE.*

Rarely may assist in differential diagnosis (e.g., AMI as opposed to angina pectoris, early acute appendicitis versus ruptured ectopic pregnancy or acute pelvic inflammatory disease, RA as opposed to osteoarthritis, acute versus quiescent gout).

Said to be useful to differentiate iron deficiency anemia (ESR normal) from anemia of acute or chronic disease alone or combined with iron deficiency, in which ESR is almost always increased.

---

[6]Jönsson G, Truedsson L, Sturfelt G, et al. Hereditary C2 deficiency in Sweden: Frequent occurrence of invasive infection, atherosclerosis, and rheumatic disease. *Medicine* 2005;84:23–34.

Table 3-3.   Changes in Erythrocyte Sedimentation Rate

Disease	Increased In	Not Increased In
Infectious	Tuberculosis (especially) Acute hepatitis Many bacterial infections	Typhoid fever Undulant fever Malarial paroxysm Infectious mononucleosis Uncomplicated viral diseases
Cardiac	Acute myocardial infraction Active rheumatic fever After open heart surgery	Angina pectoris Active renal failure with heart failure
Abdominal	Acute pelvic inflammatory disease Ruptured ectopic pregnancy Pregnancy—third month to ~3 wk postpartum Menstruation	Acute appendicitis (first 24 h) Unruptured ectopic pregnancy Early pregnancy
Joint	Rheumatoid arthritis Pyogenic arthritis	Degenerative arthritis

Miscellaneous	Significant tissue necrosis,
	   especially neoplasms (most
	   frequently malignant lymphoma,
	   cancer of colon and breast)
	 Increased serum globulins (e.g.,
	   myeloma, cryoglobulinemia,
	   macroglobulinuria)
	 Decreased serum albumin
	 Hypothyroidism
	 Hyperthyroidism
	 Acute hemorrhage
	 Nephrosis, renal disease with
	   azotemia
	 Arsenic and lead intoxification
	 Dextran and polyvinyl compounds
	   in blood
	 Temporal arteritis
	 Polymyalgia rheumatica
		Peptic ulcer
		 Acute allergy

BLOOD ANALYT

- Rarely (6 in 10,000) useful for screening of asymptomatic persons after history and physical examination. Unexplained increase with no detectable disease occurs in <3% of cases.
- ○ *Hyperviscosity syndrome should be suspected in patients with hyperproteinemia (e.g., multiple myeloma, Waldenström macroglobulinemia) with rouleaux formation but no increase of ESR.*
- ○ Extreme elevation of ESR is found particularly in association with malignancy (most frequently malignant lymphoma, carcinomas of colon and breast), hematologic diseases (most frequently myeloma), collagen diseases (e.g., RA, SLE), renal diseases (especially with azotemia), drug fever, and other conditions (e.g., cirrhosis). In patients with cancer, ESR >100 mm/hr indicates metastases. Other causes of ESR >100 mm/hr are severe infections (osteomyelitis, subacute bacterial endocarditis), giant cell arteritis, polymyalgia rheumatica, and renal diseases.

Interferences That Increase ESR
Macrocytosis
Hypercholesterolemia
Increased fibrinogen, gamma globulins, or beta globulins
Technical factors (e.g., tilted ESR tube, high room temperature)
Drugs (e.g., dextran, methyldopa, methysergide, penicillamine, theophylline, trifluperidol, vitamin A)

Interferences That Decrease ESR

Abnormally shaped RBCs, especially sickle cells; hereditary spherocytosis; acanthocytosis

Microcytosis (e.g., HbC disease)

Hypofibrinogenemia (e.g., DIC, massive hepatic necrosis)

High WBC count

Technical factors (e.g., short ESR tube, low room temperature, delay in test performance >2 hours, clotted blood sample, excess anticoagulation, bubbles in tube)

Drugs (e.g., quinine [therapeutic], salicylates [therapeutic], drugs that cause a high glucose level, high doses of adrenal steroids)

Increased In

Chronic inflammatory diseases, especially collagen and vascular diseases

Postoperative (may be increased for up to 1 month), postpartum

Decreased In

Polycythemia (vera or secondary)

Congestive heart failure

Cachexia

High doses of adrenal steroids

Factors That Do Not Affect ESR

Body temperature

Recent meal

Aspirin

Nonsteroidal anti-inflammatory drugs

Formula for normal range Westergren ESR: For men: $ESR = age\ (years) \div 2$; for women: $ESR = [age\ (years) + 10] \div 2$

Lactate, Blood

Blood lactate is an end product of anaerobic glycolysis as an alternative to pyruvate entering the Krebs cycle, enabling metabolism of glucose.

Increased Due To

Hypoxia (e.g., inadequate tissue perfusion and oxygenation)

Diabetic ketoacidosis

Treatment with Ringer lactate solution

Impaired clearance due to liver dysfunction

Deficiency of pyruvate dehydrogenase that controls entry of substrate into Krebs cycle

Lactate Dehydrogenase

LD occurs in the cytoplasm of all cells; there are five isoenzymes. The highest concentrations are found in heart, liver, skeletal muscle, kidney, and the RBCs, with lesser amounts in lung, smooth muscle, and brain. LD catalyzes the interconversion of lactate and pyruvate.

Use

Replaced by cardiac troponin (cTn) as late marker for AMI

May be a useful marker of disease activity in cryptogenic fibrosing alveolitis and extrinsic allergic alveolitis

Marker for hemolysis, in vivo (e.g., hemolytic anemias) or in vitro (artifactual)

LD is a very nonspecific test

Interferences

Artifactual hemolysis (e.g., poor venipuncture, failure to separate clot from serum, heating of blood)

Increased In

Cardiac Diseases

- AMI. Increases in 10 to 12 hours, peaks in 48 to 72 hours (~3× normal). Prolonged elevation over 10 to 14 days was formerly used for late diagnosis of AMI; now replaced by cTn. An LD reading >2,000 IU suggests a poorer prognosis. An LD-1/

LD-2 ratio >1 ("flipped" LD) may also occur in acute renal infarction, hemolysis, some muscle disorders, pregnancy, and some neoplasms.
- Congestive heart failure. LD isoenzymes are normal, or LD-5 may be increased due to liver congestion.
- Insertion of intracardiac prosthetic valves consistently causes chronic hemolysis, with increase of total LD, LD-1, and LD-2. This is also often present before surgery in patients with severe hemodynamic abnormalities of cardiac valves.
- Cardiovascular surgery. LD is increased ≤2× normal without cardiopulmonary bypass and returns to normal in 3 to 4 days; with extracorporeal circulation, it may increase ≤4 to 6× normal; this increase is more marked when the transfused blood is older.
- Increases have been described in acute myocarditis and rheumatic fever.

Liver Diseases

- Cirrhosis, obstructive jaundice, and acute viral hepatitis show moderate increases.
- Hepatitis—Most marked increase is of LD-5, which occurs during prodromal stage and is greatest at time of onset of jaundice; total LD is also increased in 50% of the cases. LD increase is isomorphic in infectious mononucleosis. An ALT:LD or AST:LD ratio within 24 hours of admission ≥1.5 favors acute hepatitis over acetaminophen or ischemic injury.
- Acute and subacute hepatic necrosis. LD-5 is also increased with other causes of liver damage (e.g., chlorpromazine hepatitis, carbon tetrachloride poisoning, exacerbation of cirrhosis, or biliary obstruction) even when total LD is normal.
- Metastatic carcinoma to the liver may show marked increases. It has been reported that an LD-4/LD-5 ratio <1.05 favors diagnosis of hepatocellular carcinoma, compared to a ratio above 1.05, which favors liver metastases in >90% of cases.[7]
- *If liver disease is suspected but total LD is very high and isoenzyme pattern is isomorphic, rule out cancer.*
- Liver disease, per se, does not produce marked increase of total LD or LD-5.
- Various inborn metabolic disorders affecting the liver (e.g., hemochromatosis, Dubin-Johnson syndrome, hepatolenticular degeneration, Gaucher disease, McArdle disease).

Hematologic Diseases

- Untreated pernicious anemia and folic acid deficiency show some of the greatest increases, chiefly in LD-1, which is >LD-2 ("flipped"), especially with Hb <8 g/dL.
- Increased in all hemolytic anemias, which can probably be ruled out if LD-1 and LD-2 are not increased in an anemic patient. Normal in aplastic anemia and iron-deficiency anemia, even when the anemia is very severe.

Diseases of Lung

- Pulmonary embolus and *infarction—pattern of moderately increased LD with increased LD-3 and normal AST 24 to 48 hours after onset of chest pain* (see heading "Lactate Dehydrogenase Isoenzymes")
- Sarcoidosis

Malignant Tumors

- Increased in ~50% of patients with various solid carcinomas, especially in advanced stages.
- In patients with cancer, a higher LD level generally indicates a poorer prognosis. Whenever the total LD is increased and the isoenzyme pattern is nonspecific or cannot be explained by obvious clinical findings (e.g., myocardial infarction, hemolytic anemia), cancer should always be ruled out. LD is moderately increased in ~60% of patients with lymphomas and lymphocytic leukemias and ~90% of patients with acute leukemia; degree of increase is not correlated with WBC counts; levels are relatively low in lymphatic types of leukemia. LD is increased in 95% of patients with chronic myelogenous leukemia, especially LD-3 (see Chapter 11).

[7]Castaldo G, Oriani G, Cimino L, et al. Serum lactate dehydrogenase isoenzyme 4/5 ratio discriminates between hepatocellular and secondary liver neoplasia. *Clin Chem* 1991;37:1419–1423.

BLOOD ANALYT

Diseases of Muscle (see Chapter 10)

- Marked increase of LD-5, likely due to anoxic injury of striated muscle
- Electrical and thermal burns and trauma; marked increase of total LD (about the same as in myocardial infarction) and LD-5

Renal Diseases

- Renal cortical infarction may mimic pattern of AMI. *Rule out renal infarction if LD-1 (>LD-2) is increased in the absence of myocardial infarction or anemia or if increased LD is out of proportion to AST and ALP levels.*
- May be slightly increased (LD-4 and LD-5) in nephrotic syndrome. LD-1 and LD-2 may be increased in nephritis.

Miscellaneous Conditions

These conditions may be related to hemolysis, involvement of liver, striated muscle, heart, etc.

- Various infectious and parasitic diseases
- Hypothyroidism, subacute thyroiditis
- Collagen vascular diseases
- Acute pancreatitis
- Intestinal obstruction
- Sarcoidosis
- Various CNS conditions (e.g., bacterial meningitis, cerebral hemorrhage, or thrombosis)
- Drugs

Decreased In

Irradiation

Lactate Dehydrogenase Isoenzymes

% Activity Distribution of LD Isoenzymes in Tissue

	LD-1	LD-2	LD-3	LD-4	LD-5
Heart	60	30	5	3	2
Liver	0.2	0.8	1	4	94
Kidney	28	34	21	11	6
Cerebrum	28	32	19	16	5
Skeletal muscle	3	4	8	9	76
Lung	10	18	28	23	21
Spleen	5	15	31	31	18
RBCs	40	30	15	10	5
Skin	0	0	4	17	79

Use

To delineate tissue source of elevated serum total LD.
Interpretation of this test must be correlated with clinical status of the patient. Do serial determinations to obtain maximum information.

Condition	LD Isoenzyme(s) Increased
AMI	1 > 2
Acute renal cortical infarction	1 > 2
Pernicious anemia	1
Sickle cell crisis	1 and 2
Electrical and thermal burn, trauma	5
Mother carrying erythroblastotic child	4 and 5
AMI with acute congestion of liver	1 and 5
Early hepatitis	5 (may become normal, even when ALT is still rising)
Malignant lymphoma	3 and 4 (2 may also increase) (reflects effect of chemotherapy)
Active chronic granulocytic leukemia	3 increased in >90% of cases but normal during remission

Carcinoma of prostate	5; 5:1 ratio >1
Dermatomyositis	5
SLE	3 and 4
Collagen disorders	2, 3, and 4
Pulmonary embolus and infarction	2, 3, and 4
Pulmonary embolus with acute cor pulmonale causing acute congestion of liver	3 and 5
Congestive heart failure	2, 3, and 4
Viral infections	2, 3, and 4
Various neoplasms	2, 3, and 4
Strenuous physical activity	4 and 5
Leptomeningeal carcinomatosis	5

Abnormally migrating macroenzymes (circulating complexes of LD with IgA or IgG immunoglobulins) may be found in some autoimmune conditions, cancer, and some miscellaneous conditions, but not in amounts that are useful for diagnosis.

Increased total LD with normal distribution of isoenzymes may be seen in myocardial infarction, arteriosclerotic heart disease with chronic heart failure, and various combinations of acute and chronic diseases (this may represent a general stress reaction).

About 50% of patients with malignant tumors have altered LD patterns. This change often is nonspecific and of no diagnostic value. Solid tumors, especially those of germ cell origin, may increase LD-1.

In megaloblastic anemia, hemolysis, renal cortical infarction, and some patients with cancer, the isoenzyme pattern may mimic that of myocardial infarction, but the time to peak value and the increase help to differentiate these conditions.

Leucine Aminopeptidase

LAP, a protease, is present in all tissues but especially in the biliary epithelium of the liver.

Use
Is rarely used.
Parallels serum ALP except that:

- LAP is usually normal in the presence of bone disease or malabsorption syndrome.
- LAP is a more sensitive indicator of choledocholithiasis and of liver metastases in anicteric patients.

When serum LAP is increased, urine LAP is almost always increased, but when urine LAP is increased, serum LAP may have already returned to normal.

Increased In
Obstructive, space-occupying, or infiltrative lesions of the liver.
SLE, in correlation with disease activity.
Various neoplasms (even without liver metastases) (e.g., breast, endometrium, and germ cell tumors).
Preeclampsia, between 33 and 39 weeks of pregnancy.

LIPIDS

Cholesterol, High-Density Lipoproteins, Low-Density Lipoproteins, Triglycerides
See Disorders of Lipid Metabolism (Chapter 5).

Lipoproteins

Apolipoprotein AI

Use
Decreased levels of apolipoprotein AI (apo AI) are associated with an increased risk of coronary heart disease (CHD).

Increased In
Familial hyperalphalipoproteinemia
Pregnancy
Estrogen therapy
Alcohol consumption
Exercise
Decreased In
Tangier disease
"Fish-eye" disease
Familial hypoalphalipoproteinemia
Familial lecithin-cholesterol acyltransferase (LCAT) deficiency
Types I and V hyperlipoproteinemia
Diabetes mellitus
Cholestasis
Hemodialysis
Infection
Drugs (e.g., diuretics, β-blockers, androgenic steroids, glucocorticoids, cyclosporine)

Apolipoprotein AII

Increased In
Alcohol consumption
Decreased In
Tangier disease
Cholestasis
Cigarette smoking

Apolipoprotein AIV

Increased In
Postprandial lipemia
Decreased In
Abetalipoproteinemia
Chronic pancreatitis
Malabsorption
Obstructive jaundice
Acute hepatitis
Total parenteral nutrition

Apolipoprotein (a)

Use
Increased risk of CHD with serum levels >0.03 g/L
Increased In
Pregnancy
Patients who have had acute myocardial infarction (AMI)
Decreased In
Drugs (e.g., nicotinic acid, neomycin, anabolic steroids)

Apolipoprotein B48

Apo B48 is normally absent during fasting.
Increased In
Hyperlipoproteinemia (types I, V)
Apo E deficiency
Decreased In
Liver disease
Hypolipoproteinemia and abetalipoproteinemia
Malabsorption

Apolipoprotein B100

Use
Increased levels are associated with an increased risk of CHD.

Increased In
Hyperlipoproteinemia (types IIa, IIb, IV, V)
Familial hyperapobetalipoproteinemia
Nephrotic syndrome
Pregnancy
Biliary obstruction
Hemodialysis
Cigarette smoking
Drugs (e.g., diuretics, β-blockers, cyclosporine, glucocorticoids)
Decreased In
Hypolipoproteinemia and abetalipoproteinemia
Type I hyperlipoproteinemia (hyperchylomicronemia)
Liver disease
Exercise
Infections
Drugs (e.g., cholesterol-lowering drugs, estrogens)

Apolipoprotein CI

Increased In
Hyperlipoproteinemia (types I, III, IV, V)
Decreased In
Tangier disease

Apolipoprotein CII

Increased In
Hyperlipoproteinemia (types I, III, IV, V)
Decreased In
Tangier disease
Hypoalphalipoproteinemia
Apo CII deficiency
Nephrotic syndrome

Apolipoprotein CIII

Use
With combined hereditary apo AI and apo CIII deficiency, increased risk of premature
    CHD
Increased In
Hyperlipoproteinemia (types III, IV, V)
Decreased In
Tangier disease
Combined with hereditary deficiency apo AI

Apolipoprotein E

Increased In
Hyperlipoproteinemia (types I, III, IV, V)
Pregnancy
Cholestasis
Multiple sclerosis in remission
Drugs (e.g., dexamethasone)
Decreased In
Drugs (e.g., adrenocorticotropic hormone [ACTH])

Magnesium[8]

Mg is primarily an intracellular ion associated with GI absorption and renal excretion.

[8]Lum G. Clinical utility of magnesium measurement. *Lab Med* 2004;35:106.

BLOOD ANALYT

Use

Diagnosis and monitoring of hypomagnesemia and hypermagnesemia, especially in renal failure or GI disorders

Increased In (>2.4 mg/dL)

Iatrogenic (is usual cause; most often with impaired renal function).

- Diuretics (e.g., furosemide >80 mg/day, thiazides)
- Antacids or enemas containing Mg
- Laxative and cathartic abuse
- Parenteral nutrition
- Mg for eclampsia or premature labor
- Lithium carbonate intoxication

Renal failure (when GFR approaches 30 mL/min); in chronic renal failure, hypermagnesemia is inversely related to residual renal function. Increase is rarely observed with normal renal function.

Dehydration with diabetic coma before treatment.

Hypothyroidism.

Addison disease and after adrenalectomy.

Controlled diabetes mellitus in older patients.

Accidental ingestion of large amount of sea water.

Signs	Approximate Mg Serum Levels in Adults (mg/dL)
Normal adult	1.7–2.3
Neuromuscular depression, hypotension	>4–6
Difficulty in urination	>5
CNS depression	6–8
Nausea, vomiting, cutaneous flushing	6
Hyporeflexia, drowsiness	8
Coma	12–17
Electrocardiographic changes	>10
Complete heart block	30
Cardiac arrest	34–40

Decreased In (<1.8 mg/dL)

Almost always caused by GI or renal disturbance. Chronic Mg deficiency produces hypocalcemia secondary to decreased production and effectiveness of PTH.

GI Disease

- Malabsorption (e.g., sprue, small bowel resection, biliary and intestinal fistulas, abdominal irradiation, celiac disease and other causes of steatorrhea; familial Mg malabsorption)
- Abnormal loss of GI fluids (chronic ulcerative colitis, Crohn disease, villous adenoma, carcinoma of colon, laxative abuse, prolonged aspiration of GI tract contents, vomiting, etc.)

Renal Disease

A level above 2 mEq/day in urine during hypomagnesemia indicates excessive renal loss.

- Chronic GN
- Chronic pyelonephritis
- Renal tubular acidosis
- Diuretic phase of acute tubular necrosis
- Postobstructive diuresis
- Drug injury
    Diuretics (e.g., mercurials, ammonium chloride, thiazides, furosemide)
    Antibiotics (e.g., aminoglycosides, gentamicin, tobramycin, carbenicillin, ticarcillin, amphotericin B)
    Digitalis (in 20% of patients taking digitalis)
    Antineoplastic (e.g., cisplatin)
    Cyclosporine

- Tubular losses due to ions or nutrients
  Hypercalcemia
  Diuresis caused by glucose, urea, or mannitol
  Phosphate depletion
  Extracellular fluid volume expansion
  Primary renal Mg wasting

Nutritional

- Prolonged parenteral fluid administration without Mg (usually >3 weeks)
- Acute and chronic alcoholism and alcoholic cirrhosis
- Starvation with metabolic acidosis
- Kwashiorkor, protein-calorie malnutrition

Endocrine

- Hyperthyroidism
- Aldosteronism (primary and secondary)
- Hyperparathyroidism and other causes of hypercalcemia
- Hypoparathyroidism
- Diabetes mellitus (in ≤39% of patients; caused by osmotic diuresis)

Metabolic

- Excessive lactation
- Third trimester of pregnancy
- Insulin treatment of diabetic coma

Other

- Toxemia of pregnancy or eclampsia
- Lytic tumors of bone
- Active Paget disease of bone; caused by increased uptake by bone
- Acute pancreatitis
- Transfusion of citrated blood
- Severe burns
- Sweating
- Sepsis
- Hypothermia

Mg deficiency frequently coexists with other electrolyte abnormalities; it may cause apparently unexplained hypocalcemia and hypokalemia and should always be measured in such cases. About 40% of cases have coexisting hypokalemia.
About 90% of patients with high or low serum Mg levels are not clinically recognized; therefore, routine inclusion of Mg with electrolyte measurements has been suggested.
Digitalis sensitivity and toxicity frequently occur with hypomagnesemia.
Ionized Mg is decreased in only ~70% of critically ill patients with decreased total Mg.
Because deficiency can exist with normal or borderline serum Mg levels, a 24-hour urine test may be indicated by frequent concomitant disorders (see previous).
A 24-hour urine level <25 mg suggests Mg deficiency (in the absence of conditions or agents that promote magnesium excretion). If caused by renal loss, urine Mg should be >3.65 to 6 mg/day.
If level is <2.4 mg/day, collect 24-hour urine sample during IV administration of 72 mg of MgCl. Some 60% to 80% of the load is excreted by patients with normal Mg stores ᴗ50% excretion suggests nonrenal Mg depletion.

Osmolality

***Osmolality* is the concentration of a solution expressed in osmoles of solute particles per kilogram of solvent, or the property of a solution that depends on concentration of solute per unit *(mass)* of solvent. Osmolality is measured with an osmometer by freezing point depression or vapor pressure elevation techniques, or it can be calculated from a formula.**
***Osmoles* refers to the molecular weight of a solute (in grams) divided by the number of ions or particles into which it dissociates in solution.**

Osmolarity **is the osmotic concentration of solution expressed as osmoles of solute per liter of solution, or the property of solution that depends on the concentration of solute per unit of total** *volume* **of solvent.**

Usual reference values:

- Serum osmolality: 280 to 300 mOs/kg of water
- Urine osmolality: 100 to 1,200 mOs/kg of water
- Urine specific gravity: 1.001 to 1.035

Use
Diagnosis of nonketotic hyperglycemic coma
To monitor fluid and electrolyte balance

- Determine serum water deviation from normal for evaluation of hyponatremia (see Table 13-27)
- *Urine and plasma osmolality are more useful to diagnose state of hydration than changes in Hct, serum proteins, and BUN, which are more dependent on factors other than hydration.*

Increased In
Hyperglycemia
Diabetic ketoacidosis (*osmolality should be determined routinely in grossly unbalanced diabetic patients*)
Nonketotic hyperglycemic coma
Hypernatremia with dehydration

- Diarrhea, vomiting, fever, hyperventilation, inadequate water intake
- Diabetes insipidus—central
- Nephrogenic diabetes insipidus—congenital or acquired (e.g., hypercalcemia, hypokalemia, chronic renal disease, sickle cell disease, effect of some drugs)
- Osmotic diuresis—hyperglycemia, administration of urea or mannitol

Hypernatremia with normal hydration—caused by hypothalamic disorders

- Insensitivity of osmoreceptors (essential hypernatremia)—water loading does not return serum osmolality to normal; chlorpropamide may lower serum sodium toward normal
- Defect in thirst (hypodipsia)—forced water intake returns serum osmolality to normal

Hypernatremia with overhydration—iatrogenic or accidental (e.g., infants given feedings with high sodium concentrations or given $NaHCO_3$ for respiratory distress or cardiopulmonary arrest)
Alcohol ingestion, which is the commonest cause of hyperosmolar state and of coexisting coma and hyperosmolar state

Decreased In (Equivalent to Hyponatremia)
Hyponatremia with hypovolemia (urine sodium is usually >20 mEq/L)

- Adrenal insufficiency (e.g., salt-losing form of congenital adrenal hyperplasia, congenital adrenal hypoplasia, hemorrhage into adrenals, inadequate replacement of corticosteroids, inappropriate tapering of steroids)
- Renal losses, (e.g., osmotic diuresis; proximal renal tubular acidosis; salt-losing nephropathies, usually tubulointerstitial diseases such as GU tract obstruction; pyelonephritis; medullary cystic disease; polycystic kidneys)
- GI tract loss (e.g., vomiting, diarrhea)
- Other losses (e.g., burns, peritonitis, pancreatitis)

Hyponatremia with normal volume or hypervolemia (dilutional syndromes)

- Congestive heart failure, cirrhosis, nephrotic syndrome
- SIADH

Formulas for *calculation* or *prediction* of serum osmolality for emergency use (not meant to supplant measured osmolality):

$$mOsm/L = (1.86 \times serum\ Na) + (serum\ glucose \div 18) + (BUN \div 28) + 9\ (in\ mg/dL)$$

or

$$in\ SI\ units: = (1.86 \times serum\ Na) + serum\ glucose\ (mmol/L) + BUN\ (mmol/L) + 9$$

More simply: $NA^+ + K^+ + (BUN \div 28) + (glucose \div 18)$. Because K^+ is relatively small, and BUN has no influence on water distribution, the formula can be simplified to $2Na^+ + (glucose \div 18)$.

Osmolal Gap

The osmolal gap is the difference between measured and calculated values; in healthy persons it is <10.

Use

Osmolal gap has been used to estimate the blood alcohol. Since serum osmolality increases 22 mOsm/kg for every 100 mg/dL of ethanol, estimated blood alcohol (mg/dL) = osmolal gap $\times$ 100 $\div$ 22.

Osmolal Gap >10 Because Of

Decreased serum water content

- Hyperlipidemia (serum will appear lipemic)
- Hyperproteinemia (total protein >10 g/dL)

Additional low-molecular-weight substances in the serum (measured osmolality will be >300 mOsm/kg water)

- Ethanol; an especially large osmolal gap with a low or only moderately elevated ethanol level should raise the possibility of another low-molecular-weight toxin (e.g., methanol).
- Methanol
- Isopropyl alcohol
- Mannitol (osmolal gap can be used to detect accumulation of infused mannitol in serum)
- Ethylene glycol, acetone, ketoacidosis, paraldehyde result in relatively small osmolal gaps, even at lethal levels

Severely ill patients, especially those in shock, acidosis (lactic, diabetic, alcoholic), renal failure
Laboratory analytic error

- Random error from all measurements could add or subtract $\leq$15 mOsm/kg
- Use of incorrect blood collection tubes

Phosphate

Phosphate is used in the synthesis of phosphorylated compounds. It accompanies glucose into cells. About 80% of phosphate is contained in bones.

See Figure 3-1.

Use

Monitor blood phosphate level in renal and GI disorders, effect of drugs

Increased In

Most causes of hypocalcemia, except vitamin D deficiency, in which it is usually decreased
Acute or chronic renal failure (most common cause) with decreased GFR
Increased tubular reabsorption or decreased glomerular filtration of phosphate

- Hypoparathyroidism (idiopathic, surgical, irradiation)
- Secondary hyperparathyroidism (renal rickets)
- Pseudohypoparathyroidism types I and II
- Other endocrine disorders (e.g., Addison disease, acromegaly, hyperthyroidism)
- Sickle cell anemia

Increased cellular release of phosphate

- Neoplasms (e.g., myelogenous leukemia, lymphomas)
- Excessive breakdown of tissue (e.g., chemotherapy for neoplasms, rhabdomyolysis, malignant hyperthermia, lactic acidosis, acute yellow atrophy, thyrotoxicosis)
- Bone disease, (e.g., healing fractures, multiple myeloma [some patients], Paget disease (some patients), osteolytic metastatic tumor in bone [some patients])
- Childhood

Increased phosphate load

- Exogenous phosphate (oral or IV) from:
  Phosphate enemas, laxatives or infusions

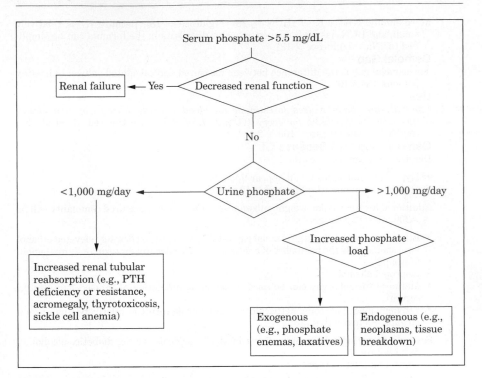

Fig. 3-1. Algorithm for hyperphosphatemia. PTH, parathyroid hormone.

> Excess vitamin D intake
> IV therapy for hypophosphatemia or hypercalcemia
> Milk-alkali (Burnett) syndrome (some patients)
> Massive blood transfusions
> *Hemolysis of blood*

Miscellaneous

- High intestinal obstruction
- Sarcoidosis (some patients)

Decreased In
Primary hypophosphatemia
Decreased GI absorption

- Decreased dietary intake
- Decreased intestinal absorption, e.g., malabsorption, steatorrhea, secretory diarrhea, vomiting, vitamin D deficiency, drugs (antacids, alcohol, glucocorticoids)

Decreased renal tubular reabsorption (>100 mg/day in urine during hypophosphatemia indicates excessive renal loss)

- Primary (e.g., Fanconi syndrome, rickets [vitamin D-deficient or dependent or familial], idiopathic hypercalciuria)
- Secondary or acquired tubular disorders (e.g., hypercalcemia, excess PTH, primary hyperparathyroidism, hypokalemia, hypomagnesemia, diuresis, glycosuria, metabolic or respiratory acidosis, metabolic alkalosis, volume expansion, acute gout, dialysis, etc.)

Intracellular shift of phosphate

- Alcoholism*
- Diabetes mellitus*

*Indicates conditions that may be associated with severe hypophosphatemia (<1 mg/dL). Moderate hypophosphatemia = 1 to 2.5 mg/dL.

- Acidosis (especially diabetic ketoacidosis)
- Hyperalimentation*
- Nutritional recovery syndrome* (rapid refeeding after prolonged starvation)
- IV administration of glucose* (e.g., recovery after severe burns, hyperalimentation)
- Respiratory alkalosis* (e.g., gram-negative bacteremia) or metabolic
- Salicylate poisoning
- Administration of anabolic steroids, androgens, epinephrine, glucagon, insulin
- Cushing syndrome (some patients)
- Prolonged hypothermia (e.g., open heart surgery)

Sepsis

Often more than one mechanism is operative, usually associated with prior phosphorus depletion.

Plasma, Discolored

Discolored plasma is differentiated by spectrophotometric analysis of plasma.
Caused by
Total bilirubin (causes of jaundice)
Lipemia
Free hemoglobin (hemolysis) (pink)
Ceruloplasmin (green color)
Excess drugs, medications, diet (e.g., sun tanning agents [orange-pink color caused by canthaxanthin]), carotenoids
Bacterial contamination
Diseases

Potassium

Potassium is a primary intracellular ion; <2% is extracellular. In acidemia, potassium moves out of cells; in alkalemia, potassium moves into cells. Hypokalemia inhibits aldosterone production; hyperkalemia stimulates aldosterone production. Plasma sodium and potassium control potassium reabsorption.

See Table 3-4 and Figures 3-2 and 3-3.
Use
Diagnosis and monitoring hyperkalemia and hypokalemia in various conditions, e.g., treatment of diabetic coma, renal failure, severe fluid and electrolyte loss, effect of certain drugs
Diagnosis of familial hyperkalemic periodic paralysis and hypokalemic paralysis
Increased In
Potassium Retention
GFR <3 to 5 mL/min

- Oliguria caused by any condition (e.g., renal failure)
- Chronic nonoliguric renal failure associated with dehydration, obstruction, trauma, or excess potassium
- Drugs
  Renal toxicity, e.g., amphotericin B, methicillin, tetracycline

GFR >20 mL/min

- Decreased (aldosterone) mineralocorticoid activity
  Addison disease
  Hypofunction of renin-angiotensin-aldosterone system
    Hyporeninemic hypoaldosteronism with renal insufficiency (GFR 25 to 75 mL/min)
    Various drugs (e.g., nonsteroidal anti-inflammatory drugs, angiotensin-converting enzyme inhibitors, cyclosporine, pentamidine)

---

*Indicates conditions that may be associated with severe hypophosphatemia (<1 mg/dL). Moderate hypophosphatemia = 1 to 2.5 mg/dL.

BLOOD ANALYT

Table 3-4.   Urine and Blood Changes in Electrolytes, pH, and Volume in Various Conditions

Measurement	Pulmonary Emphysema	Congestive Heart Failure	Excessive Sweating	Diarrhea	Pyloric Obstruction	Dehydration	Starvation	Malabsorption	Salicylate Intoxication	Primary Aldosteronism
Blood										
Sodium	N	N or D	D	D	D	I	N	D	N	I
Potassium	N	N	N	D	D	N	D	D	N or D	D
Bicarbonate	I	N	N	D	I	N or D	D	N or D	D	I
Chloride	D	D	D	D	D	I	N	N	I	D
Volume	N or I	I	N	D	D	D	N or D	D	N	N
Urine										
Sodium	D	D	D	D	D	I	N or I	D	I	D
Potassium	N	N	N	N or D	N	I	I or N	D	N or I	I
pH	D	N	N	D	I	D	D	N or D	I	N or D
Volume	N	D	N	D	D	D	I	N	N	I

Measurement	Adrenal Cortical Insufficiency	Diabetes Insipidus	Diabetic Acidosis	Mercurial Diuretic Administration	Thiazide Diuretic Administration	Ammonium Chloride Administration	Acetazolamide (Diamox) Administration	Renal Tubular Acidosis	Chronic Renal Failure	Acute Renal Failure
Blood										
Sodium	D	N or I	D	D	D	D	D	D	D	D
Potassium	I	N	N or I	D	D	D	D	D	N or D	I
Bicarbonate	N or D	N	D	I	D	D	D	D	D	D
Chloride	D	I	D	D	D	I	I	I	D or N	I
Volume	D	D	D	D	D	D	D	D	V	I
Urine										
Sodium	I	N	I	I	I	I	I	I	I	D
Potassium	N or D	N	I	I	I	I	I	I	I	D
pH	N or I	N	D	D	N or I	I	I	I	I	N or I
Volume	N or D	I	I	I	I	I	I	I	V^a	D

N, normal; D, decreased; I, increased; V, variable.
^{a}Usually increased.

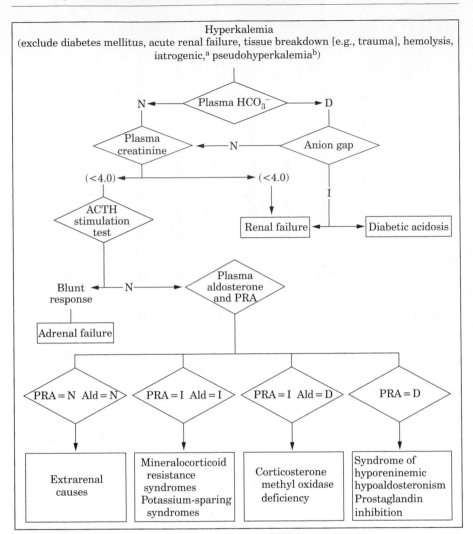

Fig. 3-2. Algorithm for hyperkalemia. ACTH, adrenocorticotropic hormone; Ald, aldosterone; D, decreased; HCO_3^-, bicarbonate; I, increased; N, normal; PRA, plasma renin activity.
[a]Potassium (K)-sparing diuretics, administration of K (e.g., blood transfusions, salt substitutes, potassium penicillin).
[b]Pseudohyperkalemia = WBC >100,000/μL or platelet count >1,000,000/μL (serum K > plasma K).

Decreased aldosterone production
    Pseudohypoaldosteronism
    Aldosterone antagonist drugs (e.g., spironolactone, captopril, heparin)
• Inhibition of tubular secretion of potassium
    Drugs (e.g., spironolactone, triamterene, amiloride)
    Hyperkalemic type of distal renal tubular acidosis (e.g., sickle cell disease, obstructive uropathy)
• Mineralocorticoid-resistant syndromes (increased renin and aldosterone may be low in those marked with an asterisk; see following)
    Primary tubular disorders

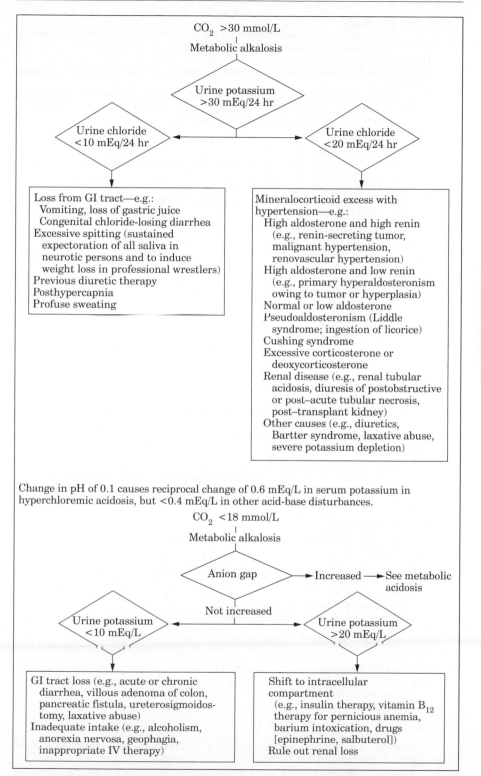

CO$_2$ >30 mmol/L
Metabolic alkalosis

Urine potassium
>30 mEq/24 hr

Urine chloride
<10 mEq/24 hr

Urine chloride
<20 mEq/24 hr

Loss from GI tract—e.g.:
  Vomiting, loss of gastric juice
  Congenital chloride-losing diarrhea
Excessive spitting (sustained
  expectoration of all saliva in
  neurotic persons and to induce
  weight loss in professional wrestlers)
Previous diuretic therapy
Posthypercapnia
Profuse sweating

Mineralocorticoid excess with
hypertension—e.g.:
  High aldosterone and high renin
    (e.g., renin-secreting tumor,
    malignant hypertension,
    renovascular hypertension)
  High aldosterone and low renin
    (e.g., primary hyperaldosteronism
    owing to tumor or hyperplasia)
  Normal or low aldosterone
  Pseudoaldosteronism (Liddle
    syndrome; ingestion of licorice)
  Cushing syndrome
  Excessive corticosterone or
    deoxycorticosterone
  Renal disease (e.g., renal tubular
    acidosis, diuresis of postobstructive
    or post–acute tubular necrosis,
    post–transplant kidney)
  Other causes (e.g., diuretics,
    Bartter syndrome, laxative abuse,
    severe potassium depletion)

Change in pH of 0.1 causes reciprocal change of 0.6 mEq/L in serum potassium in
hyperchloremic acidosis, but <0.4 mEq/L in other acid-base disturbances.

CO$_2$ <18 mmol/L
Metabolic alkalosis

Anion gap

Increased → See metabolic
acidosis

Not increased

Urine potassium
<10 mEq/L

Urine potassium
>20 mEq/L

GI tract loss (e.g., acute or chronic
  diarrhea, villous adenoma of colon,
  pancreatic fistula, ureterosigmoidostomy, laxative abuse)
Inadequate intake (e.g., alcoholism,
  anorexia nervosa, geophagia,
  inappropriate IV therapy)

Shift to intracellular
compartment
  (e.g., insulin therapy, vitamin B$_{12}$
  therapy for pernicious anemia,
  barium intoxication, drugs
  [epinephrine, salbuterol])
Rule out renal loss

BLOOD ANALYT

Fig. 3-3. Algorithm for hypokalemia.

Hereditary

Acquired (e.g., SLE, amyloidosis, sickle cell nephropathy,* obstructive uropathy, renal allograft transplant, chloride shift)

Potassium Redistribution

Familial hyperkalemic periodic paralysis (Gamstorp disease, adynamia episodica hereditaria)

Acute acidosis (especially hyperchloremic metabolic acidosis; less with respiratory; little with metabolic acidosis due to organic acids) (e.g., diabetic ketoacidosis, lactic acidosis, acute renal failure, acute respiratory acidosis)

* Decreased insulin
* Beta-adrenergic blockade
* Drugs (e.g., succinylcholine, great excess of digitalis, arginine infusion)
* Use of hypertonic solutions (e.g., saline, mannitol)
* Intravascular hemolysis (e.g., transfusion reaction, hemolytic anemia), rhabdomyolysis
* Rapid cellular release (e.g., crush injury, chemotherapy for leukemia or lymphoma, burns, major surgery)

Increased Supply of Potassium

Laboratory artifacts (e.g., hemolysis during venipuncture, conditions associated with thrombocytosis [>1,000,000/μL] or leukocytosis [>100,000/μL], incomplete separation of serum and clot.)

Potassium value can be elevated ~15% in slight hemolysis (Hb ≤50 mg/dL) and elevated ~30% to 50% in moderate hemolysis (Hb >100 mg/dL). Thus, potassium status can be assessed in those with slight hemolysis but not in those with moderate hemolysis.

Prolonged tourniquet use and hand exercise when drawing blood.

Excess dietary intake or rapid potassium infusion.

Drugs with high potassium content (e.g., 1 million units of penicillin G potassium contains 1.7 mEq of potassium).

Transfusion of old blood.

Urinary Diversion

Ureteral implants into jejunum

In neonates—dehydration, hemolysis (e.g., cephalohematoma, intracranial hemorrhage, bruising, exchange transfusion), acute renal failure, congenital adrenal hyperplasia, adrenocortical insufficiency

Decreased In

See Table 12-3 and see Figure 3-3.

Each 1 mEq/L decrease of serum potassium reflects a total deficit of <200 to 400 mEq; a serum potassium <2 mEq/L may reflect a total deficit >1,000 mEq.

In patients with hypokalemia, urine potassium, >25 mEq in 24 hours or >15 mEq/L implies at least a renal component.

Excess Renal Excretion

Osmotic diuresis of hyperglycemia (e.g., uncontrolled diabetes)

Nephropathies

* Renal tubular acidosis (proximal and especially distal)
* Bartter syndrome
* Liddle syndrome
* Mg depletion due to any cause
* Renal vascular disease, malignant hypertension, vasculitis
* Renin-secreting tumors

Endocrine

* Hyperaldosteronism (primary, secondary)
* Cushing syndrome especially caused by ectopic ACTH production
* Congenital adrenal hyperplasia
* Hyperthyroidism (especially in Asian persons)

Drugs

* Diuretics (e.g., thiazides, ethacrynic acid, furosemide); assay for diuretics should be done if urine chloride >40 mEq/L
* Mineralocorticoids (e.g., fluorocortisone)

- High-dose glucocorticoids
- High-dose antibiotics (e.g., penicillin, nafcillin, ampicillin, carbenicillin)
- Substances with mineralocorticoid effect (e.g., glycyrrhizic acid [licorice], carbenoxolone, gossypol)
- Drugs associated with Mg depletion (e.g., aminoglycosides, cisplatin, amphotericin B, foscarnet)

Acute myelogenous, monomyeloblastic, or lymphoblastic leukemia

Nonrenal Causes of Excess Potassium Loss

In patients with hypokalemia, urine potassium <25 mEq/24 h <15 mEq/L implies extrarenal loss.

GI

- Vomiting
- Diarrhea (e.g., infections, malabsorption, radiation)
- Drugs (e.g., laxatives [phenolphthalein], enemas, cancer therapy)
- Neoplasms (e.g., villous adenoma of colon, pancreatic VIPoma that produces vasoactive intestinal polypeptide >200 pg/mL, Zollinger-Ellison syndrome)
- Excessive spitting (sustained expectoration of all saliva in neurotic persons and to induce weight loss in professional wrestlers)

Skin

- Excessive sweating
- Cystic fibrosis
- Extensive burns
- Draining wounds

Cellular shifts

- Respiratory alkalosis
- Classic periodic paralysis
- Insulin
- Drugs (e.g., bronchodilators, decongestants)
- Accidental ingestion of barium compounds
- Treatment of severe megaloblastic anemia with vitamin B_{12} or folic acid
- Physiologic (e.g., highly trained athletes)

Diet

- Severe eating disorders (e.g., anorexia nervosa, bulimia)
- Dietary deficiency

Delirium tremens

In neonates—asphyxia, alkalosis, renal tubular acidosis, iatrogenic (glucose and insulin), diuretics

Major causes of *hypokalemia with hypertension*:

- Diuretic drugs (e.g., thiazides)
- Primary aldosteronism
- Secondary aldosteronism (renovascular disease, renin-producing tumors)
- Cushing syndrome
- Malignant hypertension
- Renal tubular acidosis

"Pregnancy" Test

See Chapter 14.

Protein

Proteins are a diverse group of molecules with multiple functions.

See also Chapter 8.

Total Protein (Table 3-5)

Use

Screening for nutritional deficiencies and gammopathies

BLOOD ANALYT

Table 3-5. Serum Protein Electrophoretic Patterns in Various Diseases[a]

Condition	Total Protein	Albumin	Alpha₁ Globulin	Alpha₂ Globulin	Beta Globulin	Gamma Globulin	Comment
Multiple myeloma	I	D		Dyscrasia of beta$_{2A}$ or gamma$_2$ Ig			Total globulin, marked I; Variable location of M globulin
Macroglobulinemia	I	D		Dyscrasia of beta$_{2M}$		Marked I	Electrophoresis same as multiple myeloma
Hodgkin disease	D	D	I	I		V	
Lymphatic leukemia and lymphoma	D	D			D	D	
Myelogenous and monocytic leukemia	D	D			D	I	Gamma globulin to differentiate types of acute leukemias
Hypogamma-globulinemia	D	N	N	N	N	D	
Analbuminemia	Marked D	Marked D	N	I	I	I	
GI diseases							
Peptic ulcer	D	D	May be I	May be I			
Ulcerative colitis	D	D	May be I	May be I			
Protein-losing enteropathy	Marked D	Marked D	I	I	D	D	
Acute cholecystitis	D	D				N	
Nephrosis	D	D		D	D, I (N)	D (N, I)	Typical pattern
Chronic GN	D	D	N	I	N	N	
Laënnec cirrhosis	D, N, I	D	N	D	Characteristic pattern of beta-gamma "bridging"		
Acute viral hepatitis	D, N	D (indicates acute hepatocellular damage)		D	D	V, I	

Condition	Albumin	α₁-Globulin	α₂-Globulin	β-Globulin	γ-Globulin	Comments
Stress	D		I		I	
Hypersensitivity					I	"Three-fingered" pattern
Sarcoidosis	D				I	"Sarcoid steps" help differentiate from other lung disease; Gamma globulin levels of prognostic value
Collagen disease						Stepwise increase of alpha₂, beta, and gamma
SLE	D		I		I	
Polyarteritis nodosa	D		I		N	
RA	D		I		I	
Scleroderma	D			I	V	No significant changes
Acute rheumatic fever	D		I		I	No significant changes
Essential hypertension						No significant changes
Congestive heart failure	D					Albumin D because of hemodilution (Hemodilution, diminished hepatic synthesis, and possible excessive enteric loss)
Metastatic carcinomatosis	D		I	D	I	
Certain infections (meningitis, pneumonia, osteomyelitis)	D		I	D	I	Nonspecific patterns
Myxedema						Changes due to hemodilution
Hyperthyroidism	D		N		N	
Diabetes mellitus	D		I		N	

I, increased or elevated; D, decreased or diminished; V, variable; N, normal; blank, no significant change.

[a]Nonspecific changes of decreased albumin and increased globulin occur in many conditions (e.g., infections, neoplasms, metabolic diseases).

Sources: Sunderman FW Jr. Recent advances in clinical interpretation of electrophoretic fractionations of the serum proteins. In Sunderman FW, Sunderman JC, eds. Serum Proteins and the Dysproteinemias. Philadelphia: Lippincott, 1964. Harrison HH, Levitt MH. Serum protein electrophoresis: basic principles, interpretations, and practical considerations. ASCI Check Sample. Core Chemistry NO. PTS 87-7 (PTS-25). Chicago: ASCP; 1987.

Increased In
Hypergammaglobulinemias (monoclonal or polyclonal; see following sections)
Hypovolemic states
Decreased In
Nutritional deficiency (e.g., malabsorption, Kwashiorkor, marasmus)
Decreased or ineffective protein synthesis (e.g., severe liver disease, agammaglobu-
    linemia)
Increased loss

- Renal (e.g., nephrotic syndrome)
- GI disease (e.g., protein-losing enteropathies, surgical resection)
- Severe skin disease (e.g., burns, pemphigus vulgaris, eczema)
- Blood loss, plasmapheresis

Increased catabolism (e.g., fever, inflammation, hyperthyroidism, malignancy, chronic
    diseases)
Dilutional (e.g., IV fluids, SIADH, water intoxication)

Albumin

Albumin levels generally parallel total protein levels, except when total protein
    changes are due to gamma globulins.
Use
Marker of disorders of protein metabolism (e.g., nutritional, decreased synthesis,
    increased loss)
Increased In
Dehydration (relative increase)
IV albumin infusions
Decreased In
Inadequate intake (e.g., malnutrition)
Decreased absorption (e.g., malabsorption syndromes)
Increased need (e.g., hyperthyroidism, pregnancy)
Impaired synthesis (e.g., liver diseases, chronic infection, hereditary analbuminemia)
Increased breakdown (e.g., neoplasms, infection, trauma)
Increased loss (e.g., edema, ascites, burns, hemorrhage, nephrotic syndrome, protein-
    losing enteropathy)
Dilutional (e.g., IV fluids, SIADH, psychogenic diabetes/water intoxication)
Congenital deficiency

Protein Separation (Immunodiffusion, Immunofixation, Electrophoresis)
Use
Diagnosis of specific diseases

- Multiple myeloma
- Waldenström macroglobulinemia
- Hypogammaglobulinemia
- Agammaglobulinemia
- Agamma-A-globulinemia
- Analbuminemia
- Bisalbuminemia
- Afibrinogenemia
- Atransferrinemia
- α_1-Antitrypsin variant
- Cirrhosis
- Acute-phase reactant

Other Changes
Nonspecific changes in serum proteins
Protein pattern changes in urine, cerebrospinal fluid, peritoneal fluid, etc.

Beta-2 Microglobulin

Beta-2 microglobulin is a **light-chain component of the human leukocyte antigen class I molecule. This polypeptide is present on membranes of all**

nucleated cells; its function is unknown. Levels are usually measured by immunoassay, with an upper reference limit of 2.0 mg/L.

See Chapter 4.

Use

Index of GFR

Prognostic marker for some lymphoproliferative diseases (e.g., adult acute lymphocytic leukemia, AIDS); as a tumor marker, reflects burden of tumor cells in multiple myeloma

Increased In

Decreased creatinine clearance

Inflammatory disorders

Some viral infections (e.g., AIDS, hepatitis)

Malignancies (e.g., lymphomas, certain leukemias, multiple myeloma)

Autoimmune disorders (e.g., RA, SLEr)

Others (e.g., sarcoidosis)

Sodium

Sodium is the major extracellular cation and exerts a major influence on plasma osmolality. It is adjusted by ADH and the thirst receptors to maintain plasma osmolality and volume. Aldosterone causes tubular reabsorption of sodium. Atrial natriuretic peptide hormone decreases sodium reabsorption.

See Chapter 13 and Table 3-4.

Use

Diagnosis and treatment of dehydration and overhydration. *Changes in serum sodium most often reflect changes in water balance rather than sodium balance. If a patient has not received large load of sodium, hypernatremia suggests need for water, and values <130 mEq/L suggest overhydration.* Determinations of blood sodium and potassium levels are not useful in diagnosis or in estimating net ion losses but are performed to monitor changes in sodium and potassium during therapy.

Interference

Hyperglycemia—serum sodium decreases 1.7 mEq/L for every increase of serum glucose of 100 mg/dL)

Hyperlipidemia and hyperproteinemia, which cause spurious results only with flame photometric but not with specific ion electrode techniques for measuring sodium

Transaminases[9]

The transaminases are widely distributed in the tissues, except for brain and smooth muscle.

See Chapter 8.

Alanine Aminotransferase or Serum Glutamic-Pyruvic Transaminase (SGPT)

ALT shows a day-to-day variation ≤30%. Its diurnal variation is 45%; levels are higher in afternoon than early morning.

Use

Differential diagnosis of diseases of hepatobiliary system and pancreas

Repeat testing to establish chronicity of viral hepatitis

Generally parallels but lower than AST in alcohol-related diseases

Screening for liver disease

Increased In

See AST (following section)

Obesity (not AST; modest increase to 1× to 3× ULN)

Severe preeclampsia (both)

Rapidly progressing acute lymphoblastic leukemia (both)

Levels in women ~75% of those in men

[9]Dufour DR, Lott JA, Nolte FS, et al. Diagnosis and monitoring of hepatic injury. I. Performance characteristics of laboratory tests. *Clin Chem* 2000;46:2027–2049.

BLOOD ANALYT

Decreased In
GU tract infection

Malignancy

Pyridoxal phosphate deficiency states (e.g., malnutrition, pregnancy, alcoholic liver disease)

Others

Aspartate Aminotransferase or Serum Glutamic-Oxaloacetic Transaminase (SGOT)

AST shows a **day-to-day variation ≤10%. It is widely distributed in tissues, with the highest concentrations in heart, liver, and skeletal muscle; lower concentrations are present in kidney, pancreas, and RBCs.**

Use
Differential diagnosis of diseases of hepatobiliary system and pancreas

Formerly surrogate test for screening blood donors for hepatitis

Interferences
Increase due to hemolysis, lipemia

Increase due to calcium dust in air (e.g., construction in laboratory)

Increased (because enzymes are activated during test) in:

- Therapy with oxacillin, ampicillin, opiates, erythromycin

Decreased (because of increased serum lactate-consuming enzyme during test) in:

- Diabetic ketoacidosis
- Beriberi
- Severe liver disease
- Chronic hemodialysis (reason unknown)
- Uremia—proportional to BUN level (reason unknown)

Increased In
Liver diseases (see Chapter 8)

- Active necrosis of parenchymal cells is suggested by extremely high levels. Acute viral hepatitis shows greatest increases; may be 20× to 100×.
- Rapid rise and decline suggests extrahepatic biliary disease.
- Administration of opiates to patients with diseased biliary tract or previous cholecystectomy causes increase in LD and especially AST. AST increases by 2 to 4 hours and peaks in 5 to 8 hours; the increase may persist for 24 hours, with an elevation may be 2.5 to 65 times normal.
- Congestion, e.g., heart failure, cirrhosis, biliary obstruction, primary or metastatic cancer, granulomas, hepatic ischemia
- Eclampsia
- Hepatotoxic drugs (e.g., carbon tetrachloride)

Musculoskeletal diseases (see Chapter 10) including trauma, surgery, and IM injections

- Myoglobinuria

For AMI, now replaced by CK-MB and cTn

Interpretation
- AST is increased in >95% of patients when blood is drawn at the appropriate time.
- Increase appears within 6 to 8 hours, peaks in 24 hours, and usually returns to normal in 4 to 6 days.
- Peak level is usually ~200 units (5× normal); level >300 units, along with a more prolonged increase, suggests a poorer prognosis.
- Reinfarction is indicated by a rise following a return to normal.

Others

- Acute pancreatitis
- Intestinal injury (e.g., surgery, infarction)
- Local irradiation injury
- Pulmonary infarction (relatively slight increase)
- Cerebral infarction (increased in following week in 50% of patients)
- Cerebral neoplasms (occasionally)

- Renal infarction (occasionally)
- Drugs (e.g., heparin therapy, salicylates, opiates, tetracycline, chlorpromazine, isoniazid)
- Burns
- Heat exhaustion
- Mushroom poisoning
- Lead poisoning (not useful for screening)
- Hemolytic anemia

Marked Increase (>3,000 IU/L)
Acute hypotension (e.g., AMI, sepsis, postcardiac surgery)
Toxic liver injury (e.g., drugs)
Viral hepatitis
Liver trauma
Liver metastases
Rhabdomyolysis

Decreased In
Azotemia
Chronic renal dialysis
Pyridoxal phosphate deficiency states (e.g., malnutrition, pregnancy, alcoholic liver disease)

Normal In
Angina pectoris
Coronary insufficiency
Pericarditis
Congestive heart failure without liver damage
Level can vary by <10 units/d in the same person.

AST:ALT (SGOT:SGPT) Ratio
AST is present in the liver microsomes and mitochondria; ALT is in the liver microsomes. With a great deal of necrosis, AST exceeds ALT, but in hepatic inflammation without much necrosis, ALT exceeds AST. Normal ratio is between 0.7 and 1.4, depending on methodology.

Use
Differential diagnosis of diseases of hepatobiliary system and pancreas

Increased In
Drug hepatotoxicity (>2.0)
Alcoholic hepatitis (>2.0 is highly suggestive; may be ≤6.0)
Cirrhosis (1.4 to 2.0)
Intrahepatic cholestasis (>1.5)
Hepatocellular carcinoma
Chronic hepatitis (slightly increased; 1.3)

Decreased In
Acute hepatitis caused by virus, drugs, toxins (with AST increased 3 to 10× ULN) (usually ≤0.65; ratio of 0.3 to 0.6 is said to be a good prognostic sign, but a higher ratio of 1.2 to 1.6 is a poor prognostic sign)
Extrahepatic cholestasis (normal or slightly decreased; 0.8)

Urea Nitrogen
Urea nitrogen is synthesized mainly in the liver. It is mostly the end product of protein metabolism.

Use
Diagnosis of renal insufficiency. Filtered freely in glomerulus; ≤50% is reabsorbed.
Correlates with uremic symptoms better than serum creatinine.
A low BUN of 6 to 8 mg/dL is frequently associated with states of overhydration or liver disease.
A BUN of 10 to 20 mg/dL almost always indicates normal glomerular function.
A BUN of 50 to 150 mg/dL implies serious impairment of renal function.

BLOOD ANALYT

A markedly increased BUN (150 to 250 mg/dL) is virtually conclusive evidence of severely impaired glomerular function.
In chronic renal disease, BUN correlates better with symptoms of uremia than does serum creatinine.
Provides evidence of hemorrhage into upper GI tract.
Assessment of patients requiring nutritional support for excess catabolism, e.g., burns, cancer.

Increased In
Impaired kidney function (see "Creatinine")
Prerenal azotemia—any cause of reduced renal blood flow

- Congestive heart failure
- Salt and water depletion (vomiting, diarrhea, diuresis, sweating)
- Shock

Postrenal azotemia—any obstruction of urinary tract (increased BUN:creatinine ratio)
Increased protein catabolism (serum creatinine remains normal)

- Hemorrhage into GI tract
- AMI
- Stress

Methodologic interference

- Nesslerization (chloral hydrate, chloramphenicol, ammonium salts)
- Berthelot (aminophenol, asparagine, ammonium salts)
- Fearon (acetohexamide, sulfonylureas)

Decreased In
Diuresis (e.g., with overhydration, often associated with low protein catabolism)
Severe liver damage (e.g., drugs, poisoning, hepatitis, other)
Increased utilization of protein for synthesis (e.g., late pregnancy, infancy, acromegaly, malnutrition, anabolic hormones)
Diet (e.g., low-protein and high-carbohydrate, IV feedings only, impaired absorption [celiac disease], malnutrition)
Nephrotic syndrome (some patients)
SIADH
Inherited hyperammonemias (urea is virtually absent in blood)
Methodologic interference (e.g., Berthelot, chloramphenicol, streptomycin)

BUN:Creatinine Ratio
See Chapter 3, 14.
Use
Because of considerable variability, the BUN:creatinine ratio should only be used as a rough guide. Usual range for most people on normal diet is 12 to 16.
Differentiate prerenal and postrenal azotemia from renal azotemia.

Increased Ratio (>10:1) with Normal Creatinine In:
Prerenal azotemia (BUN rises without increase in creatinine), (e.g., heart failure, salt depletion, dehydration, blood loss) due to decreased GFR
Catabolic states with increased tissue breakdown
GI hemorrhage; a ratio ≥36 is reported to distinguish upper from lower GI hemorrhage in patients with negative gastric aspirate
High protein intake
Impaired renal function plus

- Excess protein intake or production or tissue breakdown (e.g., GI bleeding, thyrotoxicosis, infection, Cushing syndrome, high-protein diet, surgery, burns, cachexia, high fever)
- Urine reabsorption (e.g., ureterocolostomy)
- Patients with reduced muscle mass (subnormal creatinine production)

Certain drugs (e.g., tetracycline, glucocorticoids)
Selective increase in plasma urea (diuretic-induced azotemia) during use of loop diuretics

Increased Ratio (>10:1) with Elevated Creatinine In

Postrenal azotemia (BUN rises disproportionately more than creatinine) (e.g., obstructive uropathy)

Prerenal azotemia superimposed on renal disease

Decreased Ratio (<10:1) with Decreased BUN In

Acute tubular necrosis

Low-protein diet, starvation, severe liver disease, and other causes of decreased urea synthesis

Repeated dialysis (urea rather than creatinine diffuses out of extracellular fluid)

Inherited deficiency of urea cycle enzymes (e.g., hyperammonemias—urea is virtually absent in blood)

SIADH (due to tubular secretion of urea)

Pregnancy

Decreased Ratio (<10:1) with Increased Creatinine In

Phenacemide therapy (accelerates conversion of creatine to creatinine)

Rhabdomyolysis (releases muscle creatinine)

Muscular patients who develop renal failure

Inappropriate Ratio

Diabetic ketoacidosis (acetoacetate causes false increase in creatinine with certain methodologies, resulting in normal or decreased ratio when dehydration should produce an increased BUN:creatinine ratio)

Cephalosporin therapy (interferes with creatinine measurement)

Uric Acid

Most uric acid is synthesized in the liver and intestinal mucosa. Two thirds is excreted by the kidneys, and one third is excreted via the GI tract. Uric acid is an end product of purine catabolism; it is released as DNA and RNA are degraded by dying cells. Levels are very labile and show day-to-day and seasonal variation in same person; levels are also increased by emotional stress, total fasting, and increased body weight. Normal levels are >7.0 mg/dL in men and >6.0 mg/dL in women.

Use

Monitor treatment of gout

Monitor chemotherapeutic treatment of neoplasms to avoid renal urate deposition with possible renal failure

Increased In

Renal failure (does not correlate with severity of kidney damage; urea and creatinine should be used)

Gout

Twenty-five percent of the relatives of patients with gout

Asymptomatic hyperuricemia (e.g., incidental finding with no evidence of gout; clinical significance is not known but people so afflicted should be rechecked periodically for gout); the higher the level of serum uric acid, the greater the likelihood of an attack of acute gouty arthritis

Increased destruction of nucleoproteins

- Leukemia, multiple myeloma
- Polycythemia
- Lymphoma, especially postirradiation; other disseminated neoplasms
- Cancer chemotherapy (e.g., nitrogen mustards, vincristine, mercaptopurine, prednisone)
- Hemolytic anemia
- Sickle cell anemia
- Resolving pneumonia
- Toxemia of pregnancy (serial determinations to follow therapeutic response and estimate prognosis)
- Psoriasis (one-third of patients)

Drugs, for example:

- Intoxicants (e.g., barbiturates, methyl alcohol, ammonia, carbon monoxide); some patients with alcoholism
- Decreased renal clearance or tubular secretion (e.g., various diuretics [thiazides, furosemide, ethacrynic acid], and all diuretics except spironolactone and ticrynafen)
- Nephrotoxic effect (e.g., mitomycin C)
- Low-dose salicylates (<4 g/day)
- Other effects (e.g., levodopa, phenytoin sodium)
- Methodologic interference (e.g., ascorbic acid, levodopa, methyldopa)

Metabolic acidosis
Diet

- High-protein weight-reduction diet
- Excess nucleoprotein (e.g., sweetbreads, liver) may increase level ≤1 mg/dL
- Alcohol consumption

Miscellaneous

- von Gierke disease
- Chronic lead poisoning
- Lesch-Nyhan syndrome
- Maple syrup urine disease
- Down syndrome
- Polycystic kidneys
- Calcinosis universalis and circumscripta
- Hypoparathyroidism
- Primary hyperparathyroidism
- Hypothyroidism
- Sarcoidosis
- Chronic berylliosis
- Patients with arteriosclerosis and hypertension *(serum uric acid is increased in 80% of patients with elevated serum triglycerides)*
- Certain population groups (e.g., Blackfoot and Pima Indians, Filipinos, New Zealand Maoris)

Most common causes in hospitalized men are azotemia, metabolic acidosis, diuretics, gout, myelolymphoproliferative disorders, other drugs, unknown causes

Duffy, et al. stated: "It is difficult to justify therapy in asymptomatic persons with hyperuricemia to prevent gouty arthritis, uric acid stones, urate nephropathy or risk of cardiovascular disease."[10]

Decreased In
Drugs

- ACTH
- Uricosuric drugs (e.g., high doses of salicylates, probenecid, cortisone, allopurinol, coumarin)
- Various other drugs (radiographic contrast agents, glyceryl guaiacolate, estrogens, phenothiazines, indomethacin)

Wilson disease
Fanconi syndrome
Acromegaly (some patients)
Celiac disease (slightly)
Pernicious anemia in relapse (some patients)
Xanthinuria
Neoplasms (occasional cases) (e.g., carcinomas, Hodgkin disease)
Healthy adults with isolated defect in tubular transport of uric acid (Dalmatian dog mutation)
Decreased in ~5% of hospitalized patients; most common causes are postoperative state (GI surgery, coronary artery bypass), diabetes mellitus, various drugs, and SIADH in association with hyponatremia

[10]Duffy WB, Senekjian HO, Knight TF, et al. Management of asymptomatic hyperuricemia. *JAMA* 1981;246:2215–2216.

Unchanged In
Colchicine administration

Vitamin D

Use
Diagnosis of rickets and vitamin D toxicity
Differential diagnosis of hypercalcemias

Serum/Urine Calcium Level	1,25-(OH)$_2$D*	25-(OH)D*
Increased		
Hyperparathyroidism	N	N, I
PTH-related peptide-associated conditions	N	D
Lymphoma	N	D, I
Granulomatous conditions (e.g., sarcoidosis)	N	I
Idiopathic hypercalciuria	N	N, I
Osteoporosis	N	N, I
Vitamin D and 25-(OH)D intoxication	I	N
1,25-(OH)$_2$D and dihydrotachysterol intoxication	N	I
Decreased		
Hypoparathyroidism	N	D, N
Pseudohyperparathyroidism	N	D, N
Vitamin D deficiency	D	D, N, I
Vitamin D–dependent rickets		
Type I	N	D
Type II	N	I
Severe liver disease	D	D, N
Nephrotic syndrome	D	D, N
Renal failure	N	D
Hyperphosphatemia	N	D
Hypomagnesemia	N	D, N
Normal		
Pregnancy, lactation	N	I
Growing children	N	I
Elderly	D, N	D, N, I
Summertime	N	N
Wintertime	D	N
Increased latitude	D	N

I = increased; D = decreased; N = normal.
*1,25-dihydroxy-vitamin D [1,25(OH)$_2$D] is formed from 25-hydroxy-vitamin D [25(OH)D].

BLOOD ANALYT

Normal Values

Addis count	No longer performed
Red blood cells (RBCs)	≤1,000,000/24 h
Casts	≤100,000/24 h
White blood cells (WBCs) + epithelial cells	≤2,000,000/24 h
Ammonia	30–50 mEq/L
Amylase	<400 IU/L
Calcium	<300 mg/24 h
Chloride	110–250 mEq/L
Creatine	Female: <100 mg/24 h (<6% of creatinine)
	Male: <100 mg/24 h (<6% of creatinine)
	Higher in children <1 y: may equal creatinine
	In older children: ≤30% of creatinine
	During pregnancy: ≤12% of creatinine
Creatinine	1.0–1.6 g/24 h
Cystine	10–100 mg/24 h
Delta-aminolevulinic acid	0–5.4 mg/24 h
Eosinophils	<100/mL
Glucose	Qualitative = 0
	≤0.5 g/24 h
Hemoglobin	0.0–1.0 mg/24 h
Hemosiderin	Negative
Iron	100–300 ng/24 h
Myoglobin	<35 ng/mL
Ketones	Qualitative = 0
Lysozyme (muramidase)	<2 μg/mL
Lead	<0.08 μg/mL or 120 μg/24 h
Microscopic examination	≤1–2 RBC, WBC, epithelial cells/HPF; <5 hyaline cast/LPF. Other casts = 0.

URINE

Osmolality		300–1,090 mOsm/kg
Oxalate		2–60 mg/24 h
pH		5–8.0; >9 indicates old specimen
Phenylpyruvic acid		Qualitative 0
Phosphorus		400–1,300 mg/24 h, depending on diet
Potassium		25–100 mEq/L depending on diet
Porphobilinogen		0–2 mg/24 h
Porphyrins, qualitative		0
Porphyrins, fractionation		
Uroporphyrin		Males: <45 μg/24 h; Females: <23 μg/24 h
Heptacarboxylporphyrin		<13 μg/24 h
Hexacarboxylporphyrin		<6 μg/24 h
Pentacarboxylporphyrin		<5 μg/24 h
Coproporphyrin		<110 μg/24 h
Protein		Qualitative = 0; <150 mg/24 h
Microalbumin		30–300 mg/24 h or albumin: creatinine = 30–300 mg/g Or excretion rate = 20–200 μg/min
Sodium		100–260 mEq/L depending on diet
Specific gravity		1.001–1.035
Total solids		30–70 g/L (average = 50) To estimate: multiply last two figures of specific gravity by 2.66 (Long's coefficient)
Urea nitrogen		66–17 g/24 h
Uric acid		250–800 mg/24 h
Urobilinogen		<4 mg/24 h
Volume	Adults	600–2,000 mL/24 h (average = 1,200) Night volume usually ~400 mL with specific gravity <1.018 or osmolality >825 mOsm/kg of body weight in children Ratio of night to day volume 1:2–1:4
	Infants	
	Premature	1–3 mL/kg/h
	Full-term	15–60 mL/24 h
	2 weeks	250–400 mL/24 h
	8 weeks	250–400 mL/24 h
	1 year	500–600 mL/24 h

Bacteriuria

See Chapter 14.

Bilirubinuria

See Chapter 8.

Calciuria

Use

Diagnosis of hypercalciuria causing renal calculi.

Increased In

Hyperparathyroidism (see Chapter 13)
Idiopathic hypercalciuria
High-calcium diet
Excess milk intake
Immobilization (especially in children)
Lytic bone lesions (e.g., metastatic tumor, multiple myeloma, osteoporosis [primary or secondary to hyperthyroidism, Cushing syndrome, acromegaly])

Drugs

- Diuretics (e.g., ammonium chloride, mercurials)
- Androgens, anabolic steroids
- Cholestyramine
- Dihydrotachysterol, vitamin D, parathyroid injections
- Viomycin

Fanconi syndrome
Glucocorticoid excess from any cause
Paget disease
Renal tubular acidosis
Rapidly progressive osteoporosis
Sarcoidosis

Decreased In
Hypoparathyroidism
Rickets, osteomalacia
Familial hypocalciuric (benign) hypercalcemia
Steatorrhea
Renal failure
Metastatic carcinoma of prostate
Drugs (e.g., sodium phytate, benzothiadiazides)

Hypercalciuria Without Hypercalcemia

Caused By
Idiopathic hypercalciuria
Sarcoidosis
Glucocorticoid excess from any cause
Hyperthyroidism
Rapidly progressive bone diseases, Paget disease, immobilization, malignant tumors
Renal tubular acidosis
Medullary sponge kidney
Furosemide administration

Casts

Type of Cast	Disorder
Hyaline	Does not indicate renal disease
RBC	Blood of glomerular origin
WBC	Glomerulonephritis, interstitial nephritis, pyelonephritis
Renal tubular epithelial	Acute tubular necrosis, glomerulonephritis, tubulointerstitial disease
Granular, waxy	Degenerative cellular elements
Broad	Chronic renal failure

Chyluria

Use
Diagnosis of injury or obstruction of lymphochylous system of chest or abdomen

Caused By
Obstruction of the lymphochylous system, usually filariasis. Microfilariae appear in the urine for 6 weeks after acute infection, then disappear unless endemic.
Trauma to chest or abdomen.
Abdominal tumors or lymph node enlargement.
Milky urine is caused by chylomicrons recognized as fat globules by microscopy (this is almost entirely neutral fat). Protein is normal or low. Hematuria is common. Specific gravity is low, and reaction is acid.
A test meal of milk and cream may cause chyluria in 1 to 4 hours.
Laboratory findings due to pyelonephritis that is often present.

URINE

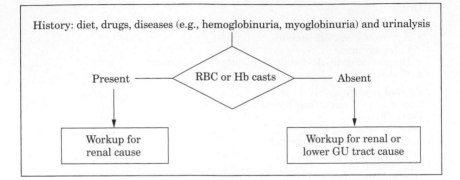

Fig. 4-1. Algorithm for red or brown urine.

Color, Abnormal[1]

Red (often includes colors from pink to red-brown)

- No specific test (chlorzoxazone, ethoxazene, oxamniquine, phenothiazines, rifampin)
- Acid urine only (phenolphthalein)

Red-orange

- No specific test (butazopyridine, chlorzoxazone, ethoxazene, mannose, oxamniquine, phenothiazines, rifampin)
- Alkaline urine only (phenindione)
- Acid urine only (phenolphthalein)

Red or pink

- No specific test (aminopyrine, aniline dyes, antipyrine, doxorubicin, fuscin, ibuprofen, phenacetin, phenothiazines, phensuximide, phenytoin)
- Acid urine only (beets, blackberries, anisindione)
- Alkaline urine only (anthraquinone laxatives, rhubarb, santonin, phenolsulfonphthalein, sulfobromophthalein sodium [bromsulphalein]; eosin produces green fluorescence)
- Darkens on standing (porphyrins)
- Presence of urates and bile
- On contact with hypochlorite bleach (toilet bowl cleaner) (aminosalicylic acid)
- Centrifuged specimen shows RBCs in base (blood)
- Test strips for blood (hemoglobin [Hb], RBCs, myoglobin)

Purple

- Alkaline urine only (phenolphthalein)
- Darkens on standing (porphyrins; fluoresces with ultraviolet light)
- No specific test (chlorzoxazone)

Red-brown

- Acid urine only (methemoglobin, metronidazole, anisindione) (see Fig. 4-1)
- Alkaline urine only (anthraquinone laxatives, levodopa, methyldopa, parahydroxyphenylpyruvic acid, phenazopyridine)
- Positive o-toluidine test for blood
    Centrifuged urine shows RBC in base if blood; centrifuged blood shows pink supernatant plasma if Hb but clear plasma if myoglobin
- Green in reflected light (antipyrine)
- Orange with addition of hydrochloric acid (HCl) (phenazopyridine)
- No specific test (chloroquine, deferoxamine, ethoxazene, ibuprofen, iron sorbitex, pamaquine, phenacetin, phenothiazines, phensuximide, phenytoin, trinitrophenol)

[1]Raymond JR, Yarger WE. Abnormal urine color: differential diagnosis. *South Med J* 1988;81: 837–841.

Brown-black

- Darkens on standing (homogentisic acid, melanin, melanogen, nitrobenzene, parahydroxyphenyl-pyruvic acid [alkaline urine only], phenol, cresol, naphthol)
- Does not darken on standing
    Ferric chloride test
    Color fades (Argyrol)
    Blue-green (homogentisic acid)
    Black (nitroprusside test is red with melanin, black with melanogen)

Yellow-brown

- Darkens on standing in acid urine (anthraquinone laxatives, rhubarb)
- Positive test for bile (bilirubin, urobilin)
- No specific test (niridazole, nitrofurantoin, pamaquine, primaquine, sulfamethoxazole)

Yellow

- Acid urine only (quinacrine, santonin)
- Alkaline urine only (beets)
- Positive test for bile (bilirubin, urobilin)
- No specific test (fluorescein dye, phenacetin, riboflavin, trinitrophenol)
- Acriflavine (green fluorescence)

Yellow-orange

- Alkaline urine only (anisindione, sulfasalazine)
- Positive test for bile (bilirubin, urobilin)
- Color increases with HCl (phenazopyridine)
- Ether soluble (carrots, vitamin A)
- High specific gravity (dehydration)
- No specific test (aminopyrine, warfarin)

Yellow-green or brown-green

- Darkens on standing (cresol, phenol [Chloraseptic], methocarbamol [Robaxin], resorcinol)
- Positive test for bile (biliverdin)

Blue-green

- Darkens on standing (methocarbamol, resorcinol)
- Blue fluorescence in acid urine (triamterene)
- Bacteriuria, pyuria (*Pseudomonas* infection [rare])
- Decolorizes with alkali (indigo-carmine dye)
- Obermayer test positive (indican)
- No specific test (chlorophyll breath mints [Clorets], Evans blue dye, guaiacol, magnesium salicylate [Doan's pills], methylene blue, thymol [Listerine])
- Biliverdin due to oxidation of bilirubin in poorly preserved specimens
    Gives negative diazo tests for bilirubin (Ictotest), but oxidative tests (Harrison spot test) may still be positive

Milky

- Lipiduria (nephrosis), chyluria (lymphatic obstruction) (ether soluble)
- Many polymorphonuclear leukocytes (PMNs) (microscopic examination; insoluble in dilute acetic acid)

White cloud is caused by excessive oxalic acid and glycolic acid in urine; occurs in oxalosis (primary hyperoxaluria)

Cloudy

- Phosphates, carbonates (dissolves in dilute acetic acid)
- Uric acid, urates (dissolves in alkali and at 60°C)
- Bacteria, yeast, sperm (insoluble in dilute acetic acid)

Colorless
    Specific gravity
        High (diabetes mellitus with glycosuria; positive test for glucose)
        Low (diabetes insipidus, recent fluid intake)
        Variable (diuretics, ethyl alcohol, hypercalcemia)

URINE

Clear to deep yellow

- Normal (due to urochrome pigment)

Blue diaper syndrome results from indigo blue in urine because of familial metabolic defect in tryptophan absorption associated with idiopathic hypercalcemia and nephrocalcinosis.

Red diaper syndrome is caused by a chromobacterium (*Serratia marcescens*) that produces a red pigment when grown aerobically at 25°C to 30°C.

Darkening of urine on standing, alkalinization, or oxygenation is nonspecific and may be caused by melanogen, Hb, indican, urobilinogen, porphyrins, phenols, salicylate metabolites (e.g., gentisic acid), homogentisic acid (due to alkaptonuria), or administration of metronidazole (Flagyl). In acid pH, urine may not darken for hours (e.g., tyrosinosis).

- Sickle cell crises produce a characteristic dark brown color independent of volume or specific gravity that becomes darker on standing or on exposure to sunlight because of the increase in porphyrins.

Creatine

Creatine is synthesized in the liver. It is the chief source of high-energy phosphocreatine for muscle metabolism. It loses water to become creatinine, all of which is excreted.

Increased In
Physiologic States

- Growing children
- Pregnancy
- Puerperium (2 weeks)
- Starvation
- Raw meat diet

Increased Formation

- Myopathy
  Amyotonia congenita
  Muscular dystrophy
  Poliomyelitis
  Myasthenia gravis
  Crush injury
  Acute paroxysmal myoglobinuria
- Endocrine diseases
  Hyperthyroidism
  Addison disease
  Cushing syndrome
  Acromegaly
  Diabetes mellitus
  Eunuchoidism
  Therapy with adrenocorticotropic hormone (ACTH), cortisone, or deoxycorticosterone acetate (DOCA)

Increased Breakdown

- Infections
- Burns
- Fractures
- Leukemia
- Systemic lupus erythematosus (SLE)

Decreased In
Hypothyroidism

Creatinine

Creatinine is derived from creatine, which is synthesized in the liver.

Use

Measure renal function (see Creatinine Clearance, Chapter 14).

Determine urine concentration of various substances when 24-hour urine cannot be obtained.

Recently marketed commercial reagent strips can semiquantitatively measure protein-to-creatinine ratio or albumin-to-creatinine ratio.

Detect artifactual dilution of urine in drug abuse testing.

In healthy young men on a meat-free diet, can be used to calculate muscle mass[2]:

$$\text{Total muscle mass (in kg)} = \text{creatinine (g) excreted/24 h} \times 21.8$$

Crystalluria

Disorder	Substance
Cystinuria, cystinosis	Cystine (crystals are also found in WBCs, cornea, and rectal mucosa)
Fanconi syndrome	Leucine
Hyperoxaluria, oxalosis	Calcium oxalate
Lesch-Nyhan syndrome	Uric acid
Orotic aciduria	Orotic acid
Xanthinuria	Xanthine
Massive hepatic necrosis (acute yellow atrophy) tyrosinemia, tyrosinosis	Tyrosine (cystine and tyrosine crystals are also found in marrow)

Crystalluria is diagnostically useful when there are cystine crystals (occurs only in homozygous or heterozygous cystinuria) or struvite crystals. Calcium oxalate, phosphate, and uric acid should arouse suspicion about possible cause of stones, but they may occur in normal urine.

Cytology

Use

Screen persons exposed to urothelial or bladder carcinogens

Detect urothelial dysplasia and carcinomas (see Chapter 14); poor sensitivity for renal cancer

Monitor effects of radiation or chemotherapy

Detect nonbacterial infections (parasitic, fungal, viral)

Characterize cells with viral inclusions

Characterize inflammatory conditions

Confirm abnormal routine urinalysis microscopy findings

Flow cytometry and DNA analysis are used for diagnosis, prognosis, and to monitor therapy but not for screening

Diagnostic Indices

See Table 14-12.

Electrolytes

Use

Diagnosis of causes of hyponatremia and hypokalemia

Suspected disorders of adrenal cortex

Aid diagnosis of causes of acute renal failure (Table 15-3)

Interferences

Value may be limited due to failure to obtain 24-hour excretion levels rather than random samples or administration of diuretics.

Eosinophiluria[3]

Eosinophiluria refers to >1% of urinary leukocytes as eosinophils.

[2]Wang Z-M, Gallagher D, Nelson ME, et al. Total-body skeletal muscle mass: evaluation of 24-h urinary creatinine excretion by computerized axial tomography. *Am J Clin Nutr* 1996;63:863–869.
[3]Corwin HL, Bray BA, Haber MH. The detection and interpretation of urinary eosinophils. *Arch Pathol Lab Med* 1989;113:1256–1258.

URINE

Use
May be useful to distinguish acute interstitial nephritis from acute tubular necrosis, in which it is absent

Caused By
Acute interstitial nephritis (drug-induced); sensitivity/specificity (S/S): 60% to 90%/>85%; positive predictive value: ~50%; negative predictive value: 98%
Acute glomerulonephritis (rapidly progressive; acute including poststreptococcal)
IgA nephropathy (Henoch-Schönlein purpura)
Chronic pyelonephritis
Acute rejection of renal allograft (small numbers)
Obstructive uropathy
Prostatitis
Eosinophilic cystitis
Schistosoma hematobium infestation
Bladder cancer
Cholesterol embolization to kidney

Ferric Chloride Test
The ferric chloride test was formerly used as a screening test for phenylketonuria. It has since been replaced by more specific tests for amino acid disorders, other metabolites, and drugs. *A positive test should always be followed by other tests (e.g., chromatography of blood and urine) to rule out genetic metabolic disorders.*

Glucose, Tests For
See Reducing Substances.

Gonadotropins, Chorionic
See also Pregnancy Test, Chapter 3.

Increased In
Normal pregnancy (secreted first by trophoblastic cells of conceptus and later by placenta). Becomes positive as early as 4 days after expected date of menstruation; it is >95% reliable by the 10th to the 14th day. Human chorionic gonadotropin (hCG) increases to a peak between the 60th and 70th days then decreases progressively. A slower rate of rise (2-day doubling of titer or increase <66%) suggests ectopic pregnancy.
Hydatidiform mole, choriocarcinoma: Test is negative 1 or more times in >60% and negative at all times in >20% of these patients, for whom more sensitive methods (e.g., radioimmunoassay) should be used. Quantitative titers should be performed for diagnosis and for following the clinical course of patients with these conditions. Serum is preferred test.

False-Positive Result Caused By
Drugs, e.g., chlorpromazine, phenothiazines, promethazine, methadone
Bacterial contamination
Protein or blood in urine

False-Negative Result Caused By
Drugs, e.g., Promethazine (DAP test)
Dilute urine
Missed abortion
Dead fetus syndrome
Home pregnancy and point of care (POC) tests that do not measure hyperglycosylated hCG

With the LA type of test, only urine should be used if patient has rheumatoid arthritis.

Normal In
Nonpregnant state
Fetal death

Hematuria[4]

Use
Screening and diagnosis of disorders of genitourinary tract (Fig. 4-2)
Screening for excess anticoagulation medication

---

[4]Froom P, Etzion R, Barak M. What is an abnormal urinary erythrocyte count as measured by test strips? *Clin Chem* 2004;50:673–675.

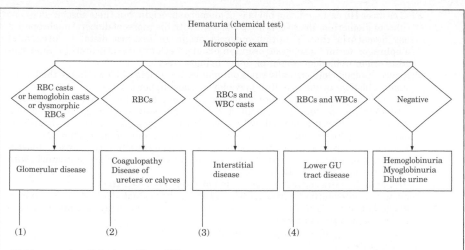

(1) Hypertension, diabetes mellitus, GN, immune-complex or postinfectious glomerular disease, drug reaction, endocarditis, embolic diseases. Tests: ASOT, ANA, C3, HB$_s$Ab, renal biopsy.
(2) Calculi, papillary necrosis, polycystic disease, sickle cell disease; GU tract trauma, neoplasm, or parasites. Tests: Cytology, CT scan, ultrasonography, IVP.
(3) Pyelonephritis, tuberculosis, sarcoidosis, drug reaction. Tests: Urine cultures, lymph node biopsy.
(4) GU tract infection (e.g., prostatitis, urethritis, vaginitis), reflux, GU tract carcinoma. Tests: Urine cultures, cytology, cystoscopy, ultrasonography.

Fig. 4-2. Algorithm for diagnosis of microhematuria.
ASOT, antistreptolysin O titer; ANA, antinuclear antibodies; CT, computed tomography; IVP, intravenous pyelogram.

Interpretation

<3% of normal persons have ≥3 RBCs/HPF or >1,000 RBCs/mL (no easy conversion formula between these two methods). Abnormal range is >3 RBCs/HPF. Hematuria is found in 18% of persons after very strenuous exercise. By flow cytometry, upper limit is ~25 RBCs/mL.

Centrifuged fresh urine sediment should be examined under high dry magnification. Urine does not show any red color at <5,000,000 RBCs/mL.

Reagent strips (orthotolidine or peroxidase) detect heme peroxidase activity in RBCs, Hb, or myoglobin with reported S/S of 91% to 100%/65% to 99%; may miss 10% of patients with microscopic hematuria. Orthotolidine test strips are sensitive to ~3 to 10 RBCs/HPF. Is more reliable in hypotonic urine (lyses RBCs) than hypertonic urine. For detection of hematuria, specificity is 65% to 99% compared to microscopy; positive predictive value (PPV) for significant disease is 0% to 2% and for possibly significant disease, it is 6% to 58%. Reagent strips exposed to air (uncapped bottles) for a week or more may give false-negative results for blood.

In microscopic hematuria, the number of RBCs is not related to the significance of the causative lesion. The source of microscopic hematuria remains obscure in ~70% of cases after workup.

Phase microscopy of urine sediment showing >5% acanthocytes (doughnut-like cells with membrane blebs) is reported to have S/S of 52% to 73%/98% to 100%. Crenated cells form in concentrated urine and are not diagnostic. Dysmorphic changes are said to indicate a glomerular source.

With an automated RBC counter that produces size distribution curves, urine RBC size distribution has been reported as less than venous RBCs in glomerulonephropathy (GN) and either greater than venous RBCs (nonglomerular) or both (mixed) types in lower genitourinary (GU) tract lesions.

Immunocytochemical staining (against human Tamm-Horsfall protein) is positive in >80% of RBCs of renal origin and <13.1% of RBCs of nonrenal origin.

URINE

RBC casts or Hb casts indicate blood is of glomerular origin, but their absence does not rule out glomerular disease. Is *not* consistent with diagnosis of diabetic nephropathy.

Gross hematuria that is initial suggests origin in urethra distal to urogenital diaphragm; terminal suggests origin in bladder neck or prostatic urethra; total suggests origin in bladder proper or upper urinary tract.

Presence of blood clots virtually rules out glomerular origin of blood. Large thick clots suggest bladder origin; small stringy clots suggest upper tract.

Proteinuria may occur with gross hematuria. In nonglomerular hematuria, sufficient proteinuria to produce 2+ reagent strips requires equivalent of 25 mL of blood/L urine (if hematocrit is normal), which would cause gross hematuria; in glomerular hematuria, proteins filter through the glomerulus out of proportion to RBCs. Therefore, microscopic hematuria with 2+ protein on reagent strips favors glomerular origin; one exception is papillary necrosis, which may show 2+ proteinuria with nonglomerular type of RBCs.

Pyuria or WBC casts suggest inflammation or infection of GU tract.

Persistent or intermittent hematuria should always be evaluated; one episode of microscopic hematuria usually does not require full evaluation (may be caused by viral infection, mild trauma, exercise, etc.).

Routine screening of all adults is not recommended.

Interferences
False-positive results

* Vaginal bleeding
* Factitious
* Bacteriuria (due to catalase production by Gram-negative bacteria and *Staphylococcus* sp., whose action on reagent strips is similar to that of Hb peroxidase)
* Red diaper syndrome
* Drugs (e.g., rifampin, phenolphthalein, iodides, bromides, copper, oxidizing agents, permanganate)
* Foods (e.g., beets, blackberries, rhubarb)
* Pigmenturia (porphyria, hemoglobinuria, myoglobinuria)
* Oxidizing contaminants (e.g., bacterial peroxidases, povidone, hypochlorite)

False-negative results

* Reducing agents (e.g., high doses of ascorbic acid [vitamin C])
* pH <5.1

Nonglomerular Hematuria Caused By
Trauma
Hemoglobinopathies (especially sickle cell trait and sickle cell Hb disease)
Hypercalciuria
Polycystic disease
GU tract tumors, infections

Some Causes of Hematuria in Adults[5]

	Gross (%)	Microscopic (%)
GU tract cancer	22.5	5.1
Kidney	3.6	0.5
Prostate	2.4	0.5
Ureter	0.8	0.2
Bladder	15.0	4.0
Other lesions		
GU tract infection	33.0	4.3
Calculi	11.0	5.0
Benign prostatic hypertrophy	13.0	13.0
Renal	—	2.2
Systemic (e.g., hemophilia, thrombocytopenia, dicumarol overdose)	1.0	—
No source found	8.4	43.0

[5]Sutton JM. Evaluation of hematuria in adults. *JAMA* 1990;263:2475–2480.

Hematuria in Children
Caused By

Glomerular Causes
Acute postinfectious GN
Membranoproliferative GN
IgG-IgA nephropathy (Berger disease)
Hereditary nephritis (Alport syndrome)
SLE
Renal infarction
Henoch-Schönlein purpura
Benign familial hematuria

Nonglomerular Causes
Polycystic kidneys
Renal tumors
Renal tuberculosis
Vascular abnormalities (e.g., renal hemangioma, essential hematuria)
Hematologic conditions (e.g., sickle cell trait, coagulation disorders)
Hydronephrosis
GU tract infection, foreign body, calculi, etc. (usually symptomatic)

Hematuria, Benign Familial or Recurrent
Benign familial or recurrent hematuria (may be same as thin basement membrane disease).
Asymptomatic hematuria without proteinuria.
Other laboratory and clinical findings are normal.
Renal biopsy is normal on light microscopy, electron microscopy, and immunofluorescence.
Other family members may also have asymptomatic hematuria.
Should gradually clear spontaneously; annual screening for other abnormalities should be performed until condition clears.

Hemoglobinuria
The renal threshold for hemoglobinuria is 100 to 140 mg/dL plasma.

Use
Confirms hemolyzed blood in urine from either the GU tract or a significant intravascular cause.
Caused By
Hematuria (any cause) with hemolysis in urine
Infarction of kidney
Intravascular hemolysis caused by, e.g.,

* Parasites (e.g., malaria, Oroya fever caused by *Bartonella bacilliformis*)
* Infection (e.g., *Clostridium*, *E. coli* bacteremia from transfused blood)
* Immune-mediated (e.g., transfusion reactions, acquired hemolytic anemia, paroxysmal cold hemoglobinuria, paroxysmal nocturnal hemoglobinuria, thrombotic thrombocytopenic purpura/hemolytic uremic syndrome)
* Disseminated intravascular coagulation
* Inherited hemolytic disorders (e.g., sickle cell disease, thalassemias, glucose-6-PD deficiency, pyruvate kinase deficiency, hereditary spherocytosis)
* Fava bean sensitivity
* Mechanical (e.g., prosthetic heart valve)
* Hypotonicity (e.g., transurethral prostatectomy with irrigation of bladder with water, hemodialysis accidents)
* Chemicals (e.g., naphthalene, sulfonamides) and drugs
* Thermal burns injuring RBCs
* Strenuous exercise and march hemoglobinuria

URINE

Interferences
False-positive (Occultest) results may occur in the presence of pus, iodides, or bromides. Serum is pink with free Hb but clear when myoglobin is present.

Hemosiderinuria

Hemosiderinuria is diagnosed when a centrifuged specimen of random urine stained with Prussian blue stain shows granules. The granules are located in casts or in cells, but if the cells have disintegrated, free granules may be predominant. In normal urine, granules are absent.

Use
Present several days after intravascular hemolysis even when hemoglobinuria is absent (e.g., paroxysmal nocturnal hemoglobinuria)

Ketonuria

Ketonuria is diagnosed when ketone bodies (acetone, beta-hydroxybutyric acid, acetoacetic acid) appear in urine.

Use
Screening for ketoacidosis, especially in diabetes mellitus when blood is not immediately available
Confirm fasting in testing for insulinoma
Interferences (Reagent Strips)
False-positive results (e.g., from drugs such as levodopa)
False-negative (e.g., volatilization of acetone, breakdown of acetoacetic acid)
Occurs In
Metabolic conditions (e.g., diabetes mellitus, renal glycosuria, glycogen storage disease)
Dietary conditions (e.g., starvation, high-fat diets)
Increased metabolic requirements (e.g., hyperthyroidism, fever, pregnancy and lactation)

Lipuria

Lipids in the urine include all fractions. Double refractile (cholesterol) bodies can be seen. There is a high protein content. This test is rarely used.

May Occur In
Hyperlipidemia due to

- Nephrotic syndrome
- Severe diabetes mellitus
- Severe eclampsia

Extensive trauma with bone fractures
Phosphorus poisoning
Carbon monoxide poisoning

Melanogenuria

Use
In some patients with metastatic melanoma, when the urine is exposed to air for several hours, colorless melanogens are oxidized to melanin, and the urine becomes deep brown and later black. Melanogenuria occurs in 25% of patients with malignant melanoma; it is said to be more frequent with extensive liver metastasis. It is not useful for judging completeness of removal or early recurrence.
Melanogenuria is also said to occur in some patients with Addison disease or hemochromatosis and in intestinal obstruction in black persons.
Confirmatory Tests
- Ferric chloride test
- Thormählen test
- Ehrlich test

None of these is consistently more reliable or sensitive than observation of urine for darkening.
Interferences
Beware of false-positive red-brown or purple suspension caused by salicylates.

Myoglobinuria

The renal threshold for myoglobinuria is 20 mg/dL plasma.

Caused By
Hereditary

- Phosphorylase deficiency (McArdle syndrome)
- Metabolic defects, e.g., associated with muscular dystrophy

Sporadic

- Ischemic (e.g., arterial occlusion) (is earliest finding in acute myocardial infarction; see Chapter 5); levels >5 mg/mL occur within 1 to 2 hours).
- Crush syndrome
- Exertional (e.g., exercise, some cases of march hemoglobinuria, electric shock, convulsions, and seizures)
- Metabolic myoglobinuria (e.g., Haff disease, alcoholism, sea snake bite, carbon monoxide poisoning, diabetic acidosis, hypokalemia, malignant hyperpyrexia, systemic infection, barbiturate poisoning)
- Up to 50% of patients with progressive muscle disease (e.g., dermatomyositis, polymyositis, SLE, others) in active stage
- Various drugs and chemicals, especially illicit (e.g., cocaine, heroin, methadone, amphetamines, diazepam)

Use
Indicates recent necrosis of skeletal or cardiac muscle
Interpretation
Diagnosis based on

- Positive benzidine or o-toluidine test of urine that contains few or no RBCs when urine is red (fresh) or brown (after standing). This is the simplest and most practical initial test. Tests may be positive even when urine is normal in color.
- Serum is clear (not pink) unless renal failure is present, in contrast to hemoglobinemia.
- Serum haptoglobin is normal (in contrast to hemoglobinemia).
- Serum enzymes of muscle origin (e.g., creatine kinase) are increased.
- Identification of myoglobin in urine by various means:
    Immunochemical tests using antisera to human myoglobin offer best S/S.
    Ultracentrifugation and electrophoresis lack specificity.
    Spectrophotometry shows similar peaks for myoglobin and hemoglobin.
    Precipitation by ammonium sulfate may give false-negative results.

Odors (of Urine and Other Body Fluids)
Use
Clues to various metabolic disorders.

Condition	Odor
Maple syrup urine disease	Maple syrup, burned sugar
Oast house disease, methionine malabsorption	Brewery, oast house
Methylmalonic, propionic, isovaleric, glutaric, and butyric/hexanoic acidemia	Sweaty feet
Tyrosinemia	Cabbage-like, fishy, rancid
Trimethylaminuria	Stale fish
Hypermethioninemia	Rancid butter, rotten cabbage
Phenylketonuria	Musty, mousy
Ketosis	Sweet
Cystinuria, homocystinuria	Sulfurous
3-Oxothiolase deficiency	Sweet
3-Methylcrotonyl-CoA carboxylase deficiency	Cat urine
Hawkinsinuria	Swimming pool

Osmolality

Osmolality (mOsm/kg = freezing point depression °C ÷ 0.00186) reflects the degree of concentration of urine.

See Osmolality, Chapter 3.

Specific gravity compares weight of a solution to an equal volume of distilled water, which depends on the total number of particles and their relative size and density. Thus a solution of glucose with MW = 180 daltons is equal in osmolality to solution of urea with MW = 60 daltons, but glucose solution has a higher specific gravity.

Osmolality measures the number of solute particles and is a constant weight:weight relationship. It is not influenced by temperature, presence of protein, or radiographic contrast medium.

Osmolarity is 1 Osm of nonelectrolyte in 1 L of water and varies with the volume-expanding effect of the dissolved substance and the proportional effect of temperature on the fluid volume. Osmolality is the preferred unit of measure.

Decreased volume of concentrated urine (specific gravity >1.030 and osmolality >500 mOsm/kg) is diagnostic of prerenal azotemia.

Urine:plasma osmolality ratio is more accurate than urine osmolality or specific gravity to distinguish prerenal azotemia (with increased ratio) from acute tubular necrosis (with decreased ratio that is rarely >1.5).

Urine osmolality of 50 mOsm/kg water = specific gravity of ~1.000 to 1.001.

Urine osmolality of 300 mOsm/kg water = specific gravity of ~1.010.

Urine osmolality of 800 mOsm/kg water = specific gravity of ~1.020.

See also Urine Concentration and Dilution Tests, Chapter 14.

Porphyrinuria

Porphyrinuria is caused mainly by coproporphyrin.

Use

Porphyrias (see Chapter 12)

Lead poisoning

Cirrhosis

Infectious hepatitis

Passive in newborn of mother with porphyria; lasts for several days

Proteinuria

See Table 14-2 and Figures 4-3 and 4-4.

Use

Detection of various renal disorders and Bence-Jones proteinuria

Interpretation

Protein excretion >1,000 mg/day makes a diagnosis of renal parenchymal disease very likely. Excretion of >2,000 mg/day in adults or >40 mg/m^2 in children usually indicates glomerular etiology. Excretion of >3,500 mg/day or protein:creatinine ratio >3.5 points to nephrotic syndrome.

The 24-hour urine test is the gold standard. If it cannot be reliably collected, a spot urine for urine protein:creatinine ratio (especially after first morning specimen and before bedtime and if renal function is not severely impaired) often correlates well. Normal <0.2; low-grade proteinuria = 0.2 to 1.0; moderate proteinuria = 1.0 to 5.0; >5 is typical of nephrosis.

Positive reagent strips should always be followed by the sulfosalicylic acid test.

- For detection of proteinuria, reagent strips have S/S of 95% to 99%; PPV for renal disease is 0% to 1.4% (in young populations).
- *When sulfosalicylic acid test shows a significantly higher concentration than the reagent strips in an adult, Bence-Jones proteinuria should be ruled out.*
- *Association with hematuria indicates high likelihood of disease.*

Comparison and Interferences (False-Positive or False-Negative Results)

	Reagent Strips	Sulfosalicylic Acid
Sensitivity	10–30 mg/dL of protein	5–10 mg/dL of protein
Gross hematuria*	+	+
Highly concentrated urine	False +	False +
Dilute urine	False –	False –
Highly alkaline urine (pH >8) (e.g., GU tract infection with urea-splitting bacteria)	False +	False –
Predominantly low-molecular-weight or nonalbumin proteins	False –	

Antiseptic contamination (e.g., benzalkonium, chlorhexidine)	False +	No effect
Phenazopyridine	+	–
Radiopaque contrast media	No effect	False +
Tolbutamide metabolites	No effect	False +
High levels of cephalosporin or penicillin analogs	No effect	False +
Sulfonamide metabolites	No effect	False +

*Protein excretion >500 mg/m^2/day is significant. With microscopic hematuria, any amount more than an occasional trace of protein is abnormal.

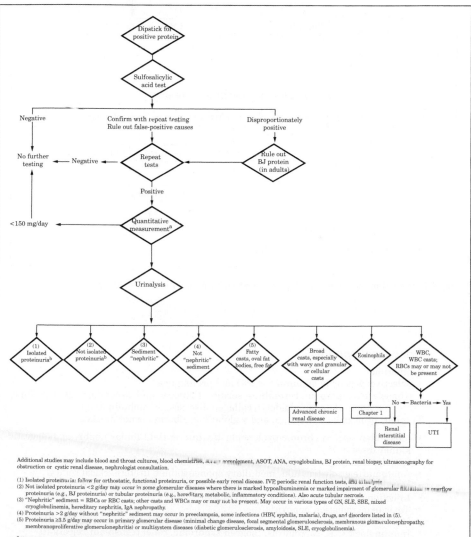

URINE

Additional studies may include blood and throat cultures, blood chemistries, serum complement, ASOT, ANA, cryoglobulins, BJ protein, renal biopsy, ultrasonography for obstruction or cystic renal disease, nephrologist consultation.

(1) Isolated proteinuria: follow for orthostatic, functional proteinuria, or possible early renal disease. IVP, periodic renal function tests, and urinalysis.
(2) Not isolated proteinuria <2 g/day may occur in some glomerular diseases where there is marked hypoalbuminemia or marked impairment of glomerular filtration; in overflow proteinuria (e.g., BJ proteinuria) or tubular proteinuria (e.g., hereditary, metabolic, inflammatory conditions). Also acute tubular necrosis.
(3) "Nephritic" sediment = RBCs or RBC casts; other casts and WBCs may or may not be present. May occur in various types of GN, SLE, SBE, mixed cryoglobulinemia, hereditary nephritis, IgA nephropathy.
(4) Proteinuria >2 g/day without "nephritic" sediment may occur in preeclampsia, some infections (HBV, syphilis, malaria), drugs, and disorders listed in (5).
(5) Proteinuria ≥3.5 g/day may occur in primary glomerular disease (minimal change disease, focal segmental glomerulosclerosis, membranous glomerulonephropathy, membranoproliferative glomerulonephritis) or multisystem diseases (diabetic glomerulosclerosis, amyloidosis, SLE, cryoglobulinemia).

[a]Check creatinine to assure 24-hour sample collection.
[b]Isolated proteinuria = no findings of GU tract abnormalities, renal manifestations of systemic disease, hypertension, decreased renal function, or abnormal renal sediment.

Fig. 4-3. Algorithm for diagnosis of proteinuria.
BJ, Bence-Jones; ASOT, antistreptolysin O titer; ANA, antinuclear antibodies; SLE, systemic lupus erythematosus; SBE, subacute bacterial endocarditis; HBV, hepatitis B virus; UTI, urinary tract infection.

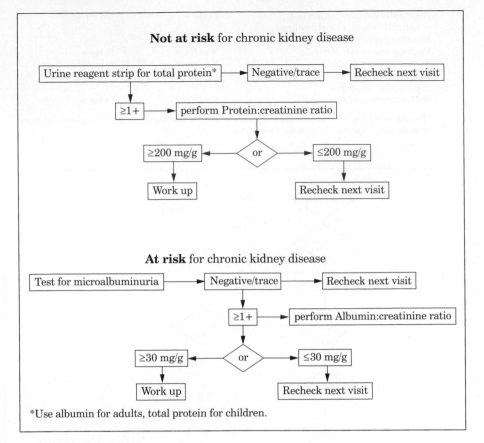

Fig. 4-4. Algorithm for diagnosis of patients at risk for chronic kidney disease.

Urine Electrophoresis

Glomerular
    Selective: primarily albumin (>80%) and proteinuria
    Nonselective: pattern resembles serum. Primary and secondary glomerulone-
        phropathies (DM, amyloidosis, collagen diseases, dysglobulinemia)
Tubular: principally α-1, α-2, β, and γ globulins; albumin is not marked.

* Most often seen in chronic pyelonephritis, interstitial tubular nephritis, polycystic
    kidney disease
* Genetic (e.g., polycystic kidney disease, medullary cystic disease)
* Anatomic (e.g., obstruction, medullary sponge kidney, ureterovesical reflux)
* Metabolic (e.g., diabetes mellitus, crystals [uric acid, calcium oxalate, cystine])
* Infection (e.g., pyelonephritis, tuberculosis)
* Toxic (e.g., radiation nephritis)
* Drugs (e.g., analgesic abuse, lithium, proteinuria, cisplatinum, aminoglycosides)
* Immunologic (e.g., sarcoidosis, Sjögren syndrome, renal transplant rejection)
* Others (e.g., sickle cell disease, multiple myeloma, amyloidosis, medullary sponge
    disease)

Overflow: Disparity between small amount with dipstick and much larger amount on 24-
    hour specimen. Most often due to monoclonal light chains (e.g., multiple myeloma,
    amyloidosis, lymphoproliferative disease); also hemoglobinuria, myoglobinuria.

Caused By

Orthostatic (Postural)

- First morning urine before arising shows high specific gravity but no protein (protein:creatinine ratio <0.1). Protein only appears after person is upright; usually <1.5 g/day (protein:creatinine ratio usually 0.1–1.3).
- Urine microscopy is normal.
- Is usually considered benign and slowly disappears over time, but is still present in 50% of persons 10 years later.
- Progressive renal insufficiency does not occur.
- Occurs in 15% of apparently healthy young men and 3% of otherwise healthy persons and some patients with resolving acute pyelonephritis or GN.
- Renal biopsy, electron microscopy, and immunofluorescent stains show pathologic changes in some patients.

Transient

- Commonly found in routine urinalysis of asymptomatic healthy children and young adults initially but not subsequently.
- Progressive renal disease is not present.
- Functional occurs in 10% of hospital medical patients; associated with high fever, congestive heart failure, hypertension, stress, exposure to cold, strenuous exercise, seizures. Usually <2 g/d; disappears with recovery from precipitating cause.

Persistent

- Glomerular (composed of large proteins [e.g., albumin, α-1-antitrypsin, proteinuria])
   Idiopathic (e.g., membranoproliferative GN, membranous glomerulopathy, minimal change disease, focal segmental glomerulosclerosis, amyloidosis)
   Secondary
   Infection (e.g., poststreptococcal, hepatitis B, bacterial endocarditis, malaria, infectious mononucleosis, pyelonephritis)
   Vascular (e.g., thrombosis of inferior vena cava or renal vein, renal artery stenosis)
   Drugs (e.g., nonsteroidal anti-inflammatory drugs, heroin, gold, captopril, penicillamine)
   Autoimmune (e.g., SLE, rheumatoid arthritis, dermatomyositis, polyarteritis, Goodpasture syndrome, Henoch-Schönlein purpura, ulcerative colitis)
   Neoplasia
   Hereditary and metabolic (e.g., polycystic kidney disease, diabetes mellitus, Fabry disease, Alport syndrome of progressive interstitial nephritis and nerve deafness)
- Decreased tubular reabsorption (composed of low-molecular-weight proteins, e.g., α and β microglobulins, free Ig light chains, retinol-binding protein, lysozyme; usually <1.5 g/d)
   Acquired
   Drugs (e.g., high-dose analgesics, phenacetin, aminoglycoside, cephalosporins, cyclosporine, lithium, methicillin)
   Heavy metal (e.g., lead, mercury, cadmium)
   Sarcoidosis
   Acute tubular necrosis
   Interstitial nephritis
   Renal tubular acidosis
   Acute and chronic pyelonephritis
   Renal graft rejection
   Congenital (e.g., Fanconi syndrome, oculo-cerebral-renal syndrome)
   Hereditary (e.g., Wilson disease, sickle cell disease, medullary cystic disease, oxalosis, cystinosis)
- Increased plasma levels of normal or abnormal proteins (e.g., Bence-Jones proteins, myoglobin, lysozyme in monocytic or myelocytic leukemias)

Microalbuminuria

Microalbuminuria is defined as persistent proteinuria that is below detection by routine reagent strips but greater than normal.

URINE

Use
In patients with diabetes mellitus (DM), should test for microalbumin even if routine reagent strips are negative

Interpretation
Albumin/creatinine ratio >30 mg/g predicts overnight excretion rate >30 μg/min.
Albuminuria $\leq$0.3 g/day, formerly detected only by sensitive assays (e.g., nephelometry, electrophoresis), can now be assayed by point-of-care methods.
Is independent risk predictor of diabetes, kidney failure, stroke, myocardial infarction, death. Indicates early stage and/or risk of cardiovascular or renal disease.

Albumin Excretion	Normal	Microalbuminuria*	Clinical Albuminuria
Albumin excretion (mg/d)	<20	30–300	>300
Albumin/g creatinine	<30	30–300	>300

*American Diabetes Association. Standards of medical care in diabetes. *Diabetes Care* 2004; 27(suppl 1):S79.

Interferences
Do not test urine during periods of exercise or prolonged upright posture, in presence of hematuria or blood contamination or GU tract infection, congestive heart failure (CHF), uncontrolled hyperglycemia or hypertension or in glass containers (albumin adheres to glass).
False-positive results may occur if pH $\geq$8, temperature >77°F, or Tamm-Horsfall protein is present.

Interpretation
The American Diabetes Association recommends that proteinuria high-risk patients be tested three times within a 3- to 6-month period; if two of three measurements are >20 mg/L, intervention should be initiated.[6] (See Chapters 13 and 14.)

• Present in ~25% of type 1 and 36% of type 2 patients with negative reagent strip test. In insulin-dependent DM, microalbuminuria has S/S of 82%/96%, respectively, and has PPV = 75% for subsequent overt nephropathy; lower values in non–insulin-dependent DM. Compared to normal, microalbuminuria is associated with longer duration of diabetes, poorer glycemic control, higher blood pressure, development of more advanced retinopathy and neuropathy, and overt nephropathy, subsequent renal failure, and increased vascular damage and risk for cardiovascular disease.

Common Causes of Low-Grade Proteinuria (<1 g/24 h)
• Kimmelstiel-Wilson syndrome
• Idiopathic low-grade proteinuria—normal history and physical exam, renal function, and urine sediment, with no hematuria
• Nephrosclerosis
• Polycystic kidney disease
• Medullary cystic disease
• Chronic obstruction of urinary tract
• Chronic interstitial nephritis (e.g., analgesic abuse, uric acid, oxalate, hypercalcemia, hypokalemia, lead, cadmium)

Bence-Jones Proteinuria

Use
Detection of various gammopathies
80% of tests are true positive due to:

• Myeloma (70% of all positive tests)
• Cryoglobulinemia
• Waldenström macroglobulinemia
• Primary amyloidosis
• Adult Fanconi syndrome
• Hyperparathyroidism
• Benign monoclonal gammopathy

[6]American Diabetes Association. Standards of medical care in diabetes. *Diabetes Care* 2004; 27(suppl 1):S79.

About 20% of results will be false-positive (i.e., urine electrophoresis does not show a spike, and immunoelectrophoresis does not show a monoclonal light chain) due to:

- Connective tissue disease (e.g., rheumatoid arthritis, SLE, scleroderma, polymyositis, Wegener granulomatosis)
- Chronic renal insufficiency
- Lymphoma and leukemia
- Metastatic carcinoma of lung, gastrointestinal, or GU tracts
- High doses of penicillin and aminosalicylic acid
- Presence of radiographic contrast media

Positive test for Bence-Jones proteinuria by heat test should always be confirmed by electrophoresis and immunoelectrophoresis/immunofiltration of concentrated urine. The heat test is not reliable and should not be used for diagnosis. The reagent strips test for albumin does not detect Bence Jones protein.

Beta₂ Microglobulin

A normal β_2 microglobulin reading is 0.2 mg/L or <1 mg/d by enzyme-linked immunosorbent assay or radioimmunoassay.

Use
Detection of various renal disorders
Increased In
Tubulointerstitial disease (>50 mg/d):

- Heavy metal poisoning (e.g., mercury, cadmium, cisplatinum)
- Drug toxicity (e.g., aminoglycosides, cyclosporine)
- Hereditary (e.g., Fanconi syndrome, Wilson disease, cystinosis)
- Pyelonephritis
- Renal allograft rejection
- Others (e.g., nephrocalcinosis)

Levels will also increase with increased production in hepatitis, sarcoidosis, Crohn disease, vasculitis, and certain malignancies, preventing diagnostic utility.
See also Chapter 3.
Interferences
Need for 24-hour timed collection
Unstable at room temperature, acid urine, and presence of pyuria
Differentiation

Precipitated by 5% Sulfosalicylic Acid

On Boiling, Precipitate Remains
Albumin
Globulin
Pseudo-Bence-Jones protein

On Boiling, Precipitate Disappears
Bence-Jones protein
A "proteose"

Precipitated at 40° to 60°C

Resuspend precipitate in normal urine and equal volume 5% sulfosalicylic acid and boil:

- Precipitate dissolves: Bence-Jones protein
- Precipitate does not dissolve: Pseudo-Bence-Jones protein

Now replaced by electrophoretic and immunologic procedures.
Globulin (Predominantly) Rather than Albumin
Multiple myeloma
Macroglobulinemia
Primary amyloidosis
Adult Fanconi syndrome (some patients)
Postrenal Proteinuria
Primarily associated with epithelial tumors of bladder or renal pelvis
Degree of proteinuria is related to size and invasiveness; generally <1 g/d (similar to pyelonephritis) and includes IgM
Renal Diseases in Which Proteinuria May Be Absent
Congenital abnormalities

Renal artery stenosis
Obstruction of GU tract
Pyelonephritis
Stone
Tumor
Polycystic kidneys
Hypokalemic nephropathy
Hypercalcemic nephropathy
Prerenal azotemia

Reducing Substances

Use
Screening for DM; however, this is not recommended as a primary screening modality
  because of its poor sensitivity

Caused By
Glycosuria

- Hyperglycemia
    Endocrine (e.g., DM, pituitary, adrenal, thyroid disease)
    Nonendocrine (e.g., liver, central nervous system diseases)
    Administration of hormones (e.g., ACTH, corticosteroids, thyroid, epinephrine) or
      drugs (e.g., morphine, anesthetic drugs, tranquilizers)
- Renal
    Tubular origin (serum glucose <180 mg/dL; oral and intravenous glucose
      tolerance tests are normal; ketosis is absent)
    Fanconi syndrome
    Toxic renal tubular disease (e.g., because of lead, mercury, degraded tetracycline)
    Inflammatory renal disease (e.g., acute GN, nephrosis)
    Glomerular due to increased glomerular filtration rate without tubular damage
- Idiopathic
    Melituria; 5% of cases of melituria in the general population are caused by renal
      glycosuria (incidence = 1:100,000), pentosuria (incidence = 1:50,000), essential
      fructosuria (incidence = 1:120,000)
- Hereditary (e.g., galactose, fructose, pentose, lactose)
    Galactose (classic and variant forms of galactosemia, galactokinase deficiency,
      severe liver disease with secondary galactose intolerance)
    Fructose (fructosemia, essential fructosuria, hereditary fructose intolerance)
    Lactose (lactase deficiency, lactose intolerance)
    Phenolic compounds (phenylketonuria, tyrosinosis)
    Xylulose (pentosuria)
- Lactosuria (e.g., during lactation and late in normal pregnancy, neonatal, sepsis,
  gastroenteritis, hepatitis)
- Xylose (excessive ingestion of fruit)

Lactose, galactose, fructose, maltose, pentose, sucrose, strong reducing substances
  (e.g., ascorbic acid, gentisic acid) may be positive with copper reduction tablets (e.g.,
  Clinitest) but negative with glucose oxidase strips (e.g., Clinistix and Tes-Tape)
Nonsugar-reducing substances (e.g., ascorbic acid, glucuronic acid, homogentisic acid
  in alkaptonuria, salicylates, phenolic compounds in phenylketonuria and tyrosinemia)
  may also be positive with copper reduction tablets (e.g., Clinitest) but negative with
  glucose oxidase strips (e.g., Clinistix and Tes-Tape)

Interferences (Glucose Oxidase Reagent Strips)
False-positive results

- Exposed to air (uncapped bottles) for a week or more
- Peroxidase contamination
- Oxidizing agents

False-negative results (found in >1% of routine urine analyses in hospital)

- Ascorbic acid >25 mg/dL
- Drugs (e.g., aspirin)
- Specific gravity >1.020
- High pH

Renal Enzyme Excretion

Renal enzyme excretion is a nonspecific but sensitive indicator of renal injury or disease activity.

Brush-border enzymes (e.g., γ-glutamyl transpeptidase and alanine aminopeptidase) represent minimal tissue injury.

Lysosomal enzymes (arylsulfatase A, β-glucuronidase, N-acetylglucosaminidase) represent more severe tissue injury.

Cytosolic enzymes (e.g., ligandin) represent severe damage or cell necrosis.

Specific Gravity

Specific gravity reflects the degree of concentration of the urine.

Use

Test of renal function (concentrate or dilute urine)

Increased In

Proteinuria

Glucosuria

Sucrosuria

Radiographic contrast medium (frequently 1.040–1.050)

Mannitol

Dextran

Diuretics

Antibiotics

Detergent

Temperature

Urinometer readings should come to room temperature or be corrected by adding (or subtracting) 0.001 to the specific gravity reading for each 3°C above (or below) calibration temperature (respectively). Subtract 0.003 for each 1 g/dL of protein and 0.004 for each 1 g/dL of glucose from temperature-compensated specific gravity. Reagent strips do not correlate well if the urine is alkaline or contains large amounts of protein.

The reagent strip method detects only ionic solutes and does not measure density; therefore it does not measure radiographic dyes or sugar. Readings are slightly increased by urine pH >7 or protein >100 mg/dL.

Uric Acid/Creatinine Ratio

The uric acid/creatinine ratio is above 1.0 in most patients with acute renal failure caused by hyperuricemia but lower in those with acute renal failure from other causes.

Urobilinogenuria

Use

Quantitative determination is not as useful as simple qualitative test; is seldom performed

Rarely useful instead of measuring direct and indirect bilirubin in blood or simple reagent strips test, which detects ~0.1 mg/dL

Interferences

False-positive reagent strip

Increased pH

Some drugs (e.g., procaine, 5-hydroxyindoleacetic acid, sulfonamides)

Increased In

Increased hemolysis (e.g., hemolytic anemias) with absent bilirubin

Hemorrhage into tissues (e.g., pulmonary infarction, severe bruises)

Hepatic parenchymal cell damage (e.g., acute hepatitis caused by viruses, toxins, drugs)

Cholangitis, since bilirubin is present

Absent In

Complete biliary obstruction; associated with pale stools

URINE

Volume

Anuria

Anuria is defined as the excretion of less than 100 mL of urine in 24 hours.

Caused By

Bilateral complete urinary tract obstruction
Acute cortical necrosis
Necrotizing glomerulonephritis
Certain causes of acute tubular necrosis

Acute Oliguria

Acute oliguria is usually defined as excretion of less than 400 mL of urine in 24 hours, or ~20 mL/h; in children, this is defined as less than 15 to 20 mL/kg/24 h.

Caused By

See Acute Renal Failure, Chapter 8.
Prerenal causes (e.g., CHF, shock)
Postrenal causes (e.g., GU tract obstruction)
Renal causes
    Glomerular: urine protein >2+ (>1.5 g/24 h), RBCs, RBC casts
    Tubulointerstitial: urine protein ≤2+ (≤1.5 g/24 h), WBCs, WBC casts

Polyuria

Polyuria is defined as a urine volume over 2,000 mL per day.

Caused By

Osmotic diuresis, including DM
Polydipsia, including diabetes insipidus (see Chapter 13)
Diuretic drugs, including alcohol, caffeine
Chronic renal failure
Partial obstruction of urinary tract with impaired urinary concentration function
Some types of acute tubular necrosis (e.g., that caused by aminoglycosides)

Other Procedures

For more information on urine findings in various diseases, see Kidney Disease, Chapter 14 and Table 14-2.
See also specific tests on urine in Chapters 7, 11, 12, and 13.

III

Diseases of Organ Systems

5 Cardiovascular Diseases

CARDIOVASC

Diseases Principally of Endocardium

Löffler Parietal Fibroplastic Endocarditis

Löffler parietal fibroplastic endocarditis may represent part of the spectrum of hypereosinophilic syndrome.

Eosinophilia ≤70% (or >1,500/µL) without other cause; may be absent at first but appears sooner or later
White blood cell (WBC) counts are frequently increased
Laboratory findings due to frequent:
    Mural thrombi in heart and embolization of spleen and lung
    Mitral and tricuspid regurgitation

Myxoma of Left Atrium

○ Anemia (mechanical, hemolytic) caused by local turbulence of blood may occur and may be severe. Bizarre poikilocytes may be seen in blood smear. Other findings may reflect the effects of hemolysis or compensatory erythroid hyperplasia. The anemia is recognized in ~50% of patients with this tumor. Increased serum lactate dehydrogenase (LD) reflects hemolysis.
Serum γ globulin is increased in ~50% of patients. IgG may be increased.
Increased erythrocyte sedimentation rate (ESR) is a reflection of abnormal serum proteins.
Platelet count may be decreased (possibly mechanical) with findings due to thrombocytopenia.
Negative blood cultures differentiate this tumor from infective endocarditis.
Occasionally WBC is increased, and C-reactive protein (CRP) may be positive.
Laboratory findings due to complications (e.g., emboli to various organs, congestive heart failure [CHF], valve obstruction).
These findings are reported much less frequently in myxoma of the right atrium, which is more likely to be accompanied by secondary polycythemia than anemia.
♦ Echocardiography is definitive.

Rheumatic Fever, Acute[1]

Acute rheumatic fever (RF) is an inflammatory multisystem immunologic disease occurring 10 days to 6 weeks following an episode of group A *Streptococcus* infection.

◆ **Diagnostic Criteria**
Laboratory confirmation of preceding group A *Streptococcus* infection by
◆ Positive throat culture for group A *Streptococcus* or recent scarlet fever (is often negative) *or*
◆ Increased serologic titer of antistreptococcal antibodies (e.g., anti-DNAse B, others) or streptococcal antigens. One titer is elevated in 95% of patients with acute RF; if all are normal, a diagnosis of RF is less likely *plus* two major or one major and two minor criteria
Minor Criteria: High ESR or CRP, prolonged P-R interval, fever, arthralgia
Major Criteria: Carditis, arthritis, Sydenham chorea, subcutaneous nodules, erythema marginatum

---

◆ Acute-phase reactants (ESR, CRP, increased WBC)
- ESR increase is a sensitive test of rheumatic activity.
  - Returns to normal with adequate treatment with adrenocorticotropic hormone (ACTH) or salicylates
  - May remain increased after WBC becomes normal
  - Said to become normal with onset of CHF, even in the presence of rheumatic activity
  - Normal in uncomplicated chorea alone
- CRP parallels ESR.
- WBC may be normal but usually is increased (10,000 to 16,000/μL) with shift to the left; increase may persist for weeks after fever subsides. Count may decrease with salicylate and ACTH therapy.

To determine clinical activity—follow ESR, CRP, and WBC. Return to normal should be seen in 6 to 12 weeks in 80% to 90% of patients; it may take ≤6 months. Normal findings do not prove inactivity if patient is receiving hormone therapy. When therapy is stopped after findings have been suppressed for 6 to 8 weeks, there may be a mild rebound for 2 to 3 days and then a return to normal. Relapse after cessation of therapy occurs within 1 to 8 weeks.

Serum proteins are altered, with decreased serum albumin and increased α_2 and γ globulins. (*Streptococcus A infections do not increase α_2 globulin*.) Fibrinogen is increased.

Anemia (hemoglobin [Hb] usually 8 to 12 g/dL), microcytic type is common; gradually improves as activity subsides.

Urine: There is a slight febrile albuminuria. Often mild abnormality of protein, casts, RBCs, WBCs indicates mild focal nephritis. Concomitant glomerulonephritis (GN) appears in ≤2.5% of cases.

Blood cultures are usually negative. Occasional positive culture is found in 5% of patients (bacteria usually grow only in fluid media, not on solid media), in contrast to bacterial endocarditis.

Increased serum cardiac troponin (cTn) implies some myocardial necrosis due to myocarditis.

Serum aspartate aminotransferase (AST) may be increased, but alanine aminotransferase (ALT) is normal unless the patient has cardiac failure with liver damage.

Transplant Rejection (Acute) of Heart

◆ Endocardial biopsy to determine acute rejection and follow effects of therapy has no substitute.

---

[1]Ferrieri P. Jones Criteria Working Group. Proceedings of the Jones Criteria workshop. *Circulation* 2002;106:2521–2523.

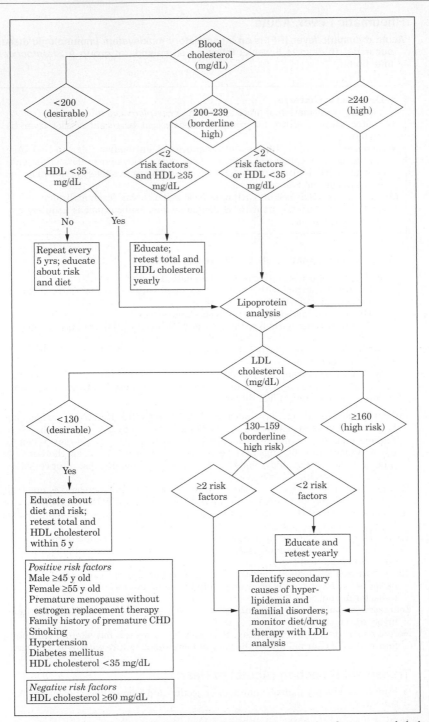

Fig. 5-1. Algorithm of recommended testing and treatment of increased serum total cholesterol (TC) and high-density lipoprotein cholesterol (HDL-C) in adults without evidence of coronary heart disease. Measure serum TC, HDL-C, and triglycerides after 12- to 14-hour fast. Average the results of two or three tests; if the difference is >30 mg/dL, repeat tests

Increasing ESR and WBC.
Increased isoenzyme LD-1 as amount (>100 IU) and percent (35%) of total LD during
first 4 weeks after surgery.
These findings are reversed with effective immunosuppressive therapy. Total LD continues to be increased even when LD-1 becomes normal.
Chronic rejection is accelerated coronary artery atherosclerosis.

Diseases Principally of Myocardium

Cor Pulmonale

Secondary polycythemia
Increased blood CO_2 when cor pulmonale is secondary to chest deformities or pulmonary emphysema
Laboratory findings of the primary lung disease (e.g., chronic bronchitis and emphysema, multiple small pulmonary emboli, pulmonary schistosomiasis)

Coronary Heart Disease

Laboratory markers of risk factors:
   Metabolic (e.g., dyslipidemias, homocysteine)
   Ischemia, necrosis, e.g., creatine kinase isoenzyme MB (CK-MB), cTn, ischemia-modified albumin
   Inflammation (e.g., CRP, myeloperoxidase [MPO], fibrinogen, serum amyloid A [SAA])
   Procoagulant (e.g., von Willebrand factor [vWF], activated protein C resistance, protein
      C deficiency, plasminogen deficiency, antiphospholipid syndrome [see Chapter 11])
      Impaired fibrinolysis (e.g., dysfibrinogenemia [see Chapter 11])
   Cystatin C because kidney dysfunction is associated with adverse cardiovascular
      events and death
   Others (e.g., sickle cell disease, polycythemia)

Tests of Lipid Metabolism

Blood lipid tests should not be performed during stress or acute illness (e.g., recent
   myocardial infarction [MI], stroke, pregnancy, trauma, weight loss, use of certain
   drugs); *should not be performed on hospitalized patients until 2 to 3 months after illness.*
Abnormal lipid test results should always be confirmed with a new specimen, preferably 1 week apart, before beginning or changing therapy.
A tourniquet that is in place longer than 3 minutes may cause 5% variation in lipid values.

Use

Assess risk of atherosclerosis, especially coronary heart disease and stroke
Classify hyperlipidemias

Lipid Decision Levels[2]

See Figure 5-1 and Tables 5-1 and 5-2.
Note: Measure serum total cholesterol (TC), high-density lipoprotein (HDL) cholesterol,
   and triglycerides (TG) after a 12- to 13-hour fast. Average results of two or three tests;
   if a difference of ≥30 mg/dL appears, repeat tests 1 to 8 weeks apart and average the
   results of three tests. Use TC for initial case finding and classification and monitoring
   of diet therapy. Do not use age- or sex-specific cholesterol values as decision levels.

[2]Expert Panel on Detection, Evaluation, and Treatment of High Blood Cholesterol in Adults.
Executive Summary of the Third Report of the National Cholesterol Education Program (NCEP)
Expert Panel on Detection, Evaluation and Treatment of High Blood Cholesterol in Adults (Adult
Treatment Panel III). *JAMA* 2001;285:2486–2496.

1 to 8 weeks apart and average three tests. Use TC for initial case finding and classification
and to monitor diet therapy. Do not use age- or sex-specific cholesterol values as decision
levels. Always rule out secondary and familial causes. (Adapted from Expert Panel on
Detection, Evaluation, and Treatment of High Blood Cholesterol in Adults. Executive
Summary of the Third Report of the National Cholesterol Education Program [NCEP]
Expert Panel on Detection, Evaluation, and Treatment of High Blood Cholesterol in Adults
[Adult Treatment Panel I]. *JAMA* 2001;285:2486–2496.)

CARDIOVASC

Table 5-1.   Serum Cholesterol and Triglyceride Risk Categories

	Serum Cholesterol							
Risk Category	HDL-C	TC	TC/ HDL-C	LDL/ HDL	LDL- C[a]	VLDL- C	Lp(a)	Serum TG[b]
Normal/desirable level or low risk	≥50	<200	3.3–4.4	0.5–3.0	<100	<30	<30	<150
Above optimal or average risk			4.4–7.1		≤130			150–199
Borderline high or moderate risk			200–239	7.1–11.0	3.0–6.0	≥160 (high)		200–499 (high)
Elevated level or high risk	<40	≥240	>11.0	>6.0	≥190 (very high)			≥500 (very high)

All values in mg/dL.
C, cholesterol; HDL, high-density lipoprotein; LDL, low-density lipoprotein; Lp(a), lipoprotein A; TC, total cholesterol; TG, triglycerides; VLDL, very low density lipoprotein.
[a]National Heart, Lung, and Blood Institute of NIH have suggested a therapeutic option (desirable goal) of LDL-C <70 mg/dL for patients at highest risk of heart disease.
[b]Expert Panel on Detection, Evaluation, and Treatment of High Blood Cholesterol in Adults. Executive Summary of The Third Report of the National Cholesterol Education Program (NCEP) Expert Panel on Detection, Evaluation, and Treatment of High Blood Cholesterol in Adults (Adult Treatment Panel III). *JAMA* 2001;285:2486–2497.

Use

Screening for primary and secondary hyperlipidemias; should include TC, HDL-C, low-density lipoprotein C (LDL-C), TG

Monitoring for increased risk for atherosclerosis, especially coronary heart disease (CHD) and stroke

Monitoring treatment of hyperlipidemias

Values should be considered in association with clinical risk factors (e.g., age, gender, obesity, smoking, hypertension, family history) and treatment goals and have recently been changed

Ratios are meant for population studies; not applied to patient care

Generally, HDL-C is inversely related to TC and LDL-C

Table 5-2.   National Cholesterol Education Program[a]

Risk Category	LDL-C Goal	Initiate Therapeutic Lifestyle Changes	Consider Drug Therapy
Lower risk (0–1 risk factors)	<160	≥160	≥190 (if 160–189, LDL-lowering drug optional)
Moderate risk (≥2 risk factors; 10-y risk<10%)	<130	≥130	≥160
Moderately high risk (≥2 risk factors; 10-y risk 10%–20%)	<130	≥130	≥130 (if 100–129, LDL-lowering drug optional)
High risk (CHD or CHD risk equivalents; 10-y risk >20%)	<100 (optional goal <70)	≥100	<100 (if <100, LDL-lowering drug optional)

All values in mg/dL.
[a]Adult Treatment Panel III guidelines have suggested a therapeutic option (desirable goal) of LDL-C <70 mg/dL for patients at highest risk of heart disease.

Cholesterol, Total, Serum

Interferences

Note effect of illness, intra-individual variation, position, season, drugs, etc., when these values are used to diagnose and treat hyperlipidemias.

Intra-individual variation may be about 4% to 10% for serum TC. Repeat TC values should be within 30 mg/dL.

TC values are up to 8% higher in winter than summer, 5% lower if bled when sitting compared to when standing, and 10% to 15% different when recumbent compared to when standing.

TC values of ethylenediaminetetraacetic acid plasma can be multiplied by 1.03 to make them comparable to serum values.

Serum TC and HDL-C can be nonfasting.

Increased In

Certain primary hyperlipoproteinemias (see Table 5-3).

Secondary hyperlipoproteinemias (e.g., diabetes mellitus, hypothyroidism, etc.) (see Chapter 12)

Secondary causes should always be ruled out.

Decreased In

Severe liver cell damage, hyperthyroidism, malnutrition (e.g., starvation, neoplasms, uremia, malabsorption), myeloproliferative diseases, chronic anemias, infection, inflammation, drugs

Primary lipoproteinemias (e.g., hypobetalipoproteinemia and abetalipoproteinemia), Tangier disease

Cholesterol, High-Density Lipoprotein, Serum

Intra-individual variation may be ~3.6% to 12.4%.

Increased In

(Value ≥60 mg/dL is negative risk factor for CHD)

Moderate consumption of alcohol, insulin, estrogens

Familial lipid disorders with protection against atherosclerosis (importance of measuring HDL-C to evaluate hypercholesterolemia)

Hyperalphalipoproteinemia (HDL-C excess)

Hypobetalipoproteinemia (see Table 13-6)

Decreased In

(<40 mg/dL)

Inversely related to risk of CHD. For every 1 mg/dL decrease in HDL-C, the risk for CHD increases by 2% to 3%.

Secondary causes: stress and recent illness (such as acute MI [AMI], stroke, surgery, trauma), starvation (nonfasting sample is 5%–10% lower), diabetes mellitus, hypothyroidism, liver disease, nephrosis, uremia, various chronic anemias and myeloproliferative disorders, certain drugs (see Chapter 12).

Genetic disorders (see Chapter 12).

Cholesterol, Low-Density Lipoprotein, Serum

(Directly related to risk of CHD.)

Increased In

Primary (e.g., familial hypercholesterolemia, familial combined hyperlipidemia) (see Chapter 12)

Secondary (e.g., diabetes mellitus, hypothyroidism, nephrosis, chronic renal failure, diet, certain drugs)

Decreased In

Severe illness, certain drugs, abetalipoproteinemia.

LDL-C is measured by ultracentrifugation and by analysis after antibody separation from HDL-C and very low-density lipoprotein (VLDL).

Can estimate LDL by Friedewald equation:

$$LDL\text{-}C = TC - (HDL\text{-}C - VLDL)$$

$$and\ VLDL = TG/5$$

Formula underestimates LDL-C (e.g., chronic alcoholism), is unsuitable for monitoring, misclassifies 15% to 40% of patients when TG = 200 to 400 mg/dL, and fails if fasting TG >400 mg/dL. Not reliable if suspect type III dyslipidemia or chylomicrons are present.

CARDIOVASC

Table 5-3. Comparison of Types of Hyperlipoproteinemia

Point of Comparison	I Rarest	II-a Common	II-b Common	III Rare	IV Most Common	V Uncommon
Age	Usually <10 y			Not known younger than 25 y	Only occasionally in children	
Etiology	Lipoprotein lipase deficiency	Familial hypercholesterolemia. Familial combined hyperlipidemia. Diabetes mellitus, hypothyroidism, nephrosis.		Homozygous apo E2. Diabetes mellitus, nephrosis.	Familial combined hyperlipidemia. Familial hypertriglyceridemia. Drugs, e.g., glucocorticoids androgens, growth hormone. Diabetes mellitus, hypothyroidism, nephrosis, Cushing syndrome.	
Increased particle	Chylomicron	LDL	LDL, VLDL	IDL	VLDL	VLDL, chylomicron
Blood lipids (mg/dL)	TG >1,000	LDL >130	TG >125 LDL >130	TG >125 TC >200	TG >125	TG >1,000

HDL, high-density lipoprotein (synthesized by liver and intestine; also derived from surface of chylomicrons and VDL during lipolysis; major lipid is phospholipid and cholesterol); IDL, intermediate-low-density lipoprotein (derived from VLDL by lipase hydrolysis of TG; precursor of LDL; major lipid is TG and cholesterol); LDL, low-density lipoprotein (derived from VLDL and IDL by lipase hydrolysis of TG; major lipid is cholesterol); TC, total cholesterol; TG, triglycerides (chylomicrons are synthesized by small intestine; major lipid is TG); VLDL, very low-density lipoprotein (apo B-100 produced from *APOB* gene is required for synthesis by liver; major lipid is TG; transports TG and cholesterol from liver to various tissues).

Triglycerides, Serum

(80% is present in VLDL, 15% is present in LDL.)

Interferences

Serum for TG and for calculating LDL-C should follow a 12-hour fast.
Diurnal variation causes TG to be lowest in the morning and highest around noon.

Increased In

Certain genetic hyperlipidemias (e.g., familial hypertriglyceridemia, von Gierke disease).

Secondary hyperlipidemias (e.g., diabetes mellitus, hypothyroidism, nephrosis, chronic renal failure, diet, certain drugs).

Concentrations associated with certain disorders:

- <150 mg/dL not associated with any disease state
- 250 to 500 mg/dL associated with peripheral vascular disease; may be a marker for patients with genetic forms of hyperlipoproteinemias who need specific therapy
- >500 mg/dL associated with high risk of pancreatitis
- >1,000 mg/dL associated with hyperlipidemia, especially type I or type V; substantial risk of pancreatitis
- >5,000 mg/dL associated with eruptive xanthoma, corneal arcus, lipemia retinalis, enlarged liver and spleen

Decreased In

Certain primary lipoproteinemias, e.g., abetalipoproteinemia, malnutrition, diet, recent weight loss, vigorous exercise (transient), certain drugs.

Total and HDL-C levels are similar when fasting or nonfasting, but TG should be measured after 12 to 14 hours of fasting. Serum levels are ~3% to 5% higher than plasma levels.

TG levels are inversely related to HDL-C levels.

Increased Risk Factors

♦ • Increased serum TC and LDL-C (>100 mg/dL; 2× if >160 mg/dL), decreased HDL-C (<40 mg/dL in men, <45 mg/dL in women) and various ratios, especially TC/HDL-C ratio

Atherogenic Index is a combination of the ratio of LDL-C to HDL-C × apo B with ratio of apo B to apo AI:

$$\text{Atherogenic Index} = \frac{(\text{TC} - \text{HDL-C}) \times \text{apo B}}{(\text{apo AI} \times \text{HDL-C})}$$

♦ • Increased high-sensitivity CRP (hsCRP) may be a more important independent risk factor (for cardiovascular events and higher mortality) than all other factors except the TC/HDL-C ratio. Predicts future cardiovascular events, acute complications and clinical restenosis in patients undergoing angioplasty. Risk increases incrementally[3] as well for peripheral vascular disease and stroke. Increase in other acute inflammatory reactants, especially fibrinogen, also may be important, but fewer data are available (see Chapter 3).

    Relative risk categories:
        Low risk CRP, <1.0 mg/L
        Average risk CRP, 1.0 to 3.0 mg/L
        High risk CRP, >3.0 mg/L

○ • Increased total serum bilirubin (0.58 mg/dL or 10 μmol/L) is related to lower risk of cardiovascular events (e.g., coronary artery disease [CAD], acute coronary syndrome [ACS], AMI) in men for unknown reasons.

○ • Increased serum homocysteine >15.9 μmol/L (normal is 5 to 15 μmol/L) triples risk of AMI. Each increase of 5 μmol/L increases risk equivalent to increased TC of 20 mg/dL.

CARDIOVASC

[3]Pearson TA, Mensah GA, Alexander RW, et al. Markers of inflammation and cardiovascular disease: application to clinical and public health practice: A statement for healthcare professionals from the Centers for Disease Control and Prevention and the American Heart Association. *Circulation* 2003;107:499–511.

○ • *Increased in* Vitamin B deficiency or genetic deficiency of methylene-tetrahydrofo-
late reductase enzyme, end-stage renal disease dialysis patients, hypothyroidism,
drugs (e.g., methotrexate [transient], phenytoin and carbamazepine [mild], theo-
phylline, nitrous oxide), and cigarette smoking
○ • Low plasma vitamin B12 and folate levels are each independent risk factors for CHD
○ • Syndrome X: Onsulin resistance, low HDL, high VLDL, and TG
○ • Various procoagulant abnormalities of blood clotting mechanisms (e.g., fibrino-
gen, factor VII, antithrombin III, antiphospholipid antibodies, protein C, protein
S, vWF)
○ • Clinical factors that increase risk: Obesity, hypertension, smoking, etc.

Apolipoproteins, Serum

**An apolipoprotein is a protein component of lipoprotein that regulates their metab-
olism; each of four major groups consists of a family of two or more immunologically distinct proteins.**

Apolipoprotein A (apo A) is the major protein of HDL; apo AI and AII constitute 90%
of total HDL protein, in a ratio of 3 to 1. Apo A comprises HDL and chylomicrons.
Apo B is the major protein in LDL; it is important in regulating cholesterol synthesis
and metabolism. Apo B is decreased by severe illness and abetalipoproteinemia.
Apo CI, apo CII, and apo CIII are associated with all lipoproteins except LDL; apo CII
is important in TG metabolism.
Serum apo AI and apo B levels are more highly correlated with severity and extent of
CHD than TC and TG.
Apo AI:apo B ratio showed greater sensitivity/specificity (S/S) for CHD than LDL-
C:HDL-C ratio, HDL-C:TG ratio, or any of the individual components.
Since apo B is the only protein in LDL-C and apo AI is the major protein constituent of
HDL-C and VLDL, the ratio apo B:apo AI reflects the ratio LDL-C:HDL-C and may
be a better discriminator of CHD than the individual components, but data on
apolipoproteins are still limited.

Chylomicrons, Serum

**Apo B-48, produced from the *APOB* gene, is required for chylomicron production in
small intestine.**

Increased In
Type V hyperlipoproteinemia
Lipoprotein lipase deficiency (autosomal recessive disorder or due to deficient cofactor
for lipoprotein lipase) presenting in children with pancreatitis, xanthomas,
hepatosplenomegaly
Apo CII deficiency (rare autosomal recessive disorder caused by absence of or presence
of defective apo CII); accumulation of VLDL and chylomicrons, increasing risk of
pancreatitis

Lipoprotein Electrophoresis

**Lipoproteins are macromolecules that transport lipids through aqueous plasma.
Shows a specific abnormal pattern in <2% of Americans (usually types II, IV). See
Table 5-3.**

Use
Identify rare familial disorders (e.g., types I, III, V hyperlipidemias) to anticipate prob-
lems in children.
May be indicated if:

• Serum TG >300 mg/dL
• Fasting serum is lipemic
• Significant hyperglycemia, impaired glucose tolerance, or glycosuria is present
• Increased serum uric acid >8.5 mg/dL
• Strong family history of premature CHD
• Clinical evidence of CHD or atherosclerosis in patient <40 years of age

If lipoprotein electrophoresis is abnormal, tests should be performed to rule out secondary hyperlipidemias (see following).

Lipoprotein-Associated Phospholipase A2

Lipoprotein-associated phospholipase A2 (Lp-PLA2) is made by macrophages and released into the blood when CAD is present.

Increased Lp-PLA2 with low LDL-C increases risk of heart disease by two times.
Increased Lp-PLA2 with high CRP increases risk of heart disease by three times.

Coronary Syndromes, Acute

The term "acute coronary syndromes" includes the continuous spectrum from silent ischemia, stable angina, unstable angina (pain without apparent cause), non-ST wave elevation, and "non-Q wave" infarction, to typical AMI. Unstable angina is probably not one entity but a combination of syndromes classified clinically into crescendo angina, non-Q wave MI, new-onset angina with accelerating symptoms, and post-MI angina.
See "Coronary Heart Disease."

Myocardial Infarction, Acute

See Figures 5-2 and 5-3 and Tables 5-4 to 5-6.
Caused By
Coronary artery atherosclerosis is usual cause
Embolization
Trauma
Arteritis

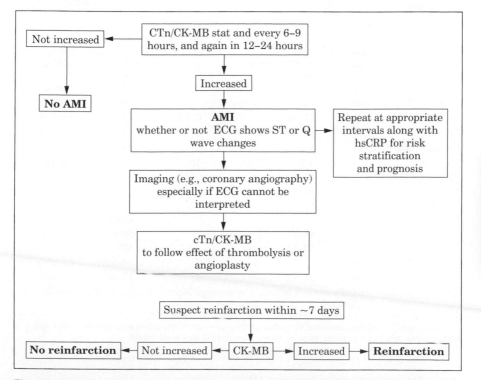

Fig. 5-2. Algorithm for diagnosis of acute myocardial infarction (AMI). (Adapted from Alpert JS, Thygesen K, Antman E, et al. Myocardial infarction redefined—a consensus document of the Joint European Society of Cardiology/American College of Cardiology Committee for the redefinition of myocardial infarction. *J Am Coll Cardiol* 2000;36:959–969.)

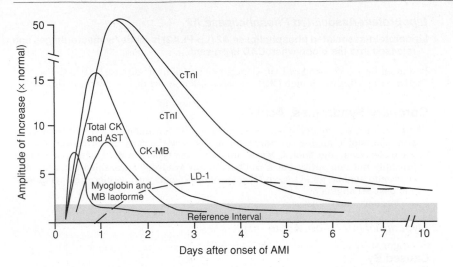

Fig. 5-3. Serial serum cardiac markers after acute myocardial infarction (AMI).

Table 5-4.	Summary of Increased Serum Marker Levels After Acute Myocardial Infarction (AMI)					
Serum Marker	Earliest Increase (hrs)[a]	Peak (hrs)[a]	Duration of Increase (hrs)[a]	Amplitude of Increase (× normal)	Specificity (%)[b]	Sensitivity at Peak(%)[b]
Troponin T	3–4	10–24	10–14 days		80%	>98%
Troponin I	4–6	10–24	4–7 days		95%	>98%
CK total	4–8	24–36	36–48	6–12	57–88%	93–100%
CK-MB	3–4	15–24	24–36	16	93–100%	94–100%
CK-MB-2/MB-1	2–4	4–6	16–24		94%	95%
Myoglobin	1–3	6–9	12–24	10	70%	75–95%
CK-MM-3/MM-1	6	10	~2			
Myosin light chain	3–8	24–35	10–15			
ECG					100%	63–84%
LD[c]	10–12	48–72	11	3	88%	87%
LD-1[c]	8–12	72–144	8–14		85%	40–90%
LD-1/LD-2[c]	>6		>3		94–99%	61–90%
AST[d]	6–8	24–48	4–6	5	48–88%	89–97%
ALT[d]	Usually normal unless liver damage is present (e.g., congestive heart failure)					

High degree of myocardial perfusion in cardiac surgery or contusion patients may lead to earlier and higher peaks and faster washout, causing shorter duration of increased values.
[a]Time periods represent average reported values.
[b]Depends on time after onset of AMI. Sensitivity is lower at earlier or later times after myocardial damage.
[c]Replaced by cardiac troponin for diagnosis of AMI.
[d]Not used for diagnosis of AMI.
Note: Range of reported values because different studies used different time periods after onset of symptoms, size of infarct, benchmarks for establishing the diagnosis, patient populations, instrumentation, etc.

Table 5-5.   Interpretation of Markers for Diagnosis of Acute Myocardial Infarction (AMI)

ECG	cTn	CK Total	CK-MB	Myoglobin	Interpretation
+	+	+	+	+	AMI.
+	±	±	±	±	AMI. Confirm with cTn for risk stratification and to monitor angioplastic/thrombolytic therapy.
−	+	−	−	−	AMI or unstable angina with increased risk of subsequent coronary event.
−	−	−	+	−	AMI or unstable angina. Confirm with serial CK-MB, ECG, and cTn.
−	+	±	±	±	AMI or unstable angina.
−	−	−	−	+	Follow up cTn or CK-MB to rule out early AMI. See elsewhere in this chapter for other causes of increased myoglobin.
−	−	+	−	−	Not AMI. See Chapter 3 for other causes of increased total CK.

+ indicates increased; − indicates not increased.

Hypercoagulable state
Substance abuse (e.g., cocaine)
Congenital anomalies (e.g., anomalous origin of left coronary from pulmonary artery or sinus of Valsalva)
Metabolic diseases (e.g., homocystinuria, Hurler syndrome, Fabry disease)
Others (coronary artery spasm, aortic dissection, carbon monoxide poisoning, poly-cythemia vera, thrombocytosis, amyloidosis, anemia)

◆ Redefinition of Myocardial Infarction[4]
Criteria for Acute, Evolving, or Recent MI

• Typical rise and gradual fall in cTn or more rapid rise and fall in CK-MB *with* ≥1 of the following:

  (a) ischemic symptoms
  (b) development of pathologic Q waves in electrocardiogram (ECG)
  (c) ECG changes indicative of ischemia (ST elevation or depression) *or*
  (d) coronary artery intervention (e.g., coronary angioplasty)

• Pathologic findings of acute MI

Criteria for Established MI

• Any of the following:

  (a) Development of new pathologic Q waves on serial ECG
  (b) Patient may or may not remember previous symptoms
  (c) Biochemical markers of myocardial necrosis may have become normal depending on time interval *or*
  (d) Pathologic findings of healed or healing MI

---

[4]Alpert JS, Thygesen K, Antman E, et al. Myocardial infarction redefined—a consensus document of The Joint European Society of Cardiology/American College of Cardiology Committee for the redefinition of myocardial infarction. *J Am Coll Cardiol* 2000;36:959–969.

CARDIOVASC

Table 5-6.   Characteristics of Serum Markers for Myocardial Damage

Early appearance: Myoglobin, CK isoforms, glycogen phosphorylase isoenzyme BB, heart
   fatty acid-binding protein
High specificity: cTnI, cTnT, CK-MB, CK isoforms
Wide diagnostic window: cTnT, cTnI, LD, myosin hight and heavy chains
Risk stratification: cTnT, cTnI, CK-MB
Predicts reperfusion: Myoglobin, cTnI, cTnT, CK isoforms
Indicates reinfarction after 2–4 d: CK-MB

◆ Use of Laboratory Determinations

For differential diagnosis and triage of chest pain in ER: false-positive ECG occurs in
   >10% to 20% of AMI cases. Nondiagnostic in ~50% of cases.
Risk stratification in patients with chest pain: Detectable cTn is a sensitive marker for
   myocardial injury in unstable angina patients with chest pain, even with normal
   CK-MB and nondiagnostic ECG, and have greater risk of cardiovascular events and
   higher mortality. Any increased cTn increases risk of adverse clinical events. Degree
   of cTn increase is related to patient prognosis.
Treatment: identify ACS patients with nonST wave elevation who would benefit from
   early coronary angiography and intervention or antithrombotic/antiplatelet therapy.
   Serial measurements can assess reperfusion after thrombolytic therapy. Peak cTn
   after reperfusion is related to infarct size. Patients undergoing heart surgery or
   coronary angioplasty are likely to have increased cTn, indicating ischemic cell death.
The utility of each marker depends on the time of specimen collection after onset of AMI.
Serial changes and combination of markers (e.g., serum cTn, CK-MB, myoglobin
   [Myg]) may be most effective because of uncertainty as to the actual duration of
   myocardial damage. *A single assay of one analyte should not be used to rule out AMI.*

◆ *Plasma Cardiac Troponins T and I*[5]

Troponin is a protein involved in heart muscle contraction.

Use/Interpretation

Increased cTn establishes the diagnosis of some irreversible myocardial necrosis (e.g.,
   anoxia, contusion, inflammation), even when ECG changes or CK-MB are nondiagnostic (which occurs in ≤50% of ACS patients). Serial normal cTn rules out myocardial necrosis.
cTn replaces CK-MB as the gold standard and replaces LD for late diagnosis of AMI.
   cTn is as sensitive as CK-MB during the first 48 hours after AMI (>85% concordance
   with CK-MB); sensitivity = 33% from 0 to 2 hours, 50% from 2 to 4 hours, 75% from
   4 to 8 hours, and approaching 100% from 8 hours after onset of chest pain. May take
   ≤12 hours for all patients to show an increase. Specificity close to 100%. High sensitivity for 6 days. cTnI may remain increased for ≤9 days; cTnT may remain
   increased for ≤14 days.
cTnI is 13 times more abundant in myocardium than CK-MB, providing a better
   signal-to-noise ratio.
The long duration of increased cTn provides a longer diagnostic window than CK-MB
   but may make it difficult to recognize reinfarction.
Rapid (20-minute) test kits using whole blood can now measure serum cTn, CK-MB,
   total CK, and Myg on site in the ER. These results may not be comparable to core
   lab values, since different values can result from different assay methods.
Serial cTn values may be indicator of cardiac allograft rejection.
Differential diagnosis of skeletal muscle injury.
Normal cTn values exclude myocardial necrosis in patients with increased CK of skele-
   tal muscle origin (e.g., arduous physical exercise).
Useful for diagnosis of perioperative AMI when CK-MB may be increased by skeletal
   muscle injury.

[5]For reference values for cardiac troponin and CK-MB for different instruments, see Apple F, Quist
HE, Doyle PJ, et al. Plasma 99th percentile reference limits for cardiac troponin and creatine
kinase MB mass for use with European Society of Cardiology/American College of Cardiology consensus recommendations. *Clin Chem* 2003;49:1331–1336.

May also be increased in <50% of patients with acute pericarditis.

A level <0.5 ng/mL indicates no myocardial damage; >2.0 ng/mL indicates some myocardial necrosis.

Not increased by electrical cardioversion or by pulmonary or orthopedic surgery.

In selecting heart donors, cTnT >1.6 μg/L predicts early graft failure with S/S = 73%/94%; cTnT >0.1 μg/L predicts early graft failure with S/S = 64%/>98%.

Interferences

Heterophile antibodies may cause false-positive results.

cTnT may be increased in some patients with skeletal muscle injury and myotonic dystrophy but not in third-generation assays.

cTnI is not increased by skeletal muscle injury, making it more highly specific for myocardial injury. Both may be detected in 10% to 30% of patients with chronic renal failure.

Presence of fibrin due to incomplete clot retraction can cause false-positive reactions.

♦ Serum Creatine Kinase Isoenzyme MB

Use

Increasingly replaced by cTn as gold standard for diagnosis within 24 hours of onset of symptoms.

Detect reinfarction or extension of MI after 72 hours.

Document reperfusion after thrombolytic therapy.

Interpretation

In AMI, CK-MB usually is evident at 4 to 8 hours, peaks at 15 to 24 hours (mean peak = 16× normal), with S/S >97% within the first 48 hours. By 72 hours, two-thirds of patients still show some increase in CK-MB. Sampling every 6 hours is more likely to identify a peak value. False-negative results may be caused by poor sample timing (e.g., only once in 24 hours or sampling <4 hours or >72 hours after AMI).

Diagnosis of AMI is usually confirmed by 8 to 12 hours, and sampling beyond 24 hours is usually not needed except to detect early reinfarction (especially in patients receiving thrombolytic therapy).

Diagnosis of AMI should not be based on only a single enzyme value. One criterion for AMI is serial CK-MB readings 4 hours apart that show ≥50% increase, with at least one sample greater than the upper reference value.

In ~5% of AMI patients (especially in sedentary, bedridden, or older patients), a peak CK-MB may be the only abnormality, with total CK and CK-MB still within reference ranges. This is because normal serum total CK values decline with decreased muscle mass.

Rapid return to normal makes CK-MB a poor marker >72 hours after symptoms.

Increased CK-MB with normal total CK may represent patients with nonQ wave AMI.

MB index (CK-MB/total CK) should be calculated; normal <2.5. For example, with extreme skeletal muscle injury (e.g., trauma, perioperative), total CK may be >4,000 IU/L and CK-MB may be ≤40 IU/L.

CK-MB should be reported in units as well as percentages, since if there is injury of both cardiac and skeletal muscle (e.g., perioperative AMI), the %CK-MB may not appear increased.

CK-MB mass immunoassays (preferred method) at 0, 3, and 6 hours can measure small but significant serial changes that may still be within the normal range. CK-MB mass ≥10 μg/L indicates AMI.

Thrombolytic therapy should be given within 4 to 6 hours of the acute event, at which time CK-MB may not yet be increased. CK-MB, cTn, and Myg measured initially and at 60 and/or 90 minutes after thrombolytic therapy can document *failed* reperfusion.[6]

Creatine Kinase and CK Isoenzyme MB May Also Be Increased

Diagnostic value of CK-MB and total CK are diminished after cardiac surgery. A diagnosis of AMI cannot be made until >12 to 24 hours after cardiac surgery; cTn should be used in such cases. Commonly increased after angioplasty of coronary arteries; may indicate reperfusion.

[6]Stewart JT, French JK, Theroux P, et al. Early noninvasive identification of failed reperfusion after intravenous thrombolytic therapy in acute myocardial infarction. *J Am Coll Cardiol* 1998; 31:1499–1505.

Cardiac trauma and contusions, electrical injury, and myocarditis may produce enzyme changes that cannot be distinguished from AMI. CK-MB and total CK can be increased in chronic exercise and chronic disease.

No significant increase after pacemaker implantation or electrical cardioversion.

If CK-MB >20% or persists >48 to 72 hours, consider atypical CK-MB.

Other causes of CK and CK-MB changes are noted in Chapter 3.

CK-MB in pericardial fluid may be helpful for postmortem diagnosis of AMI.

Serum Total Creatine Kinase

Use

Replaced by serum cTn, CK-MB, and Myg in various combinations

May allow early diagnosis because increased levels appear at 3 to 6 hours after onset and persists ≤48 hours

Sensitive indicator because of large amplitude of change (6 to 12× normal)

Interpretation

Serial total CK has sensitivity of 98% early in course of MI but a false-positive rate of 15% because of the many causes of increased CK.

Returns to normal by third day; a poorer prognosis is suggested if the increase lasts more than 3 to 4 days. Reinfarction is indicated by an elevated level after the fifth day that had previously returned to normal.

Useful in differential diagnosis of chest pain caused by diseases often associated with MI or difficult to distinguish from MI.

Creatine Kinase Isoforms

Methodology for rapid turnaround time is not widely available.

Interpretation

CK-MM and CK-MB isoforms parallel CK-MB but rise and peak earlier.

Diagnostic MM isoform changes are independent of amount of tissue damage. MB-2/MB-1 and MM-3/MM-1 isoform ratios appear to be the most useful.

MM-3/MM-1 ratio shows a large change because MM-1 is continually cleared from the blood. Ratio = 1.0 is useful cutoff value (~1.3 in controls but >14 in AMI). Because serum MM-3 is normally so low, its release from damaged cardiac muscle is readily evident.

MB-2 >1.0 IU/L and MB-2/MB-1 ratio >1.5 (normal ratio = 1) is specific for AMI within 4 to 8 hours of infarct. Within 2 to 4 hours, the ratio is >1.5 in >50% of patients; this ratio is reached within 4 to 6 hours in 92% of patients and by 8 hours in 100%. By 4 to 6 hours, an MB-2/MB-1 ratio ≤1.0—or a normal CK-MB by 10 hours—rules out AMI in 95% of cases.

MM-3 and the MM-3/MM-1 ratio also increase 2 hours after intense brief exercise and in marathon runners.

CK-MB subforms may also be increased in severe skeletal muscle damage (e.g., rhabdomyolysis) and muscular dystrophy.

Isoform ratios return to normal by 24 hours in most patients.

Serum Myoglobin

Myg is an oxygen-carrying respiratory protein found only in skeletal and cardiac muscle.

Use

Earliest marker for AMI.

Interpretation

Increased within 1 to 3 hours in >85% of AMI patients, peaks in about 8 to 12 hours (may peak within 1 hour) to about 10× upper reference limit and becomes normal in about 24 to 36 hours or less; reperfusion causes a peak 4 to 6 hours earlier.

May precede release of CK-MB by 2 to 5 hours.

Sensitivity >95% within 6 hours of onset of symptoms.

Myoglobinuria often occurs.

Simultaneous increase of carbonic anhydrase III shows that muscle is the origin of Myg.

Disadvantages

Blood samples should be drawn two—or times at about 1-hour intervals (Myg may be released in multiple short bursts).

There is a wide range of normal (6 to 90 ng/mL).

The test displays a low specificity for AMI (may also be increased in renal failure, shock, open heart surgery, skeletal muscle damage or exhaustive exercise, and patients and carriers of progressive muscular dystrophy, but not by cardioversion, cardiac catheterization, or CHF). Values are usually much higher in patients with uremia and muscle trauma compared to AMI.

B-type Natriuretic Peptide for Risk Stratification of ACS

C-Reactive Protein

Appears within 24 to 48 hours, peaks at 72 hours, and becomes negative after 7 days; correlates with peak CK-MB levels, but CRP peak occurs 1 to 3 days later. Failure of CRP to return to normal indicates tissue damage in the heart or elsewhere. Absence of a CRP increase raises question of a necrosis in prior 2 to 10 days. CRP is usually normal in unstable angina patients in absence of tissue necrosis who have a normal cTnT (<0.1 μg/L). CRP may remain increased for at least 3 months after AMI. Peak CRP correlates with peak CK-MB in AMI.

May also be increased in infections, inflammation, tissue injury, or necrosis.

Newer Markers Being Studied as Independent Predictors of Cardiac Risk

Ischemia-Modified Albumin, Serum[7]

Measures ischemia-modified albumin (IMA) (by binding with cobalt) in blood that occurs when blood perfuses an ischemic vascular bed.

Increases within 6 to 10 minutes of ischemia (in any site), remains increased for 2 to 4 hours, returns to baseline by 6 hours; becomes positive before cTn, CK-MB, or Myg.

High negative predictive value (NPV) ($>99\%$) makes it especially useful to use with simultaneous cTn and ECG as an aid to rule out ACS in patients presenting with chest pain; not indicated as stand-alone test.

	S/S (%/%)	NPV (%)	PPV (%)
At 80 IU/mL	100/20	100	16
At 85 IU/mL	93/23	93	17
At 100 IU/mL	64/66	82	24

May also be increased in stroke, end-stage renal disease, some neoplasms, acute infections, cirrhosis, gangrenous bowel; not increased in autoimmune disease, hypoxia, trauma, skeletal muscle ischemia.

Glycogen Phosphorylase BB

Glycogen phosphorylase BB (GPBB) is a glycolytic enzyme involved in carbohydrate metabolism.

Peaks earlier than CK-MB or cTn. More sensitive early marker for AMI and unstable angina within 4 hours after onset of pain than CK-MB, cTnT, and Myg. Returns to normal within 24 to 36 hours.

Sensitive marker of irreversible myocardial damage.

May be unreliable in presence of renal impairment or cerebral injury.

Not widely available. Additional studies are needed.

Plasma Myeloperoxidase[8]

Plasma myeloperoxidase (MPO) is an enzyme stored in granules of polymorphonuclear leukocytes (PMNs) and macrophages. It is released from WBC granules; marker of inflammation. Said to indicate atheromatous plaque instability.

Single initial increase of plasma MPO independently predicts risk of MI, of adverse cardiac events, of sudden death in next 1 and 6 months, even in the absence of ischemic necrosis (e.g., increased cTn) or increase of other inflammatory markers (e.g., CRP).

Low MPO markedly improves NPV of normal troponin in unstable angina.

[7]Anwaruddin S, Januzzi JL Jr, Baggish AL, et al. Ischemia-modified albumin improves the usefulness of standard cardiac biomarkers for the diagnosis of myocardial ischemia in the emergency department setting. *Am J Clin Pathol* 2005;123:140–145.

[8]Brennan M, Penn MS, Van Lente F, et al. Prognostic value of myeloperoxidase in patients with chest pain. *N Engl J Med* 2003;349:1595–1604.

CARDIOVASC

RBC Glutathione Peroxidase 1 Activity[9]

Decreased RBC glutathione peroxidase 1 activity is independently associated with an increased risk of adverse cardiovascular events.

Pregnancy-Associated Plasma Protein-A

Pregnancy-associated plasma protein-A (PAPP-A) is a zinc-binding matrix metalloproteinase synthesized by syncytiotrophoblast and abundantly expressed in eroded or ruptured plaques in ACS.

A reading >12.6 mIU/L is said to indicate increased risk in ACS patients.

Laboratory Markers Indicating Stages of Acute Coronary Syndrome[10]

Proinflammatory cytokines (e.g., interleukin 6, tumor necrosis factor α) $\longrightarrow$ Plaque destabilization (e.g., MPO) $\longrightarrow$ Plaque rupture (PAPP-A) $\longrightarrow$ Acute-phase reactant (e.g., CRP) $\longrightarrow$ Ischemia (e.g., IMA) $\longrightarrow$ Necrosis (cTn) $\longrightarrow$ Myocardial dysfunction (B-type natriuretic peptide [BNP])

Other Laboratory Findings

Serum AST and LD are increased; no longer used for diagnosis of AMI.
Serum ALT is usually not increased unless there is liver damage due to CHF, drug therapy, etc.
Serum alkaline phosphatase (ALP) (from vascular endothelium) is increased during the reparative phase (4 to 10 days after onset). Serum γ-glutamyltransferase is also increased.
Leukocytosis is almost invariable; it is commonly detected by second day but may occur as early as 2 hours. WBC count is usually 12,000 to 15,000; ≤20,000 is not rare, and sometimes the WBC count is very high. Usually comprises 75% to 90% PMNs, with only a slight shift to the left; is likely to develop before fever.
ESR is increased, usually by second or third day (may begin within a few hours); peak rate is in 4 to 5 days and persists for 2 to 6 months. Increased ESR may be more sensitive than WBC, as it may occur before fever and it persists after temperature and WBC have returned to normal. Degree of increase of ESR does not correlate with severity or prognosis.
Glycosuria and hyperglycemia occur in ≤50% of patients. Glucose tolerance is decreased.
Laboratory findings due to sequelae (e.g., increased BNP predicts CHF and increased risk of death because of pump failure, rupture of papillary muscle, rupture of myocardium; thromboembolism in 2% to 5% of cases).

Heart Failure, Congestive[11–14]

Caused By

Left ventricular dysfunction (ECG is the gold standard for this diagnosis)
Right ventricular dysfunction
Arrhythmias

- Metabolic abnormalities should always be ruled out prior to committing to long-term antiarrhythmic therapy, e.g., hypokalemia, hypomagnesemia, anemia, hypoxemia, hypothyroidism, or hyperthyroidism.
- Laboratory findings due to emboli to various organs.

[9]Blankenberg S, Rupprecht HJ, Bickel C, et al. Glutathione peroxidase 1 activity and cardiovascular events in patients with coronary artery disease. *N Engl J Med* 2003;349:1605.
[10]Apple FS, et al. Biomarkers for detection of ischemia and risk stratification in acute coronary syndrome. *Clin Chem* 2005;51:810. CAP Today 2005;19:1
[11]Clerico A, Emdin M. Diagnostic accuracy and prognostic relevance of the measurement of cardiac natriuretic peptides: a review. *Clin Chem* 2004;50:33–50.
[12]Wang TJ, Larson MG, Levy D, et al. Plasma natriuretic peptide levels and the risk of cardiovascular events and death. *N Engl J Med* 2004;350:655–663.
[13]Bhalla V, Lee S, Maisel AS. Biomarkers of CHF. *Advance/Laboratory* April 2004:64.
[14]Winter WE, Elin RJ. The role and assessment of ventricular peptides in heart failure. *Clin Lab Med* 2004;24:235–274.

Valve disease

Systolic heart failure (60% to 75% of cases of left ventricular dysfunction caused by loss of effective contractility)

Caused By

- Ischemic heart disease (69%)
- Hypertension (7%)
- Cardiomyopathy (13%), e.g.:

    Drugs, e.g., alcohol, cocaine, amphetamines, Herceptin (trastuzumab), anthracycline, chemotherapeutic agents

    Toxins, e.g., carbon monoxide, arsenic, lead

    Infections, e.g., viral, bacterial, rickettsial, protozoal

    Inflammation, e.g., collagen diseases, giant cell myocarditis, transplant rejection

    Metabolic, e.g., deficiencies of calcium, phosphorus, magnesium, thiamine

    Endocrinopathies, e.g., diabetes, thyroid disease, pheochromocytoma

    Systemic diseases, e.g., amyloidosis, hemochromatosis, sarcoidosis

    Valve defects (acquired, congenital)

    Inherited disorders, e.g., muscular dystrophy

Diastolic heart failure with preserved systolic function (25% to 40% of cases of left ventricular dysfunction; due to stiff, noncompliant myocardium)

Caused By

- Left ventricular hypertrophy, e.g., hypertension, aortic stenosis
- Myocardial ischemia
- Infiltrative diseases, e.g., amyloidosis—stiff myocardium does not fill normally

◆ *B-type Natriuretic Peptide, Blood*[9–12]

BNP is a hormone secreted by myocytes in the ventricles in response to pressure overload/myocyte stretch, with potent diuretic, natriuretic, and vascular smooth muscle-relaxing effects. Two commercial assays are available and are highly correlated: BNP and N-terminal (NT) proBNP. The C-terminal form is the active hormone, and the N-terminal (NT-proBNP) form is the inactive precursor; both are cleaved from proBNP; each is detected by different commercial assays.

Use

Aids in screening and diagnosis of CHF; enhances clinical diagnostic accuracy. High NPV (>95%) makes it a very useful rule-out test.

Differential diagnosis of dyspnea (e.g., chronic obstructive pulmonary disease).

Determination of severity: Higher values correlate closely with increasing N.Y. Heart Association classes I to IV. Prognostic tool for classes III and IV.

Risk stratification and prognosis: increased levels, even within "normal range" (>20 pg/mL in men; >23 pg/mL in women), predict risk of death and cardiac events (e.g., CHF, auricular fibrillation, stroke) but not coronary events. Significant correlation between BNP levels and low, intermediate, or high risk.

Diagnosis of left ventricular dysfunction.

Monitoring effectiveness of drug therapy, e.g., angiotensin-converting enzyme inhibitors, β-blockers.

Screening patients with risk factors, e.g., ischemic heart disease.

Interpretation

Both assays are dependent on age and gender.

- Recommended cutoff values (values are not interchangeable): BNP: 80 to 100 pg/mL; NT-proBNP: 125 pg/mL for age <75, 450 pg/mL for age >75.
- At appropriate cutoff values, BNP and NT-proBNP have similar S/S = 70%/70% and NPV = 80%.
- Reading <100 pg/mL rules out CHF as cause of dyspnea.
- Reading >400 pg/mL indicates 95% likelihood of CHF.
- Reading between 100 and 400 pg/mL warrants further workup.
- Greater increases predict worse adverse outcomes in patients with CHF.
- Increase values after AMI predict poorer prognosis.
- Increase in BNP in right heart failure is less than in left ventricular dysfunction.
- BNP increases with arrhythmias that are less marked.
- BNP and NT-proBNP can be increased in renal failure, especially if dialysis is needed.

CARDIOVASC

- Reading >480 pg/mL = 51% chance of cardiac/noncardiac events in next 6 months.
- Reading <230 pg/mL = 2.5% chance of cardiac/noncardiac events in next 6 months.
- Reading >130 pg/mL = 19% chance of sudden death.
- Reading <130 pg/mL = 1% chance of sudden death.
- Abnormal echocardiogram without symptoms: mean value = ~300 pg/mL.
- With rapid test in ER, reading >100 pg/mL makes a diagnosis of CHF regardless of age, gender, or race. *Much more data are needed.*

Not Increased In
Chronic obstructive pulmonary disease
Hypertension
Diabetes mellitus
Renal insufficiency
Renal changes:

- Slight albuminuria (<1 g/d) is common.
- Isolated RBCs and WBCs, hyaline, and (sometimes) granular casts.
- Urine is concentrated, with specific gravity >1.020.
- Moderate azotemia (blood urea nitrogen [BUN] usually <60 mg/dL) is evident with severe oliguria; may increase with vigorous diuresis. *(Primary renal disease is indicated by proportionate increase in serum creatinine and low specific gravity of urine, despite oliguria.)*
- Oliguria is a characteristic feature of right-sided failure.

ESR may be decreased because of decreased serum fibrinogen.
Serum albumin and total protein are decreased.
Liver function changes.
Laboratory findings due to underlying disease, e.g., rheumatic fever, viral myocarditis, infective endocarditis, chronic severe anemia, hypertension, hyperthyroidism.

Hypertension

Hypertension is present in 18% of adults in the United States.
Systolic hypertension

- Hyperthyroidism
- Chronic anemia with Hb <7 g/dL
- Arteriovenous fistulas—advanced Paget disease of bone; pulmonary arteriovenous varix
- Beriberi

Diastolic hypertension

- Hypothyroidism

Systolic and diastolic hypertension

- Essential (primary) hypertension
- Secondary hypertension

Caused By
Primary hypertension causes >90% of cases of hypertension.
Secondary hypertension causes <10% of cases of hypertension.

- Endocrine diseases
  Adrenal, e.g., pheochromocytoma, aldosteronism, Cushing syndrome, congenital adrenal hyperplasia
  Pituitary disease, e.g., acromegaly
  Hyperthyroidism, hyperparathyroidism, etc.
- Renal diseases (see Fig. 14-5)
  Vascular (4% of cases of hypertension), e.g., renal artery stenosis, nephrosclerosis, embolism
  Parenchymal, e.g., glomerulonephritis, pyelonephritis, polycystic kidneys, amyloidosis, Kimmelstiel-Wilson syndrome, collagen diseases, renin-producing renal tumor, urinary tract obstructions

- Central nervous system diseases, e.g., cerebrovascular accident, brain tumors, poliomyelitis
- Other, e.g., toxemia of pregnancy, polycythemia, acute porphyria
- Drugs, e.g., oral contraceptives, tricyclic antidepressants, licorice
- Toxic substances, e.g., poisoning by lead or cadmium

In children <18 years of age, caused by:

Renal disease	61%–78%
Cardiovascular disease (e.g., coarctation of aorta)	13%–15%
Endocrine (e.g., mineralocorticoid excess, pheochromocytoma, hyperthyroidism, hypercalcemia)	6%–9%
Miscellaneous (e.g., induced by traction, after genitourinary tract surgery, associated with sleep apnea)	2%–7%
Essential	1%–16%

Laboratory findings due to the underlying disease. These conditions are often unsuspected and should always be ruled out, since many of them represent curable causes of hypertension.

Laboratory tests to indicate the functional renal status (e.g., microalbuminuria, BUN, creatinine, uric acid). The higher the uric acid in uncomplicated essential hypertension, the lower the renal blood flow.

Laboratory findings due to complications of hypertension (e.g., CHF, uremia, stroke, MI).

Laboratory findings due to administration of some antihypertensive drugs, e.g.:

- Oral diuretics (e.g., benzothiadiazines): hyperuricemia, hypokalemia, or hyperglycemia or aggravation of preexisting diabetes mellitus; less commonly, bone marrow depression, aggravation of renal or hepatic insufficiency, cholestatic hepatitis, or toxic pancreatitis.
- Hydralazine: Syndrome may not be distinguishable from systemic lupus erythematosus (SLE). Antinuclear antibody may be found in ≤50% of asymptomatic patients.
- Methyldopa: ≤20% of patients may have positive direct Coombs test, but relatively few have hemolytic anemia. When drug is discontinued, Coombs test may remain positive for months, but anemia usually reverses promptly. Abnormal liver function tests indicate hepatocellular damage without jaundice. RF and SLE tests may occasionally be positive (see Chapter 17).
- Monoamine oxidase inhibitors (e.g., pargyline hydrochloride); wide range of toxic reactions, most serious of which are blood dyscrasias and hepatocellular necrosis.
- Diazoxide: Sodium and fluid retention, hyperglycemia.

When hypertension is associated with decreased serum potassium, rule out:

- Primary aldosteronism
- Pseudoaldosteronism (caused by excessive ingestion of licorice)
- Secondary aldosteronism, e.g., malignant hypertension
- Hypokalemia caused by diuretic administration
- Potassium loss caused by renal disease
- Cushing syndrome

Myocardial Trauma

Caused By

May be penetrating (e.g., bullet or stab wound) or nonpenetrating (usually, motor vehicle accident). May be associated with coronary dissection, laceration, or thrombosis or rupture of aorta.

♦ Increased serum CK-MB (>3%) alone in 15% of cases; combined with ECG changes in 20% of cases; ECG changes alone in 65% of cases.

♦ Increased serum cTnI implies some myocardial necrosis and differentiates increased CK-MB caused by skeletal muscle damage. S/S = 90%/30%; PPV is only 16%. cTnT may be increased due to muscle necrosis (not in third-generation assay).

CARDIOVASC

Myocarditis[15]

Caused By

Infections

Viruses, e.g., Coxsackie B (responsible for most cases in United States) and A, echovirus, poliomyelitis, influenza A and B, cytomegalovirus, Epstein-Barr, adenovirus, rubeola, mumps, rubella, variola, vaccinia, varicella zoster, rabies, lymphocytic choriomeningitis, chikungunya, dengue, yellow fever, HIV

Chlamydia, e.g., *C. psittaci*

Rickettsia, e.g., *R. typhi*

Bacteria, e.g., diphtheria, meningococcus, Lyme disease

Fungi, e.g., *Candida*

Protozoa (trypanosomiasis [Chagas disease], toxoplasmosis)

Helminths, e.g., trichinosis

Immune-mediated, e.g., postviral, rheumatic fever, SLE, drugs (methyldopa, sulfonamides), transplant rejection

Unknown, e.g., sarcoidosis, giant cell myocarditis

◆ Endomyocardial biopsy of right ventricular muscle remains the gold standard, despite limited S/S, to establish diagnosis of infectious myocarditis and other lesions (e.g., sarcoidosis).

◆ Serologic tests for antigens, IgM antibody, or changed titer using acute and convalescent paired sera.

○ Increased serum markers of myocardial damage are common only in early stages.

- cTn S/S = 53%/93%
- CK-MB and CK-total <10% sensitivity

Increased acute-phase reactants (e.g., ESR, CRP, mild to moderate leukocytosis)

Shock

Shock is a syndrome of failure of circulation to maintain cellular perfusion and function due to cardiac, hypovolemic, toxic/infectious, or other causes.

Leukocytosis is common, especially with hemorrhage. There may be leukopenia when shock is severe, as in Gram-negative bacteremia. Circulating eosinophils are decreased.

Hemoconcentration (e.g., dehydration, burns) or hemodilution (e.g., hemorrhage, crush injuries, and skeletal trauma) takes place.

Blood pH is usually relatively normal but may be decreased.

BUN and creatinine may be increased.

Acidosis appears when shock is well developed, with increased blood lactate, low serum sodium, low CO_2-combining power with decreased alkaline reserve.

Hypoxemia.

Serum potassium may be increased.

Hyperglycemia occurs early.

Urine examination:

Volume: Normovolemic patients have output $\geq$50 mL/hour; should investigate cause if <25 to 30 mL/hour. In hypovolemia, the normal kidney may lower 24-hour urine output to 300 to 400 mL.

Specific gravity: >1.020 with low urine output suggests that the patient is fluid-depleted. Specific gravity <1.010 with low urine output suggests renal insufficiency. Specific gravity depends on weight rather than concentration of solutes; therefore it is more affected than osmolarity by high-molecular-weight substances such as urea, albumin, and glucose.

Osmolarity: Hypovolemia is suggested by high urine osmolarity and urine:plasma osmolarity ratio 1:2. Renal failure is suggested by low urine osmolarity with oliguria and urine:plasma osmolarity ratio 1:1.

Laboratory findings due to complications or sequelae (e.g., acute respiratory distress syndrome, disseminated intravascular coagulation, acute renal failure).

---

[15]Leeper NJ, Wener LS, Dhaliwal G, et al. Clinical problem-solving. One surprise after another. *N Engl J Med* 2005;352:1474–1479.

Systemic Capillary Leak Syndrome[16]

Systemic capillary leak syndrome is a very rare recurring idiopathic disorder in adults with sudden transient extravasation of ≤70% of plasma. It displays a very high morbidity and mortality; hypotension is part of the triad.

Hemoconcentration (e.g., leukocytosis; Hb may be ~25 g/dL).
Hypoalbuminemia.
Monoclonal gammopathy (especially IgG with κ or λ light chain) without evidence of multiple myeloma) is often present. Some patients may progress to multiple myeloma.
Laboratory findings due to complications, e.g., rhabdomyolysis, acute tubular necrosis, pleural/pericardial effusion.

Diseases Principally of Pericardium

Pericarditis, Acute, and Pericardial Effusion[17]

Acute pericarditis and pericardial effusion may cause abnormal diastolic filling.
See Table 6-2 on body fluids.

Laboratory Findings Caused by Underlying Disease

Active rheumatic fever (40% of patients)
Bacterial infection (20% of patients; e.g., tuberculosis, *Streptococcus pneumoniae*, staphylococci, Gram-negative bacilli)
Other infections (e.g., viral [especially Coxsackie B], rickettsial, parasites, mycobacteria, fungi); viruses are most common infectious causes
Uremia (11% of patients)
Benign nonspecific pericarditis (10% of patients)
Neoplasms (3.5% of patients)
Collagen disease (e.g., SLE) (2% of patients)
AMI, postcardiac injury syndrome
Trauma
Myxedema
Others, e.g., hypersensitivity
Rarely caused by severe anemia, scleroderma, polyarteritis nodosa, Wegener granulomatosis, rheumatoid arthritis, radiation, mycotic infections, endomyocardial fibrosis of Africa, idiopathic causes
WBC is usually increased in proportion to fever; normal or low in viral disease and tubercular pericarditis; markedly increased in suppurative bacterial pericarditis
Examination of aspirated pericardial fluid, e.g., serologic tests for infectious agents, collagen diseases, cultures for infectious agents, cytology, etc. (see Table 6-1)

Valvular Heart Disease

Laboratory findings due to associated or underlying or predisposing disease, e.g., syphilis, rheumatic fever, carcinoid syndrome, genetic disease of mucopolysaccharide metabolism, congenital defects
Laboratory findings due to complications, e.g., heart failure, infective endocarditis, embolic phenomena

Endocarditis, Infective[18–23]

Infective endocarditis (IE) is a noncontagious infection of the heart valves or lining. It may be acute or subacute.

[16]Tahirkheli NK, Greipp PR. Treatment of the systemic capillary leak syndrome with terbutaline and theophylline. *Ann Intern Med* 1999;130:905–909.
[17]Levy PY, Cory R, Berger P, et al. Etiologic diagnosis of 204 pericardial effusions. *Medicine* 2003; 82:385–391.
[18]Mylonakis E, Calderwood, SB. Infective endocarditis in adults. *N Engl J Med* 2001;345:1318–1330.
[19]Werner M, Andersson R, Oliason L, et al. Clinical study of culture-negative endocarditis. *Medicine* 2003;82:263–273.
[20]Podglajen I, Bellery F, Poyart C, et al. Comparative molecular and microbiologic diagnosis of bacterial endocarditis. *Emerg Infect Dis* 2003;9:1543–1547.
[21]Moreillon P, Que Y-A. Infective endocarditis. *Lancet* 2004;363:139–149.
[22]Millar BC, Moore JE. Emerging issues in infective endocarditis. *Emerg Infect Dis* 2004;10:1110–1116.
[23]Houpikian P, Raoult D. Blood culture-negative endocarditis in a reference center. etiologic diagnosis of 348 cases. *Medicine* 2005;84:162–173.

CARDIOVASC

See following section, "Prosthetic Heart Valves."

♦ Diagnostic Criteria

Definite: (1) two major criteria, (2) one major plus three minor criteria, (3) five minor criteria, or (4) pathologic findings (vegetation or intracardiac abscess confirmed histologically showing active endocarditis).

Possible: one major and one minor or three minor criteria.

Rejected: Alternate diagnosis or resolution of IE with antibiotic therapy ≤ 4 days or no pathologic evidence after antibiotic therapy.

Major Criteria

* Typical organism (*Streptococcus viridans* [~50% of cases], *S. bovis, Staphylococcus aureus,* HACEK [*Haemophilus, Actinobacillus, Cardiobacterium, Eikenella, Kingella*], enterococci) in ≥2 blood cultures in absence of primary focus, or persistently positive blood cultures drawn >1 hour apart
* Involvement of endocardium by echocardiogram or valve regurgitation
* Positive serology for *Coxiella burnetii* (IgG >1:800)
* Bacterial or fungal DNA in blood or valve (including *Bartonella* sp., *Tropheryma whipplei,* other new or unusual organisms)
* *S. aureus* bacteremia, even if nosocomial or removable source of infection is present
* Positive echocardiogram (e.g., oscillating intracardiac mass)

Minor Criteria

* Risk factors: predisposing heart condition or intravenous (IV) drug abuse
* Fever >38°C (100.4°F)
* Vascular phenomena: septic pulmonary infarcts, major arterial emboli, Janeway lesions (not petechiae or splinter hemorrhages)
* Immunologic phenomena: Osler nodes, Roth spots, RF, glomerulonephritis
* Microbiologic evidence: positive blood culture other than major criteria or positive serologic findings (*Bartonella* sp. or *Chlamydia* sp.)
* Clinical: newly diagnosed clubbing or splinter hemorrhages or petechiae or purpura or microscopic hematuria (ruled out bacteriuria, menstruation, urinary catheters, end-stage renal disease) or presence of central nonfeeding venous lines or peripheral venous line (minor)
* Biochemical: CRP >100 mg/L or ESR >30 mm/h if <60 years old or >50 mm/h if >60 years old
* ECG consistent with IE but not meeting major criteria

Risk Factors

* Preexisting valve disease (e.g., rheumatic) and congenital heart diseases
* Nosocomial: most are caused by enterococci and staphylococci. Case fatality >50%:
  —Prosthetic valves (≤5% of IE)
  —Catheters, medicosurgical procedures
  —Bone marrow transplants (5% of IE) and other immunocompromised patients
  —IV lines; S. aureus is common in patients with central venous catheters, parenteral lines for feeding or chemotherapy
  —Hemodialysis patients: >50% are caused by *S. aureus*
* *S. bovis* in patients with colon cancer causes 20% of cases
* *Enterococcus faecalis* in patients: genitourinary procedures, pelvic infections, prostate disease

♦ Blood culture is positive in 80% to 90% of patients:

* *Streptococcus viridans* causes 40% to 50% of cases
* *Staphylococcus aureus* (from skin sites) ≤30% of cases
* *Streptococcus pneumoniae* 5% of cases
* *Enterococcus* (from gastrointestinal tract) 5% to 10% of cases
* Other causes may be Gram-negative bacteria (~10% of cases—e.g., *Escherichia coli, Pseudomonas aeruginosa, Klebsiella, Proteus*) and fungi (e.g., *Candida, Histoplasma, Cryptococcus*)
* *Bartonella* has been reported to cause 3% of cases, which may be culture-negative.

- HACEK organisms cause ≤10% of cases

♦ In IV drug users, *S. aureus* causes 50% to 60% of cases and ~80% of tricuspid infections and have no preexisting valve disease. Gram-negative bacteria cause 10% to 15% of cases; polymicrobial and unusual organisms appear to be increasing. Seventy-five percent or fewer patients may be HIV positive.

♦ *Proper blood cultures require adequate volume of blood, at least five cultures taken during a period of several days with temperature 101°F or higher (preferably when highest), anaerobic as well as aerobic growth, variety of enriched media, prompt incubation, and prolonged observation (growth is usual in 1 to 4 days but may require 2 to 3 weeks).*

- Beware of negative culture due to recent antibiotic therapy.
- Beware of transient bacteremia following dental procedures, tonsillectomy, etc., which do not represent bacterial endocarditis (in these cases, streptococci usually grow only in fluid media; in bacterial endocarditis, many colonies also occur on solid media).
- Positive cultures may be more difficult to obtain in right-sided endocarditis, uremia, long-standing endocarditis, and prosthetic valve endocarditis, or the presence of unusual and fastidious organisms.
- A single positive culture must be interpreted with extreme caution.
- Blood cultures remain negative in ~10% of cases (Table 5-7). When routine blood cultures are negative, special techniques may be needed to identify some organisms.
- Aside from the exceptions noted in this paragraph, the diagnosis should be based on ≥2 cultures that are positive for the same organism.

♦ DNA of organisms in blood, excised vegetations, or systemic emboli or immunohistology

Serum bactericidal test measures the ability of serial dilutions of patient's serum to sterilize a standardized inoculum of the infecting organisms; it is sometimes useful to demonstrate inadequate antibiotic levels or to avoid unnecessary drug toxicity.

Progressive normochromic normocytic anemia is a characteristic feature; in 10% of patients, Hb <7 g/dL. Rarely, there is a hemolytic anemia with a positive Coombs test. Serum iron is decreased. Bone marrow contains abundant hemosiderin.

WBC count is normal in ~50% of patients and elevated ≤15,000/μL in the rest, with 65% to 86% neutrophils. A higher WBC count indicates presence of a complication

Table 5-7.	Diagnostic Procedures for Unusual Organisms That May Cause Negative Blood Cultures						
				Excised Specimen			
	Blood culture	Serology	Antigen	Culture	PCR	Immuno-histology	Histology
Brucella sp.	+	+		+	+	+	
Coxiella burnetii	+	+		+	+	+	
Bartonella sp.	+	+		+	+	+	
Chlamydia sp.				+	+	+	
Mycoplasma sp.		+		+	+	+	
Legionella sp.	+	+		+	+	+	
Tropheryma whippelii				+			+
Histoplasma capsulatum			In urine				
Cryptococcus neoformans			In serum				
Candida albicans	+			+			+

PCR, polymerase chain reaction.

(e.g., cerebral, pulmonary). Occasionally there is leukopenia. Monocytosis may be pronounced. Large macrophages may occur in peripheral blood.
Platelet count is usually normal, but occasionally it is decreased; rarely, purpura occurs.
Serum proteins are altered, with an increase in γ globulin; therefore positive ESR, cryoglobulins, RF, etc., are found. There is often a direct correlation between ESR and the course and severity of disease.
Hematuria (usually microscopic) occurs at some stage in many patients due to glomerulitis or renal infarct or focal embolic or diffuse GN.
Albuminuria is almost invariable, even without these complications. Renal insufficiency with azotemia and fixed specific gravity is infrequent now. Nephrotic syndrome is rare.
Cerebrospinal fluid (CSF) findings in various complications, meningitis, brain abscess.
Laboratory findings due to underlying or predisposing diseases or complications, e.g., mitral valve prolapse, rheumatic valve disease, congenital heart disease, nosocomial infections (gastrointestinal or genitourinary systems, long-term indwelling IV catheters especially in HIV patients), mycotic aneurysms.

Prosthetic Heart Valves

Complications
Hemolysis: increased serum LD, decreased haptoglobin, reticulocytosis is usual. Severe hemolytic anemia is uncommon and suggests leakage caused by partial dehiscence of valve or infection.
Prosthetic valve infection occurs in ≤4% of patients with prosthetic valves.
Early (<60 days after valve replacement). Usually caused by *S. epidermidis*, *S. aureus*; also gram-negative bacteria, diphtheroids, fungi; occasionally caused by *Mycobacteria* and *Legionella*; 30% to 80% mortality.
Late (>60 days postoperatively). Usually caused by streptococci. *S. epidermidis* is common up to 12 months after surgery; 20% to 40% mortality.
♦ Blood culture positive in >90% of patients unless they received antibiotic therapy or a fastidious organism is present (e.g., HACEK, which are Gram-negative, nonenteric organisms) or require special technique (e.g., rickettsia, fungi, mycobacteria, legionella). Surgery is indicated if blood culture is still positive after 5 days of appropriate antimicrobial therapy or recurrent infection. Infection with organisms other than *Streptococcus* usually requires valve replacement.
Complications of anticoagulant therapy.
Valve dysfunction.

Rheumatic Heart Disease, Chronic

Late sequel of acute rheumatic fever
Valve distortion causing stenosis or insufficiency that may ultimately cause CHF
Valve susceptible to nonbacterial thrombotic endocarditis, resulting in emboli
Valve susceptible to infective endocarditis
Embolization from thrombi in atria or appendages, especially with auricular fibrillation:

70% of emboli lodge in arteries of lower limbs
13% of emboli lodge in arteries of upper limbs
5% to 10% of emboli lodge in arteries of viscera, e.g., kidney, spleen, brain, bowel

Laboratory findings due to CHF

Syphilitic Aortitis and Aortic Valve Regurgitation

Syphilitic aortitis is an obliterative endarteritis of vasa vasorum of thoracic aorta that can lead to aneurysm formation.

Aortitis is the most common expression of late syphilis.
Changes are caused by coronary ostial stenosis (which occurs in >25% of cases) and MI.
♦ A positive treponemal test is seen in ~90% of cases.

Vasculitis

Vasculitis, Classification

Classification by Etiology
Primary
  Polyarteritis nodosa
  Wegener granulomatosis
  Giant cell arteritis
  Hypersensitivity vasculitis
Secondary
  Infections: Bacteria (e.g., septicemia caused by *Gonococcus* or *Staphylococcus*),
    mycobacteria, viruses (e.g., cytomegalovirus, hepatitis B), rickettsia (e.g., Rocky
    Mountain spotted fever), spirochetes (e.g., syphilis, Lyme disease)
  Associated with malignancy, e.g., multiple myeloma, lymphomas
  Connective tissue diseases, e.g., RA, SLE, Sjögren syndrome
  Diseases that may simulate vasculitis, e.g., ergotamine toxicity, cholesterol emboliza-
    tion, atrial myxoma

Classification of Noninfectious Vasculitis by Size of Involved Vessel
Large Vessel:
Dissection of aorta (dissecting aneurysm)
Takayasu arteritis
Giant cell (temporal) arteritis
Medium-sized Vessel:
Polyarteritis nodosa (or small)
Kawasaki disease
Primary granulomatous central nervous system (CNS) vasculitis
Small Vessel:
Antineutrophil cytoplasmic antibodies (ANCA)–associated vasculitis (Wegener granu-
  lomatosis, Churg-Strauss syndrome, drug-induced, microscopic polyangiitis)
Immune complex-type vasculitis (Henoch-Schönlein purpura, cryoglobulinemia,
  rheumatoid vasculitis [or medium], SLE, Sjögren syndrome, Goodpasture syndrome,
  Behçet syndrome, drug-induced, serum sickness)
Paraneoplastic vasculitis (lymphoproliferative, myeloproliferative, carcinoma)
Inflammatory bowel disease
Any Size Vessel (Pseudovasculitis):
Antiphospholipid syndrome
Emboli, e.g., myxomas, cholesterol emboli, bacterial or nonbacterial endocarditis
Drugs, e.g., amphetamines

Behçet Syndrome
**Behçet syndrome is a systemic vasculitis involving arteries and veins characterized
by a triad of recurrent aphthous ulcers of mouth and genitalia, and relapsing
panuveitis.**

No definitive laboratory tests are available.
Laboratory findings due to involvement of various organ systems, e.g.:
  Large vessel occlusion, e.g., aneurysms, arthritis, meningitis
  Skin lesions

Churg-Strauss Syndrome (Allergic Granulomatosis and Angiitis)
**Churg-Strauss syndrome is a granulomatous necrotizing vasculitis involving the
respiratory tract. It resembles polyarteritis nodosa, but with involvement of the
pulmonary arteries.**

◆ A biopsy showing granulocytes around an arteriole and venule establishes the diagnosis.[24]
Increased WBC count and ESR are present in 80% of cases.

[24]Included in Hunder GG, Arend WP, Bloch DA, et al. American College of Rheumatology 1990
Criteria for Classification of Vasculitis. Introduction. *Arthritis Rheum* 1990;33:1065–1067.

CARDIOVASC

○ Eosinophilia (>10% or >1,500/mL^3) is present in ~90% of cases and seems to correlate with disease activity.
Enzyme-linked immunosorbent assay (ELISA) for antimyeloperoxidase specificity is usually positive.
Serum IgE is often increased.
p-ANCA is found in ≤60% of patients; c-ANCA is rarely present.
Laboratory findings due to associated asthma.

Dissection of Aorta (Dissecting Aneurysm)[25]

Dissection of the aorta is caused by cystic medial degeneration or unknown causes.
◆ Rapid electroimmunoassay of smooth-muscle myosin heavy-chain protein >2.5 µg/L is reported to have S/S >90%/98% during first 3 hours and rapidly decreases thereafter. Higher values for proximal than distal dissection.
Laboratory changes due to complications/sequelae (e.g., rupture or infarcts of brain, kidney, gut, limbs) or of predisposing conditions (e.g., Marfan syndrome, hypertension, arterial cannulation, unknown).

Giant Cell (Temporal) Arteritis[26–28]

Giant cell arteritis (GCA) is a systemic panarteritis of the large and medium arteries, especially the carotid arteries. It typically affects the extracranial rather than the intracranial arteries.

◆ Biopsy of the involved segment of temporal artery is diagnostic,[29] but a negative biopsy does not exclude GCA because of skip lesions. Therefore, the surgeon should remove at least 20 mm of artery, paraffin sections of which must be examined at multiple levels. Biopsy findings remain positive for at least 7 to 14 days after onset of therapy. Biopsy is negative in ~50% of cases with GCA of subclavian or axillary arteries.
○ The classic triad of increased ESR (≥50 mm/h),[27] anemia, and increased serum ALP is strongly suggestive of GCA.
    ESR is markedly increased in ~80% of patients; average Westergren = 107. A normal ESR excludes the diagnosis when there is little clinical evidence for temporal arteritis.
    CRP is more sensitive than ESR.
    Mild to moderate normocytic normochromic anemia is present in 20% to 50% of cases and is a rough indicator of degree of inflammation.
The WBC count is usually normal or slightly increased with shift to the left.
Platelet counts may be increased nonspecifically.
Serum protein electrophoresis may show increased γ globulins. Rouleaux may occur.
Serum CK is normal.
Laboratory findings reflecting specific organ involvement:
    Kidney (e.g., GN)
    CNS, e.g., intracerebral artery involvement may cause increased CSF protein, stroke, mononeuritis of brachial plexus
    Heart and great vessels, e.g., myocardial infarction, aortic dissection, Raynaud disease
    Mildly increased AST and ALP in 20% to 35% of patients
    Syndrome of inappropriate antidiuretic hormone secretion (SIADH)
    Microangiopathic hemolytic anemia
40% of patients with GCA have polymyalgia rheumatica, and 10% of patients with isolated polymyalgia rheumatica have histologic evidence of vasculitis.

[25]Suzuki T, Katoh H, Tsuchio Y, et al. Diagnostic implications of elevated levels of smooth-muscle myosin heavy-chain protein in acute aortic dissection. The smooth muscle myosin heavy chain study. *Ann Intern Med* 2000;133:537–541.
[26]Salvarani C, Cantini F, Boiardi L, et al. Polymyalgia rheumatica and giant-cell arteritis. *N Engl J Med* 2002;347:261–271.
[27]Weyand CM, Goronzy JJ. Giant cell arteritis and polymyalgia rheumatica. *Ann Intern Med* 2003;139:505–515.
[28]Weyand CM, Goronzy JJ. Medium- and large-vessel vasculitis. *N Engl J Med* 2003;349:160–169.
[29]Included in Hunder GG, Arend WP, Bloch DA, et al. American College of Rheumatology 1990 criteria for classification of vasculitis. Introduction. *Arthritis Rheum* 1990;33:1065–1067.

Henoch-Schönlein Purpura[30]

Henoch-Schönlein purpura is a hypersensitivity systemic vasculitis of the small vessels with IgA deposition. It is called Henoch purpura when abdominal symptoms are predominant and Schönlein purpura when joint symptoms are predominant.

See Chapter 14.

Diagnosis is made clinically; there are no pathognomonic laboratory findings. Coagulation tests are normal.

♦ Renal or skin biopsy supports the diagnosis; it will show focal segmental necrotizing GN that becomes more diffuse and crescentic with IgA and C3 deposition.

The urine contains RBCs, casts, and slight protein in 25% to 50% of patients. Gross hematuria and proteinuria are uncommon.

The renal picture varies from minimal urinary abnormalities for years to end-stage renal disease within months.

BUN and creatinine may be increased.

In nonthrombocytopenic purpura, hematologic tests are normal and the serum complement is usually normal.

Kawasaki Syndrome (Mucocutaneous Lymph Node Syndrome)

Kawasaki syndrome is a variant of childhood polyarteritis of unknown etiology, with a high incidence of coronary artery complications. Diagnosis is based on clinical criteria.

♦ Diagnosis is confirmed by histologic examination of the coronary artery (same as polyarteritis nodosa).

♦ Laboratory changes due to AMI.

Acute-phase reactants are increased (e.g., ESR. CRP, α-1-antitrypsin); these usually return to normal after 6 to 8 weeks.

Leukocytosis (20,000 to 30,000/μL) with shift to left occurs during first week; lymphocytosis appears thereafter, peaking at the end of the second week, and is a hallmark of this illness.

Anemia occurs in ~50% of patients, reaches nadir about the end of the second week, and improves during recovery.

CSF shows increased mononuclear cells with normal protein and sugar.

Increased mononuclear cells in urine; dipstick negative.

Increased WBC (predominantly PMNs) in joint fluid in patients with arthritis.

Polyarteritis Nodosa

Polyarteritis nodosa (PN) is a systemic necrotizing vasculitis of the medium and small arteries causing thrombosis, infarction, aneurysm, and rupture. There is no vasculitis in the arterioles, capillaries, or venules. PN causes renal and visceral involvement in but lungs are not involved.

♦ Tissue biopsy is the basis for diagnosis.

Findings are performed on a biopsy of a small or medium artery.

Findings in random skin and muscle biopsy are confirmatory in 25% of patients; they are most useful when taken from an area of tenderness; if no symptoms are present, the pectoralis major is the most useful site.

Testicular biopsy is useful when local symptoms are present.

Lymph node and liver biopsies are usually not helpful.

Renal biopsy is not specific; 30% have glomerulitis and 70% have vasculitis.

Increased BUN or creatinine; uremia occurs in 15% of patients.

○ Hepatitis B surface antigen is present in ≤20% of adult patients who usually have decreased serum complement.

○ p-ANCA is positive in 70% of patients; this rarely reflects disease activity.

○ Increased WBC count (≤40,000/μL) and PMNs are seen in >75% of cases. Increased eosinophils are found in 25% of patients, sometimes very marked; this usually occurs in patients with pulmonary manifestations.

[30]Calviño MC, Llorca J, Garcia-Porrua C, et al. Henoch-Schönlein purpura in children from northwestern Spain. *Medicine (Baltimore)* 2001;80:279–290.

CARDIOVASC

ESR and CRP are increased.

Mild anemia is frequent; may be hemolytic anemia with positive Coombs test.

Urine is frequently abnormal:

Albuminuria (60% of patients)
Hematuria (40% of patients)
"Telescoping" of sediment (variety of cellular and noncellular casts)

Abnormal serum proteins may occur (e.g., increased globulins, biologic false-positive test for syphilis, circulating anticoagulants, cryoglobulins, macroglobulins).

Laboratory findings because of organ involvement by arteritis may be present—e.g., cardiac, gastrointestinal, renal, neurologic in >75% of patients. Pulmonary arteries are *not* involved.

Takayasu Syndrome (Arteritis)

Takayasu syndrome is the term for granulomatous arteritis of the aorta.

◆ Diagnosis is established by characteristic arteriographic changes or histologic examination.

Increased ESR is found in ~75% of cases during active disease but is normal in only 50% of cases during remission.

WBC count is usually normal.

Serum proteins are abnormal, with increased γ globulins (mostly composed of IgM).

Female patients have a continuous high level of urinary total estrogens (rather than the usual rise during the luteal phase after a low excretion during follicular phase).

Laboratory findings due to involvement of coronary or renal vessels.

Laboratory tests are not useful for diagnosis or to guide management.

Thromboangiitis Obliterans (Buerger Disease)

Thromboangiitis obliterans is the vascular inflammation and occlusion of medium and small arteries and veins of limbs; it is related to smoking.

Laboratory tests are usually normal.

◆ Histology shows characteristic inflammatory and proliferative lesions.

Thrombophlebitis, Septic

Laboratory findings due to associated septicemia

- Increased WBC count (often >20,000/μL), with marked shift to left and toxic changes in neutrophils
- Disseminated intravascular coagulation may be present.
- Respiratory alkalosis occurs due to ventilation-perfusion abnormalities with hypoxia. Significant acidosis indicates shock.
- Azotemia.
- Positive blood culture (*S. aureus* is most frequent organism; others are *Klebsiella, Pseudomonas aeruginosa*, enterococci, *Candida*).

Laboratory findings due to complications, e.g., septic pulmonary infarction

Laboratory findings due to underlying disease

Wegener Granulomatosis[31]

Wegener granulomatosis (WG) is a rare autoimmune systemic necrotizing or granulomatous vasculitis most often affecting the respiratory tract and kidneys.

See Chapter 14.

◆ Diagnosis is established by biopsy of affected tissue with cultures and special stains that exclude mycobacterial and fungal infection together with antimyeloperoxidase antibodies.

---

[31]Included in Hunder GG, Arend WP, Bloch DA, et al. American College of Rheumatology 1990 Criteria for Classification of Vasculitis. Introduction. *Arthritis Rheum* 1990;33:1065–1067.

Antineutrophil Cytoplasmic Antibodies

Use

Aids in diagnosis and classification of various vasculitis-associated and autoimmune disorders.

Interpretation

♦ c-ANCA (anti-proteinase 3; coarse diffuse cytoplasmic pattern) is highly specific (>90%) for active WG. Sensitivity is >90% in systemic vasculitic phase, ~65% in predominantly granulomatous disease of respiratory tract, and ~30% during complete remission. Height of ELISA titer does not correlate with disease activity; a high titer may persist during remission for years. c-ANCA is also occasionally found in other vasculitides (polyarteritis nodosa, microscopic polyangiitis [e.g., lung, idiopathic crescentic and pauci-immune GN], Churg-Strauss vasculitis).

p-ANCA (against various proteins, e.g., myeloperoxidase, elastase, lysozyme; perinuclear pattern) occurs only with fixation in alcohol, not formalin. A positive result should be confirmed by ELISA. The test has poor specificity and 20% to 60% sensitivity in a variety of autoimmune diseases (microscopic polyangiitis, Churg-Strauss vasculitis, SLE, inflammatory bowel disease, Goodpasture syndrome, Sjögren syndrome, idiopathic GN, chronic infection). However, pulmonary small vessel vasculitis is strongly linked with myeloperoxidase antibodies.

Both p-ANCA and c-ANCA may be found in non–immune-mediated polyarteritis and other vasculitides.

Atypical pattern (neither c-ANCA or p-ANCA; unknown target antigens) has poor specificity and unknown sensitivity in various conditions, e.g., HIV infection, endocarditis, cystic fibrosis, Felty syndrome, Kawasaki disease, ulcerative colitis, Crohn disease).

Electroimmunoassay kits provide results similar to immunofluorescence assay.

Laboratory findings reflecting specific organ involvement:

Renal disease in ~80% of cases. Hematuria, proteinuria, azotemia. Nephrosis or chronic nephritis may occur. Most patients develop renal insufficiency. Biopsy is important to define extent of disease.

Also may involve CNS, respiratory tract, heart.

Nonspecific laboratory findings:

- Normochromic anemia of chronic disease, thrombocytosis, and mild leukocytosis occur in 30% to 40% of patients; eosinophilia may occur but is not a feature. Leukopenia or thrombocytopenia occurs only during cytotoxic therapy.
- ESR is increased in 90% of cases, often to very high levels; CRP correlates with disease activity even better than ESR. Both are useful to follow course and therapeutic effects.
- Serum globulins (IgG and IgA) are increased in ≤50% of cases.
- Serum C3 and C4 complement levels may be increased.
- Rheumatoid factor may be present in low titer in two thirds of cases.
- Antinuclear antibody is negative.

Laboratory findings due to secondary respiratory infection (usually staphylococcal).

Laboratory findings due to cyclophosphamide therapy, e.g., bladder cancer and sterility.

CARDIOVASC

Diseases of the Upper Respiratory Tract

Croup (Laryngotracheitis), Epiglottitis

Croup or laryngotracheitis refers to inflammation of the upper airway below the glottis.

Caused by

Group B *Haemophilus influenzae* causes >90% of cases of epiglottitis; other bacteria include β-hemolytic streptococci and pneumococci. The clinical picture in infectious mononucleosis or diphtheria may resemble epiglottitis.

Laryngotracheitis is usually viral (especially parainfluenza) but rarely bacterial in origin.

Tuberculosis (TB) may cause chronic laryngitis.

Cultures, smears, and tests for specific causative agents.
Blood cultures should be taken at the same time as throat cultures.
White blood cell (WBC) count is usually normal in croup; increased in epiglottitis.

Diseases of Larynx

♦ Biopsy for diagnosis of visible lesions (e.g., leukoplakia, carcinoma)
♦ Culture and smears for specific organisms (e.g., tubercle bacilli, fungi)
Infection may be caused by any respiratory viruses.

Nasopharyngeal Carcinoma

Caused by Epstein-Barr virus (EBV).

Nasopharyngitis and Rhinitis, Acute

Due To

Viruses (e.g., EBV, cytomegalovirus [CMV], adenovirus, respiratory syncytial virus [RSV], herpes simplex virus [HSV], Coxsackie virus) in most cases

• Acute rhinitis (common cold) usually viral, especially adenovirus

Bacteria

• Group A β-hemolytic streptococci (causes 10%–30% of cases seen by doctors), *Haemophilus influenzae, Mycoplasma pneumoniae, Chlamydia pneumoniae,* etc.). Mere presence of staphylococci, pneumococci, or α- and β-hemolytic streptococci (other than groups A, C, and G) in throat culture does not establish them as cause of pharyngitis and does not warrant antibiotic treatment.
• Streptococci may have sequelae of rheumatic fever, glomerulonephritis.
• Bacterial infection may be superimposed on viral or allergic rhinitis. Most commonly caused by streptococci, staphylococci, or *H. influenzae.*
• *Chlamydia trachomatis* and *Neisseria gonorrhoeae* infections are sexually transmitted.

Allergic: eosinophils in nasal secretions and eosinophilia
Fungal, foreign body, trauma, neoplasm
Idiopathic (no cause is identified in ~50% of cases)

Microscopic Examination of Stained Nasal Smear

○ Large numbers of eosinophils suggest allergy. Does not correlate with blood eosinophilia. Eosinophils and neutrophils suggest chronic allergy with superimposed infection.
○ Large numbers of neutrophils suggest infection.
○ Gram stain and culture of pharyngeal exudate may show significant pathogen.

Sinusitis, Acute

Often precipitated by obstruction due to viral upper respiratory infection, allergy, polyps, foreign body.

Due To

Streptococcus pneumoniae and *H. influenzae* cause >50% of cases; also anaerobes, *Staphylococcus aureus, Streptococcus* pyogenes (group A).
Moraxella (Branhamella) catarrhalis causes ~20% of cases in children.
Immunocompromised patients and nosocomial infections have a higher incidence of aerobic Gram-negative bacteria.

RESPIRATORY

Viruses cause ~10% to 20% of cases.

Pseudomonas aeruginosa and *H. influenzae* are predominant organisms in cystic fibrosis patients.

Mucor sp. and *Aspergillus* sp. should be ruled out in patients with diabetes or acute leukemia and renal transplant recipients.

Mixed anaerobes streptococci and *Bacteroides* sp. occur in ~50% of cases of chronic (≥12 weeks) sinusitis, suggesting dental origin.

Needle aspiration of sinus is required for determination of organism. Cultures of nose, throat, and nasopharynx do not correlate well.

Mucosal biopsy may be indicated if aspirate is not diagnostic in unresponsive patient with acute infection.

Laboratory Tests for Respiratory System Diseases

Pulmonary function tests and radiologic procedures are often essential to diagnosis.

Bronchoscopy, Bronchoalveolar Lavage, and Endobronchial Biopsy

These procedures involve saline lavage of the lung subsegments via fiberoptic bronchoscope.

Use

Biopsy of endobronchial tumor in which obstruction may cause secondary pneumonia with effusion but still a resectable tumor

To obtain bronchial washings for

- Diagnosis of nonresectable tumors that may be treated with radiation (e.g., oat cell carcinoma, Hodgkin disease), metastatic tumors, peripheral lesions that cannot be reached by bronchoscope.
- Diagnosis of pulmonary infection, particularly in immunocompromised patients, especially where sputum examination is not diagnostic. Quantitative bacterial culture and cytocentrifugation for staining slides provides overall diagnostic accuracy of 79% for pulmonary infection. Negative predictive value is 94%.
- Evaluation of various interstitial diseases, especially sarcoidosis, hypersensitivity pneumonitis, idiopathic pulmonary fibrosis (Table 6-1).

Table 6-1.	Differential Cell Count in Bronchoalveolar Lavage (BAL) in Interstitial Lung Diseases[a]				
	Abnormal BAL	Alveolar Macrophages	Neutrophils	Eosinophils	Lymphocytes
Normal		>90%	Smokers 1%–5% Nonsmokers 1%	<1%	5%–10%
Sarcoidosis	>60%		Normal to slight increase	1%–5%	20%–60%
Hypersensitivity pneumonitis	>80%		1%–10%	1%–5%	40%–80%[b]
Pulmonary fibrosis, idiopathic	>60%		10%–20%	1%–10%	5%–20%
Eosinophilic pneumonia	>95%		1%–5%	>20%	10%–20%
Connective tissue diseases	>50%		1%–20%	1%–5%	5%–30%

[a]Robinson-Smith TM, et al. Interpretation of the Wright-Giemsa stained bronchoalveolar lavage specimens. *Lab Med* 2004;35:553.
[b]Virtually all are CD3$^+$ with relative increase in CD8$^+$; ratio of CD4$^+$ to CD8$^+$ ≤1.

Giemsa stain
- Normal persons show <3% neutrophils, 8% to 18% lymphocytes, 80% to 89% alveolar macrophages.
- >10% neutrophils: Acute inflammation (e.g., bacterial infection [including Legionella, adult respiratory distress syndrome (ARDS)], drug reaction).
- >1% squamous epithelial cells: Indicates that a positive culture may reflect saliva contamination.
- >80% macrophages: Common in pulmonary hemorrhage. Aspergillosis is the only infection associated with significant alveolar hemorrhage that may also be found in >10% of patients with hematologic malignancies.
- >30% lymphocytes: May indicate hypersensitivity pneumonitis (often ≤50%–60% with more cytoplasm and large irregular nucleus).
- >10% neutrophils and >3% eosinophils is characteristic of idiopathic pulmonary fibrosis; alveolar macrophages predominate. Lymphocyte percentage may be increased.
- >10^5 colony-forming bacteria/mL indicates bacterial infection if <1% squamous epithelial cells are present on Giemsa stain.
- For fungal or parasitic infections.

Gram stain
- Many bacteria suggests bacterial infection if there are <1% squamous epithelial cells, especially if culture shows >10^4 bacteria/mL.
- No bacteria suggests bacterial infection is unlikely but should rule out *Legionella* with direct fluorescent antibody (DFA) test if Giemsa stain shows increased neutrophils.
- Combined with methenamine silver or Pap stain, shows 94% sensitivity for diagnosis of *Pneumocystis* infection; this increases to 100% when bronchoalveolar lavage (BAL) is combined with transbronchial biopsy.

Acid-fast stain—positive may indicate *Mycobacterium tuberculosis* or *M. avium-intracellulare* infection.

Methenamine silver for fungal infections (e.g., *Candida* sp., aspergillosis, cryptococcosis, coccidioidomycosis, histoplasmosis, blastomycosis) and filamentous bacterial pneumonia.

Toluidine blue stain may show *Pneumocystis jiroveci (carinii)* cysts in *Pneumocystis* pneumonia or *Aspergillus* hyphae in immunocompromised host with invasive aspergillosis.

Prussian blue–nuclear red stain strongly positive indicates severe alveolar hemorrhage; moderate positive indicates some hemorrhage; absent indicates no evidence of alveolar hemorrhage.

DFA stain for *Legionella*, HSV I and II (stains bronchial epithelial cells and macrophages), and CMV (stains mononuclear cells) may indicate infection with corresponding organism.

Pap stain: Atypical cytology may be caused by cytotoxic drugs, radiation therapy, viral infection (intranuclear inclusions of herpes or CMV) as well as tumor; also actinomycosis, nocardiosis.

Oil red O stain shows many large intracellular fat droplets in one third to two thirds of cells in some patients with fat embolism due to bone fractures but in <3% of patients without embolism.

Gases, Blood

See "Acid-Base Disorders," Chapter 12.

	Degree of Hypoxemia	Age		
		<60 Years	70–79 Years	>79 Years
Arterial O$_2$ tension (mm Hg) (breathing room air)	Mild	<80	<70	<60
	Moderate	<60	<50	
	Severe	<40	<40	<40
Arterial O$_2$ tension (mm Hg) (breathing supplemental O$_2$)	Uncorrected	<80	<70	<60
	Corrected	80–100	70–100	60–100
	Excessively corrected	>100 for all ages		

Use

To evaluate patients with pulmonary or acid-base disturbances.

To monitor patients with carbon monoxide poisoning, methemoglobinemia, or hemoglobin variant for O_2 saturation.

To manage patients on mechanical respirators.

Prior to thoracic or general surgery.

Decreased Pressure of Oxygen (Hypoxemia) Caused By

Hypoventilation (e.g., chronic airflow obstruction): caused by increased alveolar CO_2 that displaces O_2.

Alveolar hypoxia (e.g., high altitude, gaseous inhalation).

Pulmonary diffusion abnormalities (e.g., interstitial lung disease): Supplemental O_2 usually improves partial pressure of O_2 (pO_2).

Right-to-left shunt: supplemental O_2 has no effect; requires positive end-expiratory pressure.

* Congenital anomalies of heart and great vessels
* Acquired (e.g., ARDS)

Ventilation-perfusion mismatch: supplemental O_2 usually improves pO_2

* Airflow obstruction (e.g., chronic obstructive pulmonary disease [COPD], asthma)
* Interstitial inflammation (e.g., pneumonia, sarcoidosis)
* Vascular obstruction (e.g., pulmonary embolism)

Decreased venous oxygenation (e.g., anemia)

Cyanosis is clearly visible at pO_2 <40 mm Hg; may be seen at 50 mm Hg depending on skin pigmentation.

Increased Pressure of Oxygen (Hypercapnia) Caused By

Decreased ventilation

* Airway obstruction
* Drug overdose
* Metabolic disorders (e.g., myxedema, hypokalemia)
* Neurologic disorders (e.g., Guillain-Barré syndrome, multiple sclerosis)
* Muscle disorders (e.g., muscular dystrophy, polymyositis)
* Chest wall abnormalities (e.g., scoliosis)

Increased dead space in lungs (perfusion decreased more than ventilation decreased)

* Lung diseases (e.g., COPD, asthma, pulmonary fibrosis, mucoviscidosis)
* Chest wall changes affecting lung parenchyma (e.g., scoliosis)

Increased production (e.g., sepsis, fever, seizures, excess carbohydrate loads)

Lymph Node (Scalene) Biopsy

A biopsy of scalene fat pad, even without palpable lymph nodes, is often useful.

Positive in 15% of bronchogenic carcinomas. A lymph node biopsy may also be positive in various granulomatous diseases (e.g., TB, sarcoidosis, pneumoconiosis), other metastases, and lymphomas.

Pleura, Needle Biopsy (Closed Chest)

A needle biopsy of the pleura is performed whenever the clinician cannot make a diagnosis otherwise.

Use

To evaluate lymphocyte-predominant pleural effusion.

To diagnose an exudative pleural effusion that is undiagnosed after cytologic examination (diagnostic in 40%–75% of cases).

The test is positive for tumor in ~6% of malignant mesotheliomas and ~60% of other cases of malignancy.

The test is positive for tubercles in two thirds of cases on first biopsy, with increased yield on second and third biopsies; therefore repeat biopsy if suspicious clinically. Acid-fast stain or granulomas can be found in 50% to 80% of cases, and culture of biopsy material for TB is positive in ≤75% of cases. A fluid culture alone establishes a diagnosis of TB in 25% of cases.

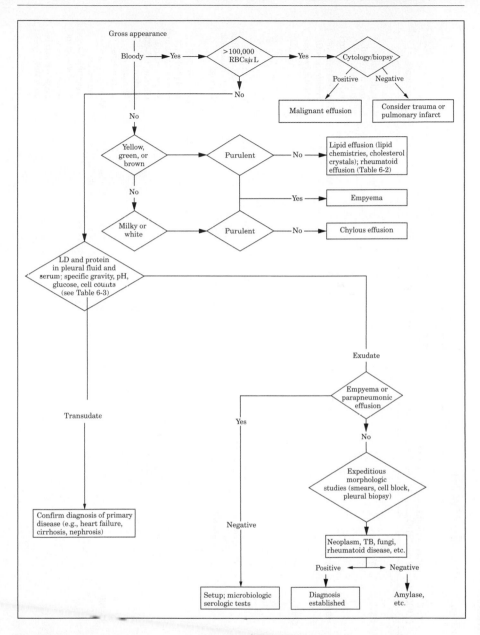

Figure 6-1. Algorithm for pleural effusion. LD, lactate dehydrogenase; TB, tuberculosis; RBCs, red blood cells.

Pleural Effusion[1]

See Figure 6–1 and Tables 6–2 and 6–3.

[1]Light RW. *Pleural Diseases*. 4th Ed. Philadelphia: Lippincott Williams & Wilkins; 2001.

Table 6-2. Pleural Fluid Findings in Various Clinical Conditions

Disease	Appearance	Total WBC (1,000/μL)	Predominant Type WBC	Total RBC (1,000/μL)	pH	Glucose mg/dL	Glucose PF:S	Protein PF:S	LD PF:S	LD IU/L	Amylase PF:S	Comments
Transudates												
Congestive heart failure	Clear, straw	<1	M	0–1	>7.4	>60	1	<0.5	<0.6	<200	≤1	If right side not involved, rule out, pulmonary infarct.
Cirrhosis	Clear, straw	<0.5	M	<1	>7.4	>60	1	<0.5	<0.6	<200	≤1	Occurs in 5% of cirrhotics with clinical ascites.
Pulmonary embolus; atelectasis	Clear, straw	5–15	M	<5	>7.3	>60	1	<0.5	<0.6		≤1	
Exudates												
Pulmonary embolus: infarction	Turbid to hemorrhagic Small volume	5–15	P May show many mesothelial cells	Bloody in one third to two thirds of patients	>7.3	>60	1	>0.5	>0.6		≤1	Occurs in 15% of patients; often no characteristic findings.
Pneumonia[a]	Turbid	5–40	P	<5	≥7.3	>60	1	>0.5	>0.6		≤1	Occurs in 50% bacterial pneumonias and Legion/naires disease, 5%–20% of viral and Mycoplasms pneumonias.
Empyema[b]	Turbid to purulent	25–100	P	<5	5.50–7.29	<60	<0.5	>0.5	>0.6	May be >1,000/L	≤1	Most commonly caused by anaerobic bacteria, Staphylococcus aureus, Gram-negative aerobic bacteria.

TB	Straw, serosanguineous 15%	M	≤10	<10	<7.3 in 20%	30–60 in 20%	1	>0.5	>0.6	≤1	AFB stain positive in 15%–20% and culture of fluid positive in 30% of cases. Biopsy for histologic examination and culture of pleura are diagnostic in 75%–85% of cases. Often presents as effusion; pulmonary disease may be absent.
Malignancy[c]	Straw to turbid to bloody	M	<10	1 to >100	<7.3 in 30%	<60 in 30%	1	>0.5	>0.6	≤1	
RA effusion[d]	Turbid or green or yellow	P in acute M in chronic	1–20	<1	<7.3; usually ~7.0	<30 in 95%		>0.5	>0.6	Often >1,000/L	Biopsy is useful, especially in men with rheumatoid nodules and high RF titer.
SLE	Straw to turbid	P in acute M in chronic			<7.3 in 30%	<60 in 30%		>0.5	>0.6	>2	PF may show LE cells, ANA titer, and low complement. Usually found only when lupus is active.
Rupture of esophagus	Purulent	P			6.0	N or D		>0.5	>0.6	salivary type	

(continued)

Table 6-2. (Continued)

Disease	Appearance	Total WBC (1,000/μL)	Predominant Type WBC	Total RBC (1,000/μL)	pH	Glucose		Protein	LD		Amylase	Comments
						mg/dL	PF:S	PF:S	PF:S	IU/L	PF:S	
Pancreatitis	Serous to turbid to serosanguineous	5–20	P	1–10	>7.3	>60	1	>0.5	>0.6		>2	Occurs in 15% of acute cases. Left-sided in 70% of cases.

Note: Blood specimens should always be drawn at the same time as serous fluid for determination of glucose, protein, LD, amylase, pH, etc. Pleural fluid for pH should be collected in the same way as arterial blood samples (i.e., heparinized syringe, maintained anaerobically on ice, analyzed promptly). Pleural fluid pH should normally be at least 0.15 greater than arterial blood pH. Normal pH is alkaline and may approach 7.6.

PF:S, ratio of pleural fluid to serum; M, mononuclear cells; P, polymorphonuclear leukocytes; PE, pleural fluid; TB, tuberculosis; WBC, white blood cell; RBC, red blood cell; LD, lactate dehydrogenase; RA, rheumatoid arthritis; SLE, systemic lupus erythematosus; RF, rheumatoid factor, ANA, antinuclear antibodies.

Parapneumonic effusions (exudate type of effusion associated with lung abscess, bronchiectasis; ~5% of bacterial pneumonias).

    Aerobic Gram-negative organisms (*Klebsiella, Escherichia coli, Pseudomonas*) are associated with a high incidence of exudates (with 5,000–40,000/μL, high protein, and normal glucose, normal pH) and resolve with antibiotic therapy.

    Nonpurulent fluid with positive Gram stain, positive blood culture, or low pH suggests that effusion will become or behave like empyema.

    Streptococcus pneumoniae causes parapneumonic effusions in 50% of cases, especially with positive blood culture.

    Staphylococcus aureus has effusion in 90% of infants, 50% of adults.

    Streptococcus pyogenes in 90% of cases; massive effusion, greenish color.

    Haemophilus influenzae has effusion in 50%–75% of cases.

[b]pH <7.0 and glucose <40 mg/dL indicate need for closed chest tube drainage even without grossly purulent fluid. pH of 7.0–7.2 is a questionable indication and should be repeated in 24 h, but tube drainage is favored if pleural fluid LD >1,000 IU/L. Tube drainage is also indicated if there is grossly purulent fluid or positive Gram stain or culture.

In *Proteus mirabilis* empyema, high ammonia level may cause a pH ~8.0.

[c]Usually is large; frequently hemorrhagic (50% have RBC >10,000/μL).

    Cytology establishes the diagnosis in approximately 50% of patients. Cytology plus biopsy is diagnostic in about 90% of cases.

    Lung and breast cancer and lymphoma cause 75% of malignant effusions; in 6%, no primary tumor is found. Pleural or ascitic effusion occurs in 20%–30% of patients with malignant lymphoma.

    In some instances of suspected lymphoma with negative conventional test results, flow cytometry of pleural fluid showing a monoclonal lymphocyte population can establish the diagnosis.

    Mucopolysaccharide level may be increased in mesothelioma.

[d]Decreased glucose is the most useful finding clinically; may be 0.

    RA cells may be found. RF may be present but may also be found in other effusions (e.g., TB, cancer, bacterial pneumonia).

    Needle biopsy usually may show characteristic rheumatoid nodule.

    Protein level is >3 g/dL.

Table 6-3. Comparison of "Typical"[a] Findings in Transudates and Exudates[b]

Findings	Transudates	Exudates
Specific gravity[c]	<1.016	>1.016
PF[d]	<3.0	>3.0
PF:serum ratio[e]	<0.5	>0.5
LD[f]		
IU	<200	>200
PF:serum ratio	<0.6	>0.6
Ratio PF:ULN serum[e]	<2:3	>2:3
WBC count (/μL)	<1,000 in 80%; >10,000 is rare	>1,000
	Mainly lymphocytes	May be grossly purulent
RBCs (/μL)	Few	Variable; few or may be grossly bloody
Glucose	Equivalent to serum	May be decreased due to bacteria or many WBCs
Cholesterol (mg/dL)	<45	Usually >45
PF:serum ratio	<0.32	>0.32
pH	Usually 7.4–7.5	Usually 7.35–7.45
Appearance	Clear	Usually cloudy
Color	Pale yellow	Variable

PF, pleural fluid; LD, lactate dehydrogenase; ULN, upper limits of normal; WBC, white blood cell; RBC, red blood cell.
[a]Typical means 67%–75% of patients.
[b]Isoenzymes not useful for differentiating.
[c]Long-standing transudates, however, can produce a high specific gravity. The only value of specific gravity is for rapid bedside estimate of protein; otherwise is superfluous.
[d]Protein level of 3.0 g/dL misclassifies ~10% of effusions if it is the only criterion.
Use of [d] and [e] will correctly differentiate 99% of exudates and transudates. Transudate meets none of these criteria, and *exudate meets at least one criterion*. Unequivocal criteria of transudate precludes the need for pleural biopsy in most cases unless two mechanisms are suspected (e.g., nephritic syndrome with miliary tuberculosis, congestive heart failure with malignancy). It would be uncommon for use of diuretics in congestive heart failure to change characteristics of transudate to that of exudate. Borderline fluids should be classified as exudates.
[f]If nonhemolyzed, nonbloody effusion.

Normal Values
Total protein
Albumin   0.3–4.1 g/dL
Globulin   50%–70%
Fibrinogen   30%–45%
pH   6.8–7.6
Specific gravity (no longer ordered)   1.010–1.026

The underlying cause of an effusion is usually determined by first classifying the fluid as an exudate or a transudate. A transudate does not usually require additional testing, but *exudates always do*.
Pleural fluid (PF) analysis results in a definitive diagnosis in ~25% and a probable diagnosis in another 50% of patients; it may help to rule out a suspected diagnosis in 30%. No diagnosis is established in ~15% of exudates.

Transudate
Due To
Congestive heart failure (causes 15% of cases); acute diuresis can result in pseudoexudate
Cirrhosis with ascites (pleural effusion in ~5% of these cases)—rare without ascites
Nephrotic syndrome
Early (acute) atelectasis
Pulmonary embolism (some cases)

RESPIRATORY

Superior vena cava obstruction
Hypoalbuminemia
Peritoneal dialysis—occurs within 48 hours of initiating dialysis
Early mediastinal malignancy
Misplaced subclavian catheter
Myxedema (rare cause)
Constrictive pericarditis—effusion is bilateral
Urinothorax—due to ipsilateral genitourinary tract obstruction

Exudate

Caused by

Pneumonia, malignancy, pulmonary embolism, and gastrointestinal conditions (especially pancreatitis and abdominal surgery) cause 90% of all exudates. The cause is unknown in ~10% to 15% of all exudates.
Infection (causes 25% of cases)

* Bacterial pneumonia
* Parapneumonic effusion (empyema)
* TB
* Abscess (subphrenic, liver, spleen)
* Viral, mycoplasmal, rickettsial
* Parasitic (ameba, hydatid cyst, filaria)
* Fungal effusion (*Coccidioides, Cryptococcus, Histoplasma, Blastomyces, Aspergillus*; in immunocompromised host, *Aspergillus, Candida, Mucor*)

Pulmonary embolism/infarction
Neoplasms (metastatic carcinoma, especially breast, ovary, and lung; lymphoma; leukemia; mesothelioma; pleural endometriosis) (cause of 42% of cases)
Trauma (penetrating or blunt)

* Hemothorax, chylothorax, empyema, associated with rupture of diaphragm

Immunologic mechanisms

* Rheumatoid pleurisy (5% of cases)
* Systemic lupus erythematosus (SLE)
* Other collagen vascular diseases occasionally cause effusions (e.g., Wegener granulomatosis, Sjögren syndrome, familial Mediterranean fever, Churg-Strauss syndrome, mixed connective tissue disease)
* Following myocardial infarction or cardiac surgery
* Vasculitis
* Hepatitis
* Sarcoidosis (rare cause; may also be transudate)
* Familial recurrent polyserositis
* Drug reaction (e.g., nitrofurantoin hypersensitivity, methysergide)

Chemical mechanisms

* Uremic
* Pancreatic (pleural effusion occurs in ~10% of these cases)
* Esophageal rupture (high *salivary* amylase and pH <7.30 that approaches 6.00 in 48–72 hours)
* Subphrenic abscess

Lymphatic abnormality (e.g., irradiation, Milroy disease)
Injury (e.g., asbestosis)
Altered pleural mechanics (e.g., late [chronic] atelectasis)
Endocrine (e.g., hypothyroidism)
Movement of fluid from abdomen to pleural space

* Meigs syndrome (protein and specific gravity are often at transudate–exudate border but usually not transudate)
* Urinothorax
* Cancer
* Pancreatitis, pancreatic pseudocyst

Cirrhosis, pulmonary infarct, trauma, and connective tissue diseases are responsible for ~9% of all cases.

Exudates That Can Present As Transudates
Due To
Pulmonary embolism (>20% of cases)—caused by atelectasis
Hypothyroidism—caused by myxedema heart disease
Malignancy—because of complications (e.g., atelectasis, lymphatic obstruction)
Sarcoidosis—Stage II and III

Location
Typically left-sided: Ruptured esophagus, acute pancreatitis, rheumatoid arthritis.
    Pericardial disease is left-sided or bilateral; it is rarely exclusively right-sided.
Typically right-sided or bilateral: Congestive heart failure (CHF) (if only on left, con-
    sider that right pleural space may be obliterated or patient has another process [e.g.,
    pulmonary infarction]).
Typically right-sided: Rupture of amebic liver abscess.

Gross Appearance
Clear, straw-colored fluid is typical of transudate.
Turbidity (cloudy, opaque appearance) may be caused by lipids or increased WBCs;
    after centrifugation, a clear supernatant indicates WBCs or debris as the cause;
    clear or white supernatant is caused by chylomicrons.
Red indicates blood; brown indicates blood has been present for a longer time.
Bloody fluid suggests malignancy, pulmonary infarct, trauma, postcardiotomy syn-
    drome; also uremia, asbestos, pleural endometriosis. Bloody fluid from traumatic
    thoracentesis should clot within several minutes, but blood present more than sev-
    eral hours will have become defibrinated and does not form a good clot. Nonuniform
    color during aspiration and absence of hemosiderin-laden macrophages also suggest
    traumatic aspiration. Absent platelets suggests the condition is not caused by trau-
    matic thoracentesis.
Red blood cell (RBC) count of 5,000 to 10,000/μL causes a blood-tinged color. If grossly
    bloody, hematocrit (Hct) >50% of peripheral Hct indicates a hemothorax.
White fluid suggests chylothorax, cholesterol effusion, or empyema.
Chylous (milky) is usually due to trauma (e.g., auto accident, postoperative) but may
    be obstruction of duct (e.g., especially lymphoma; metastatic carcinoma, granulomas)
    or parenteral nutrition via a central line with perforation of superior vena cava.
After centrifugation, supernatant is clear in empyema but cloudy or turbid in chylous
    effusion caused by chylomicrons, which also stain with Sudan III.
PF triglycerides (TG) >110 mg/dL or TG PF:serum ratio >2 occurs only in chylous
    effusion (seen especially within a few hours after eating). TG <50 mg/dL excludes chy-
    lothorax. Equivocal TG levels (50–10 mg/dL) may require a lipoprotein electrophore-
    sis of fluid to demonstrate chylomicrons, which are diagnostic of chylothorax.
Pseudochylous (may have lustrous sheen) appearance in chronic inflammatory con-
    ditions (e.g., rheumatoid pleurisy, TB, chronic pneumothorax therapy) is caused by
    either cholesterol crystals (rhomboid-shaped) in sediment or lipid-containing
    inclusions in leukocytes. Distinguish from chylous effusions by microscopy.
    Chylomicrons ≤50 mg/dL with cholesterol >250 mg/dL occurs in pseudochylous
    effusions.
Black fluid suggests *Aspergillus niger* infection.
Greenish fluid suggests biliopleural fistula.
Purulent fluid indicates infection.
Anchovy (dark red-brown) color is seen in amebiasis, old blood.
Anchovy paste in ruptured amebic liver abscess; amebas found in <10%.
Turbid and greenish-yellow fluid is classic for rheumatoid effusion.
Very viscous (clear or bloody) is characteristic of mesothelioma; also in pyothorax.
Debris in fluid suggests rheumatoid pleurisy; food particles indicate esophageal rupture.
Color of enteral tube food or central venous line infusion due to tube or catheter enter-
    ing pleural space.

Odor
Putrid due to anaerobic empyema.
Ammonia due to urinothorax.

Protein, Albumin, Lactate Dehydrogenase
See Table 6-3.
When exudate criteria are met by lactate dehydrogenase (LD) but not by protein, con-
    sider malignancy and parapneumonic effusions.

RESPIRATORY

Very high PF LD (>1,000 IU/L) occurs in empyema, rheumatoid pleurisy, paragonimiasis; sometimes with malignancy; rarely with TB. Level indicates degree of pleural inflammation; increasing values suggest need for more aggressive therapy. Measurement of LD isoenzymes is said to have limited value.

Glucose

Transudate has same concentration as serum.

Usually normal but 30 to 55 mg/dL or PF:serum ratio <0.5 and pH <7.30 may be found in TB, malignancy, SLE; also esophageal rupture; lowest levels may occur in empyema and rheumatoid arthritis (RA). Therefore, only helpful if very low level (e.g., <30). A level of 0 to 10 mg/dL is highly suspicious for RA. Poor prognostic sign in pneumonia. In neoplasm, lower glucose indicates greater tumor burden. Rarely found in SLE, Churg-Strauss, urinothorax, hemothorax, paragonimiasis.

pH

♦ Low pH (<7.30) always means exudate, especially empyema, malignancy, rheumatoid pleurisy, SLE, TB, esophageal rupture; may also be caused by systemic acidosis, hemothorax, urinothorax, paragonimiasis.

pH <6.0 is consistent with but not diagnostic of esophageal rupture.

Collagen vascular disease is the only other cause of pH <7.0.

In parapneumonic effusion, a pH <7.20 indicates need for tube drainage; pH >7.30 suggests that resolution with only medical therapy is possible. A pH <7.0 indicates the presence of complicated parapneumonic effusion.

pH may fall before glucose becomes decreased.

Proteus infection may increase pH because of urea splitting.

In malignant effusion, pH <7.30 is associated with short survival time, poorer prognosis, and increased positive yield with cytology and pleural biopsy; tends to correlate with PF glucose <60 mg/dL.

Generally, low pH is associated with low glucose and high LD; if low pH with normal glucose and low LD, the pH is probably a lab error.

Amylase

Increased PF:serum ratio >1.0 and may be >5 or PF > upper limit of normal for serum. Should be determined only for left pleural effusions.

• Acute pancreatitis—may be normal early with increase over time
• Pancreatic pseudocyst—always increased, may be >1,000 IU/L
• Also perforated esophageal rupture, peptic ulcer, necrosis of small intestine (e.g., mesenteric vascular occlusion); 10% of cases of metastatic cancer

Isoenzyme studies

• *Pancreatic* type of amylase in acute pancreatitis and pancreatic pseudocyst
• *Salivary* type of amylase is found in esophageal rupture and occasionally in carcinoma of ovary or lung or salivary gland tumor

Other Chemical Determinations

♦ C-reactive protein ranged from 10 to 20 mg/dL in transudates compared to 30 to 40 mg/dL in exudates in one small study. Parapneumonic effusions were highest (89 ± 16 mg/dL). The PF:serum ratio was 0.8 ± 0.5 mg/dL in transudates and 2.8 ± 0.7 mg/dL in exudates.

♦ Cholesterol and TG (see "Gross Appearance")

♦ Routine tumor markers (e.g., carcinoembryonic antigen [CEA], cancer antigen-125, acid phosphatase in prostate cancer, hyaluronic acid in mesothelioma) are not generally recommended (Table 6-4). CEA >10 ng/mL is suggestive but not diagnostic of malignant PF; usually <10 ng/mL in lymphomas, sarcomas, mesotheliomas.

Immune complexes (measured by Raji cell, C1q component, radioimmunoassay, etc.) are often found in exudates due to collagen vascular diseases (SLE, RA). Latex agglutination tests show frequent false-positive results and should not be ordered. Occasionally, latex agglutination for bacterial antigens is useful.

Cell Count

Total WBC count is almost never diagnostic.

• >10,000/μL indicates inflammation, most commonly with pneumonia, pulmonary infarct, pancreatitis, postcardiotomy syndrome
• >50,000/μL is typical only in parapneumonic effusions, usually empyema
• Chronic exudates (e.g., malignancy and TB) are usually <5,000/μL
• Transudates are usually <1,000/μL

Table 6-4. Comparison of Tumor Markers in Various Pleural Effusions		
	CA-125	CEA[a]
Benign effusion	–	–
Mesothelioma	–	–
Melanoma	–	–
Lymphoma	–	–
Carcinosarcoma	–	–
Breast	–	+
Lung	–	+
Gastrointestinal tract	–	+
Ovary (mucinous)	–	+
Ovary (serous)[b]	+	–
Fallopian tube[b]	+	–
Endometrium[b]	+	–

CA-125, C125 tumor antigen; CEA, carcinoembryonic antigen; + indicates value increased; –indicates value not increased.
[a]CEA not increased <5 mg/mL.
[b]CA-125 >1,000 units/mL has 85% sensitivity and 96% specificity.
Source: Pinto MM, Bernstein LH, Brogan DA, et al. Immunoradiometric assay of CA-125 in effusions: comparison with carcinoembryonic antigen. *Cancer* 1987;59:218.

5,000 to 6,000 RBCs/μL are needed to give a red-tinged appearance to PF

• Can be caused by needle trauma, producing 2 mL of blood in 1,000 mL of PF.

>100,000 RBCs/μL is grossly hemorrhagic and suggests malignancy, pulmonary infarct, or trauma, but is occasionally seen in CHF alone.
Hemothorax (PF:venous Hct ratio >2 suggests trauma, bleeding from a vessel, bleeding disorder, or malignancy but may be seen in same conditions as above.

Smears
Wright stain differentiates PMNs from mononuclear cells; cannot differentiate lymphocytes from monocytes.
Mononuclear cell counts >50% occur in about one third of transudates and in chronic exudates (lymphoma, TB, viral, fungal infections, malignancy, rheumatoid, uremia). Counts >50% are seen in two thirds of cases caused by cancer. Counts >85% to 90% suggests TB, lymphoma, sarcoidosis, rheumatoid pleurisy, chylothorax. Also seen after coronary artery bypass surgery.
Polymorphonuclear leukocytes (PMNs) predominate in early inflammatory effusions (e.g., pneumonia, pulmonary infarct, pancreatitis, subphrenic abscess).
Presence of eosinophils in PF (>10% of total WBCs) is not diagnostically significant.

• Not usually accompanied by striking blood eosinophilia
• May mean blood or air in pleural space (e.g., pneumothorax [most common], repeated thoracenteses, traumatic hemothorax)
• Is also said to be associated with asbestosis, pulmonary infarction, polyarteritis nodosa, Churg-Strauss syndrome
• Parasitic, fungal, drug-related (e.g., nitrofurantoin, bromocriptine, dantrolene)
• Idiopathic effusion (in about one third of cases; may be caused by occult pulmonary embolism or asbestos)
• Uncommon with malignant effusions; rare with TB
• Cause not established in ~25% of cases

Basophils >10% only in leukemic involvement of pleura.
After several days, mesothelial cells, macrophages, lymphocytes may predominate.
Large mesothelial cells >5% are said to rule out TB (must differentiate from macrophages) except in AIDS. Also absent when pleura is coated with fibrin.
Occasionally, LE cells make the diagnosis of SLE.

RESPIRATORY

Bacterial stains: Gram stain for early diagnosis of bacterial infection. Acid-fast smears are positive in only <20% of TB pleurisy.

♦ **Culture**

Often positive in empyema but not in parapneumonic effusions. Sensitivity >50% in TB. Cultures from chest tubes may be inaccurate compared to direct aspirates.

♦ **Bacterial antigens**

May detect *H. influenzae* type b, *S. pneumoniae*, several types of *N. meningitides, Legionella*. Useful when viable organisms cannot be recovered (e.g., prior antibiotic therapy).

♦ **Cytology**

♦ Neoplasms

○ Rheumatoid effusions: Cytologic triad of slender elongated and round giant multi-nucleated macrophages and necrotic background material with characteristically low glucose is said to be pathognomonic. Mesothelial cells are nearly always absent.

♦ **Cell-free DNA[2]**

Markedly increased in exudates, with sensitivity/specificity (S/S) ≥90%/~67%. Correlates with LD and protein levels in PF.

Pleural Fluid Findings in Various Clinical Conditions

See Figure 6-1.

Tuberculosis

Pleural effusions occur in ≤5% of all TB patients, >15% of patients with extrapulmonary TB, and >20% of TB patients with negative sputum smears.

Fluid is an exudate with high protein content—almost always >4.0 g/dL.

♦ Acid-fast smears are positive in only <20% and culture is positive in ~67% of cases; culture combined with histologic examination establishes the diagnosis in 95% of cases.

Sputum culture is positive in ~25% of patients. PF culture is positive in 25% of cases. BACTEC cultures have greater sensitivity and earlier results.

♦ Molecular techniques have high S/S. Polymerase chain reaction has S/S >80%/>86%.

♦ Needle biopsy can be done without hesitation; histology and culture may be needed for diagnosis. Biopsy culture is positive in ~33% when PF culture is negative.

Increased lymphocytes, especially with lymphocyte:neutrophil ratio >0.75.

Adenosine deaminase >70 IU/L without empyema or RA is said to be diagnostic of TB; >40 IU/L is suggestive of TB, and higher values are more likely to be TB.

Large mesothelial cells >5% are said to rule out TB (must differentiate from macrophages).

TB often presents as effusion, especially in youth; pulmonary disease may be absent; risk of active pulmonary TB within 5 years is 60%.

Malignancy (See Table 6-5)

Can cause exudate by metastasis to pleura or transudate by metastasis to lymph nodes obstructing lymph drainage, giving exudate-type fluid. Low pH and glucose indicate a poor prognosis with short survival time.

"Characteristic" effusion is moderate to massive, frequently hemorrhagic, with moderate WBC count with predominance of mononuclear cells; however, only half of malignant effusions have RBC count >10,000/µL.

♦ Cytology is positive in 60% of malignancies on first tap, 80% by third tap. Is more sensitive than needle biopsy. In combination with needle biopsy, sensitivity increased by <10%. Sensitivity: adenocarcinoma >70%, squamous cell carcinoma = 20%, sarcoma = 25%, mesothelioma = 10%, Hodgkin disease ~25%, diffuse histiocytic lymphoma = 75%. Lung and breast cancer and lymphoma cause 75% of malignant effusions; in 6%, no primary tumor is found. Pleural or ascitic effusion occurs in 20% to 30% of patients with malignant lymphoma.

♦ Combined cytology and pleural biopsy give positive results in 90%.

♦ See "Thoracoscopy/Open Lung Biopsy." Is diagnostic in >90% of patients with negative cytology.

○ Electron microscopy is most useful to distinguish metastatic adenocarcinoma from mesothelioma.

○ Mesothelioma cells stain with Alcian blue. Adenocarcinomas stain with periodic acid–Schiff (PAS) after diastase digestion. Mucopolysaccharide level may be increased (normal <17 mg/dL) in mesothelioma.

---

[2]Chan MH, Chow KM, Chan AT, et al. Quantitative analysis of pleural fluid cell-free DNA as a tool for the classification of pleural effusions. *Clin Chem* 2003;49:740–745.

Table 6-5.	Some Methods for Detection of Neoplasms in Effusions
Method	Advantages/Disadvantages
Microscopic morphology	Low cost. Lowest sensitivity.
Immunocytochemical staining with tumor specific antigens	Improved sensitivity/specificity.
DNA ploidy	Flow cytometry showing a monoclonal population can establish the diagnosis of lymphoma in lymphocytic effusions. May have high false-negative rates.
Cytogenetics and fluorescent in situ hybridization	Detects chromosome number, deletions, translocations.
Polymerase chain reaction and sequencing for gene mutations	Detects oncogenes and tumor suppressor gene mutations.
Genomic microarrays for cancer-specific or cancer-associated genes and pathways of expression	Limited use for early detection. May be useful for pharmacogenomics and classification. Not yet fulfilled.
Proteomics for cancer-specific or cancer-associated proteins and peptides	Not yet applied to effusions. Recent use in serum diagnosis (e.g., ovarian cancer). Too early to foretell utility.

Source: Ross JS. Emerging cancer diagnostics. *Am J Clin Pathol* 2003;120:822–824.

Pulmonary Infarction
Effusion occurs in 50% of patients with pulmonary infarct; is bloody in one third to two thirds of patients; often no characteristic diagnostic findings occur.

Small volume, serous or bloody, predominance of PMNs, may show many mesothelial cells; this "typical pattern" is seen in only 25% of cases.

Congestive Heart Failure
CHF is the most common cause of PF. Occurs in ≤70% of cases. Is typically bilateral; ≤20% are right-sided and ≤9% are left-sided. If unilateral or left-sided in patients with CHF, rule out pulmonary infarct.

◆ Increased serum B-type natriuretic peptide (BNP).

Pneumonias
Parapneumonic effusions are an exudate type of effusion associated with lung abscess, bronchiectasis, and ~5% of bacterial pneumonias.

Aerobic Gram-negative organisms (*Klebsiella, Escherichia coli, Pseudomonas*) are associated with a high incidence of exudates (with 5,000 to 40,000/L, high protein, normal glucose, normal pH) and resolve with antibiotic therapy. Nonpurulent fluids with positive Gram stain, positive blood culture, or low pH suggest that effusion will become or behave like empyema.

S. pneumoniae causes parapneumonic effusions in 50% of cases, especially with positive blood culture.

S. aureus has effusion in 90% of infants, 50% of adults; usually causes widespread bronchopneumonia.

S. pyogenes in 90% of cases; massive effusion, greenish color.

H. influenzae has effusion in 50% to 75% of cases.

Viral or mycoplasma pneumonia—pleural effusions develop in 20% of cases.

Legionnaires disease—pleural effusion occurs in up to 50% of patients; may be bilateral.

Pneumocystis jiroveci (carinii) pneumonias often have PF:serum LD ratio >1.0 and PF:serum protein ratio <0.5.

pH <7.0 and glucose <40 mg/dL indicate need for closed chest tube drainage, even without grossly purulent fluid.

pH of 7.0 to 7.2 is questionable indication and should be repeated in 24 hours, but tube drainage is favored if PF LD >1,000 IU/L. Tube drainage is also indicated with grossly purulent fluid or positive Gram stain or culture. Normal pH is alkaline and may approach 7.6.

Gas-liquid chromatography may identify the products of anaerobic acute bacterial and aerobic infections.

RESPIRATORY

Table 6-6.	Comparison of Pleural Fluid in Rheumatoid Arthritis and Systemic Lupus Erythematosus (SLE)	
Test	Rheumatoid Arthritis	SLE
pH >7.2	≤7.2	>7.2
Glucose	<30 mg/dL	Normal
Lactate dehydrogenase	>700 IU/L	<700 IU/L
Rheumatoid factor	Strongly positive	Negative or weakly positive
Ratio pleural fluid to serum	>1.0	<1.0
Rheumatoid arthritis cells (ragocytes)	May be present	Absent
Epithelioid cells	Present	Absent
C4	Markedly decreased ($<10 \times 10^5$ g/g of protein)	Moderately decreased ($<30 \times 10^6$ g/g of protein)
Clq–binding assay	Moderately positive	Weakly positive
Ratio pleural fluid to serum	>1.0	<1.0

Empyema
Usually WBCs >50,000/μL, low glucose, and low pH. Suspect clinically when effusion develops during adequate antibiotic therapy.
In *Proteus mirabilis* empyema, high ammonia level may cause a pH ~8.0.

Rheumatoid Effusion
See Table 6-6.
Found in ~70% of RA patients at autopsy.
○ Exudate is frequently turbid and may be milky. "Classic picture" is cloudy greenish fluid with 0 glucose level. Is <50 mg/dL in 80% of patients and <25 mg/dL in 66% of patients; is the most useful routine laboratory finding. Failure to increase during intravenous glucose infusion distinguishes RA from other causes. *Nonpurulent, nonmalignant effusions not caused by TB or RA almost always have glucose level >60 mg/dL.*
♦ Combination of low pH (usually 7.00), low glucose, and low C4 strongly indicate rheumatoid effusion.
○ RF titer ≥1:320 or ≥ serum titer strongly favors rheumatoid pleurisy.
○ RA cells may be found (see "Cytology" earlier in this chapter).
♦ Needle biopsy usually shows nonspecific chronic inflammation but may show characteristic rheumatoid nodule microscopically. One third of cases have parenchymal lung disease (e.g., interstitial fibrosis).
Other laboratory findings of RA are found (see Chapter 10).
Protein level is >3 g/dL.
Increased LD (usually higher than in serum) is commonly found in other chronic pleural effusions and is not useful in differential diagnosis.

Sputum Examination

Sputum Color	Condition
Rusty	Lobar pneumonia
Anchovy-paste (dark brown)	Amebic liver abscess rupture into bronchus
Caseous material	TB
Red-currant jelly	*Klebsiella pneumoniae*
Red (pigment, not blood)	*Serratia marcescens*; rifampin overdose
Black	*Bacteroides melaninogenicus* pneumonia; anthracosilicosis
Green (with WBCs, sweet odor)	Pseudomonas infection
Milky	Bronchioalveolar carcinoma
Yellow (without WBCs)	Jaundice

Smears and cultures for infections (e.g., pneumonias, TB, fungi) must be adequate samples of sputum showing ciliated cells, macrophages; neutrophils (usually >25/ low power field (LPF) in good specimen) if acute inflammation is present unless patient is neutropenic; monobacterial population if caused by bacterial infection; acute inflammation without a definite bacterial pattern may be caused by *Legionella* or RSV or influenza viruses. *Must be promptly refrigerated.* Saliva contamination may show squamous epithelial cells (>19/LPF = poor specimen; 11–19/LPF = fair specimen; <10/LPF = good specimen), extracellular strands of streptococci, clumps of anaerobic actinomyces, candidal budding yeasts with pseudohyphae. For possible anaerobic aspiration, fine-needle aspiration or alveolar lavage is needed.
Cytology for carcinoma.

Thoracoscopy/Open Lung Biopsy

A thoracoscopy or open lung biopsy allows visual inspection of the pleural surface and lung and facilitates visualization of multiple large biopsies.

Use
Supplement blind needle biopsy, especially in inaccessible sites.
Supplement bronchoscopy that has minimal diagnostic yield in pleural disease.
Evaluate exudative effusion of unknown etiology. Diagnostic yield >90%; for malignancy, diagnostic yield is ≤95%.
Combined with fluid cytology and needle biopsy, diagnostic sensitivity = 97%.
Diagnosis and stage malignant mesothelioma and other cancers and diagnosis of TB when less invasive workup has failed to make a diagnosis. Accuracy = 96%; S/S = 91%/100%; negative predictive value (NPV) = 93%.
Diagnosis of occupational diseases (asbestos, silicosis).
Semiquantitative analysis of dust content (asbestos).
Increasingly replaces needle biopsy of pleura.
Rarely establishes the diagnosis of benign disease.
Treatment of loculated or incompletely drained empyema.
Treatment of some cases of pneumothorax, hemothorax, chylothorax.
Talc pleurodesis therapy for recurrent or malignant effusions.

Pulmonary Diseases
Chronic Obstructive Pulmonary Disease[3]
Spirometry is used to test for airway obstruction.

Severity	Ratio of Forced Expiratory Volume in 1 s to Forced Vital Capacity	Predicted Forced Expiratory Volume in 1 s
At risk (e.g., smoking, pollutants)	0.7	≥80%
Mild	≤0.7	≥80%
Moderate	≤0.7	50%–80%
Severe	≤0.7	30%–50%
Very severe	≤0.7	<30%

Bronchial Asthma
Bronchial asthma is a chronic inflammatory disorder of the airways causing hyperresponsiveness, airway obstruction with wheezing, cough, and dyspnea.

Earliest change is decreased pCO_2 with respiratory alkalosis with normal pO_2. Then pO_2 decreases before pCO_2 increases.

[3]Source: Physicians Information and Education Resource. *ACP Observer* Jan–Feb 2006.

RESPIRATORY

With severe episode:

- Hyperventilation causes decreased pCO_2 in early stages (may be <35 mm Hg).
- Rapid deterioration of patient's condition may be associated with precipitous fall in pO_2 and rise in pCO_2 (>40 mm Hg).
- pO_2 <60 mm Hg may indicate severe attack or presence of complication.
- Normal pCO_2 suggests that the patient is tiring.
- Acidemia and increased pCO_2 suggest impending respiratory failure.

Mixed metabolic and respiratory acidosis occurs.

When a patient requires hospitalization, arterial blood gases should be measured frequently to assess status.

○ Eosinophilia and increased serum IgE may be present.

Sputum is white and mucoid without blood or pus (unless infection is present).

○ Eosinophils, Charcot-Leyden crystals (crystallized cationic proteins derived from eosinophils), and Curschmann spirals (casts of mucus and cell debris) may be found in sputum.

Sputum should be stained to rule out underlying bacterial infection or *Aspergillosis* colonization.

Laboratory findings caused by underlying diseases that may be primary and that should be ruled out, especially polyarteritis nodosa, parasitic infestation, bronchial carcinoid, drug reaction (especially aspirin), poisoning (especially cholinergic drugs and pesticides), hypogammaglobulinemia.

Bronchiectasis

Bronchiectasis is a permanent dilatation of airways that normally are <2 mm in diameter. A high-resolution computerized tomographic (CT) scan is noninvasive gold standard for diagnosis.

Caused By

Primary disorders of bronchial structure (e.g., cartilage defects)

Disorders of mucus clearance ($\sim3\%$, e.g., cystic fibrosis, ciliary function disorders)

Infectious ($>29\%$, e.g., severe pneumonia, especially *S. aureus, Klebsiella pneumoniae, M. pneumoniae, Bordetella pertussis,* influenza virus, adenovirus, severe measles or pertussis, mycobacteria; immunoglobulin deficiency)

Inflammatory (e.g., ulcerative colitis)

Idiopathic ($>50\%$ of cases)

WBC count usually normal unless pneumonitis is present.

Mild to moderate normocytic normochromic anemia with chronic severe infection.

Sputum abundant and mucopurulent (often contains blood); sweetish smell.

Sputum bacterial smears and cultures.

Laboratory findings due to complications (pneumonia, pulmonary hemorrhage, brain abscess, sepsis, cor pulmonale, occurs in $<29\%$ of COPD patients).

Rule out cystic fibrosis of the pancreas and hypogammaglobulinemia or agammaglobulinemia.

Bronchitis, Acute/Chronic

Due To

Viruses (e.g., RSV, rhinovirus, echovirus, coronavirus, adenovirus, parainfluenza, influenza) in most cases

Bacteria (e.g., *S. pneumoniae, M. pneumoniae, Chlamydia pneumoniae, B. pertussis, Legionella* sp., *H. influenzae)*

Fungi (e.g., *Candida* sp., *Cryptococcus neoformans, Histoplasma capsulatum, Coccidioides immitis, Blastomyces dermatitidis)*

Irritants (especially smoking)

WBC and erythrocyte sedimentation rate (ESR) normal or increased.

Eosinophil count increased if there is allergic basis or component.

Smears and cultures of sputum and bronchoscopic secretions.

Laboratory findings due to associated or coexisting diseases (e.g., emphysema, bronchiectasis).

Acute exacerbations are most commonly caused by:

- Viruses
- *M. pneumoniae*
- *H. influenzae*

- *S. pneumoniae*
- *Moraxella (Branhamella) catarrhalis*

Emphysema, Obstructive
Obstructive emphysema refers to permanent enlargement of the air spaces.

Laboratory findings of underlying disease that may be primary (e.g., pneumoconiosis, TB, sarcoidosis, kyphoscoliosis, fibrocystic disease of pancreas, α-1-antitrypsin deficiency).
Laboratory findings of associated conditions, especially duodenal ulcer.
Laboratory findings due to decreased lung ventilation:

- pO_2 decreased and pCO_2 increased; ultimate development of respiratory acidosis
- Secondary polycythemia
- ○ • Cor pulmonale

Lung Disease, Restrictive
Restrictive lung disease is characterized by decreased lung expansion with decreased total lung capacity.

Adult Respiratory Distress Syndrome[4,5]
ARDS is a unique clinical syndrome of acute lung injury causing severe unresponsive hypoxemia, pulmonary infiltrates in ≥3 lung regions not caused by volume overload or cardiovascular disease.

Due To
Noncardiac pulmonary edema and respiratory failure in the presence of the following associated events (more than one cause is often present):

- Pancreatitis, a very serious complication occurring in 20% to 50% of cases
- Sepsis: Most common; more likely caused by Gram-negative than Gram-positive organisms; occurs in 23% of cases of Gram-negative bacteremia
- Others (e.g., pneumonia, aspiration, shock, fat emboli, trauma, disseminated intravascular coagulopathy [DIC], several blood transfusions, smoke or toxic gas inhalation, certain types of drug toxicity)

Initially there is respiratory alkalosis and varying degrees of hypoxemia resistant to supplementary O_2; then profound anoxemia with pO_2 <50 mm Hg on room air.
Bronchoalveolar lavage shows increased PMNs (≤80%). Eosinophilia occurs occasionally.
Opportunistic organisms may be found if the disease presents as ARDS.
Acute onset of bilateral pulmonary infiltrates on radiographs.
Pulmonary function tests.

Goodpasture Syndrome
Goodpasture syndrome is characterized by alveolar hemorrhage and glomerulonephritis (GN) (usually rapidly progressive) associated with antibody against pulmonary alveolar and glomerular basement membranes. About 60% to 80% of cases show pulmonary and renal disease; 20% to 40% show renal disease alone; <10% show only pulmonary disease.

Proteinuria and RBCs and RBC casts in urine.
Renal function may deteriorate rapidly or renal manifestations may be mild.
- ◆ Renal biopsy may show characteristic linear immunofluorescent deposits of IgG and often complement and focal or diffuse proliferative GN.
- ◆ Serum may show antiglomerular basement membrane IgG antibodies by enzyme-linked immunosorbent assay (ELISA) (S/S ≥95%). Titer does not correlate with severity of pulmonary or renal disease but may indicate effectiveness of therapy.
Eosinophilia is absent and iron deficiency anemia more marked than in idiopathic pulmonary hemosiderosis.
Sputum or bronchoalveolar lavage showing hemosiderin-laden macrophages may be a clue to occult pulmonary hemorrhage.

[4]Esteban A, Fernandez-Segoviano P, Frutos-Vivar F, et al. Comparison of clinical criteria for the acute respiratory distress syndrome with autopsy findings. *Ann Intern Med* 2004;141:440–445.
[5]Piantadosi CA, Schwartz DA. The acute respiratory distress syndrome. *Ann Intern Med* 2004; 141:460–470.

RESPIRATORY

Other causes of combined pulmonary hemorrhage and GN are Wegener granulomatosis, hypersensitivity vasculitis, SLE, polyarteritis nodosa, endocarditis, mixed cryoglobulinemia, allergic angiitis and granulomatosis (Churg-Strauss syndrome), Behçet syndrome, Henoch-Schönlein purpura, and pulmonary-renal reactions to drugs (e.g., penicillamine).

Laboratory changes due to GN (e.g., proteinuria, hematuria, RBC casts in urine). Cytoplasmic and perinuclear antineutrophil cytoplasmic antibodies appear in ≤30% of cases sometime during the course of illness.

Hyaline Membrane Disease (Neonatal Respiratory Distress Syndrome)
See Chapter 14.

Hypersensitivity Pneumonitis
Hypersensitivity pneumonitis occurs with occupational and hobbyist exposure, (e.g., farmers, pigeon fanciers, etc.)

♦ Antibody (typically IgG, IgM, IgA) to offending materials is demonstrated in serum and often in BAL by various techniques (e.g., agar diffusion, ELISA, immunofluorescence assay IFA, CF, LA).

Others (e.g., eosinophilic granuloma [Chapter 11], sarcoidosis [Chapter 16], SLE [Chapter 16], Wegener granulomatosis [Chapter 5]).

Pneumoconiosis
♦ Biopsy of lung, scalene lymph node—histologic, chemical, spectrographic, and x-ray diffraction studies; electron microscopy (e.g., silicosis, berylliosis).

Bacterial smears and cultures of sputum (especially for tubercle bacilli).

Cytologic examination of sputum and bronchoscopic secretions for malignant cells.

Asbestos bodies are sometimes found in sputum after exposure to asbestos dust, even without clinical disease.

Increased WBC if associated infection.

Secondary polycythemia or anemia.

Acute beryllium disease may show occasional transient hypergammaglobulinemia.

Chronic beryllium disease may show:

• Secondary polycythemia
• Increased serum γ globulin
• Increased urine calcium
• Increased beryllium in urine long after beryllium exposure has ended.

Silicosis-associated conditions:

• Acute silicosis causing inexorable hypoxemic respiratory failure
• ≤25% have mycobacterial infections, half of which are nontuberculous
• Increased incidence of nocardiosis, cryptococcosis, sporotrichosis
• 10% have connective tissue diseases (e.g., progressive systemic sclerosis, RA, SLE)
• Increased incidence of antinuclear antibodies, rheumatoid factor, hypergammaglobulinemia. Angiotensin-converting enzyme increased in one third of patients.

Talc foreign body granulomas with birefringent silicate material seen with polarizing microscope.

Bentonite clay lung changes show foamy macrophages containing PAS-positive material.

Neoplasms, Lung

Carcinoid of Bronchus
See Chapter 13.

Carcinoma, Bronchogenic
Classified as:
Non-small cell lung carcinoma (NSCLC) in 70% to 75% of cases

• Squamous cell carcinoma (25%–30%)
• Adenocarcinoma (30%–35%)
• Large cell carcinoma (10%–15%)

Small cell lung carcinoma (SCLC) in 20% to 25% of cases
Combined pattern in 5% to 10% of cases

♦ Cytologic examination of sputum for malignant cells—positive in 40% of patients on first sample, 70% with three samples, 85% with five samples. False-positive tests are <1%.

♦ Sputum cytology is positive in 67% to 85% of squamous cell carcinoma, in 64% to 70% of small cell undifferentiated carcinoma, and in 55% of adenocarcinoma.
♦ Biopsy of scalene lymph nodes for metastases to indicate inoperable status—positive in 15% of patients.
♦ Biopsy of bronchus, pleura, lung, metastatic sites in appropriate cases.
♦ Cytology of pleural effusion (see "Pleural Effusion").
♦ Needle biopsy of pleura is positive in 58% of cases with malignant effusion.
♦ Transthoracic needle aspiration provides definitive cytologic diagnosis of cancer in 80% to 90% of cases; useful when other methods fail to provide a microscopic diagnosis.
♦ Thoracoscopy.
♦ Cancer cells in bone marrow and rarely in peripheral blood.
   ○ Biochemical tumor markers: Used for monitoring response to therapy and to correlate with staging.
   • Serum CEA is increased in one third to two thirds of patients with all four types of lung cancer.
     —Values <5 ng/mL correlate with survival over 3 years compared to level >5 ng/mL.
     —Values >10 ng/mL correlate with higher incidence of extensive disease and extrathoracic metastases.
     —A fall to normal suggests complete tumor removal.
     —A fall to still elevated values may indicate residual tumor.
     —An elevated unchanged value suggests residual progressive disease.
     —A value that falls and then rises during chemotherapy suggests that resistance to drugs has occurred.
   • Serum neuron-specific enolase (NSE) may be increased in 79% to 87% of patients with SCLC and in 10% of NSCLC and nonmalignant lung diseases (see Chapter 16). Pretreatment level correlates with stage of SCLC. May be used to monitor disease progression; it may fall in response to therapy and become normal in complete remission, but NSE is not useful for initial screening or detecting early recurrence. Is marker of choice in SCLC.
   • CEA, squamous cell carcinoma antigen, and NSE are increased in 25% and CYFRA 21-1 is increased in 67% of squamous cell carcinomas. CYFRA 21-1 is independent prognostic factor in earlier stages and NSE in advanced stages of squamous cell carcinoma.[6]

Paraneoplastic syndromes

• Endocrine and metabolic (primarily caused by SCLC):
   Adrenocorticotropic hormone (Cushing syndrome) is most commonly produced ectopic hormone (50% of patients with SCLC).
   Hypercalcemia occurs in >12% of patients (mostly epidermoid carcinoma); correlates with large tumor mass that is often incurable and quickly fatal (see Chapter 13.)
   Serotonin production by carcinoid of bronchus. (See "Serotonin," Chapter 13.)
   Syndrome of inappropriate secretion of antidiuretic hormone occurs in 11% of patients with SCLC.
   Prolactin usually due to anaplastic tumors.
   Gonadotropin production predominantly with large cell carcinoma.
   Renal tubular dysfunction with glycosuria and aminoaciduria.
   Hyponatremia due to massive bronchorrhea in bronchoalveolar cell carcinoma.
   Others (e.g., melanocyte-stimulating hormone, vasoactive intestinal peptides).
• Coagulopathies (e.g., DIC, migratory thrombophlebitis, chronic hemorrhagic diathesis).
• Neuromuscular syndromes (most commonly with SCLC) (e.g., myasthenia, encephalomyelitis—antineuronal antibodies and SCLC associated with limbic encephalitis).
• Cutaneous (e.g., dermatomyositis, acanthosis nigricans).

Syndromes due to metastases (e.g., functional hepatic changes, Addison disease, diabetes insipidus).

[6]Kulpa J, Wojcik E, Reinfuss M, et al. Carcinoembryonic antigen, squamous cell carcinoma antigen, CYFRA 21-1, and neuron-specific enolase in squamous cell lung cancer patients. *Clin Chem* 2002;48:1931–1937.

RESPIRATORY

Findings of complicating conditions (e.g., pneumonitis, atelectasis, lung abscess).
Normochromic, normocytic anemia in <10% of patients.

Mesothelioma[7-9]

Mesothelioma is caused most commonly caused by asbestos exposure.

♦ Cytology of pleural effusion or ascites.

♦ Histology by needle biopsy, thoracoscopy, electron microscopy, immunohistochemical staining (e.g., cytokeratin, osteopontin, calretinin, mesothelin).

♦ Serum mesothelin-related protein (soluble form of mesothelin) is increased in 84% of malignant mesothelioma patients and <2% of other lung or pleural diseases. May be useful to monitor therapy and possibly for screening.

♦ Serum osteopontin (ELISA) is increased and correlates with duration of exposure and radiographic changes. Levels may also be increased in other cancers (e.g., breast, pancreas).

♦ Restrictive pattern of pulmonary function tests is typical.

Anemia of malignancy, increased ESR, platelet count, γ globulin, hypoalbuminemia, and abnormal liver function tests are common.

Laboratory findings due to cardiac tamponade, superior vena cava syndrome, miliary spread, etc.

Pulmonary Infections

Abscess, Lung

A lung abscess is defined as a localized suppurative necrotic area >2 cm in size in the lung parenchyma.

Caused by bacteria (including tubercle bacilli). Anaerobic bacteria in ≤90% of cases, usually polymicrobial; aerobic bacteria in 50% of cases (usually with anaerobes); aerobic bacteria alone in 10% of cases. Also *Entamoeba histolytica, Paragonimus westermani*, fungi, etc.

An acute abscess (symptoms <2 weeks' duration) is less likely to have underlying neoplasm and to have infection with more virulent organism (e.g., *S. aureus*).

A chronic abscess (>4 weeks' duration) is more likely to have underlying neoplasm or to have infection with less virulent organism.

♦ Sputum—marked increase; abundant, foul, purulent; may be bloody; contains elastic fibers.

Putrid sputum is pathognomonic for anaerobic infection.

• Gram stain is diagnostic—sheets of PMNs with a bewildering variety of Gram-positive and Gram-negative organisms.

• Cytologic examination for malignant cells.

Blood culture—may be positive in acute stage.

Increased WBC in acute stages (15,000–30,000/μL).

Increased ESR.

Normochromic normocytic anemia in chronic stage.

Albuminuria is frequent.

Findings of underlying disease—especially bronchogenic carcinoma in ≤12% of cases; also aspiration pneumonia, alcoholism, drug addiction, septic embolus, postabortion state, coccidioidomycosis, amebic abscess, TB.

Associated with empyema in 30% of cases.

Allergic Bronchopulmonary Aspergillosis

Allergic bronchopulmonary aspergillosis is a hypersensitivity disorder caused by bronchial tree colonization with *Aspergillus fumigatus*.

♦ Demonstration of organism in sputum or BAL

Serologic tests

Laboratory findings due to associated conditions (e.g., bronchial asthma, bronchiectasis, cystic fibrosis)

Pneumonia

See Table 6-7. See Chapter 15 for organisms.

[7]Pass HI, Lott D, Lonardo F, et al. Asbestos exposure, pleural mesothelioma, and serum osteopontin levels. *N Engl J Med* 2005;353:1564–1573.

[8]Robinson BWS, Lake RA. Advances in malignant mesothelioma. *N Engl J Med* 2005;353:1591–1603.

[9]Cullen MR. Serum osteopontin levels: Is it time to screen asbestos-exposed workers for pleural mesothelioma? *N Engl J Med* 2005;353:1617–1618.

Table 6-7.   Causes of Pneumonia

Underlying Condition and Other Clues	Organism
Obstructive cancer	*Streptococcus pneumoniae, Haemophilus influenzae, Moraxella catarrhalis,* anaerobes
Alcoholics	*S. pneumoniae, H. influenzae, Klebsiella* sp., *Legionella* sp., anaerobes, *Mycobacterium tuberculosis,* aspiration pneumonia
Immunosuppressed conditions (e.g., AIDS, organ transplants, sickle cell disease)	**Bacteria:** Usual bacteria are *S. pneumoniae, H. influenzae, Staphylococcus aureus,* Gram-negative bacilli, *M. tuberculosis, M. avian-intracellulare, Legionella* sp. **Fungi:** *Aspergillus, Mucor,* and *Candida* sp., *Pneumocystis jiroveci (carinii), Cryptococcus neoformans, Histoplasma capsulatum, Coccidioides immitis, Blastomyces dermatitidis, Nocardia* sp. **Parasites:** *Strongyloides stercoralis* **Protozoa:** *Toxoplasma gondii* **Viruses:** Herpesviruses (especially CMV); also herpes simplex virus, respiratory syncytial virus, adenovirus, influenza virus
Atypical pneumonia	*Mycoplasma pneumoniae, Chlamydia psittaci, Chlamydia pneumoniae, Coxiella burnetii, Francisella tularensis,* many viruses
Other patients use same water-cooling facilities	*Legionella pneumophila*
Exposure to wild animals	Tularemia, plague
Exposure to farm animals	Anthrax, Q fever, severe acute respiratory syndrome
Exposure to birds	Psittacosis
Exposure to tuberculosis	*M. tuberculosis*
Travel	U.S. Southwest and deserts (coccidioidomycosis), midwestern United States (histoplasmosis), Africa (hemorrhagic fevers)
Epidemics	Typhus
Bronchopneumonia	Caused by wide range of organisms, including *S. aureus, H. influenzae, Klebsiella* sp., *Streptococcus pyogenes*
Interstitial pneumonia	Most often caused by viruses or *M. pneumoniae*

Caused By
Bacteria
S. pneumoniae causes 60% to 70% of bacterial pneumonia in patients requiring hospitalization. May cause ~25% of hospital-acquired cases of pneumonia. Blood culture positive in 25% of untreated cases during first 3 to 4 days.
Staphylococcus causes <1% of all acute bacterial pneumonia with onset outside the hospital but more frequent after outbreaks of influenza; may be secondary to measles, mucoviscidosis, prolonged antibiotic therapy, debilitating diseases (e.g., leukemia, collagen diseases), Frequent cause of nosocomial pneumonia. Bacteremia in <20% of patients.
H. influenzae is important in the 6- to 24-month age group; it is rare in adults except for middle-aged men with chronic lung disease and/or alcoholism and patients with immunodeficiency (HIV, multiple myeloma, chronic lymphocytic leukemia). Can mimic pneumococcal pneumonia; may be isolated with *S. pneumoniae.*
Klebsiella pneumoniae causes 1% of primary bacterial pneumonias, especially in alcoholics and upper lobe pneumonia; tenacious, viscid, red-brown ("currant jelly") sputum is typical. Blood culture positive in 25% of cases. WBC is variable.
Other Gram-negative bacilli (e.g., *Enterobacter, E. coli, Proteus mirabilis, Pseudomonas aeruginosa,* and *Acinetobacter*) are common causes of hospital-acquired pneumonia but unlikely outside the hospital.
Tubercle bacilli
Others (e.g., streptococcus, tularemia, plague)

Legionella pneumophila (see Chapter 15)
Mycoplasma pneumoniae is most common in the young adult male population (e.g., armed forces camps)
Chlamydia pneumoniae, Chlamydia psittaci
Viruses (e.g., influenza, parainfluenza, adenoviruses, RSV, echovirus, Coxsackievirus, reovirus, CMV, viruses of exanthems, herpes simplex, hantavirus)
Rickettsiae—Q fever is most common in endemic areas; typhus
Fungi (e.g., *Pneumocystis jiroveci [carinii], Histoplasma,* and *Coccidioides* in particular; blastomycosis, aspergillosis)
Protozoans (e.g., *Toxoplasma*)

Laboratory Findings

♦ Sputum reveals abundant WBCs in bacterial pneumonias. Gram stain shows abundant organisms in bacterial pneumonias (e.g., pneumococcal, staphylococcal). Culture sputum for appropriate bacteria. *Sputum that contains many organisms and WBCs on smear but no pathogens on aerobic culture may indicate aspiration pneumonia. Sputum is not appropriate for anaerobic culture.*
Sensitivity of sputum culture is estimated at 25% to 50%.
♦ In all cases of pneumonia, blood culture and sputum culture and smear for Gram stain should be performed before antibiotic therapy is started. Optimum specimen of sputum shows >25 PMNs and ≤5 squamous epithelial cells/LPF (10 × magnification), but >10 PMNs and <25 epithelial cells may be considered acceptable sputum specimen. Sample of >25 epithelial cells indicates unsatisfactory specimen from oropharynx and should not be submitted for culture. If good sputum specimen is obtained, further diagnostic microbiologic tests are usually not pursued.
Nasopharyngeal aspirate may identify *S. pneumoniae* with few false-positive findings, but *S. aureus* and Gram-negative bacilli often represent false-positive findings.
In *H. influenzae* pneumonia, sputum culture is negative in >50% of patients with positive cultures from blood, PF, or lung tissue, and may be present in the sputum in the absence of disease.
♦ Transtracheal aspiration (puncture of cricothyroid membrane) generally yields a faster, more accurate diagnosis.
♦ Protected brush bronchoscopy and BAL have high sensitivity.
♦ Diagnostic lung puncture to determine specific causative agent as a guide to antibiotic therapy may be indicated in critically ill children.
♦ Open lung biopsy is the gold standard, with 97% accuracy, but it has a 10% complication rate. Pleural effusions that are aspirated should also have Gram stain and culture performed.
♦ Respiratory pathogens isolated from blood, PF, or transtracheal aspirate (except patients with chronic bronchitis) or identified by bacterial polysaccharide antigen in urine may be considered the definite etiologic agent.
♦ Urine antigen for *S. pneumoniae,* type B *H. influenzae,* or *Legionella pneumophila* may be helpful.
Positive in ~90% of bacteremic pneumococcal and 40% of nonbacteremic pneumonias. May be particularly useful when antibiotic therapy has already begun.
Acute-phase serum should be stored at onset. If an etiologic diagnosis is not established, a convalescent-phase serum should be taken. A 4 × increase in antibody titer establishes the etiologic diagnosis (e.g., *L. pneumophila, Chlamydia* sp., respiratory viruses [including influenza and RSV], *M. pneumoniae*). Serologic tests to determine whether pneumonia is caused by *Histoplasma, Coccidioides,* etc.
WBC count is frequently normal or slightly increased in nonbacterial pneumonias; a considerable increase in the WBC count is more common in bacterial pneumonia. *In severe bacterial pneumonia, WBC count may be very high or low or normal. Because individual variation is considerable, it has limited value in distinguishing bacterial and nonbacterial pneumonia.*
Urine protein, WBCs, and hyaline and granular casts in small amounts are common. Ketones may occur with severe infection. *Check for glucose to rule out underlying diabetes mellitus.*

Miscellaneous Diseases

Histiocytosis X

See also Chapter 13.
♦ Diagnosis is established by open lung biopsy.

A pulmonary disorder is the major manifestation of this disease; bone involvement is seen in a minority of cases with lung disease. Pleural effusion is rare.

BAL shows increase in total number of cells; 2% to 20% are Langerhans cells, small numbers of eosinophils, neutrophils, and lymphocytes, and 70% are macrophages.

Most adults do not have positive gallium-67 scans.

Mild decrease in pO_2 is seen, which falls with exercise.

Lipoid Pneumonia

○ Sputum shows fat-containing macrophages that stain with Sudan. *They may be present only intermittently; therefore, examine sputum more than once.*

♦ Biopsy is diagnostic (performed because it mimics lung cancer and infectious disease).

Pulmonary Alveolar Proteinosis

Pulmonary alveolar proteinosis is a rare disease of unknown cause characterized by amorphous, lipid-rich, surfactant-like apoproteins in the alveoli that interfere with gas exchange. It is an idiopathic or secondary complication of AIDS, opportunistic infections, and hematologic malignancy.

○ PAS-positive material appears in sputum. Negative with Alcian blue.

○ PSP dye injected intravenously is excreted in sputum for long periods of time.

♦ Immunohistochemical stains positive for surfactant protein A and D in sputum, and BAL has been reported to be highly specific.

BAL fluid contains increased total protein, albumin, phospholipids, and CEA.

○ Serum CEA is increased and correlates with BAL. Reflects severity of disease and decreases with response to treatment.

○ Routine laboratory test findings are nonspecific.

• Serum LD increases in 80% of cases when protein accumulates in lungs and becomes normal when infiltrate resolves; correlates with serum CEA.

• Decreased arterial O_2.

• Secondary polycythemia may occur.

♦ Diagnosis usually requires open lung biopsy.

♦ Electron microscopy shows pathognomonic lamellar bodies in alveolar spaces or BAL.

Laboratory findings due to superinfection.

Pulmonary Embolism and Infarction and Phlebothrombosis

No laboratory test is diagnostic for pulmonary embolism (PE) or infarction or deep vein thrombosis (DVT). Only venography and pulmonary angiography are conclusive. Fewer than 10% of emboli lead to pulmonary infarction.

Tests that indicate recent extensive clotting of any origin (e.g., postoperative status):

• D-dimer test.

• Staphylococcal clumping test measures breakdown products of fibrin in serum; these indicate the presence of a clot that has begun to dissolve. S/S = 88%/66% using venography as the gold standard.

• Serial dilution protamine sulfate test measures the presence of a fibrin monomer that is one of the polymerization products of fibrinogen. It is less sensitive than the staphylococcal clumping test but indicates clotting earlier.

• Tests for coagulopathies; see Chapter 11.

♦ Plasma D-Dimer (Quantitative)[10,11]

Plasma D-dimer is a fibrin product generated by action of plasmin on cross-linked fibrin molecules indicating that a clot has formed. It is a direct marker of fibrinolysis (plasmin generation) and an indirect marker of coagulation (thrombin generation). Test results and cutoff values are not interchangeable between manufacturers and vary in sensitivities and specificities.

[10]Chunilal SD, Eikelboom JW, Attia J, et al. Does this patient have pulmonary embolism? *JAMA* 2003;290:2849–2858.

[11]Fedullo PF, Tapson VF. The evaluation of suspected pulmonary embolism. *N Engl J Med* 2003; 349:1247–1256.

RESPIRATORY

Use

Detects fibrin degradation products from lysis of both fibrin clot and fibrinogen.

◆ At cutoff level of 500 μg/L, newest ELISA tests have S/S >90%/~30%. NPV approaches 100%; therefore the most useful result is a normal value to *exclude* DVT and PE in patients with low to moderate pretest probability. Values lower than the cutoff level rule out this diagnosis and obviate need for other tests (e.g., pulmonary angiography).

Use only ELISA quantitative test for diagnosis of DVT/PE. Semiquantitative test (latex agglutination) is used *only* for diagnosis of DIC, not for DVT or PE. See Chapter 11.

Increased in (may remain increased for ≤7 days; usefulness decreases with time)

- DVT
- DIC with fibrinolysis
- Renal, liver, or cardiac failure
- Inflammation (e.g., arthritis), infection (e.g., pneumonia)
- Thrombolytic therapy
- Major injury or surgery
- Cancer
- Monoclonal gammopathy

○ Arterial blood gases (obtained when patient is breathing room air):
pO_2 <80 mm Hg in 88% of cases, but normal pO_2 does not rule out PE. In the appropriate clinical setting, pO_2 <88 mm Hg (even with a normal chest radiograph) is an indication for lung scans and search for DVTs. O_2 >90 mm Hg with a normal chest radiograph suggests a different diagnosis. Normal complete lung scans exclude the diagnosis. pCO_2 may be decreased because of hyperventilation and slightly elevated pH.

Serum enzymes are only indicated for differential diagnosis of acute myocardial infarction.

- Increased serum LD (due to LD isoenzymes 2 and 3) in 80% of patients rises on the first day, peaks on second day, and is normal by the tenth day.
- Increased serum alkaline phosphatase (heat-labile derived from vascular endothelium) during reparative phase 4 to 10 days after onset. Serum γ glutamyltransferase may be similarly increased.
- Serum aspartate aminotransferase is usually normal.
- Cardiac troponin is not increased.

◆ Increased BNP in the blood probably represents concomitant CHF causing or due to PE. An increase predicts adverse outcome in PE; low value has high NPV.

Increased WBC in 50% of patients is rarely >15,000/μL. Increased ESR.

"Triad" of increased LD and bilirubin with normal aspartate aminotransferase is found in only 15% of cases.

Serum indirect bilirubin is increased (as early as fourth day) to ~5 mg/dL in ≤20% of cases.

Pleural effusion occurs in one half of patients; bloody in one third to two thirds of cases; typical pattern in only one fourth of cases.

These laboratory findings depend on the size and duration of the infarction, and the tests must be performed at the appropriate time to detect abnormalities.

Laboratory findings caused by predisposing conditions:

- Malignant tumors
- Pregnancy
- Use of estrogens
- Hypercoagulable conditions (polycythemia vera, splenectomy with thrombocytosis, dysfibrinogenemias, protein C or S or antithrombin III deficiencies, anticardiolipin antibodies, lupus anticoagulant, hyperhomocysteinemia, others [see Chapter 11])
- Fat embolism (see "Diseases of Skeletal System," Chapter 10)

◆ Venography (now largely replaced by duplex ultrasonography) and spiral CT scans are rapidly replacing ventilation-perfusion scans, which were former gold standard methods to diagnose DVT and PE, respectively.

7 Gastrointestinal Diseases

Laboratory Tests of Gastrointestinal Function

Bentiromide

Bentiromide is a synthetic tripeptide. A dose of 500 mg, taken orally after an overnight fast, is cleaved by pancreatic chymotrypsin, releasing paraaminobenzoic acid (PABA) in the small intestine, which is measured in a 6-hour urine sample (normal value is >60%).

Use

Initial test gauges pancreatic exocrine (chymotrypsin) activity to rule out pancreatic disease in patients with chronic diarrhea, weight loss, or steatorrhea. Sensitivity of the 6-hour test is ≤100% in severe chronic pancreatitis (with steatorrhea) and 40% to 50% in mild to moderate chronic pancreatitis (without steatorrhea).

Accuracy may be increased with a D-xylose tolerance test or carbon-14-labeled-PABA for differentiation of pancreatic exocrine insufficiency from false-positive result (intestinal mucosal disease).

Interference

False-negative results may occur because of drugs (e.g., thiazides, chloramphenicol, sulfonamides, acetaminophen, phenacetin, sunscreens, procaine anesthetics) and certain foods (prunes, cranberries).

Decreased In

False-positive results: Renal insufficiency, diabetes mellitus gastric emptying, severe liver disease, or diffuse gut mucosal disease (malabsorption such as celiac sprue)

Biopsy, Colon

Rectal biopsy is particularly useful in diagnosis of

• Cancer of colon
• Polyps of colon

- Secondary amyloidosis
- Amebic ulceration
- Schistosomiasis (even when no lesions are visible)
- Hirschsprung disease
- Inflammatory bowel disease

Biopsy, Small Intestine

Use

Verifies mucosal lesions or establishes the diagnosis of various causes of malabsorption
Confirms deficiency of various enzymes in intestinal mucosal cells (e.g., lactase deficiency)
Diagnosis of neoplasms of small intestine
For differential diagnosis of some cases of diarrhea
For differential diagnosis of some nutritional deficiencies
Monitoring intestinal allografts

Biopsy is diagnostic (diffuse lesion, diagnostic histology):

- Whipple disease
- Agammaglobulinemia
- Abetalipoproteinemia (see Chapter 12: acanthotic red blood cells [RBCs], steatorrhea, failure of β-lipoprotein manufacture, neurologic findings)
- Celiac sprue (becomes normal after dietary gluten withdrawal and abnormal after challenge)
- *Mycobacterium avium-intracellulare* infection (organisms seen on AFB stains)

Biopsy may or may not be of specific diagnostic value (patchy lesions, diagnostic histology):

- Amyloidosis
- Intestinal lymphangiectasia
- Malignant lymphoma of small bowel
- Eosinophilic gastroenteritis
- Regional enteritis
- Systemic mastocytosis
- Hypogammaglobulinemia and dysgammaglobulinemia
- Parasitic infestations (giardiasis, coccidiosis, strongyloidiasis, capillariasis)

Biopsy may be abnormal but not diagnostic (diffuse lesions; histology not diagnostic):

- Celiac sprue
- Tropical sprue
- Severe prolonged folate and vitamin B_{12} deficiency
- Zollinger-Ellison syndrome
- Drug-induced lesions (neomycin, antimetabolites)
- Malnutrition
- Bacterial overgrowth of small bowel
- Graft-versus-host reaction
- Viral enteritis

Biopsy may be abnormal but not diagnostic (patchy lesions; histology abnormal but not diagnostic):

- Acute radiation enteritis
- Dermatitis herpetiformis enteropathy

Biopsy is normal:

- Cirrhosis
- Pancreatic exocrine insufficiency
- Postgastrectomy malabsorption without intestinal mucosal disease
- Functional bowel disease (irritable colon, nonspecific diarrhea)

During biopsy, x-ray localization, prompt fixation of tissue, proper orientation of tissue for histologic sectioning, and serial sectioning of specimen are all necessary for proper interpretation. Multiple biopsies may be necessary for patchy lesions.

D-Xylose Tolerance Test

D-xylose is a five-carbon sugar that remains intact when absorbed across intestinal mucosa; it is incompletely absorbed and is metabolized by gut bacteria. After an overnight fast, 5 or 25 g of d-xylose is given orally. Up to age 9 years, use 5-g dose and 1-hour serum sample; urine collection may not be reliable.

Normal:
>25 mg/dL in blood at 1 hour or >20 mg/dL 1 hour after 5-g dose.
With normal renal function, >4 mg/dL is excreted after 25-g dose.
Reference ranges may vary between laboratories.

Use
Screening test for diffuse small intestinal mucosal disease or bacterial overgrowth.
Follow response to gluten-free diet in celiac disease.
Replaced by biopsy except in diseases with patchy distribution of lesions.
Screening for intestinal malabsorption. Chief use is to distinguish proximal small intestinal malabsorption caused by impaired transport across diseased mucosa, which shows decreased values, from pancreatic steatorrhea (impaired digestion in lumen), which shows normal values.
Urine test has poor sensitivity in mild mucosal disease.
False-positive and false-negative rates of 20% to 30%.

Decreased In
Steatorrhea caused by proximal small intestinal malabsorption (e.g., sprue, some patients with *Giardia lamblia* infestation, bacterial overgrowth, viral gastroenteritis; may not be useful in adult celiac disease)
Decreased glomerular filtration, e.g.,

* Elderly persons
* Myxedema
* Ascites
* Increased portal pressure
* Renal insufficiency
* Delayed gastric emptying
* Vomiting
* Dehydration
* Drugs (e.g., nonsteroidal anti-inflammatory drugs [NSAIDs]), which can impair absorption or urinary excretions

Normal In
Steatorrhea caused by pancreatic disease
Postgastrectomy state
Malnutrition

Gastric Analysis

Use
Determine status of acid secretion in hypergastrinemia patients in whom a gastrinoma is suspected or who are being treated for gastrinoma
Rarely, to evaluate refractory peptic ulcer disease (e.g., determine whether patients who have undergone surgery for ulcer disease and who have complications are secreting acid).

Interpretation

1-h basal acid

<2 mEq	Normal, gastric ulcer, or carcinoma
2–5 mEq	Normal, gastric or duodenal ulcer
>5 mEq	Duodenal ulcer
>20 mEq	Z-E syndrome

1 h after stimulation by pentagastrin

0 mEq	Achlorhydria, gastritis, gastric carcinoma
1–20 mEq	Normal, gastric ulcer, or carcinoma
20–35 mEq	Duodenal ulcer
35–60 mEq	Duodenal ulcer, high normal, Z-E syndrome
>60 mEq	Z-E syndrome

Ratio of basal acid to poststimulation outputs

20%	Normal, gastric ulcer, or carcinoma
20%–40%	Gastric or duodenal ulcer
40%–60%	Duodenal ulcer, Z-E syndrome
>60%	Z-E syndrome

Z-E, Zollinger-Ellison syndrome.

Achlorhydria

Chronic atrophic gastritis (serum gastrin is frequently increased)

Pernicious anemia	100% of patients
Vitiligo	20%–25%
Alopecia areata	6%
Rheumatoid arthritis	10%–20%
Thyrotoxicosis	10%

Gastric carcinoma (50% of patients), even following pentagastrin stimulation. Hypochlorhydria occurs in 25%, hydrochloric acid is normal in 25%, hyperchlorhydria is rare in patients with gastric carcinoma.

Gastric ulcer	Common
Adenomatous polyps of stomach	85% of patients
Ménétrier disease	75%
Chronic renal failure	13% (usually normal; occasionally increased)

Iatrogenic

Postvagotomy, postantrectomy	>90%
Measure acid output after intravenous (IV) insulin to demonstrate adequacy of vagotomy (see "Insulin Test Meal")	
Medical (e.g., potent histamine 2 receptor antagonists, substituted benzimidazoles)	>80%

Occurs in normal persons: 4% of children, increasing to 30% of adults over age 60. *True achlorhydria excludes duodenal ulcer.*

Hyperchlorhydria and Hypersecretion[1]

Duodenal ulcer	40%–45%
Z-E syndrome (see Chapter 13);	100%

12-hour night secretion shows acid of >100 mEq/L and volume >1,500 mL.
Basal secretion is >60% of secretion caused by histamine or betazole stimulation.
Hyperplasia/hyperfunction of antral gastrin cells >90% (unusual condition with marked hyperchlorhydria, severe peptic ulceration, moderately increased fasting serum gastrin with exaggerated postprandial increase [>200% above fasting levels], no gastrin-secreting tumors.)

Hypertrophic hypersecretory gastropathy	100%
Massive resection of small intestine (transient)	50%
Systemic mastocytosis	Rare

When basal serum gastrin level is equivocal, serum gastrin level should be measured following stimulation with infusion of secretin or calcium.

Z-E, Zollinger-Ellison.

Gastrin, Serum

See Chapter 13
Normal levels: 0 to ≤200 pg/mL serum
Elevated levels: >500 pg/mL

---

[1]Rosenfeld L. Gastric tubes, meals, acid and analysis: rise and decline. *Clin Chem* 1997;43: 837–842.

Condition	Serum Gastrin	Serum Gastrin After Intragastric Administration of 0.1 N HCl
Peptic ulcer without Z-E syndrome	Normal range	—
Z-E syndrome	Very high	No change
Pernicious anemia	High level may approach that in Z-E syndrome	Marked decrease

Z-E, Zollinger-Ellison.

Secretin infusion (IV of 2 IU/kg body weight) with blood specimens drawn before and at intervals.

- Secretin test is preferred first test because of greater sensitivity and simplicity.
- Normal persons and patients with duodenal ulcer show no increase in serum gastrin.
- Patients with Zollinger-Ellison (Z-E) syndrome show increased serum gastrin that usually peaks in 45 to 60 minutes (usually >400 pg/mL). With fasting gastrin <1,000 pg/mL, sensitivity = 85% for an increased serum gastrin >200 pg/mL.
- With other causes of hypergastrinemia associated with hyperchlorhydria (e.g., retained antrum syndrome, gastric outlet obstruction, small bowel resection, renal insufficiency), serum gastrin is unchanged or decreases.

Calcium infusion (IV calcium gluconate, 5 mg/kg body weight/hr for 3 h) with preinfusion blood specimen compared to specimens every 30 minutes for up to 4 hours.

- Recommended when secretin test is negative in patients in whom Z-E syndrome is suspected.
- Normal patients and those with ordinary duodenal ulcer show minimal serum gastrin response to calcium.
- Patients with antral G cell hyperfunction may or may not show serum gastrin increase >400 pg/mL.
- Patients with Z-E syndrome show increase in serum gastrin >400 pg/mL in 2 to 3 hours (sensitivity = 43% for an increase of 395 pg/mL in serum gastrin). Positive in one third of patients with a negative secretin test.[2]

Indications for measurement of serum gastrin and gastric analysis include

- Atypical peptic ulcer of stomach, duodenum, or proximal jejunum, especially if multiple, in unusual location, poorly responsive to therapy, or multiple, with rapid onset, or showing severe recurrence after adequate therapy
- Unexplained chronic diarrhea or steatorrhea with or without peptic ulcer
- Peptic ulcer disease with associated endocrine conditions (see "Multiple Endocrine Neoplasia," Chapter 13)

Serum gastrin levels are indicated with any of the following:

- Basal acid secretion >10 mEq/h in patients with intact stomachs
- Ratio of basal to poststimulation output >40% in patients with intact stomachs
- All patients with recurrent ulceration after surgery for duodenal ulcer
- All patients with duodenal ulcer for whom elective gastric surgery is planned
- Patients with peptic ulcer associated with severe esophagitis or prominent gastric or duodenal folds or hypercalcemia or extensive family history of peptic ulcer disease
- Measurement for screening of all peptic ulcer patients would not be practical or cost effective

Increased Serum Gastrin without Gastric Acid Hypersecretion

Atrophic gastritis, especially when associated with circulating parietal cell antibodies PA in ~75% of patients
Some cases of carcinoma of body of stomach, a reflection of the atrophic gastritis that is present

[2]Frucht H, Howard JM, Slaff JI, et al. Secretin and calcium provocative tests in the Zollinger-Ellison syndrome. *Ann Intern Med* 1989;111:713–722.

Gastric acid inhibitor therapy
After vagotomy

Increased Serum Gastrin with Gastric Acid Hypersecretion

Z-E syndrome
Hyperplasia of antral gastrin cells
Isolated retained antrum (a condition of gastric acid hypersecretion and recurrent
    ulceration after antrectomy and gastrojejunostomy that occurs when the duodenal
    stump contains antral mucosa)

Increased Serum Gastrin with Gastric Acid Normal or Slight Hypersecretion

Rheumatoid arthritis (RA)
Diabetes mellitus
Pheochromocytoma
Vitiligo
Chronic renal failure with serum creatinine >3 mg/dL; occurs in 50% of patients
Pyloric obstruction with gastric distention
Short-bowel syndrome due to massive resection or extensive regional enteritis
Incomplete vagotomy

Insulin Test Meal

See Chapter 13.
Aspirate gastric fluid and measure gastric acid every 15 minutes for 2 hours after IV
    administration of sufficient insulin (usually 15 to 20 IU) to produce blood sugar
    <50 mg/dL.

Use
Differentiate causes of hypergastrinemia (see Table 13-14)
Supplanted by other tests; formerly used to
    Aid in distinguishing benign and malignant gastric ulcers
    Aid in diagnosis of PA
    Evaluate patients with ulcer dyspepsia but normal radiographs

Interpretation
Normal: Increased free HCl due to hypoglycemia.
Successful vagotomy produces achlorhydria.

Stool, Laboratory Examination

Normal Values

Bulk	100–200 g; 500 g on fiber-supplemented diet; >250 g is considered abnormal
Water	Up to 75%
Total osmolality	200–250 mOsm
PH	7.0–7.5 (may be acid with high lactose intake)
Nitrogen	<2.5 g/d
Potassium	5–20 mEq/kg
Sodium	10–20 mEq/kg
Magnesium	<200 mEq/kg
Coproporphyrin	400–1,000 mg/24 h
Trypsin	20–950 units/g
Urobilinogen	50–300 mg/24 h

Microscopic Examination

RBCs absent
Epithelial cells present (increased with gastrointestinal [GI] tract irritation); absence
    of epithelial cells in meconium of newborn may aid in diagnosis of intestinal obstruc-
    tion in the newborn
Few white blood cells (WBCs) present (increased with GI tract inflammation)
Crystals of calcium oxalate, fatty acid, and triple phosphate commonly present
Hematoidin crystals sometimes found after GI tract hemorrhage

Charcot-Leyden crystals sometimes found in parasitic infestation (especially amebiasis)
Some undigested vegetable fibers and muscle fibers sometimes found normally
Neutral fat globules (stained with Sudan), normal 0 to 2+

Color Changes

Normally: brown
Clay color (gray-white): biliary obstruction
Tarry: if >100 mL of blood in upper GI tract
Red: blood in large intestine or undigested beets or tomatoes
Black: blood
Silver: combination of jaundice and blood (cancer of ampulla of Vater)
Various colors: depending on diet

Due to Drugs	Resulting Color
Alkaline antacids and aluminum salts	White discoloration or speckling
Anticoagulants (excess)	Caused by bleeding
Anthraquinones	Brown staining
Bismuth salts	Black
Charcoal	Black
Diathiazine	Green to blue
Indomethacin	Green (due to biliverdin)
Iron salts	Black
Mercurous chloride	Green
Phenazopyridine	Orange-red
Phenolphthalein	Red
Phenylbutazone and oxyphenbutazone	Black (due to bleeding)
Pyrvinium pamoate	Red
Rhubarb	Yellow
Salicylates	Caused by bleeding
Santonin	Yellow
Senna	Yellow to brown
Tetracyclines in syrup (due to glucosamine)	Red

Occult Blood

See later in this chapter.

Chromium-51 Test for Bleeding

Tag 10 mL of the patient's blood with 7.4 MBq (200 μCi) of chromium-51 (^{51}Cr), and administer it IV. Collect daily stools for radioactivity measurement and also measure simultaneous blood samples.

Use

Measure GI blood loss in ulcerative diseases (e.g., ulcerative colitis, regional enteritis, peptic ulcer).

Interpretation

Radioactivity in the stool establishes GI blood loss. Comparison with radioactivity measurements of 1 mL of blood indicates the amount of blood loss.

Electrolytes

	Sodium (mEq/24 h)	Chloride (mEq/24 h)	Potassium (mEq/24 h)
Normal[a]	7.8 ± 2.0	3.2 ± 0.7	18.2 ± 2.5
Idiopathic proctocolitis	22.3	19.8	Normal
Ileostomy	30	19.0	4.1
Cholera	Increased	Increased	

[a]Average values for eight healthy individuals. Variable but considerably lower than simultaneous concentrations in serum.
Normal calcium ≅0.6 g/24 h.

Fat

See "Malabsorption."

Osmotic Gap

Osmotic Gap (OG) = measured osmolality minus $2 \times$ (Na + K) or 290 mOsm/kg H_2O
   minus $2 \times$ (Na + K)

Increased In

Osmotic diarrhea.
See "Factitious Disorders," Chapter 16.

Stool Findings	Possible Diagnosis
Osmotic gap <50 mOsm/kg H_2O and Na >90 mEq/L	Secretory diarrhea or osmotic diarrhea due to Na_2SO_4 or Na_2PO_4[a]
Osmotic gap >100 mOsm/kg H_2O and Na <60 mEq/L	Osmotic diarrhea; if fasting does not return stool volume to normal, consider factitious Mg ingestion[b]
Osmolality >375 mOsm/kg H_2O and Na <60 mEq/L	Possible contamination with concentrated urine
Osmolality <200–250 mOsm/kg H_2O	Possible contamination with dilute urine or water. Stool osmolality considerably lower than plasma osmolality; only useful if <250 mOsm/kg.

[a]Stool sulfate and phosphate increased; chloride <20 mEq/L.
[b]Mg usually >50 and often >100 mmol/L; normal during fasting <10 mmol/L; normal on regular diet = 10–45 mmol/L.

Other Procedures

Alkalinization of stool to pH of 10 turns blue due to phenolphthalein in certain laxa-
   tives. Useful in cases of laxative abuse.
Examination for ova and parasites.
Trypsin digestion (see "Cystic Fibrosis of Pancreas," Chapter 8).
See "Laboratory Diagnosis of Malabsorption."

Urobilinogen

Normal = 50 to 300 mg/24 h; 100 to 400 Ehrlich units/100 g.

Increased In

Hemolytic anemias

Decreased In

Complete biliary obstruction
Severe liver disease
Oral antibiotic therapy altering intestinal bacterial flora
Decreased hemoglobin turnover (e.g., aplastic anemia, cachexia)

Latex Agglutination Test Kit for Leukocytes

Detects fecal lactoferrin, a marker protein for fecal leukocytes; uses frozen or fresh
   stool.

Use

Detection of bowel inflammation not evident by endoscopy or radiographic studies.

Interpretation

In one study a stool dilution of 1:50 had a negative predictive value (NPV) of 94% for
   the presence of invasive enteropathogens. Positive predictive value (PPV) and NPV
   of 93% and 88%, respectively, compared to stool microscopy for leukocytes are
   reported. At 1:200 dilution, sensitivity <70%; therefore if test is negative when
   infectious must be ruled out with considerable certainty (e.g., immunocompromised
   patient), stool should be cultured.
[111]Indium-labeled leukocytes have been used as quantitative index of fecal leukocyte
   loss in research laboratory.

Microscopic Examination of Diarrheal Stools for Leukocytes

Primarily polymorphonuclear leukocytes (PMNs)—any number of PMNs found in fewer than two thirds of cases

* Shigellosis: 70% had >5 PMNs/oil immersion field
* Salmonellosis: 30% had >5 PMNs/oil immersion field
* Campylobacter: 30% had >5 PMNs/oil immersion field
* Rotavirus: 11% had >5 PMNs/oil immersion field
* Invasive *Escherichia coli* colitis
* Yersinia infection
* Ulcerative colitis
* *Clostridium difficile* (see "Colitis, Pseudomembranous")

Primarily mononuclear leukocytes

* Typhoid

Leukocytes absent

* Cholera
* Noninvasive *E. coli* diarrhea
* Other bacterial toxins (e.g., *Staphylococcus*, *Clostridium perfringens*)
* Viral diarrheas
* Parasitic infestations (e.g., *G. lamblia*, *Entamoeba histolytica*, *Dientamoeba fragilis*)
* Drug related

Fecal Calprotectin[3]

Calprotectin constitutes ~60% of the soluble cytosol proteins in neutrophils and correlates with the intensity of neutrophilic infiltration and therefore the severity of inflammation.

Concentrations (assayed by enzyme-linked immunosorbent assay [ELISA] antibodies) in patients with chronic diarrhea is reported to identify patients with inflammatory bowel disease (IBD) with these characteristics:

	Sensitivity[a]	Specificity[a]	PPV[a]	NPV[a]
Cutoff = 50 μg/g stool	55%–77%	77%–91%	76%–90%	58%–78%
Cutoff = 100 μg/g stool	33%–59%	88%–100%	84%–96%	47%–71%

PPV, positive predictive value; NPV, negative predictive value.
[a]95% confidence limits.

Also increased by: Drugs (e.g., aspirin, NSAIDs), hepatitis C virus infection, and cirrhosis.
In children, increased in cow's milk and other food allergies.

Disorders of the Gastrointestinal Tract

Disorders of the Esophagus

Carcinoma of the Esophagus

♦ Cytologic examination of esophageal washings is positive for malignant cells in 75% of patients. It is falsely positive in <2% of patients.
♦ Diagnosis is confirmed by biopsy of tumor.

Diaphragmatic Hernia

Microcytic anemia (because of blood loss) may be present.
Stool may be positive for blood.

[3]Carroccio A, Iacono G, Cottone M, et al. Diagnostic accuracy of fecal calprotectin assay in distinguishing organic causes of chronic diarrhea from irritable bowel syndrome. *Clin Chem* 2003;49: 861–867.

Esophageal Varices[4]

Varices are portal-systemic collaterals formed after preexisting vascular channels are dilated by portal hypertension. They do not form unless the hepatic venous pressure gradient is at least 12 mmHg.

Varices occur in 40% to 60% of patients with cirrhosis. Variceal hemorrhage occurs in 25% to 35% of patients. Initial bleeds are fatal in ≤30%. The 1-year survival rate ranges from 32% to 80%.

Varices cause 80% to 90% of episodes of GI bleeding in patients with cirrhosis.

Increased risk of bleeding with increasing severity of cirrhosis (see Chapter 8).

Infections of Esophagus

Caused By
Fungi

* *Candida albicans* is most common; other *Candida* species
* *Torulopsis glabrata*
* *Aspergillus* species
* *Histoplasma capsulatum*
* *Blastomyces dermatitidis*

Viruses

* Herpes simplex virus (especially in AIDS patients)
* Cytomegalovirus (CMV) (especially in AIDS patients)
* HIV-1
* Epstein-Barr
* Varicella-zoster

Bacteria

* Gram-positive, usual oral flora (e.g., *Streptococcus viridans*, *Staphylococcus*)
* Gram-negative cocci, rods, enteric bacilli
* Tubercle bacilli (rare; usually no evidence of active pulmonary disease)
* *Actinomyces israelii*
* *Treponema pallidum*

Predisposing factors

* Immunosuppression (e.g., HIV)
* Drugs (e.g., corticosteroids, anticancer chemotherapy, radiation, broad-spectrum antibiotics)
* Debilitating illnesses (e.g., diabetes mellitus, chronic renal failure, burns, elderly persons)
* Trauma (e.g., nasogastric tubes, tracheal intubation)

◆ Diagnosis by endoscopy: cytologic brushings, biopsy, bacterial smears, and cultures

Mallory-Weiss Syndrome

Mallory-Weiss syndrome is characterized by spontaneous cardioesophageal laceration, usually caused by retching.

Laboratory findings due to hemorrhage from cardioesophageal laceration.

Perforation of Esophagus, Spontaneous

◆ In spontaneous perforation of the esophagus, gastric contents will be found in thoracocentesis fluid.

Plummer-Vinson Syndrome

Plummer-Vinson syndrome is an iron-deficiency anemia associated with dysphagia, atrophic gastritis, glossitis, etc. It carries an increased risk of cancer of the esophagus and hypopharynx.

---

[4]Sharara AI, Rockey DC. Gastroesophageal variceal hemorrhage. *N Engl J Med* 2001;345:669–681.

Primary Systemic Diseases, Esophagus Involvement In

Scleroderma *(esophageal involvement in >50% of patients with scleroderma)*
Esophageal varices (cirrhosis of liver)
Malignant lymphoma
Bronchogenic carcinoma
Infections (see previous section)
Sarcoidosis
Crohn disease (CD)
Behçet disease
Graft-versus-host disease
Pemphigus vulgaris
Bullous pemphigoid
Benign mucous membrane pemphigoid
Epidermolysis bullosa dystrophica

Disorders of the Stomach

Dumping Syndrome

Dumping syndrome is the term used to describe clinical manifestations of abnormally rapid gastric emptying. Occurs in some patients with Z-E syndrome, pancreatic insufficiency patients, and ≤15% of postvagotomy or other gastric surgery patients.

There are no specific laboratory findings. During symptoms, patients may have:

• Rapid prolonged alimentary hyperglycemia
• Decreased plasma volume
• Decreased serum potassium
• Increased blood and urine serotonin
• Hypoglycemic syndrome (occurs in <5% of post-subtotal gastrectomy patients)
  Prolonged alimentary hyperglycemia followed after 2 hours by precipitous hypoglycemia
  Late hypoglycemia shown by 6-hour oral glucose tolerance test

Laboratory findings due to complications of gastric or duodenal ulcer or surgery, e.g., hemorrhage, perforation, obstruction:

• Stomal gastritis—anemia caused by chronic bleeding
• Postgastrectomy malabsorption
• Postgastrectomy anemia (due to chronic blood loss, malabsorption, vitamin B_{12} deficiency, etc.)
• Afferent-loop obstruction—marked increase in serum amylase

Gastritis, Benign Giant Hypertrophic (Ménétrier Disease)

Ménétrier disease is a rare idiopathic diffuse enlargement of the gastric folds in the antrum.
○ Protein-losing enteropathy causing decreased serum protein and albumin due to loss of plasma proteins through gastric mucosa; γ globulins may be decreased. Protein loss is nonselective, in contrast to loss through the glomerular membrane, in which there is greater loss of low-molecular-weight versus high-molecular-weight proteins.
♦ Diagnosis is confirmed by full-thickness gastric biopsy; superficial biopsy may appear normal.
○ Serum calcium may be low because of decreased serum albumin.
Hypochlorhydria is diagnosed by gastric analysis in 75% of cases. Gastric fluid taken during endoscopy shows increased protein concentration (normal = 0.8–2.5 g/L), and protein electrophoresis resembles pattern of serum electrophoresis. Increased pH of gastric fluid (normal <2).
Protein loss can also be determined by injecting radiolabeled ^{51}Cr-albumin and measuring radioactivity in stool. Can also use α_1-antitrypsin clearance (calculated by measuring trypsin in blood and stool; normal <13) to measure protein loss, since this resists digestion by trypsin; can only be used if there is acid hyposecretion since it is destroyed by pH <3.

Laboratory findings due to complications (e.g., iron deficiency anemia caused by chronic GI hemorrhage, edema caused by hypoalbuminemia).
Liver function tests are normal.
Proteinuria is absent.

Gastritis, Chronic

♦ A diagnosis of chronic gastritis depends on biopsy of gastric mucosa.

Atrophic (Type A Gastritis; Autoimmune Type; Gastric Antrum Is Spared)

Parietal cell antibodies and intrinsic factor antibodies help identify those patients prone to PA.
Achlorhydria
Vitamin B_{12} deficient megaloblastosis
Hypergastrinemia (due to hyperplasia of gastrin-producing cells)
Gastric carcinoids
Low serum pepsinogen I concentrations
Laboratory findings due to other autoimmune diseases (e.g., Hashimoto thyroiditis, Addison disease, Graves disease, myasthenia gravis, hypoparathyroidism, insulin-dependent diabetes mellitus)

Nonatrophic (Type B Gastritis; Gastric Antrum Is Involved)

Anemia caused by iron deficiency and malabsorption may occur.
Helicobacter pylori infection; is detectable in ~80% of patients with peptic ulcer and chronic gastritis. Diagnosis by biopsy, culture, direct Gram stain, urease test, serologic tests. (See Chapter 15.)
Hypogastrinemia (caused by destruction of gastrin-producing cells in antrum).
Chronic antral gastritis is consistently present in patients with benign gastric ulcer.
Gastric acid studies are of limited value. Severe hypochlorhydria or achlorhydria after maximal stimulation usually denotes mucosal atrophy.

Others

Infections (other bacteria [syphilis], viral [e.g., CMV], parasitic [e.g., anisakiasis], fungal)
Chemical (e.g., NSAIDs, bile reflux, drugs)
Lymphocytic gastritis
Eosinophilic gastroenteritis
Noninfectious granulomatous (e.g., sarcoidosis, CD)
Ménétrier disease
Radiation

Neoplasms, Gastric

♦ Diagnosis is confirmed by biopsy of tumor.
♦ Lymph node biopsy for metastases; needle biopsy of liver, bone marrow, etc.

Adenomatous Polyps

Accounts for 10% to 20% of polyps that are premalignant; most are hyperplastic (not premalignant).
May occur in familial adenomatous polyposis, Gardner syndrome, Ménétrier disease.
Gastric analysis reveals achlorhydria in 85% of patients.
Sometimes there is evidence of bleeding.
Polyps occur in 5% of patients with pernicious anemia (PA) and 2% of patients with achlorhydria.

Carcinoma

♦ Exfoliative cytology positive in 80% of patients; false-positive result in <2%
Tumor markers are not useful for early detection.

• Increased serum carcinoembryonic antigen (CEA) (>5 ng/dL) in 40% to 50% of patients with metastases and 10% to 20% of patients with surgically resectable

disease. May be useful for postoperative monitoring for recurrence or to estimate metastatic tumor burden.
• Increased serum α-fetoprotein and cancer antigen (CA) 19-9 in 30% of patients, usually incurable.

Gastric analysis

• Achlorhydria following histamine or betazole in 50% of patients
• Hypochlorhydria in 25% of patients
• Normal in 25% of patients
• Hyperchlorhydria rare

Anemia due to chronic blood loss
Occult blood in stool
○ *Carcinoma of the stomach should always be searched for by periodic prophylactic screening in high-risk patients, especially those with PA, gastric atrophy, gastric polyps.*

Leiomyoma, Leiomyosarcoma, Lymphoma

These neoplasms may show evidence of bleeding.

Carcinoid

See Chapter 13.

Peptic Ulcer Disease

Duodenal Ulcer and Gastric Peptic Ulcer

♦ *H. pylori*–associated gastritis is present in ~95% of all patients with duodenal ulcer except those with Z-E syndrome. (See Chapter 15.)

Laboratory Findings Caused by Associated Conditions

• Z-E syndrome, multiple endocrine neoplasia (MEN) type I, hyperparathyroidism
• Various drugs (e.g., adrenocorticotropic hormone and adrenal steroids, NSAIDs)
• Chronic renal failure
• Kidney stones
• α antitrypsin deficiency
• Systemic mastocytosis
• Chronic pancreatitis
• Mucoviscidosis
• RA
• Chronic pulmonary disease (e.g., pulmonary emphysema)
• Cirrhosis
• CD
• Polycythemia vera

Laboratory Findings Caused by Treatment

• Milk-alkali (Burnett) syndrome: alkalosis, hypercalcemia, azotemia, renal calculi, or nephrocalcinosis
• Vagotomy (dumping syndrome)

Laboratory Findings Caused by Underlying Conditions

• *Curling ulcer—hemorrhage 8 to 10 days and perforation 30 days after burn; causes death in 15% of fatal burn cases*
• Cerebrovascular accidents and trauma and inflammation (Cushing ulcer)

Laboratory Findings Due to Complications

Gastric retention—dehydration, hypokalemic alkalosis.
Perforation—increased WBC count with shift to the left, dehydration, increased serum amylase, increased amylase in peritoneal fluid.
Hemorrhage.

Recurrent ulcer after partial gastrectomy (≤3% of patients) may be caused by adequacy of operation, but acid secretory syndrome should be considered (e.g., gastrinoma, retained antrum syndrome) and serum gastrin should be assayed.
*Peptic ulcer is absent in patients with ulcerative colitis (unless under steroid therapy),
carcinoma of stomach, pernicious anemia, and pregnancy.*

Diseases of the Intestine

Appendicitis, Acute

Twenty percent of acute appendicitis patients have atypical clinical findings.
Increased WBC count (12,000 to 14,000/μL) with shift to the left in acute catarrhal
stage; higher and more rapid rise with suppuration or perforation.
Erythrocyte sedimentation rate (ESR) may be normal during first 24 hours.
It has been said that a c-reactive protein (CRP) <2.5 mg/dL at 12 hours after onset of
symptoms excludes acute appendicitis.
Later: laboratory findings due to complications (e.g., dehydration, abscess formation,
perforation with peritonitis)
○ Urine may contain WBC, RBCs, bacteria in ≤40% of patients in emergency room
with acute abdominal pain. More than 30 RBCs/high-power field (hpf) or >20 WBC/
hpf suggests genitourinary (GU) tract disorder.
♦ Plain radiograph, ultrasound, and computed tomographic (CT) scan are very useful,
especially if patient is obese, elderly, immunosuppressed, or has a right lower quad-
rant mass.

Bacterial Overgrowth

Due To
Decreased gastric acid (e.g., PA, atrophic gastritis, gastric surgery, drugs such as
proton-pump inhibitors)
Structural changes (e.g., adhesions, diverticula, fistulas, surgical anastomoses)
Motility syndromes (e.g., diabetes mellitus, acute infections, scleroderma)
Deficient host defenses
Anemia may be megaloblastic or macrocytic because of cobalamin deficiency.
Decreased cobalamin (bacteria consume cobalamin) but increased folate (which is a
product of bacterial fermentation).
Deficiency of water-soluble vitamins (thiamine, nicotinamide) and fat-soluble vitamins
(A, D, E, K).
Fecal fat is increased.
Schilling test with intrinsic factor test is decreased.
Radiolabeled breath tests use D-xylose (catabolized by Gram-negative aerobes and
absorbed in the proximal small bowel) or bile acids deconjugated by glycolic acid bac-
teria).
Fasting breath H$_2$ test is increased with early increase after glucose or lactulose chal-
lenge reflects increased bacterial fermentation. Insufficient sensitivity/specificity
(S/S).
Jejunal aspirate for bacterial count and identification may show >10^5/mL with colonic
organisms.
Usual bacterial counts

• Stomach <10^4/mL
• Ileum <10^6/mL
• Jejunum <10^5/mL
• Colon <10^{10}/mL

Celiac Disease (Gluten-Sensitive Enteropathy, Nontropical Sprue, Idiopathic Steatorrhea)[5,6]

**Celiac disease is an autoimmune multisystem disorder (principally manifested in
the GI tract) in genetically susceptible persons that may be caused by mucosal**

[5]Farrell RJ, Kelly CP. Celiac sprue. *N Engl J Med* 2002;346:180–188.
[6]Mäki M, Mustalahti K, Kokkonen J, et al. Prevalence of celiac disease among children in Finland.
N Engl J Med 2003;348:2517–2524.

injury by a complex of gliadin (a protein from dietary gluten in wheat, rye, barley, or oats) with tissue transglutaminase (tTG), a cross-linking enzyme. Findings are caused by malabsorption and autoimmunity.

See Figure 7-1.

Diagnostic Criteria

Presumptive

- Positive serologic test
- Biopsy diagnostic of celiac disease

Definite

- On gluten-free diet, resolution of symptoms, disappearance of serology titer, and reversal of biopsy findings (optional)

♦ Serologic tests (not performed on gluten-free diet)[7,8]:

- Anti-IgA endomysial antibodies (EMA) by ELISA or if S/S >85%/>95% and is antibody test of choice to support the diagnosis and to screen populations at risk. (Endomysium is sheath of reticular fibrils around muscle fibers.)
- Anti-IgA tTG antibodies (by ELISA) has S/S = >90%/>95%. False-negative results may occur in patients with IgA deficiency (present in 2.5% of patients with celiac disease for whom corresponding IgG antibody tests may be useful). More reproducible than EMA test.
- Antigliadin IgA antibodies (by ELISA) have been superseded by these more sensitive tests; has S/S = 80%/80%–90%. IgA antigliadin antibodies becomes undetectable 3 to 6 months after gluten abstinence; may be used to monitor dietary compliance. May be most effective marker for children <3 years of age. Gliadin is a component of gluten.
- False-negative results may occur in patients on immunosuppressive therapy.
- If patient is IgA deficient, serology using IgG-tTG or IgG-EMA should be used.

♦ Biopsy of jejunum is the diagnostic gold standard; shows characteristic although not specific mucosal lesions. Establishing the diagnosis is essential; patients should not be committed to lifelong gluten-free diet without first assessing intestinal mucosal histology. False-negative results may occur because of patchy distribution of pathology.

♦ Firm diagnosis requires definite clinical response to gluten-free diet in 3 to 9 months, preferably with histologic documentation that the mucosa has reverted to normal by repeat biopsy. If patient fails to respond to rigid dietary control, biopsy should be repeated to rule out GI lymphoma, giardiasis, hypogammaglobulinemia and other causes of villous atrophy; and diet should be rechecked.

♦ Gluten challenge is no longer considered essential to establish the diagnosis. It is done if the diagnosis is uncertain and not documented by biopsy before gluten withdrawal, to determine if symptoms and mucosal changes occur.

○ Steatorrhea demonstrated by positive Sudan stain on ≥2 stool samples or quantitative determination of fat in 72-hour pooled stool sample.

○ Xylose tolerance test distinguishes malabsorption caused by impaired transport across diseased mucosa from that caused by impaired digestion in lumen. Normal in many patients with mild to moderate disease.

○ Malabsorption may cause folate deficiency with megaloblastic bone marrow and iron deficiency with mild hypochromic macrocytic anemia. Celiac disease should always be considered in cases of iron deficiency or macrocytic anemia. May also have coagulopathy due to vitamin K deficiency and hypocalcemia and vitamin D deficiency causing osteomalacia. In patients with unexplained diarrhea or malabsorption celiac sprue should be ruled out by small bowel biopsy.

---

[7]Alaedini A, Green PHR. Narrative review: celiac disease: understanding a complex autoimmune disorder. *Ann Intern Med* 2005;142:289–298.
[8]Van Meensel B, Hiele M, Hoffman I, et al. Diagnostic accuracy of ten second-generation (human) tissue transglutaminase antibody assays in celiac disease. *Clin Chem* 2004;50:2125–2135.

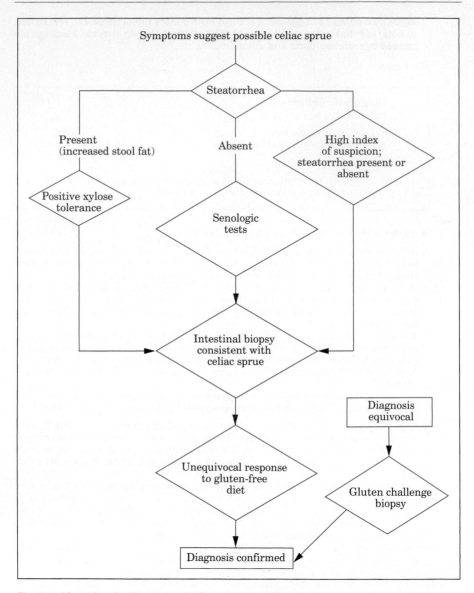

Fig. 7-1. Algorithm for diagnosis of celiac sprue.

○ Laboratory findings due to frequently associated autoimmune diseases ([e.g., thyroid, liver], type 1 diabetes mellitus, dermatitis herpetiformis [≤20% of celiac patients], Addison disease, arthritis) and other diseases (e.g., selective IgA deficiency; hyposplenism, T-cell lymphoma of small intestine; also Down syndrome, IgA nephropathy, inflammatory bowel disease). Patients who should be screened include those with steatorrhea, malabsorption, or autoimmune diseases.

Human leukocyte antigen (HLA) variation DQ2 is expressed in ~95% of patients; HLA-DQ8 is expressed in ~5% of patients; absence of these virtually excludes this diagnosis.

See Figure 7-2.

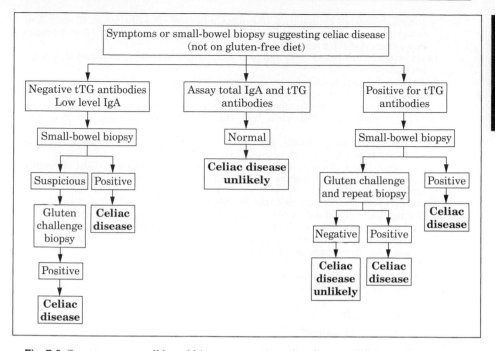

Fig. 7-2. Symptoms or small bowel biopsy suggesting celiac disease. tTG, transglutaminase.

Chloridorrhea, Congenital

Congenital chloridorrhea is a rare autosomal recessive condition of profound watery diarrhea beginning at birth caused by a Cl^-/HCO_3^- transport defect in the ileum and colon.

♦ Hypochloremia, hypokalemia, hyponatremia, metabolic alkalosis, dehydration.
♦ Copious, acidic, chloride-rich (>100 mEq/L) diarrhea.
Normal intestinal mucosal histology.
There is also a similar but rarer autosomal recessive condition of congenital diarrhea with sodium-rich (sodium > chloride), alkaline stool, increased fecal HCO_3^-, and metabolic acidosis.

Colitis, Collagenous

Collagenous colitis is a syndrome of chronic nonbloody diarrhea. The incidence is ~3/1,000 in such patients.

♦ Diagnosis is established by biopsy of colon in patients thought to have irritable bowel syndrome.
ESR is increased, and anemia, hypoalbuminemia occur in some patients.
Eosinophil count is increased in some patients.

Colitis, Pseudomembranous

Pseudomembranous colitis is an antibiotic-related diarrhea and colitis caused by _C. difficile_.

♦ Tissue culture assay is gold standard (S/S >94%/99%). Level of toxin is not related to clinical severity.

♦ Diagnosis depends on detection of cytotoxin in stool. Demonstration of toxin A or antigens by rapid immunoassays shows good S/S = 64%–87%/99%. Rapid results make these useful for screening.

Latex agglutination has variable and poor sensitivity and is not recommended as a single test.

Detection of glutamate dehydrogenase enzyme by latex agglutination or immunoassay lacks good specificity (enzyme found in other organisms). Stool assay for glutamate dehydrogenase enzyme combined with toxin A assay in one test may be more useful.

For *C. difficile*–associated diarrhea, both culture and cytotoxin assay should be performed.

Counterimmune electrophoresis, gas-liquid chromatography, and Gram stain of stool have high false-negative and false-positive results.

Stool culture is less efficient, since some strains are nontoxinogenic; >50% of healthy neonates, 2% to 5% of healthy adults, and ≤25% of adults recently treated with antibiotics are carriers.

Nontoxinogenic strains may be found in 10% to 20% of hospitalized patients. Toxin testing alone will not detect 20% to 30% of *C. difficile*–associated diarrhea.

Polymerase chain reaction of stool for toxin A and/or B may be available.

Fecal leukocytes in stool (see "Stool, Laboratory Examination"); large numbers in 50% of cases; bloody diarrhea in ≤10% of cases.

WBC count >15,000/μL in <50% of cases.

Hypoalbuminemia in ≤24% of cases.

Laboratory findings due to dehydration and electrolyte imbalance in severe cases.

Diarrhea, Acute

See Table 7-1 and Figure 7-3.

Osmotic (Malabsorptive) Diarrhea

Osmotic diarrhea is defined as diarrhea with a <3-week (upper limit 6–8 weeks) duration. Increased osmotically active solutes in bowel; diarrhea usually stops during fasting.

Due To
Exogenous

• Laxatives (e.g., magnesium sulfate, milk of magnesia, sodium sulfate [Glauber's salt], sodium phosphate, polyethylene glycol/saline)
• Drugs (e.g., lactulose, colchicine, cholestyramine, neomycin, PAS)
• Foods (e.g., mannitol, sorbitol [in diet candy, chewing gum, soda])

Endogenous
Congenital malabsorption

• Specific (e.g., lactase deficiency, fructose malabsorption)
• General (e.g., abetalipoproteinemia and hypobetalipoproteinemia, congenital lymphangiectasia, cystic fibrosis)

Acquired malabsorption

• Specific (e.g., pancreatic disease, celiac sprue, parasitic infestation, rotavirus enteritis, metabolic disorders [thyrotoxicosis, adrenal insufficiency], jejunoileal bypass, bacterial overgrowth, short-bowel syndrome, inflammatory disease [e.g., mastocytosis, eosinophilic enteritis])

Secretory (Abnormal Electrolyte Transport) Diarrhea

Secretory diarrhea is caused by increased water and chloride secretion; normal water and sodium absorption may be inhibited.

Caused By
Exogenous
Drugs

• Laxatives (e.g., aloe, anthraquinones, bisacodyl, castor oil, dioctyl sodium sulfosuccinate, phenolphthalein, senna)

Table 7-1. Comparison of Acute Infectious Diarrhea

Community-Acquired/Traveler's Diarrhea	Nosocomial with Onset >3 Days After Hospitalization	Persistent Diarrhea (>7 d)	Immunocompromised, Especially if HIV+
Salmonella,[a,b] *Yersinia,*[a] *Cyclospora*[a] *Shigella*[b,c] *Campylobacter*[b,d] Toxin-producing *E. coli* O157:H7[b,e] *C. difficile* toxins A/B[f] *E. histolytica* *Vibrio*[b,h] Norwalk virus[b,j] (viral antigen in stool) Rotavirus (EIA of stool for antigen) Adenovirus (EIA of stool) Cytomegalovirus *Staphylococcus aureus,*[k] *Bacillus cereus*[k,l]	*Clostridium difficile* toxins A/B *Salmonella* *Shigella* *Campylobacter* Toxin-producing *E. coli*	Consider: protozoa, e.g., *Cyclospora*[a,b] *Cryptosporidium*[b,g] *Giardia*[b,i] *Isospora belli*	Consider: Microsporidia *Mycobacterium avium-intracellulare* Culture from biopsy of colon

EIA, electroimmunoassay.
[a]Consider food-borne; community-acquired.
[b]Consider if onset in 16 to 72 hours.
[c]Consider person-to-person; community-acquired.
[d]Consider undercooked poultry; community-acquired.
[e]Consider food-borne, especially undercooked hamburger or raw seed sprouts; community-acquired.
[f]Consider recent antibiotic use.
[g]Consider waterborne, especially in immunocompromised patients.
[h]Consider seafood ingestion.
[i]Consider waterborne, especially in IgA deficient patients, day care centers.
[j]Consider on cruise ships, nursing homes, schools, families, eating undercooked shellfish.
[k]Consider if onset within 6 hours.
[l]Consider if onset in 6 to 24 hours.
Adapted from: Thielman NM, Guerrant RL. Clinical practice. Acute infectious diarrhea. *N Engl J Med* 2004;350:38–47.

- Diuretics (e.g., furosemide, thiazides), asthma (theophylline), thyroid drugs
- Cholinergic drugs, e.g.,
  Myasthenia gravis (cholinesterase inhibitors)
  Cardiac (quinidine) and antihypertensives (angiotensin-converting enzyme inhibitors)
  Antidepressants (clozapine)
  Gout (colchicine)

Toxins (e.g., arsenic, mushrooms, organophosphates, alcohol)
Viral or bacterial toxins (e.g., *S. aureus*, *E. coli*, *Vibrio cholerae*, *Bacillus cereus*, *Campylobacter jejuni*, *Yersinia enterocolitica*, *C. botulinum*, *C. perfringens*)
Endogenous
Hormones

- Serotonin (carcinoid)
- Calcitonin (medullary carcinoma of thyroid)
- Villous adenoma
- VIPoma

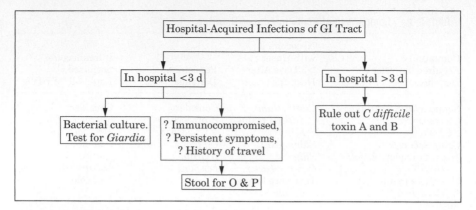

Fig. 7-3. Abbreviated sequence of tests for diarrhea in hospitalized adult patients. O & P, ova and parasites.

Gastric hypersecretion

- Z-E syndrome
- Systemic mastocytosis
- Basophilic leukemia
- Short-bowel syndrome

Bile salts (e.g., disease or resection of terminal ileum)
Fatty acids (e.g., disease of small intestine mucosa, pancreatic insufficiency)
Congenital (e.g., congenital chloridorrhea, congenital sodium diarrhea)
Watery stool
Volume >1 L/d
Blood and pus are absent
Stool osmolality close to plasma osmolality with no anion gap
Diarrhea usually continues during 24–48 hour fasting except for fatty acid malabsorption

Exudative Diarrhea

Active inflammation of the bowel mucosa.
Caused by
Inflammation

- Infectious (e.g., *Shigella, Salmonella, Campylobacter, Yersinia, C. difficile*, tuberculosis [TB], amebae)
- Idiopathic (e.g., ulcerative colitis, CD)
- Injury (e.g., radiation)
- Ischemia (e.g., mesenteric thrombosis)
- Vasculitis
- Abscess (e.g., diverticulitis)

Stool contains blood and pus.
Some features of osmotic diarrhea may be present.
20% to 40% of cases of acute infectious diarrhea remain undiagnosed.

Motility Disturbances

Caused By
Decreased small intestinal motility (e.g., hypothyroidism, diabetes mellitus, amyloidosis, scleroderma, postvagotomy)
Increased small intestinal motility (e.g., hyperthyroidism, carcinoid syndrome)
Increased colonic motility (e.g., irritable bowel syndrome)

Malabsorption

Caused By

Defective digestion or absorption
Infectious (e.g., *G. lamblia* causing impaired absorption)
Decreased small bowel surface area (e.g., surgery)
Lymphatic obstruction

Diarrhea, Chronic

Diarrhea is defined as chronic when it is of at least 4 weeks' duration and possibly 6 to 8 weeks' duration.

Caused By

Infection (e.g., giardiasis, amebiasis, *Cryptosporidium, Isospora, Strongyloides, C. difficile*)
IBD (e.g., CD, ulcerative colitis, collagenous colitis)
Carbohydrate malabsorption (e.g., lactase or sucrase deficiency)
Foods (e.g., ethanol, caffeine, sweeteners such as sorbitol, fructose)
Drugs (e.g., antibiotics, antihypertensive, antiarrhythmic, antineoplastic, colchicine, cholestyramine; see previous section on acute diarrhea)
Laxative abuse (see Chapter 16); factitious
Endocrine (e.g., diabetes mellitus, adrenal insufficiency, hyperthyroidism, hypothyroidism)
Hormone-producing tumors (e.g., gastrinoma, VIPoma, villous adenoma, medullary thyroid carcinoma, pheochromocytoma, ganglioneuroma, carcinoid tumor, mastocytosis, somatostatinoma, ectopic hormone production by lung or pancreas carcinoma)
Injury caused by radiation, ischemia, etc.
Infiltrations (e.g., scleroderma, amyloidosis, lymphoma)
Colon carcinoma
Previous surgery (e.g., gastrectomy, vagotomy, intestinal resection)
Immune system disorders (e.g., systemic mastocytosis, eosinophilic gastroenteritis)
Intraluminal maldigestion
    Bile duct obstruction, cirrhosis
    Bacterial overgrowth
    Pancreatic exocrine insufficiency
Celiac sprue
Whipple disease
Abetalipoproteinemia
Dermatitis herpetiformis
Intestinal lymphangiectasia
Allergy
Idiopathic

Diverticulosis, Colon

Laboratory findings due to complications, e.g.,

- Hemorrhage occurs in 5% of patients (hypochromic microcytic anemia, occult blood in stool)
- Infection including diverticulitis, abscess formation, peritonitis (increased WBC and ESR)
- Obstruction

Enterocolitis, Necrotizing, in Infancy

Necrotizing enterocolitis is a syndrome of acute intestinal necrosis of unknown etiology; it is especially associated with prematurity and exchange transfusions.

No specific laboratory tests are available.
Bloody stools feature no characteristic organisms; significant organisms are often found by frequent repeated cultures of blood, urine and stool.
There may be oliguria, neutropenia, and anemia.
Persistent metabolic acidosis, severe hyponatremia, and disseminated intravascular coagulation are a common triad in infants.

Enteropathy, Protein-Losing

Protein-losing enteropathy refers to the GI loss of plasma protein in abnormal amounts.

Secondary (i.e., disease states in which clinically significant protein-losing enteropathy may occur as a manifestation)

- Giant hypertrophy of gastric rugae (Ménétrier disease; see "Gastritis, Benign Giant Hypertrophic")
- Eosinophilic gastroenteritis
- Gastric neoplasms
- Infections (e.g., Whipple disease, bacterial overgrowth, enterocolitis, shigellosis, parasitic infestation, viral infections, *C. difficile* infection)
- Nontropical sprue
- Inflammatory and neoplastic diseases of small and large intestine, including ulcerative colitis, regional enteritis
- Constrictive pericarditis
- Immune diseases (e.g., systemic lupus erythematosus [SLE])
- Lymphatic obstruction (e.g., lymphoma, sarcoidosis, mesenteric TB)

Primary (i.e., hypoproteinemia is the major clinical feature)

- Intestinal lymphangiectasia
- Nonspecific inflammatory or granulomatous disease of small intestine

Proteinuria absent
Serum total protein, albumin, γ globulin, and calcium are decreased
Serum α and β globulins normal
Serum cholesterol usually normal
Mild anemia
Eosinophilia (occasionally)
Steatorrhea with abnormal tests of lipid absorption
Increased permeability of GI tract to large molecular substances shown by IV iodine-131-polyvinylpyrrolidone (^{131}I-PVP) test (see "Malabsorption")

Gallstone Ileus

Laboratory findings caused by preceding chronic cholecystitis and cholelithiasis
Laboratory findings caused by acute obstruction of terminal ileum *(accounts for 1%–2% of patients)*

Gastroenteritis, Eosinophilic

♦ Diagnosis requires histologic evidence of predominant eosinophilic (>20 eosinophils/hpf) infiltration of GI tract in absence of parasitic infection or extraintestinal disease.
Laboratory findings due to:

- Diarrhea, malabsorption, protein-losing enteropathy or GI tract obstruction with predominant disease of muscular layer
- Eosinophilic ascites with predominant disease of serosal layer

Eosinophilia in 80% of cases. IgE may be increased, especially in children.

Hirschsprung Disease (Aganglionic Megacolon)

Hirschsprung disease, or aganglionic megacolon, is caused by the congenital failure of the neural crest cells to complete caudal migration to anus, causing failure of the aganglionic segment to relax. It involves the rectosigmoid in ≤80% of cases and the whole colon and parts of small intestine in ≤10% of cases.

♦ Rectal biopsy to include muscle layers shows absence of myenteric plexus ganglia in muscle layers. This is only diagnostic if ganglia are present to rule out this diagnosis.

○ *Up to 15% of all infants with delayed passage of meconium will have Hirschsprung disease.*

Infarction of the Intestine

Due To
Primary (idiopathic)
Secondary (~75% of cases) to:
Emboli (e.g., from subacute bacterial endocarditis (SBE), nonbacterial valve vegetations, left atrium or ventricle, atherosclerotic vascular disease) or
Venous thrombosis (acute, subacute, or chronic)

- Prothrombotic states (including pregnancy, oral contraceptive use [<18% of cases], neoplasms); see Chapter 11
- Hematologic disorders (including polycythemia vera, essential thrombocythemia, paroxysmal nocturnal hemoglobinuria); see Chapter 11
- Cirrhosis and portal hypertension
- Inflammatory states (e.g., pancreatitis, peritonitis and abdominal sepsis, IBD)
- Postoperative state (e.g., abdominal surgery, splenectomy)
- Others (e.g., blunt abdominal trauma)

Routine blood tests are not usually helpful.
Hematemesis, hematochezia, or melena are present in ~15% and occult blood in <50% of cases.
Ascites is serosanguineous.
Metabolic acidosis with increased serum lactate is a late finding.
CT scan, magnetic resonance imaging, angiography.

Inflammatory Bowel Disease[9]

IBD refers to a chronic relapsing spectrum of disorders of unknown cause with destructive mucosal immune reaction in a genetically susceptible host. It is caused by an aberrant immune response and loss of tolerance to normal intestinal flora, leading to chronic inflammation of the gut.

Regional Enteritis (Crohn Disease)
CD is a systemic inflammatory disease with predominantly GI tract involvement.

There are no pathognomonic findings for CD or to distinguish it from ulcerative colitis (UC).
○ Endoscopic biopsy may show granulomas in >60% of cases of CD but in only 6% of cases of UC.
○ Anti-*Saccharomyces cerevisiae* (baker's or brewer's yeast) antibodies (ASCA) are found in ~60% of CD cases, but found in only ~10% of cases in UC.
Atypical perinuclear-staining antineutrophil cytoplasmic antibodies (P-ANCA) are found in <15% of cases of CD but in ≤70% of UC patients.
Increased WBC, ESR, CRP, and other acute-phase reactants correlate with disease activity. Mild increase of WBC indicates activity, but a marked increase suggests suppuration (e.g., abscess). ESR tends to be higher in disease of colon than of ileum.
Anemia due to iron deficiency or vitamin B_{12} or folate deficiency or chronic disease.
Decreased serum albumin, increased γ globulins.
Diarrhea may cause hyperchloremic metabolic acidosis, dehydration, decreased sodium, potassium, magnesium.
Mild liver function test changes due to pericholangitis (especially increased serum alkaline phosphatase [ALP]).
Laboratory changes due to complications or sequelae (e.g., malabsorption, perforation and fistula formation, abscess formation, arthritis, sclerosing cholangitis, iritis, uveitis, etc.).

[9]Bossuyt X. Serologic markers in inflammatory bowel disease. *Clin Chem* 2006;52:171–181.

Ulcerative Colitis, Chronic Nonspecific

There are no pathognomonic findings for this disease; nor are there findings that distinguish it from CD.

⊃ ASCA in ~10% in cases of UC but in ~60% of cases of CD.

P-ANCA are found in 70% of UC patients but only occasionally in cases of CD.

Laboratory findings parallel severity of the disease. With diarrhea and fever, hemoglobin (Hb) <7.5 g/dL, increased neutrophil count, and ESR >30 mm/h indicate severe disease.

Stools are positive for blood; negative for usual enteric pathogens and parasites.

Changes in liver function: serum ALP often increased slightly. Other liver function tests are usually normal.

Laboratory changes due to complications or sequelae (e.g., hemorrhage, carcinoma, electrolyte disorders, toxic megacolon with perforation).

The lower sensitivity of combined serologic tests only modestly influences pretest and posttest probability in IBD but is very useful in distinguishing CD from UC. Serial measurements are not useful and do not correlate with disease activity; titers are stable over time.

Assays lack standardization.

* ASCA$^+$/P-ANCA$^-$ predicts CD in 80% of cases with S/S = 67%/78%.
* ASCA$^-$/P-ANCA$^+$ predicts UC in 64% of cases with S/S = 78%/67%.
* ASCA$^-$/P-ANCA$^-$ predicts indeterminate disease. Occurs in ≤50% of IBD patients.
* ASCA$^+$ is associated in CD with penetration, strictures, ileal rather than colonic disease, and treatment-resistance to left-sided UC.
* ASCA$^+$ in ≤25% of first-degree relatives.
* Exocrine pancreatic antibodies are specific for IBD but have low sensitivity (30%).

Inflammatory Disorders of the Intestine

Infectious

Idiopathic (e.g., ulcerative colitis, regional enteritis, colitis of indeterminate type [e.g., collagenous colitis])

Motility disorders (e.g., diverticulitis, solitary rectal ulcer syndrome)

Circulatory disorders (e.g., ischemic colitis, associated with obstruction of colon)

Iatrogenic

* Enemas, laxatives, drugs
* Radiation
* Following small intestinal bypass and diversion of fecal stream
* Graft-versus-host disease

Specific disease association

* Chronic granulomatous disease of childhood
* Immunodeficiency syndromes
* Hemolytic uremic syndrome
* Behçet disease

Miscellaneous

* Collagenous colitis
* Eosinophilic colitis and allergic proctitis
* Necrotizing enterocolitis
* Idiopathic ulcer of colon

WBC is normal early. Later, it tends to rise, with increase in PMNs; counts of 15,000 to 25,000/μL suggest strangulation; a level >30,000/μL suggests mesenteric thrombosis.

Hb and hematocrit concentrations are normal early but later increase, with dehydration.

Urine specific gravity increases, with deficit of water and electrolytes. unless preexisting renal disease is present. Urinalysis helps rule out renal colic, diabetic acidosis, etc.

Gastric contents

* Positive guaiac test suggests strangulation; there may be gross blood if strangulated segment is high in jejunum.

Rectal contents—gross rectal blood suggests carcinoma of colon or intussusception.
Decreased serum sodium, potassium, chloride, and pH and increased CO_2 are helpful
    indications for following the course of the patient and to guide therapy.
Increased blood urea nitrogen suggests blood in intestine or renal damage.
Serum amylase may be moderately increased in absence of pancreatitis.
Increased serum lactate dehydrogenase (LD), aspartate aminotransferase, creatine
    kinase, phosphorus may indicate infarction of small intestine.

In Neonate

Caused By

Congenital mechanical

* Intrinsic (e.g., pyloric stenosis, meconium ileus, atresia, imperforate anus)
* Extrinsic (e.g., volvulus, malrotation, congenital bands, hernia)

Acquired mechanical (e.g., intussusception, necrotizing enterocolitis, meconium plugs,
    adhesions, mesenteric thrombosis)
Functional

* Hirschsprung disease
* Paralytic ileus (e.g., sepsis, Pseudomonas enteritis, maternal drugs such as heroin,
    hypermagnesemia)
* Endocrine (e.g., hypothyroidism, adrenal insufficiency)
* Other (e.g., sepsis, central nervous system disease, meconium plug syndrome)

Laboratory Findings in Neonate

Gastric aspirate >15 mL or is bile stained.
Vomitus is colorless when obstruction proximal to ampulla of Vater (e.g., pyloric atre-
    sia) but bile stained and alkaline with obstruction distal to ampulla. *Bile-stained
    vomitus in a neonate is always abnormal and is to be considered a surgical problem
    until proved otherwise.*
Findings due to complications (e.g., perforation, infarction, enterocolitis, peritonitis,
    changes in fluid and electrolytes).
Laboratory findings due to associated conditions:

* Duodenal atresia is associated with
    Down syndrome (30% of cases)
    Intestinal malrotation (20% of cases)
    Congenital heart disease (17% of cases)
    Annular pancreas (20% of cases)
    Renal anomalies (5% of cases)
    Tracheoesophageal anomalies (7% of cases)
* Polyhydramnios in 50% of cases of duodenal obstruction; 40% show hyperbiliru-
    binemia
* Cystic fibrosis is associated with
    Meconium ileus
    Increased incidence of intestinal atresia

Lymphangiectasia, Intestinal

♦ A biopsy of the small bowel or lymphangiography will confirm a diagnosis of intesti-
    nal lymphangiectasia.
Decreased serum protein.
IV infusion of ^{51}Cr-labeled albumin demonstrates excessive protein loss in stools.
May manifest in abnormal lymph nodes (inguinal, pelvic, retroperitoneal) and lymph-
    edema between early infancy and childhood.
Laboratory evidence of steatorrhea and malabsorption.

Malabsorption

See Figure 7-4 and Table 7-2.

Caused By

Inadequate mixing of food with bile salts and lipase (e.g., pyloroplasty, subtotal or total
    gastrectomy, gastrojejunostomy)

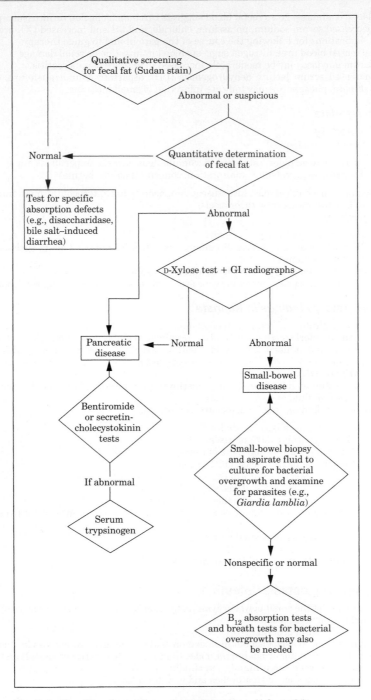

Fig. 7-4. Algorithm for workup of malabsorption. (Adapted from Roberts IM. Workup of the patient with malabsorption. *Postgrad Med* 1987;8:32–33, 37–42.)

Table 7-2.   Comparison of Types of Malabsorption

Test	Mucosal Disease	Pancreatic Disease	Bacterial Overgrowth	Lymphatic Obstruction
		Impaired Digestion in Lumen		
Biopsy of intestine	A	N	Sl A	Usually A
Stool fat	I	Markedly I	Sl I	I
Screening blood tests				
Prothrombin	N/I	N/I	N/I	N/I
Carotene	D	D	N/D	D
Cholesterol	D	D	D	D
Albumin	D	N	N/D	D
Iron	D	N	N	N
Folate	D	N	N	N
Vitamin B_{12}	N	N	N/D	N
Specific tests for malabsorption				
^{14}C triolein breath	D	D	D	D
D-xylose absorption	D	N	D/N	N
Schilling	N	D	D	N
Other breath tests H_2 ^{14}C-xylose or ^{14}C-cholyglycine	N/A	N	A	N
Bentiromide	N/D	N/D		N
Small-bowel radiograph	A	N	N	A

A, abnormal; N, normal; D, decreased; I, increased; Sl, slightly.

Inadequate lipolysis due to lack of lipase (e.g., cystic fibrosis of the pancreas, chronic pancreatitis, cancer of the pancreas or ampulla of Vater, pancreatic fistula, vagotomy)

Inadequate emulsification of fat due to lack of bile salts (e.g., obstructive jaundice, severe liver disease, bacterial overgrowth of small intestine, disorders of terminal ileum)

Primary absorptive defect in small bowel

Inadequate absorptive surface due to extensive mucosal disease (e.g., regional enteritis, tumors, amyloid disease, scleroderma, irradiation)

Biochemical dysfunction of mucosal cells (e.g., celiac sprue syndrome, severe starvation, or administration of drugs such as neomycin sulfate, colchicine, or PAS)

Obstruction of mesenteric lymphatics (e.g., by lymphoma, carcinoma, intestinal TB)

Inadequate length of normal absorptive surface (e.g., surgical resection, fistula, shunt)

Miscellaneous (e.g., "blind loops" of intestine, diverticula, Z-E syndrome, agammaglobulinemia, endocrine and metabolic disorders)

Infection (e.g., acute enteritis, tropical sprue, Whipple disease [*Tropheryma whippelii*]; in common variable hypogammaglobulinemia, 50% to 55% of patients have chronic diarrhea and malabsorption caused by a specific pathogen such as *G. lamblia* or overgrowth of bacteria in small bowel)

Factitious (see Chapter 16).

♦ *Fat Absorption Indices (Steatorrhea)*

Direct qualitative stool examination

≥ 2 random stool samples are collected on diet of >80 g of fat daily

Interpretation

• Gross—oil droplets, egg particles, buttery materials.
• Microscopic examination after staining for fat (e.g., Oil Red O, Sudan).

Sensitivity >94% with moderate/severe fat malabsorption (>10% of ingested fat excreted); ~75% in mild/moderate fat malabsorption (6%–10% of ingested fat excreted); positive in ~14% of normal persons.

- 4+ fat in stool means excessive fat loss.

Interference
Neutral fat
Mineral and castor oil ingestion
Dietetic low-calorie mayonnaise ingestion
Rectal suppository use
Quantitative determination of fecal fat is the gold standard test to establish the diagnosis of fat malabsorption.

Interpretation
Normal is <7 g/24 h when a 3-day pooled stool sample is collected on a diet of 80 to 100 g of fat/day or <6 g/24 h (or <4% of measured fat intake) on diet of <50 g of fat/d for a 3-day period.
Determination parallels but is more sensitive than triolein ^{131}I test in chronic pancreatic disease.

Increased In
Chronic pancreatic disease (>9.5 g/24 h).
May also be increased in:

- High-fiber diet (>100 g/d)
- When dietary fat is ingested in solid form (e.g., whole peanuts)
- Neonatal period
- If weight is much heavier than normal (>300 g/24 h; normal weight is <200 g/24 h or normal fecal solids of 25–30 g/24 h).

Serum trypsinogen <10 ng/mL in 75% to 85% of patients with severe chronic pancreatitis (those with steatorrhea) and 15% to 20% of those with mild to moderate disease; occasionally low in cancer of pancreas; normal (10–75 ng/mL) in nonpancreatic causes of malabsorption.
Bentiromide used to differentiate pancreatic exocrine insufficiency (abnormal result) from intestinal mucosal disease (normal result) (see "Bentiromide").
♦ Secretin-cholecystokinin is the most sensitive and reliable test of chronic pancreatic disease.
Indirect indices of fat absorption include the following; these lack sensitivity and specificity for routine screening.

- Serum cholesterol may be decreased.
- Prothrombin time (PT) may be prolonged because of malabsorption of vitamin K.
- Serum carotene is always abnormal in steatorrhea unless therapy is successful. Not recommended for screening; poor precision at lower end of reference range. May also be low in liver disease, high fever, hyperthyroidism, chronic illness, and decreased dietary intake (blood level falls within 1 week but vitamin A level is unaffected by dietary change for 6 months because of much larger body stores). May be increased in hyperlipidemia and hypothyroidism. Normal is 70 to 290 μg/dL. A reading of 30 to 70 μg/dL indicates mild depletion; <30 indicates severe depletion.
- Carotene tolerance test: Measure serum carotene following daily oral loading of carotene for 3 to 7 days. Low values for serum carotene levels are usually associated with steatorrhea. Increase of serum carotene by >35 μg/dL indicates previously low dietary intake of carotene and/or fat.
- Patients with sprue in remission with normal fecal fat excretion may still show low carotene absorption.

Interference
Mineral oil interferes with carotene absorption. On a fat-free diet, only 10% is absorbed.

- Vitamin A tolerance test (for screening steatorrhea)
  Measure plasma vitamin A level 5 hours after ingestion.
  Normal rise is 9× fasting level.
  Flat curve in liver disease.
  Not useful after gastrectomy.
  With vitamin A as ester of long-chain fatty acid, flat curve occurs in both pancreatic disease and intestinal mucosal abnormalities; when water-soluble forms of

vitamin A are used, the curve becomes normal in patients with pancreatic disease but remains flat in intestinal mucosal abnormalities.

* Triolein ^{131}I and oleic acid ^{131}I absorption with measurement of blood, breath, or fecal radioactivity; sensitive and specific for screening but may not be routinely available.

Triolein ^{131}I absorption test used to screen patients with steatorrhea.

* Normal: $\geq$10% of administered radioactivity appears in the blood within 6 hours; <5% appears in the feces; indicates that digestion of fat in the small bowel and absorption of fat in the small bowel are normal.
* Abnormal: do an oleic acid ^{131}I absorption test.

Triolein ^{14}C breath test
^{14}C-labeled triolein is administered and ^{14}CO$_2$ is measured in collected breath. Said to have S/S >85% for fat malabsorption.

Interferences
False-positive results with:

* Poor gastric emptying (e.g., gastric surgery, diabetes mellitus)
* CO_2 retention (e.g., chronic lung disease)
* Impaired metabolism (e.g., severe liver disease)
* Dilution of ^{14}CO$_2$ (e.g., hyperlipidemia, ascites, obesity)
* Apparently healthy persons

False-negative results with:

* Increased CO_2 production (e.g., hyperthyroidism, fever)
* Mild degree of fat malabsorption

Oleic acid ^{131}I absorption test: Normal values same as for the triolein absorption test.
Interpretation
An abnormal result indicates a defect in small bowel mucosal absorption function (e.g., sprue, Whipple disease, regional enteritis, TB enteritis, collagen diseases involving the small bowel, extensive resection). Abnormal pancreatic function does not affect the test.

Most common laboratory abnormalities are decreased serum carotene, albumin, and iron; increased ESR; increased stool weight (>300 g/24 h) and stool fat (>7 g/24 h); anemia.

Normal D-xylose test, low serum trypsinogen, pancreatic calcification on radiograph of abdomen establish diagnosis of chronic pancreatitis. If calcification is absent (as occurs in 70%–80% of cases), abnormal contents of pancreatic secretion after secretin-cholecystokinin stimulation or abnormal bentiromide tests establish diagnosis of chronic pancreatitis.

Anemia is caused by deficiency of iron, folic acid, vitamin B$_{12}$, or various combinations, depending on their decreased absorption.

Carbohydrate Absorption Indices

* Oral glucose tolerance test is of limited value; flat curve or delayed peak occurs in celiac disease and nontropical sprue. Curve is normal in pancreatic insufficiency.
* D-Xylose tolerance test of carbohydrate absorption:
  Measure total 5-hour urine excretion; may also measure serum levels at 2 hours.
  Accuracy is 90% in distinguishing normal levels in pancreatic disease from decreased levels in intestinal mucosal disease and intestinal bacterial overgrowth, but opinions vary on usefulness. Also decreased in renal disease, myxedema, and the elderly, although absorption is normal.
* Disaccharide malabsorption
Due To
Primary malabsorption (congenital or acquired) because of absence of specific disaccharidase in brush border of small intestine mucosa

* Isolated lactase deficiency (also called milk allergy, milk intolerance, congenital familial lactose intolerance, lactase deficiency) (is most common of these defects; occurs in ~10% of whites and 60% of blacks; infantile type shows diarrhea, vomiting, failure to thrive, malabsorption, etc.; often appears first in adults; become asymptomatic when lactase is removed from diet).

- Sucrose-isomaltose malabsorption (inherited recessive defect)
    Oral sucrose tolerance curve is flat, but glucose plus fructose tolerance test is normal. Occasionally there is an associated malabsorption with increased stool fat and abnormal D-xylose tolerance test, although intestinal biopsy is normal.
    Hydrogen breath test after sucrose challenge.
    Intestinal biopsy with measurement of disaccharidase activities.
    Sucrose-free diet causes cessation of diarrhea.
- Glucose-galactose malabsorption (inherited autosomal-recessive defect that affects kidney and intestine)
    Oral glucose or galactose tolerance curve is flat, but IV tolerance curves are normal.
    Glucosuria is common. Fructose tolerance test is normal.

Secondary malabsorption

- Resection of >50% of disaccharidase activity
    Lactose is most marked, but there may also be sucrose. Oral disaccharide tolerance (especially lactose) is abnormal, but intestinal histology and enzyme activity are normal.
- Diffuse intestinal disease—especially celiac disease in which activity of all disaccharidases may be decreased, with later increase as intestine becomes normal on gluten-free diet; also cystic fibrosis of pancreas, severe malnutrition, ulcerative colitis, severe *Giardia* infestation, blind-loop syndrome, β-lipoprotein deficiency, effect of drugs (e.g., colchicine, neomycin, birth control pills)
    Oral tolerance tests (especially lactose) are frequently abnormal, with later return to normal with gluten-free diet. Tolerance tests with monosaccharides may also be abnormal because of defect in absorption as well as digestion.
- Bacterial overgrowth—See Figure 7-6 and Table 7-3.
    Culture of duodenal aspirate showing $>10^5$ colony-forming units of anaerobic organisms is considered diagnostic.
    ^{14}C-D-xylose breath test has good specificity.
    Hydrogen breath tests (glucose-H_2, lactulose-H_2)—not recommended because of limited sensitivity and specificity.

Laboratory Tests for Lactase Deficiency

(Similar tests for other disaccharide deficiencies can be performed.)

- Oral lactose tolerance curve is flat (blood drawn 15, 30, 60, and 90 minutes after a 50-g dose of lactose) but tolerance test is normal using constituent monosaccharides (25 g each of glucose and galactose), indicating isolated lactase deficiency rather than general mucosal absorptive defect.
    Normal: Blood glucose increases >20 mg/dL above fasting level; may increase >20 to 25 mg/dL in diabetics despite impaired lactose absorption.
    Abnormal: Glucose increases <20 mg/dL above fasting level. False abnormal test may be caused by delayed gastric emptying or small bowel transit or delayed blood collection. Poor sensitivity—largely replaced by breath hydrogen lactose test.
- Hydrogen breath test measures (by gas chromatography; based on production of H_2 by bacteria in colon from unabsorbed lactose) amount of H_2 exhaled at 2 hours after ingestion of 50 g of lactose in fasting state. Normal = 0 to 0.11 mL/min.
    Lactase deficiency: Rise in breath hydrogen = 0.31 to 2.50 mL/min (>20 ppm). Peak or cumulative 4-hour values also differentiates these patients. False-negative results caused by absence of H_2-producing bacteria in colon or prior antibiotic therapy in ~20% of patients. False-positive results caused by bacterial overgrowth. Similar test can be used to detect disaccharidase deficiency.
- Stool examination
    After ingestion of 50 g of lactose, frothy diarrheal stools typically show low pH (4.5 to 6.0; normal >7.0), high osmolality, positive test for reducing substances (e.g., Clinitest tablets; >0.5% is abnormal; 0.25%–0.5% is suspicious; 0.25% is normal); found in children but rarely in adults.
    Chromatography detects specific carbohydrates.
    Fecal studies are of limited value.
- Endoscopic intestinal biopsy for histologic examination and lactase enzyme activity assay is now considered obsolete.

Table 7-3. Infectious Food-borne Diseases

Organism	Identification	Cases of Food-borne Gastroenteritis (%)
Bacterial[a]		88.6
Bacillus cereus gastroenteritis	Isolation of $\geq 10^5$ *B. cereus*/g of suspected food Isolation of same-serotype *B. cereus* from other ill patients but not from control persons Detection of enterotoxin by special tests (e.g., immunogel diffusion)	0.03
Botulism	Isolation of *Clostridium botulinum* from stool of patients Detection of toxin in stool, serum, or food by mouse test	0.4
Brucellosis	Isolation of *Brucella* organism from blood	0.1
Campylobacteriosis	Increase in blood agglutination titer of fourfold or greater at onset and 3–6 wk later Isolation of same strain of organism from patient's stool Isolation of organism from suspected food Increase in blood agglutination titer of fourfold or greater at onset and 2–4 wk later	
Cholera	Isolation of organism from vomitus or stool Isolation of organism from suspected food Demonstration that organism is enterotoxigenic by special biologic tests	
Clostridium perfringens enteritis	Isolation of same serotype of *C. perfringens* from food and from patients but not from control persons Isolation of $\geq 10^5$ organisms from suspected food Fecal spore count $> 10^6$/g in most patients within a few days of onset Demonstration of toxin in feces (fluorescent antibody test)	18.5
Escherichia coli	Isolation of same serotype of *E. coli* from suspected food and from patients but not from control persons Demonstration that organism strain is enteropathogenic	
Listeriosis	Isolation of organism from tissue of fatal case Isolation of same phage type and serogroup from patient and food	

(continued)

Table 7-3. Continued

Organism	Identification	Cases of Food-borne Gastroenteritis (%)
	Demonstration of virulence by biologic tests	
Salmonellosis	Isolation of organism from stool or rectal swab, urine, or blood Isolation of same organism serovar from suspected food	31.9
Shigellosis	Isolation of organism from stool or rectal swab Isolation of same organism serovar from suspected food	18.0
Staphylococcal poisoning or intoxication	Detection of enterotoxin in suspected food (serologic assay) Isolation of same phage type of organism from patient and suspected food Isolation of $\geq 10^5$ organisms/g of suspected food	16.5
Streptococcus, Group A	See Chapter 15	3.2
Vibrio parahaemolyticus	See Chapter 15	0.03
Yersiniosis	Isolation of *Yersinia enterocolitica* or *Y. pseudotuberculosis* from stool or blood or from suspected food	5.5
Viral[b]		
Hepatitis A and E	See Tables 8.5, 8.6	
Norwalk and parvo-like	Fourfold or greater increase of blood antibody titer from acute to convalescent phase Immunoelectron microscopy	
Rotavirus		
Chemical (scombroid)	See footnote	
Amebae (e.g., *Entamoeba histolytica, Blastocystis hominis*)	Identification of cysts or trophozoites in feces, biopsy, aspirate; serology	5.1
Parasitic		0.8
Cryptosporidiosis	Demonstration of organisms in stool or suspected food Detection of antigen in stool	
Giardiasis	Recognition of organism in stool, duodenal contents, or small bowel Detection of antigen in stool	
Balantidium coli infestation	Recognition of organism in stool, tissue biopsy Rarely recovered in United States	
Helminthic		
Cestodiasis (e.g., caused by *Diphyllobothrium latum, Taenia saginata, Taenia solium*)	Eggs and proglottids in stool	
Trichinosis	Recognition of cysts in muscle biopsy	

(*continued*)

Table 7-3.	Continued	

Organism	Identification	Cases of Food-borne Gastroenteritis (%)
	Demonstration of larvae in suspected food Demonstration of adults and larvae in stool only during first 1–2 wk Detection of antigen in stool Serologic tests for antibody	
Trematodiasis (e.g., caused by *Clonorchis sinensis, Fasciola hepatica, Paragonimus westermani*)	Eggs in stool	
Fungal		
Mushroom poisoning	Demonstration of toxin in urine and suspected gathered mushrooms	

[a]Confirm by culture of food, patient's stool, or food handler's stool.
[b]Suspected by exclusion by negative tests for other causes of the symptoms (e.g., failure to find *Entamoeba histolytica, Shigella, Salmonella*). Fecal white blood cells in 20% of rotavirus cases; absent in Norwalk, Norwalk-like, and adenovirus cases.
Antigen detection: Commercial monoclonal-based antibody kits for rotavirus (enzyme immunoassay [EIA], latex agglutination, enzyme-linked immunosorbent assay) are inexpensive, permit rapid diagnosis, and require only small amounts of stool, which may be frozen until testing. Detection of viral antigen in stool may be negative due to brief period of excretion. Sensitivities of 70%–100% and specificities of 50%–100% are reported. False-positive rates are high in newborns and in breast-feeding children. Less useful in adults and outside of rotavirus season, when confirmatory testing should be performed. Kits also available for adenovirus. Rapid assays for other viruses are under development.
Antibody detection (e.g., to Norwalk virus, especially caused by ingestion of raw oysters) can be diagnosed by presence of serum IgM or by 4× rise in specific IgG antibody titers (EIA) drawn at the first week (acute-phase serum) and after the second week (convalescent serum). Patient will have long since recovered from self-limited illness. Chief use is to identify cause of an outbreak. Stool antigen and serum antibody assay for Norwalk virus are only available in research laboratories at present. Monoclonal antibodies for adenovirus 40 and 41.
Direct electron microscopy of stool can detect (≤90% sensitivity) and identify all the morphologic types of enteric viruses (e.g., rotaviruses, adenoviruses, astrovirus, calicivirus, Norwalk virus) by characteristic morphology. Detection requires ≥1 million viruses/mL of stool; usually present only during first 48 hours of viral diarrhea. Required for conclusive diagnosis of Norwalk virus. Immune electron microscopy improves sensitivity by 10 to 100 times, but technology limits this to few laboratories.
Culture: Rotavirus, adenovirus, astrovirus culture available in research centers; not useful for routine diagnosis. Other viruses cannot be cultured.
Electropherotyping: Detection of rotavirus RNA in stool by gel electrophoresis pattern is 100% specific and >90% sensitive in first days of illness; chiefly research tool in United States.
Dot-hybridization probes for rotavirus are more sensitive and specific than antigen detection but are only available in research centers.
Polymerase chain reaction techniques are being developed.
See appropriate sections in Chapter 15.
Source: Steele JCH Jr, ed. Food-borne diseases. *Clin Lab Med* 1999;19:469–703.

Protein Absorption Indices

- Normal fecal nitrogen is <2 g/d. There is marked increase in sprue and severe pancreatic deficiency.
- Measure plasma glycine or urinary excretion of hydroxyproline after gelatin meal. Plasma glycine increases 5× in 2 hours in normal persons. In those with cystic fibrosis of the pancreas, the increase is <2.5×.
- Serum albumin may be decreased.

^{131}I-PVP test: Give 0.55 to 0.925 MBq (15 to 25 μCi) of ^{131}I-PVP via IV and collect all stools for 4 to 5 days.

Interpretation
Normally <2% is excreted in feces when the mucosa of the GI tract is intact. In protein-losing enteropathy, >2% of administered radioactivity appears in stool.

Electrolyte Absorption Indices

• Serum calcium, magnesium, potassium, and vitamin D may be decreased.

^{51}Cr albumin test (IV dose of 1.11 to 1.85 MBq [30 to 50 μCi]) shows increased excretion in 4-day stool collection due to protein-losing enteropathy.

♦ Biopsy of small intestine mucosa is excellent for verification of sprue, celiac disease, and Whipple disease.

Culture for bacterial overgrowth should be considered in malabsorption associated with abnormal intestinal motility (e.g., scleroderma) or anatomic abnormalities (e.g., diverticula). Positive if >10^5 to 10^6 organisms/mL from upper intestinal contents, but may vary from one location to another; should be collected for anaerobic and aerobic culture. Perform with peroral intestinal biopsy. If breath tests using ^{14}C-bile acid or ^{14}C-D-xylose or hydrogen are available, they are more sensitive and specific for bacterial overgrowth.

Breath test for bile acid malabsorption: oral radiolabeled ^{14}C-glycocholate undergoes bacterial deconjugation in the colon. ^{14}CO$_2$ derived from glycine is absorbed in the bowel, excreted by the lungs, and measured in breath. This simulates the secretion of bile acids into duodenum and 95% resorption in terminal ileum. It identifies bacterial overgrowth or impaired ileal absorption of bile acids.

Interpretation
Normal: ~5% enters the colon.
Increased:

• Bacterial overgrowth in small intestine allows earlier bacterial deconjugation and therefore more ^{14}CO$_2$ appears in breath.
• Disease or resection of terminal ileum allows more bile acids into the colon, where they undergo bacterial conjugation.

Schilling test. Performed before and after administration of antibiotics, it is a useful adjunct to intestinal culture to detect bacterial overgrowth.

Meckel Diverticulum

Laboratory findings caused only by complications:

• GI hemorrhage
• Intestinal obstruction
• Perforation or intussusception (~20% of patients; the other 80% of patients are asymptomatic)

○ Should be suspected when GI bleeding and symptoms of appendicitis occur together.

Megacolon, Toxic

Toxic megacolon is a life-threatening complication of IBD. It is characterized by atonic dilatation of the colon due to transmural inflammation.

Caused By
Severe UC is most common cause
CD
Pseudomembranous colitis
Ischemic colitis
Bacterial colitis
Amebiasis
Laboratory findings caused by sepsis (e.g., increased WBC and PMNs), dehydration.
Bloody diarrhea.

Neoplasms, Colon[10,11]

Blood in stool (occult or gross). Annual screening for occult blood detects <50% of cancers and 10% of adenomas.

Comparison of Fecal DNA and Hemoccult II

	Sensitivity for Detection of Advanced Neoplasia	Sensitivity for Detection of Adenoma	Specificity for Detection of Adenoma	Specificity for Detection of Advanced Neoplasia	Cost/Test	Cost/y of of Life Gained (US$)
Hemoc-cult II	13%	11%		95%	$3–40	$5,700–$17,800
Fecal DNA	35%–68%	15% (much higher with high-grade dysplasia)	†	94%	$400–800	$47,700

Evidence of inflammation (e.g., increased WBC and ESR)
Anemia—usually hypochromic

- May be the only symptom of carcinoma of right side of colon (present in >50% of these patients)
- Stools sometimes negative for occult blood

Laboratory evidence of liver metastases (see Chapter 8)
Serum CEA (see Chapter 16)
Laboratory findings due to underlying condition (e.g., hereditary polyposis, chronic nonspecific ulcerative colitis)
Laboratory findings due to complications (e.g., hemorrhage, perforation, obstruction, intussusception)
♦ Biopsy of lesion establishes the diagnosis

Carcinoid Tumors

Carcinoid tumors may cause increased 5-hydroxyindoleacetic acid in urine (see Chapter 13).

Colon Cancer Syndromes[12]

See Table 7-4.

Nonpolyposis Syndromes

Hereditary nonpolyposis colon cancer (Lynch syndrome)
Muir-Torre syndrome
Turcot syndrome associated with glioblastoma
Z-E syndrome with MEN-I

Polyposis Syndromes

- Adenomatous polyposis syndromes:
    Gardner syndrome
    Turcot syndrome associated with medulloblastoma
    Attenuated familial adenomatous polyposis
    Occasional discrete polyps of colon and rectum
- Hamartomatous polyposis syndromes:
    Peutz-Jeghers syndrome

[10]Imperiale TF, Ransohoff DF, Itzkowitz SH, et al. Fecal DNA versus fecal occult blood for colorectal-cancer screening in an average-risk population. *N Engl J Med* 2004;351:2704–2714.
[11]Woolf SH. A smarter strategy? Reflections on fecal DNA screening for colorectal cancer. *N Engl J Med* 2004;351:2755–2758.
[12]Baudhuin LM, Donner WH. Hereditary colorectal cancer. diagnostic strategies for the clinical laboratory. *Clin Lab News* July 2004:14.

Table 7-4.	Comparison of Some Inherited Gastrointestinal Polyps				
Syndrome	Type	Location	Cancer Predisposition and Mode of Inheritance	Associated Abnormalities
Familial polyposis	Adenoma	Colon; also stomach, small bowel	Yes (~100%) AD	Osteomas of mandible
Gardner syndrome	Adenoma	Colon; also stomach, small bowel; may develop before puberty; 100% become malignant	Yes (~100%) AD	Multiple osteomas of jaw and skull, fibrous and fatty tumors of skin and mesentery, epidermoid inclusion cysts of skin
Turcot syndrome	Adenoma	Colon	Yes AR	Brain tumors usually within first two decades of life
Peutz-Jeghers syndrome	Hamartoma	Small bowel; also stomach, colon	Yes (risk <3%–6%, especially stomach, duodenum AD	Pigmented foci on buccal and perianal mucosa, hands, feet are characteristic; bladder and nasal polyps
Juvenile polyps	Hamartoma, Adenoma	Colon; also stomach small bowel	Rare AD	
Neurofibromatosis	Neurofibroma	Stomach, small bowel	No	Skin
Cronkhite-Canada syndrome	Inflammatory	Small bowel; also stomach, colon	~15% risk Sporadic	Alopecia, dystrophic nails, hyperpigmentation, enteropathy

AD, autosomal dominant; AR, autosomal recessive.
Source: Eastwood GL, Avunduk C. *Manual of Gastroenterology*. 2nd ed. Boston: Little, Brown; 1994.

> Juvenile polyposis
> Cowden syndrome

Laboratory findings due to intestinal polyps and associated lesions
Laboratory findings due to complications (e.g., bleeding, obstruction, malignancy)

Villous Adenoma of Rectum

○ *Villous tumor of rectum may cause secretory diarrhea with potassium loss and decreased serum potassium.*

Neoplasms Caused by Primary Diseases of Small Intestine

See Table 7-5.
♦ Biopsy of lesions confirms the diagnosis.
Laboratory findings due to complications (e.g., hemorrhage, obstruction, intussusception, malabsorption).
Laboratory findings due to underlying conditions (e.g., Peutz-Jeghers syndrome, carcinoid syndrome).

Table 7-5. Comparison of Two Major Types of Lymphoma

	Western Type	Alpha Chain Disease
Population	Western world	Middle East
Sex distribution	Equal	Preponderance in males
Age	<10 or >50 y	10–30 y
Location	Ileum	Duodenum, jejunum
Therapy	Excision, radiation, chemotherapy	Antibiotics, chemotherapy
Laboratory findings	Anemia, obstruction, intussusception, perforation	Paraproteinemia, anemia, steatorrhea

Laboratory findings caused by conditions with increased risk of small bowel tumor.

GI Condition	Tumor
Celiac sprue	Non-Hodgkin lymphoma, adenocarcinoma
CD	Adenocarcinoma
Familial adenomatous polyposis	Adenocarcinoma, adenoma
Postcolectomy ileostomy	Adenocarcinoma
Neurofibromatosis	Adenocarcinoma, leiomyoma
AIDS	Non-Hodgkin lymphoma
Nodular lymphoid hyperplasia	Non-Hodgkin lymphoma
Immunoproliferative small bowel disease	Non-Hodgkin lymphoma

GI, gastrointestinal; CD, Crohn disease.

Pyloric Stenosis

Serum HCO_3^- ≥29 mmol/L or chloride ≤98 mmol/L has high S/S in vomiting in early infancy.

Sprue, Tropical

Tropical sprue is a disease of the entire small intestine in persons who visit or reside in various tropical regions. It is probably an infectious disease caused by persistent toxigenic coliform bacteria in the small intestine (e.g., *Klebsiella pneumoniae, Enterobacter cloacae, E. coli*) responds to antibiotic therapy.

Characterized by an initial bout of acute watery diarrhea followed by persistent, progressive course if untreated.
Malabsorption (see "Malabsorption"), e.g.:

* Steatorrhea in 50% to 90% of cases
* Deficiency of folate and vitamin B_{12} after 6 months (not corrected by adding intrinsic factor)
* Abnormal xylose tolerance in most cases
* Oral glucose tolerance test abnormal in ~50% of cases

Histologic changes can be seen in a jejunal biopsy.

Vascular Occlusion, Mesenteric

Chronic (mesenteric arterial insufficiency)

* Laboratory findings caused by malabsorption and starvation

Acute

* Marked increase in WBC count (≥15,000–25,000/μL) with shift to the left.
* Infarction of intestine may cause increased serum LD, aspartate aminotransferase, ALP, creatine kinase, blood urea nitrogen, amylase, and phosphorus.
* Increased plasma lactate with metabolic acidosis has been suggested as an indicator for surgery in patients with acute abdomen.

- Laboratory findings caused by intestinal hemorrhage, obstruction, shock.
- Laboratory findings due to preexisting heart disease, atherosclerosis, or coagulopathy.

Disorders of the Peritoneum

Ascites

See also "Pleural Effusion," Chapter 6, for differential diagnosis of effusions.
Due To

Chronic parenchymal liver disease	81.0%
Cancer	10.0%
Heart failure	3.0%
TB	1.7%
Dialysis	1.0%
Others (e.g., pancreatic, fulminant liver failure, biliary origin, lymphatic injury, chlamydia infection, nephrotic syndrome, Meigs syndrome, myxedema, SLE)	<1.0% each

TB, tuberculosis; SLE, systemic lupus erythematosus.

Chronic Liver Disease differs from ascites caused by malignancy:

♦ • Albumin gradient (serum albumin minus ascitic fluid [AF] albumin) reflects portal pressure.
Almost always ≥1.1 in cirrhosis (most common cause), alcoholic hepatitis, massive liver metastases, fulminant hepatic failure, portal vein thrombosis, Budd-Chiari syndrome, cardiac ascites, acute fatty liver of pregnancy, myxedema, mixed (e.g., cirrhosis with peritoneal TB). May be falsely low if serum albumin <1.1 g/dL or patient in shock. May be falsely high with chylous ascites (lipid interferes with albumin assay).
<1.1 g/dL in >90% of cases of peritoneal carcinomatosis (most common cause) or TB, pancreatic or biliary ascites, nephrotic syndrome, bowel infarction or obstruction, serositis in patients without cirrhosis.

- AF/serum albumin ratio <0.5 in cirrhosis (>90% accuracy).
- AF total protein >2.5 mg/dL in cancer is only 56% accurate because of high protein content in 12% to 19% of these ascites as well as changes caused by albumin infusion and diuretic therapies.
- AF/serum ratio of LD (>0.6) or protein (>0.5) are not more accurate (~56%) than only total protein for diagnosis of exudate.
- AF cholesterol <55 mg/dL in cirrhosis (94% accuracy).
- Total WBC count is usually <300/μL (50% of cases) and PMN <25% (50% of cases).
- Chemical findings do not distinguish neoplasia from TB etiology.
- Liver function tests are abnormal.
- Cirrhosis findings are similar with or without hepatocellular carcinoma.

♦ *Cardiac Ascites* is associated with a blood-AF albumin gradient >1.1 g/dL, but malignant AF shows blood-AF albumin gradient <1.1 g/dL in 93% of cases.

Infected AF

♦ • WBC count >250/μL: sensitivity = 85%, specificity = 93%) and neutrophils >50% are presumptive of bacterial peritonitis.
♦ • pH <7.35 and arterial-AF pH difference >0.10; both these findings are virtually diagnostic of bacterial peritonitis and absence of the above findings virtually excludes bacterial peritonitis.
- AF lactate >25 mg/dL and arterial-AF difference >20 mg/dL are often present.
- AF LD is markedly increased.
- AF glucose is unreliable for diagnosis.
- AF phosphate, potassium, and gamma-glutamyltransferase may also be increased.

♦ • Gram stain shows few bacteria in spontaneous bacterial peritonitis (SBP) but many when caused by intestinal perforation. Culture sensitivity = 50% for SBP and ~80% for secondary peritonitis.

♦ • AF in *blood culture bottles* has 85% sensitivity.

♦ • TB acid-fast stain sensitivity = 20% to 30% and TB culture sensitivity = 50% to 70%.

• Total protein <1.0 g/dL indicates high risk for SBP.

Secondary Peritonitis shows polymicrobial infection, total protein ≥1.0 g/dL, AF LD > serum upper limit of normal, glucose <50 mg/dL compared to SBP. SBP has prevalence 15%; due to E. coli ~50%, Klebsiella, and other Gram-negative bacteria, Gram-positive ~25% (especially streptococci).

Continuous Ambulatory Peritoneal Dialysis: monitor dialysate for the following (Figures 7-5 and 7-6):

♦ • Infection: Peritonitis is defined as WBC count >100/μL, usually with >50% PMNs (normal is <50 WBC/μL , usually mononuclear cells), or positive Gram stain or culture (most prevalent: coagulase-negative staphylococci, *S. aureus, Streptococcus* sp.; multiple organisms, especially mixed aerobes and anaerobes occur with bowel perforation). Successful therapy causes fall in WBC count within first 2 days and a return to <100/μL in 4 to 5 days; differential returns to predominance of monocytes in 4 to 7 days with increased eosinophils in 10% of cases. Patients check outflow bags for turbidity. Turbid dialysate can occasionally occur without peritonitis during first few months of placing catheter (due to catheter hypersensitivity) with WBC count 100 to 8,000/μL, 10% to 95% eosinophils, sometimes increased PMNs, and negative cultures. Occasional RBCs may be seen during menstruation or with ovulation at mid-cycle. *Because of low WBC decision level, manual hemocytometer count rather than an automated instrument must be used.*

• Metabolic change: assay dialysate for creatinine and glucose; calculate ultrafiltrate volume by weighing dialysate fluid after 4-hour dwell time and subtracting it from preinfusion weight using specific gravity of 1.0.

♦ **Pancreatic Disease:** AF amylase > serum amylase is virtually specific for pancreatic disease, but both levels are normal in 10% of cases. Methemalbumin in serum or AF and total protein >4.5 g/dL indicate poor prognosis.

♦ **Chylous Ascites:** Triglyceride is 2 × to 8 × serum level. Protein = 2 to 3 g/dL. Due to lymphatic obstruction (e.g., lymphoma or carcinoma [60% of cases]), inflammation or obstruction of small intestine, trauma to chest or abdomen, filariasis; in pediatric patients, is often caused by congenital lymphatic defects.

♦ **Malignant Ascites:** increased fluid cholesterol (>45 mg/dL) and fibronectin (>10 mg/dL) has S/S = 90%/82%. Positive cytology has S/S = 70%/100%. Increased AF CEA (>2.5 mg/dL) has S/S = 45%/100%.
Abdominal Trauma

♦ Criteria to diagnose *penetrating* abdominal wounds by peritoneal lavage;

• >10,000 RBC/μL (>5,000 RBC/μL for gunshot wounds)
• >500 WBC/μL or
• Bacteria, fecal or vegetable matter on Gram stain or bile (Ictotest)
• Detection of endotoxin by limulus amoebocyte lysate assay for ileocolic perforation
• Amylase or ALP to detect small bowel or pancreas injury has been used
• Increased WBC, amylase, and ALP are often delayed >3 hours
• RBC and WBC counts of lavage fluid have most clinical utility

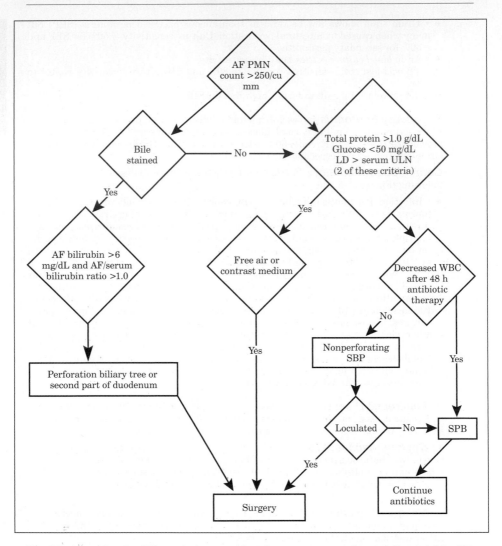

Fig. 7-5. Algorithm for differentiating secondary from spontaneous bacterial peritonitis. AF, ascitic fluid; PMN, polymorphonuclear leukocytes; LD, lactate dehydrogenase; ULN, upper limit of normal; WBC, white blood cell; SBP, spontaneous bacterial peritonitis.

Peritoneal Fluid Bicarbonate Value to Differentiate Site of Penetrating Wounds of GI Tract

Wound Site	Effect on Bicarbonate Value
Stomach or duodenum proximal to pancreatic duct	Decrease
Duodenum just distal to pancreatic duct	Increase
Third part of duodenum, jejunum, or ileum	Probably no effect

Fluid Source	Bicarbonate Values (mEq/L) (Reference Values)
Peritoneal	24.0–29.0
Pancreatic	66.0–127.0
Duodenal	4.0–21.0
Jejunal	2.0–32.0
Ileal	2.3
Gastric	–
Plasma/venous blood	20.0–30.0

GI

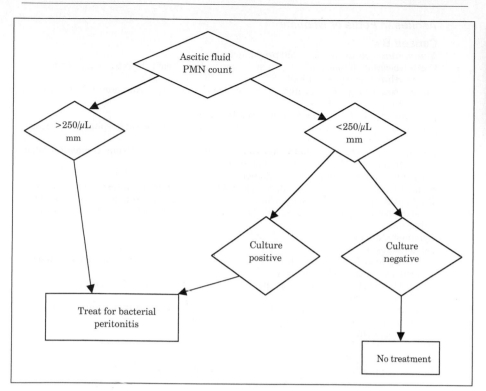

Fig. 7-6. Algorithm for spontaneous bacterial peritonitis. PMN, polymorphonuclear leukocytes.

♦ Criteria to diagnose *blunt* abdominal trauma by peritoneal lavage with 10,000 mL of normal saline; falsely low RBC count if <600–800 mL of fluid is recovered:

- Grossly bloody fluid or
- >100,000 RBC/μL (newspaper print is unreadable through lavage tubing if RBC count is this high); negative test <50,000 RBC/μL; equivocal results = 50,000–100,000 RBC/μL; or
- >500 WBC/μL or
- Amylase >2.5 × normal

♦ Criteria to diagnose *intestinal injury* in blunt abdominal trauma by peritoneal lavage with 10,000 mL of normal saline, especially 3 to 18 hours after injury:

- Absence of bloody ascites may signal solid organ injury
- >10,000 WBC/μL and WBC/μL = (RBC/μL divided by 150)

♦ To differentiate urine from ascitic or pleural fluid (in cases of possible GU tract fistula or accidental aspiration of bladder):

- Urine creatinine is >2× the serum level
- Uncontaminated ascitic or pleural fluid creatinine is usually same as serum level but always <2× serum level
- Urea nitrogen also greater in urine

Increased serum inorganic phosphate in 25% of cases of ischemic bowel disease; >5.5 mg/dL
indicates extensive bowel injury, acute renal failure, or metabolic acidosis and poorer prognosis.

Ascites in Fetus or Neonate

Caused By
Nonimmune (occur in 1 in 3,000 pregnancies)

Cardiovascular abnormalities causing congestive heart failure (e.g., structural, arrhythmias) (40% of cases)

Chromosomal (e.g., Turner and Down syndromes are most common; trisomy 13, 15, 16, 18) (10%–15% of cases)

Hematologic disorders (any severe anemia) (10% of cases)

Inherited (e.g., α-thalassemia, hemoglobinopathies, glucose-6-phosphate dehydrogenase deficiency)

Acquired (e.g., fetal-maternal hemorrhage, twin-to-twin transfusion, congenital infection [parvovirus B19], methemoglobinemia)

Congenital defects of chest and abdomen

Structural (e.g., diaphragmatic hernia, jejunal atresia, volvulus, intestinal malrotation)

Peritonitis caused by GI tract perforation, congenital infection (e.g., syphilis, TORCH [*t*oxoplasmosis, *o*ther agents, *r*ubella, *C*MV, *h*erpes simplex], hepatitis), meconium peritonitis

Lymphatic duct obstruction

Biliary atresia

Nonstructural (e.g., congenital nephrotic syndrome, cirrhosis, cholestasis, hepatic necrosis, GI tract obstruction)

Lower GU tract obstruction (e.g., posterior urethral valves, urethral atresia, ureterocele) is most common cause

Inherited skeletal dysplasias (enlarged liver causing extramedullary hematopoiesis)

Fetal tumors, most often teratomas and neuroblastomas

Vascular placental abnormalities

Genetic metabolic disorders (e.g., Hurler syndrome, Gaucher disease, Niemann-Pick disease, G_{M1} gangliosidosis type I, I-cell disease, β-glucuronidase deficiency)

Immune (maternal antibodies reacting to fetal antigens [e.g., Rh, C, E, Kell])

Peritonitis, Acute

See Figures 7-5 and 7-6.

Primary

♦ Gram stain of direct smear and culture of peritoneal fluid usually shows streptococci in children. In adults is caused by *E. coli* (40%–60%) or *S. pneumoniae* (15%), other Gram-negative bacilli and enterococci; usually one organism. May be caused by *M. tuberculosis*.

♦ Diagnostic peritoneal lavage fluid shows WBC count >200/μL in 99% of cases.

Marked increase in WBC (≤50,000/μL) and PMN (80%–90%).

Laboratory findings due to nephrotic syndrome and postnecrotic cirrhosis and occasionally bacteremia in children and cirrhosis with ascites in adults.

Secondary

Laboratory findings due perforation of hollow viscus (e.g., appendicitis, perforated ulcer, volvulus). Usually more than one organism is found.

♦ Occurs and recurs very frequently in continuous ambulatory peritoneal dialysis. Suggested by turbid dialysate (indicates >300 WBC/(μL); Gram stain, culture, and leukocytosis may be absent. Caused by Gram-positive bacteria in ~70%, enteric Gram-negative bacilli and *Pseudomonas aeruginosa* in 20% to 30%, others in 10% to 20%, sterile in 10% to 20%. *If more than one pathogen is found, rule out perforated viscus.*

Systemic Disorders

Genetic Gastrointestinal Diseases

Disease	Mode of Inheritance
Atrophic gastritis (PA)	
MEN types I and II	AD

Gastric cancer	
Colon cancer	
Cancer family syndrome (cancer of colon, breast, endometrium)	AD
Familial polyposes (see "Hereditary Polyposis")	
Celiac disease	
Cystic fibrosis	AR
Shwachman syndrome	AR
Hereditary hemorrhagic telangiectasia (Osler-Weber-Rendu syndrome)	AD
Hereditary pancreatitis	AD
Ehlers-Danlos type IV (bowel rupture)	AD
Tylosis (esophageal cancer; hyperkeratosis palms and soles)	AD
Hereditary hollow visceral myopathy (intestinal pseudoobstruction)	AD
Familial Mediterranean fever (recurrent polyserositis)	AR
Hermansky-Pudlak syndrome (IBD, platelet dysfunction, oculocutaneous albinism, pulmonary fibrosis)	AR
Lactase deficiency	AR
Sucrase-isomaltase deficiency	AR
Hartnup disease	AR
Cystinuria	AR
Pancreatic lipase deficiency	AR
Congenital PA	AR
Imerslünd-Grasbeck syndrome	AR
Congenital chloride diarrhea	AR
Hirschsprung megacolon	
Acrodermatitis enteropathica	AR

PA, pernicious anemia; MEN, multiple endocrine neoplasia; IBD, inflammatory bowel disease; AR, autosomal recessive; AD, autosomal dominant.

Gastrointestinal Diseases with Systemic Manifestations

Anemia (e.g., caused by bleeding occult neoplasm)
Arthritis, uveitis, etc., in ulcerative colitis
Carcinoid syndrome
Endocrine manifestations due to replacement by metastatic tumors of GI tract
Vitamin deficiency (e.g., sprue, malabsorption)

Gastrointestinal Manifestations of Some Systemic Diseases

Allergy
Amyloidosis
Autoimmune/connective tissue diseases (e.g., SLE, RA, scleroderma, Sjögren syndrome, PA, Addison disease)
Bacterial infection (lymphogranuloma venereum)
Cirrhosis (esophageal varices, hemorrhoids, peptic ulcer)
Collagen diseases (e.g., scleroderma, polyarteritis nodosa, SLE)
Cystic fibrosis of pancreas
Down syndrome (various anomalies, atresias, malrotation)
Embolic accidents (e.g., rheumatic heart disease, bacterial endocarditis)
Endocrinopathies (e.g., hyperparathyroidism, hypoparathyroidism, Addison disease, etc.)
Heavy metals (e.g., arsenic, gold, lead)
Hematologic disorders (e.g., sickle cell crises, Henoch purpura, lymphomas and leukemias, hemolytic uremic syndrome, thrombotic thrombocytopenic purpura)
Hereditary angioedema
Hirschsprung disease
Infections (e.g., AIDS and other immunodeficiency disorders; see previous section)
Ischemic vascular disease
Metastatic carcinoma
Neurofibromatosis (involves GI tract in 25% of cases)

Osler-Weber-Rendu disease (GI bleeding in 10%–40% of patients)
Parasitic infestation
Peptic ulcer associated with other diseases (in 8%–22% of patients with hyperparathyroidism, 10% of patients with pituitary tumor, Z-E syndrome)
Porphyrias (e.g., acute intermittent porphyria)
Tangier disease (yellow-orange patches in colon mucosa)
Turner syndrome (GI hemorrhage caused by vascular malformations)
Uremia

Gastrointestinal Tract Conditions with No Useful Laboratory Findings

Chronic esophagitis
Diverticula of esophagus and stomach
Esophageal spasm
Prolapse of gastric mucosa
Foreign bodies in stomach

Hemorrhage, Gastrointestinal

Caused By

Duodenal ulcer (25% of patients)
Esophageal varices (18% of patients)
Gastric ulcer (12% of patients)
Gastritis (12% of patients)
Esophagitis (6% of patients)
Mallory-Weiss syndrome (5% of patients)
Other (22% of patients)
Anticoagulant therapy: Hemorrhage into GI tract occurs in 3% to 4% of patients on anticoagulant therapy; may be spontaneous or secondary to unsuspected disease (e.g., peptic ulcer, carcinoma, diverticula, hemorrhoids). Occasionally there is hemorrhage into the wall of the intestine with secondary ileus. PT may be in the therapeutic range or, more commonly, is increased. *Coumarin drug action is potentiated by administration of aspirin, antibiotics, phenylbutazone, and thyroxine and by T-tube drainage of the common bile duct, especially if pancreatic disease is present.*
In addition to the main cause of bleeding, 50% of patients have an additional lesion that could cause hemorrhage (especially duodenal ulcer, esophageal varices, hiatus hernia). *With previously known GI tract lesions, 40% of patients bled from a different lesion.*

Occult Bleeding[13]

Caused By

Mass (e.g., carcinoma, adenoma)
Inflammation (e.g., IBD, CD, erosive esophagitis)
Vascular disorders (e.g., varices, hemangioma)
Infections (e.g., TB, amebiasis, hookworm, whipworm, strongyloidiasis, ascariasis)
Other sites (e.g., hemoptysis, epistaxis, oropharynx)
Others (e.g., factitious, coagulopathies, long distance running)

Use

Screening for asymptomatic ulcerated lesions of GI tract is generally recommended now, especially carcinoma of the colon and large adenomas.

Interpretation

Kits (e.g., Hemoccult cards) utilize guaiac (uses pseudoperoxidase activity of Hb); will detect blood losses of ~20 mL/d. Normal amount of blood lost in stool daily is ~0.5 to 1.5 mL/d or 2 mg Hb/g of stool (not detected by occult blood tests). Fecal Hb must be >10 mg/g of stool (10 mL of daily blood loss) to give positive Hemoccult 50% of the time. Only ~50% of colon cancers shed enough blood to produce a positive test.
Requires two smears from three consecutive stool samples.

---

[13]Rockey DC. Occult gastrointestinal bleeding. *N Engl J Med* 1999;341:38–46.

Hemoccult will give 1% to 3% false-positive results, even with strict protocol for stool collection.

Sensitivity of Hemoccult and HemoQuant is only ~20% to 30% for colorectal cancer and ~13% for polyps; most of these lesions will be missed.

Benzidine reaction is too sensitive; yields too many false-positive results. Guaiac test yields too many false-negative results.

Comparison of Fecal Occult Blood Tests

	Test		
Characteristic	Guaiac (Hemoccult II Hemoccult II Sensa)	Heme-porphyrin (HemoQuant)	Immunochemical (HemeSelect, FlexSure)
Point of care	++++	0	0 to ++
Testing time	1 min	1 h	5 min to 1 d
False-positive results caused by:			
Nonhuman Hb	++++	++++	0
Dietary peroxidase	+++	0	0
Rehydration	+++	0	0
Iron	0	0	0
False-negative results caused by:			
Hb degradation	+++	0	+++
Storage	++	0	++
Vitamin C	++	0	0

Hb, hemoglobin.

In various screening programs, 2% to 6% of participants have positive tests; of these, carcinoma is found in 5% to 10% and adenoma in 20% to 40%. Sensitivity = 81% for left colon cancer, 47% for colon and cecum cancer, 45% for rectal cancer. About 90% of positive results are false-positive results.

Recommendations for Guaiac Testing:

• Test two areas from each of three consecutive stool samples.
• Test all samples within 7 days of collection.
• Rehydration of slide prior to development is controversial.
• Use of fecal sample obtained by digital rectal exam is not recommended.
• For 3 days before test, avoid large doses of aspirin (>325 mg/d) and other NSAIDs or ascorbic acid (false-negative result may occur with >500 mg/d); red meat, poultry, fish, and certain fruits and vegetables that contain catalases and peroxidases (e.g., cucumbers, horseradish, cauliflower), especially if slides are rehydrated.
• Even one positive is considered a positive test even without dietary restriction.

Other Tests for Occult Blood:

• Quantitative HemoQuant test kit (uses fluorescence to assay stool-derived porphyrins) doubles sensitivity of guaiac tests; may be affected by red meat and aspirin (for up to 4 days) but not by these other substances; manual test is performed in a laboratory and requires 90 minutes; normal <2 mg/g, >4 mg/g is increased, and 2 to 4 mg/g is borderline.
• Immunochemical tests (e.g., HemeSelect) specifically detect human Hb, do not require diet or chemical restrictions (do not react with animal heme or foods), are stable for up to 30 days, and can detect ~0.3 mg Hb/g of stool compared to 5× to 10× this amount to cause a positive guaiac test.
• Samples from the *upper* GI tract should not be tested for blood using urine dipsticks or stool occult blood test kits (low pH may cause false-negative and oral drugs false-positive results).

Adenomas <2 cm in size are less likely to bleed. Upper GI tract bleeding is less likely than lower GI tract bleeding to cause a positive test.

Long distance running is associated with positive guaiac test in ≤23% of runners.

Stools may appear grossly normal with GI bleeding of 100 mL/d.

Consistent melena requires 150 to 200 mL blood in the stomach.

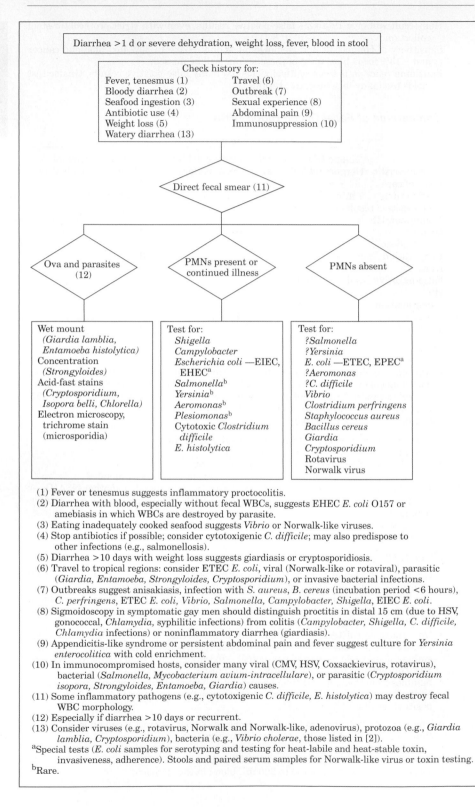

Diarrhea >1 d or severe dehydration, weight loss, fever, blood in stool

Check history for:
Fever, tenesmus (1)   Travel (6)
Bloody diarrhea (2)   Outbreak (7)
Seafood ingestion (3)   Sexual experience (8)
Antibiotic use (4)   Abdominal pain (9)
Weight loss (5)   Immunosuppression (10)
Watery diarrhea (13)

Direct fecal smear (11)

Ova and parasites (12)   PMNs present or continued illness   PMNs absent

Wet mount
*(Giardia lamblia,
Entamoeba histolytica)*
Concentration
(Strongyloides)
Acid-fast stains
*(Cryptosporidium,
Isopora belli, Chlorella)*
Electron microscopy,
trichrome stain
(microsporidia)

Test for:
Shigella
Campylobacter
Escherichia coli —EIEC,
EHEC[a]
Salmonella[b]
Yersinia[b]
Aeromonas[b]
Plesiomonas[b]
Cytotoxic *Clostridium
difficile*
E. histolytica

Test for:
?*Salmonella*
?*Yersinia*
E. coli —ETEC, EPEC[a]
?*Aeromonas*
?*C. difficile*
Vibrio
Clostridium perfringens
Staphylococcus aureus
Bacillus cereus
Giardia
Cryptosporidium
Rotavirus
Norwalk virus

(1) Fever or tenesmus suggests inflammatory proctocolitis.
(2) Diarrhea with blood, especially without fecal WBCs, suggests EHEC *E. coli* O157 or amebiasis in which WBCs are destroyed by parasite.
(3) Eating inadequately cooked seafood suggests *Vibrio* or Norwalk-like viruses.
(4) Stop antibiotics if possible; consider cytotoxigenic *C. difficile*; may also predispose to other infections (e.g., salmonellosis).
(5) Diarrhea >10 days with weight loss suggests giardiasis or cryptosporidiosis.
(6) Travel to tropical regions: consider ETEC *E. coli*, viral (Norwalk-like or rotaviral), parasitic (*Giardia, Entamoeba, Strongyloides, Cryptosporidium*), or invasive bacterial infections.
(7) Outbreaks suggest anisakiasis, infection with *S. aureus*, *B. cereus* (incubation period <6 hours), *C. perfringens*, ETEC *E. coli*, *Vibrio*, *Salmonella*, *Campylobacter*, *Shigella*, EIEC *E. coli*.
(8) Sigmoidoscopy in symptomatic gay men should distinguish proctitis in distal 15 cm (due to HSV, gonococcal, *Chlamydia*, syphilitic infections) from colitis (*Campylobacter, Shigella, C. difficile, Chlamydia* infections) or noninflammatory diarrhea (giardiasis).
(9) Appendicitis-like syndrome or persistent abdominal pain and fever suggest culture for *Yersinia enterocolitica* with cold enrichment.
(10) In immunocompromised hosts, consider many viral (CMV, HSV, Coxsackievirus, rotavirus), bacterial (*Salmonella, Mycobacterium avium-intracellulare*), or parasitic (*Cryptosporidium isopora, Strongyloides, Entamoeba, Giardia*) causes.
(11) Some inflammatory pathogens (e.g., cytotoxigenic *C. difficile, E. histolytica*) may destroy fecal WBC morphology.
(12) Especially if diarrhea >10 days or recurrent.
(13) Consider viruses (e.g., rotavirus, Norwalk and Norwalk-like, adenovirus), protozoa (e.g., *Giardia lamblia, Cryptosporidium*), bacteria (e.g., *Vibrio cholerae*, those listed in [2]).
[a]Special tests (*E. coli* samples for serotyping and testing for heat-labile and heat-stable toxin, invasiveness, adherence). Stools and paired serum samples for Norwalk-like virus or toxin testing.
[b]Rare.

Infections of the Gastrointestinal Tract[14]

See Figure 7-7 and Chapter 15.

Bacteria (e.g., *E. coli O157:H7, Shigella* sp., *Salmonella* sp., *Campylobacter* sp., *Listeria monocytogenes, Yersinia enterocolitica, Vibrio cholerae, V. parahaemolyticus, C. difficile* [major nosocomial colitis after antibiotics alter bowel flora], *C. perfringens* type A, *S. aureus, B. cereus)*

Viruses (e.g., adenovirus, CMV, Norwalk, rotavirus [symptomatic usually only in very young, children], astrovirus, HIV)

Protozoa (e.g., Microsporidia, *Entamoeba histolytica, Giardia lamblia, Balantidium coli, Cryptosporidium* spp., *Isospora belli)*

Helminths (e.g., *Diphyllobothrium latum, Echinococcus granulosus* and *multilocularis, Taenia saginata, Taenia solium, Ascaris lumbricoides, Enterobius vermicularis)*

AIDS, Gastrointestinal Involvement

Mouth—Candida

Esophagus—CMV, Candida, herpes simplex

Small intestine—CMV, *cryptosporidia, Giardia, Isospora belli, microsporidia, M. avium-intracellulare*

Colon—*Candida*, amebae, *Campylobacter, Chlamydia trachomatis*, *C. difficile*, CMV, *Histoplasma, M. avium-intracellulare, Salmonella, Shigella*

Proctitis, Acute

♦ Rectal Gram stain shows >1 PMN/hpf (1,000×)

In homosexual men, specific etiology can be found in 80% of cases completely studied. The most common causes are *C. trachomatis* (non-lymphogranuloma venereum strains) in >75% of cases, *Neisseria gonorrhoeae*, lymphogranuloma venereum, herpes simplex virus type 2, *Treponema pallidum*.

- *Histopathology of rectal biopsy in acute proctocolitis caused by* C. trachomatis *is indistinguishable from CD; culture and serologic tests for* C. trachomatis *and serologic tests for lymphogranuloma venereum strains should be performed in such cases.*
- *Primary or secondary syphilitic proctitis may be very severe and of variable appearance; serologic test for syphilis should be performed.*

Liver and biliary tract—CMV hepatitis, ampullary stenosis, cryptosporidiosis, *M. avium-intracellulare*

Oral Manifestations of Systemic Diseases

Hematologic diseases

- Acute leukemia—edema and hemorrhage
- Granulocytopenia—ulceration and inflammation
- Iron-deficiency anemia—atrophy
- PA—glossitis
- Polycythemia—erosions

Infections

- Bacterial (e.g., diphtheria, scarlet fever, syphilis, Vincent angina)
- Fungal (e.g., actinomycosis, histoplasmosis, mucormycosis, moniliasis)
- Viral (e.g., herpes simplex, herpangina, measles, infectious mononucleosis)

Systemic diseases (e.g., SLE, primary amyloidosis, hereditary hemorrhagic telangiectasia [Osler-Weber-Rendu disease])

Nutritional deficiencies (e.g., pellagra, riboflavin deficiency, scurvy, PA)

Fig. 7-7. Algorithm for etiology of infectious diarrhea. Bacteria cause the severest forms of infectious diarrhea; viruses (e.g., rotaviruses, Norwalk viruses) are the most common causes. CMV, cytomegalovirus; EHEC, enterohemorrhagic; EIEC, enteroinvasive; EPEC, enteropathogenic; ETEC, enterotoxigenic; HSV, herpes simplex virus; PMNs, polymorphonuclear neutrophil leukocytes; WBC, white blood cell. (Adapted from Guerrant RL, Bobak DA. Bacterial and protozoal gastroenteritis. *N Engl J Med.* 1991;325:327–340.)

[14]Acheson D, Fiore A. Preventing foodborne disease—what clinicians can do. *N Engl J Med* 2004; 350:437–440.

8

Hepatobiliary Diseases and Diseases of the Pancreas

LIVER/PANCR

Laboratory Tests for Diseases of Liver

Liver Function Tests and Common Test Patterns

See Table 8–1.
See Figures 8-1–8-3.
Patterns of abnormalities rather than single test changes are particularly useful despite sensitivities of only 65% in some cases.
Abnormal test results may occur in systemic diseases that are not primarily hepatic (e.g., heart failure, SLE, sarcoidosis, TB, sickle cell disease, sepsis, infections such as brucellosis, subacute bacterial endocarditis). Individual tests are normal in high proportions of patients with proven specific liver diseases; normal values may not rule out liver disease.
A confusing pattern may occur in mixed forms of jaundice (e.g., sickle cell disease producing hemolysis and complicated by pigment stones causing duct obstruction).

1. Bilirubin, serum and urine
2. Ratio of conjugated to total bilirubin
3. Enzyme tests that detect injury to hepatocytes (AST, ALT)
4. Ratio of enzymes
5. Enzyme tests that detect cholestasis (ALP, 5'-nucleotidase, γ-glutamyl transpeptidase [GGT], leucine aminopeptidase [LAP])
6. Tests of metabolism and biosynthesis (total protein, albumin, prothrombin time, cholesterol)
7. Tests to detect chronic inflammation (immunoglobulins)

Total Serum Bilirubin

- Not a sensitive indicator of hepatic dysfunction; may not reflect degree of liver damage
- Must exceed 2.5 mg/dL to produce clinical jaundice
- >5 mg/dL seldom occurs in uncomplicated hemolysis unless hepatobiliary disease is also present.
- Is generally less markedly increased in hepatocellular jaundice (<10 mg/dL) than in neoplastic obstructions (≤20 mg/dL) or intrahepatic cholestasis
- In extrahepatic biliary obstruction, bilirubin may rise progressively to a plateau of 30 to 40 mg/dL (due in part to balance between renal excretion and diversion of bilirubin to other metabolites). Such a plateau tends not to occur in hepatocellular jaundice and bilirubin may exeed 50 mg/dL (partly due to concomitant renal insufficiency and hemolysis).
- Concentrations are generally higher in obstruction due to carcinoma than due to stones.
- In viral hepatitis, higher serum bilirubin suggests more liver damage and longer clinical course.
- In acute alcoholic hepatitis, >5 mg/dL suggests a poor prognosis.
- Increased serum bilirubin with normal ALP suggests constitutional hyperbilirubinemias or hemolytic states.
- Due to renal excretion, maximum bilirubin = 10 to 35 mg/dL; if renal disease is present may reach 75 mg/dL.
- Conjugated bilirubin >1.0 mg/dL in an infant always indicates disease.

Table 8-1. Increased Serum Enzyme Levels in Liver Diseases

Serum Enzyme	Acute Viral Hepatitis		Complete Biliary Obstruction		Cirrhosis		Liver Metastases	
	Frequency[a]	Amplitude[b]	Frequency	Amplitude	Frequency	Amplitude	Frequency	Amplitude
AST	>95%	14	>95%	3	75%	2	50%	1–2
ALT	>95%	17	>95%	4	50%	1	25%	1–2
ALP	60%	1–2	>95%	4–14	55%	1–2	50%	1–10 (TB)
							40%	1–3 (sarcoidosis)
							80%	1–14 (carcinoma)
							Frequently	1–20 (amyloidosis)
Leucine aminopeptidase	80%	1–2	85%	3	30%	1	70%	2–3
Isocitrate dehydrogenase	>95%	6	10%	1	20%	1	40%	2
5'-Nucleotidase	70%	1–2	>95%	6	50%	1–2	65%	3–4

[a]Frequency, average percentage of patients with increased serum enzyme level when blood taken at optimal time.
[b]Amplitude, average number of times normal that serum level is increased.

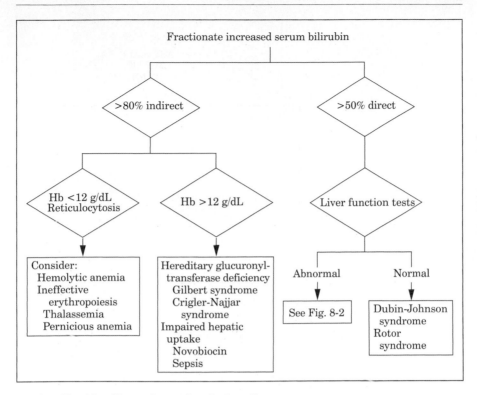

Fig. 8-1. Algorithm illustrating workup for jaundice.

Serum Bilirubin (Conjugated:total)

- <20% conjugated
  Constitutional (e.g., Gilbert disease, Crigler-Najjar syndrome)
  Hemolytic states
- 20% to 40% conjugated
  Favors hepatocellular disease rather than extrahepatic obstruction
  Disorders of bilirubin metabolism (e.g., Dubin-Johnson, Rotor syndromes)
- 40% to 60% conjugated: Occurs in either hepatocellular or extrahepatic type
- >50% conjugated: Favors extrahepatic obstruction rather than hepatocellular disease

AST and ALT

In cytoplasm of liver cells, 1 1/2–2× as much AST as ALT. Half-life of AST is ~18 hours, half-life of ALT is ,48 hours. Thus, in early acute hepatitis, AST is usually higher initially, but by 48 hours, ALT is usually higher. AST is also found in mitochondria

- Most sensitive tests for acute hepatocellular injury (e.g., viral, drug); precedes increase in serum bilirubin by ~1 week
- >500 U/L suggests acute hepatocellular injury; seldom >500 U/L in obstructive jaundice, cirrhosis, viral hepatitis, AIDS, alcoholic liver disease.
- Most marked increases (thousands U/L) occur with extensive hepatocellular damage (e.g., viral hepatitis, acute heart failure, exposure to carbon tetrachloride, drug injury [e.g., acetaminophen]).
- AST soaring to peak of 1,000 to 9,000 U/L, declining by 50% within 3 days and to <100 U/L within a week, suggests shock liver with centrolobular necrosis (e.g., due to congestive heart failure, arrhythmia, sepsis, GI hemorrhage); serum bilirubin and ALP reflect underlying disease.

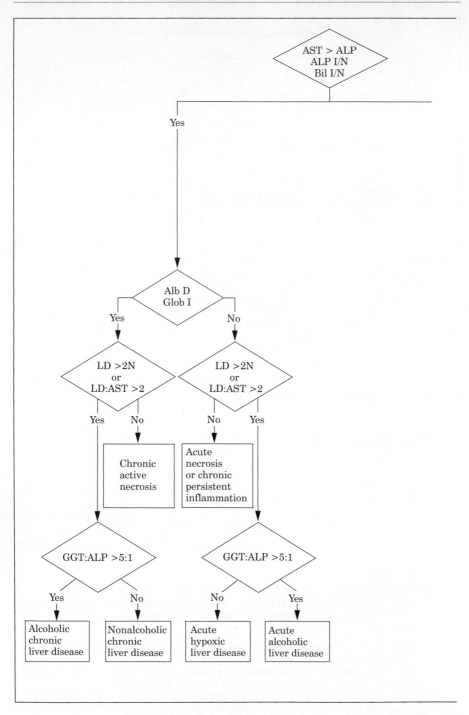

Fig. 8-2. Algorithm illustrating sequential abnormal liver function test interpretation. (N, normal; I, increased; Bil, bilirubin; Alb, albumin; Glob, globulin; ALP, alkaline phosphatase; LD, lactate dehydrogenase; GGT, gamma-glutamyltransferase; CHF, congestive heart failure. Enzymes all in same U/L.) (Adapted from JB Henry, *Clinical diagnosis and management by laboratory methods,* 16th ed. Philadelphia: Saunders, 1979.)

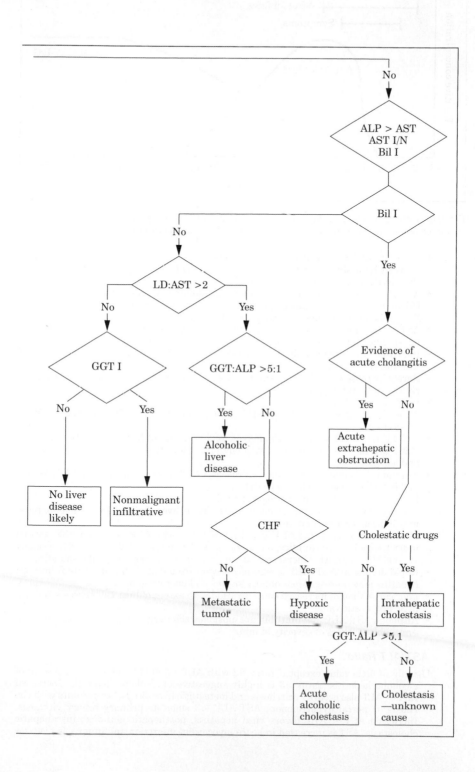

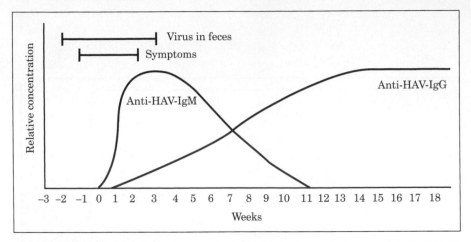

Fig. 8-3. Antibody markers in hepatitis A virus (HAV) infection. (IgG, immunoglobulin G; IgM, immunoglobulin M.) (Reproduced with permission of Abbott Laboratories, Pasadena, CA.)

- Rapid rise of AST and ALT to very high levels (e.g., >600 U/L and often >2,000 U/L) followed by a sharp fall in 12 to 72 hours is said to be typical of acute bile duct obstruction due to a stone.
- Abrupt AST rise may also be seen in acute fulminant viral hepatitis (rarely >4,000 U/L and declines more slowly; positive serological tests) and acute chemical injury.
- Patient is rarely asymptomatic with level >1,000 U/L.
- AST >10× normal indicates acute hepatocellular injury but lesser increases are nonspecific and may occur with virtually any form of liver injury.
- Increases ≤8× upper limit of normal (ULN) are nonspecific; may be found in any liver disorder.
- Rarely increased >500 U/L (usually <200 U/L) in posthepatic jaundice, AIDS, cirrhosis, and viral hepatitis
- Usually <50 U/L in fatty liver
- <100 U/L in alcoholic cirrhosis; ALT is normal in 50% and AST is normal in 25% of these cases.
- <150 U/L in alcoholic hepatitis (may be higher if patient has delirium tremens)
- <200 U/L in ~50% of patients with cirrhosis, metastatic liver disease, lymphoma, and leukemia
- Normal values may not rule out liver disease: ALT is normal in 50%, and AST is normal in 25% of cases of alcoholic cirrhosis.
- Degree of increase has poor prognostic value.
- Serial determinations reflect clinical activity of liver disease. Persistent increase may indicate chronic hepatitis.
- Mild increase of AST and ALT (usually <500 U/L) with ALP increased >3× normal indicates cholestatic jaundice, but more marked increase of AST and ALT (especially >1,000 U/L) with ALP increased <3× normal indicates hepatocellular jaundice.
- Rapid decline in AST, ALT is sign of recovery from disease but in acute fulminant hepatitis may represent loss of hepatocytes and poor prognosis.
- Poor correlation of increased concentration with extent of liver cell necrosis and has little prognostic value
- Although AST, ALT, and bilirubin are most characteristic of acute hepatitis, they are unreliable markers of severity of injury.

AST/ALT Ratio

Usually of little value except if ratio >2 with ALT <300 U/L, which is suggestive of alcoholic hepatitis; ratio >3 is highly suggestive of alcoholic hepatitis. Increased AST > ALT also occurs in cirrhosis and metastatic liver disease. In patients with cirrhosis or portal hypertension, AST/ALT ≥3 suggests primary biliary cirrhosis. Increased AST < ALT favors viral hepatitis, posthepatic jaundice, intrahepatic cholestasis. AST is increased in acute myocardial infarction and in muscle diseases

(≤300 U/L), but ALT is usually normal unless there is liver congestion. ALT is more specific for liver disease than AST.

Enzyme Tests That Detect Cholestasis (ALP, 5'-nucleotidase, GGT, LAP)

- Increased ALP in liver diseases (due to increased synthesis from proliferating bile duct epithelium) is the best indicator of biliary obstruction but does not differentiate intrahepatic cholestasis from extrahepatic obstruction. In cholestasis is increased out of proportion to other liver function tests.
- Increases before jaundice occurs
- High values (>5× normal) favor obstruction and normal levels virtually exclude this diagnosis.
- Markedly increased in infants with congenital intrahepatic bile duct atresia but is much lower in extrahepatic atresia
- Increased 10× normal: carcinoma of head of pancreas, choledocholithiasis, drug cholestatic hepatitis
- 15 to 20× increase: primary biliary cirrhosis, primary or metastatic carcinoma
- Increase (3–10× normal) with only slightly increased transaminases may be seen in biliary obstruction and converse in liver parenchymal disease (e.g., cirrhosis, hepatitis); increased >3× normal in <5% of acute hepatitis.
- Increased (2–10× normal; usually 1.5–3× increase) serum ALP and LD in early infiltrative (e.g., amyloid) and space-occupying diseases of the liver (e.g., tumor, granuloma, abscess)
- Increase <3 to 4× normal is nonspecific and may occur in all types of liver diseases (e.g., congestive heart failure, infiltrative liver diseases, cirrhosis, acute [viral, toxic, alcoholic] or chronic hepatitis, acute fatty liver).
- Increased 5× normal: Infectious mononucleosis, postnecrotic cirrhosis
- Increased ALP (of liver origin) and LD with normal serum bilirubin, AST, ALT, suggests obstruction of one hepatic duct, or metastatic or infiltrative disease of liver.

GGT/ALP ratio >5 favors alcoholic liver disease.

Isolated increase of GGT is a sensitive screening and monitoring test for alcoholism. Increased GGT due to alcohol or anticonvulsant drugs is not accompanied by increased ALP.

Serum 5'-nucleotidase (5'-N) and LAP parallel the increase in ALP in obstructive type of hepatobiliary disease, but the 5'-N is increased only in the latter and is normal in pregnancy and bone disease, whereas the LAP is increased in pregnancy but is usually normal in bone disease. GGT is normal in bone disease and pregnancy. Therefore, these enzymes are useful in determining the source of increased serum ALP. Although serum 5'-N usually parallels ALP in liver disease, it may not increase proportionately in individual patients.

Serum Enzyme	Biliary Obstruction	Pregnancy	Childhood; Bone Disease
ALP	Increased	Increased	Increased
GGT	Increased	Normal	Normal
5'-N	Increased	Normal	Normal
LAP	Increased	Increased	Normal

Bilirubin ("bile") in urine implies increased serum conjugated bilirubin and excludes hemolysis as the cause. Often precedes clinical icterus. May occur without jaundice in anicteric or early hepatitis, early obstruction or liver metastases. (Tablets detect 0.05–0.1 mg/dL; dipsticks are less sensitive; test is negative in normal persons.)

Complete absence of urine urobilinogen strongly suggests complete bile duct obstruction; is normal in incomplete obstruction. Decreased in some phases of hepatic jaundice. Increased in hemolytic jaundice and subsiding hepatitis. Increase may evidence hepatic damage even without clinical jaundice (e.g., some patients with cirrhosis, metastatic liver disease, congestive heart failure). Presence in viral hepatitis depends on phase of disease (normal is <1 mg or 1 Ehrlich unit/2 hour specimen).

Tests of Metabolism and Biosynthesis

Serum albumin reflects liver damage more slowly.

- Is usually normal in hepatitis and cholestasis
- Increase toward normal by 2 to 3 g/dL in treatment of cirrhosis implies improvement and more favorable prognosis than if no increase with therapy.

Prothrombin time

- May be prolonged due to lack of vitamin K absorption in obstruction or lack of synthesis in hepatocellular disease. Not useful when only slightly prolonged.
- Corrected within 24 to 48 hours by parenteral administration of vitamin K (10 mg/day for 3 days) in obstructive but not in hepatocellular disease. Failure to correct suggests poor prognosis; extensive hepatic necrosis should be considered.
- Markedly prolonged PT is a good index of severe liver cell damage in hepatitis and may herald onset of fulminant hepatic necrosis.

Serum cholesterol

- May be normal or slightly decreased in hepatitis
- Markedly decreased in severe hepatitis or cirrhosis
- Increased in posthepatitic jaundice or intrahepatic cholestasis
- Markedly increased in primary biliary cirrhosis

Tests to Detect Chronic Inflammation or Autoimmunity

Serum gamma globulin

- Tends to increase with most forms of chronic liver disease
- Increases are not specific; found in other chronic inflammatory and neoplastic diseases.
- Moderate increases (e.g., >3 g/dL) are suggestive of chronic active hepatitis; marked increases are suggestive of autoimmune chronic hepatitis.
- Polyclonal increases in IgG and IgM are found in most types of cirrhosis; are non-specific.
- Increased IgM alone may suggest primary biliary cirrhosis.
- Increased IgA may occur in alcoholic cirrhosis.
- Ig are usually normal in obstructive jaundice.

Test for antimitochondrial antibodies to rule out primary biliary cirrhosis in females (present in >90% of cases) and radiologic studies to rule out primary sclerosing cholangitis (see Table 8–18).

Liver Biopsy[1]

Use
Diagnose, grade, and stage alcoholic, nonalcoholic, and autoimmune liver diseases
Diagnose, grade, and stage chronic hepatitis (HBV, HCV). Assess disease progression and indication for antiviral therapy. No consistent correlation between serum ALT and severity of liver pathology; significant liver damage can occur with normal ALT.
Evaluate abnormal or inconclusive biochemical or serological tests; cholestasis in primary biliary cirrhosis or primary sclerosing cholangitis
Diagnose hemochromatosis and quantitate amount of iron present
Diagnose Wilson disease and quantitate amount of copper present
Exclude coexisting or alternative diseases
Diagnose a mass in the liver
In liver transplant, evaluate donor liver before procedure or recepient after transplant
Evaluate effect of therapy on liver morphology
Culture tissue in patients with fever of unknown etiology

Contraindications
Bleeding tendency (e.g., hemophilia,* NSAID within prior 10 days, platelet count <50,000/μL, BT >10 minutes, PT >3–5 seconds above control, possible vascular tumor such as hemangioma),[†] or blood not available for possible transfusion
Possible echinococcal cysts in liver
Infection in right pleural space or abdomen*
Uncooperative patient
Marked obesity or ascites*[†]

---

[1]Bravo AA, et al. Liver biopsy. *N Engl J Med* 2001;344:495.
*Relative contraindication
[†]May use transjugular liver biopsy

Diseases of the Liver

Hepatocellular Disease

Cirrhosis of Liver

♦ Criteria for diagnosis by liver biopsy or ≥3 of the following:

- Hyperglobulinemia, especially with hypoalbuminemia
- Low-protein (<2.5 g/dL) ascites
- Evidence of hypersplenism (usually thrombocytopenia, often with leukopenia and less often Coomb's negative hemolytic anemia)
- Evidence of portal hypertension (e.g., varices)
- Characteristic "cork screw" hepatic arterioles on celiac arteriography
- Shunting of blood to bone marrow on radioisotope scan
- *Abnormality of serum bilirubin, transaminases, or ALP is often not present and therefore not required for diagnosis.*

○ Serum bilirubin is often increased; may be present for years. Fluctuations may reflect liver status due to insults to the liver (e.g., alcoholic debauches). Most bilirubin is of the unconjugated type unless cirrhosis is of the cholangiolitic type. Higher and more stable levels occur in postnecrotic cirrhosis; lower and more fluctuating levels occur in Laennec cirrhosis. Terminal icterus may be constant and severe.

○ Serum AST is increased (<300 units) in 65% to 75% of patients. Serum ALT is increased (<200 U) in 50% of patients. Transaminases vary widely and reflect activity or progression of the process (i.e., hepatic parenchymal cell necrosis).

Serum ALP is increased in 40% to 50% of patients.

○ Serum total protein is usually normal or decreased. Serum albumin parallels functional status of parenchymal cells and may be useful for following progress of liver disease; but it may be normal in the presence of considerable liver cell damage. Decreasing serum albumin may reflect development of ascites or hemorrhage. Serum globulin level is usually increased; it reflects inflammation and parallels the severity of the inflammation. Increased serum globulin (is usually gamma) may cause increased total protein, especially in chronic viral hepatitis and posthepatitic cirrhosis.

Serum total cholesterol is normal or decreased. Progressive decrease in cholesterol, HDL, LDL with increasing severity. Decrease is more marked than in chronic active hepatitis. LDL may be useful for prognosis and selecting patients for transplantation. Decreased esters reflect more severe parenchymal cell damage.

Urine bilirubin is increased; urobilinogen is normal or increased.

BUN is often decreased (<10 mg/dL); increased with GI hemorrhage.

Serum uric acid is often increased.

Electrolytes and acid–base balance are often abnormal and reflect various combinations of circumstances at the time, such as malnutrition, dehydration, hemorrhage, metabolic acidosis, respiratory alkalosis. In cirrhosis with ascites, the kidney retains increased sodium and excessive water, causing dilutional hyponatremia.

Blood ammonia is increased in liver coma and cirrhosis and with portacaval shunting of blood.

Anemia reflects increased plasma volume and some increased destruction of RBCs. If more severe, rule out hemorrhage in GI tract, folic acid deficiency, excessive hemolysis, etc.

WBC is usually normal with active cirrhosis; increased (<50,000/μL) with massive necrosis, hemorrhage, etc.; decreased with hypersplenism.

Laboratory findings due to complications or sequelae, often in combination

- Portal hypertension
  Ascites
  Esophageal varices
  Portal vein thrombosis
- Liver failure
- Hepatocarcinoma

Table 8-2.   Classification of Liver Disease by Mechanism of Jaundice

	Chief Mechanism[1]	Causes Page #	Examples of Diseases	Enzymes	Other Chemicals	Urine
Hepato-cellular	Necrosis of liver cells	Drugs Toxins Viruses	Hepatitis	↑	↑Bilirubin: Conjugated > unconjugated	↑Bile and urobilin-ogen
			Alcohol	V	V, depending on duration	
			Cirrhosis	↑AST (<300 ≤3/4 of cases) >ALT (<200 U in 1/2 of cases)	↑TP, globulin ↓albumin	
		Bacteria Amebae	Abscess	↑ALP	↑Bilirubin ↑globulin ↓albumin	
	Fatty infiltration	Alcohol Drugs Nutritional Metabolic Infection	Fatty liver	Sl. ↑ALT > AST N ALP	↑ferritin (≤5×) and transfer-rin saturation in ~60% of cases	
Obstruc-tive[2]	Obstruction or impaired excretion of bile	Neoplasms	Bile ducts, head of pancreas	↑ALP	↑Bilirubin is mostly conjugated ↑Cholesterol	0 bile or uro-bilinogen, depend-ing on complete-ness of obstruc-tion
		Strictures	Sclerosing cholangitis Primary biliary cirrhosis	V, depending on duration	Antimito-chondrial antibodies for	
		Stones	Stones		primary biliary	
		Biliary atresia	Congenital		cirrhosis in females	
		Cholestasis	Drugs Focal lesions (e.g., metas-tases, gran-ulomas, amyloid, abscess, etc.)	↑ALP, GGT	(present in >90% of cases) Radiologic studies for primary sclerosing cholangitis	
Metabolic (inherited)	Crigler-Najjar Syndrome	Failure of bilirubin-glucuronide conjugation	—	N	↑Unconju-gated bilirubin No conjugated bilirubin	No conju-gated bili
	Gilbert Disease	Impaired excretion of conjugated bilirubin	—	N	Transient ↑Unconju-gated bilirubin	N Bile and urobilino-gen

(continued)

Table 8-2. *(continued)*

	Chief Mechanism[1]	Causes Page #	Examples of Diseases	Enzymes	Other Chemicals	Urine
	Dubin-Johnson Syndrome	Inability to transport bilirubin-glucuronide through hepatocytes into canaliculi	—	N	↑Conjugated bilirubin	N Bile and urobilinogen
	Rotor Syndrome	Impaired excretion of conjugated bilirubin	—	N	↑Conjugated bilirubin	
	Breast-milk jaundice	Mother's milk contains pregnanediol, which inhibits glucuronyltransferase activity	—	N	↑Unconjugated bilirubin	
	Hemochromatosis	See Fig. 8–14.	—			
	Wilson disease		—			
	Alpha₁-antitrypsin deficiency					
Vascular	Budd-Chiari	Prothrombotic states; see Ch. 11	—	↑		
	Portal vein thrombosis	Prothrombotic states; see Ch. 11	—	↑		
	Congestive heart failure, constrictive pericariditis, effusion, etc.		—		Unconjugated > conjugated	
	Hepatic venoocclusive disease	High dose chemotherapy and stem cell transplant	—	AST >4× normal		
Hemolytic	Increased production of bilirubin	Hemolysis Ineffective erythropoiesis	Hemolytic anemias, PA, thalassemias, etc.	N or due to underlying disease ↑LD	↑Unconjugated bilirubin N TP, albumin	↑Urobilinogen ↓Hb, ↓haptoglobin

Indirect bilirubin is synonomous with unconjugated bilirubin and *direct* is synonomous with conjugated bilirubin. Unconjugated bilirubin is not water soluble and therefore does not appear in urine.
↑, increased; ↓, decreased; N, normal; V, variable
[1]Often more than one mechanism is present (e.g., stones due to underlying hemolytic disease, obstructive disease that secondarily also develops liver necrosis).
[2]Obstruction may first be incomplete and become complete later (e.g., neoplasms).

Table 8-3.   Comparison of Different Mechanisms of Jaundice

	Cholestasis	Hepatocellular	Infiltration
Disease example	Common duct stone Drugs	Acute viral hepatitis	Metastatic tumor, granulomas, amyloid
Serum bilirubin	6–20 mg/dL*	4–8 mg/dL	Usually <4 mg/dL, often normal
AST, ALT (U/mL)	May be slightly I, <200	Markedly I, often 500–1,000	May be slightly I, <100
Serum ALP	3–5 × N†	1–2 × N	2–4 × N
Prothrombin time	I in chronic cases	I in severe disease	N
Response to parenteral vitamin K	Yes	No	

N = normal, I = increase
*Serum bilirubin >10 mg/dL is rarely seen with common duct stone and usually indicates carcinoma.
†Increased serum ALP <3× normal in 15% of patients with extrahepatic biliary obstruction, especially if obstruction is incomplete or due to benign conditions. Occasionally AST and LD are markedly increased in biliary obstruction or liver cancer.

- Abnormalities of coagulation mechanisms (see Chapter 11), e.g.,
  Prolonged PT (does not respond to parenteral vitamin K as frequently as in patients with obstructive jaundice)
  Prolonged bleeding time in 40% of cases due to decreased platelets and/or fibrinogen
- Hepatic encephalopathy (neurologic and mental abnormalities in some patients with liver failure or portosystemic shunt)
  ♦ Diagnosis is clinical; characteristic laboratory findings are supportive but not specific.
  ○ CSF is normal except for increased glutamine levels, which reflect brain ammonia levels (due to conversion from ammonia). Glutamine >35 mg/dL is always associated with hepatic encephalopathy (normal = 20 mg/dL); correlates with depth of coma and is more sensitive than arterial ammonia.

Table 8-4.   Comparison of Three Main Types of Liver Disease Due to Drugs

	Predominantly Cholestatic	Predominantly Hepatocellular	Mixed Biochemical Pattern
Example of drugs	Anabolic steroids,* estrogens* Organical arsenicals, antithyroid drugs (e.g., methimazole), chlorpromazine, PAS, erythromycin, sulfonylurea derivatives (including sulfonamides, phenothiazine tranquilizers, oral diuretics, antidiabetic drugs)	Cinchophen Isonicotinic acid hydrazide Monamine oxidase inhibitors (particularly iproniazid)	Phenylbutazone Phenytoin PAS and other anti-tuberculosis agents
Serum bilirubin	May be ≥30 mg/dL		
AST, ALT, LD (U/mL)	Mild to moderate increase	More markedly increased	
Serum ALP, LAP	More markedly increased; may remain increased for years after jaundice has disappeared	Less markedly increased	

*ALP, AST, ALT are not increased as much compared with other drugs.

○ Blood ammonia is increased in 90% of patients but does not reflect the degree of coma. Normal level in comatose patient suggests another cause of coma. Not reliable for diagnosis but may be useful to follow individual patients. Arterial specimens are preferable; must be iced and analyzed within 20 minutes.

Respiratory alkalosis due to hyperventilation is frequent.

Hyponatremia and iatrogenic hypernatremia are frequent complications and are associated with a higher mortality rate.

Hypokalemic metabolic alkalosis may occur due to diuretic excess.

Serum amino acid profile is abnormal. All serum amino acids are markedly increased in coma due to acute liver failure.

• Spontaneous bacterial peritonitis—in 10% to 30% of cirrhosis cases with ascites. 70% have positive blood culture; usually single organism, especially *E. coli, pneumococcus, Klebsiella*. ≥250 PMNs/μL is diagnostic. May precipitate hepatorenal syndrome.
• Hepatorenal syndrome (see Chapter 14)
• Most commonly die of liver failure, bleeding, infections

Laboratory findings due to causative/associated diseases or conditions	Frequency in United States
Alcoholism	60%–70%
Biliary disease (e.g., primary biliary cirrhosis, sclerosing cholangitis)	5%–10%
Cryptogenic	10%–15%
Chronic viral hepatitis (HBV with or without HDV; HCV)	10%
Hemochromatosis	5%
Wilson disease	Rare
Alpha$_1$-antitrypsin deficiency	Rare
Autoimmune chronic active hepatitis	
Mucoviscidosis	
Glycogen-storage diseases	
Galactosemia	
Porphyria	
Fructose intolerance	
Tyrosinosis	
Infections (e.g., congenital syphilis, schistosomiasis)	
Gaucher disease	
Ulcerative colitis	
Osler-Weber-Rendu disease	
Venous outflow obstruction (e.g., Budd-Chiari syndrome, venoocclusive disease, congestive heart failure)	

Markers that may indicate progression to cirrhosis

• Decreased albumin
• AST/ALT ratio >1
• Increased bilirubin, mainly inconjugated
• Increased globulins
• Decreased platelt count
• Increased PT

Fatty Liver

Due To[2]
• Nutritional* (e.g., alcoholism, malnutrition, starvation, rapid weight loss)
• Drugs (e.g., aspirin,[†] glucocorticoids,* synthetic estrogens,* some antiviral agents,*[†] calcium-channel blockers,[†] cocaine,[†] methotrexate,* valproic acid[†])
• Metabolic/genetic (e.g., acute fatty liver of pregnancy,[†] dysbetalipoproteinemia,* Weber-Christian disease,* cholesterol ester storage,[‡] Wolman disease[‡])
• Other (e.g., HIV infection,* *Bacillus cereus* toxins,[†] liver toxins [o.g , organic solvents, phosphorus[†]], small bowel disease [inflammatory, bacterial overgrowth],* fatty liver of pregnancy [see below])

---

[2]Data from: P Angulo. Nonalcoholic Fatty Liver Disease. *N Engl J Med* 2002;346:1221.

*May principally cause macrovesicular steatosis due to imbalance in hepatic synthesis and export of lipids

[†]May principally cause microvesicular steatosis due to defective mitochondrial function

[‡]May principally cause accumulation of phospholipids in lysosomes

Laboratory findings are due to underlying conditions (most commonly alcoholism; nonalcoholic fatty liver [NAFL] is commonly associated with NIDDM diabetes mellitus [≤75%], obesity [69%–100%], hyperlipidemia [20%–81%]; malnutrition, toxic chemicals)
♦ Biopsy of liver establishes the diagnosis.
NAFL is distinguished by neglible history of alcohol consumption and negative random blood alcohol assays.
Liver function tests
   Most commonly, serum AST and ALT are increased 2 to 3×; usually ALT > AST in NAFL.
   Serum ALP is normal or slightly increased in <50% of patients.
   Increased serum ferritin (≤5×) and transferrin saturation occur in ~60% of cases.
   Other liver function tests are usually normal.
   Serologic tests for viral hepatitis are negative.
Cirrhosis occurs in ≤50% of alcoholic and ≤17% of nonalcoholic cases.
Biochemically different form occurs in acute fatty liver of pregnancy, Reye syndrome, tetracycline administration.
Fatty liver may be the only postmortem finding in cases of sudden, unexpected death.

Fatty Liver of Pregnancy, Acute

Incidence of ≤1 per 15,000 deliveries; usually occurs >35th week of pregnancy. Medical emergency because of high maternal and fetal mortality that is markedly improved by termination of pregnancy.

Often associated with preeclampsia (see Chapter 15)
Increased AST and ALT to ~300 U (rarely >500 U) is used for early screening in suspicious cases; ratio is not helpful in differential diagnosis.
Increased WBC in >80% of cases (often >15,000/μL)
Evidence of DIC in >75% of patients (see Fig. 11–19)
Serum uric acid is increased disproportionately to BUN and creatinine, which may also be increased.
Serum bilirubin may be normal early but will rise unless pregnancy terminates.
Blood ammonia is usually increased.
Blood glucose is often decreased, sometimes markedly.
Neonatal liver function tests are usually normal but hypoglycemia may occur.
♦ Biopsy of liver confirms the diagnosis.

Table 8-5.   Comparison of Types of Acute Hepatitis

	Viral	Due to Drugs	Toxic/Ischemia	Alcoholic
Peak ALT (× URL)	8–40×	3–40×	10–100× or more	3–5×
AST/ALT	<1 ≤40× URL	<1	>1 for first 1–2 days, then ALT > AST; usually >40× URL	AST > ALT >2 ≤8× URL
Duration of increase	5	<2 if stop drug	1–2	3–5×
ALP (× URL)	<3× in ≤95%	>3× in 50%	<2×	>3× in 25%
PT (sec > URL)	<3×	<3×	>4×	<3×
Incidence of jaundice	10%–70%	20%–30%	<10%	50%–70%
Serum bilirubin	Increase is variable		Usually <5 mg/dL (<2 mg/dL in 80%)	>5 mg/dL suggests a poor prognosis
Viral serology	+	−	−	−

URL, upper reference limit. PT increased >4 sec suggests a poor prognosis.

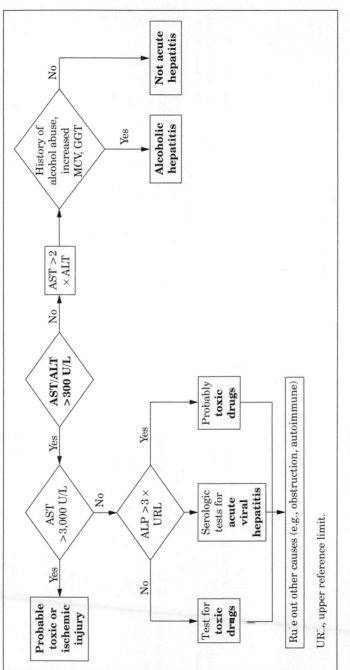

Fig. 8-4 Algorithm for suspected acute hepatic injury.

URᴸ, upper reference limit.

Table 8-6. Comparison of Different Types of Viral Hepatitis

	A	B	C	D	E
Genome	ssRNA	dsDNA	ssRNA	ssRNA	ssRNA
Classification	Picornaviridae	Hepadnaviridae	Flaviviridae	Unclassified	Caliciviridae?
Cause of hepatitis (% in United States)	~30	~40	~20	Always associated with HBV; 4% of acute HBV cases have HDV coinfection	Rare; occurs in travelers to endemic areas
Incubation period (days)	15–60	45–160	14–180	42–180	15–64
Transmission					
Enteric	Yes	No	No	No	Yes
Sexual	No	Yes	Possible	Possible	No
Perinatal	No	Yes	Possible	Possible	No
Parenteral	Rare	Yes	Yes	Yes	No
Posttransfusion incidence (%)	None	0.002	1–4		None
Viremia	Transient	Prolonged	Prolonged	Prolonged	Transient?
Fecal excretion of virus	+	–	–	–	+
Onset	Abrupt	Insidious	Insidious	Abrupt	Abrupt
Course	Mild, often subclinical	Most children; 50% adults[b]	See text		Mild, self-limited[a]
Asymptomatic	Most children		~75%	Rare	Often

Jaundice	Child: 10% Adult: 70%–80%	15%–40%[c]	10%–25%	Varies	25%–50%
Fulminant	1% Causes 5% of fulminant cases	0.2%–2.0%	~0.5%	High	May cause one-third, fulminant cases with 90% mortality
Carrier state	No	Adult: 6%–10% Child: 25%–50% Infant: 70%–90% ≤1% of U.S. donors	50%–70% ≤1% of U.S. donors addicts and hemophiliacs	10%–15% 1%–10% of drug	No Unknown
Chronic hepatitis	No	5%–10% of acute infections	>50%	<5% coinfection; 80% superinfection	No
Hepatocellular	No	Yes	Yes	Yes	Unknown; not likely
Mortality	1%–2%	1%–2%	1%–2%	≤30% in chronic cases	1%–2%; 20% in pregnancy

[a]Resembles hepatitis A. Case fatality 1%–2% except ≤20% in pregnancy. Usually milder infection and biochemical abnormalities than HBV or HAV infection.
[b]≤20% have serum sickness-like prodroma.
[c]Nonicteric patient is more likely to progress to chronic hepatitis. 1% of icteric cases become fulminant (<8 wks) and 90% die within 2–4 wks; associated with encephalopathy; renal, electrolyte, acid-base imbalances; hypoglycemia; coagulation derangements.

Infections

Abscess of Liver, Pyogenic

Due To
Biliary tract infection secondary to obstruction especially neoplastic
Direct extension
Trauma
Hepatic artery route
Bacteremia
Portal vein pyelophlebitis (especially due to appendicitis)
Unknown
♦ Gram stain and culture from blood or bile

* Gram-negative bacilli (e.g., *E. coli, Klebsiella* spp.)
* Anaerobes (e.g., *Bacteroides fragilis*)
* *Staph. aureus* or streptococci are found in children with bacteremia.
* Pseudomonas, streptococcal, fungal species due to increased use of biliary stents and broad-spectrum antibiotics
* Amebic

Abnormalities of liver function tests

* Decreased serum albumin in 50% of cases; increased serum globulin
* Increased serum ALP in 75% of cases
* Increased serum bilirubin in 20% to 25% of cases; >10 mg/dL usually indicates pyogenic rather than amebic and suggests poorer prognosis because of more tissue destruction
* See Space-Occupying Lesions of Liver.

Most patients have increased WBC due to increase in granulocytes and anemia.
Ascites is unusual compared to other causes of space-occupying lesions.
Laboratory findings due to complications (e.g., right pleural effusion in 20% of cases, subphrenic abscess, pneumonia, empyema, bronchopleural fistula)
♦ Patients with amebic abscess of liver due to *Entamoeba histolytica* also show positive serologic tests for ameba.
Stools may be negative for cysts and trophozoites.
Needle aspiration of abscess may show *Entamoeba histolytica* in 50% of patients.
    Characteristic brown or anchovy-sauce color may be absent; secondary bacterial infection may be superimposed.
See *Echinococcus granulosus* cyst.
♦ Abscesses can be visualized by ultrasound, CT, MRI, etc.

Hepatitis

Non-Viral

Due To (e.g., miliary TB, staphylococcal bacteremia, salmonelloses, amebiasis, leishmaniasis, malaria, candidasis, drugs, etc.)

Acute Viral

See Table 8-6 and Fig. 8-5.
Cannot distinguish different types of viral hepatitis by clinical features or routine chemistries; serologic tests are needed.
Due To
Epstein-Barr virus (infectious mononucleosis)
Hepatitis A, B, C, D, E, G
CMV or herpesvirus infection, especially in immunosuppressed patients or newborns
Yellow fever
Rubella, adenovirus, enterovirus occur infrequently in immunosuppressed patients or children.

Prodromal Period

♦ Serologic markers appear in serum (Table 8-6).
Bilirubinuria occurs before serum bilirubin increases.
Increase in urinary urobilinogen and total serum bilirubin just before clinical jaundice occurs

Table 8-7.   Serologic Markers of Viral Hepatitis

Stage of Infection	HAV	HBV	HCV	HDV	HEV
Acute disease	Anti-HAV-IgM	HBcAb-IgM	Anti-HCV	HDAg	Anti-HEV[a]
Chronic disease	NA	HBsAg	Anti-HCV	Anti-HDV	NA
Infectivity	HAV-RNA[b]	HBeAg, HBsAg, HBV-DNA[c]	Anti-HCV, HCV-RNA	Anti-HDV, HDV-RNA[b]	HEV-RNA[b]
Recovery	None	HBeAb, HBeAb	None	None	None
Carrier state	NA	HBeAg	None	Anti-HDV, HDAg	NA
Immunity screen	Anti-HAV-total (includes anti-HAV-IgG)	HBsAb, HBcAb-total	None	None	Anti-HEV[a]

[a]Not available in United States.
[b]Only available in research laboratories.
[c]Only for investigational use.

○ Serum AST and ALT both rise during the preicteric phase and show very high peaks (>500 U) by the time jaundice appears.
ESR is normal.
Leukopenia (lymphopenia and neutropenia) is noted with onset of fever, followed by relative lymphocytosis and monocytosis; may find plasma cells and <10% atypical lymphocytes (in infectious mononucleosis is >10%).

Asymptomatic Hepatitis: Biochemical evidence of acute hepatitis is scant and often absent.

Acute Icteric Period

Tests show parenchymal cell damage

Conjugated serum bilirubin is 50% to 75% in the early stage; later, unconjugated bilirubin is proportionately higher.
Serum AST and ALT fall rapidly in the several days after jaundice appears and become normal 2 to 5 weeks later.

• In *hepatitis associated with infectious mononucleosis*, peak levels are usually <200 units and peak occurs 2 to 3 weeks after onset, becoming normal by the fifth week.
• *In toxic hepatitis*, levels depend on severity; slight elevations may be associated with therapy with anticoagulants, anovulatory drugs, etc.; poisoning (e.g., carbon tetrachloride) may cause levels ≤300 units.
• *In severe toxic hepatitis (especially CCl4 poisoning)*, serum enzymes may be 10 to 20× higher than in acute hepatitis and show a different pattern, i.e., increase in LD > AST > ALT.
• *In acute hepatitis*, ALT > AST > LD.

Other liver function tests are often abnormal, depending on severity of the disease—bilirubinuria, abnormal serum protein electrophoresis, ALP, etc.
Serum cholesterol:ester ratio is usually depressed early; total serum cholesterol is decreased only in severe disease.
Serum phospholipids are increased in mild but decreased in severe hepatitis. Plasma vitamin A is decreased in severe hepatitis.
Urine urobilinogen is increased in the early icteric period; at peak of the disease it disappears for days or weeks; urobilinogen simultaneously disappears from stool.
ESR is increased; falls during convalescence.
Serum iron is often increased.
Urine: Cylindruria is common; albuminuria occurs occasionally; concentrating ability is sometimes decreased.

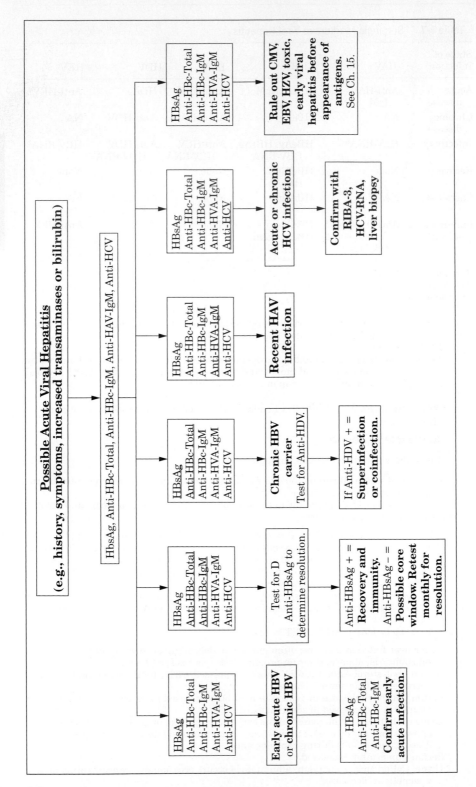

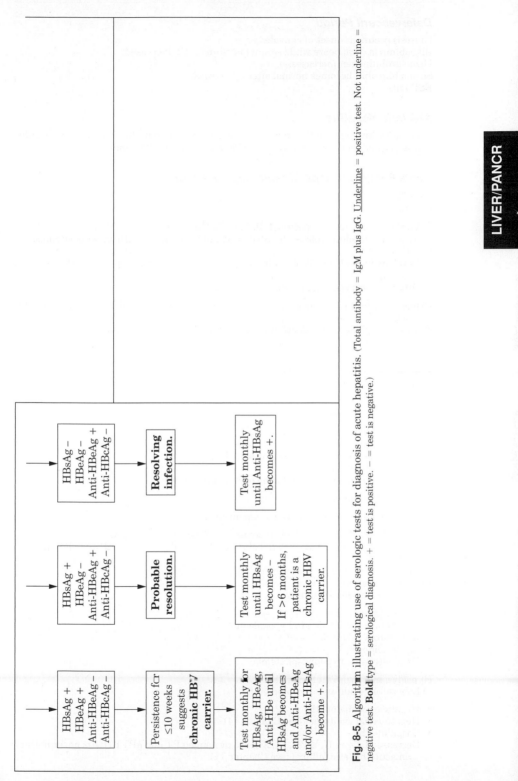

Fig. 8-5. Algorithm illustrating use of serologic tests for diagnosis of acute hepatitis. (Total antibody = IgM plus IgG. Underline = positive test. Not underline = negative test. **Bold** type = serological diagnosis. + = test is positive. − = test is negative.)

243

Defervescent Period

Diuresis occurs at onset of convalescence.
Bilirubinuria disappears while serum bilirubin is still increased.
Urine urobilinogen increases.
Serum bilirubin becomes normal after 3 to 6 weeks.
ESR falls.

Anicteric Hepatitis

Laboratory findings are the same as in the icteric type, but abnormalities are usually
less marked and there is slight or no increase of serum bilirubin.

Acute Fulminant Hepatitis with Hepatic Failure

Due To
Infection

- Viral hepatitis (e.g., hepatitis A, B, C, D, E; HSV 1, 2, 6; EBV, CMV)
  Acute liver failure related to HSV is usually associated with immunosuppressive
  therapy.
  Develops in ~1% to 3% of adults with acute icteric type B hepatitis with resultant
  death.
- Other rare causes (e.g., amebic abscesses, disseminated TB)

Drugs (e.g., acetaminophen, methyltestosterone, isoniazid, halothane, idiosyncratic
reaction)
Toxins (e.g., phosphorus, death-cap mushroom [*Amanita phalloides*])
Acute fatty liver

- Pregnancy
- Reye syndrome
- Drugs (e.g., tetracycline)

Autoimmune
Ischemic liver necrosis

- Shock
- Budd-Chiari syndrome (acute)
- Wilson disease with intravascular hemolysis
- Congestive heart failure
- Extracorporeal circulation during open heart surgery

Marked infiltration by tumor

- Acute leukemia, lymphomas, malignant histiocytosis

❍ Serum bilirubin progressively increases; may become very high.
Increased serum AST, ALT, may fall abruptly terminally; serum ALP and GGT may be
increased.
Serum cholesterol and esters are markedly decreased.
Decreased albumin and total protein
Electrolyte abnormalities, e.g.,

- Hypokalemia (early)
- Metabolic alkalosis due to hypokalemia
- Respiratory alkalosis
- Lactic acidosis
- Hyponatremia, hypophosphatemia

Hypoglycemia in ~5% of patients
❍ Laboratory findings associated with:

- Hepatic encephalopathy
- Hepato-renal syndrome (see Chapter 14)
- Coagulopathy
  Decreased factors II, V, VII, IX, X cause prolonged PT and aPTT (PT is never normal
  in acute hepatic failure) (see Chapter 11).

Decreased antithrombin III
Platelet count <100,000 in two thirds of patients
* Hemorrhage, especially in GI tract
* Bacterial and fungal infections, especially streptococci and *Staph. aureus*
* Ascites

As patient deteriorates, titers of HBsAg and HBeAg often fall and disappear.

Cholangiolitic Hepatitis

Same as acute hepatitis, but evidence of obstruction is more prominent (e.g., increased
serum ALP and conjugated serum bilirubin), and tests of parenchymal damage are
less marked (e.g., AST increase may be 3–6× normal).

Hepatitis, Alcoholic

♦ Diagnosis is established by liver biopsy and history of alcohol intake. Liver biopsy
should be done in any alcoholic with enlarged liver as the only way to make definite
diagnosis of alcoholic hepatitis. Many alcoholics have normal liver biopsy.
○ Increased serum GGT and MCV >100 together or separately are useful clues for
occult alcoholism.
Ratio of desialylated transferrin to total transferrin >0.013 has been recently reported
to have S/S = 81%/98% for ongoing alcohol consumption.
Serum AST is increased (rarely >300 U/L), but ALT is normal or only slightly elevated.
AST and ALT are more specific but less sensitive than GGT. Levels of AST and ALT do
not correlate with severity of liver disease. AST:ALT ratio >1 associated with AST
<300 U/L will identify 90% of patients with alcoholic liver disease; is particularly
useful for differentiation from viral hepatitis, in which increase of AST and ALT are
about the same.
Cholestasis in ≤35% of patients
In acute alcoholic hepatitis, GGT level is usually higher than AST level. GGT is often
abnormal in alcoholics even with normal liver histology. Is more useful as index of
occult alcoholism (particularly with increased MCV) or to indicate that elevated
serum ALP is of bone or liver origin than to follow course of patient for which AST
and ALT are most useful.
Serum ALP may be normal or moderately increased in 50% of patients and is not useful as a diagnostic test.
Serum bilirubin may be mildly increased except with cholestasis; is not useful as a
diagnostic test. However, if bilirubin continues to increase during a week of therapy
in the hospital, it indicates a poor prognosis.
Decreased serum albumin and increased polyclonal globulin with disproportionately
increased IgA are frequent. Decreased albumin means long-standing or relatively
severe disease.
Increased PT that is not corrected by parenteral administration of 10 mg/day of vitamin K for 3 days is best indicator of poor prognosis.
Discriminant function to assess severity of alcoholic hepatitis = 4.6 × (PT (seconds)
minus control PT) + serum bilirubin. DF >32 is equated with severe disease.
Increased WBC (>15,000) in up to one third of patients with shift to left (WBC is
decreased in viral hepatitis); normal WBC may indicate folic acid depletion.
Anemia in >50% of patients may be macrocytic (folic acid or vitamin B_{12} deficiency),
microcytic (iron or pyridoxine deficiency), mixed, or hemolytic.
Metabolic alkalosis may occur due to K^+ loss with pH normal or increased, but pH
<7.2 often indicates disease is becoming terminal.
In terminal stage (last week before death) of chronic alcoholic liver disease, there is
often decrease of serum sodium and albumin and increase of PT and serum bilirubin; AST and LD decrease from previously elevated levels.
Indocyanine green (50 mg/kg) is abnormal in 90% of patients.
Compared to nonalcoholics, alcoholics as a group show an increase in a number of
blood components (e.g., AST, phosphorus, ALP, GGT, MCV, MCH, Hb, WBC) and a
decrease in others (e.g., total protein, BUN); however these variations usually
remain within the reference range. These changes may last for >6 weeks after
abstaining from alcohol.

Laboratory findings due to sequelae or complications

- Fatty liver
- Cirrhosis
- Portal hypertension
- Infections (e.g., GU tract, pneumonia, peritonitis)
- DIC
- Hepatorenal syndrome
- Encephalopathy

Hepatitis, Chronic Active

Progressive hepatitis >6 months duration of unknown etiology affecting patients of all ages possibly due to an external agent [e.g., viruses, drugs] and genetic susceptibility that triggers a cascade of T- cell-mediated events against liver antigens.

Due To
Viruses

- HBV (with or without HDV)
- HCV (with or without HGV)
- CMV, others

Metabolic

- Wilson disease
- Alpha$_1$-antitrypsin deficiency
- Hemochromatosis
- Primary biliary cirrhosis
- Sclerosing cholangitis

Drugs (e.g., methyldopa, nitrofurantoin, isonizid, oxyphenacetin) and chemicals
Nonalcoholic fatty liver
Alcoholic hepatitis
Autoimmune causes

- Type I (lupoid) (anti-smooth muscle; antiactin)
- Type II (anti-kidney-liver-microsomal)
- Type III (anti-soluble liver antigen)

Occurs in 5–10% of adults with acute HBV.

♦ Criteria for Diagnosis (all must be present for definite diagnosis)*	Probable	Definite
Increased serum AST[1] or ALT concentrations	X	X
Increased serum ALP <3× normal concentration		X
Increased serum total or gamma globulin or IgG		
>1.5× upper limit of normal		X
1.0–1.5× upper limit of normal	X	
Antibody titers to nucleus, smooth muscle or liver/kidney microsome type 1 >1:80 (adults) or >1:20 (children)		X
Lower titers or presence of other autoantibodies	X	
Absence of markers for viral hepatitis (e.g., HAV, HBV, HCV, CMV, EBV)	X	X
Absence of excess alcohol consumption		
<25 gm/day (women) or <35 gm/day (men)		X
<40 gm/day (women) or <50 gm/day (men)	X	
Exposure to blood products		
No		X
Yes, but unrelated to disease	X	
Exposure to hepatotoxic drugs		
No		X
Yes, but unrelated to disease	X	

| Compatible histologic findings and absence of biliary lesions, copper deposits or other changes suggestive of other causes of lobular hepatitis. | X | X |

[1]AST increase is more prominent than increase in ALP or bilirubin.
*Czaja AJ. The variant forms of autoimmune hepatitis. *Ann Int Med* 1996;125:588.

Hepatitis A

Due to a nonenveloped, single-stranded RNA picornavirus

Serum bilirubin usually 5 to 10× normal. Jaundice lasts few days to 12 weeks. Usually not infectious after onset of jaundice.
Serum AST and ALT increased to hundreds for 1 to 3 weeks.
Relative lymphocytosis is frequent.

Serologic Tests for Viral Hepatitis A (HAV)[3]

See Tables 8-6 and 8-7; Figs. 8-3, 8-5, 8-6.

♦ Anti-HAV-IgM appears at the same time as symptoms in >99% of cases, peaks within first month, becomes nondetectable in 12 (usually 6). Presence confirms diagnosis of recent acute infection.
♦ Anti-HAV-total is predominantly IgG except immediately after acute HAV infection when it is mostly IgM and IgA. Almost always positive at onset of acute hepatitis and is usually detectable for life; found in ~50% of adult population in USA; indicates previous exposure to HAV, recovery, and immunity to type A hepatitis. Negative anti-HAV-total effectively excludes acute HAV. Positive anti-HAV-total does not distinguish recent from past infection for which anti-HAV-IgM test is needed. Test for anti-HAV-total is relatively insensitive (minimum detection amount = 100 mU/mL) and may not detect protective antibody response after one dose of inactivated HAV vaccine (minimum protective antibody is <10 mU/mL).
Serial testing is usually not indicated.
Tests for anti-HAV-total and anti-HAV-IgM are not influenced by normal doses of immune globulin.
HAV-Ag and HAV-RNA are only available as research tools.
Carrier and chronic hepatitis do not occur. Fulminant hepatitis <0.4%.

Hepatitis B

Due to an enveloped, double-stranded, DNA hepadnavirus.

HBV hepatitis is generally divided into three stages:

• Stage of acute hepatitis: usually lasts 1–6 months with mild or no symptoms.
    AST and ALT are increased > tenfold.
    Serum bilirubin is usually normal or only slightly increased.
    HBsAg gradually arises to high titers and persists; HBeAg also appears.
    Gradually merges with next stage.

• Stage of chronic hepatitis: transaminases increased >50% for >6 months duration; may last only 1 year or for several decades with mild or severe symptoms; most cases resolve, but some develop cirrhosis and liver failure
    AST and ALT fall to ?–10× normal range.
    HBsAg usually remains high, and HBeAg remains present.

• Chronic carrier stage: are usually, but not always, healthy and asymptomatic.
    AST and ALT fall to normal or <2× normal.
    HBeAg disappears, and anti-HBe appears.

[3]Lemon SM. Type A Viral Hepatitis: Epidemiology, Diagnosis, and Prevention. *Clin Chem* 1997; 43:1494.

Table 8-8.	Comparison of Type 1 and Type 2 Autoimmune Hepatitis*	
	Type 1 Autoimmune Hepatitis	Type 2 Autoimmune Hepatitis
Characteristic autoantibodies are absent in ~10% of patients	Antinuclear antibodies (ANA), and smooth muscle antibodies titer ≥1:80	Liver-kidney microsome 1 (LKM-1)
	Antiactin antibodies are more specific	Liver cytosol
	Atypical perinuclear antineutrophilic cytoplasmic (pANCA) antibodies	
Presence of other autoimmune diseases (e.g., thyroiditis, type I diabetes, RA, ulcerative colitis, celiac disease) is an important clue.	Autoantibodies against soluble liver antigen and liver-pancreas antigen (SLA/LP) found in 10%–30% of patients are most specific for Type 1	

*Krawitt, EL. Autoimmune hepatitis. *N Engl J Med* 2006;354:54. Czaja AJ. The variant forms of autoimmune hepatitis. *Ann Int Med* 1996; 125:588.

HBsAg titer falls although may still be detectable; anti-HBs subsequently develops, marking the end of carrier stage.

Anti-HBc is usually present in high titer (>1:512).

Laboratory findings due to sequellae e.g.,

• GN or nephrotic syndrome due to deposition of HBeAg or HBcAg in glomeruli which often progresses to chronic renal failure.

Serologic Tests for HBV

See Tables 8-7 and 8-10 through 8-14.

Use

Differential diagnosis of hepatitis

Screening of blood and organ donors

Determine immune status for possible vaccination

Hepatitis B Surface Antigen (HBsAg)

♦ Earliest indicator of active HBV infection. Usually appears in 27 to 41 days (as early as 14 days). Appears 7 to 26 days before biochemical abnormalities. Peaks as ALT

Table 8-9.	Comparison of Viral Hepatitis			
Virus	Family	Genome	Source	Transmission
HAV	Picornaviridae	RNA	Stool	Fecal-oral
HBV	Hepadnavirus	DNA	Blood, body fluids except stool	Parenteral, sexual, perinatal
HCV	Flaviviridae	RNA	Blood, body fluids	Parenteral; sexual: rare, if ever
HDV	Satellite	Defective RNA	Blood, body fluids except stool	Parenteral; ? sexual
HEV	Calciviridae	RNA	Stool	Fecal-oral
HGV	Flaviviridae	RNA	Blood, body fluids	Parenteral

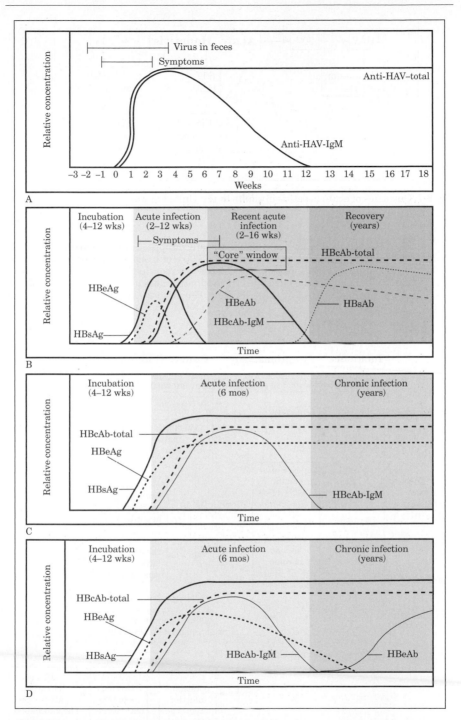

Fig. 8-6. Hepatitis serologic profiles. **A:** Antibody response to hepatitis A. **B:** Hepatitis B core window identification. **C, D:** Hepatitis B chronic carrier profiles: no seroconversion **(C)**; late seroconversion **(D)**. (Reproduced with permission of Hepatitis Information Center, Abbott Laboratories, Abbott Park, IL.)

LIVER/PANCR

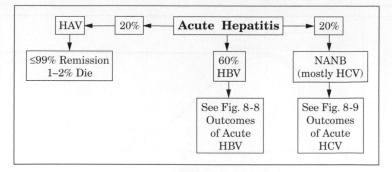

Fig. 8-7. Outcomes of acute hepatitis in adults in the United States.

rises. Persists during the acute illness. Usually disappears 12 to 20 weeks after onset of symptoms or laboratory abnormalities in 90% of cases. Is the most reliable serologic marker of HBV infection. Persistence >6 months defines carrier state. May also be found in chronic infection. HB vaccination does not cause a positive HBsAg. Titers are not of clinical value. Present sensitive assays detect <1.0 ng/mL of

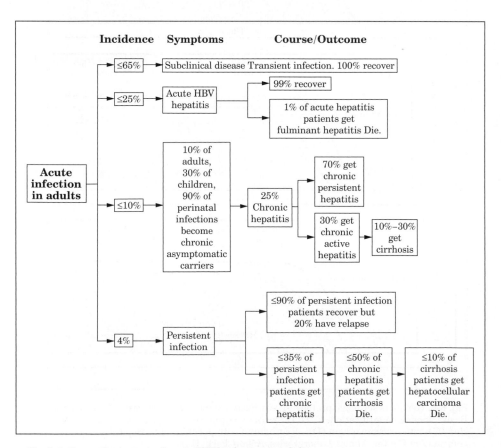

Fig. 8-8. Course/outcomes of acute HBV infection in adults.

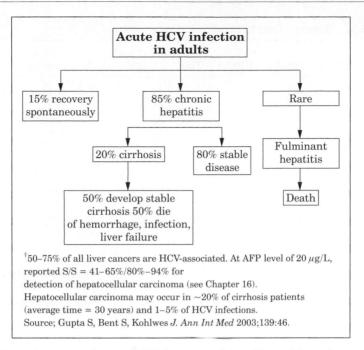

Fig. 8-9. Course/outcomes of acute HCV infection in adults with or without abnormal ALT values.

circulating antigen, which is the level needed to find 10% to 15% of reactive blood donors who carry antigen but express only low levels. Is never detected in some patients and diagnosis is based on presence of HBc-IgM.

HBsAg and Blood Transfusions

Transfusion of blood containing HBsAg causes hepatitis or appearance of HBsAg in blood in >70% of recipients; needle-stick from such blood causes hepatitis in 45% of cases. When HBsAg carrier is discovered (e.g., in screening program), 60% to 80% show some evidence of hepatic damage.

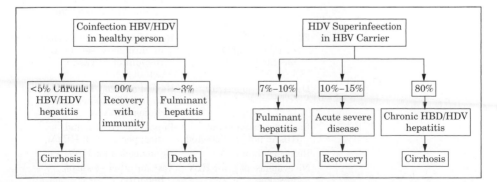

Fig. 8-10. Course/outcomes of hepatitis B and D infection in adults.

Table 8-10.   Serologic Tests for Hepatitis B Virus Infection

HBsAg	HBsAb	HBeAg	HBeAb	HBcAb-Total	HBcAb-IgM	Interpretation
+	−	−	−	−	−	Late incubation or early acute HBV
+	−	+	−	−	−	Early acute HBV Highly infectious
+	−	+	−	+	+	Acute HBV
+	−	−	+	+	+	"Serologic window/gap" or acute HBV
−	−	−	−	+	+	"Serologic gap"
−	−	−	+	+	+	Convalescence
−	+	−	+	+	+	Early recovery
−	+	−	+	+	−	Recovery[a]
+	−	±	±	+	−	Chronic infection (chronic carrier)[a]
						May also have increased ALT and HBV-DNA
−	+	−	−	−	−	Old previous HBV with recovery and immunity or HBV vaccination or passive transfer antibody[b]
−	−	−	−	−	−	Not HBV infection
						Susceptible

+ = positive; − = negative; ± = positive or negative.
[a]Chronic carriers of HBV may have clinical hepatitis due to other causes (e.g., non-A, non-B hepatitis) rather than only HBV. By definition, carriers of only HBV have HbsAg for >6 months and normal ALT.
[b]Various serologic patterns may occur after blood transfusion or injection of immune (gamma) globulin by passive transfer. Anti-HBs can be found for up to 6 to 8 months after injection of high-titer HB immunoglobulin because of 25-day half life.

Table 8-11.   Serologic Tests for Hepatitis B Virus Infection Follow-Up

HBsAg	HBsAb	HBeAg	HBeAb	Interpretation	Follow-up
+	−	−	−	Acute HBV infection	Repeat serology for resolution of chronicity; serum ALT to monitor disease activity
+	−	+	−	Early acute HBV infection; highly infectious	Repeat serology for resolution or chronicity; serum ALT to monitor disease activity
+	−	+	+	Decreasing infectivity	Repeat serology for resolution; serum ALT to monitor disease activity
+	−	−	+	Early seroconversion; HBsAb not yet detected	Repeat for HBsAb and disappearance of HBsAg
−	+	−	+	Recovery; immune	None needed for HBV
−	−	−	−	No evidence of prior HBV infection	Test for other cause of hepatitis

+, positive; −, negative.

Table 8-12. Serologic Tests for Prenatal Screening for Hepatitis B Virus

Test				
HBsAg	HBeAg	HBsAb	Interpretation	Follow-Up
−	−	+	Mother is HBV immune	Not needed
−	−	−	No evidence of HBV infection	Not needed unless other evidence of hepatitis
+	+	−	Mother is HBV carrier Infant at high risk of acquiring HBV infection during delivery and developing chronic hepatitis	Infant must be vaccinated within 12 hrs of birth
+	−	−	Mother is HBV carrier Infant at high risk of acquiring HBV infection during delivery and developing chronic hepatitis	Infant must be vaccinated within 12 hrs of birth

Persons with a positive test for HBsAg should never be permitted to donate blood or plasma.

HBsAg is found in:

Chronic persistent hepatitis	50%
Chronic active hepatitis	25%
Cirrhosis	3%
Prevalence in U.S.	0.25%
Multiple transfused patients	3.8%
Drug addicts	4.2%
Blood donor population	<0.1%

◆ *Antibody to HBsAg (Anti-HBsAg)*

Presence of antibody (titer ≥10 mU/mL) without detectable HBsAg indicates recovery from HBV infection, absence of infectivity, immunity from future HBV infection, and does not need gamma globulin administration if exposed to infection; this blood can be transfused.

• May also occur after transfusion by passive transfer.
• Found in 80% of patients after clinical cure. Appearance may take several weeks or months after HBsAg has disappeared and after ALT has returned to normal, causing a "serologic gap" during which time (usually 2–6 week "window") only IgM-anti-HBsAg can identify patients who are recovering but may still be infectious.

Table 8-13. Serologic Tests for Candidate for Hepatitis B Virus Vaccination

Test				
HBsAg	HBsAb	HBcAb	Interpretation	Follow-Up
+	−		Acute HBV infection	See Table 8-12
−	−	+	Acute HBV or carrier	Previous HBV infection; vaccinate
−	+	+	Immune; previous HBV infection or vaccination	None
+	−	+	Previous HBV infection; may not be immune	Vaccinate
−	−	−	Not immune	Vaccinate

+, positive; −, negative.

Table 8-14.	Serologic Tests for Hepatitis B Virus Vaccination Follow–Up	
HBsAb	Interpretation	Follow-Up
+	Effective immunization	Repeat in future years to ensure immunity
−	No evidence of immunity	Await appearance of HBsAb or repeat vaccination

+, positive; −, negative.

- Only antibody produced in response to vaccine. Presence can be used to show efficiency of immunization program. Appears in ~90% of healthy adults after three-dose deltoid muscle immunization; 30% to 50% of these lose antibodies in 7 years and require boosters.
- Revaccination of nonresponders produces adequate antibody in <50% after 3 additional doses.
- A few persons acquire HBV infection after developing high titers of anti-HBsAg due to a mutant HBV virus.

In fulminant hepatitis—antibody is produced early and may coexist with low antigen titer. In chronic carriers—no IgM antibody is present but antigen titers are very high.

♦ Hepatitis Be Antigen (HBeAg)

Is subparticle of core antigen

Indicates highly infectious state. Appears within 1 week after HBsAg; in acute cases disappears prior to disappearance of HBsAg; is found only when HBsAg is found. Occurs early in disease before biochemical changes and disappears after serum ALT peak. Usually lasts 3 to 6 weeks. Is a marker of active HBV replication in liver; with few exceptions, is present only in persons with circulating HBV-DNA and is used as alternative or surrogate marker for HBV-DNA assay.
Best predictor of maternal infectivity (90%) to untreated neonates at time of delivery.
Is useful to determine resolution of infection. Persistence >20 weeks suggests progression to chronic carrier state and possible chronic hepatitis. Presence in HBsAg-positive mothers indicates 90% chance of infant acquiring HBV infection.
Loss of HBeAg is associated with fulminant hepatitis.
≤15% in US and >50% in Asia, Africa, southern Europe may be HBeAg negative and HBV-DNA positive in patients infected with a HBV mutant.

♦ Antibody to HBe (Anti-HBe) appears after HBeAg disappears and remains

detectable for years. Indicates decreasing infectivity, suggesting good prognosis for resolution of acute infection. Association with anti-HBc in absence of HBsAg and anti-HBs confirms recent acute infection (2–16 weeks).

♦ Antibody to Core Antigen-Total (Anti-HBc-Total) is first antibody to appear

4 to 10 weeks after appearance of HBsAg; at same time as clinical illness; persists for years or for lifetime.
Anti-HBc-total and HBsAg are always present and anti-HBsAg is absent in chronic HBV infection.

♦ Anti-HBc-IgM is the earliest specific antibody; usually within 2 weeks after HBsAg.

Is found in high titer for a short time during the acute disease stage that covers the serologic window and then declines to low levels during recovery (see Fig. 8–6); may be detectable ≤6 months. May be the only serologic marker present after HBsAg and HBeAg have subsided but before these antibodies have appeared ("serologic gap" or "window"). Because this is the only test unique to recent infection, it can differentiate acute from chronic HBV. It is the only serologic test that can differentiate recent and remote infection with one specimen. However, because some patients with chronic HB infection become positive for anti-HBc-IgM during flares, it is not an absolutely reliable marker of acute illness. Before anti-HBc-IgM disappears, anti-HBc-IgG appears and lasts indefinitely.

Anti-HBc detects virtually all persons who have been previously infected with HBV and can therefore serve as surrogate test for other infectious agents (e.g., NANB). Exclusion of anti-HBc positive donors reduces the incidence of post-transfusion hepatitis and possibly of other virus infection (e.g., AIDS) due to the frequency of dual infection. Present without other serological markers and with normal AST in ~2% of routine blood donors; 70% of these are due to recovery from subclinical HBV (and may be infectious) and the rest are considered false positive. False-positive anti-HBc can be confirmed by immune response pattern to hepatitis B vaccination. Anti-HBc is not protective (unlike anti-HBsAg) and therefore cannot be used to distinguish acute from chronic infection.

◆ *HBV-DNA* (by PCR) indicates active infection. Is the most sensitive and specific assay for early diagnosis of HBV and may be detected when all other markers are negative (e.g., in immunocompromised patients). May become negative before HBeAg becomes negative. Measures HBV replication even when HBeAg is not detectable. Marked decrease in patients who respond to therapy; concentrations <200 ng/L are more likely to respond to therapy. Increased risk for development of hepatocellular carcinoma if >10,000 copies/mL. In typical HBV chronic carrier there are 1,000,000 virions for every HCV virion, explaining why HBV is much more contagious than HCV.
Dane particle (complete virion) is detected only in liver tissue, not in blood.

Other Laboratory Findings

○ Very high serum ALT and bilirubin are not reliable indicators of patient's clinical course, but prolonged PT, especially >20 seconds, indicates the likely development of acute hepatic insufficiency; therefore the PT should be performed when patient is first seen.

• Acute fulminant hepatitis may be indicated by triad of prolonged PT, increased PMNs, and nonpalpable liver with likely development of coma.
• Acute viral hepatitis B completely resolves in 90% of patients within 12 weeks with disappearance of HBsAg and development of anti-HBs.
• Relapse, usually within 1 year, has been recognized in 20% of patients by some elevation of ALT and changes in liver biopsy.
• Chronic hepatitis (disease for >6 months and ALT >50% above normal)

Current Term	Old Term	Grade/Stage	Hepatic Activity (Knodell Score) (0–22 combination of grade and stage)
Mild liver disease	Benign chronic persistent hepatitis in 70%	Grade 0–2 inflammation and Stage 1 scarring	3–6
Moderate liver disease	Chronic active hepatitis in 30%	Grade 3 inflammation and Stage 2 scarring	7–8
Severe liver disease	Severe chronic active hepatitis	Grade 3–4 inflammation and Stage 3 scarring	9–11
Advanced liver disease (cirrhosis)		Any grade Stage 4	12+

• Effective treatment of chronic HBV hepatitis causes ALT, HBeAg, and HBV-DNA to become normal.
• HBV patients with normal ALT levels have normal liver biopsies and need not be referred for treatment but should monitor ALT every 6 to 12 months for increase >1.5× and HBsAg every 1 to 2 years.
• Chronic carrier has also been defined as either: HBsAg positive on 2 occasions >6 months apart, or one specimen that is HBsAg positive, anti-HBc-IgM negative, but anti-HBc-positive.

LIVER/PANCR

- 10% of adults and 90% of children ≤4 years old become chronic carriers, 25% of whom develop cirrhosis and increased risk of hepatoma. HBV carriers should be screened periodically with serum alpha-fetoprotein and ultrasound or CT scan of liver for hepatoma.
- Platelet count <150,000/μL suggests fibrosis is occurring.

Laboratory indicators for favorable response to interferon

- Pretreatment serum ALT >100 U/L (high ALT may indicate better host immune response to HBV)
- HBV-DNA <200 ng/L (pg/mL)
- Absence of HIV
- Also <4 years' duration and acquiring infection after 6 years of age

Laboratory effects of interferon treatment

- Serum ALT may increase to >1,000 U/L .
- 10% of patients show sustained disappearance of HBV-DNA and clearance of HbeAg.
- If serum ALT is persistently increased despite HBeAg, presence of an HBeAg-negative mutant that may emerge during treatment is suggested.
- 5% to 10% of patients with seroconversion due to therapy will have reactivation in next 10 years; this is usually transitory.

Laboratory contraindications to interferon therapy for chronic HB

- Liver decompensation
    Serum albumin <3.0 gm/L
    Serum bilirubin >3.0 mg/dL
    PT increased >3×
- Portal hypertension (e.g., ascites, bleeding esophageal varices, encephalopathy)
- Hypersplenism
    WBC <2,000/μL
    Platelet count <70,000
- Autoimmune disease (e.g., rheumatoid arthritis, polyarteritis nodosa)
- Major system impairment
- Others (e.g., pregnancy, current IV drug abuser, psychiatric)

Hepatitis C (Formerly Non-A, Non-B Hepatitis; NANB)[4]

Due to an enveloped, single-stranded, RNA flavivirus

See Fig. 8-11 and Tables 8-6 and 8-7.

♦ **Diagnostic Criteria**
Acute
Clinical criteria *and*

- Acute illness with discrete onset of symptoms
- Jaundice or increased ALT

Laboratory criteria

- ALT >7× normal
- IgM anti-HAV negative or HBsAg negative, *and* anti-HCV positive by EIA confirmed by more specific test (e.g., RIBA, PCR) *or* anti-HCV positive by EIA with signal to cutoff ratio of >3.8

Chronic
Clinical criteria *and*

- Usually asymptomatic

Laboratory criteria

- Anti-HCV positive by EIA, confirmed by more specific test (e.g., RIBA, PCR) *or* anti-HCV positive by EIA with signal to cutoff ratio of >3.8

---

[4]Guidelines for laboratory testing and result reporting of antibody to hepatitis C virus. *MMWR.* Feb 7, 2003/52/#RR-3. Consensus Statement of Management of Hepatitis C. *NIH.* 2002;19(#3), June 10–12.

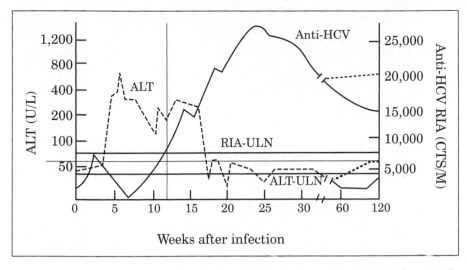

Fig. 8-11. Comparison of serum ALT and anti-hepatitis C virus findings in acute hepatitis C. Chronic infection is indicated by broken lines. (CTS/M, counts/minute; RIA, radioimmunoassay; ULN, upper limit of normal.)

Can remain infectious for years. ≤80% become chronic with viremia.
Routine screening for HCV should be performed and HCV should be ruled out in these persons:

- History of IV drug abuse, tattoos, body piercing, multiple sexual partners, household contacts of HCV carriers
- Received blood product transfusions produced before 1990 (>70% of severe hemophiliacs are infected with HCV)
- Ever on long-term hemodialysis
- Ever received blood from donor who later tested positive for HCV (2%–7% of blood donors in the United States are asymptomatic carriers)
- Persistently abnormal serum ALT

Causes ≤25% of sporadic cases of acute viral hepatitis in adults, 90% of posttransfusion hepatitis

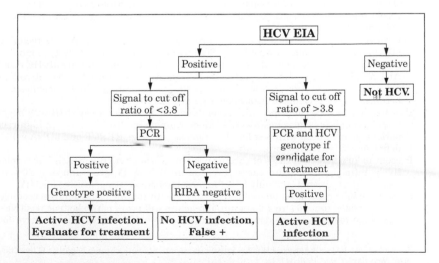

Fig. 8-12. Sequence of tests for diagnosis of HCV.

Source of infection: injecting-drug use = 42%; occupational exposure = ~5%; transfusion = <1%; dialysis = 0.6%; household contact = 3%; heterosexual transmission = 6% (cumulative risk may = 18%); unidentified = 42%

Perinatal infection at time of birth occurs in 5% of infants of HCV-infected mothers.

Biochemical and histologic evidence of abnormality occurs in 7% of sporadic cases, ≤60% of posttransfusion cases, and ≤80% of immunosuppressed patients.

Occult HBV infection is present in about one third of patients with chronic HCV liver disease by HBV-DNA analysis of liver biopsy.[5]

○ May be associated with mixed cryoglobulinemia with vasculitis (see Chapter 11), thyroiditis, Sjögren syndrome, membranoproliferative GN, and porphyria cutanea tarda, which should be ruled out in cases of hepatitis C, and HCV infection should be ruled out in patients with those disorders. Patients with alcoholic liver disease have more rapidly progressive disease with higher ALT values and more severe histological changes. ~40% of liver transplantations in United States are done for chronic hepatitis C with cirrhosis.

Increased Serum Transaminases

○ Increases 2 to 8 weeks after infection. Characteristically shows unpredictable waxing and waning pattern returning to almost-normal levels (formerly called *acute "relapsing" hepatitis*); is highly suggestive but only occurs in 25% of cases. ALT is poorer predictor of histology in HCV than in HBV.

Patients with monophasic ALT response usually recover completely with no biopsy evidence of residual disease.

May be extreme (>10× normal).

ALT is usually <800 U. ALT cannot be relied upon when deciding whether to perform liver biopsy in chronic hepatitis C; biopsy is needed to define severity. Is primary marker to monitor therapy. In chronic HCV, AST:ALT >1 has S/S = 52%/100% and PPV = 100% for cirrhosis. Ratio does not correlate with serum ALP, bilirubin, albumin, or PT. Continuously normal suggests lower likelihood of fibrosis.

Anicteric patients with ALT >300 U/L are at high risk for progressing to chronic hepatitis.

○ **Liver Biopsy**

See later in Chapter.

♦ Antibody to Hepatitis C Virus (anti-HCV) (by EIA)

Use

Screening low- and high-prevalence populations including blood donors

Initial evaluation of patients with liver disease including increased serum ALT

Interpretation

Indicates past or present infection but does not differentiate between acute, chronic, or resolved infection. Sensitivity ≥97%; only ~80% in chronic carriers. Low PPV in low-prevalence population.

Seroconversion: average time after exposure = 2 to 3 weeks with EIA-3. Detected in 80% of patients within 15 weeks, in >90% within 5 months, in >97% by 6 months after exposure or 2 to 3 months after increase in ALT. Therefore serial anti-HCV and ALT for up to 1 year after suspected acute hepatitis may be needed. Negative EIA rules out HCV infection in low-risk group. In 30% of cases, gradually declines and becomes negative, completely disappearing in 10 to 20 years.

Positive EIA must be confirmed with recombinant immunoblot assay (RIBA-2); negative RIBA indicates false-positive EIA; indeterminate in ≤10% of cases. In high-risk patients may confirm with test for HCV nucleic acid (e.g., RT-PCR and bDNA which define active HCV infection).

Present in 70% to 85% of cases of chronic posttransfusion NANB hepatitis but is relatively infrequent in acute cases. Present in 70% of IV drug abusers, 20% of hemodialysis patients, and only 8% of homosexual men testing positive for HIV.

Prevalence in normal blood donors is 0.5% to 2.0%. In routine blood donor screening, it is estimated that 40% to 70% of initial reactors will prove not to be true positives. Surrogate markers fail to detect one third to one half of blood units positive for

---

[5]Cacciola I, et al. Occult hepatitis B virus infections in patients with chronic hepatitis C liver disease. *New Engl J Med* 1999;341:22.

anti-HCV. Found in 7% to 10% of transfusion recipients. Only one third of anti-HCV donors had increased ALT and 54% were positive for anti-HBc.

In one study, anti-HCV was positive in 75% of patients with hepatocellular carcinoma, 56% of patients with cirrhosis, and 7% of controls.

May still be present in various quality assurance and calibration sera, and proficiency samples

Because resolves slowly is considered chronic only with evidence of activity >12 months

Interferences
False Positive

- Autoimmune diseases (≤80% of cases of autoimmune chronic active hepatitis)
- EIA and RIBA are also found in polyarteritis nodosa (~10%) and SLE (~2%).
- Rheumatoid factor
- Hypergammaglobulinemia
- Paraproteinemia
- Passive antibody transfer
- Anti-idiotypes
- Anti-superoxide dismutase (a human enzyme used in the cloning process)
- Repeat freezing and thawing or prolonged storage of blood specimens

False negative

- Early acute infection
- Immunosuppression
- Immunoincompetence
- Repeat freezing and thawing or prolonged storage of blood specimens

Recombinant Immunoblot Assay (RIBA)
Use
Confirms positive EIA in >50% of cases; in high-risk population RIBA confirms diagnosis >88% of cases.
Interpretation
Positive RIBA indicates past or previous exposure but does not distinguish between them. Increasingly replaced by HCV-RNA assay

HCV-RNA Assay (Viral Load) (by RT-PCR)
After incubation period rapidly increases ≤10^8 U/mL. Cleared in <50% in acute phase; never develops in 30%.
Qualitative Tests
Most sensitive test. Lower limit of detection = 50 U/mL (100 RNA copies/mL); reported as positive or negative for HCV-RNA.
Use
Diagnose acute HCV infection prior to seroconversion; detects virus as early as 1 to 2 weeks after exposure

Detection may be intermittent; one negative RT-PCR is not conclusive.

Monitor patients' response on antiviral therapy

To confirm initial quantitative test or to evaluate indeterminate RIBA

False-positive and false-negative results may occur.
Quantitative Tests
Lower limit of detection = 200 U/mL (500 RNA copies/mL). Determines concentration of HCV-RNA. Quantitative tests from different manufacturers do not yield identical results.

Large spontaneous fluctuations in RNA level can occur, therefore should measure ≥2 times to evaluate changes due to therapy.

RT-PCR is positive in 75% to 85% of persons positive for anti-HCV and >95% of persons with acute or chronic HCV hepatitis.

More sensitive nucleic acid tests can detect low levels of HCV-RNA in serum, lymphocytes, liver tissue.
Use
May be used to assess likelihood of response to antiviral therapy and to assess this response. Patients with pretreatment level <2 million copies/mL (by PCR or

quantitative bDNA) are most likely to respond to interferon therapy. Positive test after 12 weeks of interferon therapy predicts failed response; negative test has ~30% predictive value for sustained response. Negative result 6 months after treatment indicates cure in >99% of cases. Not used to determine treatment endpoint.

Less sensitive than qualitative test RT-PCR

Can use to confirm diagnosis of chronic HCV with positive antibody screening test

Can use for diagnosis of acute infection and in immunodeficient patients with negative antibody screening test but suspected of having HCV infection

Not used to exclude diagnosis of HCV infection

Earliest marker for diagnosis of fulminant hepatitis C. Negative test in patient with fulminant hepatitis rules out HCV infection.

Confirms persistent HCV infection after liver transplantation when anti-HCV is positive and serum ALT is normal. Helps distinguish recurrent disease from other causes of inflammation (e.g., rejection).

Diagnose chronic hepatitis patients with:
Negative anti-HCV
False-positive serological tests due to autoantibodies

HCV Genotyping

Using PCR and subsequent nucleic acid sequencing

At least 6 genotypes and >90 subtypes. There may be a correlation between genotype and disease. Mixed infections often occur.

HCV Genotype in USA*	Occurrence (%)	
1a	37	Higher rate of chronic hepatitis; poorer response to interferon therapy and more likely to relapse
1b	30	More severe liver disease; higher risk of hepatocellular carcinoma
2a, 2b, or 3		Greater likelihood of response; need to treat for 24 rather than 48 weeks

*Other genotypes have various geographic distribution.

Use

Evaluate patient before starting treatment. May not be possible with low viral load (<1,000 RNA copies/mL) or due to mixed genotypes.

Determine dose, drug and length of treatment.

Assess likelihood of response to treatment.

May aid in identifying source of infection.

Antiviral therapy is recommended for patients with greatest risk of progression to cirrhosis

• Positive anti-HCV with
    Persistently increased ALT
    Detectable HCV-RNA
    Liver biopsy showing at least moderate inflammation and necrosis or fibrosis

Response to antiviral therapy indicated

• ~50% show normal serum ALT
• 33% lose detectable HCV-RNA in serum; is associated with remission. Presence after sustained response to interferon indicates late relapse.
• 50% relapse after therapy ends

Decreased interferon response occurs in <15% of patients indicated

• Higher serum HCV-RNA titers
• HCV genotype 1

Laboratory contraindications to interferon therapy

• Persistently increased serum ALT
• Cytopenias
• Hyperthyroidism

- Renal transplantation
- Evidence of autoimmune disease

No tests are routinely available for other NANB viruses.

Hepatitis D (Delta) (HDV)

Due to a single-stranded enveloped RNA virus

See Tables 8-5, 8-6, and 8-7.
Hepatitis D virus depends upon HBV for expression and replication. It may be found in the serum for 7 to 14 days during acute infection. Can cause acute or chronic hepatitis. The course depends upon the presence of HBV infection. Is often severe with relatively high mortality in acute disease and frequent development of cirrhosis in chronic disease. Chronic HDV infection is more severe and has higher mortality than other types of viral hepatitis. Prevalence in United States is 1% to 10% of HBsAg carriers principally in high-risk groups of IV drug abusers and multiple-transfused patients but uncommon in other groups at risk for HBV infection (e.g., health care workers, male homosexuals).

Serologic Tests for HDV

See Tables 8-6, 8-7, 8-15, and 8-16.
Serum HDVAg and HDV-RNA appear during incubation period after HBsAg and before rise in ALT, which often shows a biphasic elevation. HBsAg and HDVAg are transient; HDVAg resolves with clearance of HBsAg. Anti-HDV appears soon after clinical symptoms but titer is often low and short lived.
♦ Diagnosis of HDV hepatitis is made by presence of anti-HDV in patient with HBsAg-positive hepatitis. Anti-HDV should not be done unless there is confirmed diagnosis of HBV.
Coinfection means simultaneous acute HBV and acute HDV infection; usually causes acute self-limited illness with additive liver damage due to each virus followed by recovery. <5% become chronic. ~3% have fulminant course.
Superinfection means acute HDV infection in a chronic HBV carrier. Mortality = 2% to 20%; >80% develop chronic hepatitis. Serum anti-HDV appears and rises to high sustained titers indicating continuing replication of HDV; intrahepatic HDAg is present. HDV-RNA persists in low titers.
♦ Acute coinfection is distinguished from superinfection by presence of serum HBsAg and anti-HBc-IgM, which indicate acute HBV.

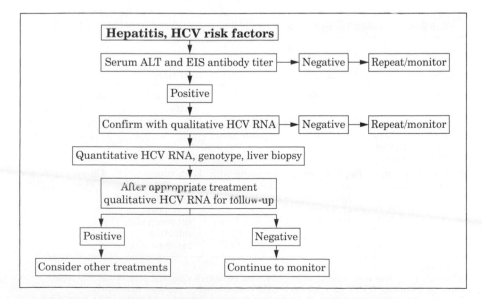

Fig. 8-13. Laboratory diagnosis of HCV.

Table 8-15. Comparison of Types of Hepatitis D Virus (HDV) Infections

	Coinfection	Superinfection	Chronic HDV
HBV infection	Acute	Chronic	Chronic
HDV infection	Acute	Acute to chronic	Chronic
Chronicity rate	<5%	>75%	Cirrhosis in >70%
Serology			
HBsAg	+	Usually persistent	Persistent
HBcAb-IgM	+	Negative	Negative
Anti-HDV-total	Negative or low titer	+	+
Anti-HDV-IgM*	Transient +	Transient	High titer
HDV-RNA (HDAg)	Transient +	Usually persistent	Persistent
Liver HDAg	Transient +	Usually persistent	Persistent

+, positive.
*Decrease in anti-HDV-IgM usually predicts resolution of acute HDV. Presistent anti-HDV-IgM typically predicts progression to chronic HDV infection. High titer correlates with active liver inflammation.

♦ Chronic HDV infection occurs in ≤80% of acute cases; shows presence of HBsAg and high titer of both IgM- and IgG-HDV (titer >1:100 suggests chronic HDV hepatitis) and absence of anti-HBc-IgM in serum. Confirm by liver biopsy showing HDAg by FA. IgA-HDV is almost exclusively associated with chronic HDV and correlates with more severe histological changes.
♦ Serum anti-HDV-IgM documents acute HDV infection; a decrease usually predicts resolution of acute infection; low levels will remain in persistent infection.
Western blot can demonstrate serum HDV-Ag when RIA is negative. Persistence correlates with development of chronic HDV hepatitis and viral antigen in liver biopsy.
Serum HDV-RNA is used for diagnosis and to monitor response to therapy. RT-PCR can detect down to 10 genome copies/sample.

Table 8-16. Serologic Diagnosis of Hepatitis B Virus (HBV) and Hepatitis D Virus (HDV)

Test				
HBsAg	HBcAb-IgM	Anti-HDV-IgM	Anti-HDV-IgG	Interpretation
Transient+	+ High titer	Transient +	Transient low titer	Acute HBV and acute HDV[a]
Transient decrease due to inhibitory effect of HDV on HBV synthesis	Negative or low titers	High titer first, low titer later	Increasing titers	Acute HDV and chronic HBV[b]
May remain + in chronic HBV	Replaced by anti-HBc-IgG in chronic HBV	+ correlates with HDAg in hepatocytes	High titers correlate with active infection; may remain+ for years after infection resolves	Chronic HDV and chronic HBV[c]

+, positive.
[a]Clinically resembles acute viral hepatitis; fulminant hepatitis is rare, and progression to chronic hepatitis is unlikely. If HBV does not resolve, HDV can continue to replicate indefinitely.
[b]Clinically resembles exacerbation of chronic liver disease or of fulminant hepatitis with liver failure.
[c]Clinically resembles chronic liver disease progressing to cirrhosis.

Serum anti-HDV may be sought in patients with HBsAg-positive chronic or acute hepatitis in high-risk group or with severe disease or with biphasic acute hepatitis or acute onset in chronic hepatitis.

Serum ALT is significantly higher in HBV carriers than in those without concomitant HDV infection.

Hepatitis E

Due to unenveloped, single-stranded RNA virus of Calciviridae family; HGV-RNA found in ~1%–2% of blood donors in United States

See Tables 8-6 and 8-7.

◆ Antibody to hepatitis E establishes diagnosis. IgM antibodies indicate recent infection.

◆ Serologic markers for HVA, HVB, HVC, and other causes of acute hepatitis (e.g., EMB, CMV) are absent.

Recent travel to endemic areas (e.g., Mexico, India, Africa, Burma, Russia)

Hepatitis G (HGV)[6–8]

Due to single-stranded RNA virus of Flaviviridae family. HGV-RNA found in ~1%–2% of American blood donors; higher in multiple-transfused persons, those with hepatitis B or C, drug addicts. Benign course; not known to cause acute, chronic, or fulminant hepatitis.

◆ Detected by RT-PCR for HGV-DNA.

○ Serum ALT is persistently normal; increase is due to concomitant HCV infection. Serological assays are under development.

In hemodialysis patients

*   ≤5% are HGV positive
*   ~25% have anti-HCV and ~15% are PCR positive for HCV
*   ~5% are HBsAg positive
*   >50% had anti-HBs or anti-HBc (representing resolved HBV infection)

Infection tends to persist for many years.

Has protective effect on HIV coinfection

Pylephlebitis, Septic

Inflammation of portal vein or any of its branches

Increased WBC and PMNs in >90% of patients; usually >20,000/μL
Anemia of varying severity
Moderate increase in serum bilirubin in ~33% of patients
Other liver function tests positive in ~25% of patients
Needle biopsy of liver not helpful; contraindicated
Blood culture may be positive
Laboratory findings due to preceding disease (e.g., acute appendicitis, diverticulitis, ulcerative colitis)
Laboratory findings due to complications (e.g., portal vein occlusion)

Lesions, Space-Occupying

Due To
Neoplasms (e.g., primary hepatocellular carcinoma, metastatic)
Cysts

*   Echinococcus
*   ≤40% of patients with autosomal dominant polycystic renal disease

[6]Masuko K, et al. Infection with hepatitis GB virus C in patients on maintenance hemodialysis. *New Eng J Med* 1996;334:1485.

[7]Alter HJ. The cloning and clinical implications of HGV and HGBV-C. *New Eng J Med* 1996; 334:1536.

[8]de Lamballerie X, Charrel RN, Dussol B. Hepatitis GB virus C in patients on hemodialysis. *New Eng J Med* 1996;334:1549.

LIVER/PANCR

Abscesses (amebic, pyogenic)
Granulomas

- Sarcoidosis
- Infections (e.g., TB, cat-scratch disease, Q fever, Lyme disease, secondary syphilis)
- Drugs (e.g., gold, quinidine, dilatiazem, hydralazine, methimazole, tocainide)

○ Increased serum ALP is the most useful index of partial obstruction of the biliary tree in which serum bilirubin is usually normal and urine bilirubin is increased.

- Increased in 80% of patients with metastatic carcinoma
- Increased in 50% of patients with TB
- Increased in 40% of patients with sarcoidosis
- Increased in >85% of patients with amyloidosis

Increased serum LAP parallels ALP but is not affected by bone disease.
Whenever the ALP is increased, a simultaneous increase of 5'-N establishes biliary disease as the cause of the elevated ALP.
AST is increased in 50% of patients (≤300 units).
ALT is increased less frequently (≤150 units).
○ Detection of metastases by panel of blood tests (ALP, LD, transaminase, bilirubin) has sensitivity of 85%. ALP or GGT alone has S/S = 25% to 33%/≤75%. Serum LD is often increased in cancer even without liver metastases.
Radioactive scanning of the liver has 65% sensitivity.
♦ Blind needle biopsy of the liver is positive in 65% to 75% of patients.
○ Laboratory findings due to primary disease (e.g., increased serum CEA in colon carcinoma, carcinoid syndrome, pyogenic liver abscess)

Neoplasms of Liver

Hepatocellular Carcinoma (Hepatoma)

♦ Serum alpha-fetoprotein (AFP) (see Chapter 16) may be increased for up to 18 months before symptoms; is sensitive indicator of recurrence in treated patients but a normal postoperative level does not ensure absence of metastases. Levels >500 ng/dL in adults strongly suggest hepatoma. Levels >100× URL have S/S = 60%/100%. In ≤30% of hepatoma cases, AFP <4× URL; such increases are common in chronic HBC and HCV.
♦ Serum GGT hepatoma-specific band (HSBs I', II, II') by electrophoresis activity >5.5 U/L has S/S = 85%/97%, accuracy = 92%. Does not correlate with AFP or tumor size.[9]
♦ Hemoperitoneum—ascites in ~50% of patients but tumor cells found irregularly
Hepatoma almost always occurs in patients with cirrhosis, which may not be recognized.
Laboratory findings associated with underlying disease

- Hemochromatosis (≤20% of patients die of hepatoma).
- HBV, HCV; look for viral DNA
- More frequent in postnecrotic than in alcoholic cirrhosis
- Cirrhosis associated with alpha$_1$-antitrypsin deficiency and other inborn errors of metabolism (e.g., tyrosinemia)
- *Clonarchis sinensis* infection is associated with cholangiosarcoma.
- Relative absence of hepatoma associated with cirrhosis of Wilson disease

Sudden progressive worsening of laboratory findings of underlying disease (e.g., increased serum ALP, LD, AST, bilirubin)
Laboratory findings due to obstruction of hepatic (Budd-Chiari syndrome) or portal veins or inferior vena cava may occur.
Occasional marked hypoglycemia unresponsive to epinephrine injection; occasional hypercalcemia
ESR and WBC sometimes increased

---

[9]Yao DF, et al. Diagnosis of hepatocellular carcinoma by quantitative detection of hepatoma-specific bands of serum γ-glutamyltransferase. *AJCP* 1998;110:743.

Anemia is common; polycythemia occurs occasionally.

Serologic markers of viral hepatitis are frequently present.

CEA in bile is increased in patients with cholangiocarcinoma and intrahepatic stones but not in patients with benign stricture, choledochal cysts, sclerosing cholangitis. Increases with progression of disease and declines with tumor resection. Does not correlate with serum bilirubin or ALP.

Serum CEA is usually normal.

After resection, additional tumors often develop, requiring continuing surveillance.

Benign (e.g., hemangioma, adenoma, focal nodular hyperplasia, hamartoma, others)

Metabolic (Inherited)

Alpha$_1$-Antitrypsin (AAT) Deficiency

Autosomal recessive deficiency of AAT [chromosome 14], a serine protease inhibitor, the principal substrate of which is neutrophil elastase, which when unchecked is associated with familial pulmonary emphysema and liver disease. The heterozygous state occurs in 10%–15% of general population who have serum levels of AAT ~60% of normal; homozygous state occurs in 1:2,000 persons who have serum levels ~10% of normal; there are >70 genetic variants of AAT.

See Table 11-30.

♦ Absent alpha$_1$ peak on serum protein electrophoresis. Should be confirmed by assay of serum AAT (electroimmunoassay) and Pi phenotyping (isoelectric focusing on polyacrilamide gel). Designated as M (normal), S (at risk for emphysema in homozygotes), and Z (at risk for chronic liver disease in homozygotes)

DNA analysis also permits prenatal diagnosis and functional analysis of total trypsin inhibitory capacity (90% is due to AAT activity).

AAT May Be Decreased In

Typically <50 mg/dL

Prematurity

Severe liver disease

Malnutrition

Renal losses (e.g., nephrosis)

GI losses (e.g., pancreatitis, protein-losing diseases)

Exudative dermopathies

AAT deficiency should be ruled out in children with neonatal hepatitis, giant cell hepatitis, chronically abnormal liver chemistries, or juvenile cirrhosis, and in adults with chronic hepatitis without serologic markers, cryptogenic cirrhosis, hepatoma.

AAT Increased In (is an acute phase reactant)

Acute or chronic infections

Neoplasia (especially cervical cancer and lymphomas)

Pregnancy

Use of birth control pills

○ Liver biopsy supports the diagnosis and helps stage extent of liver damage. Shows characteristic intracytoplasmic inclusions (in both heterozygotes and homozygotes) that may be found in patients with emphysema without liver disease and in asymptomatic heterozygous relatives, but must be searched for and stained specifically, since the rest of the pathology in the liver is not specific. ~9% of adults with nonalcoholic cirrhosis are MZ phenotype. Hepatoma may occur in cirrhotic livers.

AAT mutant Z gene encodes a mutant protein that accumulates in endoplasmic reticulum of hepatocytes.

Liver disease occurs in 10% to 20% of children with this deficiency. Clinical picture may be neonatal hepatitis (in 15% of those with ZZ phenotype), prolonged obstructive jaundice during infancy, cirrhosis, or asymptomatic. 5% to 10% of infants with undefined cholestasis have AAT deficiency. In ~25% of these patients, clinical and biochemical abnormalities become normal by age 3 to 10 years; ~25% have abnormal liver function tests with or without clinical cirrhosis; ~25% survive first decade with

confirmed cirrhosis; 25% die of cirrhosis between 6 months and 17 years of age. Hepatocellular carcinoma occurs in 5%.
○ Pulmonary emphysema occurs. Associated with phenotypes Pi ZZ and probably Pi SZ, but not Pi MZ. See Chapter 6.

Breast-Milk Jaundice

Due to the presence in mother's milk of pregnanediol, which inhibits glucuronyl-transferase activity

Severe unconjugated hyperbilirubinemia. Develops in 1% of breast-fed infants by fourth to seventh day. May reach peak of 15 to 25 mg/dL by second to third week; then gradually disappears in 3 to 10 weeks in all cases. If nursing is interrupted, serum bilirubin falls rapidly by 2 to 6 mg/dL in 2 to 6 days and may rise again if breast feeding is resumed; if interrupted for 6 to 9 days, serum bilirubin becomes normal.
No other abnormalities are present.
Kernicterus does not occur.

Cholestasis, Neonatal

Due To
Idiopathic neonatal hepatitis	50%–60%
Extrahepatic biliary atresia	20%
Metabolic disease	
Alpha1 antitrypsin deficiency	15%
Cystic fibrosis	
Tyrosinemia	
Galactosemia	
Nieman-Pick disease	
Defective bile acid synthesis	

Infection (e.g., CMV, syphilis, sepsis, GU tract infection)
Toxic (e.g., drugs, parenteral nutrition)
Other conditions, e.g.,
    Paucity of bile ducts (Alagile syndrome)
    Indian childhood cirrhosis
    Hypoperfusion/shock

Crigler-Najjar Syndrome (Hereditary Glucuronyl-Transferase Deficiency)

Rare familial autosomal recessive disease due to marked congenital deficiency or absence of glucuronyl-transferase which conjugates bilirubin to bilirubin glucuronide in hepatic cells [counterpart is the homozygous Gunn rat]

See Table 8-17.

Type I

Unconjugated serum bilirubin is increased; it appears on first or second day of life, rises in 1 week to peak of 12 to 45 mg/dL, and persists for life. No conjugated bilirubin in serum or urine.
Fecal urobilinogen is very low.
Liver function tests are normal; BSP is normal.
Liver biopsy is normal.
There is no evidence of hemolysis.
Untreated patients often die of kernicterus by age 18 months.
Nonjaundiced parents have diminished capacity to form glucoronide conjugates with menthol, salicylates, and tetrahydrocortisone.
Type I should always be ruled out when there is persistent unconjugated bilirubin levels of 20 mg/dL after 1 week of age without obvious hemolysis and especially after breast-milk jaundice has been ruled out.

Table 8-17. Differential Diagnosis of Hereditary Jaundice with Normal Liver Chemistries and No Signs or Symptoms of Liver Disease

	Conjugated Hyperbilirubinemias		Unconjugated Hyperbilirubinemias		
				Crigler-Najjar Syndrome	
	Dubin-Johnson Syndrome	Rotor Syndrome	Gilbert Disease	Type I	Type II
Incidence	Uncommon	Rare	≤7% of population	Very rare	Uncommon
Inheritance mode	AR	AR	AD	AR	AD
Serum bilirubin usual total (mg/dL)	2–7; ≤25 Direct ~60%	2–7; ≤20 Direct ~60%	<3; ≤6 Mostly indirect; increases with fasting	>20 All indirect	<20 All indirect
Defect in bilirubin metabolism	Impaired biliary excretion of conjugated organic anions and bilirubin		Hepatic UDP-glucuronyl transferase activity Decreased	Absent	Marked decrease
Impaired excretion of dyes requiring conjugation (e.g., BSP)	Yes; initial rapid fall, then rise in 45–90 mins	Yes; slow clearance; no later increase	May be slightly impaired in ≤40% of patients		
Effect of phenobarbital			Decrease to normal	None	Marked decrease
Urine coproporphyrin Total I/III*	Normal >80%	Increased <80%			
Age at onset of jaundice	Childhood, adolescence	Adolescence, early adulthood	Adolescence	Infancy	Childhood, adolescence
Usual clinical features	Asymptomatic jaundice in young adults	Asymptomatic jaundice	Appear in early adulthood; often first recognized with fasting; very mild hemolysis in ≤40% of patients	Jaundice, kernicterus in infants, young adults	Asymptomatic jaundice; kernicterus rare
Oral cholecystogram	GB usually not visualized	Normal	Normal	Normal	Normal
Liver biopsy	Characteristic pigment	No pigment	Normal		
Treatment	Not needed	None	Not needed	Liver transplant; no response to phenobarbital	Phenobarbital
Animal model	Corriedale sheep			Gunn rat	

AD, autosomal dominant; AR, autosomal recessive; BSP, sulfobromsulfophthalein; GB, gallbladder; UDP-glucuronyl transferase, uridine-diphosphate glucuronosyl-transferase.
*Normally coproporphyrin III, 75% of total.

This syndrome has been divided into two groups:

	Type I	Type II
Transmission	Autosomal recessive	Autosomal dominant
Hyperbilirubinemia	More severe (usually >20 mg/dL)	Less severe and more variable (usually <20 mg/dL)
Kernicterus	Frequent	Absent
Bile	Essentially colorless	Normal color
Bilirubin-glucuronide	Totally absent	Present
Bilirubin concentration	Very low (<10 mg/dL) Only traces of conjugated bilirubin	Nearly normal (50–100 mg/dL)
Stool color	Pale yellow	Normal
Parents	Normal serum bilirubin in both parents	One parent usually shows minimal to severe icterus
	Partial defect (~50%) in glucuronide conjugation in both parents	Defect in glucuronide conjugation may be present only in one parent

Type II

Patients have partial deficiency of glucuronyl transferase (autosomal dominant with incomplete penetrance). Not related to Type I syndrome; may be homozygous form of Gilbert disease. May not become jaundiced until adolescence. Neurologic complications are rare.

Serum unconjugated bilirubin = 6 to 25 mg/dL. Increases with fasting or removal of lipid from diet. May decrease to <5 mg/dL with phenobarbital treatment.

Dubin-Johnson Syndrome (Sprinz-Nelson Disease)

Autosomal recessive disease [gene located on chromosome 10q24] due to inability to transport bilirubin-glucuronide through hepatocytes into canaliculi but conjugation of bilirubin-glucuronide is normal. Characterized by mild chronic, recurrent jaundice. May have hepatomegaly and right upper-quadrant abdominal pain. Usually is compensated except in periods of stress. Jaundice [innocuous and reversible] may be produced by estrogens, birth control pills, or last trimester of pregnancy. May resemble mild viral hepatitis.

See Table 8-17.
○ Serum total bilirubin is increased (1.5–6.0 mg/dL); rarely ≤25 mg/dL during intercurrent illness; significant amount is conjugated. Normal in heterozygotes.
Urine contains bile and urobilinogen.
○ Other liver function tests are normal. No evidence of hemolysis.
♦ Urine total coproporphyrin is usually normal but ~80% is coproporphyrin I (normally 25% is coproporhyrin I and 75% is coproporhyrin III); diagnostic of Dubin-Johnson syndrome. Not useful to detect individual heterozygotes. Fecal coproporphyrins are normal.
○ Liver biopsy shows large amounts of yellow-brown or slate-black pigment in centrolobular hepatic cells (lysosomes) and small amounts in Kupffer cells.
♦ BSP excretion is impaired with late (normal at 45 minutes; increased at 90 and 120 minutes); virtually pathognomonic but is no longer performed.

Gilbert Disease

Chronic, benign, intermittent, familial [autosomal dominant with incomplete penetrance], nonhemolytic unconjugated hyperbilirubinemia with evanescent increases of unconjugated serum bilirubin, which is usually discovered on routine laboratory examinations; due to defective transport and conjugation of unconjugated bilirubin. Jaundice is usually accentuated by pregnancy, fever, exercise, and various drugs, including alcohol and birth control pills. Rarely identified before puberty. May be mildly symptomatic. 3%–7% prevalence in total population.

See Table 8-17.

♦ Presumptive diagnostic criteria
Exclusion of other diseases
Unconjugated hyperbilirubinemia on several occasions
Liver chemistries and hematologic parameters are normal.
♦ Unconjugated serum bilirubin is increased transiently and has been previously normal at least once in ≤33% of patients. It may rise to 18 mg/dL but usually is <4 mg/dL. Considerable daily and seasonal fluctuation. Fasting (<400 calories/day) for 72 hours causes elevated unconjugated bilirubin to increase >100% in Gilbert disease but not in healthy persons (increase <0.5 mg/dL) or those with liver disease or hemolytic anemia. Fasting bilirubin returns to baseline 12 to 24 hours after resumption of normal diet.
Combination of basal total bilirubin >1.2 mg/dL and fasting increase of unconjugated bilirubin >1 mg/dL has S/S = 84%/78%, PPV = 85%, NPV = 76%. Provocative tests are rarely needed. Conjugated serum bilirubin is normal but may give elevated results using liquid diazo methods but not by dry methods or chromatography. Enzyme inducers (e.g., phenobarbital) normalize unconjugated bilirubin in 1 to 2 weeks. Prednisone administration reduces bilirubin concentration.
Liver function tests are usually normal.
Fecal urobilinogen usually normal but may be decreased.
Urine shows no increased bilirubin.
Liver biopsy is normal.

Hemochromatosis[10–12]

Increased iron stores associated with tissue damage [cirrhosis, diabetes, cardiomyopathy]

See Fig. 8-14.
Due To
Hereditary hemochromatosis (HH) is HLA-linked autosomal recessive defect causing increased duodenal absorption of iron (2–4 mg/day compared to normal 1 mg/day in men) leading to excess iron deposition (~1 gram/year) in various organs; abnormal gene present in 10% of white Americans; frequency of homozygosity 5:1000 of north European descent. 1% to 3% of heterozygotes develop iron overload; due to coincidental condition with altered iron absorption or metabolism. Causes ≤90% of HH cases. May be C282Y homozygosity or C282Y/H63D compound heterozygosity.
Other primary causes of iron overload (may have one hemochromatosis allele)

• Neonatal hemochromatosis (severe iron overload disorder with onset in utero). Death usually soon after birth. Marked hepatic and extrahepatic (e.g., heart, pancreas, adrenal; not spleen) siderosis with relative lack in RE cells. Fulminant liver failure including increased alpha-fetoprotein. Variable fibrinogen consumption, thrombocytopenia, anemia, acanthocytosis. Oligohydramnios or less commonly polyhydramnios may indicate intrauterine growth retardation or fetal hydrops. Liver iron analysis is not useful because high in normal newborn.
• Juvenile hereditary hemochromatosis
• Aceruloplasminemia (loss of plasma ferroxidase activity impairing cell efflux of iron) that may cause hypochromic microcytic anemia
• Others (e.g., mutations in receptor-22 or ferroportin-1, and African iron overload)

Secondary

• Increased intake (e.g., excessive medicinal iron ingestion, long-term frequent transfusions)
• Anemias with ineffective erythropoiesis (especially thalassemia syndromes, sideroblastic anemias, etc.) or increased erythropoiesis (chronic hemolytic anemias)

[10]Biasiotto G, et al. Identification of new mutations of the HFE, hepcidin, and transferrin receptor 2 genes by denaturing HPLC analysis of individuals with biochemical indications of iron overload. *Clin Chem* 2003;49:1981.
[11]Pietrangelo A. Hereditary hemochromatosis: a new look at an old disease. *N Engl J Med* 2004;350:2383.
[12]Swinkels DW, et al. Hereditary hemochromatosis: genetic complexity and new diagnostic approaches. *Clin Chem* 2006;52:950.

Others

- Chronic hemodialysis
- Porphyria cutanea tarda (minor)
- Alcoholic liver disease (minor; deposited in Kupfer cells, not hepatocytes) and other chronic liver diseases
- Following portal-systemic shunt
- Congenital atransferrinemia

◆ Increased transferrin saturation (TS) (= serum iron/TIBC × 100) is earliest detectable biochemical abnormality in classic HH. Is usually >70% and frequently approaches 100%; repeat fasting TS >60% in men and >50% in women without other known causes detects >90% of cases and probably represents hemochromatosis. 50% to 62% usually indicates heterozygous state but occasionally found in homozygous persons. Most heterozygotes have no detectable changes unless there is a secondary cause (e.g., thalassemia). TS of 50% has S/S = 52%/91%. An increased value should be repeated (fasting) twice at weekly intervals. Screening will discover hemochromatosis in 2 to 3/1,000 persons; should be sought especially in patients with diabetes mellitus, bronze skin ("bronze diabetes"), congestive heart failure, idiopathic cardiomyopathy, arthritis, cirrhosis, hypogonadism. >45% is an indication for genetic testing. Surrogate marker is used because measuring transferrin for TS is an immunologic procedure too costly and time consuming for most laboratories.

◆ Increased serum ferritin (usually >1,000 μg/L); increased in ~two-thirds of patients with hemochromatosis. Increasing levels indicate tissue accumulation of iron. Is good index of total body iron but has limited value for screening because may be increased in acute inflammatory conditions and is less sensitive than TS in early cases.

- >350 μg/L in fasting men and >250 μg/L in women is recommended for screening.
- Level of 200 μg/L in women and 250 μg/L in men has S/S = 70%/80%. May not be increased in patients who have not yet accumulated excess amounts of iron (e.g., children, young adults, premenopausal women).
- <40-year-old patient with serum ferritin <1,000 μg/L in HH is not likely to have hepatic fibrosis; can omit liver biopsy before starting treatment.
- >1,000 μg/L may indicate cirrhosis in C282Y homozygotes.
- >5,000 μg/L indicates tissue damage (e.g., liver degeneration) with release of ferritin into circulation.

Critical threshold associated with cirrhosis is unknown. Liver biopsy is probably not indicated if serum ferritin is normal.

◆ Serum iron is increased (usually >200 μg/dL in women and >300 μg/dL in men and typically >1,000 μg/dL) but should not be only screening test because of many other conditions in which it occurs. Confirm by repeat fasting sample at least two more times. *Serum iron may show marked diurnal variation with lowest values in evening and highest between 7 AM and noon.*

◆ Total iron-binding capacity (TIBC) is decreased (~200 μg/dL; often approaches zero; generally higher in secondary than in primary type).

◆ Liver biopsy is needed to confirm or refute diagnosis, grade amount of iron, and assess tissue damage (presence of fibrosis/cirrhosis, other liver diseases). Is indicated when repeat fasting serum ferritin (>750 mg/L) and TS are increased after 4 to 6 weeks of abstinence from alcohol. Histologic exam confirms increased stainable iron (special stain) in perilobular hepatocytes and biliary epithelium in HH with little in Kupffer cells (in contrast to secondary iron overload) or bone marrow; with or without inactive cirrhosis. In later stages, liver biopsy alone does not distinguish HH from secondary hemochromatosis. Liver iron is increased (normal 200–2,000 μg/gram in men and 200–1,600 in women). >1,000 μg/100 mg of dry liver is consistent with homozygous state but may reach 5,000. Some heterozygotes may reach 1,000 μg/100 mg but do not progress beyond this level. Fibrosis or cirrhosis usually does not occur at levels <2,000 μg/100 mg dry liver unless alcoholism is also present. For chemical analysis of iron, should use acid-washed needle and place specimen in iron-free container. Liver iron and serum ferritin may also be increased in alcoholic cirrhosis but levels are not as abnormal (<2× normal) as in hemochromatosis. Liver iron must be related to patient age: Hepatic iron index (μg/gram divided by 55.8 × age) in homozygotes, ≥1.9; in heterozygotes, usually ≤1.5. False negative may be due to phlebotomy treatment; false positive may be due to secondary hemosiderosis. Another calculation is liver iron (μmoles/g dry weight) divided by patient age:

homozygotes, >2; <2 in heterozygotes, healthy persons, and patients with alcoholic liver disease.

○ Presence of excess iron in other tissue biopsy sites (e.g., synovia, GI tract) should arouse suspicion of HH; iron stains should be done.

Bone marrow biopsy stained for iron is not useful for diagnosis of HH.

Other tests to assess iron stores (when liver biopsy is not possible)

• Chelating agent (0.5 g IM deferoxamine mesylate) causes urinary excretion >5 mg/24 hrs in HH but <2 mg/24 hrs in normal persons. Measures only chelatable iron rather than total iron stores so may underdiagnosis HH; not a useful diagnostic test.

• Weekly phlebotomy 5 to 10× causes iron deficiency in alcoholic liver disease but >50 weekly phlebotomies are required in HH.

○ Slightly increased serum ALT values may be a clue to unsuspected hemochromatosis. Liver function tests depend on presence and degree of liver damage (e.g., cirrhosis).

On average, women have serum ferritin concentrations 1000 μg/L less than men; men have 2× incidence of cirrhosis (25%) and diabetes (15%) compared to women.

Laboratory findings due to involvement of various organs and hemochromatosis should be ruled out in patients with these unexplained findings:

• Diabetes mellitus (IDDM) in 40% to 75% of cases; glucose intolerance
• Osteoarthritis and chrondrocalcinosis (pseudogout) in 50% of cases
• Hypogonadism/pituitary dysfunction in ~50% of cases
• Skin pigmentation ("bronze diabetes")
• Cardiomyopathy in 33% of cases (congestive heart failure)
• Cirrhosis in 69% of cases; does not resolve with phlebotomy; associated alcoholism
• Portal hypertension
• Hepatocellular carcinoma develops in ≤30% of cases and has become the chief cause of death in HH.

○ Laboratory findings due to complications and sequelae

• Increased susceptibility to bacterial infections, especially *Yersinia, Listeria monocytogenes, Yersinia enterocolitica, Salmonella typhimurium, Klebsiella pneumoniae, E. coli* (also occurs in other iron overload conditions)

• Macrocytosis[13] and increased MCV (not due to cirrhosis) have recently been noted in HH and resolve when weekly phlebotomies reduce Hb and ferritin.

○ When diagnosis of HH is established, other family members should be screened; one fourth of siblings will have the disease; 5% of patients' children will be homozygous for hemochromatosis gene. Negative relatives should be rescreened every 5 years.

○ Genotyping is not used for screening to discover sporadic cases but useful to identify patients' siblings at risk since HLA-identical sibs will almost always also be homozygous for hemochromatosis gene and at high risk for developing clinical disease. May be useful to distinguish primary HH from cirrhotic patients with secondary iron overload and siderosis. HPLC is fast enough to be used for large population screening. Genetic testing with *HFE* mutation analysis has replaced HLA typing; preferred for family testing.

♦ DNA test for HH genes by direct exonic sequencing or HPLC. C282Y or H63D mutations present in 69% to 97% of affected patients; would not identify ≤31% of clinically affected patients. Genetic mutations plus iron overload establishes the diagnosis.

Ideally should begin therapy when serum ferritin is >200 μg/dL. Adequate treatment with phlebotomy (1–2 units/week) is indicated by serum ferritin <50 ng/dL and TS <30%, which may take ≤2 to 3 years, and maintained at serum ferritin <100 ng/dL and TS <50%. Insulin requirement decreases in > one third of diabetics; liver function tests often improve; arthritis, impotence, and sterility usually do not improve. Removal of 500 mL of blood causes loss of 200 to 250 mg of iron.

Can proceed with phlebotomy without liver biopsy if ferritin <1,000 ng/dL and normal liver enzymes until Hgb or Hct do not recover before next phlebotomy.

Evaluate for cardiac disease before liver transplant for decompensated cirrhosis.

Hyperbilirubinemia, Neonatal[14]

Scleral/facial jaundice becomes visible at serum bilirubin of 6 to 8 mg/dL.
Shoulder/trunk jaundice becomes visible at serum bilirubin of 8 to 10 mg/dL.

[13] Amidon P, Jankovich R. Letter to editor. *Ann Intern Med* 2001;135:1091.
[14] Wood A. Neonatal hyperbilirubinemia. *N Engl J Med* 2001;344:581.

LIVER/PANCR

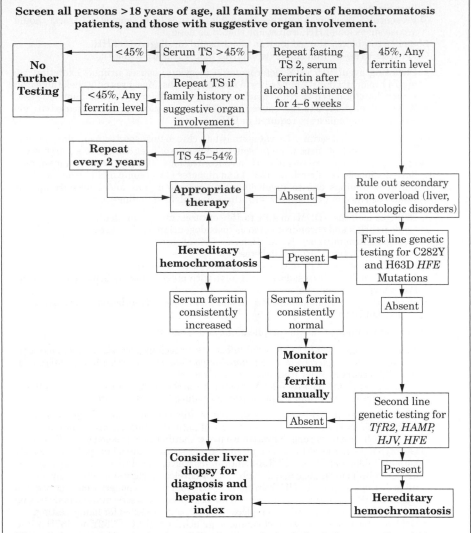

Screen all persons >18 years of age, all family members of hemochromatosis patients, and those with suggestive organ involvement.

If heterozygotes, rule out associated conditions (e.g., porphyria, viral and other types of hepatitis).
If homozygotes with normal TS and serum ferritin, retest serum ferritin annually.
TS threshold may be lower for African Americans than for whites.

Fig. 8-14. Sequence of tests for hemochromatosis screening and treatment.

Lower-body jaundice becomes visible at serum bilirubin of 10 to 12 mg/dL.
General jaundice becomes visible at serum bilirubin of 12 to 15 mg/dL.
Various classifications are illustrated below (e.g., physiologic or nonphysiologic, unconjugated or conjugated, infectious, genetic, etc.)

Physiologic

Transient unconjugated hyperbilirubinemia ["physiologic jaundice"] that occurs in almost all newborns

In normal full-term neonate, average maximum serum bilirubin is 6 mg/dL (≤12 mg/dL is in physiologic range) that occurs during the second to fourth day and then rapidly falls to ~2.0 mg/dL by fifth day (phase I physiologic jaundice). Declines slowly to <1.0 mg/dL during fifth to tenth day, but may take one month to fall to <2 mg/dL (phase II physiologic jaundice). Phase I due to deficiency of hepatic bilirubin-glucuronyl transferase activity and six-fold increase in bilirubin load presented to liver. In Asian and American Indian newborns, the average maximum serum levels are approximately double (10–14 mg/dL) the levels in non-Asians, and kernicterus is more frequent. Serum bilirubin >5 mg/dL during first 24 hours of life is indication for further workup because of risk of kernicterus.

In older children (and adults) icterus is apparent clinically when serum bilirubin is >2 mg/dL, but in newborns clinical icterus is not apparent until serum bilirubin is >5 to 7 mg/dL; therefore only half of the full-term newborns show clinical jaundice during first 3 days of life.

In premature infants—average maximum serum bilirubin is 10 to 12 mg/dL and occurs during the fifth to seventh day. Serum bilirubin may not fall to normal until thirtieth day. Further workup is indicated in all premature infants with clinical jaundice because of risk of kernicterus in some low-birth weight infants with serum levels of 10 to 12 mg/dL.

In postmature infants and half of small-for-dates infants—serum bilirubin is <2.5 mg/dL and physiologic jaundice is not seen. When mothers have received phenobarbital or used heroin, physiologic jaundice is also less severe.

When a pregnant woman has unconjugated hyperbilirubinemia, similar levels occur in cord blood but when the mother has conjugated hyperbilirubinemia (e.g., hepatitis), similar levels are not present in cord blood.

Nonphysiologic

Cause should be sought for underlying pathologic jaundice if:

* Total serum bilirubin >7 mg/dL during first 24 hours or increases >5 mg/dL/day or visible jaundice
* Peak total serum bilirubin >12.5 mg/dL in white or black full-term or >15 mg/dL in Hispanic or premature infants
* Conjugated serum bilirubin >1.5 mg/dL
* Clinical jaundice longer than 7 days in full-term or 14 days in premature infants or before age 36 hours or with dark urine (containing bile)

Initial tests in unconjugated hyperbilirubinemia

* Serial determinations of total and conjugated bilirubin
* CBC including RBC morphology, platelet count, normoblast, and reticulocyte counts
* Blood type mother and infant, Coomb's test, maternal blood for antibodies
* Blood cultures
* Urine microscopy and culture
* Serologic tests for infection
* Serum TSH and T_4
* Urine for nonglucose-reducing substances

Unconjugated

Increased destruction of RBCs

* Isoimmunization (e.g., incompatibility of Rh, ABO, other blood groups)
* Biochemical defects of RBCs (e.g., glucose 6-PD deficiency, pyruvate deficiency, hexokinase deficiency, congenital erythropoietic porphyria, alpha and gamma thalassemias)

- Structural defects of RBCs (e.g., hereditary spherocytosis, hereditary elliptocytosis, infantile pyknocytosis)
- Infection
  Viral (e.g., adenovirus, CMV, Coxsackie B, HAV, HBV, HSV, rubella, varicella zoster)
  Bacterial (e.g., syphilis, listeria)
  Protozoal (e.g., toxoplasmosis)
- Extravascular blood (e.g., subdural hematoma, ecchymoses, hemangiomas)
- Erythrocytosis (e.g., maternal-to-fetal or twin-to-twin transfusion, delayed clamping of umbilical cord)

Increased enterohepatic circulation

- Any cause of delayed bowel motility
  Pyloric stenosis—unconjugated hyperbilirubinemia >12 mg/dL develops in 10% to 25% of infants usually during second to third week, at which time vomiting begins; jaundice is due to decreased hepatic glucuronyl transferase activity of unknown mechanism.
  Duodenal and jejunal obstruction may also be associated with exaggerated unconjugated hyperbilirubinemia, which becomes normal 2 to 3 days after surgical relief.
  In Hirschsprung disease, unconjugated hyperbilirubinemia is usually more mild.
  Meconium ileus, meconium plug syndrome
  Hypoperistalis (e.g., drug-induced, fasting)

Endocrine and metabolic

- Neonatal hypothyroidism—associated with prolonged and exaggerated unconjugated hyperbilirubinemia in 10% of cases and is promptly alleviated by thyroid hormone therapy. *Always rule out congenital hypothyroidism in cases of unexplained persistent or excessive unconjugated hyperbilirubinemia; may be the only manifestation of hypothyroidism.*
- Infants of diabetic mothers—associated with higher incidence of prolonged and exaggerated unconjugated hyperbilirubinemia of unknown mechanism; not related to severity or duration of diabetes.
- Drugs and hormones (e.g., breast-milk jaundice, Lucey-Driscoll syndrome, novobiocin)
- Galactosemia
- Tyrosinosis
- Hypermethionemia
- Heart failure
- Hereditary glucuronyl-transferase deficiency (Crigler-Najjar Syndrome)
- Gilbert disease
- Breast-milk jaundice

Interference of albumin binding of bilirubin

- Drugs (e.g., aspirin, sulfonamides)
- Severe acidosis
- Hematin
- Free fatty acids (e.g., periods of stress, inadequate caloric intake)
- Prematurity (serum albumin may be 1–2 g/dL less than in full-term infants)

Neonatal physiologic hyperbilirubinemia

Conjugated

Premature infants with these conditions will have more severe hyperbilirubinemia than full-term infants.
Biliary obstruction—usually due to extrahepatic biliary atresia but may be due to choledochal cyst, obstructive inspissated bile plugs, or bile ascites; congenital biliary atresia
Neonatal hepatitis
Sepsis, especially *E. coli pyelonephritis* (moderate azotemia, acidosis, increased serum bilirubin, slight hemolysis, normal or slightly increased AST)
Hereditary diseases (e.g., galactosemia, alpha$_1$-antitrypsin deficiency, cystic fibrosis, hereditary fructose intolerance, tyrosinemia, infantile Gaucher disease, familial intrahepatic cholestasis [Byler disease], neonatal hemosiderosis)
In the course of hemolytic disease of the newborn—due to liver damage of unknown cause

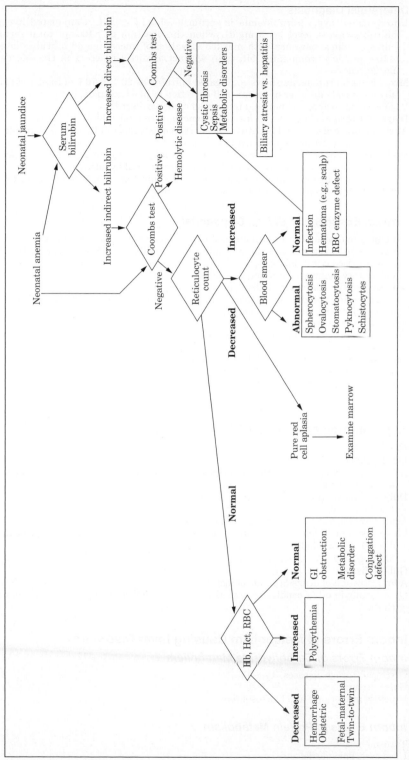

Fig. 8.15 Algorithm for workup of neonatal jaundice and anemia.

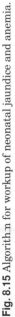

Differential Diagnosis

Unconjugated hyperbilirubinemia is serum level >1.5 mg/dL. Conjugated hyperbilirubinemia is level >1.5 mg/dL when this fraction is >10% of total serum
bilirubin (since newborn with marked elevation of unconjugated bilirubin level,
≤10% of the unconjugated bilirubin will act as direct-reacting in the van den
Bergh reaction).

Mixed hyperbilirubinemia shows conjugated bilirubin as 20% to 70% of total and usually represents disorder of hepatic cell excretion or bile transport.

Visible icterus before 36 hours old indicates hemolytic disorder.

Diagnostic studies should be performed whenever serum bilirubin >12 mg/dL.

After hemolytic disease and hepatitis, the most frequent cause of hyperbilirubinemia is
enterohepatic circulation of bilirubin.

Visible icterus persisting after seventh day is usually due to impaired hepatic excretion, most commonly due to breast feeding or congenital hypothyroidism.

Increase in conjugated bilirubin usually indicates infection or inflammation of liver,
but can also be seen in galactosemia and tyrosinosis.

Atresia, Extrahepatic Biliary, Congenital

○ Conjugated serum bilirubin increased in early days of life in some infants but not
until second week in others. Level is often <12 mg/dL during first months, with subsequent rise later in life.

○ Laboratory findings as in Complete Biliary Obstruction

♦ Liver biopsy to differentiate from neonatal hepatitis

Laboratory findings due to sequelae (e.g., biliary cirrhosis, portal hypertension, frequent infections, rickets, hepatic failure)

^{131}I-rose bengal excretion test

Most important to differentiate this condition from neonatal hepatitis, for which
surgery may be harmful.

>90% of cases of extrahepatic biliary obstruction in newborns are due to biliary atre-
sia; occasional cases may be due to choledochal cyst (causes intermittent jaundice in
infancy), bile plug syndrome, or bile ascites (associated with spontaneous perforation of the common bile duct).

Hyperbilirubinemia, Older Children

Due To
Conjugated

*All cases of conjugated hyperbilirubinemia also show some increase of unconjugated
serum bilirubin.*

Dubin-Johnson syndrome

Rotor syndrome

Acute viral hepatitis causes most cases in children

Cholestasis due to chemicals and drugs or associated with other diseases (e.g., Hodgkin
disease, sickle cell disease)

Unconjugated

Gilbert disease

Administration of drugs (e.g., novobiocin)

Occasionally in other conditions (e.g., thyrotoxicosis, following portacval shunt in cirrhosis)

Inborn Errors of Metabolism Causing Liver Disorders

Inborn Errors of Carbohydrate Metabolism

Glycogen storage diseases, Type IV

Galactosemia

Fructose intolerance and fructosemia

Inborn Errors of Protein Metabolism

Tyrosinemia

Urea cycle enzyme defects

Inborn Errors of Lipid Metabolism

Gaucher disease
Gangliosidosis
Cholesterol ester storage disease
Neimann-Pick disease
Lipodystrophy
Wolman disease

Others

Alpha$_1$-antitrypsin deficiency—causes 20% to 35% of cases of neonatal liver disease
Byler disease
Cystic fibrosis rarely presents as prolonged neonatal jaundice.
Hemochromatosis
Hepatic porphyria
Histiocytosis-X
Hypothyroidism
Hypopituitarism
Leprechaunism
Mucopolysaccharidoses
Wilson disease
Zellweger syndrome

Jaundice in infants receiving parenteral alimentation—many are premature and have
   various complications (e.g., RDS, septicemia, acidosis, congenital heart disease)

- Increased AST, ALT, ALP
- Serum proteins normal
- Increased serum bile acids
- Increased serum ammonia
- Abnormal plasma amino acid patterns (increased threonine, serine, methionine)

Associated with Hemolytic Disease of Newborn

Occurred in 10% of cases ("inspissated bile" syndrome) prior to modern prevention of
   Rh disease

- Cord blood conjugated bilirubin ≥2 mg/dL indicates that syndrome will develop.
- Jaundice may persist for 3 to 4 weeks.
- Most cases have required exchange transfusion.

Clinical and Laboratory Findings

Jaundice at birth, or days or weeks later. Both conjugated and unconjugated bilirubin
   levels are increased in variable proportions.
Mild hemolytic anemia is typical.
Increased AST, ALT, etc., may be marked and is usually greater than in biliary atresia,
   but increases are not useful for differentiating the two conditions.
Laboratory findings as in acute viral hepatitis (see Table 8–9)
Liver biopsy to differentiate from biliary atresia and to avoid unnecessary surgery is
   useful in ~65% of patients but it may be misleading.
[131]I-rose bengal excretion test indicates complete biliary obstruction if <10% of the
   radioactivity is excreted in stools during 48 to 72 hours and incomplete obstruction if
   >10%. Complete obstruction is found in all infants with biliary atresia and in ~20%
   with neonatal hepatitis and severe cholestasis. Administration of phenobarbital and
   cholestyramine increases the ^{131}I-rose bengal excretion in neonatal hepatitis but not
   in extrahepatic atresia. Some authors have suggested a repeat test in 3 to 4 weeks
   prior to exploratory surgery if rose bengal test indicates complete obstruction.
Laboratory tests for various etiologic agents
Laboratory findings of chronic liver disease, which develops in 30% to 50% of these infants
Whenever mother has hepatitis during pregnancy or is HBsAg positive, test cord blood
   and baby's blood every 6 months. If baby develops HBsAg or anti-HBs, do liver
   chemistries at periodic intervals. Infants who acquire hepatitis in utero or at time of

birth may develop clinical acute hepatitis with abnormal liver chemistries, benign course, or development of HBsAb. Infants who are asymptomatic but develop HBsAg often become chronic carriers with biochemical and liver biopsy evidence of chronic hepatitis and increased likelihood of hepatoma (see Serologic Tests for Hepatitis).

Lucey-Driscoll Syndrome (Neonatal Transient Familial Hyerbilirubinemia)

Syndrome is due to some factor in mother's serum only during last trimester of pregnancy that inhibits glucuronyltransferase activity; disappears about 2 weeks postpartum.

Newborn infants have severe nonhemolytic unconjugated hyperbilirubinemia usually ≤20 mg/dL during first 48 hours and a high risk of kernicterus.

Rotor Syndrome

Autosomal recessive, familial, asymptomatic, benign defective uptake and storage of conjugated bilirubin and possibly in transfer of bilirubin from liver to bile or in intrahepatic binding; usually detected in adolescents or adults. Jaundice may be produced or accentuated by pregnancy, birth control pills, alcohol, infection, surgery.

See Table 8-17.
○ Mild chronic fluctuating nonhemolytic conjugated hyperbilirubinemia (usually <10 mg/dL)
○ Urine coproporphyrins are markedly increased especially coprophyrin I (increased > III).
Other liver function tests are normal.
Liver biopsy is normal; no pigment is present.
BSP excretion is impaired.

Wilson Disease[15]

Autosomal recessive defect that impairs copper excretion by liver, which may cause copper accumulation in liver and brain resulting in cirrhosis, neuropsychiatric disease, and corneal pigmentation.

Heterozygous gene for Wilson disease occurs in 1 of 200 in the general population; 10% of these have decreased serum ceruloplasmin; liver copper is not increased (<250 μg/g of dry liver). Serum copper and ceruloplasmin and urine copper are inadequate to detect heterozygous state.
Homozygous gene (clinical Wilson disease) occurs in 1 of 200,000 in the general population.
○ Liver biopsy may show no abnormalities, moderate to marked fatty changes with or without fibrosis, or active or inactive mixed micronodular-macronodular cirrhosis.
♦ Findings of liver function tests may not be abnormal, depending on the type and severity of disease. *In patients presenting with acute fulminant hepatitis, Wilson disease is suggested if there is a disproprotionately low serum ALP and relatively mild increase in AST and ALT.* ALP is frequently decreased; ALP/bilirubin ratio <2.0 is said to distinguish Wilson disease as cause of fulminant liver failure with S/S = 100%/100%.
○ *Should also be ruled out in any patient with hepatitis with negative serology for viralhepatitis, Coombs-negative hemolysis* (due to copper released from necrotic liver cells)*, or neurologic symptoms to allow for early diagnosis and treatment of Wilson disease.*
♦ Radiocopper incorporation into ceruloplasmin is significantly reduced compared with heterozygotes or normal persons. ^{64}Cu is administered IV or PO and serum concentration is plotted against time. Serum ^{64}Cu disappears within 4 to 6 hours

[15]Ferenci, P. Diagnosis and current therapy of Wilson's disease. *Aliment Pharmacol Ther* 2004; 19:157.

Table 8-18. Tests for Diagnosis of Wilson Disease

Test	May Also Be Increased In	May Also Be Decreased In	Comment
Decreased serum ceruloplasmin[1] (normal range = 20–50 mg/dL)	• Acute inflammatory reactions (e.g., infection, rheumatoid arthritis) • Pregnancy, use of estrogen or birth control pills • Thyrotoxicosis • Cirrhosis • Cancer *May cause green color of plasma.*	• Wilson disease (*It is normal in ≤5% of homozygous Wilson disease patients.*) • May not be decreased in Wilson disease with acute or fulminant liver involvement • Rare homozygotes >30 mg/dL • 10%–20% of persons heterozygous for Wilson disease • Normal infants (therefore cannot use this test for Wilson disease in first year of life) • Hypoproteinemia (e.g., renal protein loss [e.g., nephrosis], malabsorption [e.g., sprue] malnutrition, severe decompensated liver disease • Aceruloplasminaemia (rare) • Menkes' disease	*Serum ceruloplasmin (<20 mg/dL) with increased hepatic copper (>250 µg/g) occurs only in Wilson disease or normal infants <6 months of age.*
24-hour urine copper (normal <50 µg/24 hours)	Urinary copper is increased (>100 µg/ 24h); may be normal in presymptomatic patients	• False-positive with significant proteinemia • Other liver diseases with extensive hepato-cellular necrosis	
Total serum copper is decreased and generally parallels serum ceruloplasmin (normal = 80–120 µg/dL)			Not a good indicator because changes during course of disease
Increased serum *free (noncerulo-plasmin)* copper (normal = <10 µg/dL)	Usually >25 µg/dL S/S = virtually 100%		Calculated from difference between total serum copper and ceruloplasmin-bound copper. Free copper (µg/dL) = total serum copper (µg/dL) minus ceruloplasmin (mg/dL) × 3

(continued)

LIVER/PANCR

Table 8-18. *(continued)*

Test	May Also Be Increased In	May Also Be Decreased In	Comment
Liver copper (normal <50)	• Increased in >80% of cases • Usually >250 μg/g of dry liver • May also be elevated in chronic cholestatic syndromes (e.g., primary biliary cirrhosis, primary sclerosing cholangitis, extrahepatic biliary and Indian childhood cirrhosis), which are easily differentiated from Wilson disease by increased serum ceruloplasmin • Neonates, young children • Lower cutoff of 75 μg/g has NPV = 97%		• Copper concentrations may vary between nodules; thus extensive sampling may be necessary to confirm diagnosis.
Histochemical staining of paraffin-embedded liver specimens for copper and copper-associated protein.	May be present in other hepatic disorders	May be negative in Wilson disease	• Focal copper deposits by rodanine stain is said to be pathognomonic but occurs in 10% of patients.
Electron microscopy			Shows pathognomonic mitochondrial changes that distinguish homozygotes
Kayser-Fleischer rings (slit lamp)	Are present in 95% of cases with, and ≤60% of cases without, neurological disease but may be absent in younger patients with only liver manifestations; present in 10% of asymptomatic siblings		

[1]Is a serum glycoprotein containing 6 copper atoms/molecule, synthesized mostly in liver; is an acute phase reactant
All specimens should be collected in copperfree containers.

and than reappears in persons without Wilson disease; secondary reappearance is absent in Wilson disease because incorporation of ^{64}Cu into ceruloplasmin is decreased. Useful when liver biopsy is contraindicated but rarely used since advent of transjugular liver biopsy. Can use mass spectroscopy rather than radioactive Cu.
  Chelating agent (e.g., D-penicillamine) produces urine Cu excretion of 2 to 4 mg/day.

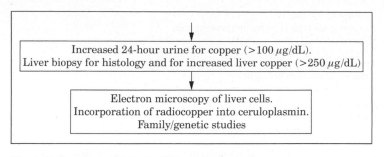

Fig. 8-16. Sequence of tests for Wilson disease.

Other tests that have been used in diagnosis of heterozygotes may not be available locally

* D-penicillamine administration induces increased urinary copper excretion.
* Copper content of cultured fibroblasts
* Family screening: diagnosis in index patient odds of finding homozygote in siblings is 25%; among children is 0.5%. Mutation analysis is only reliable to screen families.
* Molecular genetic studies but most common mutation is present in <30% of populations and many are compound heterozygotes.

Laboratory findings due to complications and sequelae

* Cirrhosis (e.g., ascites, esophageal varices, liver failure)
* Hypersplenism (e.g., anemia, leukopenia, thrombocytopenia). Coombs-negative nonspherocytic hemolytic anemia may occur.
* Renal proximal tubular dysfunction may cause aminoaciduria (especially cystine and threonine), glucosuria; distal renal tubular acidosis is less common; nephrocalcinosis (hypercalciuria, hyperphosphaturia), uricosuria with decreased serum uric acid.

Laboratory findings due to effects of therapeutic agents

* Long-term treatment with copper-depleting agents may sometimes cause a mild sideroblastic anemia and leukopenia due to copper deficiency.
* Penicillamine toxicity (e.g., nephrotic syndrome, thrombocytopenia, lupus, etc.)

All transplant recipients have complete reversal of underlying defects in copper metabolism.

Miscellaneous Disorders

Transplant of Liver

Indications
Liver Failure Due To
Arterial thrombosis
Autoimmune liver disease
Chronic cholestasis, e.g., biliary atresia (infants), sclerosing cholangitis with serum bilirubin >8 to 10 mg/dL, or recurrent bacterial cholangitis
Venoocclusive disease, e.g., Budd-Chiari syndrome
Cirrhosis (e.g., alcoholic, postnecrotic, primary or secondary biliary) with ≥2 signs of liver insufficiency
Hepatitis
Fulminant hepatic failure with coma Grade 2
Certain inborn errors of metabolism, e.g.,

* Alpha$_1$-antitrypsin deficiency
* C-protein deficiency
* Crigler-Najjar syndrome type I
* Cystic fibrosis
* Erythropoietic protoporphyria
* Glycogen storage diseases type I and IV

- Hemophilia A and B
- Homozygous type II hyperlipoproteinemia
- Hyperoxaluria type I
- Niemann-Pick disease
- Tyrosinemia
- Urea cycle enzyme deficiencies
- Wilson disease

Liver trauma
Polycystic liver disease
Rejection of liver transplant (cause of 20% of retransplants)
Reye syndrome
Unresectable liver neoplasms confined to liver and <5 cm in size
Laboratory indications, e.g.,

- Poor synthesis function (e.g., albumin <3.5 g/dL, fibrinogen, prolonged PT >3 seconds above control or INR >1.3)
- Progressive hyperbilirubinemia >2 mg/dL
- Evidence of hypersplenism and/or bleeding esophageal varices, portal hypertension with intractable ascites, encephalopathy, hepatorenal syndrome, spontaneous bacterial peritonitis

Contraindications
Positive serology for HBsAg, HBcAb, HIV
Sepsis other than of hepatobiliary system
Stage 4 hepatic coma
Unrelated failure or advanced disease of other organ systems
Extrahepatic neoplasms (other than skin cancer)
Active alcohol or substance abuse
Irreversible brain damage

Postoperative Complications

	Reported Incidence
Early	
Primary nonfunction due to graft ischemia	5%–10%
Portal vein thrombosis	
Hepatic artery thrombosis	5%–10%
Hyperacute rejection	
Early acute rejection	
Immunosuppressant therapy toxicity	
Hepatorenal syndrome	≤9.8%
Hepatopulmonary syndrome	13.2%
Infection/sepsis	

Later
Acute and chronic rejection
Side effects of immunosuppressant therapy
Biliary stenosis
Recurrence of disease (especially hepatitis B,
    hepatitis C, EBV-associated lymphoproliferative
    disorders)
Vanishing bile duct syndrome

Rejection
May be due to hepatic artery and portal vein thrombosis, ischemic reperfusion injury, infection and sepsis, biliary tract strictures, recurrence of HCV and HBV
Usually liver enzymes and PT begin to improve within 48 hours. Hypoglycemia, progressive coagulopathy, severe progressive lactic acidosis, failure to improve AST and ALT are early indicators of rejection.
Most episodes occur within first 3 months; patients are usually asymptomatic.
Electrolytes must be monitored rapidly to treat cardiac arrest due to sudden release of large amounts of potassium from perfused liver and to monitor IV fluid replacement.

Ionized calcium is lost due to chelation by citrate in transfused blood; left ventricular dysfunction may occur when serum level <1.2 mEq/L. Serum sodium is monitored to avoid postoperative neurologic complications due to rapid increase during transplant and post operative periods (e.g., central pontine myelinolysis). Normalization of serum HCO3⁻ and anion gap signifies early function of liver transplant and of kidneys.

○ Serum GGT is the most sensitive marker for rejection; rises early during rejection before serum ALP and bilirubin. Is more specific than other markers because other complications (e.g., CMV infection) cause relatively low levels compared with AST and ALT.

○ Serum ALP lags behind serum GGT and bilirubin indicators of rejection.

In uncomplicated cases, serum ALP and GGT remain within reference range.

○ AST and ALT rise after reperfusion of the allograft; increase to >4 to 5× upper limit of reference range, even in uncomplicated cases. Persistent or late increases may be due to rejection or to other causes such as viral infections (e.g., CMV, HSV, adenovirus), occlusion of hepatic artery, liver abscess.

○ Serum total and conjugated bilirubin are monitored with enzymes and are useful to help differentiate between biliary obstruction (suggesting rejection) and hepato-cellular disease. Increase may be early sign of rejection but is less useful than enzymes.

Serum cyclosporine monitoring is important because it is metabolized in the liver and proportion of cyclosporine and its metabolites may be altered when postoperative liver function is not maintained.

PT and aPTT monitor synthesis of coagulation factors; specific factor measurements are not needed.

Cultures from appropriate sites for evidence of infection

♦ Liver biopsy is gold standard for diagnosis

- Distinguish causes of rejection that have no specific biochemical pattern (e.g., acute rejection, chronic rejection, opportunistic viral infection, recurrence of HBV infection, CMV, changes in hepatic blood perfusion, unrecognized disease in donor liver)
- Differentiate from cholangitis, hepatitis, ischemic injury, which may mimic rejection
- Substantial numbers of false positives occur.

Laboratory findings due to immunosuppression therapy:

- Nephrotoxicity
- Liver toxicity (e.g., serum cyclosporine concentration >1,200 ng/dL)
- Infection (e.g., bacterial, fungal, HBV, CMV, HSV, EBV)
- Cancer (e.g., non-Hodgkin lymphoma; Kaposi sarcoma; carcinomas of cervix, perineum, lip)
- Complications of hypertension

In rare cases, genetic defects (e.g., Factor XI deficiency) can be transmitted to the recipient and cause postoperative complications.

Trauma

May be laceration, hematoma, or vascular

Serum LD is frequently increased (>1,400 units) 8 to 12 hours after major injury. Shock due to any injury may also increase LD.

Other serum enzymes and liver function tests are not generally helpful.

Findings of abdominal paracentesis

- Bloody fluid (in ~75% of patients) confirming traumatic hemoperitoneum and indicating exploratory laparotomy
- Nonbloody fluid (especially if injury occurred >24 hours earlier)

Microscopic—some red and white blood cells

Determine amylase, protein, pH, presence of bile.

Obstructive Disease

Cholestasis

See Table 8-19.

Table 8-19. Comparison of Various Types of Cholestatic Disease

Disorder	Bilirubin (mg/dL)	ALP	AST	ALT	Albumin
			Serum Values*		
CBD obstruction					N
Stone	0–10	N–10	N–10	N–10	N
Cancer	5–20	2–10	N	N	N
Intrahepatic					
Drug–induced	5–10	2–10	N–5	10–50	
Acute viral hepatitis	0–20	N–3	10–50	10–50	N
Alcoholic liver disease	0–20	5	<10	<50% of AST	N/sl D

CBD, common bile duct; N, normal; sl D, slightly decreased.
*Serum value, times normal.

○ Increased serum ALP
○ Increased GGT; 5′-N and LAP parallel ALP and confirm the hepatic source of ALP
○ Increased serum cholesterol and phospholipids but not triglycerides
○ Increased fasting serum bile acid (>1.5 μg/mL) with ratio of cholic acid: chenodeoxycholic acid >1 in primary biliary cirrhosis and many intrahepatic cholestatic conditions but <1 in most chronic hepatocellular conditions (e.g., Laennec cirrhosis, chronic active hepatitis) *(There is relatively little experience with this test.)*
Cholestasis may occur without hyperbilirubinemia.
Due To
Intrahepatic Obstruction
Space-occupying lesions (e.g., amyloidosis, sarcoidosis, metastases; non-Hodgkin lymphoma more often than Hodgkin disease)
Drugs (e.g., estrogens, anabolic steroids)—most common cause (see Table 8-19)
Normal pregnancy
Alcoholic hepatitis
Infections, e.g.,

• Acute viral hepatitis
• Gram-negative sepsis
• Toxic shock syndrome
• AIDS
• Parasitic, fungal

Sickle cell crisis
Postoperative state following long procedure and multiple transfusions
Benign recurrent familial intrahepatic cholestasis—rare condition
Hepatocellular
Sclerosing pericholangitis (associated with inflammatory bowel disease)
Primary biliary cirrhosis
Postnecrotic cirrhosis (20% of cases)
Congenital intrahepatic biliary atresia
Multifocal lesions (e.g., metastases, lymphomas, granulomas)
Sclerosing cholangitis
Intraductal stones
Intraductal papillomatosis
Cholangiocarcinoma
Caroli disease (congenital biliary ectasia)
Extrahepatic Ducts
Carcinoma (e.g., pancreas, ampulla, bile ducts, gallbladder), lympomas
Stricture (e.g., primary sclerosing cholangitis), stone, cyst, atresia, etc., of ducts
Pancreatitis (acute, chronic), pseudocysts

Parasites
AIDS
Increased risk of cholangiocarcinoma in progressive cholestatic diseases

Cholestasis, Benign Recurrent Intrahepatic

Autosomal recessive condition; attacks begin after age 8, lasts weeks to months, complete resolution between episodes, may recur after months or years; exacerbated by estrogens

Increased serum ALP but GGT is usually normal
Transaminase usually <100 U
Serum direct bilirubin may be normal or ≤10 mg/dL.
Liver biopsy shows centrolobular cholestasis without inflammation, bile pigment in hepatocytes and canaliculi; little or no fibrosis.

Cirrhosis, Primary Biliary[16] (Cholangiolitic Cirrhosis, Hanot Hypertrophic Cirrhosis, Chronic Nonsuppurative Destructive Cholangitis, etc.)

Slow progressive multisystem autoimmune disease; chronic nonsuppurative inflammation and asymmetric destruction of small intrahepatic bile ducts producing chronic cholestasis, cirrhosis, and ultimately liver failure

---

♦ **Diagnostic criteria**
(*Definite* diagnosis requires all 3 criteria.)

• Antimitochondrial autoantibodies present
• Cholestatic pattern (increased ALP) of long duration (>6 months) not due to known cause (e.g., drugs)
• Compatible histologic findings on liver biopsy

Probable diagnosis requires 2 of these 3 criteria.

♦ Serum ALP is markedly increased; is of liver origin. Reaches a plateau early in the course and then fluctuates within 20% thereafter; changes in serum level have no prognostic value. 5'-N and GGT parallel the ALP. *This is one of the few conditions that will elevate both serum ALP and GGT to striking levels.*
♦ Serum mitochondrial antibody titer is strongly positive in ~95% of patients (1:40 to 1:80) and is hallmark of disease (98% specificity); titer >1:160 is highly predictive of PBC even in absence of other findings. Does not correlate with severity or rate of progression. Titers differ greatly in patients. Similar titers occur in 5% of patients with chronic hepatitis; low titers occur in 10% of patients with other liver disease; rarely found in normal persons. Titer may decrease after liver transplantation but usually remains detectable.
♦ Serum bilirubin is normal in early phase but increases in 60% of patients with progression of disease and is a reliable prognostic indicator; an elevated level is a poor prognostic sign. Conjugated serum bilirubin is increased in 80% of patients; levels >5 mg/dL in only 20% of patients; levels >10 mg/dL in only 6% of patients. Unconjugated bilirubin is normal or slightly increased.
♦ Laboratory findings show relatively little evidence of parenchymal damage

• AST and ALT may be normal or slightly increased (≤1–5× normal), fluctuate within a narrow range, and have no prognostic signficance.
• Serum albumin, globulin, and PT normal early; abnormal values indicate advanced disease and poor prognosis; not corrected by therapy.

[16]Data from: P Angulo. Nonalcoholic fatty liver disease. *N Engl J Med* 2002;346:1221.

♦ Marked increase in total cholesterol and phospholipids with normal triglycerides; serum is not lipemic; serum triglycerides become elevated in late stages. Associated with xanthomas and xanthelasmas. In early stages, LDL and VLDL are mildly elevated and HDL is markedly elevated (thus atherosclerosis is rare). In advanced stage, LDL is markedly elevated with decreased HDL and presence of lipoprotein-X (non-specific abnormal lipoprotein seen in other cholestatic liver disease).

○ Serum IgM is increased in ~75% of patients; levels may be very high (4–5× normal). Other serum immunoglobulins are also increased.

Hypocomplementemia

Polyclonal hypergammaglobulinemia. Serum IgM is increased in ~75% of patients with failure to convert to IgG antibodies; levels may be very high (4–5 × normal). Other serum immunoglobulins are also increased.

♦ Biopsy of liver categorizes the four stages and helps assess prognosis but needle biopsy is subject to sampling error since the lesions may be spotty; findings consistent with all four stages may be found in one specimen.

○ Serum ceruloplasmin is characteristically elevated (in contrast to Wilson disease).

Liver copper may be increased 10 to 100× normal; correlates with serum bilirubin and advancing stages of disease.

ESR is increased 1 to 5× normal in 80% of patients.

Urine contains urobilinogen and bilirubin.

Laboratory findings of steatorrhea

• Serum 25-hydroxyvitamin D and vitamin A are usually low.
• PT is normal or restored to normal by parenteral vitamin K.

Laboratory findings due to associated diseases

• >80% have one, and >40% have at least two, other circulating antibodies to autoimmune disease (e.g., RA, autoimmune thyroiditis [hypothyroidism in 20% of patients], Sjögren syndrome, scleroderma) although not useful diagnostically.

Laboratory findings due to sequelae and complications

• Portal hypertension, hypersplenism
• Treatment-resistant osteopenia
• Hepatic encephalopathy, liver failure
• Renal tubular acidosis (due to copper deposition in kidney) is frequent but usually subclinical.
• Increased susceptibility to urinary tract infection is associated with advanced disease.

Should be ruled out in an asymptomatic female with elevated serum ALP without obesity, diabetes mellitus, alcohol abuse, some drugs.

Vascular Disorder of Liver

Budd-Chiari Syndrome[17]

Heterogeneous group of disorders due to obstruction of hepatic venous outflow

Due To

Thrombosis due to hypercoagulable states (e.g., polycythemia vera [10%–40% of cases], essential thrombocythemia, myelofibrosis; antiphospholipid syndrome; deficiencies of protein C, protein S, antithrombin III, etc.) See Chapter 11, Paroxysmal nocturnal hemoglobinuria.

Membranes and webs

Others (e.g., neoplasms, collagen vascular diseases, cirrhosis, polycystic liver disease, etc.)

○ Laboratory findings of parenchymal cell necrosis and malfunction, e.g., increased serum AST, ALT may be increased >5× in acute and fulminant forms. ALP and bilirubin may be increased and serum albumin decreased. Ascitic fluid total protein usually >2.5 g/dL.

○ Laboratory findings of portal hypertension

[17] Menon KVN, et al. The Budd-Chiari syndrome. *N Engl J Med* 2004;350:578.

♦ Radiologic visualization (e.g., ultrasound, CT scan, MRI, hepatic angiography)
♦ Liver biopsy

Congestive Heart Failure

Pattern of abnormal liver function tests is variable depending on severity of heart failure; the mildest show only slightly increased ALP and slightly decreased serum albumin; moderately severe also show slightly increased serum bilirubin and GGT; one fouth to three fourths of the most severe will also show increased AST and ALT ($\leq$200 U/L) and LD ($\leq$400 U/L). All return to normal when heart failure responds to treatment. Serum ALP is usually the last to become normal, and this may be weeks to months later.
Serum bilirubin is increased in $\leq$70% of cases (unconjugated more than conjugated); usually <3 mg/dL but may be >20 mg/dL. It usually represents combined right- and left-sided failure with hepatic engorgement and pulmonary infarcts. Serum bilirubin may suddenly rise rapidly if superimposed myocardial infarction occurs.
AST and ALT may be increased 2 to 3× normal in < one third of cases but much higher in severe acute heart failure.
PT may be slightly increased in 80% of cases, with increased sensitivity to anticoagulant drugs.
Fails to correct with vitamin K
Serum albumin is slightly decreased in <50% of patients but is rarely <2.5 mg/dL.
Serum cholesterol and esters may be decreased.
Serum ammonia may be increased.
Urine urobilinogen is increased. Urine bilirubin is increased in the presence of jaundice.
These findings may occur with marked liver congestion due to other conditions (e.g., Chiari syndrome [occlusion of hepatic veins] and constrictive pericarditis).
Constrictive pericarditis produces changes similar to Budd-Chiari syndrome.

Hepatic Infarction

Is rare due to dual blood supply

Due To
Hypercoagulable states
Emboli
Vascular disease (e.g., polyarteritis nodosa, aortic dissection)
Hematologic disorders (e.g., sickle cell disease, polycythemia vera)
Others (e.g., surgery, drugs, toxemia of pregnancy)

Increased WBC count may be marked.
Increased serum AST is often seen.

Ischemic Hepatitis

Diffuse hepatic injury due to acute decreased liver perfusion; also called shock liver; usually as part of congestive heart failure; usually benign, self-limited

PT may be slightly increased $\leq$3 seconds.
Mildly increased serum AST usually resolves in <10 days if no other factors are present.

Portal Hypertension

Due To
Prehepatic (e.g., portal vein thrombosis, splenic arteriovenous fistula)
Intrahepatic

• Presinusoidal (e.g., metastatic tumor, granulomas such as sarcoid, schistosomiasis)
• Sinusoidal (e.g., cirrhosis)
• Postsinusoidal (e.g., hepatic vein thrombosis, alcoholic hepatitis)

Posthepatic (e.g., pericarditis, tricuspid insufficiency, inferior vena cava web)

Veno-Occlusive Disease of Liver[18]

Syndrome of painful hepatomegaly, jaundice, weight gain of >5%, and fluid avidity

Due To
Injury to sinusoidal endothelial cells and hepatocytes, most commonly caused by:

* High dose chemotherapy with or without irradiation
* Stem cell transplantation especially with HLA disparity between donor and recipient
* Drinking bush tea in Jamaica

♦ Transvenous liver biopsy and wedged hepatic venous pressure gradient >10 mm Hg is gold standard for diagnosis
♦ Increased serum AST >4× normal and bilirubin
Exclusion of other causes (e.g., pericardial effusion, constrictive pericarditis, mass lesions of liver, Budd-Chiari syndrome)

Diseases of the Gallbladder and Biliary Tree

Biliary Obstruction, Complete (Intrahepatic or Extrahepatic)

○ Typical pattern of extrahepatic obstruction includes increased serum ALP (>2–3× normal), AST <300 U/L, conjugated serum bilirubin.
In extrahepatic type, the increased ALP is related to the completeness of obstruction. Normal ALP is extremely rare in extrahepatic obstruction. Very high levels may also occur in cases of intrahepatic cholestasis. Serum LAP parallels ALP.
AST is increased (≤300 U), and ALT is increased (≤200 U); they usually return to normal within 1 week after relief of obstruction. In *acute* biliary duct obstruction (e.g., due to common bile duct stones or acute pancreatitis), AST and ALT are increased >300 U (and often >2,000 U) and decline 58% to 76% in 72 hours without treatment; simultaneous serum total bilirubin shows less marked elevation and decline and ALP changes are inconsistent and unpredictable.
Conjugated serum bilirubin is increased; unconjugated serum bilirubin is normal or slightly increased.
Serum cholesterol is increased (acute, 300–400 mg/dL; chronic, ≤1,000 mg/dL).
Serum phospholipids are increased.
PT is prolonged, with response to parenteral vitamin K more frequent than in hepatic parenchymal cell disease.
Urine bilirubin is increased; urine urobilinogen decreased.
There is decreased stool bilirubin and urobilinogen (clay-colored stools).
Laboratory findings due to underlying causative disease are noted (e.g., stone, carcinoma of duct, metastatic carcinoma to periductal lymph nodes).

Bile Duct Obstruction (One)

○ Characteristic pattern is serum bilirubin that remains normal in the presence of markedly increased serum ALP.

Cancer of Gallbladder and Bile Ducts

Laboratory findings reflect varying location and extent of tumor infiltration that may cause partial intrahepatic duct obstruction or obstruction of hepatic or common bile duct, metastases in liver, or associated cholangitis; 50% of patients have jaundice at the time of hospitalization.
Laboratory findings of duct obstruction are of progressively increasing severity in contrast to the intermittent or fluctuating changes due to duct obstruction caused by stones. A papillary intraluminal duct carcinoma may undergo periods of sloughing, producing the findings of intermittent duct obstruction.
Anemia is present.
♦ Cytologic examination of aspirated duodenal fluid may demonstrate malignant cells.

---

[18] Wadleigh M, et al. Hepatic veno-occlusive disease: pathogenesis, diagnosis and treatment. *Curr Opin Hematol* 2003;10:451.

○ Silver-colored stool due to jaundice combined with GI bleeding may be seen in carcinoma of duct or ampulla of Vater.

Cholangitis, Acute

Infection of bile ducts usually due to gram-negative [e.g., E. coli, Klebsiella sp], gram-positive, and anaerobic [Streptococcus fecalis, enterococcus, Bacteroides fragilis] organisms usually associated with obstruction

○ Marked increase in WBC (≤30,000/μL) with increase in granulocytes
○ Blood culture positive in ~30% of cases; 25% of these are polymicrobial.
○ Laboratory findings of incomplete duct obstruction due to inflammation or of preceding complete duct obstruction (e.g., stone, tumor, scar). See Choledocholithiasis.
○ Laboratory findings of parenchymal cell necrosis and malfunction
Increased serum AST, ALT, etc.
Increased urine urobilinogen

Cholangitis, Primary Sclerosing

Chronic fibrosing cholestatic inflammation of intra- and extrahepatic bile ducts predominantly in men under age 45, rare in pediatric patients; ≤75% are associated with inflammatory bowel disease, especially ulcerative colitis. Slow, relentless, progressive course of chronic cholestasis to death [usually from liver failure]. 25% of patients are asymptomatic at time of diagnosis.

◆ **Diagnostic criteria**
1. Cholestatic biochemical profile for >6 months
   • Serum ALP may fluctuate but is always increased (usually ≥3× upper limit of normal).
   • Serum GGT is increased.
   • Serum AST is mildly increased in >90%. ALT > AST in 3/4 of cases.
   • Serum bilirubin is increased in 50% of patients; occasionally is very high; may fluctuate markedly; gradually increases as disease progresses. Persistent value >1.5 mg/dL is poor prognostic sign that may indicate irreversible medically untreatable disease.
2. Compatible clinical history (e.g., inflammatory bowel disease) and exclusion of other causes of sclerosing cholangitis (e.g., previous bile duct surgery, gallstones, suppurative cholangitis, bile duct tumor or damage due to floxuridine, AIDS, congenital duct anomalies).
3. Characteristic cholangiogram to distinguish from primary biliary cirrhosis.

Increased gamma globulin in 30% and increased IgM in 40% to 50% of cases
Anti-neutrophil cytoplasmic (ANCA) in ~65% and antinuclear antibodies <35% of cases are present at higher levels than in other liver diseases but diagnostic significance is not yet known.
In contrast to primary biliary cirrhosis, antimitochondrial antibody, smooth-muscle antibody, rheumatoid factor, ANA are negative in >90% of patients.
HBsAg is negative.
○ Liver biopsy provides only confirmatory evidence in patients with compatible history, laboratory, and X-ray findings. Liver copper is usually increased but serum ceruloplasmin is also increased.
Laboratory findings due to sequelae
○ Cholangiocarcinoma in 10% to 15% of patients may cause increased serum CA 19-9
○ Portal hypertension, biliary cirrhosis, secondary bacterial cholangitis, steatorrhea and malabsorption, cholelithiasis, liver failure
Laboratory findings due to underlying disease, e.g.,

• ≤7.5% of ulcerative colitis patients have this disease; much less often with Crohn disease. Associated with syndrome of retroperitoneal and mediastinal fibrosis

Cholecystitis, Acute

Increased ESR, WBC (average 12,000/μL; if >15,000, suspect empyema or perforation), and other evidence of acute inflammatory process
Serum AST is increased in 75% of patients.
Increased serum bilirubin in 20% of patients (usually >4 mg/dL; if higher, suspect associated choledocholithiasis)
Increased serum ALP (some patients) even if serum bilirubin is normal
Increased serum amylase and lipase in some patients
Laboratory findings of associated biliary obstruction if such obstruction is present
Laboratory findings of preexisting cholelithiasis (some patients)
Laboratory findings of complications (e.g., empyema of gallbladder, perforation, cholangitis, liver abscess, pyelophlebitis, pancreatitis, gallstone ileus)

Cholecystitis, Chronic

May be mild laboratory findings of acute cholecystitis or no abnormal laboratory findings
May be laboratory findings of associated cholelithiasis
Laboratory findings of sequelae (e.g., carcinoma of gall bladder)

Choledocholithiasis

Gallstones in bile ducts due to passage from gall bladder or anatomical defects [e.g., cysts, strictures]

During or soon after an attack of biliary colic

• Increased WBC
• Increased serum bilirubin in about one third of patients
• Increased urine bilirubin in about one third of patients
• Increased serum and urine amylase
• Increased serum ALP

○ Laboratory evidence of fluctuating or transient cholestasis. Persistent increase of WBC, AST, ALT suggests cholangitis.
Laboratory findings due to secondary cholangitis, acute pancreatitis, obstructive jaundice, stricture formation, etc.
In duodenal drainage, crystals of both calcium bilirubinate and cholesterol (some patients); 50% accurate (only useful in nonicteric patients)

Cholelithiasis

Laboratory findings of underlying conditions causing:

• Hypercholesterolemia (e.g., diabetes mellitus, malabsorption)
• Chronic hemolytic disease (e.g., hereditary spherocytosis)

Laboratory findings due to complications (e.g., cholecystitis, choledocholithiasis, gall stone ileus)

Laboratory Tests for Pancreatic Disease

Amylase, Serum

Composed of pancreatic and salivary types of isoamylases distinguished by various methodologies; nonpancreatic etiologies are almost always salivary; both types may be increased in renal insufficiency

See Fig. 8-17.
Increased In
Acute pancreatitis (e.g., alcoholic, autoimmune). Urine levels reflect serum changes by a time lag of 6 to 10 hours.
Acute exacerbation of chronic pancreatitis
Drug-induced acute pancreatitis (e.g., aminosalicylic acid, azathioprine, corticosteroids, dexamethasone, ethacrynic acid, ethanol, furosemide, thiazides, mercaptopurine, phenformin, triamcinolone)

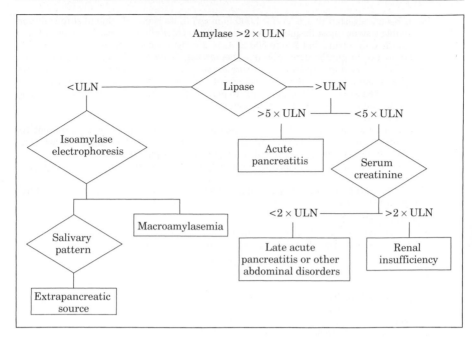

Fig. 8-17. Algorithm for increased serum amylase and lipase. (ULN, upper limit of normal.)

Drug-induced methodologic interference (e.g., pancraozymin [contains amylase], chloride and fluoride salts [enhance amylase activity], lipemic serum [turbidimetric methods])

Obstruction of pancreatic duct by:

- Stone or carcinoma
- Drug-induced spasm of sphincter of Oddi (e.g., opiates, codeine, methyl choline, cholinergics, chlorothiazide) to levels 2 to 15× normal
- Partial obstruction + drug stimulation (see Cholecystokinin-Secretin Test)

Biliary tract disease

- Common bile duct obstruction
- Acute cholecystitis

Complications of pancreatitis (pseudocyst, ascites, abscess)
Pancreatic trauma (abdominal injury; following ERCP)
Altered GI tract permeability

- Ischemic bowel disease or frank perforation
- Esophageal rupture
- Perforated or penetrating peptic ulcer
- Postoperative upper abdominal surgery, especially partial gastrectomy (≤2× normal in one third of patients)

Acute alcohol ingestion or poisoning
Salivary gland disease (mumps, suppurative inflammation, duct obstruction due to calculus, radiation)
Malignant tumors (especially pancreas, lung, ovary, esophagus; also breast, colon); usually >25× URL (upper ref limit) which is rarely seen in pancreatitis
Advanced renal insufficiency; often increased even without pancreatitis
Macroamylasemia
Others, such as chronic liver disease (e.g., cirrhosis; ≤2× normal), burns, pregnancy (including ruptured tubal pregnancy), ovarian cyst, diabetic ketoacidosis, recent thoracic surgery, myoglobinuria, presence of myeloma proteins, some cases of intracranial bleeding (unknown mechanism), splenic rupture, dissecting aneurysm

It has been suggested that a level >1,000 Somogyi units is usually due to surgically correctable lesions (most frequently stones in biliary tree), the pancreas being negative or showing only edema; but 200 to 500 units is usually associated with pancreatic lesions that are not surgically correctable (e.g., hemorrhagic pancreatitis, necrosis of pancreas).

Increased serum amylase with low urine amylase may be seen in renal insufficiency and macroamylasemia. Serum amylase ≤4× normal in renal disease only when creatinine clearance is <50 mL/min due to pancreatic or salivary isoamylase; but rarely >4× normal in absence of acute pancreatitis.

Decreased In
Extensive marked destruction of pancreas (e.g., acute fulminant pancreatitis, advanced chronic pancreatitis, advanced cystic fibrosis). Decreased levels are clinically significant only in occasional cases of fulminant pancreatitis.

Severe liver damage (e.g., hepatitis, poisoning, toxemia of pregnancy, severe thyrotoxicosis, severe burns)

Methodologic interference by drugs (e.g., citrate and oxalate decrease activity by binding calcium ions)

- Normal: 1% to 5%
- Macroamylasemia: <1%; very useful for this diagnosis
- Acute pancreatitis: >5%; use is presently discouraged for this diagnosis

$$\text{Amylase:creatinine clearance ratio} =$$
$$(\text{urine amylase/serum amylase}) \times (\text{serum creatinine/urine creatinine}) \times 100$$

May Be Normal In
Relapsing chronic pancreatitis
Patients with hypertriglyceridemia (technical interference with test)
Frequently normal in acute alcoholic pancreatitis

Lipase, Serum

Glycoprotein enzyme filtered by glomeruli and completely reabsorbed by proximal tubules; method should always include colipase in reagent

See Fig. 8-17.

Increased In
Acute pancreatitis
Perforated or penetrating peptic ulcer, especially with involvement of pancreas
Obstruction of pancreatic duct by:

- Stone
- Drug-induced spasm of sphincter of Oddi (e.g., codeine, morphine, meperidine, methacholine, cholinergics) to levels 2 to 15× normal
- Partial obstruction + drug stimulation

Chronic pancreatitis
Acute cholecystitis
Small bowel obstruction
Intestinal infarction
Acute and chronic renal failure (increased 2–3× in 80% of patients and 5× in 5% of patients)
Organ transplant (kidney, liver, heart), especially with complications (e.g., organ rejection, CMV infection, cyclosporin toxicity)
Alcoholism
Diabetic ketoacidosis
After endoscopic retrograde cholangiopancreatography
Some cases of intracranial bleeding (unknown mechanism)
Macro forms in lymphoma, cirrhosis
Drugs

- Induced acute pancreatitis (see preceding section on serum amylase)
- Cholestatic effect (e.g., indomethacin)
- Methodologic interference (e.g., pancreozymin [contains lipase], deoxycholate, glycocholate, taurocholate [prevent inactivation of enzyme], bilirubin [turbidimetric methods])

Chronic liver disease (e.g., cirrhosis) (usually ≤2× normal)

Decreased In
Methodologic interference (e.g., presence of Hb, quinine, heavy metals, calcium ions)
Usually Normal In
Mumps
Macroamylasemia
(Values are lower in neonates.)

Glycoprotein 2, Serum[19]

Protein present in zymogen exocrine secretion by acinar cells; ELISA assay

Increased In
Acute pancreatitis: at cutoff value of 4.5 pmol/L, S/S was superior to serum amylase and lipase
Chronic pancreatitis or carcinoma of pancreas; may be increased secondary to duct obstruction or acinar cell destruction

Diseases of the Pancreas

Carcinoma of Pancreas

Body or Tail

Laboratory tests are often normal.
○ Serum markers for tumor CA 19-9, CEA, etc. (see Chapter 16)

- In carcinoma of pancreas, CA 19-9 has S/S = 70%/87%, PPV = 59%, NPV = 92%. No difference in sensitivity between local disease and metastatic disease. Often normal in early stages, therefore *not useful for screening*. Increased value may help differentiate benign disease from cancer. Declines to normal in 3 to 6 months if cancer is completely removed so may be useful for prognosis and follow-up. Detects tumor recurrence 2 to 20 weeks before clinical evidence. Not specific for pancreas since high levels may also occur in other GI cancers, especially those affecting colon and bile duct.
- Testosterone:dihydrotestosterone ratio <5 (normal ~10) in >70% of men with pancreatic cancer (due to increased conversion by tumor). Less sensitive but more specific than CA 19-9; present in higher proportion of Stage I tumors.

♦ The most useful diagnostic tests are ultrasound or CT scanning followed by endoscopic retrograde cholangiopancreatography (ERCP) (at which time fluid is also obtained for cytologic and pancreatic function studies). This combination will correctly diagnose or rule out cancer of pancreas in ≥90% of cases. ERCP with brush cytology has S/S = ≤25%/ ≤100%.
CEA level in bile (obtained by percutaneous transhepatic drainage) was reported increased in 76% of a small group of cases.
Serum amylase and lipase may be slightly increased in early stages (<10% of cases); with later destruction of pancreas, they are normal or decreased. They may increase following secretin-pancreozymin stimulation before destruction is extensive; therefore, the increase is less marked with a diabetic glucose tolerance curve. Serum amylase response is less reliable. See serum glycoprotein 2.
○ Glucose tolerance curve is of the diabetic type with overt diabetes in 20% of patients with pancreatic cancer. Flat blood sugar curve with IV tolbutamide tolerance test indicates destruction of islet cell tissue. *Unstable, insulin-sensitive diabetes that develops in an older man should arouse suspicion of carcinoma of the pancreas.*
Serum LAP is increased (>300 units) in 60% of patients with carcinoma of pancreas due to liver metastases or biliary tract obstruction. *It may also be increased in chronic liver disease.*
♦ Triolein ^{131}I test demonstrates pancreatic duct obstruction with absence of lipase in the intestine, causing flat blood curves and increased stool excretion.
Radioisotope scanning of pancreas may be done (^{75}Se) for lesions >2 cm.
♦ Ultrasound guided needle biopsy has reported sensitivity of 80% to 96%; false positives are rare.

[19]Ying Hao, et al. Determination of plasma glycoprotein 2 levels in patients with pancreatic disease. *Arch Pathol Lab Med* 2004;128:668.

LIVER/PANCR

Head

The abnormal pancreatic function tests and increased tumor markers that occur with carcinoma of the body of the pancreas may be evident.

♦ Laboratory findings due to complete obstruction of common bile duct

* Serum bilirubin increased (12–25 mg/dL), mostly conjugated (increase persistent and nonfluctuating)
* Serum ALP increased
* Urine and stool urobilinogen absent
* Increased PT; normal after IV vitamin K administration
* Increased serum cholesterol (usually >300 mg/dL) with esters not decreased

♦ Secretin-cholecystokinin stimulation evidences duct obstruction when duodenal intubation shows decreased volume of duodenal contents (<10 mL/10 minute collection period) with usually normal bicarbonate and enzyme levels in duodenal contents. Acinar destruction (as in pancreatitis) shows normal volume (20–30 mL/10-minute collection period), but bicarbonate and enzyme levels may be decreased. Abnormal volume, bicarbonate, or both is found in 60% to 80% of patients with pancreatitis or cancer. In carcinoma, the test result depends on the relative extent and combination of acinar destruction and of duct obstruction. Cytologic examination of duodenal contents shows malignant cells in 40% of patients. Malignant cells may be found in up to 80% of patients with periampullary cancer.

Other liver function tests are usually normal.

See serum glycoprotein 2.

Cystic Fibrosis (CF) of Pancreas (Mucoviscidosis)[20,21]

Autosomal recessive disorder with abnormal ion transport due to (>1,000) chromosome 7 mutations transmembrane conductance regulator (CFTR gene) that controls salt, especially chloride, entry/exit into cells; incidence of 1:2,500 in non-Hispanic whites in North America with a carrier frequency of 1:20; 1:17,000 in African Americans; marked heterogeneity among patients

---

♦ **Diagnostic criteria**

At least one characteristic clinical feature (respiratory, sweat, GI, GU) *or*
sibling with CF *or*
positive neonatal screening
and sweat chloride ≥60 mEq/L *or*
presence of 2 *CFTR* genes *or*
positive nasal transmembrane potential difference.

♦ *Quantitative Pilocarpine Iontophoresis Sweat Test (Properly Performed)*

Striking increase in sweat chloride concentration (>60 mEq/L) is consistent with CF.
Increased sweat sodium (>60 mEq/L) and, to a lesser extent, potassium is present in virtually all homozygous patients; value is 3 to 5× higher than in healthy persons or with other diseases. Is consistently present throughout life from time of birth and degree of abnormality is not related to severity of disease or organ involvement. S/S = 98%/83%; PPV = 93%. Sweat volume is not increased.

Sweat chloride 40 to 59 mEq/L is considered borderline and requires further investigation; <40 mEq/L is considered normal. May be normal in nonclassic form of CF. 2% of CF patients have values ≤60 mEq/L.

Rare patients with borderline values have only mild disease.

[20]Richards CS, Haddow JE. Prenatal screening for cystic fibrosis. *Clin Lab Med* 2003;23:503.
[21]Lyon E, Miller C. Current challenges in cystic fibrosis screening. *Arch Pathol Lab Med* 2003; 127:1133.

Sweat potassium is not diagnostically valuable because of overlap with normal controls.

Increased sweat chloride and sodium is not useful for detection of heterozygotes (who have normal values) or for genetic counseling.

A broad range of sweat concentrations is seen in CF and in normal persons but there is minimal overlap.

Sweat values (mEq/L)

| | Chloride | | Sodium | | Potassium | |
	Mean	Range	Mean	Range	Mean	Range
Cystic Fibrosis	115	79–148	111	75–145	23	14–30
Normal	28	8–43	28	16–46	10	6–17

Note that some instruments measure sweat conductivity, not sweat chloride concentration, which are not equivalent. *Sweat conductivity is considered only a screening test*; values ≥50 mEq/L should have quantitative sweat chloride. Conductivity values are ~15 mEq/L higher than sweat concentrations.

Sweat Chloride Concentration

≥60 mEq/L on ≥2 occasions has sensitivity = 90%; with characteristic clinical manifestations or family history, confirm diagnosis of CF

Interferences

Sweat testing is fraught with problems and technical and laboratory errors are very frequent; should be performed in duplicate and repeated at least once on separate days on samples >100 mg of sweat.

Values may be increased to CF range in healthy persons when sweat rate is rapid (e.g., exercise, high temperature) but pilocarpine test does not increase sweating rate.

Mineralocorticoids decrease sodium concentration in sweat by ~50% in normal subjects and 10% to 20% in CF patients whose final sodium concentration remains abnormally high.

Increased In

Endocrine disorders (e.g., untreated adrenal insufficiency, hypothyroidism, vasopressin-resistant diabetes insipidus, familial hypoparathyroidism, pseudohypoaldosteronism)

Metabolic disorders (e.g., malnutrition, gycogen storage disease Type I, mucopolysaccharidosis IH and IS, fucosidosis)

Genitourinary disorders (e.g., Klinefelter syndrome, nephrosis)

Allergic/immunologic disorders (e.g., hypogammaglobulinemia, prolonged infusion with prostaglandin E1, atopic dermatitis)

Neuropsychologic disorders (e.g., anorexia nervosa)

Others (e.g., ectodermal dysplasia, G6PD deficiency)

○ Laboratory changes secondary to complications which *should also suggest diagnosis of CF*

Respiratory abnormalities

* Chronic lung disease (especially upper lobes) with laboratory changes of decreased pO_2, accumulation of CO_2, metabolic alkalosis, severe recurrent infection, secondary corpulmonale, etc; nasal polyps, pansinusitis; normal sinus X-rays are strong evidence against CF.
* Bronchoalveolar lavage usually shows increased PMNs (>50% in CF; ~3% in normal persons) with high absolute neutrophil count; is strong evidence of CF even in absence of pathogens.
* Bacteriology: Special culture techniques should be used in these patients. Before year of age, *Staphylococcus aureus* is found in 25% and *pseudomonas* in 20% of respiratory tract cultures; in adults *pseudomonas* grows in 80% and *S. aureus* in 2 *H. influenzae* is found in 3.4% of cultures. *Pseudomonas aeruginosa* is found inc ingly often after treatment of staph and special identification and susceptibilit should be performed on *P. aeruginosa*. *P. cepacia* is becoming more impor Older children. Increasing serum antibodies against *P. aeruginosa* can d probable infection when cultures are negative.

Gastrointestinal abnormalities

- Chronic or acute and recurrent pancreatitis
- Pancreatic insufficiency frequency by age 1 year >90%; in adults >95%. Protein-calorie malnutrition, hypoproteinemia; fat malabsorption of with vitamin deficiency. Stool and duodenal fluid show lack of trypsin digestion of X-ray film gelatin; useful screening test up to age 4; decreased chymotrypsin production (see Bentiromide Test). (See Malabsorption).
- Impaired glucose intolerance in ~40% of patients with glycosuria, and hyperglycemia in 8% precedes diabetes mellitus.
- Overt liver disease including cirrhosis, fatty liver, bile duct strictures, cholelithiasis, etc. in ≤5% of cases. Neonatal cholestasis in ≤20% of affected infants may persist for months.
- Meconium ileus during early infancy; causes 20% to 30% of cases of neonatal intestinal obstruction; present at birth in 8% of these children. Almost all of them will develop the clinical picture of CF.
- Increased incidence of GI tract cancers

Salt loss syndromes

- Hypochloremic metabolic alkalosis and hypokalemia due to excessive loss of electrolytes in sweat and stool
- Acute salt depletion

GU tract abnormalities

- Aspermia in 98% due to obstructive changes in vas deferens and epididymis is confirmed by testicular biopsy.

Serum chloride, sodium, potassium, calcium, and phosphorus are normal unless complications occur (e.g., chronic pulmonary disease with accumulation of CO_2; massive salt loss due to sweating may cause hyponatremia). Urine electrolytes are normal. Submaxillary saliva has slightly increased chloride and sodium but not potassium; considerable overlap with normal results prevents diagnostic use.

Submaxillary saliva is more turbid, with increased calcium, total protein, and amylase. These changes are not generally found in parotid saliva.

Serum protein electrophoresis shows increasing IgG and IgA with progressive pulmonary disease; IgM and IgD are not appreciably increased.

Serum albumin is often decreased (because of hemodilution due to cor pulmonale; may be found before cardiac involvement is clinically apparent).

- ◆ DNA genotyping (using blood; can use buccal scrapings) to confirm diagnosis based on 2 mutations is highly specific but not very sensitive. Supports diagnosis of CF but failure to detect gene mutations does not exclude CF because of large number of alleles. Substantial number of CF patients have unidentified gene mutations. Should be done when sweat test is borderline or negative. Can also be used for carrier screening.

Identical genotypes can be associated with different degrees of disease severity. Genotype should not be used as sole disgnostic criterion of CF.

Prevalence of the 25 most common genes in the panel account depends on population group:

	Detection Rate of Panel (%)	Frequency of Carriers
Ashkenazi Jew	97	1/25
North European	90	1/25
South European	68–70	1/29
Black	69	1/60
Hispanic	55–57	1/45
Asian	30	1/90

- ◆ Neonatal screening using dried filter paper blood that measures immunoreactive trypsin has been used for screening with confirmation by sweat test and genotyping. Normal in ~15% of CF infants. Increased false-negative rate in meconium ileus. Doctors cannot diagnose CF in 30% of affected children until >1 year old.
- ◆ Prenatal screening by chorionic villus sampling in first trimester or amniocentesis in second or third trimester. >1,000 mutations of CFTR (cystic fibrosis transmembrane conductance regulator) gene but the 25 most common account for ~90% of

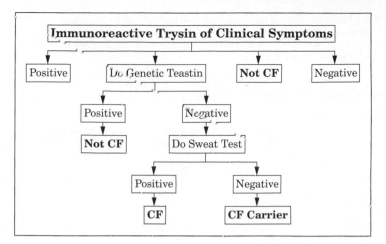

Fig. 8-18. Algorithm for prenatal screening for cystic fibrosis.

carriers. 52% are homozygous for ΔF508 and 36% are heterozygous for ΔF508/other CF mutation.
♦ Nasal electrical potential-difference measurements may be more reliable than sweat tests but are much more complex; mean = −46 mV in affected persons but −19 mV in unaffected persons.

Macroamylasemia

Complex of amylase with IgA, IgG, or other high-molecular weight plasma proteins that cannot filter through glomerulus due to large size

♦ Serum amylase *persistently* increased (often 1–4× normal) without apparent cause
Serum lipase is normal; normal pancreatic to salivary amylase ratio
Urine amylase normal or low
○ Amylase-creatinine clearance ratio <1% with normal renal function is very useful for this diagnosis; should make the clinician suspect this diagnosis.
♦ Macroamylase is identified in serum by special gel filtration or ultracentrifugation technique.

Table 8-20. Comparison of Classic and Nonclassic Forms of CF*

Classic CF (No functional CFTR protein)	Nonclassic CF (Some functional CFTR protein)
Sweat chloride usually 90–110 mEq/L May be 60–90 mEq/L	Sweat chloride usually 60–90 mEq/L May be normal
Pancreatic exocrine insufficiency	Usually adequate pancreatic exocrine function; pancreatitis in 5%–20% of cases
Severe chronic bacterial infection of airways	Variable chronic bacterial infection of airways with later onset
Severe hepatobiliary disease in 5%–10% of cases	—
Meconium ileus at birth in 15%–20% of cases	—
Chronic sinusitis	Chronic sinusitis
Obstructive azoospermia	Obstructive azoospermia

*Knowles MR, Durie PR. *N Eng J Med* 2002;347:439.

LIVER/PANCR

May be found in ~1% of randomly selected patients and 2.5% of persons with increased serum amylase. Same findings may also occur in patients with normal molecular-weight hyperamylasemia in which excess amylase is principally salivary gland isoamylase types 2 and 3.

Pancreatitis, Acute[22–24]

♦ Serum Lipase

- Increases within 3 to 6 hours with peak at 24 hours and usually returns to normal over a period of 8 to 14 days. Is superior to amylase; increases to a greater extent and may remain elevated for up to 14 days after amylase returns to normal.
- In patients with signs of acute pancreatitis, pancreatitis is highly likely (clinical specificity = 85%) when lipase ≥5× URL, if values change significantly with time, and if amylase and lipase changes are concordant. (*Lipase should always be determined whenever amylase is determined.*) New methodology improves clinical utility.
- Urinary lipase is not clinically useful.
- It has been suggested that a lipase:amylase ratio >3 (and especially >5) indicates alcoholic rather than nonalcoholic pancreatitis).
- If lipase ≥5× URL, acute pancreatitis or organ rejection is highly likely but unlikely if <3× URL. (See Fig. 8-17.)

♦ Serum amylase

- Increase begins in 3 to 6 hours, rises rapidly within 8 hours in 75% of patients, reaches maximum in 20 to 30 hours, and may persist for 48 to 72 hours. >95% sensitivity during first 12 to 24 hours. The increase may be ≤40× normal, but the height of the increase and rate of fall do not correlate with the severity of the disease, prognosis, or rate of resolution.
- In patients with signs of acute pancreatitis, amylase >3× ULN or >600 Somogyi units/dL is very suggestive of acute pancreatitis.
- An increase >7 to 10 days suggests an associated cancer of pancreas or pseudocyst, pancreatic ascites, nonpancreatic etiology. *Similar high values may occur in obstruction of pancreatic duct; they tend to fall after several days. ≤19% of patients with acute pancreatitis (especially when seen more than 2 days after onset of symptoms) may have normal values, especially with an alcoholic etiology and longer duration of symptoms, even when dying of acute pancreatitis.*
- May also be normal in relapsing chronic pancreatitis and patients with hypertriglyceridemia (technical interference with test)
- Frequently normal in acute alcoholic pancreatitis
- Acute abdomen due to GI infarction or perforation rather than acute pancreatitis is suggested by only moderate increase in serum amylase and lipase (<3× URL), evidence of bacteremia.
- 10% to 40% of patients with acute alcoholic intoxication have elevated serum amylase (about half are salivary type); they often present with abdominal pain but increased serum amylase is usually <3× URL. Levels >25× URL indicate metastatic tumor rather than pancreatitis.

♦ Serum pancreatic isoamylase can distinguish elevations due to salivary amylase that may account for 25% of all elevated values. (In healthy persons, 40% of total serum amylase is pancreatic type and 60% is salivary type.)

Only slight increase in serum amylase and lipase values suggests a different diagnosis than acute pancreatitis. *Many drugs increase both amylase and lipase in serum.*

Serum calcium is decreased in severe cases 1 to 9 days after onset (due to binding to soaps in fat necrosis). The decrease usually occurs after amylase and lipase levels

[22]Ranson JHC. Etiological and prognostic factors in human acute pancreatitis: a review. *Am J Gastroenterol* 1982;77:633.
[23]Papachristou GI, Whitcomb DC. Inflammatory markers of disease severity in acute pancreatitis. *Clin Lab Med* 2005;25:17.
Whitcomb DC. Acute pancreatitis. *N Engl J Med* 2006;354:2142.

have become normal. Tetany may occur. (*Rule out hyperparathyroidism if serum calcium is high or fails to fall in hyperamylasemia of acute pancreatitis.*)

Increased urinary amylase tends to reflect serum changes by a time lag of 6 to 10 hours, but sometimes increased urine levels are higher and of longer duration than serum levels. The 24-hour level may be normal even when some of the 1-hour specimens show increased values. Amylase levels in hourly samples of urine may be useful. Ratio of amylase clearance to creatinine clearance is increased (>5%) and avoids the problem of timed urine specimens; also increased in any condition that decreases tubular reabsorption of amylase (e.g., severe burns, diabetic ketoacidosis, chronic renal insufficiency, multiple myeloma, acute duodenal perforation). Considered not specific and now discouraged by some but still recommended by others.

Serum bilirubin may be increased when pancreatitis is of biliary tract origin but is usually normal in alcoholic pancreatitis. Serum ALP, ALT, and AST may increase and parallel serum bilirubin rather than amylase, lipase, or calcium levels. Marked amylase increase (e.g., >2,000 U/L) also favors biliary tract origin. Fluctuation >50% in 24 hours of serum bilirubin, ALP, ALT, AST suggests intermittent biliary obstruction.

○ Serum trypsin is increased. High sensitivity makes a normal value useful for excluding acute pancreatitis. But low specificity (increased in large proportion of patients with hepatobiliary, bowel, and other diseases and renal insufficiency; increased in 13% of patients with chronic pancreatitis, 50% with pancreatic carcinoma) and RIA technology limit utility.

○ Serum CRP peaks 3 days after onset of pain; at 48 hours, sensitivity = 65% to 100%, PPV = 37% to 77%. Level of 150 mg/L distinguishes mild from severe disease.

♦ Laboratory criteria for severe disease or predictor of mortality

- PaO_2 <60
- Creatinine >2 mg/dL after rehydration
- Blood glucose >250 mg/dL
- Hemoconcentration (Hct >47% or failure to decrease in 24 hours after admission), but Hct may be decreased in severe hemorrhagic pancreatitis
- GI bleed >500 mL/24 hours
- Presence, volume, and color of peritoneal fluid

Methemalbumin may be increased in serum and ascitic fluid in hemorrhagic (severe) but not edematous (mild) pancreatitis; may distinguish these two conditions but not useful in diagnosis of acute pancreatitis.

WBC is slightly to moderately increased (10,000–20,000/μL).

Glycosuria appears in 25% of patients.

Hypokalemia, metabolic alkalosis, or lactic acidosis may occur.

Laboratory findings due to predisposing conditions (may be multiple)

- Alcohol abuse accounts for ~36% of cases.
- Biliary tract disease accounts for 17% of cases.
- Idiopathic accounts for >36% of cases.
- Infections (especially viral such as mumps and coxsackie, CMV, AIDS)
- Trauma and postoperative accounts for >8% of cases
- Drugs (e.g., steroids, thiazides, azathioprine, estrogens, sulfonamides; children taking valproic acid) account for >5% of cases.
- Hypertriglyceridemia (Hyperlipidemia—Types V, I, IV) accounts for 7% of cases
- Hypercalcemia from any cause
- Tumors (pancreas, ampulla)
- Anatomic abnormalities of ampullary region causing obstruction (e.g., annular pancreas, Crohn disease, duodenal diverticulum)
- Hereditary
- Renal failure; renal transplantation
- Miscellaneous (e.g., collagen vascular disease, pregnancy, ischemia, scorpion bites, parasites obstructing pancreatic duct [*Ascaris*, fluke], Reye syndrome, fulminant hepatitis, severe hypotension, cholesterol embolization)

Laboratory findings due to complications

- Pseudocysts of pancreas

- Pancreatic infection or abscess diagnosed by increased WBC, Gram stain, and culture of aspirate
- Polyserositis (peritoneal, pleural, pericardial, synovial surfaces). Ascites may develop cloudy or bloody or "prune juice" fluid, 0.5 to 2.0 L in volume, containing increased amylase with a level higher than that of serum amylase. No bile is evident (unlike in perforated ulcer). Gram stain shows no bacteria (unlike infarct of intestine). Protein >3 g/dL and marked increase in amylase.
- Adult respiratory distress syndrome (with pleural effusion, alveolar exudate, or both) may occur in ~40% of patients; arterial hypoxemia is present.
- DIC
- Hypovolemic shock
- Others

Prognostic laboratory findings
- On admission
    WBC >16,000/μL
    Blood glucose >200 mg/dL
    Serum LD >350 U/L
    Serum AST >250 units/L
    Age >55 years
- Within 48 hours
    >10% decrease in HCT
    Serum calcium <8.0 mg/dL
    Decrease in Hct >10 points
    Increase in BUN >5 mg/dL
    Arterial pO_2 <60 mmHg
    Metabolic acidosis with base deficit >4 mEq/L
- Mortality
    1% if 3 signs are positive
    15% if 3 to 4 signs are positive
    40% if 5 to 6 signs are positive
    100% if ≥7 signs are positive
- Degree of amylase elevation has no prognostic significance

♦ CT scan, MRI, ultrasound are useful for confirming diagnosis or identifying causes or other conditions.

Pancreatitis, Chronic

See also Malabsorption
Laboratory findings are often normal.
♦ Cholecystokinin-secretin test measures the effect of IV administration of cholecystokinin and secretin on volume, bicarbonate concentration, and amylase output of duodenal contents and increase in serum lipase and amylase. This is the most sensitive and reliable test ("gold standard") for chronic pancreatitis especially in the early stages. Is technically difficult and is often not performed accurately; gastric contamination must be avoided. Some abnormality occurs in >85% of patients with chronic pancreatitis. Amylase output is the most frequent abnormality. When all three are abnormal, there is a greater frequency of abnormality in the tests listed below.
Normal duodenal contents

- Volume: 95 to 235 mL/hour
- Bicarbonate concentration: 74 to 121 mEq/L
- Amylase output: 87,000 to 267,000 mg

Serum amylase and lipase increase after administration of cholecystokinin and secretin in ~20% of patients with chronic pancreatitis. They are more often abnormal when duodenal contents are normal. Normally serum lipase and amylase do not rise above normal limits.
Fasting serum amylase and lipase are increased in 10% of patients with chronic pancreatitis.
Serum pancreolauryl test: Fluorescein dilaurate with breakfast is acted on by a pancreas-specific cholesterol ester hydrolase-releasing fluorescein, which is absorbed

from gut and measured in serum; preceded by administration of secretin and followed by metoclopramide. Reported S/S = 82%/91%.[25]

Diabetic oral glucose tolerance test (GTT) in 65% of patients with chronic pancreatitis and frank diabetes in >10% of patients with chronic relapsing pancreatitis. When GTT is normal in the presence of steatorrhea, the cause should be sought elsewhere than in the pancreas.

♦ Laboratory findings due to malabsorption (occurs when >90% of exocrine function is lost) and steatorrhea

* Bentiromide test is usually abnormal with moderate to severe pancreatic insufficiency but often normal in early cases.
* Schilling test may show mild malabsorption of Vitamin B_{12}.
* Xylose tolerance test and small bowel biopsy are not usually done but are normal.

Chemical determination of fecal fat demonstrates steatorrhea. It is more sensitive than tests using triolein [131]I.

* Triolein ^{131}I is abnormal in one third of patients with chronic pancreatitis.
* Starch tolerance test is abnormal in 25% of patients with chronic pancreatitis.

Laboratory findings due to causes of chronic pancreatitis and pancreatic exocrine insufficiency

* Alcohol in 60% to 70%
* Idiopathic in 30% to 40%
* Obstruction of pancreatic duct (e.g., trauma, pseudocyst, pancreas divisum, cancer, or obstruction of duct or ampulla)
* Others occasionally (e.g., cystic fibrosis, primary hyperparathyroidism, heredity, malnutrition, miscellaneous [Z-E syndrome, Schwachman syndrome, $alpha_1$-antitrypsin deficiency, trypsinogen deficiency, enterokinase deficiency, hemochromatosis, parenteral hyperalimentation]).

Radioactive scanning of pancreas (selenium) yields variable findings in different clinics.
♦ CT, ultrasound, endoscopic retrograde pancreatography are most accurate for diagnosing and staging chronic pancreatitis.

Pseudocyst of Pancreas

Serum conjugated bilirubin is increased (>2 mg/dL) in 10% of patients.
Serum ALP is increased in 10% of patients.
Fasting blood sugar is increased in <10% of patients.
Duodenal contents after secretin-pancreozymin stimulation usually show decreased bicarbonate content (<70 mEq/L) but normal volume and normal content of amylase, lipase, and trypsin.
♦ Findings of pancreatic cyst aspiration[26]

* Best when panel of tests is used
* High fluid viscosity and CEA indicate mucinous differentiation and exclude pseudocyst, serous cystadenoma, other nonmucinous cysts or cystic tumors.
* Increased CA 72-4, CA 15-3, and tissue polypeptide antigen (TPA) are markers of malignancy; if all are low, pseudocyst or serous cystadenoma is most likely.
* CA 125 is increased in serous cystadenoma.
* Pancreatic enzymes, leukocyte esterase, and NB/70K are increased in pseudocyst fluid.
* Cytological examination

Laboratory findings of preceding acute pancreatitis are present (this is mild and unrecognized in one third of patients). Persistent increase of serum amylase and lipase after an episode of acute pancreatitis may indicate formation of a pseudocyst.

[25]Dominguez-Munoz JE, Malfertheiner P. Optimized serum pancreolauryl test for differentiating patients with and without chronic pancreatitis. *Clin Chem* 1998;44:869.
[26]Centeno BA. Fine needle aspiration biopsy of the pancreas. *Clin Lab Med* 1998;18:401.

Laboratory findings due to conditions preceding acute pancreatitis are noted (e.g., alcoholism, trauma, duodenal ulcer, cholelithiasis). Develops in 10% of patients with acute pancreatitis.

Laboratory findings due to complications

- Infection
- Perforation
- Hemorrhage by erosion of blood vessel or into a viscus

Detected by ultrasound or CT scan

9

Central and Peripheral Nervous System Disorders

Laboratory Tests for Disorders of the Nervous System

Normal CSF Values

Measurement of these components should always be performed on simultaneously drawn blood samples.

Appearance	Clear, colorless: no clot
Total cell count	
Adults, children	0–6/μL (all mononuclear cells)
Infants	<19/μL
Neonates	<30/μL
Glucose	
Lumbar fluid	45–80 mg/dL (20 mg/dL < blood level)
Ventricular fluid	5–10 mg/dL > lumbar fluid
Total protein	
Cisternal	15–25 mg/dL
Ventricular	5–15 mg/dL
Lumbar	
Neonates	≤150 mg/dL
2–3 weeks	20–80 mg/dL
3 months–60 years	15–45 mg/dL
>60 years	15–60 mg/dL
Protein electrophoresis	
Transthyretin (Prealbumin)	2%–7%
Albumin	56%–76%
Alpha-1 globulin	2%–7%
Alpha-2 globulin	4%–12%
Beta globulin	8%–18%
Gamma globulin	3%–12%
IgG	<4.0 mg/dL
	<10% of total CSF protein
Albumin index (ratio)	<9.0
IgG synthesis rate	0.0–8.0 mg/day
IgG index (ratio)	0.28–0.66
CSF IgG–albumin ratio	0.09–0.25
Oligoclonal bands	Negative
Myelin basic protein	0.0–4.0 ng/mL
Chloride	120–130 mEq/L (20 mEq/L > serum values)
Sodium	142–150 mEq/L
Potassium	2.2–3.3 mEq/L
Carbon dioxide	25 mEq/L
pH	7.35–7.40
Transaminase (AST)	7–49 units
Lactate dehydrogenase (LD)	~10% of serum level
LD-1	38%–58% (LD-1 > LD-2)
LD-2	26%–36%
LD-3	12%–24%
LD-4	1%–7%
LD-5	0%–5%
Creatine kinase (CK)	0–5 IU/L
Bilirubin	0
Urea nitrogen	5–25 mg/dL
Amino acids	30% of blood level
Xanthochromia	0
Total volume	
Adults	90–150 mL
Neonates	10–60 mL
Generation rate	0.35 mL/min = 500 mL/d

CNS

Conditions in which Normal CSF Is Found

Found In
Korsakoff syndrome
Wernicke encephalopathy
Jakob-Creutzfeldt disease
Tuberous sclerosis (protein is rarely increased)
Idiopathic epilepsy (if protein is increased, rule out neoplasms; if cell count is
    increased, rule out neoplasm or inflammation)
Narcolepsy, cataplexy, etc.
Parkinson disease
Hereditary cerebellar degenerations
Migraine
Ménière syndrome
Psychiatric conditions (e.g., neurocirculatory asthenia, hysteria, depression, anxiety,
    schizophrenia) *(Rule out psychiatric condition as a manifestation of primary disease,
    e.g., drugs, porphyria, primary endocrine diseases.)*
Transient cerebral ischemia
Amyotrophic lateral sclerosis
Muscular dystrophy
Progressive muscular atrophy
Syringomyelia
Deficiency diseases (e.g., Vitamin B_{12} deficiency with subacute combined degeneration
    of spinal cord, pellagra, beriberi)
Subacute myelo-opticoneuropathy (SMON)
Minimal brain dysfunction of childhood
Cerebral palsies
Febrile convulsions of childhood
See Chapter 12 for metabolic and hereditary diseases that affect the nervous system
    (e.g., gangliosidosis, mucopolysaccharidoses, glycogen storage disease).

Utility of Lumbar Puncture for Various Conditions

	High Specificity	**Moderate Specificity**
High Sensitivity	Bacterial, TB, fungal meningitis	Viral meningitis, subarachnoid hemorrhage, MS, CNS syphilis, infectious polyneuritis, paraspinal abscess
Moderate Sensitivity	Meningeal tumor	Viral encephalitis, intracranial hemorrhage, subdural hematoma

Abnormal Cerebrospinal Fluid (CSF)

See Table 9-1.

Gross Appearance

Viscous CSF may occur with metastatic mucinous adenocarcinoma (e.g., colon), large
    numbers of cryptococci, severe meningeal infection or, rarely, injury to annulus
    fibrosus with release of nucleus pulposus fluid.
Turbidity may be due to increased WBC ($>200/\mu L$), RBC ($>400/\mu L$), presence of bac-
    teria ($>10^5/mL$), or of other microorganisms (fungi, amebae), contrast media,
    epidural fat aspirated during lumbar puncture.
Clots or pellicles indicates protein >150 mg/dL.
Protein >100 mg/dL usually causes CSF to look faintly yellow.
CSF with RBC $>6,000/\mu L$ appears grossly bloody; with RBC $= 500$ to $6,000/\mu L$ appears
    cloudy, xanthochromic, or pink tinged (in bright light in clear glass tubes containing >1
    mL of CSF). RBC count that decreases between first and last tube indicates traumatic
    tap (occurs in $\leq 20\%$ of cases). HSV infection should be considered if CSF RBC
    $>500/\mu L$.
Xanthochromia caused by breakdown of Hb-producing bilirubin, oxyHB, metHb; may
    be due to:
    Bleeding within 2 to 36 hours. Is detected visually or by spectrophotometer.
    Can often be detected in <6 hours.

Table 9-1. Cerebrospinal Fluid (CSF) Findings in Various Conditions

	Appearance	Protein (mg/dL)	Glucose (mg/dL)	WBC/µL	Microbiology/Serology/Other
Normal					
Ventricular	C, colorless no clot	5–15	45–80	0–10; ≤32 in term neonates; <10 at 1 month	
Cisternal		10–25			
Lumbar		10–45			
TB meningitis	O, sl yellow, delicate clot	45–500; usually 100–200	<45 in 75% of cases; N in ≤20%	Usually 25–100; rarely >500; chiefly L	Acid fast stain: 25% sensitive Culture: 75% sensitive PCR: 100% specific
Tuberculoma		I	N	Small number of cells	
Acute pyogenic meningitis	O to Pu, sl yellow; delicate clot; if bloody, rule out anthrax	50–1,500; usually 100–500	Usually 0–45	Usually 1,000–5,000, chiefly P; range 100–>10,000	Gram stain 60%–90% sensitive Culture: S/S = 80%/100% Direct antigen/PCR: S/S = 50%–90%/100%
Aseptic meningitis[a]	C, T, or X	20 to >200	N	≤500, occ 2,000; first PMNs; later mononuclear cells	Identification techniques (e.g., bacterial cultures, PCR) negative
Viral meningitis	Usually clear	N or I	N	10–1,000; mostly L	PCR Specific IgM antigens Culture: 40%–70% sensitive Seroconversion
AIDS	N	50–100	N	≤300	Culture: 40%–70% sensitive HIV antibodies, antigens
Acute anterior polio	C or sl O, may be sl yellow, may be delicate clot	20–350	N	10 to >500, P first, then L	Serologic tests Stool culture AST in CSF is always I
Mumps	N or O	20–125	N	0 to >2,000	IgM and IgG in blood and CSF Culture of CSF
Measles	N or O	sl I	N	≤500	Blood serology

(continued)

Table 9-1. *(continued)*

	Appearance	Protein (mg/dL)	Glucose (mg/dL)	WBC/μL	Microbiology/Serology/Other
Herpes zoster	N	20–110	N	≤300 in 40% of patients	PCR
Equine, St. Louis encephalitis, choriomeningitis	N or sl T	20 to >200	N	10–200; occ to 3,000	Blood serologic tests
Herpes simplex		I	N	10–1,000, chiefly L; RBCs are usually present	PCR of CSF has S/S = 98%/>94%; replaces brain biopsy CSF culture in congenital infection CSF serologic tests
Rabies		N or sl I	N	N or ≤100 mononuclear cells	Culture, antigen detection, PCR of saliva, CSF, tears, brain, or animal brain Tissue exam
West Nile meningoencephalitis	N		N	≤525; mean 40	IgM in serum and CSF PCR of CSF (sens. = 57%) and serum (sens. = 15%) Brain autopsy antigen detected in all
Postinfectious	N	15–75	N	5–200, rarely ≤1,000	Serologic tests for specific viruses
Rickettsia Rocky Mountain spotted fever	N	Often N	N	I in 20–50%	DFA of skin biopsy Serology: paired serum for IgM and IgG PCR
Fungal Coccidioidomycosis		I	N early; then D	≤200 early; may be higher later; I eosinophils	Culture 50% sensitive CF in CSF = 75%–90% sensitive Wet prep in 20% KOH Antigen assay

Disease	Appearance/Pressure	Protein	Glucose	Cells	Comments
Cryptococcal meningitis	N	≤500 in 90%; average = 100	D in 55%; average = 30	≤800; average = 50 (L > P)	India ink ≤50% sensitive; Cryptococcal antigen assay ~90% sensitive; Culture ~90% sensitive
Histoplasmosis					See Chapter 15
Toxoplasmosis	X	≤2,000	N	50–500; chiefly monocytes	Serologic tests in serum; PCR; Organism identified in sediment smear
Syphilis					Positive serologic test in blood; CSF VDRL and PCR for treponemal DNA have high S/S = 40%–60%
Tabes dorsalis	N	25–100; IgG less marked than in general paresis	N	10–80	Early: VDRL titer may be low; Late: ~25% of patients may have normal CSF and negative VDRL in blood and CSF
General paresis[b]	N	≤100; marked I in gamma globulin	N	≤175, mononuclear	VDRL titer usually high
Meningovascular syphilis	N	≤260 in 66%; IgG in 75% of cases	N	10–100; N in 60%	
Syphilitic meningitis				≤2,000 L	
Asymptomatic CNS lues		I protein and cell count are index of activity			Serologic test may be negative in blood but positive in CSF
Leptospirosis	N	I ≤80	N	≤500 monos	
Lyme disease		I IgG and oligoclonal bands		450 L; usually ~100	B. burgdorferi antibodies in CSF > serum PCR for DNA
Primary amebic (Naegleria, Acanthamoeba) meningitis	Sanguino–Pu, may be T or Pu	I	Usually D	400–21,000; mostly P; also RBC	Amoebas seen on Wright stain of CSF; Culture

(continued)

Table 9-1. *(continued)*

	Appearance	Protein (mg/dL)	Glucose (mg/dL)	WBC/μL	Microbiology/Serology/Other
Cysticercosis (*Taenia soleum*)		Usually 50–200	D in 20% of cases	I P and L ≤7% eosinophils in 50% of cases	
Chronic meningitis.[c] Symptoms for 1–4 weeks		Moderate to marked I	D	100–400, mostly L	
Cavernous sinus thrombophlebitis	Usually N; may be B	Usually N or I	Usually N	Usually N or I	N unless meningitis or empyema
Brain abscess[d]		May be ≤75–300	N	25–300; PMN, L, RBCs	CSF cultures sterile Positive blood cultures in 10% Can be caused by almost any organism including fungi, *Nocardia*
Extradural abscess		100–400	N	Relatively few PMNs and L	
Subdural empyema		I	N	≤Few hundred; mostly PMNs	Negative smears and cultures Peripheral WBC is I (≤25,000/μL)
Cord tumor	C, occ X	≤3,500 in 85%; N in 15%	N	≤100, chiefly L; N in 60%	
Brain tumor	C, occ X; B if hemorrhage into tumor	≤500[e]	May be D if cells are present	≤150; N in 75%	Tumor cells in 20%–40% of solid tumors; absence does not exclude tumor
Leukemia		I	D to 50% of blood		Tumor cells identified by special molecular methods
Pseudotumor cerebri	N	N	N	N	Increased pressure

Cerebral thrombosis	N	≤100, N in 60%	N	≤50; N in 75%; rarely ≤2,000	
Cerebral embolism[f] Bland	Sl X in 1/3 of cases in few days; may be B			May be 10,000 RBC	
Septic	Sl X	I	N	≤200 with varying L and PMNs; ≤1,000 RBCs	Negative culture
Cerebral hemorrhage	N in 15%, X in 10%, B in 75%	Usually ≤2,000	N	Same as in blood; N in 10%	
Subarachnoid hemorrhage	B; X within 12 hrs; no clot	Usually ≤1,000	N	Same as in blood	
Hypertensive encephalopathy	I pressure	≤100	N	N	
Postoperative neurosurgery (especially posterior fossa)	I	I	<40	1,000–2,000; mostly PMNs	CSF sterile unless postoperative infection
Traumatic tap	B	I by blood	N	Same as in blood	
Head trauma	N, B, or X	I if bloody	N	Same as in blood	
Acute epidural hemorrhage	C unless associated injuries	N	N	N	
Subdural hematoma, acute	C, B, or X, depending on associated injuries	N or sl I			Infants are often anemic
Chronic subdural hematoma	Usually X	300–2,000			
Multiple sclerosis	N	N	N	Always >50	

(continued)

311

Table 9-1. *(continued)*

	Appearance	Protein (mg/dL)	Glucose (mg/dL)	WBC/µL	Microbiology/Serology/Other
Polyneuritis					
Polyarteritis; porphyria; beriberi; alcohol effect; arsenic poisoning	N; X if protein very I	Usually N	N	N but albumino-cytologic dissociation in Guillain-Barré syndrome that may occur in heavy metal poisoning, infection, etc.	
Diabetes mellitus	Same as polyarteritis, etc.	Often ≤300	I	Same as polyarteritis, etc.	
Acute infection	Same as polyarteritis, etc.	≤1,500	N	Same as polyarteritis, etc.	
Lead encephalopathy	N or sl yellow	≤100	N	0–100	
Sarcoidosis (findings in ≤50%)		sl I; oligoclonal bands may be present	D in 50%	I in 40% Typically 10–100 but ≤6,000	I ACE in serum or CSF in 50%–70%
Behçet disease (25% have meningoencephalitis)		I	N	I	
Alcoholism	N	N	N	Usually N	
Diabetic coma	N	N	I	Usually N	
Uremia	N	N or I in ~50%	N or I	N or I in ~50%	

Epilepsy	N	May be B	N	N	N
Eclampsia				May be RBCs	Uric acid I ≤3× N reflecting marked I in serum
Guillain-Barré syndrome	Usually ≤200		50–100 average; albumino-cytologic dissociation	N	N

B, bloody; C, clear; D, decreased; I, increased; L, lymphocytes; N, normal; O, opalescent; occ, occasionally; Pu, purulent; sl, slightly; T, turbid; X, xanthochromic.

aPossible underlying disorders: infections (e.g., viral, bacterial [e.g., incompletely treated or very early bacterial meningitis], spirochetes [e.g., leptospirosis, syphilis. Lyme disease], TB, fungal, amebic, mycoplasma, rickettsia, helminthic); chemical or drug-induced meningitis; systemic disorders (e.g., vasculitis, collagen vascular disease, SLE, sarcoidosis); neoplasm (e.g., leukemia, metastatic carcinoma

bCSF is always abnormal in untreated general paresis.

cPossible underlying disorders: Infections (TB [most common cause], bacteria, spirochetes, fungi, protozoa, amebae, mycoplasma, rickettsia, helminthes); systemic disorders (e.g., vasculitis, collagen vascular disease, sarcoid, neoplasm)

dFindings depend on stage and duration of abscess.

e*Protein is particularly increased with meningioma of the olfactory groove and with acoustic neuroma. Usually N in brain stem gliomas and "diencephalic syndrome" of infants due to glioma of hypothalamus.*

fUsually same as in cerebral thrombosis.

Neonates, elderly, immunocompromised, alcoholics more likely to develop meningitis due to *Listeria monocytogenes, Streptococcus agalactiae*, group B streptococcus; gram-negative bacilli (e.g., *E. coli, Klebsiella* spp, *Serratia marcescens, Pseudomonas aeruginosa, Salmonella* spp.)

Post-trauma, postoperative neurosurgical, CSF shunts—*Staphylococcus* spp.

Infants, children—enteroviruses (e.g., echovirus, coxsackievirus).

- Traumatic lumbar puncture >1 to 2 hours earlier
- Hemorrhage into CSF (e.g., subarachnoid or intracerebral hemorrhage); is present in all patients for ≤2 weeks and 70% of patients at 3 weeks

Bilirubin >6 mg/dL

WBCs

CSF WBC may be corrected for presence of blood (e.g., traumatic tap, subarachnoid hemorrhage) by subtracting 1 WBC for each 700 RBCs/μL counted in CSF if the CBC is normal.
   If significant anemia or leukocytosis is present:

$$\text{Corrected WBC} = \text{WBC in bloody CSF} - \frac{[\text{WBC (blood)} \times \text{RBC (CSF)}]}{[\text{RBC (blood)}]}$$

   (RBC and WBC are cells/μL)
In normal CSF, ratio of WBC/RBC is <1:500. Minimal blood contamination may cause ≤2 PMN/25 RBCs, or ≤10 PMN/25–100 RBCs.
CSF WBC count (>3,000/μL) with predominantly PMNs strongly suggests bacterial cause and >2,000/μL in 38% of cases. When WBC <1,000/μL in bacterial meningitis, one third of cases have >50% lymphocytes or mononuclear cells. *However, WBCs are usually PMNs in early stages of all types of meningitis; mononuclear cells only appear in a second specimen 18 to 24 hours later in nonbacterial cases.* Predominantly, lymphocytes occur in ≤10% of ABM cases; may be due to early stages or antibiotic treatment or *Listeria* meningitis.
May be falsely low due to delay in counting.
Neutrophilic leukocytes are found in:

- Bacteria (e.g., *Nocardia, Actinomyces, Arachnia, Brucella*)
- Fungal infections (*Blastomyces, Coccidioides, Candida, Aspergillus, Zygomycetes, Cladosporium, Allescheria*)
- Chemical meningitis
- Other conditions (e.g., SLE)
- Half-life of neutrophils in CSF is ~2 hours

Lymphocytic cells are found in:

- Bacterial infections (e.g., *Treponema pallidum, Leptospira, Actinomyces israelii, Arachnia propionica*, 90% of *Brucella* cases, *Borrelia burgdorferi* [Lyme disease], *M. tuberculosis*)
- Fungal infections (e.g., *Cryptococcus neoformans, Candida* species, *Coccidioides immitis, Histoplasma capsulatum, Blastomyces dermatitides, S. schenckii, Allescheria boydii, Cladosporium trichoides*)
- Parasitic diseases (e.g., toxoplasmosis, cysticercosis)
- Viral infections (e.g., mumps, lymphocytic choriomeningitis, HTLV-III, echovirus). Atypical lymphocytes may be seen in EBV infection and less often in CMV or HSV infection.
- Parameningeal disorders (e.g., brain abscess)
- Noninfectious disorders (e.g., neoplasms, sarcoidosis, multiple sclerosis, granulomatous arteritis)

Eosinophils may be found in:

- Lymphoma
- Helminth infection (e.g., angiostrongyliasis, cysticercosis)
- Rarely, other infections (e.g., TB, syphilis, Rocky Mountain spotted fever, coccidioidomycosis)
- >5% (or >10% neutrophils or significant pleocytosis) may indicate malfunction or infection of a ventriculoperitoneal shunt[1]

CSF Chemistries

CSF glucose
   Decreased by utilization by bacteria (pyogens or tubercle bacilli), WBCs, or occasionally cancer cells in CSF

---

[1]Novak R. Cerebrospinal fluid shunts. *CAP Today* 2004:93.

Lags behind blood glucose by about 1 hour

May rapidly become normal after onset of antibiotic therapy

Is decreased in only ~50% of cases of bacterial meningitis

<45 mg/dL is almost always abnormal; <40 mg/dL is always abnormal

Normally is ~50% to 65% of blood glucose, which should *always* be drawn immediately before

Normal CSF:serum ratio of glucose = 0.6. In acute bacterial meningitis (ABM), is usually <0.5; a ratio <0.4 has S/S = 80%/96% for distinguishing ABM from acute viral meningitis (AVM); a ratio <0.25 is found in <1% of AVM cases and 44% of ABM cases, even when CSF glucose is normal. A ratio of <8.0 is significant in infants.

<40 mg/dL in 50% to 60% of ABM cases; <15 mg/dL in 30% of ABM cases

May also be decreased in acute infection due to syphilis, Lyme disease, 10% to 20% of cases of lymphocytic choriomeningitis, and encephalitis due to mumps or herpes simplex but generally rare in viral infections or parameningeal processes. May also be decreased in rheumatoid meningitis, lupus myelopathy, and other causes of chronic meningitis such as bacteria (e.g., *Brucella, Mycobacterium tuberculosis*), syphilis, fungi (*Cryptococcus, Coccidioides*), parasites (e.g., cysticercosis), granulomatous meningitis (e.g., sarcoid), chemical meningitis, carcinomatous meningitis, hypoglycemia, and subarachnoid hemorrhage.

CSF protein is least specific parameter

Total protein may be corrected for presence of blood (e.g., due to traumatic tap or intracerebral hemorrhage) by subtracting 1 mg/dL of protein for each 1,000 RBCs/μL if serum protein and CBC are normal and CSF protein and cell count are determined on same tube of CSF. *Serum protein levels must be normal in order to interpret any CSF protein values and should therefore always be measured concurrently.*

May not be increased in early stages of many types of meningitis

Normal in 10% of patients with ABM (20% of cases of meningococcal meningitis)

Usually >150 mg/dL in ABM; increase occurs especially with *S. pneumoniae*

<100 mg/dL is usual in nonbacterial meningitis (S/S = 82%/98%)

>172 mg/dL occurs in 1% of AVM and 50% of ABM cases

>500 mg/dL is infrequent and occurs chiefly in bacterial meningitis, bloody CSF, or cord tumor with spinal block and occasionally in polyneuritis and brain tumor

>1,000 mg/dL suggests subarachnoid block; with complete spinal block, the lower the level of the cord tumor, the higher the protein concentration

When antibiotic treatment of bacterial meningitis is started before CSF obtained, protein may be only slightly elevated

May show mild-to-moderate elevation in myxedema (25% of cases), uremia, connective tissue disorders, Cushing syndrome

Decreased CSF protein (3–20 mg/dL) may occur in hyperthyroidism, one third of patients with benign intracranial hypertension, after removal of large volumes of CSF (e.g., during pneumoencephalography, traumatic leaks), in children 6 to 24 months old

Combination of CSF protein, glucose, and WBC levels is more useful than individual parameters.

CSF protein, glucose, and WBC levels may not return to normal in ~50% of patients with clinically cured bacterial meningitis and therefore are not recommended as a test of cure.

CSF lactate has been reported useful to differentiate bacterial from viral meningitis; is independent of serum concentrations. Due to sequelae of increased WBC.

If <3 mmol/L (normal range), viral meningitis is most likely.

If >4.2 mmol/L, bacterial (including TB) or fungal meningitis is most likely.

If 3 to 6 mmol/L with negative Gram stain and prior antibiotic therapy, partially treated bacterial meningitis is most likely. In bacterial meningitis, level is still high after 1 to 2 days of antibiotic therapy.

Mild symptoms with negative Gram stain, few PMNs: CSF lactate may differentiate mild bacterial from very early viral meningitis

May also be increased in non-Hodgkin lymphoma with meningeal involvement, severe cerebral malaria, head injury, and anoxia

CSF and serum ACE are increased in 50% to 70% of cases of neurosarcoidosis; CSF ACE is increased 2×

Reported to be increased in meningitis and Behçet disease and decreased in Alzheimer disease, Parkinson disease, others

CNS

CSF chloride reflects only blood chloride level, but in TB meningitis a decrease of 25% may exceed the serum chloride decrease because of dehydration and electrolyte loss. It is not useful in diagnosis of TB meningitis.

CSF glutamine >35 mg/dL is associated with hepatic encephalopathy (due to conversion from ammonia).

CSF IL-6 (marker of inflammation) is increased in bacterial meningitis but not in viral or aseptic meningitis or those without meningitis.

CSF tuberculostearic acid (cell wall component of *Mycobacterium tuberculosis*) by gas–liquid chromatography has been reported to have good S/S.

CSF Enzymes

Normal CSF is not permeable to serum enzymes. Changes in AST are irregular and generally of limited diagnostic value. If determinations of AST, LD, and CK in CSF are all performed, at least one shows marked increase in 80% of patients with cortical stroke (usually due to emboli) but this is not noted in lacunar strokes (usually due to small vessel hypertensive disease). Generally are not useful in CNS diseases.

Transaminase (AST)
Increased In

Large infarcts of brain during first 10 days. In severe cases, serum AST may also be increased; occurs in ~40% of patients.

~40% of CNS tumors (various benign, malignant, and metastatic), depending on location, growth rate, etc.; chiefly useful as indicator of organic neurologic disease

Some other conditions (e.g., head injury, subarachnoid hemorrhage)

Lactate Dehydrogenase (LD)
Increased In

Cerebrovascular accidents—increase occurs frequently, reaches maximum level in 1 to 3 days, and is apparently not related to xanthochromia, RBC, WBC, protein, sugar, or chloride levels. Subarachnoid and subdural hemorrhage cause increase of all LD isoenzymes especially LD-3, 4, 5 (not due only to hemolysis).

CNS tumors—LD-5 >9% and decreased LD-1:LD-5 ratio <2.5 in absence of infection or hemorrhage suggests tumor in meninges. LD-5 >10% suggests higher-grade malignancy. Increase in LD-3, LD-4 and occasionally LD-5 may occur in leukemic and lymphomatous infiltration.

Meningitis—is sensitive indicator of meningitis (in specimen with no blood); normal or mild increase in viral meningitis; more marked increase in bacterial meningitis. Bacterial meningitis shows increase of LD-4 and LD-5; viral meningitis shows increase of LD-1 and LD-2; TB meningitis shows increase of LD-1, LD-2, LD-3, (especially LD-3); HIV alone does not alter LD isoenzyme pattern; isoenzyme changes may only appear in later stage and are of low sensitivity.

Creatine Kinase (CK total) is Not Useful
CSF CK-BB Levels Association with Neurologic Injury

In global anoxic or ischemic brain insults due to respiratory or cardiac arrest, CK-BB levels 24 to 72 hours after injury can be used to estimate overall extent of brain damage; good correlation with neurologic prognosis after resuscitation. Less correlation with outcome in head trauma and stroke. Not recommended for estimating stroke size.

- >40U/L: Correlates with poorer prognosis
- <5 IU/L: Only mild injury; most patients will awaken, some minimal deficit
- >10 IU/L: Substantial brain injury; guarded prognosis
- 5 to 20 IU/L: Mild to moderate; often moderate to severe impairment; guarded prognosis
- 21 to 50 IU/L: Severe impairment; poor prognosis; few patients awaken; most die in hospital
- >50 IU/L: Rarely regain minimal reflexes or responsiveness; poor prognosis; usually die in hospital

CSF CK-MM is Normally Absent; If Present, Indicates Blood Contamination Due to Traumatic Tap or Subarachnoid Hemorrhage.

Mitochondrial-CK is Found With High CK-BB Levels; Not Used to Estimate Prognosis or Brain Damage.

Adenosine Deaminase (Enzyme Elaborated by Activated T Lymphocytes) is Increased (>30 U/L); May Aid in Early Diagnosis of TB Meningitis.

Tumor Markers

Increased CSF CEA has been reported helpful in diagnosis of suspected metastatic carcinoma (from breast, lung, bowel) with negative cytology.

Beta-glucuronidase has been reported to be increased in 75% of patients with metastatic leptomeningeal adenocarcinoma and 60% of patients with acute myeloblastic leukemia involving CNS. Normal <49 mU/L, indeterminate = 49 to 70 mU/L, suspicious >70 mU/L.

Lysozyme (muramidase) is increased in various CNS tumors especially myeloid and monocytic leukemias, but is also increased when neutrophils are increased (e.g., ABM).

Minimal residual leukemic disease is detected by flow cytometry since immature leukocytes with these markers (CD10+, TdT+ or CD34+ cells) are not normally present in CSF.

Gamma-aminobutyric acid is decreased in CSF in Huntington disease.

Colloidal gold test is no longer used; replaced by electrophoresis/immunofixation of CSF. IgG in CSF is increased 14% to 35% in two thirds of patients with neurosyphilis. IgG oligoclonal bands may be seen in neurosyphilis and multiple sclerosis.

In eclampsia, CSF shows gross or microscopic blood and increased protein ($\leq$200 mg/dL) in most cases. Glucose is normal. Uric acid is increased (to 3$\times$ normal level), in all cases reflecting the marked increase in serum level. In normal pregnancy, CSF values have same reference range as in nonpregnant women.

Dexamethasone Suppression Test (DST)

Blood is drawn at 11 PM, 8 AM, 12 noon, 4 PM, and 11 PM for plasma cortisol levels. One mg of dexamethasone is given immediately after the first sample is taken. An abnormal test result is failure of suppression of plasma cortisol to level $\leq$5 μg/dL in any sample after the first. Plasma dexamethasone should also be measured to avoid false values due to aberrant clearance of dexamethasone.

Use

A positive DST will "rule in" the diagnosis of endogenous depression but a negative DST will not rule it out, since it may be positive in only 40% to 50% of such patients.

In the presence of a positive DST, appropriate drug treatment (e.g., tricyclic antidepressants) that results in normalization of DST with clinical recovery is a good prognostic sign whereas failure of DST to normalize suggests a poor prognosis and the need for continued antidepressant therapy. Despite clinical improvement, treatment should be continued until DST becomes negative (usually within 10 days). With relapse, DST may become abnormal when symptoms are still mild, before fully developed syndrome develops. The need to continue treatment is indicated if a positive DST that became negative with therapy reverts to positive after drug treatment is discontinued or the drug dosage is lowered.

Interference

Certain drugs or substances that cause nonsuppression, especially phenytoin, barbiturates, meprobamate, carbamazepine, and alcohol (chronic high doses or withdrawal within 3 weeks) can interfere with DST.

Enhanced suppression may be caused by benzodiazepines (high doses), corticosteroids (spironolactone, cortisone, artificial glucocorticoids such as prednisone, [topical and nasal forms]), and dextroamphetamine.

Other drugs that are said to interfere include estrogens (not birth control pills), reserpine, narcotics, and indomethacin.

Medical conditions including weight loss to 20% below ideal body weight, pregnancy or abortion within 1 month, endocrine diseases, systemic infections, serious liver disease, cancer, and other severe physical illnesses, may also cause false-positive test results.

Lithium maintenance therapy will not interfere with DST.

With a 50% prevalence of melancholia in the population studied and fulfillment of certain medical criteria, DST was found to have a S/S = 67%/96%, and a confidence level of 94% in determining diagnosis. Using only the 4 PM blood, the sensitivity was ~50%. However, there are still no clear indications for routine use of DST in clinical psychiatry, and many of the routine methods are not accurate at the decision level.

Response of TSH to administration of thyrotropin-releasing hormone (TRH) has also been suggested as useful in the diagnosis of unipolar depression and prediction of relapse. These patients have a maximum rise in serum TSH level of $<7\ \mu U/mL$ (normal $= 17 \pm 9$). Use of this test with DST is said to add confidence to diagnosis of major unipolar depression; abnormal response to either test before treatment suggests that patient is particularly liable to have early relapse, unless there is laboratory proof as well as clinical evidence of recovery after treatment.

Diseases of the Nervous System

See Table 9-1.

Autoimmune Disorders

Autoimmune Autonomic Failure, Primary[2]

Autoimmune disorder possibly due to anti–ganglionic acetylcholine receptor antibodies causing dysfunction of efferent sympathetic and parasympathetic pathways resulting in orthostatic hypotension, anhydrosis, decreased production of saliva and tears, erectile dysfunction, impaired bladder emptying and responsive to plasma exchange

Due To
Diabetes mellitus
Amyloidosis
Idiopathic
♦ Detection of antibodies binding to neuronal ganglionic acetylcholine receptors detected by radioimmunoprecipitation
Decreased plasma norepinephrine levels

Guillain–Barré Syndrome[3]

Acute [<2 months' duration] demyelinating paralyzing symmetrical polyneuropathy due to autoantibodies [70% is reversible, 10% die, 20% have residual defects]

♦ CSF shows albumino-cytologic dissociation with normal cell count and increased protein (average 50–100 mg/dL). Protein increase parallels increasing clinical severity; increase may be prolonged. CSF may be normal at first.
♦ Biopsy of nerve shows evidence of demyelination and remyelination.
♦ Electrophysiological changes may be negative for first 1 to 2 weeks.
Laboratory findings due to associated disease may be present (e.g., evidence of recent infection with *Campylobacter jejuni* in 15% to 40%, and CMV in 5% to 20% of cases; EBV and *Mycoplasma pneumoniae* in <2% of cases in western nations, other viral and rickettsial infections, immune disorders, diabetes mellitus, exposure to toxins [e.g., lead, alcohol], neoplasms). No agent was identified in ≤70% of cases.[4]

Multiple Sclerosis (MS)

♦ Diagnosis should not be made not on the basis of CSF findings unless there are *multiple clinical lesions in time* (by clinical history) and *anatomic location* (by MRI, evoked potentials, or physical examination).
♦ CSF changes are found in >90% of MS patients. Oligoclonal IgG bands or elevated IgG index are the 2 CSF findings recognized as positive.[5]
♦ Qualitative test of IgG on unconcentrated CSF is single most informative test.[6]

---

[2]Schroeder C, et al. Plasma exchange for primary autoimmune autonomic failure. *N Engl J Med* 2005;353:1585.
[3]Köller H, Kieseier BC, Jander S, Hartung HP. Chronic inflammatory demyelinating polyneuropathy. *N Engl J Med* 2005;352:1343–1356. Review.
[4]Sivadon-Tardy V, et al. Guillain-Barré syndrome, greater Paris area. *Emerg Infect Dis* 2006;12:990.
[5]McDonald WI, Compston A, Edan G, et al. Recommended diagnostic criteria for multiple sclerosis: guidelines from the International Panel on the diagnosis of multiple sclerosis. *Ann Neurol* 2001;50:121–127.
[6]Barclay L. New guidelines for standards for CSF analysis in MS. *Arch Neurol* 2005;62:865–870. Available at: http://wwwmedscape.com. Accessed May 2005.

Best performed using IEF with immunodetection by blotting or fixation run with simultaneous serum sample on adjacent track with positive and negative controls. Should show one of five recognized staining patterns of oligoclonal banding.

Quantitative IgG analysis is informative complementary test but not considered a substitute for qualitative test, which has highest S/S.

90% of MS patients have oligoclonal bands in CSF, at least 2 of which are not present in simultaneously examined serum. A few patients with definite MS may have normal CSF immunoglobulins and lack oligoclonal bands.

Found in 85% to 95% of patients with definite MS and 30% to 40% with possible MS (specificity = 79%); it is the most sensitive marker of MS.

Positive results also occur in ≤10% of patients with noninflammatory neurologic disease (e.g., meningeal carcinomatosis, cerebral infarction), and ≤40% of patients with inflammatory CNS disorders (e.g., neurosyphilis, viral encephalitis, progressive rubella encephalitis, subacute sclerosing panencephalitis, bacterial meningitis, toxoplasmosis, cryptococcal meningitis, inflammatory neuropathies, trypanosomiasis).

Oligoclonal bands in serum may occur in leukemias, lymphomas, some infections and inflammatory diseases, immune disorders.

Not known to correlate with severity, duration, or course of MS.

Persists during remission

During steroid treatment, prevalence of oligoclonal bands and other gamma globulin abnormalities may be reduced by 30% to 50%.

Evaluation of light chains may help in cases of equivocal oligoclonal IgG patterns.

○ IgG index indicates IgG synthesis in CNS. >0.7 occurs in 90% of MS patients; may also occur in other neurological diseases (e.g., meningitis). CSF IgM and IgA may also be increased but are not useful for diagnosis.

○ Myelin basic protein

Indicates recent myelin destruction; increased in 70% to 90% of MS patients during an acute exacerbation and usually returns to normal within 2 weeks. Weakly reactive (4–8 ng/mL) indicates active lesion >1 week old. Normal = <1 ng/mL.

Useful for following course of MS but not for screening

May be helpful very early in course of MS before oligoclonal bands have appeared or in ~10% of patients who do not develop these bands

Is frequently increased in other causes of demyelination and tissue destruction (e.g., meningoencephalitis, leukodystrophies, metabolic encephalopathies, SLE of CNS, brain tumor, head trauma, amyotrophic lateral sclerosis, cranial irradiation and intrathecal chemotherapy, 45% of patients with recent stroke) and other disorders (e.g., diabetes mellitus, chronic renal failure, vasculitis, carcinoma of vasculitis, immune complex diseases, pancreas)

Falsely increased by contamination with blood

Increased association with certain histocompatibility antigens (e.g., whites with B7 and Dw2 antigen)

○ Albumin index (ratio of albumin serum/CSF) is measure of integrity of blood/CSF barrier. Avoids misinterpreting falsely increased CSF IgG concentrations. Increase indicates CSF contaminated with blood (e.g., traumatic tap) or increased permeability of blood brain barrier (e.g., aged persons, obstruction of CSF circulation, diabetes mellitus, SLE of CNS, Guillain- Barré syndrome, polyneuropathy, cervical spondylosis).

CSF total protein

Normal or may be mildly increased in ~25% of patients; not very useful test by itself

Decreased values or values >100 mg/dL should cast doubt on diagnosis

CSF gamma globulin is increased in 60% to 75% of patients regardless of whether the total CSF protein is increased. Gamma globulin ≥12% of CSF total protein is abnormal if there is not a corresponding increase in serum gamma globulin; but may also be increased in other CNS disorders (e.g., syphilis, subacute panencephalitis, meningeal carcinomatosis) and may also be increased when serum electrophoresis is abnormal due to non-CNS diseases (e.g., RA, sarcoidosis, cirrhosis, myxedema, multiple myeloma).

CSF IgG concentration

♦ Increased (reference range <4.0 mg/dL) in ~70% of cases, often when total protein is normal

♦ Increase in *production* of IgG is expressed as ratio of CSF to serum albumin to rule out increased IgG due to disruption of blood–brain barrier

CSF IgG does not correlate with duration, activity, or course of MS.

May also be increased in other inflammatory demyelinating diseases (e.g., neurosyphilis, acute Guillain-Barré syndrome), 5% to 15% of patients with miscellaneous neurologic diseases, and a few normal persons; recent myelography is said to invalidate the test.

○ CSF IgG-albumin ratio indicates in situ production of IgG. Abnormal in 90% of MS patients and 18% of non-MS neurologic patients.

○ CSF IgG synthesis rate (3.3 mg/day) is increased in 90% of MS patients and 4% of non-MS patients.

○ PCR demonstrates expansion of B-cell clones.

Peripheral blood studies and routine CSF tests yield no changes of diagnostic value.

CSF WBC is slightly elevated in ~25% of patients but usually <20 mononuclear cells/μL; >25 cells/μL in <1% of cases. *>50 cells/μL should cast doubt on diagnosis.* Albumin, glucose, and pressure are normal.

CNS Trauma

Laboratory findings due to single or various combinations of brain injuries (e.g., contusion, laceration, subdural hemorrhage, extradural hemorrhage, subarachnoid hemorrhage)

Laboratory findings due to complications (e.g., pneumonia, meningitis)

In possible skull fractures

♦ Immunofixation electrophoresis with antitransferrin-precipitating antibody is performed to differentiate CSF (desialated) transferrin, found only in CSF, perilymph, aqueous and vitreous humor of eye, from nasal secretions.

♦ IgM, prealbumin (transthyretin), and transferrin are higher in CSF than in serum. It has been recommended that nasal secretions may be differentiated from CSF by absence of glucose (using test tapes or tablets) in nasal secretions but this is not reliable because nasal secretions may normally contain glucose. Tears may taste salty to the patient.

Acute Epidural Hemorrhage

CSF is usually under increased pressure; it is clear unless there is associated cerebral contusion, laceration, or subarachnoid hemorrhage.

Subdural Hematoma

CSF findings are variable—clear, bloody, or xanthochromic, depending on recent or old associated injuries (e.g., contusion, laceration).

Chronic subdural hematoma fluid is usually xanthochromic; protein content is 300 to 2,000 mg/dL.

Anemia is often present in infants.

Infections

Abscess, Brain

Localized collection of pus. Aspirate should include performance of Gram stain, aerobic and anaerobic cultures, fungal and acid-fast stains and culture, serum IgG for toxoplasmosis.

Due to

Source	Usual Location	Usual Organism
Penetrating trauma, postoperative	Site of injury or surgery	*Staphylococcus aureus,* coagulase negative; *Staphylococcus* spp.; *Clostridium* spp.; gram-negative organisms*
Teeth, paranasal sinus	Frontal lobe	Aerobic/anaerobic streptococci†; *Staphylococcus aureus;* anaerobes; gram-negative organisms*
Otitis media, mastoiditis	Temporal lobe, cerebellum	Aerobic/anaerobic streptococci; other anaerobes; gram-negative organisms*

| Hematogenous (e.g., congenital/acquired heart disease; pulmonary disease) | Middle cerebral artery distribution | *Streptococcus* spp.; sometimes with other organisms |

*Gram-negative species (e.g., *Proteus, Klebsiella, Pseudomonas*)
†Mixed anaerobic (e.g., *Streptococci* or *Bacteroides*) and aerobic organisms (e.g., *Streptococci, Staphylococci,* or *S. pneumoniae*). *Toxoplasma* and *Nocardia* may be due to underlying AIDS. May be caused by almost any organism, including fungi, and *Nocardia*. 20% of cultures are sterile.

○ CSF shows WBC ~25 to 300/µL and increased neutrophils, lymphocytes, and RBCs.

• Lumbar puncture risks brain herniation.
• Protein may be increased (75–300 mg/dL).
• Glucose is normal.
• Bacterial cultures are negative.
• Findings depend on stage and duration of abscess.
• ♦ *With rupture, acute purulent meningitis with many organisms*

○ Positive blood cultures in ~10% of patients.
○ Laboratory findings due to associated primary disease

• 10% of cases are due to penetrating skull trauma
• 50% of cases are due to contiguous spread from sinuses, mastoids, middle ear
• 20% of cases are cryptogenic
• 20% of cases are due to hematogenous spread of:
  Dental infections
  Primary septic lung disease (e.g., lung abscess, bronchiectasis, empyema)
  Cyanotic congenital heart disease (e.g., septal defects)
  Other causes

Abscess, Epidural, of Spinal Cord

CSF protein is increased (usually 100–400 mg/dL), and there are relatively few WBCs (lymphocytes and neutrophils).
Most common organism is *Staphylococcus aureus*, followed by *Streptococcus* and gram-negative bacilli.
Laboratory findings due to preceding condition (e.g., adjacent osteomyelitis; bacteremia due to dental, respiratory, or skin infections)

Acquired Immune Deficiency Syndrome (AIDS), Neurologic Manifestations

See AIDS (Chapter 15).
Dementia (also called subacute encephalitis) is most common neurologic syndrome with AIDS—in >50% of cases; may be initial or later manifestation.
CSF abnormalities in 85%:

• Increased protein (50–100 mg/dL) in 60% of patients
• Mild mononuclear pleocytosis (5–50 cells/µL) in 20% of patients
• HIV antibodies

Aseptic meningitis—may occur early, late, or chronic recurrent
CSF may show:

• 20 to 300 cells/µL
• Increased protein (may be 50–100 mg/dL)
• ♦ HIV culture is usually positive
• ♦ Increased CSF:serum antibody ratio, indicating local antibody production

Myelopathy—gradual onset; usually associated with dementia
Polymyositis is most common type.
Peripheral neuropathies, some of which may resemble Guillain-Barré syndrome
CSF may show increased protein (50–100 mg/dL) and pleocytosis of 10 to 50 cells/µL.

CNS

Opportunistic CNS infections
- Viral (c.g., CMV, HSV I and II, papovavirus, EBV)
- Nonviral (e.g., cryptococcal, toxoplasmosis, *Aspergillus fumigatus*, *Candida albicans*, *Coccidioides immitis*, *Mycobacterium avium-intracellulare* and *M. tuberculosis*, *Nocardia asteroides*, *Listeria*)

Neoplasms (e.g., Kaposi sarcoma, non-Hodgkin lymphoma)
Vascular (e.g., infarction, hemorrhage, vasculitis)
Associated diseases (e.g., neurosyphilis)

Cerebral Subdural Empyema

Due to

Source	Usual Organism
Penetrating trauma†, postoperative intracranial surgery	*Staphylococcus aureus,* coagulase-negative; *Staphylococcus* spp.; *Clostridium* spp.; gramnegative organisms*
Acute sinusitis	Aerobic/anaerobic streptococci†; anaerobic organisms; gram-negative organisms*
Otitis media	Aerobic/anaerobic streptococci; other anaerobes; gram-negative organisms*
Hematogenous	Varies with site of primary infection

*Gram-negative species, e.g., *Proteus, Klebsiella, Pseudomonas*
†Mixed anaerobic (e.g., *Streptococci* or *Bacteroides*) and aerobic organisms (e.g., *Streptococci, Staphylococci,* or *S. pneumoniae*). *Toxoplasma* and *Nocardia* may be due to underlying AIDS. May be caused by almost any organism, including fungi, and *Nocardia.*

CSF
- Cell count is increased to a few hundred, with predominance of PMNs.
- Protein is increased.
- Glucose is normal.
- Bacterial smears and cultures are negative.

WBC is usually increased ($\leq$25,000/μL).
Laboratory findings due to preceding diseases.

Encephalitis

Inflammation of brain of various etiologies

See Table 9-1.
Due to
Virus

- Flaviviridae (e.g., West Nile, Japanese, St. Louis)
- Togaviridae (e.g., Eastern and Western and Venezuelan equine)
- Bunyaviridae (e.g., Rift Valley fever)
- Herpesviridae (e.g., HSV, CMV, VZV)
- Others (e.g., retrovirus [e.g., HIV], adenovirus, influenza, rabies, mumps, influenza, adenovirus, enterovirus [e.g., coxsackievirus, echovirus, poliovirus])

Bacteria (e.g., listeria, mycoplasma, Lyme disease, Whipple disease, rickettsia, syphilis, TB); see Table 15-2
Fungal (e.g., *Cryptococcus*, coccidioidomycosis)
Amoebae (e.g., *Naegleria, Acanthamoeba*)
Protozoa (e.g., malaria, toxoplasmosis)
Prion
♦ CSF findings (see Table 9-1)
♦ Appropriate culture and serologic tests for specific organism identification and additional laboratory tests—see separate sections for each agent

Meningitis, Aseptic

Inflammation of meninges without identifiable cause; is usually viral

Due to
Infections

- Viral (especially poliomyelitis, coxsackievirus A and B, echovirus, HIV, EBV, lymphocytic choriomeningitis, and many others); culture positive in~40% of cases, especially with enteroviruses (see Chapter 15)
- Bacterial (e.g., incompletely treated or very early bacterial meningitis, bacterial endocarditis, parameningeal infections such as brain abscess, epidural abscess, paranasal sinusitis)
- Spirochetes (e.g., leptospirosis, syphilis, Lyme disease)
- Tuberculous (CSF glucose levels may not be decreased until later stages)
- Fungal (e.g., *Candida, Coccidioides, Cryptococcus*)
- Protozoan (e.g., *Toxoplasma gondii*)
- Amebic (e.g., *Naegleria, Acanthamoeba*)
- Mycoplasma
- Rickettsia (e.g., Rocky Mountain spotted fever)
- Helminths

Chemical meningitis
Drug-induced meningitis (e.g., ibuprofen, trimethoprim, immune globulin, sulfadiazine, azathioprine, antineoplastic drugs)—onset usually within 24 hours of drug ingestion
Systemic disorders

- Vasculitis, collagen vascular disease (e.g., SLE)
- Sarcoid
- Behçet syndrome
- Vogt-Koyanagi syndrome
- Harada syndrome
- Neoplasm (e.g., leukemia, metastatic carcinoma)

CSF

- Protein is normal or slightly increased.
- Increased cell count shows predominantly PMNs at first, mononuclear cells seen later.
- Glucose is normal.
- Bacterial cultures and bacterial stains are negative.

If glucose levels are decreased, rule out TB, cryptococcosis, leukemia, lymphoma, metastatic carcinoma, sarcoidosis, drug-induced.

Meningitis, Bacterial, Acute (ABM)

See Tables 9-1, 9-2, and Chapter 15.
♦ Gram stain is positive in ~70% of patients; sensitivity is increased by cytocentrifugation of specimen (sensitive to 10^4 organisms/mL). Smears for Gram and acid-fast stains must be routinely *centrifuged* on all CSF specimens because other findings may be normal in meningitis. When Gram stain is positive, CSF is more likely to show decreased glucose, increased protein, and increased WBCs.
75% of cases are caused by *N. meningitidis, S. pneumoniae, H. influenzae.*
In community-acquired cases in adults, 51% are caused by *S. pneumoniae*, 37% are caused by *H. influenzae*, and 4% are caused by *Listeria monocytogenes*. Over age 50, aerobic gram-negative bacilli are also common.
Gram stain of scrapings from petechial skin lesions demonstrate pathogen in ~70% of patients with meningococcemia; Gram stain of buffy coat of peripheral blood, and less often, peripheral blood smear may reveal this organism.
Gram stain of CSF sediment is negative in cases of ABM because at least 10^5 bacteria/ mL CSF must be present to demonstrate 1 to 2 bacteria/100× microscopic field. Gram stain is positive in 90% of cases owning to pneumococci, 85% of cases owning to *H. influenzae*, 75% of cases owning to meningococci, but only 30% to 50% of cases owning to gram negative enteric bacilli. If antibiotics have been given before CSF obtained, Gram stain may be negative.
In 50% of cases owning to *Listeria monocytogenes*, the Gram stain may be negative and the cellular response is usually monocytic, which may cause this meningitis to be mistakenly diagnosed as viral, syphilis, TB, Lyme disease, etc. Identified by PCR.

CNS

Table 9-2. Etiology of Bacterial Meningitis by Age

	Newborns	<1 year	1–5 years	5–14 years	>15 years	Elderly
Most frequent	Escherichia coli		Streptococcus pneumoniae	Neisseria meningitides	S. pneumoniae	S. pneumoniae N. meningitidis
Common	Enterobacter aerogenes/ Klebsiella pneumoniae β-hemolytic streptococcus Listeria monocytogenes Staphylococcus aureus		N. meningitides S. pneumoniae	H. influenzae S. pneumoniae	N. meningitides S. aureus	Gram-negative bacilli L. monocytogenes
Uncommon	Paracolon bacilli Pseudomas spp. H. influenzae		Pseudomas spp. S. aureus β-hemolytic streptococcus E. coli	β-hemolytic streptococcus	E. coli Pseudomas spp.	
Rare	N. meningitides		Enterobacter aerogenes/ Klebsiella pneumoniae paracolons various other gram-negative organisms		H. influenzae	

The frequency of different organisms may vary from year to year; in presence of epidemics, or by geographic location. Occasionally more than one organism is recovered. H. influenzae formerly caused most cases between 6 months and 3 years (but was unusual before 2 months), but incidence has declined markedly due to effective vaccination. Enteric bacteria are so rarely found in older children that, in their presence, immunologic defect or congenital dermal sinus should be ruled out. If surgery has not been performed and S. aureus is present, congenital dermal sinus should be ruled out.
Gram stain of CSF should always be done in addition to culture because it provides a more immediate clue to the causative agent and the proper therapy and because the culture may be negative if the patient received antibiotics soon before the lumbar puncture. Cultures should also be obtained from blood and from petechial skin lesions if present. Gram stain of buffy coat of blood is often useful.
CSF glucose is very useful in differentiating bacterial from viral meningitis and is a good index to the severity of the infection, with a lower level in more severe infections.
Newborns with overwhelming pneumococcal infections may have no decrease in glucose or increase of cells.
CSF should be reexamined in 24 hours as a guide to therapeutic response; a good response shows negative gram-stained smear and culture, increased glucose, and a changing cell count from predominance of PMNs to predominance of mononuclear cells; total cell count and protein may show an initial rise. CSF should be reexamined when therapy is to be stopped; treatment should not be stopped unless CSF is normal except for slight increase of cells (≤~20 lymphocytes).

Stains are positive in <60% of cases of treated ABM, <5% of cases of TB meningitis, 20% to 70% of cases of fungal meningitis and <2% of cases of brain abscess. Sensitivity of Gram stain is increased using fluorescent techniques with acridine orange.

♦ Positive CSF bacterial culture has S/S = 92%/95%, false-negative rate = 8%, and false-positive rate = 5%. Culture is more reliable than Gram stain, although results of the stain offer a more immediate guide to therapy.

♦ Blood culture is usually positive if patient has not received antibiotics.

Limulus amebocyte lysate is a rapid specific indicator of endotoxin produced by gram-negative bacteria (*N. meningitidis, Hemophilus influenzae* type B, *E. coli, Pseudomonas*). Is not affected by prior antibiotic therapy; is more rapid and sensitive than counterimmunoelectrophoresis (CIE). Is often not routinely available.

Serological methods are often preferred (e.g., positive in 85% of coccidioidal cases compared with culture, which is positive in 37% of cases) especially in syphilis, brucellosis, Lyme disease. Higher titer in CSF than blood indicates antibody synthesis in CSF. Blood and CSF serology is positive in CNS syphilis (Table 9-1); positive in 7% to 10% of active cases of infectious mononucleosis.

Detection of bacterial antigen (rapid latex agglutination assay has largely replaced CIE) in CSF for *S. pneumoniae*, group B streptococcus (*Streptococcus agalactiae*), *H. influenzae*, some strains of *Neisseria meningitidis*. PCR for *S. agalactiae* has PPV and PNV >98%.

* Not affected by previous antimicrobial therapy that might inhibit growth in culture.
* *H. influenzae* is now rare due to routine immunization of children.
* Not likely to be useful if CSF chemistry and cell count are normal unless patient is immunocompromised.
* False positive for *H. influenza* may occur due to recent immunization; should not be performed if recently vaccinated.
* False positive for Group B Streptococcus antigen in urine is common due to its colonization of perineum.
* For these reasons and cost, is currently done much less frequently.

Opening pressure is increased (normal = 100–200 mm Hg)

Laboratory findings due to presence of infection (e.g., increased number of band forms, toxic granulations, Döhle bodies, vacuolization of PMNs)

Laboratory findings due to preceding diseases, e.g.:

* Pneumonia, otitis media, sinusitis, skull fracture prior to pneumococcal meningitis
* Neisseria epidemics prior to this meningitis
* Bacterial endocarditis, septicemia, etc.
* *Streptococcus pneumoniae* in alcoholism, myeloma, sickle cell anemia, splenectomy, immunocompromised state
* *Cryptococcus* and *M. tuberculosis* in steroid therapy and immunocompromised state
* Gram-negative bacilli in immunocompromised state
* *H. influenzae* in splenectomy
* Lyme disease

Laboratory findings due to complications (e.g., Waterhouse-Friderichsen syndrome, subdural effusion)

♦ Most frequent and important differential diagnosis is between acute bacterial meningitis (ABM) and acute viral meningitis (AVM). The most useful test results are:

* CSF identification of organism by stain or culture, specific nucleic acid or antigen by PCR
* Decreased CSF glucose and decreased CSF:serum ratio of glucose even if CSF glucose is normal
* Increased CSF protein >1.72 gm/L (1% of AVM and 50% of ABM cases)
* CSF WBC >2,000/μL in 38% of ABM cases and PMN >1,180/μL but low counts do not rule out ABM.
* Peripheral WBC is only useful if WBC (>27,200/μL) and total PMN (>21,000/μL) counts are very high, which occurs in relatively few patients; leukopenia is common in infants and elderly.

CNS

Meningitis, Chemical

Due to injection of anesthetic, antibiotic, radiopaque dye, etc., or to rupture into CSF of contents of epidermoid tumor or craniopharyngioma

CSF
  Pleocytosis is mild to moderate, largely lymphocytic.
  Protein shows variable increase.
  Glucose is usually normal.

Meningitis, Chronic

(Symptoms for >4 weeks)

Due to

Various infections
  TB (most common cause)
  Bacteria (e.g., Brucella)
  Spirochetes (e.g., leptospirosis, syphilis, Lyme disease)
  Fungal (e.g., *candida, coccidioides, cryptococcus*)
  Protozoan (e.g., *Toxoplasma gondii*)
  Amebic (e.g., *Naegleria, Acanthamoeba*)
  Mycoplasma
  Rickettsia
  Helminths
Systemic disorders
  Vasculitis, collagen vascular disease
  Sarcoid
  Neoplasm (e.g., leukemia, lymphoma, metastatic carcinoma)
CSF
  WBC 100 to 400 WBC/μL, preponderance of lymphocytes
  Glucose often decreased
  Protein usually moderately or markedly increased

Meningitis, Mollaret

Rare disorder of recurrent episodes [2–7 days each] of aseptic meningitis occuring over several years with symptom-free intervals in which other organ systems are not involved. Usually due to HSV-2 infection and has also been reported due to epidermoid cyst or anatomical defects that are discovered later by MRI or CT scan.

CSF
  ♦ During first 12 to 24 hours may contain up to several thousand cells/μL, predominantly PMNs and 66% of a large type of mononuclear cells (originally "endothelial cells") that are of unknown origin and significance and are characterized by vague nuclear and cytoplasmic outline with rapid lysis even while being counted in the hemocytometer chamber; they may be seen only as "ghosts" and are usually not detectable after the first day of illness. After the first 24 hours, the PMNs disappear and are replaced by lymphocytes, which, in turn, rapidly disappear when the attack subsides.
  Protein may be increased ≤100 mg/dL.
  Glucose is normal or may be slightly decreased.
There is mild leukopenia and eosinophilia.

Meningitis/Encephalomyelitis, Viral, Acute

For other infectious, postvaccinal, postexanthematous, postinfectious, see Chapter 15.
CSF shows increased protein and lymphocytes (see Table 9-1).
Should not be mistaken for TB, parasitic, chemical, incompletely treated bacterial meningitis, etc.
Postinfectious encephalomyelitis patients have an invariable, irreversible demyelinating syndrome; is most commonly associated with varicella and URI (especially influenza) and measles.

Vaccination has reduced the incidence of acute and postinfectious encephalitis and of poliomyelitis but a few cases of vaccine-associated infections occur.
Coxsackievirus and echovirus usually cause benign aseptic meningitis.
Laboratory findings due to preceding illness (e.g., measles) are noted.
♦ Viral culture (see Chapter 15) varies with organism; better for mumps, echovirus, and coxsackievirus than for Herpesviridae. HSV can be cultured from CSF in 50% to 75% of patients with meningitis only during first episode and <5% with encephalitis; rarely positive with recurrences. In Colorado tick fever, viral detection by culture, immunofluorescence, and RT-PCR of whole blood (virus is in RBCs).
♦ PCR to detect HSV (S/S >95%), human enteroviruses, and increasing number of organisms in CSF is more significant than in brain tissue where it may represent irrelevant latent infection. Can be confirmed by Southern blotting (S/S = 98%/97%). Brain biopsy has been gold standard for many virus encephalitides using EM, IHC, and culture. PCR has high PPV in AIDS patients with CNS lymphoma due to EBV. Quantitative PCR for determination of viral load is useful in CMV to determine clinical significance and to monitor therapy. PCR detection of HSV DNA in CSF is positive within 24 hours of onset of symptoms. Remains positive during first week of therapy. Has replaced brain biopsy, culture, immunohistochemistry as test of choice.
♦ PCR of CSF or fresh brain tissue for panel detection of HSV, varicella-zoster, enterovirus, eastern equine encephalitis, St. Louis encephalitis, CMV, EBV, California serogroup viruses, and rabies (in saliva) makes 72-hour diagnosis possible on one sample and should replace culture, mouse innoculation, immunoassay, serology, and brain biopsy.
♦ Mumps IgM antibodies in CSF and serum indicates mumps encephalitis.
♦ ELISA to detect IgM in CSF is sensitive and specific for Japanese B encephalitis; is usually present at hospitalization and almost always present by third day of illness.
♦ Paired serum samples during acute and convalescent periods may show seroconversion or 4× increase in specific antibody titers.
♦ Brain biopsy is currently reserved for patients who do not respond to acyclovir therapy and have unknown abnormality on CT scan or MRI.
♦ Brain biopsy is also required for diagnosis of progressive multifocal leukoencephalopathy.
West Nile meningoencephalitis[7]
    IgM is found in CSF and serum
    RT-PCR detects virus in CSF and serum
    Brain tissue (autopsy) is positive for antigen by immunohistochemical analysis and RT-PCR.

Meningoencephalitis, Amebic

Due to free-living ameba, Naegleria or Acanthamoeba, in contaminated water forced into nasal cavity. Rapid progression to death in 7–10 days.

Increased WBC, predominantly neutrophils.
CSF findings
    Fluid may be cloudy, purulent, or sanguinopurulent.
    Protein is increased.
    Glucose is usually decreased; may be normal.
    Increased WBCs are chiefly PMNs. RBCs are frequently present also. Motile amebas may be seen in hemocytometer chamber or on wet mount using phase or diminished light.
    ♦ Amebas are seen on Wright's, Giemsa, H&E stains. Gram stain and cultures are negative for bacteria and fungi.
    ♦ Culture of tissue or CSF on agar or tissue culture demonstrates organisms.
    ♦ Electron microscopy allows precise classification of amebas.
    ♦ IFA and immunoperoxidase are reliable methods to identify amebas in tissue sections.

[7]Nash D, Mostashari F, Fine A, et al. and the 1999 West Nile Outbreak Response Working Group. The outbreak of West Nile virus infection in the New York City area in 1999. N Engl J Med 2001;344:1807–1814.

CNS

Myelitis

CSF may be normal or may show increased protein and cells (20–1,000/μL—lymphocytes and mononuclear cells) with normal glucose.

Laboratory findings due to causative condition (e.g., poliomyelitis, herpes zoster, TB, syphilis, parasites, abscess, MS, postvaccinal myelitis, paraneoplastic)

Prion Diseases

See Chapter 15.

Tuberculoma of Brain

CSF shows increased protein with small number of cells. The tuberculoma may be transformed into TB meningitis with increased protein and cells (50–300/μL), decreased glucose and chloride.

Laboratory findings due to TB elsewhere

TB meningitis (see Chapter 15)

Inherited Conditions

Bassen-Kornzweig Syndrome

See Chapter 9.

Cerebellar Ataxia, Progressive with Skin Telangiectasis

See Tables 11-6 and 11-7.

Metachromatic Leukodystrophy

See Table 12-13 and Chapter 12 for other conditions that affect the CNS.

Refsum Disease

Rare autosomal recessive lipidosis of the nervous system due to phytanoyl-coenzyme A hydroxylase deficiency with retinitis pigmentosa, peripheral neuropathy, cerebellar ataxia, nerve deafness, and ichthyosis. Stored lipid (phytanic acid) is not synthesized in body but is exclusively dietary.

CSF shows albuminocytologic dissociation (normal cell count with protein usually increased to 100–700 mg/dL).
♦ Increased plasma phytanic acid ≥800 μmol/L (normal <19 μmol/L)

von Hippel-Lindau Disease (Hemangioblastomas of Retina and Cerebellum)

Laboratory findings due to associated conditions (e.g., polycythemia, pheochromocytomas, renal cell carcinoma, cysts of kidney and epididymis, benign cysts and nonfunctional neuroendocrine tumors of pancreas)

von Recklinghausen Disease (Multiple Neurofibromas)

CSF findings of brain tumor if acoustic neuroma occurs

Miscellaneous Conditions

Alzheimer Disease (Senile Dementia)

Most common cause of dementia. Major pathology is accumulation of Aβ peptide form of amyloid, which is cleaved from a larger protein, gene for which resides on chromosome 21.

There are no abnormal laboratory findings, but laboratory tests are useful to rule out other diseases that may resemble these syndromes but are amenable to therapy.

♦ Gold standard for diagnosis is histology of brain (biopsy or autopsy).
Tests under development:
  Increased Tau protein and decreased β-Amyloid $_{(1-42)}$ in CSF in patients with dementia may rule out other causes (e.g., vascular, tumor, endocrine) leaving Alzheimer as most likely.
  Neural thread protein detected in first morning urine and CSF.
Recommended tests in all patients with new onset of dementia should include: CBC, urinalysis, electrolyte and blood chemistry panel, screening metabolic panel, serum vitamin B_{12} and folate measurements, thyroid and other endocrine disorders, serologic test for syphilis.
In patients >age 60 with dementia, the usual causes are Alzheimer type (75%), drugs and alcohol (13%), endocrine (4%), low serum iron, folate, or cobalamin (8%), GU tract infection (2.5%).

Coma and Stupor

Due to
Poisons, drugs, or toxins
  Sedatives (especially alcohol, barbiturates)
  Enzyme inhibitors (especially salicylates, heavy metals, organic phosphates, cyanide)
  Other (e.g., paraldehyde, methyl alcohol, ethylene glycol)
Cerebral disorders
  Brain contusion, hemorrhage, infarction, seizure, or aneurysm
  Brain mass (e.g., tumor, hematoma, abscess, parasites)
  Subdural or epidural hematoma
  Venous sinus occlusion
  Hydrocephalus
  Hypoxia
    Decreased blood O_2 content and tension (e.g., lung disease, high altitude)
    Decreased blood O_2 content with normal tension (e.g., anemia, carbon monoxide poisoning, methemoglobinemia)
  Infection (e.g., meningitis, encephalitis)
Vascular abnormalities (e.g., subarachnoid hemorrhage, hypertensive encephalopathy, shock, acute myocardial infarction, aortic stenosis, Adams-Stokes, tachycardias)
Metabolic abnormalities
  Acid–base imbalance (acidosis, alkalosis)
  Electrolyte imbalance (increased or decreased sodium, potassium, calcium, magnesium)
  Porphyrias
  Aminoacidurias
  Uremia
  Hepatic encephalopathy
  Other disorders (e.g., leukodystrophies, lipid storage diseases, Bassen-Kornzweig syndrome)
Nutritional deficiencies (e.g., vitamin B_{12}, thiamine, niacin, pyridoxine)
Endocrine
  Pancreas (diabetic coma, hypoglycemia)
  Thyroid (myxedema, thyrotoxicosis)
  Adrenal (Addison disease, Cushing syndrome, pheochromocytoma)
  Panhypopituitarism
  Parathyroid (hypofunction or hyperfunction)
Psychogenic conditions that may mimic coma
  Depression, catatonia
  Malingering
  Hysteria, conversion disorder

Mental Retardation

Laboratory findings due to underlying causative condition (see appropriate separate sections)

CNS

Due to
Prenatal
Infections (e.g., syphilis, rubella, toxoplasmosis, CMV)
Metabolic abnormalities (e.g., diabetes mellitus, eclampsia, placental dysfunction)
Chromosomal disorders (e.g., Down syndrome, 18-trisomy, cri du chat syndrome, Klinefelter syndrome)
Metabolic abnormalities
    Amino acid metabolism (e.g., phenylketonuria, maple syrup urine disease, hemocystinuria, cystathioninuria, hyperglycemia, argininosuccinicaciduria, citrullinemia, histidinemia, hyperprolinemia, oasthouse urine disease, Hartnup disease, Joseph syndrome, familial iminoglycinuria)
    Lipid metabolism (e.g., Batten disease, Tay-Sachs disease, Niemann-Pick disease, abetalipoproteinemia, Refsum disease, metachromatic leukodystrophy)
    Carbohydrate metabolism (e.g., galactosemia, mucopolysaccharidoses)
    Purine metabolism (e.g., Lesch-Nyhan syndrome, hereditary orotic aciduria)
    Mineral metabolism (e.g., idiopathic hypercalcemia, pseudo- and pseudohypoparathyroidism)
    Other syndromes (e.g., tuberous sclerosis, Louis-Bar syndrome)
Perinatal
Infections (e.g., syphilis, rubella, toxoplasmosis, CMV, HIV, HSV)
Kernicterus
Prematurity
Anoxia
Trauma
Postnatal
Poisoning (e.g., lead, arsenic, carbon monoxide)
Infections (e.g., meningitis, encephalitis)
Metabolic abnormalities (e.g., hypoglycemia, malnutrition)
Postvaccinal encephalitis
Cerebrovascular accidents
Trauma

Neuritis/Neuropathy, Multiple

Laboratory findings due to causative disease
Infections:

* Epstein-Barr (mononucleosis associated: CSF shows increased protein and up to several hundred mononuclear cells)
* Diptheria: CSF protein is 50 to 200 mg/dL
* Lyme disease
* HIV
* Hepatitis associated
* Leprosy

Postvaccinal effect
Metabolic conditions (e.g., pellagra, beriberi, combined system disease, pregnancy, porphyria, diabetes mellitus). CSF usually normal. In ~70% of patients with diabetic neuropathy, CSF protein is increased to >200 mg/dL.
    Uremia: CSF protein is 50 to 200 mg/dL; occurs in a few cases of chronic uremia
        Collagen disease
        Polyarteritis nodosa: CSF usually normal; nerve involvement in 10% of patients
            SLE
    Neoplasm (leukemia, multiple myeloma, carcinoma): CSF protein often increased; may be associated with an occult primary neoplastic lesion outside CNS
    Amyloidosis
    Sarcoidosis
    Toxic conditions due to drugs and chemicals (especially lead, arsenic, etc.)
    Alcoholism—CSF usually normal
    Bassen-Kornzweig syndrome
    Refsum disease
    Chédiak-Higashi syndrome
    Immune mediated (e.g., Guillain-Barré syndrome)

Cranial Nerve, Multiple
Laboratory findings due to causative conditions
  Metabolic (e.g., diabetes mellitus, renal failure, chronic liver disease, myxedema, porphyria)
  Trauma
  Aneurysms
  Tumors (e.g., meningioma, neurofibroma, carcinoma, cholesteatoma, chordoma)
  Infections (e.g., herpes zoster)
  Benign polyneuritis associated with cervical lymph node tuberculosis or sarcoidosis

Neuritis of One Nerve or Plexus
Laboratory findings due to causative disease
  Diabetes mellitus
  Infections (e.g., HIV, diphtheria, herpes zoster, leprosy)
  Sarcoidosis
  Polyarteritis nodosa
  Tumor (leukemia, lymphoma, carcinomas)—may find tumor cells in CSF
  Trauma
  Serum sickness
  Bell's palsy
  Idiopathic
  Drugs, toxic substances

Facial Palsy, Peripheral Acute
Laboratory findings due to causative disease
  Idiopathic (Bell palsy)—occasional slight increase in cells in CSF
  Infection

  • Viral (e.g., varicella zoster, HSV, HIV, EBV, poliomyelitis, mumps, rubella)
  • Bacterial (e.g., Lyme disease, syphilis, leprosy, diphtheria, cat scratch disease, *Mycoplasma pneumoniae*)
  • Parasitic (e.g., malaria)
  • Meningitis
  • Encephalitis
  • Local inflammation (otitis media, mastoiditis, osteomyelitis, petrositis)

  Trauma
  Tumor (acoustic neuromas, tumors invading the temporal bone)
  Granulomatous (e.g., sarcoidosis) and connective tissue diseases
  Diabetes mellitus
  Hypothyroidism
  Uremia
  Drug reaction
  Postvaccinal effect
  Paget disease of bone
  Melkersson-Rosenthal syndrome
  Lyme disease and Guillain-Barré syndrome may produce bilateral palsy.

Hemianopsia, Bitemporal
Laboratory findings due to causative disease
  Usually pituitary adenoma
  Also metastatic tumor, sarcoidosis, Hand-Schuller-Christian disease, meningioma of sella, and aneurysm of circle of Willis

Ophthalmoplegia
Laboratory findings due to causative disease
  Diabetes mellitus
  Myasthenia gravis
  Hyperthyroid exophthalmos

Trigeminal Neuralgia (Tic Douloureux)
Laboratory findings due to causative disease
  Usually idiopathic
  May also stem from multiple sclerosis or herpes zoster

CNS

Retrobulbar Neuropathy

Laboratory findings due to causative disease
CSF is normal or may show increased protein and ≤200/μL lymphocytes.
○ Multiple sclerosis ultimately develops in 75% of these patients.

Autonomic Neuropathy

Laboratory findings due to causative disease
  Diabetes mellitus is most common
  Amyloidosis
  Acute porphyria
  Guillain-Barré syndrome
  Thallium poisoning

Pseudotumor Cerebri

Intracranial hypertension of unknown etiology with neurological complex of headache and papilledema without mass lesion or ventricular obstruction.

CSF is normal except for increased opening pressure.
Laboratory findings due to associated conditions (only obesity has been reported consistently)
  Addison disease
  Infection
  Metabolic (acute hypocalcemia and other "electrolyte disturbances," empty sella syndrome, pregnancy)
  Drugs (e.g., psychotherapeutic drugs, sex hormones and oral contraceptives, corticosteroid administration usually after reduction of dosage or change to different preparation)
  Immune diseases (e.g., SLE, polyarteritis nodosa, serum sickness)
  Other conditions (e.g., sarcoidosis, Guillain-Barré syndrome, head trauma, various anemias, chronic renal failure)

Reye Syndrome

Acute noninflammatory encephalopathy with fatty changes in liver and kidney and rarely heart and pancreas. Occurs typically in children recovering from influenza, varicella, or nonspecific viral illness and is associated with use of aspirin.

♦ **Diagnostic Criteria**
Markedly increased CSF pressure with no other abnormalities
Serum AST, ALT, or ammonia ≥3× ULN
Noninflammatory, panlobular fatty liver is seen histologically (see Acute Hepatic Failure)

Seizures That May Have Laboratory Abnormalities

Associated Conditions
Brain tumors, abscess, etc.
Circulatory disorders (e.g., thrombosis, hemorrhage, embolism, hypertensive encephalopathy, vascular malformations, angiitis)
Hematologic disorders (e.g., sickle cell anemia, leukemia, TTP)
Metabolic abnormalities
  Carbohydrate metabolism (e.g., hypoglycemia [<40 mg/dL], hyperglycemia [>400 mg/dL], glycogen storage disease)
  Amino acid metabolism (e.g., phenylketonuria, maple syrup urine disease)
  Lipid metabolism (e.g., leukodystrophies, lipidoses)
  Electrolytes (e.g., sodium [<120 or >145 mEq/L], calcium [<7 mg/dL], magnesium)
  Hyperosmolality (>300 mOsm/L)
  Other disorders (e.g., porphyria, eclampsia, renal failure)
Drugs (crack cocaine, amphetamines, ephedrine, etc.)
Allergic disorders (e.g., drug reaction, postvaccinal)

Infections
   Meningitis, encephalitis
   Postinfectious encephalitis (e.g., measles, mumps)
   Fetal (e.g., rubella, measles, mumps)
   Others
Degenerative brain diseases

Neoplastic Lesions
Brain Tumor
CSF
   CSF is clear, but is occasionally xanthochromic or bloody if there is hemorrhage into
      the tumor.
   WBC may be increased ≤150 cells/μL in 75% of patients; normal in others.
   Protein is usually increased. *Protein is particularly increased with meningioma of
      the olfactory groove and with acoustic neuroma.*
   ◆ Tumor cells may be demonstrable in 20% to 40% of patients with all types of solid
      tumors, but failure to find malignant cells does not exclude meningeal neoplasm.
   Atypical WBCs in leukemia or lymphoma
   Tumor antigens/markers may indicate source of some metastatic tumors.
   Glucose may be decreased if cells are present.
   Brain stem gliomas, which are characteristically found in childhood, are usually
      associated with normal CSF.
   Usually normal in "diencephalic syndrome" of infants due to glioma of hypothalamus

Glomus Jugulare Tumor
CSF protein may be increased.

Leukemic Involvement of CNS
See Chapter 11.
Intracranial hemorrhage is principal cause of death in leukemia (may be intracerebral,
   subarachnoid, subdural).
More frequent when WBC is >100,000/μL and with rapid increase in WBC, especially
   in blast crises
Platelet count frequently decreased
Evidence of bleeding elsewhere
CSF findings of intracranial hemorrhage.
◆ Meningeal infiltration of leukemic cells:

• CNS is involved in 5% of patients with ALL at diagnosis and is the major site of relapse.
• PCR is used to detect minimal residual cells that are not recognized morphologically.
• Meninges are involved in <30% of patients with malignant lymphoma; most prevalent in diffuse large cell ("histiocytic"), lymphoblastic, and immunoblastic leukemia;
   occurs in one third to one half of patients with Burkitt's lymphoma and 15% to 20%
   of patients with non-Hodgkin lymphoma.
• Hodgkin disease seldom involves CNS.
• Involvement by chronic lymphocytic leukemia, well-differentiated lymphocytic lymphoma and plasmacytoid lymphomas is very rare.

CSF may show
   Increased pressure and protein
   Glucose decreased to <50% of blood level
   ◆ Increased cells that are often not recognized as blast cells because of poor preser-
      vation and that may be identified by cytochemical, immunoenzymatic, immuno-
      fluorescent, and flow cytometry techniques
   ◆ Malignant cells found in 60% to 80% of patients with meningeal involvement
Complicating meningeal infection (e.g., various bacteria, opportunistic fungi)

Spinal Cord Tumor
◆ CSF protein is increased. It may be very high and is associated with xanthochromia
   when there is a block of the subarachnoid space.

CNS

With complete block, for cord tumors located at lower levels, protein concentration is higher.

Tumor cells may be demonstrable.

Vascular Disorders

Arteritis, Cranial

See Vasculitis, Chapter 5.

Cerebrovascular Accident (Nontraumatic, Stroke)

Blood Tests for Cerebrovascular Accidents

Plasma DNA concentration measured by PCR assay for *β–globin* gene present in all nucleated cells of the body is reported to correlate with stroke severity and predict mortality and morbidity in ER.[8]

Preliminary studies indicate S-100b (marker of astrocytic activation) and B-type neurotrophic growth factor may be a useful adjunct to CT scanning.[9]

Autoantibodies to brain-specific antigen N-methyl-D-aspartate receptor may assist diagnosis of stroke or assess risk of TIA.[10]

Due to

Hemorrhage
   Ruptured berry aneurysm (45% of patients)
   Hypertension (15% of patients)
   Angiomatous malformations (8% of patients)
   Miscellaneous causes (e.g., brain tumor, blood dyscrasia)—infrequent
   Undetermined cause (rest of patients)
Occlusion (e.g., thrombosis, embolism, etc.) in 80% of patients
Especially if blood pressure is normal, always rule out ruptured berry aneurysm, hemorrhage into tumor, angioma, and coagulopathies (see Chapter 11).

Berry Aneurysm

In early subarachnoid hemorrhage (<8 hours after onset of symptoms), the test for occult blood may be positive before xanthochromia develops. After bloody spinal fluid occurs, WBC/RBC ratio may be higher in CSF than in peripheral blood.

Bloody CSF clears by 10th day in 40% of patients. CSF is persistently abnormal after 21 days in 15% of patients. ~5% of cerebrovascular episodes due to hemorrhage are wholly within the parenchyma and CSF findings are normal.

Laboratory findings due to other diseases that occur with increased frequency in association with berry aneurysm (e.g., coarctation of the aorta, polycystic kidneys, hypertension).

Hemorrhage, Cerebral

Increased WBC (15,000–20,000/μL); higher than in cerebral infarct (e.g., embolism, thrombosis)

Increased ESR

Urine
   Transient glycosuria
   Laboratory findings of concomitant renal disease
Laboratory findings due to other causes of intracerebral hemorrhage (e.g., leukemia, aplastic anemia, polyarteritis nodosa, SLE, and other coagulopathies)
♦ CSF—See Tables 9-1, 9-3.

Thrombosis, Cerebral

♦ CSF
   Protein may be normal or increased to ≤100 mg/dL.
   Cell count may be normal or ≥10 WBC/μL during first 48 hours and rarely ≥2,000 WBC/μL transiently on third day.

---

[8]Rainer TH, Wong LK, Lam W, et al. Prognostic use of circulating plasma nucleic acid concentrations in patients with acute stroke. *Clin Chem* 2003;49:562–569.
[9]Reynolds MA, Kirchick HJ, Dahlen JR, et al. Early biomarkers of stroke. *Clin Chem* 2003;49:1733–1739.
[10]Dambinova SA, Khounteev GA, Izykenova GA, et al. Blood test detecting autoantibodies to N-methyl-D-aspartate neuroreceptors for evaluation of patients with transient ischemic attack and stroke. *Clin Chem* 2003;49:1752–1762.

Table 9-3.	Differentiation between Bloody Cerebrospinal Fluid (CSF) Due to Subarachnoid Hemorrhage and Traumatic Lumbar Puncture	

CSF Finding	Subarachnoid Hemorrhage	Traumatic Lumbar Puncture
CSF pressure	Often increased	Low or normal
Blood in tubes for collecting CSF	CSF and blood uniformly mixed in all tubes	Earlier tubes more bloody than later tubes; RBC count decreases in later tubes
CSF clotting	No clots	Often clots
Xanthochromia in supernatant	Present if >2 hrs since hemorrhage	Absent unless patient is icteric; may appear if examination is delayed >2 hrs
Immediate repeat of lumbar puncture at higher level	CSF same as initial puncture	CSF clear

Increased CRP and ESR are risk factors for development of stroke.
Increased CRP is associated with a poorer short-term prognosis.
Laboratory findings due to some diseases that may be causative
  Hematologic disorders (e.g., polycythemia, sickle cell disease, thrombotic thrombopenia, macroglobulinemia); see Chapter 11
  Vasculitis (e.g., polyarteritis nodosa, Takayasu syndrome, dissecting aneurysm of aorta, syphilis, meningitis); see Chapter 5
  Hypotension (e.g., myocardial infarction, shock)

Embolism, Cerebral
♦ CSF
  Usually findings are the same as in cerebral thrombosis.
  Hemorrhagic infarction develops in one third of patients, usually producing slight xanthochromia; some of these patients may have grossly bloody CSF (10,000 RBCs/μL).
  Septic embolism (e.g., bacterial endocarditis) may cause increased WBC (≤200/μL with variable lymphocytes and PMNs), increased RBC (≤1,000/μL), slight xanthochromia, increased protein, normal glucose, and negative culture.
Laboratory findings due to underlying causative disease
  Bacterial endocarditis
  Nonbacterial thrombotic vegetations on heart valves
  Chronic rheumatic mitral stenosis with atrial thrombi
  Mural thrombus due to underlying myocardial infarction
  Myxoma of left atrium
  Fat embolism in fracture of long bones
  Air embolism in neck, chest, or cardiac surgery

Thrombosis of Cerebral Veins and Sinuses[11]

Produces hemorrhagic infarcts in ~40% of cases

Due to
85% have prothrombotic cause or risk factors genetic (see Chapter 11) or acquired (e.g., pregnancy, nephrotic syndrome).
Infections (e.g., otitis, mastoiditis, sinusitis, meningitis)
Trauma (e.g., head injury, neurosurgery)
Inflammation (e.g., SLE, sarcoidosis, Wegener granulomatosis)
Hematologic (e.g., polycythemia, thrombocythemia)
Drugs (e.g., oral contraceptives)
Others (e.g., cancer)

Hypertensive Encephalopathy
Laboratory findings due to changes in other organ systems and to other conditions (e.g., cardiac, renal, endocrine, toxemia of pregnancy)

[11]Stam J. Thrombosis of the cerebral veins and sinuses [review]. *N Engl J Med* 2005;352:1791–1798.

CNS

Laboratory findings due to progressive changes that may occur (e.g., focal intracerebral hemorrhage)

CSF frequently shows increased pressure and protein ≤100 mg/dL.

Spinal Cord Infarction

CSF changes same as in cerebral hemorrhage or infarction

Laboratory findings due to causative condition
  Polyarteritis nodosa
  Dissecting aneurysm of aorta
  Arteriosclerosis of aorta with thrombus formation
  Iatrogenic (e.g., aortic arteriography, clamping of aorta during cardiac surgery)

Laboratory findings due to underlying causative disease
  Primary brain tumors, metastatic tumors, leukemias, and lymphomas
  Pituitary adenomas (CSF protein and pressure usually normal)
  Infections (e.g., tuberculoma)
  Parasites forming abscesses, granulomas, cysts or migrating lesions (e.g., *Taenia solium, Echinococcus*, schistosomiasis, toxoplasmosis, amebiasis, trichinosis, cryptococcosis)

Laboratory findings due to associated genetic conditions (e.g., tuberous sclerosis, neurofibromatosis)

Thrombophlebitis of Cavernous Sinus

CSF is usually normal unless there is associated subdural empyema or meningitis, or it may show increased protein and WBC with normal glucose, or it may be hemorrhagic. Mucormycosis may cause this clinical appearance in diabetic patients.

Laboratory findings due to preceding infections, complications (e.g., meningitis, brain abscess), or other causes of venous thromboses (e.g., sickle cell disease, polycythemia, dehydration)

Laboratory findings due to involvement of cranial nerves

10 Musculoskeletal and Joint Diseases

MUSCULOSKEL

Laboratory Tests for Skeletal Muscle Diseases

Creatine and Creatinine

Creatine is synthesized in the liver, taken up by muscle cells to store energy as creatine phosphate. Creatinine is formed by hydrolysis of creatine and phosphocreatine in muscle and by ingestion of meat.

See Chapter 3.

Increased creatinuria with increased creatine/creatinine ratio occurs with active muscle disease and in neurologic conditions and other disorders with muscle atrophy (e.g., Addison disease, hyperthyroidism, male eunuchoidism).

Serum Enzymes in Diseases of Muscle

See Chapter 3 and Table 10-1.

Creatine kinase (CK) is the test of choice. It is more specific and sensitive than AST and LD and more discriminating than aldolase (ALD) but AST is more significantly associated with inflammatory myopathy and more useful in these cases (see Chapter 3).

Increased In
Polymyositis
Muscular dystrophy
Myotonic dystrophy
Some metabolic disorders
Malignant hyperthermia
Prolonged exercise; peak 24 hours after extreme exercise (e.g., marathon); smaller increases in well-conditioned athletes
Wilms tumors with rhabdomyomatous features (CK-MB may also be increased)

Normal In
Scleroderma
Acrosclerosis
Discoid lupus erythematosus
Muscle atrophy of neurologic origin (e.g., old poliomyelitis, polyneuritis)
Hyperthyroid myopathy

Decreased In
Rheumatoid arthritis (RA) (~2/3 of patients)

Skeletal Muscle Disorders That May Cause Increased Serum CK-MB
Drugs (e.g., alcohol, cocaine, halothane [malignant hyperthermia], ipecac)
Dermatomyositis/polymyositis
Muscular dystrophy (Duchenne, Becker)
Exercise myopathy; slight-to-significant increases in 14% to 100% of persons after extreme exercise (e.g., marathons); smaller increases in well-conditioned athletes
Familial hypokalemic periodic paralysis
Endocrine (e.g., hypoparathyroid, acromegaly; hypothyroidism rarely increases CK-MB ≤6% of total)
Rhabdomyolysis
Infections

- Viral (e.g., HIV, EBV, influenza, picornaviruses, coxsackievirus, echovirus, adenoviruses)
- Bacterial (e.g., *Staphylococcus, Streptococcus, Clostridium, Borrelia*)
- Fungal
- Parasitic (e.g., trichinosis, toxoplasmosis, schistosomiasis, cysticercosis)

Skeletal muscle trauma (severe)

Muscle Biopsy

May be examined by
  Light microscopy, including special stains
  Electron microscopy
  Immunohistochemistry
  Assay of tissue contents (special reference laboratories), e.g., glycogen, carnitine, various enzymes (e.g., dehydrogenases, maltases, reductases, etc.)

Myoglobinemia and Myoglobinuria

See Chapters 4 and 5.

MUSCULOSKEL

Table 10-1. Increased Serum Enzyme Levels in Muscle Diseases

| Enzyme | Muscular Dystrophy | | | | | | | | Myotonic Dystrophy | Polymyositis |
| | Duchenne | | Limb–Girdle | | Facioscapulohumeral | | | | | |
	Frequency (%)	Amplitude	Frequency (%)	Amplitude	Frequency (%)	Amplitude	Frequency (%)	Amplitude	Frequency (%)	Frequency (%)
CK	>95	65	75	25	80	5			50	70
ALD	90	9	25	3	30	2			20	75
AST	90	4	25	2	25	1.5			15	25
LD	90	4	15	1.5	10	1			10	25

Frequency = average percentage of patients with increased serum enzyme level when blood is taken at optimal time. Amplitude = average number of times normal level that serum level is increased.

Diseases of Skeletal Muscles

Classification

Congenital (inherited) myopathy (nemaline, centronuclear)
Dystrophies, including Duchenne, Becker, facioscapulohumeral, limb-girdle, myotonic
Inflammatory, including infectious (e.g., trichinosis), granulomatous (e.g., sarcoidosis), and autoimmune (e.g., dermatomyositis)
Metabolic, including
  Endocrine

* Hypothyroidism (rarely associated with myotonia)
  Increased serum CK in 60% to 80% of patients to average 4x to 8× ULN; becomes
    normal 4 to 6 weeks after treatment. CK-MB is rarely increased ≤6% of total.
    Other serum enzyme levels are normal.
  Decreased urine creatine; increased creatine tolerance
* Hyperthyroidism
  Normal serum enzyme levels
  Increased urine creatine; decreased creatine tolerance
  Normal muscle biopsy findings
  Causes some cases of hypokalemic periodic paralysis
* Acromegaly
  Serum CK may be increased to average of 2× ULN.
* Cushing syndrome and adrenal corticosteroid therapy
  Increased serum enzymes—uncommon, and may be due to the primary disease
  Muscle biopsy—degenerative and regenerative changes in scattered muscle
    fibers; no inflammatory cell infiltration
  Increased urine creatine
* Other endocrinopathies (e.g., hypoadrenalism, hyperparathyroidism)
  Inherited metabolic myopathies (see Chapter 12)
* Glycogen storage diseases (Types II, III, V, VII)
* Disordered lipid metabolism (muscle carnitine deficiency)

Trauma

Metabolic Diseases of Muscle

Malignant Hyperthermia[1]

Rare autosomal dominant hypermetabolic syndrome causing abnormally increased release of calcium from membrane of sarcoplasmic reticulum; triggered by various inhalational [e.g., ether] and local anesthetic agents, muscle relaxants [e.g., succinylcholine, tubocurarine], and rarely, various types of severe heat stress or exercise intolerance causing hyperthermia, muscle rigidity, and 70% fatality

♦ Combined metabolic and respiratory acidosis is the most consistent abnormality and is diagnostic in the presence of muscle rigidity or rising temperature. pH is often <7.2, base excess [BE] >−10, hypoxia, and arterial pCO_2 of 70 to 120 torr. *Immediate* arterial blood gas analysis should be performed.
Muscle damage is reflected by:
♦ Increased serum potassium (>7 mEq/L) and calcium initially with below-normal values later
♦ Serum CK, LD, and AST markedly increased with peak in 24 to 48 hours after surgery; CK often 20,000 to 100,000 units/L

[1]Litman RS, Rosenberg H. Malignant Hyperthermia. Update on susceptibility testing. *JAMA* 2005;293:2918.

MUSCULOSKEL

Table 10-2.	Types of Periodic Paralysis		
	Hypokalemic (Familial, Sporadic, Associated with Hyperthyroidism)	Hyperkalemic (Adynamia Episodica Hereditaria)	Normokalemic
Induced by	Glucose and insulin, ACTH, DOCA, epinephrine	KCl	KCl
Serum potassium during attack	Decreased	Transiently increased	Normal or slightly decreased
Urine potassium excretion	Decreased	Normal	Decreased

ACTH, corticotropin; DOCA, deoxycorticosterone acetate; KCl, potassium chloride.

♦ Myoglobinemia and myoglobinuria due to rhabdomyolysis may be present early; oliguria with acute renal shutdown may occur later

Coagulopathy, including DIC, may occur later but is infrequent.

Resting serum CK may be elevated in relatives. However, the S/S of serum CK are too low to warrant its use for diagnosis or screening and should not be used to diagnose susceptibility to malignant hyperthermia.

♦ Gold standard for diagnosis by in vitro exposure of biopsied skeletal muscle to caffeine-halothane contracture test; S/S = 99%/94%; test is done at few laboratories—is very expensive.

♦ Ryanodine receptor gene on chromosome 19q13.1 and others; mutations are found in >50% of susceptible persons. DNA screen for 17 most common 19q13.1 mutations detects ≤25% of patients (low sensitivity).

Paralysis, Familial Periodic

See Table 10-2.

Hypokalemic

♦ Serum potassium is decreased during the attack. May contribute to rhabdomyolysis and myoglobinuria.

♦ ECG changes:

• Serum potassium ~<2.0 to 2.5 mEq/L causes prolonged ST segment mostly due to elevated U wave, flattened T waves

Urine potassium excretion decreases at the same time.

Serum enzymes are normal.

Hyperkalemic

Autosomal dominant disorder in which sudden increases in serum potassium cause muscle paralysis. May be provoked by exercise or excess in diet. Myotonia precedes or occurs between episodes.

♦ ECG changes:

• Serum potassium >~6.5 mEq/L causes peaked T waves
• Serum potassium >~7 to 8 mEq/L causes loss of P waves, prolonged PR interval
• Serum potassium >~8 to 10 mEq/L causes sine wave pattern, peaked T waves, loss of P waves; cardiac standstill can occur

Muscular Dystrophies

X-linked myopathies due to deficiency of cytoskeletal protein dystrophin. Becker is milder allelic variant of Duchenne dystrophy.

See Table 10-3 and Fig. 10-1.

Table 10-3.   Laboratory Findings in the Differential Diagnosis of Some Muscle Diseases

Disease	Complete Blood Cell Count	ESR	Thyroid Function Tests	Percentage of Patients with Increase in Various Serum Enzyme Levels	Muscle Biopsy	Comment
Myasthenia gravis	N	N	N	N	Lymphorrhages	Cancer of lung should always be ruled out; high frequency of associated diabetes mellitus, especially in older patients Serum electrolytes N
Polymyositis	Total eosinophil count frequently I	Moderately to markedly I; occasionally N	N	CK in 65%; levels may vary greatly and become N with steroid therapy; marked increase may occur in children LD in 25%, AST in 25%	Necrosis of muscle with phagocytosis of muscle fibers; infiltration of inflammatory cells	Associated cancer in ≤17% of cases (especially lung; also breast) Serum alpha$_2$ and gamma globulins may be I
Muscular dystrophy	N	N	N	In active phase, CK in 50%, LD in 10%, AST in 15%	Various degenerative changes in muscle; late muscle atrophy; no cellular infiltration	

N, normal; I, increased.

MUSCULOSKEL

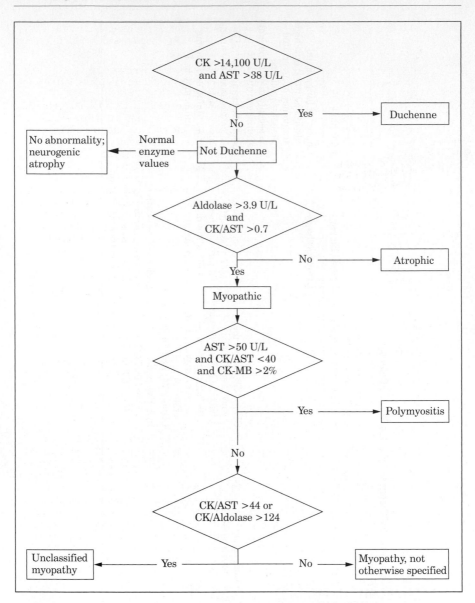

Fig. 10-1. Algorithm for serum enzymatic diagnosis of chronic muscle disease. Serum enzymes are not useful diagnostically in patients receiving immunosuppressive therapy in which the cause of muscle weakness is uncertain and muscle biopsy is required. (From Hood D, Van Lente F, and Estes M. Serum enzyme alterations in chronic muscle disease: a biopsy-based diagnostic assessment. *Am J Clin Pathol* 1991;95:402.)

♦ Serum enzymes (CK is most useful) are increased, especially in

- Young patients: Highest levels ($\leq$50× normal) are found at onset of disease in infancy or childhood, with gradual return to normal.
- The more rapidly progressive dystrophies (such as the Duchenne type): They may be slightly or inconsistently increased in the limb-girdle and facioscapulohumeral types.

* The active early phase: Increased levels are not constant and are affected by patient's age and duration of disease. Enzymes may be increased before disease is clinically evident.

Elevated serum enzyme levels are not affected by steroid therapy.

Preclinical diagnosis of Duchenne and Becker dystrophies in families with history of disease or for screening.

♦ Serum CK is always increased in affected children (5–100× ULN of adults) to peak by 2 years of age; then begin to fall as disease becomes manifest. Persistent normal CK virtually rules out this diagnosis. Begin testing at 2 to 3 months of age. (Note: Normal children have very high CK levels during first few days, which fall to 3× ULN by fourth day and fall to 2–3× adult level during first month of life; levels remain higher than adults during first 2 years.) Neonatal screening that is positive with whole blood should be confirmed with serum. CK >3× ULN for age in all boys with Duchenne dystrophy and >2× in those with Becker dystrophy. Sex-linked dystrophy is virtually only cause of high values in normal neonates. High values persist in dystrophy but false positives do not. Neonatal screening of girls has been discontinued. Prenatal screening at 18 to 20 weeks gestation by placental aspiration of fetal blood has been abandoned due to false-negative and false-positive results.

Clinical Diagnosis

CK is increased in almost all patients with Duchenne (average 30× ULN) and Becker (usually >10 × ULN) dystrophies. Diagnosis is in doubt if CK is normal. Highest levels occur in young patients and decrease with age so that levels are ~50% less by 7 years of age; usually consistently exceed 5× ULN but in terminal cases may decline further. Except for polymyositis, CK is normal or <5× ULN in other myopathies and neurogenic atrophy. CK MB is sometimes seen in Becker and limb-girdle dystrophies of up to 10% of total.

Duchenne dystrophy: Increased CK-MB (10%–15% of total) in 60% to 90% of patients; CK-BB may be slightly increased; CK-MM is chief fraction. CK-MB may be slightly increased (usually <4%) in carriers with increased total CK.

Serum aldolase is increased in ~20% of patients.

Serum LD is increased in ~10% of patients. AST is increased in ~15% of patients.

Identify Female Carriers

CK is increased in carriers with 2 affected sons or one son and one affected male relative in ~70% of cases of Duchenne and 50% of cases of Becker dystrophy. Highest levels and greatest frequency occur in younger carriers; may only be present during childhood and not in later life. Levels may be up to 10× ULN but usually <3× and average = 1.5× ULN; values overlap with those of normal females. Therefore special precautions are needed: draw blood after normal activity in afternoon or evening but not after vigorous or prolonged exercise or IM injections or during pregnancy; recheck at weekly intervals 3×; values are higher in blacks than in whites.

♦ Dystrophin protein quantitated by Western blot (WB) on biopsy of muscle is <3% in Duchenne dystrophy and ~3% to 20% or abnormally formed in Becker dystrophy.

♦ Immunofluorescence performed on biopsy of muscle is used to confirm WB results in males or to diagnose females with suspected dystrophinopathy.

♦ DNA studies show specific mutation in ~60% of patients.

* Prenatal diagnosis by chorionic villous sampling at 12th week of gestation
* Diagnosis of carriers
* Diagnosis and differential diagnosis (e.g., from limb-girdle dystrophy)

Muscle biopsy specimen shows muscle atrophy but no cellular infiltration.

Urine creatine is increased; urine creatinine is decreased. These changes are less marked in limb-girdle and facioscapulohumeral dystrophies than in Duchenne dystrophy.

ESR is usually normal.

Thyroid function tests are normal.

Laboratory findings due to myocardial damage in most female carriers after age 16 years

Facioscapulohumeral Dystrophy

Autosomal dominant slowly progressive dystrophy due to abnormality on chromosome 4q35. Begins in late adolescence; normal life span.

MUSCULOSKEL

Serum CK may be mildly increased in 75% of patients to average $3\times$ ULN; frequently normal by age 50.

Limb-Girdle Dystrophy

Heterogeneous group of disorders in both sexes; autosomal recessive disorder that begins in second decade and progresses to disability by 30 years of age and death by 50 years of age

Serum CK is increased in 70% of patients to average of $10\times$ ULN; not useful to detect carriers
Not useful to distinguish it from other autosomal recessive forms of dystrophy, myopathy, or neurologic disorders (e.g., hereditary proximal spinal muscular atrophy)
Muscle histology is nonspecific

Myotonic Dystrophy

Autosomal dominant disorder due to abnormality of chromosome 19. Begins in late adolescence; normal life span. Myotonia is impairment of muscle relaxation.

Serum CK is normal or mildly increased in 50% of patients to average of $3\times$ ULN.
Increased creatine in urine may occur irregularly.
Findings due to atrophy of testicle and androgenic deficiency are noted.
Urine 17-ketosteroids are decreased.
Thyroid function may be decreased.

Myopathies

Myasthenia Gravis (MG)[2]

See Table 10-3.
♦ Acetylcholine Receptor (AChR) Binding Antibodies is the standard assay and should be ordered first:

- Negative in ≤34% of patients with MG
- Negative ≤50% of patients with ocular MG
- May be negative in first 6–12 months
- Is more likely to be positive in severe than in mild cases of MG
- Correlates with severity ameliorated by treatment
- Specificity >99%. False positive may occur in thymoma patients without MG, lung cancer, Lambert-Eaton syndrome, patients receiving penicillamine or bone marrow transplants, primary biliary cirrhosis, AMS, and elderly persons.

♦ AChR-Blocking Antibodies

- Present in >50% of patients with generalized MG
- Present in 30% of patients with ocular MG
- Present in 19% of patients in remission
- Present in only 1% of MG patients without AChR-binding antibodies
- Not detected by AChR-modulating antibody assay
- More often associated with more severe forms of disease

♦ AChR-Modulating Antibodies

- Highest activity (>90%) in MG patients with thymoma
- Present in >70% of patients with ocular MG
- Does not distinguish between AChR-binding and blocking antibodies
- Positive in 7% of MG patients when AChR-binding antibodies are not detected

Striational antibodies to skeletal muscle cross-striations are found in

- 30% of adult MG patients
- ~90% of MG patients with thymoma; absence argues against thymoma
- ≤25% of patients with thymoma without MG; may be useful to predict risk of MG in patients with thymoma and to predict recurrence of thymoma
- ~5% of patients with Lambert-Eaton myasthenic syndrome
- Less frequent within 1 year of onset of MG
- Less frequent in patients receiving immunosuppressive drug therapy

[2]Case Records of Mass. General Hospital. *NEJM* 2000;342:508.

- Rare in MG patients <20 years old; increased frequency with each decade of disease after onset
- Absent in congenital MG
- 25% of patients treated with D-penicillamine
- Graft-versus-host disease in marrow transplant recipients; can be used for monitoring autoimmune complications of marrow transplantation
- Autoimmune liver diseases >90% of seropositive patients have more than one type of autoantibody.

Other immunologic abnormalities are frequent (e.g., thyrotoxicosis, RA, PA, SLE).

Anti-DNA (in 40% of cases), ANA anti-parietal cell, anti-smooth muscle, antimitochondrial, antithyroid antibodies, rheumatoid factor (RF), etc., may be found.

Thymic tumor develops in 15% to 20% of generalized MG patients; 70% of patients have thymic hyperplasia with germinal centers in medulla.

CBC, ESR, thyroid function tests, serum enzymes and electrolytes are normal.

High frequency of associated diabetes mellitus is seen, especially in older patients; therefore GTT should be performed with or without cortisone.

Always rule out cancer of lung.

Myopathy Associated with Alcoholism

Acute (necrotizing)

- Increased serum CK, AST, and other enzymes. Serum CK increased in 80% of patients; rises in 1 to 2 days; reaches peak in 4 to 5 days; lasts ~2 weeks. CK in CSF is normal, even when serum level is elevated.
- Gross myoglobinuria
- Acute renal failure (some patients)

Chronic—may show some or all of the following changes:

- Increased serum CK in 60% of patients to average of 2× ULN
- Increased AST and other enzymes due to liver as well as muscle changes
- Increased urine creatine
- Diminished ability to increase blood lactic acid with ischemic exercise
- Abnormalities on muscle biopsy (support the diagnosis)
- Myoglobinuria

Myotubular, Mitochondrial, and Nemaline (Rod) Myopathy

X-linked, morphologically distinct congenital myopathies. Routine laboratory studies including serum enzymes are normal.

♦ Muscle biopsy with histochemical staining establishes the diagnosis.

Polymyositis

Nongenetic primary inflammatory myopathy; may be idiopathic or due to infection or may be associated with skin disease [dermatomyositis] or collagen or malignant disease; 10%–20% of patients over 50 years of age have a neoplasm. Syndrome may include pulmonary fibrosis, Raynaud syndrome, dry cracked skin on hands ["mechanics hands"].

See Chapter 16 and Table 16-1.

○ Serum enzymes

- Serum CK is the most useful. Increased in 70% of patients. Levels may vary greatly (≤50× normal). Degree of increase is highest in children and usually reflects the activity of the disease but can be normal in active disease; decrease usually occurs 3 to 4 weeks before improvement in muscle strength and increases 5 to 6 weeks before clinical relapse; the level frequently becomes normal with steroid therapy (in ~3 months) or in chronic myositis.
- Serum aldolase is increased in 75% of patients.
- Serum LD is increased in 25% of patients.
- Serum AST is increased in ~25% of the patients.
- Serum α-hydroxybutyric dehydrogenase may parallel the increased LD.

♦ Muscle biopsy findings are definitive; also for dermatomyositis and inclusion-body myositis. They also help to exclude other types of myositis.

Total eosinophil count is frequently increased. WBC may be increased in fulminant disease.

Mild anemia may occur.

ESR is may be normal or moderately to markedly increased; not clinically useful.

Thyroid function tests are normal.

Urine shows a moderate increase in creatine and a decrease in creatinine. Myoglobinuria occurs occasionally in severe cases.

Increased ANA titers are found in 20% of patients. RF tests may be positive in 50% of patients.

Anti-Jo-1 (PM-1; histidyl-transfer RNA synthetase antibody) in ≤50% of polymyositis and 10% of dermatomyositis patients; strong association with interstitial lung disease

Rarely detected in other diseases

Serum γ globulins may be increased.

Associated carcinoma is present in ≤20% of the patients and in ≤5% of patients over 40 years of age (especially those with cancer of lung or breast). The polymyositis may antedate the neoplasm by up to 2 years.

Other types of inflammatory myositis

♦ Inclusion-body myositis shows characteristic biopsy finding on electron microscopy. Serum CK is normal or only slightly increased.

Laboratory Tests for Bone Diseases[3,4]

Use

To identify patients suitable for therapy

To estimate response to therapy for osteoporosis over a period of months to years in conjunction with bone mineral density

Bone formation markers of osteoblast activity: Bone-specific alkaline phosphatase, osteocalcin, procollagen type I

Bone resorption markers of osteoclast activity: Tartrate-resistant acid phosphatase (TRAP), hydroxyproline, pyridinoline, deoxypyridinoline, N-telopeptide, C-telopeptide, urine calcium

Because of diurnal rhythm, specimens should be collected at same time of day (preferably AM)

Acid Phosphatase, Tartrate-Resistant (TRAP), Serum

Synthesized by osteoclasts in contrast to prostatic acid phosphatase that is tartrate sensitive; also found in Kupfer cells and macrophages

Use

Marker of bone resorption

Alkaline Phosphatase (ALP), Bone-Specific (TRAP), Serum

Synthesized by osteoblasts; is involved in calcification of bone matrix. Only ~80% of total ALP is destroyed by heating along with some nonbone-specific ALP.

Use

Marker of bone formation

Increased In

Paget disease; may be more sensitive than total ALP, especially when activity is low

Primary hyperparathyroidism

Osteomalacia

Osteoporosis

Pregnancy

---

[3]Caulfield MP, Reitz RE. Biochemical markers of bone turnover and their utility in osteoporosis. *MLO Med Lab Obs* 2004;36:34–37.

[4]Hammett-Stabler C. The use of biochemical markers in osteoporosis. *Clin Lab Med* 2004;24:175.

Calcium, Serum

See Chapter 3 and Chapter 13.

Hydroxyproline, Urine

Hydrolysis product of collagen not found in proteins other than connective tissue

Use
Marker of collagen turnover (including bone resorption)
Limited diagnostic value; largely replaced by following tests

Increased In
Increased collagen catabolism (e.g., especially Paget disease; hyperparathyroidism, acromegaly, psoriasis, burns)
Certain inborn errors of metabolism (e.g., hydroxyprolinemia, familial aminoglycinuria)

Osteocalcin (Serum; Urine)

Cytosolic calcium-binding protein synthesized by osteoblasts during bone formation. Major noncollagen in bone. Excreted in urine by glomerular filtration. Assay values are not interchangeable between laboratories.

Use
Marker of bone turnover rather than just of resorption or formation
Assess patients at risk for osteoporosis
Classify patients with established osteoporosis
Determine efficacy of therapy in osteoporosis or bone metastases

Increased In
Increased bone formation (e.g., Paget disease, primary hyperparathyroidism, healing fractures, osteogenic sarcoma, hyperthyroidism, effective therapy for osteoporosis)

Decreased In
Hypoparathyroidism
Cushing syndrome

Pyridinium and Deoxypyridinoline, Cross-Links (Urine or Serum)

Stabilizing factors to Type I bone collagen within organic matrix of mineralized bone; released into circulation; measured by immunoassay; <10% from other sources—aorta, connective tissues, tendon, dentin

Use
Marker of increased osteoclastic activity (bone resorption and demineralization)
Monitor response to therapy for osteoporosis

Telopeptide, N-Terminal or C-Terminal (Urine or Serum)

Assay by antibodies to intermolecular cross-links of bone type I collagen that is major protein of matrix

Use
Markers of Type I collagen resorption and deposition
Serial changes decide course of therapy and monitor response to therapy for osteoporosis
Failure to change >30% after 4 to 8 weeks of therapy may suggest need to change therapy
More specific to bone than pyridinoline, hydroxyproline, or calcium
Not for diagnosis of osteoporosis

Increased In (indicates bone resorption)
Paget disease
Osteoporosis
Primary hyperparathyroidism
Metastatic bone cancer

MUSCULOSKEL

Diseases of Bone

Fat Embolism

Occurs after trauma [e.g., fractures, insertion of femoral head prosthesis]; also occurs in sickle cell disease

❍ Arterial blood gas values are always abnormal in clinically significant fat embolism syndrome; are the most useful and important laboratory data. Patients show decreased lung compliance, abnormal ventilation-perfusion ratios, and increased shunt effect. Decreased arterial pO_2 with normal or decreased pCO_2.

Unexplained decrease in Hb in 30% to 60% of patients

Decreased platelet count in 80% of patients, with rebound in 5 to 7 days

❍ Free fat in urine in 50% of patients and in stained blood smear

❍ Fat globules in sputum (some patients) and BAL

❍ Fat globulinemia in 42% to 67% of patients and in 17% to 33% of controls

Increased serum lipase in 30% to 50% of patients 3 to 4 days after injury; increased free fatty acids—not of diagnostic value

Increased serum triglycerides

Normal CSF

Hypocalcemia is a common nonspecific finding (due to binding to free fatty acids).

Hyperuricemia

♦ *Laboratory findings alone are inadequate for diagnosis, prognosis, or management.*

Neoplasms

Osteogenic Sarcoma

Primary bone malignancy

Marked increase in serum ALP ($\leq 40 \times$ normal); reflects new bone formation and parallels clinical course (e.g., metastasis, response to therapy); is said to occur in only 50% of patients

Laboratory findings due to metastases—80% of patients have lung metastases at time of diagnosis

Laboratory findings due to preexisting diseases (e.g., Paget disease)

♦ Histological examination of lesion establishes diagnosis.

Metastatic Tumor of Bone[5]

♦ Histological examination of lesion establishes diagnosis.

Patients can have either: Osteolytic and osteoblastic metastases, or mixed lesions containing both.

Only myeloma has purely lytic lesions. Metastases from prostate cancer are predominantly osteoblastic.

Osteolytic metastases (especially from primary tumor of bronchus, breast, kidney, or thyroid)

• Urine calcium is often increased; marked increase may reflect increased rate of tumor growth.
• Serum calcium and phosphorus may be normal or increased.
• Serum ALP is usually normal or slightly to moderately increased.
• Serum acid phosphatase is often slightly increased, especially in prostatic metastases.

Osteoblastic metastases (especially from primary tumor in prostate)

• Serum calcium is normal; it is rarely increased.
• Urine calcium is low.
• Serum ALP is usually increased.
• Serum acid phosphatase is increased in prostatic carcinoma (see Chapter 14).
• Serum phosphorus is variable.

[5]Roodman CD. Mechanisms of bone metastasis. *N Engl J Med* 2004;350:1655.

○ Increased concentration of markers of bone turnover (pyridinoline and deoxypyridi-noline and associated N-telopeptides, serum bone ALP), which may predict metas-tases in breast, prostate, lung cancers

Osteomyelitis

♦ Organism is identified by culture of bone biopsy material in 50% to 70% of patients; blood culture is positive in ~50% of patients; results of sinus drainage cultures in chronic osteomyelitis do not correlate with causative organism unless *Staphylococcus aureus* is cultured from sinus.
○ Microbiology

• *S. aureus* causes almost all infections of hip and two-thirds of infections of skull, ver-tebrae, and long bones. Other bacteria may be present simultaneously and con-tribute to infection.
• *S. aureus* causes 90% of cases of hematogenous osteomyelitis, which occurs princi-pally in children, but only 50% of blood cultures are positive.
• Group B streptococci, *S. aureus,* and *E. coli* are chief organisms in neonates. *H. influenzae* type B, *S. aureus*, group A *Streptococcus,* and *Salmonella* are chief organ-isms in older children. *S. aureus,* coagulase-negative staphylococci, gram-negative bacilli (especially *Pseudomonas aeruginosa*, *Serratia marcescens*, *E. coli*) are most frequent organisms.
• *Staphylococcus epidermidis* is the most common organism involved in total hip arthroplasty infection.
• Gram-negative bacteria cause most infections of mandible, pelvis, and small bones.
• *Salmonella* is more commonly found in patients with sickle cell and some other hemoglobinopathies.
• Diabetic patients with foot ulcers and surgical infections that extend to bone usually have polymicrobial infection, often including anaerobes.
• Most infections due to *Candida, Aspergillus,* and other fungi occur in diabetic and immunocompromised patients. *Candida* infection also occurs in patients with central and hyperalimentation lines. Patients are often on steroid and antibiotic therapy.
• Mucor occurs in poorly controlled diabetics.
• IV drug abusers frequently have osteomyelitis of sternoclavicular joints due most commonly to *P. aeruginosa* and *S. aureus*.
• Puncture wounds of calcaneus usually involve pseudomonal organisms.
• Cranial involvement in neonates following scalp fetal monitoring during labor is mainly associated with group B streptococci, *E. coli*, and staphylococci.
• Histoplasmosis is described in patients with AIDS. HSV and vaccinia have been described in immunocompromised patients.
• *Coccidioides immitis* may occur in endemic areas.

WBC may be increased, especially in acute cases.
ESR is increased in <50% of patients but may be important clue in occult cases (e.g., intervertebral disk space infection).
Laboratory findings due to underlying conditions (e.g., postoperative status, radio-therapy, foreign body, tissue gangrene, contiguous infection)
○ Vertebral osteomyelitis

• May be due to unusual organisms (e.g., *M. tuberculosis*, fungi, *Brucella*)
• Increased WBC in <50% of patients
• Increased ESR in >80% of patients
• Blood culture may be positive.
• Aspiration of involved site with stains, cultures and histologic exam
  Gram-positive cocci, especially *S. aureus* are most common.
  Gram-negative enteric bacilli, especially *E. coli* and Salmonella, cause ~30% of cases especially in sickle cell disease.
  Pseudomonas aeruginosa is associated with IV drug abuse.
  Brucella infection occurs in certain parts of the world.

Laboratory findings due to predisposing factors (e.g., diabetes, IV drug abuse, GU tract infection) or complications (e.g., epidural or subdural abscess, aortic involvement)

MUSCULOSKEL

Osteopetrosis (Albers-Schonberg Disease; Marble Bone Disease)[6]

Inherited heterogeneous group of disorders with defect in bone resorption by osteoclasts causing abnormally dense bone with increased skeletal mass; four types of autosomal recessive and one of autosomal dominant

Normal serum calcium, phosphorus, and ALP
Serum acid phosphatase and CK-MB (from osteoclasts) may be increased.
In severe form, there may be hypocalcemia with secondary hyperparathyroidism, increased serum calcitriol, rickets.
Laboratory findings due to

* Myelophthisis causing anemia, thrombocytopenia; infections commonly cause death in first decade of life.
* Hypersplenism
* Extramedullary hematopoiesis
* Fractures of brittle bones (especially in autosomal dominant type)
* Osteomyelitis

Osteoporosis (Osteopenia)[4,5]

Osteopenia is generic term for decreased mineralized bone [bone mass]. Osteoporosis indicates deterioration of microarchitecture of bone. Osteomalacia coexists with osteoporosis in 20% of patients.

Due To
Endocrine and metabolic disorders (e.g., hypogonadism, Cushing syndrome, hyperparathyroidism, hyperthyroidism, acromegaly, others)
Nutritional deficiency (e.g., diet, malabsorption)
Marrow disorders (e.g., multiple myeloma, lymphoproliferative disorders)
Renal disorders (e.g., renal insufficiency, renal osteodystrophy, renal tubular acidosis)
Disorders of connective tissue (e.g., Marfan syndrome, Ehlers-Danlos syndrome, osteogenesis imperfecta, GS diseases, homocystinuria)
Drugs (e.g., glucocorticoids, cyclosporine, diuretics, ethanol, antacid phosphate binders, anticonvulsants, lithium, cholestyramine, others)
Miscellaneous (e.g., lack of gravitational force, immobilization, space flight, pregnancy, lactation)
♦ Diagnosis is established by bone mineral density x-ray studies or by bone biopsy that may be combined with tetracycline labeling.
Laboratory tests used to evaluate response to therapy by rate of bone turnover, disease severity, fracture risk
All serum chemistry values are commonly normal in any form of osteopenia—done to rule out other conditions (e.g., bone metastases, hyperparathyroidism). A clue to diagnosis of nutritional vitamin D deficiency is very low 24-hr urine calcium (<50 mg/day).
Serum vitamin D that is below normal (e.g., 15 ng/mL of 25-hydroxy-vitamin D) suggests osteomalacia.
During therapeutic trial of calcium and vitamin D, serum and urine calcium should be monitored monthly to avoid toxicity. Urine calcium is maintained <300 mg/gm creatinine and serum calcium <10.2 mg/dL by reducing dose of vitamin D.

Paget Disease of Bone (Osteitis Deformans)

Focal bone disorder with increased bone turnover rate causing localized disorganized, enlarged, softened bone

♦ Marked increase in serum total ALP (in 90% of cases) is directly related to severity and extent of disease; sudden additional increase with development of osteogenic sarcoma occurs in ~1% of patients. May be normal in patients with monostotic dis-

[4]Hammett-Stabler C. The use of biochemical markers in osteoporosis. *Clin Lab Med* 2004;24:175.
[5]Roodman CD. Mechanisms of bone metastasis. *N Engl J Med* 2004;350:1655.
[6]Tolar J, et al. Osteopetrosis. *N Engl J Med* 2004;351:2839.

ease (~15% of symptomatic patients). Serum ALP (bone-specific isoenzyme) is more sensitive marker of bone formation and is increased in 60% of patients with normal total ALP.

Serum calcium increased during immobilization (e.g., due to intercurrent illness or fracture)

Normal or slightly increased serum phosphate

Frequently increased urine calcium; renal calculi common

Increase in urinary pyridinium cross-link pyridinoline is better indicator of bone resorption than the increase in urinary hydroxyproline which may be marked.

Osteocalcin is often normal.

Biochemical response to calcitonin therapy

* Initial decrease of serum ALP and urinary hydroxyproline followed by return to former values despite continued therapy; occurs in ~20% of cases
* Serum ALP and urinary hydroxyproline decrease 30% to 50% in 3 to 6 months and maintain those values for duration of therapy—occurs in >50% of cases
* Serum ALP and urinary hydroxyproline become normal only in previously untreated patients with only small increase in bone turnover—occurrence is unusual

♦ Radionuclide scan shows areas of heavy uptake in affected bones

Rickets and Osteomalacia

Defective mineralization of bone and cartilage in children and bone in adults with delayed cartilage maturation and disorganized arrangement of cells at epiphysis

Due To

Low serum calcium-phosphorus product

* Vitamin D deficiency (e.g., due to inadequate sunlight or diet; malabsorption, drugs)
* Hypophosphatemia, e.g.,
    Vitamin D-resistant rickets
    Fanconi syndrome
    Excess intake of phosphate-binding antacids
    Hypophosphatemic nonrachitic bone disease
    Tumor-induced osteomalacia
* Renal tubular acidosis

Normal or high serum calcium-phosphorus product

* Renal osteomalacia
* Hypophosphatasia

1,25-Dihydroxy-Vitamin D (Calcitriol)

Formed from 25-hydroxy vitamin D primarily by renal tubules; causes increased intestinal absorption of calcium and phosphate

Use

Differential diagnosis of hypocalcemic disorders

Monitor patients with renal osteodystrophy

Increased In

Hyperparathyroidism

Chronic granulomatous disorders

Hypercalcemia associated with lymphoma

Decreased In

Severe vitamin D deficiency

Hypercalcemia of malignancy (except lymphoma)

Tumor-induced osteomalacia

Hypoparathyroidism

Pseudohypoparathyroidism

Renal osteodystrophy

Type I vitamin D–resistant rickets

MUSCULOSKEL

25-Hydroxy-Vitamin D

Formed in liver from vitamin D

Use
Evaluation of vitamin D intoxication or deficiency

Increased In
Vitamin D intoxication (distinguishes this from other causes of hypercalcemia); does
not occur until >125 ng/mL

Decreased In
♦ Hypovitaminosis defined as serum <37.5 nmol/L; <20 nmol/L indicates severe defi-
ciency in adults. Infants and small children should have >25–30 nmol/L; desirable
range = 75 to 160 nmol/L.
Rickets, osteomalacia
Secondary hyperparathyroidism
Malabsorption of vitamin D (e.g., severe liver disease, cholestasis)
Diseases that increase vitamin D metabolism (e.g., TB, sarcoidosis, primary hyper-
parathyroidism)

Hypophosphatemia, Primary (Familial Vitamin D–Resistant Rickets)

**Hereditary metabolic defect in phosphate transport in renal tubules and possibly
intestine**

○ Serum phosphorus is markedly decreased.
Serum calcium is relatively normal.
Serum ALP is moderately increased.
Stool calcium is increased, and urine calcium is decreased.
♦ Administration of vitamin D does not cause serum phosphorus to increase (in con-
trast to ordinary rickets), but urine and serum calcium may be increased with suffi-
ciently large dose.
Renal aminoaciduria is absent, in contrast to ordinary rickets.
Treatment is monitored by choosing dose of vitamin D that will not increase serum
calcium to >11 mg/dL or urine calcium >200 mg/day.
Serum phosphorus usually remains low; increase >4 mg/dL may indicate renal injury
due to vitamin D toxicity.

Rickets, Vitamin D–Dependent

♦ Blood level of $1,25\text{-}(OH)_2D$ is very low in Type I (autosomal recessive deficiency of
$1\text{-}\alpha$ hydroxylase enzyme in kidney) and increased in Type II (group of genetic disorders causing increased end-organ resistance to $1,25\text{-}(OH)_2D$).
○ Serum ALP is increased. This is the earliest and most reliable biochemical abnormality; it parallels the severity of the rickets. It may remain elevated until bone
healing is complete. Serum calcium is frequently decreased, sometimes causing
tetany; is usually normal. Urine calcium is decreased.
Serum phosphorus is usually decreased but not as markedly or as consistently as in
hypophosphatemic rickets.
In some persons, serum calcium and phosphorus may be normal.
Increased serum PTH (secondary to low serum calcium) and urinary c-AMP.
♦ Serum 25-hydroxy-vitamin D is low (usually <5 ng/mL; normal = 10–20 ng/mL).
♦ Findings rapidly become normal after adequate vitamin D is given (may require very
large doses).
Generalized renal aminoaciduria is present; it disappears when adequate vitamin D
is given.
Vitamin D–deficient state is suggested by

• Low serum phosphorus
• Severe liver disease
• Malabsorption
• Anticonvulsant therapy

Laboratory Tests for Joint Diseases

Acute phase reactants (e.g., ESR, CRP in Chapter 3)
Anti-*Borrelia burgdorferi* antibodies (see Chapter 15)

Table 10-4.   Laboratory Tests in Differential Diagnosis of Rickets and Osteomalacia

	Vitamin D– Deficient Rickets	Vitamin D– Dependent Rickets Type I	Vitamin D– Dependent Rickets Type II	Chronic Renal Failure	Hypopara-thyroidism	Pseudo-hypopara-thyroidism
Blood						
Calcium	D	D	D	D	D	D
Phosphorus	N/D	N/D	N/D	I	I	I
ALP	I	I	I	I	N/I	N/I
PTH	I	I	I	I	D	I
25(OH)D	D	N	N	N/D	N	N
1–25(OH)$_2$D	I	D	I	D	D	D
Urine						
Phosphorus	I	I	I	D	D	D
Calcium	D	D	D	D	D	D

Calcium and phosphorus absorption is decreased in all of these conditions.
N = normal, D = decreased, I = increased

>   Anticardiolipin antigens
>   Anticytoplasmic antigens (see Chapter 3)
>   Antinuclear antibodies (Table 17-1)
>   Complement (C3, C4, CH50)
>   Cryoglobulins
>   Immune complexes (C1q binding, Raji cell assay)
>   RF
>   Synovial fluid examination (see Tables 10-6, 10-7)

Diseases of Joints

Autoimmune Arthropathies

Rheumatoid Arthritis (RA)[7]

Progressive systemic autoimmune disease with chronic inflammation of synovial tissues of unknown etiology

See Table 10-8.

♦ **Diagnostic Criteria:** American Rheumatism Association has 11 criteria for diagnosis of RA; 7 are required for diagnosis of classic RA, 5 for definite RA, and 3 for probable RA. 4 laboratory findings in these criteria are positive serum test for RF (by any method; positive in <5% of normal control subjects), poor mucin clotting of synovial fluid, characteristic histologic changes in synovium, and characteristic histologic changes in rheumatoid nodules.

♦ Anticyclic citrullinated peptide (anti-CCP; citrulline antibody) is newly discovered immune protein. S/S = 41% to 80%/>89%.[8] Becomes positive earlier than RF.
♦ IgM RF in 50% to 90% of RA patients. S/S = 72%/80%, but in first 6 months of illness, is only positive in ~40% of patients. Often positive in other autoimmune disorders, hepatitis, TB, and ≤5% of healthy persons (see Chapter 16). Seronegative RA incidence <0.5%.

[7]www.rheumatology.org/publications/classification/index.asp?aud=mem
[8]Hoffman IEA, et al. Diagnostic performance and predictive value of rheumatoid factor, anti-citrullinated peptide antibodies and the HLA shared epitope for diagnosis of rheumatoid arthritis. *Clin Chem* 2004;50:261.

Table 10-5.	Normal Values—Synovial Fluid
Volume	1.0–3.5 mL
pH	Parallels serum
Appearance	Clear, pale yellow, viscous, does not clot
Fibrin clot	0
Mucin clot	Mucin clot test adds little additional information to WBC count; is rarely used.
WBC /μL	<200 even in presence of leukocytosis in blood
Neutrophils	<25%
Crystals	See Table 10-9.
Fasting uric acid, bilirubin	Approximately the same as in serum
Total protein	~25%–30% of serum protein. Mean = 1.8 gm/dL
	Abnormal if >2.5 gm/dL; inflammation moderately severe if >4.5 gm/dL
Glucose	Glucose concentration may give spurious results unless obtained after prolonged fasting; differences between joint and blood samples may not be significant unless >50 mg/dL
Culture	No growth

♦ Serologic tests for RF (autoantibodies to immunoglobulins) use nephelometry, latex, bentonite, or sheep or human RBCs.

- Use slide test only for screening; confirm positive result with tube dilution (nephelometry, ELISA). Significant titer is >1:80. In RA, titers are often 1:640 to 1:5120 and sometimes ≤1:320,000. Titers in conditions other than RA are usually <1:80.
- Gives useful objective evidence of RA, but a negative result does not rule out RA. Negative in one third of patients with definite RA. Positive result in <50% during first 6 mos of disease. Various methods show S/S = 50% to 75%/75% to 90%. Positive in 80% of "typical" cases; high titers in patients with splenomegaly, vasculitis, subcutaneous nodules, or neuropathy. Titer may decrease during remission but rarely becomes negative. Progressive increases in titer during first 2 years indicate a more severe course.
- Positive in 5% to 10% of healthy population; progressive increase with age in <25% to 30% of persons older than 70 years
- Positive in 5% of rheumatoid variants (arthritis associated with IBD, Reiter syndrome, juvenile RA, rheumatoid spondylitis, tophaceous gout, pseudogout)
- Positive in 5% of cases of scleroderma, mixed connective tissue disease, polymyositis, polymyalgia rheumatica
- Positive in 10% to 15% of patients with SLE
- Positive in 90% of patients with primary Sjögren syndrome or cryoglobulinemic purpura
- Positive in 10% to 40% of patients with Waldenstrom macroglobulinemia, chronic infections (e.g., syphilis, leprosy, brucellosis, TB, SBE), viral infections (e.g., hepatitis, EBV infection, influenza, vaccinations [positive in ≤10% of cases of parvovirus B19-associated arthritis]), parasitic diseases (e.g., malaria, schistosomiasis, trypanosomiasis, filariasis), chronic liver disease, chronic pulmonary interstitial fibrosis, etc.
- Positive in ≤20% of patients of psoriatic arthritis
- Positive in 25% of patients of sarcoid arthritis
- Negative in osteoarthritis, ankylosing spondylitis, rheumatic fever, suppurative arthritis; ANA present in up to 28% of patients; low titer anti-native DNA may be present.

♦ ANA Profile: RA nuclear antigen is found in 85% to 95% of patients.
♦ RF is present in ~80% of patients. Frequently present in Sjögren syndrome; less often in other connective tissue diseases; occasionally in chronic infections (e.g., SBE, gammopathies).
Histones are found in 20% of patients.

Serum complement is usually normal except in patients with vasculitis; depressed level is usually associated with very high levels of RF and immune complexes (see Chapter 3 and Table 16-1).

Immune complexes—monoclonal RF and C1q binding assays are positive more frequently in RA than other assays but correlate poorly with disease activity. Positive test for mixed cryoglobulins indicates presence of immune complexes and is associated with increased incidence of extra-articular manifestations, especially vasculitis. Not clinically useful.

Increased ESR, CRP, and other acute phase reactants. ESR and CRP are often used as guide to activity and to therapy, but may be normal in 5% of patients. Very high ESR (>100 mm/hr) is distinctly unusual in early cases.

WBC is usually normal; there may be a slight increase early in active disease.

Mild thrombocytosis occurs frequently as an acute phase reactant.

Serum protein electrophoresis shows increase in globulins, especially in γ and α_2 globulins, and decreased albumin.

Moderate normocytic hypochromic anemia of chronic disease (see Chapter 11) with decreased serum iron, normal TIBC, and normal iron stores (serum ferritin and bone marrow iron); not responsive to iron, folic acid, vitamin B_{12}, or splenectomy. If HCT <26%, search for other cause of anemia (e.g., GI tract bleeding). Anemia diminishes as patient goes into remission or responds to therapy.

Serum CK is decreased below normal in >60% of patients; not associated with decreased serum aldolase and myosin indicating not due to general impairment of muscle function.

Serum calcium, phosphorus, ALP, uric acid, and ASOT are normal.

Synovial biopsy is especially useful in monoarticular form to rule out TB, gout, etc.

Synovial fluid glucose may be greatly decreased (<10 mg/dL), mucin clotting is fair to poor (see Table 10-6).

Laboratory findings due to extra-articular involvement (usually occur late in severe disease) (e.g., pleural or pericardial effusion, interstitial pulmonary fibrosis)

Laboratory findings due to therapeutic drugs (e.g., salicylates, NSAIDs, gold, penicillamine); see Amyloidosis.

Juvenile Rheumatoid Arthritis

Group of inflammatory arthropathies affecting patients <16 years old for ≥6 weeks and other causes have been excluded; four types based on clinical symptoms

No laboratory tests are diagnostic.

Reported incidence of RF and ANAs varies depending on clinical type and laboratory technique—may be negative.

Laboratory findings due to associated conditions (e.g., psoriasis)

Felty Syndrome

Occurs in 1% of patients with far-advanced RA associated with splenomegaly and leukopenia

♦ Serologic tests for RF are positive in high titers.

ANAs are usually present. Titers of immune complexes are high and complement levels are lower than those in patients with RA.

Leukopenia (<2,500/μL) and granulocytopenia are present.

Anemia and thrombocytopenia due to hypersplenism may occur and respond to splenectomy.

Psoriasis-Associated Arthritis

Inflammatory arthropathy that occurs in <2% of patients with psoriasis [chronic autoimmune skin disease]. There is no correlation between skin activity and joint manifestations; either one may precede the other.

Increased serum uric acid is due to increased turnover of skin cells in psoriasis.

Serologic tests for RF are negative; should not be classified as RA.

♦ No characteristic laboratory findings

Reiter Syndrome

Triad of acute inflammatory arthritis, urethritis, and conjunctivitis present in ≤33% of patients; additional features may include dermatitis, buccal ulcerations, circinate balanitis, keratosis blennorrhagica, and ocular manifestations

MUSCULOSKEL

Table 10-6. Synovial Fluid Findings in Various Diseases of Joints

Property	Normal	Noninflammatory[a]	Hemorrhagic[b]		Acute Inflammatory[c]				Septic		
					Acute Gouty Arthritis	RF	RA		TB Arthritis	Gonorrheal Arthritis	Septic Arthritis[e,f]
Volume	3.5 mL	I	I		I				I		
Appearance	Clear, colorless	Clear, straw	Blood or xanthochromic		Turbid yellow				Turbid yellow		
Viscosity	High	High	V		D				D		
Fibrin clot	0	Usually 0	Usually 0		+				+		
Mucin clot[d]	Good	Good	V		Fair to poor				Poor		
WBC (no./cu mm)[g]	<200	<5,000	<10,000	Range	750–45,000	300–98,000	300–75,000		2,500–105,000	1,500–108,000	15,600–213,000
				Average	13,500	17,800	15,500		23,500	14,000	65,400
Neutrophils (%)	<25	<25	<50	Range	48–94	8–98	5–96		29–96	2–96	75–100
				Average	83	46	65		67	64	95
Blood-synovia[h] glucose difference (mg/dL)[i]	<10	<10	<25	Range	0–41		0–88		0–108	0–97	40–122
				Average	12	6	31		57	25	71

(continued)

Property	Normal	Noninflam-matory[a]	Hemorrhagic[b]	Acute Gouty Arthritis	RF	RA	TB Arthritis	Gonorrheal Arthritis	Septic Arthritis[e,f]
Culture[j]	Neg	Neg	Neg	Neg	Neg	Neg	See Infective Arthritis.		

I, increased; D, decreased; Neg, negative; V, variable; WBC, white blood count; +, positive.

[a]For example, degenerative joint disease, traumatic arthritis, some cases of pigmented villonodular synovitis.

[b]For example, tumor, hemophilia, neuroarthropathy, trauma, some cases of pigmented villonodular synovitis.

[c]For example, RA, Reiter's syndrome, acute gouty arthritis, acute pseudogout, SLE

[d]Mucin clot test adds little additional information to WBC count.

[e]For example, pneumococcal

[f]In purulent arthropathy of undetermined cause, very high synovial fluid lactate (>2,00) mg/dL) indicates a nongonococcal septic arthritis (Gram-negative bacilli, Gram-positive cocci, fungi). Lactate is <100 mg/dL in gonococcal infection, gout, RA, osteoarthritis, trauma.

[g]Use saline instead of acetic acid, which clumps the joint fluid.

[h]Glucose concentration may give spurious results unless obtained after prolonged fasting, and differences between joint and blood samples may not be significant unless >50 mg/dL.

[i]Joint tap should be performed, preferably after the patient has been fasting for >4 hrs, and a blood glucose determination should be performed simultaneously.

[j]Material should be cultured aerobically and anaerobically. Culture for tubercle bacilli should be performed.

Synovial fluid analysis is primarily useful to diagnose or to rule out infectious arthritis, gout, or pseudogout.

To distinguish inflammatory from noninflammatory conditions, synovial fluid WBC > 2,000/cu mm and > 75% PMNs have sensitivities of 84% and 75% and specificities of 84% and 92%, respectively.

359

Table 10-7. Synovial Fluid Findings in Acute Inflammatory Arthritis of Various Etiologies[a]

Disease	WBC	Complement Activity	Rheumatoid Factor	Crystals[b]	Other Findings
Acute gouty arthritis	I	I	0	Monosodium urate; within PMNs during acute stage	
Acute chondrocalcinosis	I	I	0	Calcium pyrophosphate	
Reiter syndrome	Markedly I	Markedly I	0		Macrophages with ingested leukocytes
Rheumatoid arthritis	I	Low	Usually +		
Juvenile rheumatoid arthritis	I	Low	0		Abundant lymphocytes (sometimes >50%); immature lymphocytes and monocytes present
Systemic lupus erythematosus	Usually very low	Low or 0	V	0	LE cells may be present
Arthritis associated with psoriasis, ulcerative colitis, ankylosing spondylitis	I	I			

0, absent; +, positive; I, increased; LE, lupus erythematosus; V, variable.

[a]Measurement of rheumatoid factor and complement in synovial fluid is rarely helpful; antinuclear antibody determination is not useful.

[b]Crystals of gout and pseudogout should be identified *within* polymorphonuclear neutrophils using polarised light microscopy. Finding of characteristic crystals is diagnostic of gout and of chondrocalcinosis. Must be differentiated from crystals of corticosteroid esters and cholesterol or talc (after recent joint infections). Crystals are engulfed by WBCs during acute attack but between acute episodes may lie free in fluid.

Table 10-8.	Serologic Tests in Various Rheumatoid Diseases			
Disease[a]	ANA[b]	RF[c]	Serum Complement	LE Clot[d]
SLE	100 (H)	30–40	D	70–80
Rheumatoid arthritis				
Adult	50 (L–M)	80–90	N or I	5–15
Juvenile	<5 (L–M)	15	N	<5
Mixed connective tissue disease	100 (M–H)	50	N or I	20
Dermatomyositis	25	10–15	N	<5
Scleroderma	25–40	33	N	<5
Polyarteritis nodosa	<5 (L)	5–10	N or D	<5
Sjögren syndrome	95 (M–H)	75	N or D	20
Ankylosing spondylitis	5–10	<5	N	<5

Numbers = percentage of cases positive for each test. D, decreased; I, increased; N, normal.
[a]Normal ESR in patients with nonspecific rheumatic symptoms suggests fibromyositis rather than any of the above disorders.
[b]ANA, fluorescent antinuclear antibody; H, titer >1:200; M–H, titer 1:100–1:200; L–M, titer 1:20–1:100; ANA titer ≥1:160 with suggestive pattern and clinical setting is very helpful diagnostically, but when titer is negative, other laboratory tests are not productive. Anti–DNA antibodies correlate best with a diagnosis of SLE; they are positive in <5% of patients with other immunologic diseases. Diagnosis of SLE is barely credible without a positive ANA test.
[c]Positive rheumatoid factor (RF) test shows a significantly higher titer in RA than in other collagen diseases, but diagnosis is primarily clinical rather than serologic. Serial titers are not helpful to follow response to treatment since antiglobulins remain at constant levels despite clinical status. Frequently positive at low to moderate titers in polyclonal hypergammaglobulinemia (e.g., SLE, sarcoidosis, cirrhosis, active viral hepatitis, some acute viral infections).
Measurement of RF and complement in synovial fluid is rarely helpful; ANA determination is not useful. Crystals of gout and pseudogout should be identified *within* PMNs.
[d]Lupus erythematosus (LE) cells in peripheral blood clot preparation. Now rarely used.

Increased acute phase reactants

• Increased ESR parallels the clinical course.
• Increased CRP
• WBC is increased (10,000–20,000/μL), as is the granulocyte count.

Moderate normochromic anemia
Serum globulins are increased in long-standing disease.
Culture or serologic evidence of preceding infections (e.g., *Chlamydia, Campylobacter, Salmonella, Shigella*) is associated in ≤10% of these infections. Nonbacterial cystitis, prostatitis, or seminal vesiculitis and subclinical infection of ileum and colon occur.
Synovial fluid shows 1,000 to 8,000 WBCs; culture is negative.
HLA-B27 is found in up to 90% of white patients; not diagnostically useful.

Ankylosing Spondylitis (Marie-Strumpell Disease)

Inflammatory disorder of axial skeleton of unknown etiology; ocular involvement in ≤40%

♦ There is no diagnostic laboratory test for this disorder.
ESR is increased in ≤80% of patients.
Mild to moderate hypochromic anemia develops in ≤30% of patients.
Serologic tests for RF are positive in <15% of patients with arthritis of the vertebral region only.
CSF protein is moderately increased in ≤50% of patients.
Secondary amyloidosis develops in 6% of patients.
Laboratory findings due to carditis and aortitis with aortic insufficiency, which occur in 1% to 4% of patients
Laboratory findings of frequently associated diseases (e.g., chronic ulcerative colitis, regional ileitis, psoriasis) are noted.

MUSCULOSKEL

Histocompatibility antigen HLA-B27 is found in 95% of these white patients and in lesser numbers with variants of this condition. ~20% of carriers of HLA-B27 have ankylosing spondylitis but it is not helpful in establishing the diagnosis.

Ochronosis

See Alkaptonuria (Chapter 12).

Arthritis, Infective

◆ Joint fluid (See Table 10-6.)

* Bacterial
    In purulent arthritis, organism is recovered from joint in 90% of patients and from blood in 50% of patients. Most often due to *S. aureus* (60%) and *Streptococcus* species.
    Gram stain is positive in ~50% of patients; it is particularly useful for establishing diagnosis promptly and in cases in which cultures are negative.
    Culture may be negative because of prior administration of antibiotics.
    In TB arthritis, Gram stain and bacterial cultures are negative, but acid-fast stain, culture, and biopsy of synovia confirm the diagnosis.
    In children, most common organisms are *H. influenzae* type b, *S. aureus*, various streptococci, and gram-negative bacilli.
    In young adults, >50% of cases are due to *Neisseria gonorrhoeae*; rest are due to *S. aureus*, streptococci, or gram-negative bacilli.
* Viral (e.g., mumps, rubella, HBV, parvovirus B-19)
* Fungal (e.g., *Sporothrix schenckii*, *Coccidioides immitis*, *Candida*, *Blastomyces dermatitidis*)
* If 5 biopsies are cultured, bacterial growth in ≤2 or only in broth media indicates contamination, but growth in all 5 in solid and broth media suggests infection.

Laboratory findings due to preexisting infections (e.g., subacute bacterial endocarditis, meningococcic meningitis, pneumococcal pneumonia, typhoid, gonorrhea, Lyme disease, TB, rat-bite fever, syphilis)
Infection of prosthetic joints

* Early onset (within first 3 months)
* Delayed onset (within first 2 years—two thirds of patients)
    Due to organisms introduced during surgery or to those of nosocomial infection, which multiply slowly (50% of cases occur >1 year later). Most common are skin flora (e.g., *Staph. epidermidis*, other coagulase-negative staphylococci, *Corynebacterium* sp.)
* Late onset (after 2 years—one third of cases)
    Due to hematogenous seeding from infected focus (e.g., GU tract, dental)
* Increased WBC and ESR support diagnosis of infection rather than aseptic loosening of prosthesis.

Mucin clot test adds little additional information to WBC count; is rarely used now
Glucose concentration may give spurious results unless obtained after prolonged fasting, and differences between joint and blood samples may not be significant unless >50 mg/dL.
Crystals are engulfed by WBC during acute attack but between acute episodes may lie free in fluid.

Crystalline Arthropathy

Chondrocalcinosis ("Pseudogout")

Inflammatory mono- or polyarticular arthritis due to deposition of calcium pyrophosphate dehydrate crystals in joints

◆ Joint fluid contains crystals identified as calcium pyrophosphate dehydrate, inside and outside of WBCs, and macrophages that are differentiated from urate crystals under polarized light, which distinguishes them from gout. See Tables 10-6, 10-7, and 10-9. Crystals may also be identified by other means (e.g., chemical, x-ray diffraction).

Blood and urine findings are normal.
Laboratory findings due to associated conditions (e.g., hyperparathyroidism, hypothyroidism, acromegaly, hemochromatosis, gout, hypomagnesemia, degenerative arthritis)

Gout

Group of disorders of purine metabolism characterized by monosodium urate crystal deposits in joints and soft tissues, episodes of acute inflammatory arthritis [response to crystal deposits], and hyperuricemia. Most uric acid is synthesized in liver and intestinal mucosa. Two thirds excreted by kidney; one third excreted by bowel.

Due To
Primary (i.e., inborn) (30% of patients)
  Idiopathic
  Increased purine biosynthesis
  Lesch-Nyhan syndrome
Secondary (70% of patients)
  Overproduction (10% of secondary cases); overexcreters: >750 to 1,000 mg/day of uric acid

  • Neoplastic and hemolytic conditions (e.g., leukemia, polycythemia vera, secondary polycythemia, malignant lymphomas). Blood dyscrasias are found in ~10% of patients with clinical gout.
  • Psoriasis

  Increased breakdown of adenosine triphosphate

  • Glycogen storage diseases (I, III, V, VII)
  • Alcohol ingestion
  • Myocardial infarction
  Decreased renal function (90% of secondary cases); underexcreters: <700 mg/day of uric acid

  • Decreased renal clearance
  Chronic renal disease
  Chronic lead intoxication
  Increased organic acids (e.g., lactate, β-hydroxybutyrate in diabetic ketoacidosis, acute ethanol intoxication, toxemia of pregnancy, starvation)
Also associated with hypertension (in one third of patients with gout), familial hypercholesterolemia, obesity, acute intermittent porphyria, sarcoidosis, parathyroid dysfunction, myxedema

  • Drugs (e.g., diuretics, aspirin, cyclosporin) (≤20% of cases). May cause ≤50% of all new cases of gouty arthritis; this occurs later in life and in women is more common than primary gout.

♦ **Diagnostic Criteria:** Presence of crystals of monosodium urate from tophi or joint fluid viewed microscopically under polarized light—strongly negative birefringent needle-shaped crystals both *inside* and outside PMNs or macrophages; differentiates it from pseudogout. Found in 90% of patients during an acute attack. Found in synovial fluid in 75% of patients between attacks.

○ Increased serum uric acid

• Does *not* establish the diagnosis of gout.
• Is normal in 30% of acute attacks. Several determinations may be required to establish increased values; beware of serum levels reduced to normal range as a result of recent aspirin use. Changes in therapy may cause wide fluctuations in serum uric acid levels. The incidence of gout occurring at various uric acid levels in men was found to be: 1.1% at <6 mg/dL, 7.3% at 6 to 6.9 mg/dL, 14.2% at 7 to

MUSCULOSKEL

Table 10-9.   Birefringent Materials in Synovial Fluid

Material	Usual Shape, Size	Birefringence	Cause	Location Within or Outside of PMNs, Macrophages
Crystals				
Monosodium urate	Needle, rod, parallel edges; 8–10 μm long	Strongly −	Gout	Within or outside
Calcium pyrophosphate dihydrate	Rhomboid; may be rod, diamond, square, needle; <10 μm long	Weakly +	Pseudogout	Only within
Calcium oxalate	Bipyramidal	Strong; 0	Long-term renal dialysis	Within or outside
Hydroxyapatite, other basic calcium phosphates	Aggregates only; small, (<1 μm), round, irregular	Weak; 0	Degenerating, calcifying joint (e.g., acute or chronic arthritis)	
Cholesterol	Flat, plate, corner notch; may be needle, rectangle; often >100 μm	Variable		
Cartilage, collagen	Irregular, rodlike	Strong; +		
Charcot-Leyden	Spindle; crystalloids of eosinophil membrane protein	Variable	Eosinophilic synovitis	
Steroids			Injection into joint	
Betamethasone acetate	Rods; blunt ends; 10–20 μm	Strong; −		
Cortisone acetate	Large rods	Strong; +		
Methyl prednisone acetate	Small, pleomorphic; tend to clump	Strong; 0		
Prednisone tebutate	Small, pleomorphic, branched, irregular	Strong; +		
Triamcinolone acetonide	Small, pleomorphic fragments; tend to clump	Strong; 0		
Triamcinolone hexacetonide	Large rods, blunt ends; 15–60 μm	Strong; 0		

(continued)

Table 10-9. *(continued)*

Material	Usual Shape, Size	Birefringence	Cause	Location Within or Outside of PMNs, Macrophages
Anticoagulants			Injection into joint	
EDTA (dry)	Small, amorphous	Weak		
Lithium heparin (not sodium)	May resemble pseudogout	Weak; +		
Other Materials				
Debris	Small, irregular, nonparallel edges	Variable		
Fat (cholesterol esters)	Globules	Strong Maltese cross		
Starch granules	Round; size varies	Strong Maltese cross		

+, positive birefringence; −, negative birefringence; 0, no axis
EDTA = ethylenediaminetetraacetic acid
Crystals are best seen in fresh, wet-mount preparations examined with polarizing light.
Hydroxyapatite complexes [diagnostic of apatite disease] and basic calcium phosphate complexes can be identified only by EM and MS; most cases are suspected clinically but never confirmed.
(From Judkins SW, Cornbleet PJ. Synovial fluid crystal analysis. *Lab Med.* 1997;28:774.)

7.9 mg/dL, 18.7% at 8 to 8.9%, 83% at ≥9 mg/dL, 90% at 10 mg/dL. Many gout patients have levels <8 mg/dL and >1/3 never have an elevated level. Since the mean interval between first and second gout attacks is 11.4 years and only 25% have a second attack within 12 years, drug therapy for this group may not be cost effective.

- Serum uric acid is increased in ~25% of asymptomatic relatives.
- About 10% of adult males have increased serum uric acid.
- Only 1% to 3% of patients with hyperuricemia have gout.
- Secondary hyperuricemia usually produces much higher serum uric acid than primary type. If serum uric acid is >10 mg/dL, underlying malignancy should be considered after renal failure has been ruled out.

○ Uric acid stones develop 3 to 10× more frequently in gouty patients than in the general population even though 75% of gouty patients have normal 24-hour excretion of uric acid. When serum uric acid is <9 mg/dL or urine level is <700 mg/24 hours, risk of renal calculi is <21%; when serum uric acid is >13 mg/dL or urine level is >1,100 mg/24 hours, risk is >50%. With primary gout, 10% to 25% of patients develop uric acid stones; in 40% of them, the stones appear >5 years before an episode of gout.

24-hour urine uric acid excretion:

- If >600 mg/24 hours, it should be repeated after 5 day purine-free diet
- If <600 mg/24 hours or urine uric acid:creatinine ratio <0.6 and no history of kidney or GU tract disease, treatment of hyperuricemia is with probenecid.
- If >600 mg/24 hours or urine uric acid:creatinine ratio >0.8 or there is history of GU tract or kidney disease, allopurinol is drug of choice.
- Uric acid:creatinine ratios 0.6 to 0.8 are indeterminate; ratios of 0.2 to 0.6 are considered normal or indicate underexcretion.
- 700 to 1,000 mg/24 hours is considered borderline.
  >1,000 mg/24 hours is abnormal and is indication for treatment in patients with asymptomatic hyperuricemia.

MUSCULOSKEL

Uric acid crystals and amorphous urates are *normal* findings in urinary sediment.
Low-grade proteinuria occurs in 20% to 80% of gouty persons for many years before
    further evidence of renal disease appears.
♦ Histologic examination of gouty nodule is characteristic.
Moderate leukocytosis and increased ESR occur during acute attacks; normal at other
    times.
RF is detectable in low titers in 10% of patients with gout or pseudogout; but RA rarely
    coexists with these conditions.
Serum triglycerides are frequently increased, resulting in a high frequency of types IIb
    and IV lipoprotein patterns; HDL-cholesterol level is frequently decreased.
See Tables 10-6, 10-7, 10-9 and sections on renal disease (Chapter 14) and serum uric
    acid (Chapter 3).

Osteoarthritis

**Noninflammatory degenerative arthritis with loss of cartilage and resultant hyper-
trophic changes in adjacent bone. May be primary [idiopathic] or secondary to
metabolic, trauma, inflammation, etc.**

Laboratory tests are normal and not helpful.
Synovial fluid is yellow clear, noninflammatory (<2,000 WBC/μL), normal viscosity.

Arthritis Associated with Systemic Disease

Arthritis Associated with Hemochromatosis

Degenerative arthropathy occurs in >20% of these patients

Laboratory findings of hemochromatosis (See Chapter 8)
Negative RF
No subcutaneous nodules
Biopsy of synovia shows striking iron deposits in synovial lining but not in deeper cells
    or macrophages, differentiating it from hemarthrosis, RA
Synovial fluid is usually pale yellow, noninflammatory, adequate viscosity, low WBC
    count (mostly mononuclear cells). Iron levels comparable to serum.
May be associated with chondrocalcinosis

Arthritis Associated with Inflammatory Bowel Disease (Ulcerative Colitis/Regional Enteritis)

**Characterized by sacroiliitis with or without spondylitis [in ≤20% of patients
with Crohn disease] or acute synovitis [monoarticular or polyarticular] with
absent RF**

See Chapter 7
Joint fluid is sterile on the basis of both bacteriological and microscopical findings. It is
    similar to fluid of RA and Whipple disease (cell count, differential count, specific gravity,
    viscosity, protein, glucose, poor mucin clot formation). Joint fluid examination is princi-
    pally useful in evaluating monarticular involvement to rule out suppurative arthritis.
Synovial biopsy findings are similar to RA biopsy findings.
Absent RF and ANAs
Laboratory findings due to the bowel disease (e.g., increased CRP, ESR, WBC,
    increased platelets)

Others

Many other systemic diseases that are not primarily disorders of muscle, bone, or
    synovia are associated with arthritis/arthralgias and are too numerous to list here.
    Some examples include infections, autoimmune/connective tissue diseases,
    immunodeficiency disorders, vasculitides, etc.

Polymyalgia Rheumatica

No well-defined pathologic lesions are present; may be low-grade synovitis.

○ ESR is increased (usually >60 mm/hr) for >1 month; this is a criterion for diagnosis. Anemia of chronic disease is commonly present.

WBC may be increased in some patients.

Abnormalities of serum proteins are frequent, although there is no consistent or diagnostic pattern. Most frequently the albumin is decreased with an increase in α-1 and α-2 globulins and fibrinogen.

Cryoglobulins are sometimes present.

RF is usually negative; present in serum in 5% to 10% of patients over 60 without arthritis.

Serum enzymes (e.g., AST, ALP) may be increased in one third of patients.

○ Muscle biopsy specimen is usually normal or may show mild nonspecific changes.

○ Temporal artery biopsy findings are often positive because one third of patients with giant cell arteritis present with polymyalgia rheumatica, which ultimately develops in 50% to 90% of them (see Temporal Arteritis).

11 Hematology

HEMATOLOGY

General Hematologic Laboratory Tests

Bone Marrow Analysis[1]

Cellularity to fat ratio: 100% at birth; declines ~10% each decade; young children = 9:1; young adults 2:1; middle age = 1:1; elderly gradually decreases to 1:9.

Use

Diagnosis of some cancers (e.g., leukemias, lymphomas, multiple myeloma, metastases)

Nonhematopoietic neoplasms (e.g., neuroblastoma, other childhood tumors)

Staging of Hodgkin disease and non-Hodgkin lymphomas (NHLs)

Dysproteinemias and plasma cell disorders

Tumor involving bone marrow (may show "leukoerythroblastic" peripheral blood picture)

Aplastic anemia, agranulocytosis, cytopenia

Megaloblastic anemias, iron deficiency

Idiopathic thrombocytopenic purpura, thrombotic thrombocytopenic purpura

Myelofibrosis due to, e.g., agnogenic myeloid metaplasia and other myelodysplasias; metastatic carcinoma; miliary tuberculosis (TB); granulomatous diseases; exposure to drugs, chemicals (e.g., benzene), or radiation (e.g., for lymphoma); Paget disease; parathyroid disease

Monitor recovery in marrow-ablative chemotherapy or bone marrow transplants

Infectious diseases and fever of unknown origin (culture, identify organisms)

Lysosomal storage diseases

Amyloidosis

Unexplained anemia, splenomegaly, lymphadenopathy, hepatomegaly

Tests May Include

Smear (Wright-Giemsa, Prussian blue for iron, cytochemistry, organisms)

Touch prep (Wright-Giemsa)

Paraffin sections (hematoxylin-eosin [H&E], periodic acid–Schiff [PAS], reticulin and fibrous tissue, organisms, immunohistochemistry, molecular diagnostics)

Flow cytometry

Cytogenetics (e.g., prognosis in leukemias and lymphomas; distinguish reactive from neoplastic processes; identify various translocations, deletions, fusions)

Molecular genetics (e.g., polymerase chain reaction [PCR] detection of viral DNA and RNA; fluorescence in situ hybridization [FISH] detection of chromosome abnormalities in blood or marrow smears)

HEMATOLOGY

---

[1]Cotelingam JD. Bone marrow interpretation: the science and the art. *Pathol Case Revs* 2000; 5:239.

Microbial cultures
Cytochemistry (e.g., acid phosphatase in hairy cell leukemia)
Electron microscopy
Tissue culture

Bone Marrow Stainable Iron (Hemosiderin)

Bone marrow stainable iron is present in reticuloendothelial (RE) cells and developing normoblasts (sideroblasts).

Use
Is the gold standard for diagnosis of iron deficiency; its presence almost invariably rules out iron-deficiency anemia (IDA). Marrow iron disappears before the peripheral blood changes. Only individuals with decreased marrow iron are likely to benefit from iron therapy.
Diagnosis of iron overload.

Interferences
May be normal or increased by injections of iron dextran (which is utilized very slowly), despite other evidence of IDA

Increased In
Anemias of chronic disease (e.g., uremia, chronic infections, cirrhosis, neoplasms, rheumatoid arthritis [RA])
Megaloblastic anemias in relapse
Idiopathic hemochromatosis and hemochromatosis secondary to

- Increased intake (e.g., Bantu siderosis, excessive medicine ingestion, repeated transfusions)
- Anemias with increased erythropoiesis (especially thalassemia major; also thalassemia minor, some other hemoglobinopathies, paroxysmal nocturnal hemoglobinuria, refractory anemias with hypercellular bone marrow, etc.). In hemolytic anemias, decrease or absence may signify acute hemolytic crisis.
- Liver injury (e.g., following portal shunt surgery)
- Atransferrinemia

Sideroblastic anemia
Decreased In
Iron deficiency (e.g., inadequate dietary intake, chronic bleeding, malignancy, acute blood loss)
Rapidly disappears after hemorrhage
Polycythemia vera (usually absent in polycythemia vera but usually normal or increased in secondary polycythemia)
Pernicious anemia (PA) in early phase of therapy
Myeloproliferative diseases—iron stores may be absent without other evidence of iron deficiency
Congenital atransferrinemia
Collagen diseases (especially systemic lupus erythematosus [SLE])
Infiltration of marrow (e.g., malignant lymphomas, metastatic carcinoma, myelofibrosis, miliary granulomas)
Chronic infection (e.g., pulmonary TB, bronchiectasis, chronic pyelonephritis)
Miscellaneous conditions (e.g., old age, diabetes mellitus, newborns)
Serum iron and total iron-binding capacity (TIBC) may be normal in IDA, especially if hemoglobin (Hb) is <9 g/dL.

Bone Marrow Cellularity

Decreased In
Normal aging
Aplastic anemias (e.g., drugs, toxins, radiation)
Infections (e.g., viral)
Preleukemic states (e.g., paroxysmal nocturnal hemoglobinuria [PNH])
Congenital (e.g., Fanconi anemia)
Idiopathic
Increased In
Newborns
Myeloproliferative conditions (e.g., leukemias and preleukemias)

Lymphoproliferative conditions
Leukemoid reactions
Some anemias (e.g., PA, hemolytic anemia, some refractory anemias)
Others (e.g., hypersplenism)

Enzyme Immunoassay

The enzyme immunoassay (EIA) is a nonisotopic immunoassay using enzymes (most commonly horseradish peroxidase), coenzymes, enzyme inhibitors, or fluorogenic substrates as labels for antigens or antibodies. The enzyme-linked immunosorbent assay (ELISA) is the most commonly used type of EIA.

Use
Quantification of most clotting factors, fibrinolytic components, regulatory substances; can detect attomole quantities
Serologic tests for infectious diseases

Flow Cytometry[2,3]

Flow cytometry identifies and counts single cells labeled by fluorochrome monoclonal antibodies to specific surface or intracellular antigens associated with cell lineage (e.g., T-lymphocyte versus B-lymphocyte), cell function (presence of cytokines or other receptors), degree of maturation (e.g., pre-B or mature B cells).

Use
Suitable specimens include peripheral blood, bone marrow aspirates and core biopsies, fine-needle aspirates, fresh tissue biopsies, all body fluids.
Diagnosis, characterization, and monitoring of hematologic malignancies.

- Distinguish myeloid and lymphoid lineage in acute and minimally differentiated leukemia
- Diagnosis of immunodeficiency disorders by immunophenotyping; prognosis
- Diagnosis of PNII
- Monitor effect of therapy
- Detect minimal residual disease in cerebrospinal fluid (CSF) or bone marrow

Enumeration of lymphocyte subsets e.g., CD4[+] T-cells as surrogate marker for disease progression in AIDS.
Using anti-HbF monoclonal antibodies to detect HbF (can detect <0.05% fetal red blood cells [RBCs]):

- More accurate than Kleihauer-Betke stain for quantitation of fetal-maternal hemorrhage.
- Detect increased number of RBCs containing decreased HbF ("F" cells) in hemoglobinopathies, some patients with myelodysplasia.

Diagnosis of PNH, myelodysplasia, and systemic mastocytosis.
Diagnose DNA content (aneuploidy) and DNA synthetic activity of tumors (assessing degree of malignancy, e.g., breast cancer).
Measure apoptosis
Detect multiple drug resistance in cancer chemotherapy (e.g., due to overexpression of P-glycoprotein and other proteins).
Histocompatibility crossmatch of organs for transplantation and in stem cell transplantation.
CD34[+] stem cell counting in peripheral blood or bone marrow graft correlates with success of graft and length of hematopoietic recovery after stem cell transplantation.
Measure cell-bound antibody and sort subpopulations that differ in amount of bound antibody.
Reticulocyte counting (e.g., anemias, vitamin deficiencies, regenerative activity in bone marrow transplantation). Also, determination of reticulocyte maturation index and immature reticulocyte fraction (e.g., monitoring anemias).
Human leukocyte antigen B27 (HLA-B27) determination.

HEMATOLOGY

[2]Davis BH. Diagnostic utility of red cell flow cytometric analysis. *Clin Lab Med* 2001;21:829–840.
[3]Dunphy CH. Applications of flow cytometry and immunohistochemistry to diagnostic hematopathology *Arch Pathol Lab Med* 2004;1128:1004–1022.

Detect antineutrophil antibodies bound to granulocytes or free in plasma.
Neutrophil function studies in immunodeficiency (e.g., phagocytosis, oxidative burst, immunophenotyping), as in chronic granulomatous disease.
Mitogen stimulation evaluation of T cells.
In transfusion medicine:

- Detect and quantitate low levels of immunoglobulins bound to RBCs not detected by direct antiglobulin (Coombs) test (DAT) in patients with hemolysis
- Detect RBC chimerisms
- Accurate RBC phenotyping after multiple transfusions
- Platelet cross-matching
- Assess leukocyte contamination of blood products

In transplantation

- Stem cell transplantation: adequacy of CD34 counts in donors or pheresis
- Detection of HLA alloantibodies in solid organ transplantation

Platelet function, e.g., surface receptor measurement and distribution in diagnosis of congenital platelet function disorders (gpIIb/IIIa in Glanzmann thrombasthenia; gpIb in Bernard-Soulier disease), measure platelet-associated IgG in immune thrombocytopenia, others.
RBC survival studies using RBCs labeled with biotin instead of chromium-51 (^{51}Cr).
Detection of intracellular parasites (e.g., *Babesia, Plasmodium, Trypanosoma*) using RNA- and DNA-binding fluorochromes that bind to parasites.
In microbiology, detection of specific antibodies; detection of presence of heterogeneous populations with different responses to antimicrobial treatments.
Not recommended for diagnosis of Hodgkin lymphoma, chronic myelogenous leukemia (CML), or myelodysplastic syndrome but can use for monitoring in latter two disorders.

Molecular Diagnosis of Hematologic Disorders

Use
RBC disorders

- Hereditary spherocytosis and pyropoikilocytosis
- Hereditary nonspherocytic hemolytic anemia—pyruvate kinase deficiency
- Hemolytic anemia—glucose-6-phosphate dehydrogenase (G6PD) deficiency
- Porphyrias

Hemoglobinopathies, e.g.:

- Sickle cell anemia and HbC, SC, E, D diseases; β- and α-thalassemias
- Hemoglobinopathies with unstable hemoglobins
- Hereditary persistence of HbF

Neutrophil disorders, e.g.:

- Chronic granulomatous disease
- Myeloperoxidase deficiency
- Glutathione reductase and synthetase deficiencies

Coagulation disorders (e.g., hemophilia A and B, von Willebrand disease, inherited resistance to activated protein C)
Neoplasias

- Establish or confirm diagnosis
- Determine stage of disease
- Detect minimal residual disease
- Predict outcome

Tests of Red Blood Cell Function and Morphology

Blood Smear[4]

See Figure 11-1.

[4]Pierre RV. Red cell morphology and the peripheral blood film. *Clin Lab Med* 2002;22:25–61.

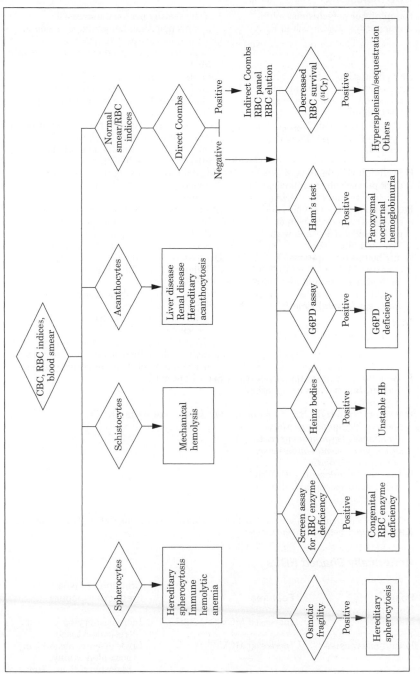

Fig. 11-1. Sequence of laboratory tests for hemolytic anemia with normal electrophoresis. CBC, complete blood count; RBC, red blood cell; Hb, hemoglobin; 51Cr, chromium-51; G6PD, glucose-6-phosphate dehydrogenase.

HEMATOLOGY

The smear may also confirm the RBC indices or indicate leukemia or other conditions.

RBC Inclusions

Basophilic or polychromatophilic macrocytes (RBCs rich in RNA)	≤15 in healthy persons. Increased erythropoiesis in hemorrhage or hemolysis. Called reticulocytes if supravital stain. Owing to polyribosomes producing Hb. Increased MCV.
Basophilic stippling (composed of ribosomes and remnants of mitochondria homogenously distributed)	Anemias (especially pyrimidine 5'-nucleotidase deficiency; megaloblastic), alcoholism, lead or arsenic poisoning. Drying artifact.
Microcytes with stippling	Thalassemia. Lead or heavy metal poisoning.
Cabot rings (mitotic spindle remnants)	Occasional in severe hemolytic and megaloblastic anemias, overwhelming infection, postsplenectomy.
Howell-Jolly bodies (one or two dark purple spherical bodies) (nuclear remnants of DNA)	Megaloblastic anemia; thalassemia; myelodysplasia, lead poisoning, postsplenectomy state.
Pappenheimer bodies (siderotic granules) nonheme iron at periphery of RBC seen with Prussian blue stain.	Anemias with defect of incorporating iron into Hb (e.g., sideroblastic anemias, thalassemia, lead poisoning, postsplenectomy state). Iron overload.
Heinz bodies (precipitates of denatured Hb attached to RBC membranes) (are not seen with Wright stain; requires supravital stain, e.g., crystal violet.)	Decreased RBC enzymes (e.g., G6PD deficiency, metHb reductase; often in >50% of RBCs). Drug-induced hemolytic anemias (e.g., dapsone, phenacetin). Unstable Hb (e.g., Zurich). After splenectomy. Artifactual (e.g., exposing blood to oxidizers such as phenylhydrazine, incubating blood at room temperature for several hours).
Plasmodium trophozoites, *Babesia microti, Babesia divergens,* other organisms.	See Chapter 15.
Wuchereria bancrofti, Brugia malayi, Loa loa; Trypanosoma brucei gambiense, Trypanosoma cruzi, and *Trypanosoma rhodesiense; Borrelia recurrentis.*	On smear; not within RBCs.
Reticulocytes (not seen with Wright stain; requires supravital stain, e.g., cresyl violet).	

MCV, mean corpuscular volume; RBC, red blood cell; Hb, hemoglobin; G6PD, glucose-6-phosphate dehydrogenase; metHb, methemoglobin.

Abnormally Shaped RBCs

Shape	Features	Condition in which Frequently Occurs
Round		
Macrocytes	Increased MCV (>100 fL).	Increased erythropoiesis (reticulocytosis).
Round macrocytes	Increased MCV.	Liver disease; alcoholism; postsplenectomy; hypothyroidism, after splenectomy.
Oval (macrooval oocytes)	Increased MCV. RBCs lack central pallor.	Megaloblastic anemia, cancer chemotherapy, myelodysplastic syndromes.

Microcytes	Decreased MCV (<80 fL).	Hypochromic anemias. Defective iron supply, absorption, release, or utilization.
Microspherocytes		Artifacts caused by shear force in marrow preparations. Also in severe frostbite.
Spherocytes (loss of membrane)	Increased MCHC (>36%), usually decreased MCV. No central pallor.	Hereditary spherocytosis, autoimmune hemolytic anemia, recent blood transfusion.
Stomatocytes	Slit-like central pallor.	Hereditary stomatocytosis. Rhesus factor null disease. Acute alcoholism (transient). Certain drugs (e.g., phenothiazines). Neoplastic, cardiovascular, hepatobiliary diseases. Artifactual.
Target cells (podocytes) (increased ratio of RBC surface area to volume; thinner RBCs)	Decreased osmotic fragility.	Hemolytic anemia, thalassemias, and hemoglobinopathies (e.g., HbC disease or trait, HbD, HbE, HbS); iron deficiency anemia; liver disease; postsplenectomy state; artifactual.
Torocytes		Doughnut-shaped artifacts caused by slow drying.
Anisocytosis		Marked in severe anemias.
Elongated		
Elliptocytes		Hereditary (>25% in smear). Microcytic anemias (<25% in smear) (e.g., iron deficiency, neoplasms). Sickle cell trait, thalassemia, PA, HbC disease.
Ovalocytes	Egg-shaped.	Megaloblastic anemia.
Teardrop (dacrocyte)		Chronic idiopathic myelofibrosis. Myelophthisis caused by tumor replacement of marrow. Occasionally in other myelodysplasias or myeloproliferative disorders (e.g., spent polycythemia). Also thalassemia (especially homozygous β type), iron deficiency, conditions with Heinz bodies.
Drepanocytes (polymerization of HbS)	Sickle cells	Sickle cell disorders (not in S trait). Normal in white-tailed deer.
HbC crystalloids		HbC trait or disease.
Spiculated		
Acanthocytes (abnormal ratio of membrane lipids)	Pointed membrane spicules of uneven length.	*Hereditary:* Acanthocytosis characterized by abetalipoproteinemia

HEMATOLOGY

		(many are present) (See Chapter 12). *Acquired:* Postsplenectomy state (few are present). Fulminating liver disease (variable number) with low serum cholesterol. Malabsorption.
Echinocytes	Blunt uniform spicules.	Difficult to distinguish from burr cells. Caused by artifact.
Burr cells	Crenated or "animal cracker" RBCs.	Not clinically specific. Upper GI bleeding. Uremia. Liver disease. Rhesus factor null cells. PK deficiency. Anorexia nervosa. Hypophosphatemia; hypomagnesemia. Hyposplenism.
Schistocytes (traumatic destruction of RBC membrane)	Helmet- or triangle-shaped.	Microangiopathic hemolytic anemia (e.g., DIC, TTP); prosthetic heart valves or severe valvular heart disease; severe burns. Renal transplant rejection; snakebite.
"Bite" cells (precipitated Hb [Heinz bodies])		Hemolysis, e.g., due to certain drugs with or without G6PD deficiency, unstable Hb.
RBC fragmentation	Seen on peripheral blood smear (>10/1,000 RBCs) and on histogram of RBC size with automated cell counters.	Cytotoxic chemotherapy for neoplasia; autoimmune hemolytic anemia; severe iron deficiency; megaloblastic anemia; acute leukemia; myelodysplasia, inherited structural abnormality of RBC membrane protein spectrin.

MCV, mean corpuscular volume; RBC, red blood cell, MCHC, mean corpuscular hemoglobin concentration; PA, pernicious anemia; Hb, hemoglobin; GI, gastrointestinal; PK, pyruvate kinase; DIC, disseminated intravascular coagulation; TTP, thrombotic thrombocytopenic purpura.

Other RBC Findings

Rouleaux ("stack of coins")	Abnormal increased proteins (e.g., multiple myeloma). Reversible by saline dilution; does not affect automated RBC counts.
RBC agglutination (due to presence of IgM antibody)	Cold agglutinins (e.g., *Mycoplasma pneumoniae*, infectious mononucleosis). Caused by antibody-antigen reaction. Not reversible by saline dilution; affects automated RBC counts.

RBC, red blood cell; IgM, immunoglobulin M.

Circulating histiocytes in peripheral blood may be seen in severe sepsis (<20% of cases of subacute bacterial endocarditis).
Endothelial cells in peripheral blood rarely may occur in cytomegalovirus infection on terminal edge of routine blood smear.

Protoporphyrin, Free Erythrocyte

A normal free erythrocyte protoporphyrin count is <100 g/dL of packed RBCs.

See Figure 12-7.

Use

Screening for lead poisoning and for iron deficiency. Hematofluorometer is used for simultaneously screening populations for both iron deficiency and lead poisoning.

Increased In

Iron deficiency (even prior to anemia; thus, is early sensitive sign and useful for screening).
Range = 100 to 1,000 μg/dL; average ~200 μg/dL.
Chronic lead poisoning.
Most sideroblastic anemias (e.g., acquired idiopathic).
Anemia of chronic diseases.

Normal or Decreased In

Primary disorders of globin synthesis:

* Thalassemia minor (therefore useful to differentiate from iron deficiency)

Pyridoxine-responsive anemia
One form of sideroblastic anemia due to block proximal to protoporphyrin synthesis.

Tests for Anemias

Tests for Classification of Anemias (Red blood Cell Indices)

Mean Corpuscular Hemoglobin

Mean corpuscular hemoglobin (MCH) is obtained by dividing Hb by RBC count. It represents the average amount of Hb per RBC (26–34 pg).

Use

Limited value in differential diagnosis of anemias
Instrument calibration

Interferences (Increased In)

Marked leukocytosis (>50,000/μL)
Cold agglutinins
In vivo hemolysis
Monoclonal proteins in blood
High heparin concentration
Lipemia

Decreased In

Microcytic and normocytic anemias

Increased In

Macrocytic anemias
Infants and newborns

Mean Corpuscular Hemoglobin Concentration

The MCH concentration (MCHC) is obtained by dividing hematocrit (Hct) by Hb. It represents the average concentration of Hb per RBC (33–37 g/dL).

Use

Instrument calibration and laboratory quality control, chiefly because changes occur very late in the course of iron deficiency when anemia is severe.
Usually better than MCH to identify hypochromasia.

Interferences

(With automated cell counters)
Decreased
  Marked leukocytosis (>50,000/μL)
Increased
  Hemolysis (e.g., sickle cell anemia, hereditary spherocytosis, some cases of autoimmune hemolytic anemia) with shrinkage of RBCs making them hyperdense.
  Conditions with cold agglutinins or severe lipemia of serum
  Rouleaux or RBC agglutinates
  High heparin concentration

HEMATOLOGY

Decreased In
(Decreased is defined as <30.1 g/dL)
Hypochromic microcytic anemias. *Normal value does not rule out any of these anemias. Low MCHC may not occur in IDA when performed with automated instruments.*

Increased In
Only in hereditary spherocytosis; should be suspected whenever MCHC >36 g/dL.
Infants and newborns.
Not increased in PA.

Mean Corpuscular Volume

Mean corpuscular volume (MCV) is calculated as Hct divided by RBC count with manual methods; it is measured directly by automated instruments. It represents the average measurement of RBC volume (82–98 fL [μm^3]).

See Figure 11-2.

Use
Classification and differential diagnosis of anemias
Useful screening test for occult alcoholism

Interferences
Marked leukocytosis (>50,000/μL) (increased values)
In vitro hemolysis or fragmentation of RBCs (decreased values)
Warm autoantibodies
Cold agglutinins (increased values)
Methanol poisoning (increased values)
Marked hyperglycemia (>600 mg/dL) (increases MCV)
Marked reticulocytosis (>50%) from any cause (increases MCV)
Presence of microcytic and macrocytic cells in same sample may result in a normal MCV.

Increased In

* Macrocytic anemias (MCV >95 fL and often >110 fL; MCHC >30 g/dL)
    Megaloblastic anemias
    PA (vitamin B_{12} or folate deficiency)
    Sprue (e.g., steatorrhea, celiac disease, intestinal resection or fistula)
    Macrocytic anemia of pregnancy
    Megaloblastic anemia of infancy
    Fish tapeworm infestation
    Carcinoma of stomach, following total gastrectomy
    Drugs:
        Oral contraceptives
        Anticonvulsants (e.g., phenytoin, primidone, phenobarbital)
        Antitumor agents (e.g., methotrexate, hydroxyurea, cyclophosphamide)
        Antimicrobials (e.g., sulfamethoxazole, sulfasalazine, trimethoprim, zidovudine, pyrimethamine)
    Orotic aciduria
    Megaloblastic disorders
    Di Guglielmo disease
    Nonmegaloblastic macrocytic anemias; are usually normocytic (MCV usually <110 fL)
    Alcoholism
    Liver disease
    Anemia of hypothyroidism
    Accelerated erythropoiesis (some hemolytic anemias, posthemorrhage)
    Myelodysplastic syndromes (aplastic anemia, acquired sideroblastic anemia)
    Myelophthisic anemia
    Postsplenectomy
Infants and newborns

Normal In
Normocytic anemias (MCV = 80–94 fL; MCHC >30 g/dL)

* Following acute hemorrhage
* Some hemolytic anemias
* Some hemoglobinopathies
* Anemias due to inadequate blood formation

Myelophthisic
Hypoplastic
Aplastic
- Endocrinopathies (hypopituitarism, hypothyroidism, hypoadrenalism, hypogonadism)
- Anemia of chronic disease (chronic infections, neoplasms, uremia)

Decreased In
Microcytic anemias (MCV <80 fL; MCHC <30 g/dL)

- Usually hypochromic
  Iron-deficiency anemia, e.g.,
    Inadequate intake
    Poor absorption
    Excessive iron requirements
    Chronic blood loss
  Pyridoxine-responsive anemia
  Thalassemia (major or combined with hemoglobinopathy)
  Sideroblastic anemia (hereditary)
  Lead poisoning
  Anemia of chronic diseases (<1/3 of patients)
  Disorders of porphyrin synthesis
- Usually normocytic
  Anemia of chronic diseases
  Hemoglobinopathies

Low MCV (in decreasing order of frequency) is caused by iron deficiency, α-thalassemia, heterozygous β-thalassemias, chronic disease, abnormal HbC and HbE. MCV <72 fL has sensitivity/specificity (S/S) of 88%/84% as a predictor of thalassemia trait.[5]

Red Cell Distribution Width

Red cell distribution width (RDW) is a quantitative measure of anisocytosis. It is a coefficient of variation of the distribution of individual RBC volume, as determined by automated blood cell counting instruments. Normal RDW is 11.5% to 14.5%. No subnormal values have been reported.

Use
Classification of anemias based on MCV and RDW (Table 11-1).
Is most useful to distinguish IDA from that of chronic disease or heterozygous thalassemia and to improve detection of early iron or folate deficiency.
The RDW is more sensitive in microcytic than macrocytic RBC conditions. Not helpful for patients without anemia.
Hb distribution width and cell Hb distribution width are two other indices of RBC heterogeneity that can be obtained from newer hematology analyzers; may be useful for further segregation of thalassemic traits.

Iron Measurements

Ferritin, Serum
Ferritin is the chief iron-storage protein in the body.

See Tables 11-2 to 11-4.
Use
Diagnosis of iron deficiency or excess; correlates with total body iron stores.

- Predict and monitor iron deficiency
- Determine response to iron therapy or compliance with treatment
- Differentiate iron deficiency from chronic disease as cause of anemia
- Monitor iron status in patients with chronic renal disease with or without dialysis

HEMATOLOGY

---

[5]Kiss TL, Ali MA, Levine M, et al. An algorithm to aid in the investigation of thalassemia trait in multicultural populations. *Arch Pathol Lab Med* 2000;124:1320–1323.

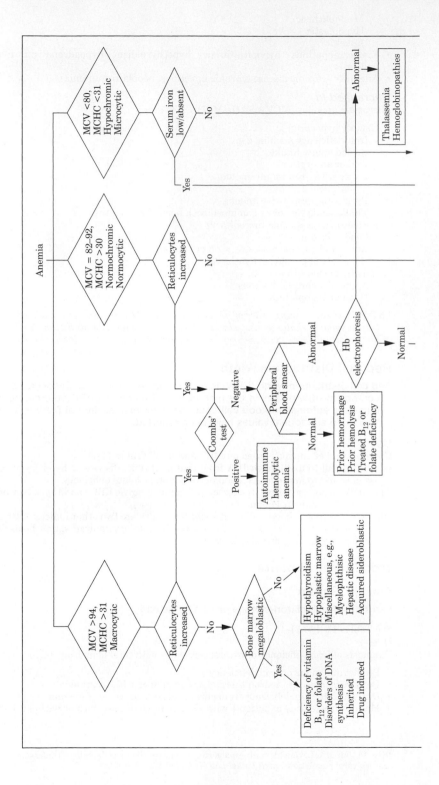

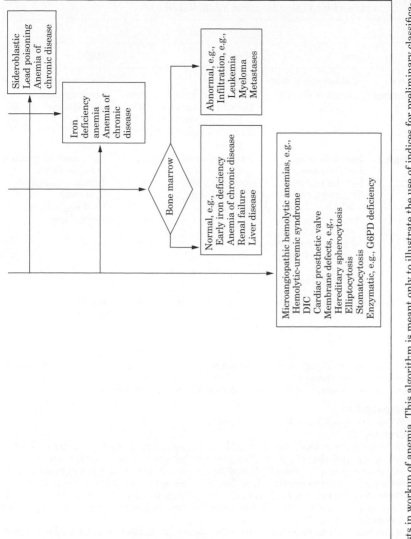

Fig. 11-2. Sequence of laboratory tests in workup of anemia. This algorithm is meant only to illustrate the use of indices for preliminary classification of anemias; many of the subsequent steps in the diagnostic workup are not included. Note also that some conditions may appear in more than one category. MCV, mean corpuscular volume; MCHC, mean corpuscular hemoglobin concentration; Hb, hemoglobin; DIC, disseminated intravascular coagulation; G6PD, glucose-6-phosphate dehydrogenase. (Adapted from Wintrobe M, et al., *Clinical Hematology.* 7th ed. Philadelphia: Lea & Febiger; 1974.)

Table 11-1.	Classification of Red Blood Cell Disorders by Mean Corpuscular Volume (MCV) and Red Blood Cell Distribution Width (RDW)		
	MCV		
	Low	Normal	High
RDW **Low** **Normal**	Thalassemia minor Anemia of chronic disease	Normal Anemia of chronic disease Hereditary spherocytosis (may also have high RDW) Some hemoglobinopathy traits (e.g., AS)	Aplastic anemia Myelodysplastic syndrome
High	Iron deficiency HbH disease S-β-thalassemia Fragmentation of RBCs Hemoglobinopathy traits (AC) Some patients with anemia of chronic disease G6PD deficiency	Early deficiency of iron, vitamin B$_{12}$, or folate Sickle cell anemia HbSC disease	Deficiency of vitamin B$_{12}$ or folate Immune hemolytic anemia Cold agglutinins Alcoholism

G6PD, glucose-6-phosphate dehydrogenase; HbH, hemoglobin H; HbSC, hemoglobin SC.

- Detect iron overload states and monitor rate of iron accumulation and response to iron-depletion therapy
- Population studies of iron levels and response to iron supplement

Decreased In
Iron deficiency (see Iron-Deficiency Anemia).

Increased In
Ferritin is an acute-phase reactant and thus is increased in many patients with various acute and chronic liver diseases, alcoholism (declines during abstinence), malignancies (e.g., leukemia, Hodgkin disease), infection and inflammation (e.g., arthritis), hyperthyroidism, Gaucher disease, acute myocardial infarction, etc. *Serum ferritin may not be decreased when iron deficiency coexists with these conditions; in such cases, bone marrow stain for iron may be the only way to detect the iron deficiency.*

Iron overload (e.g., hemosiderosis, idiopathic hemochromatosis). Can be used to monitor therapeutic removal of excess storage iron. Transferrin saturation is more sensitive to detect early iron overload in hemochromatosis; serum ferritin is used to confirm diagnosis and as indication to proceed with liver biopsy. Ratio of serum ferritin (in ng/mL) to alanine aminotransferase (ALT) (in IU/L) >10 in iron-overloaded thalassemic patients but averages ≤2 in viral hepatitis; ratio decreases with successful iron chelation therapy.

Anemias other than iron deficiency (e.g., megaloblastic, hemolytic, sideroblastic, thalassemia major and minor, spherocytosis, porphyria cutanea tarda)

Renal cell carcinoma due to hemorrhage within tumor

End-stage renal disease; values ≥1,000 μg/L are not uncommon. Values <200 μg/L are specific for iron deficiency in these patients.

Increases with age, is higher in men than women, in women who use oral contraceptives, and in persons who eat red meat compared to vegetarians.

Iron, Serum
The serum iron level reflects Fe^{3+} bound to transferrin, not free Hb in serum.

Table 11-2. Comparison of Iron-Deficiency Anemia Alone and Combined with Thalassemia Minor or Anemia of Chronic Disease

	Iron-Deficiency Anemia Alone	Anemia of Chronic Disease Alone	Combined Anemias of Iron Deficiency and Chronic Disease	Thalassemia Minor Alone	Combined Anemias of Iron Deficiency and Thalassemia Minor
MCV	D	N or D	D	**Very D**	Very D
RDW	I	I or N	I	I or N	I
RBC count	**D**	D	D	**N or I**	N or D
Serum iron	**D**	D	D	N	D
Serum ferritin	D	**I or N**	N or I	N	D
Marrow iron stain	D to 0	N or I	D to 0	N	D to 0
TIBC	I	**D**	I or N	N	I
Hb electrophoresis	N	N	N	**Ab**^{a}	**Ab**^{a}
sTfR	I	**N**	I	I	I

0, absent; Ab, abnormal; D, decreased; I, increased; N, normal; MCV, mean corpuscular volume; RDW, red blood cell distribution width; RBC, red blood cell; TIBC, total iron-binding capacity; Hb, hemoglobin; sTfR, serum transferrin receptor. Bold type indicates most useful differences.
^{a}Hemoglobin electrophoresis abnormal in *beta* thalassemia but not *alpha* thalassemia.

Table 11-3.   Red Blood Cell Indices[a]

Type of Anemia	MCV[b] (fL)	MCH[c] (pg)	MCHC[d] (g/dL)
Normal	82–92	27–31	32–36
Normocytic	82–92	25–30	32–36
Macrocytic	95–150	30–50	32–36
Microcytic (usually hypochromic)	50–80	12–25	25–30

Use: Classification and differential diagnosis of anemias.
MCV, mean corpuscular volume; MCH, mean corpuscular hemoglobin; MCHC, MCH concentration;
Hct, hematocrit; RBC, red blood cell; Hb, hemoglobin.
MCV (fL) = Hct/RBC.
MCH (pg) = Hb/RBC count, represents average amount of Hb per RBC.
MCHC (gm/dL) = Hb/Hct, represents average concentration of Hb per RBC.
MCV (fL [μm^3]) Hct/RBC count with manual methods; measured directly by automated instruments.
Average measurement of RBC volume.
Formula for estimating Hct from Hb:
Hct = Hb (gm/dL) $\times$ 2.8 + 0.8 or Hct = 3 $\times$ Hb

Use

Differential diagnosis of anemias
Diagnosis of hemochromatosis and hemosiderosis
Should always be measured with TIBC for evaluation of iron deficiency
Diagnosis of acute iron toxicity, especially in children

Interferences

Falsely increased by hemolysis or iron contamination of glassware or reagents
Falsely decreased in lipemic specimens
Diurnal variation causes increases late in the day
Iron dextran administration causes increase for several weeks (may be >1,000 $\mu g/dL$)

Table 11-4.   Some Common Causes of Leukemoid Reaction

Cause	Myelocytic	Lymphocytic	Monocytic
Infections	Endocarditis Pneumonia Septicemia Leptospirosis Other	Infectious mononucleosis Infectious lymphocytosis Pertussis Varicella Tuberculosis	Tuberculosis
Toxic conditions	Burns Eclampsia Poisoning (e.g., mercury)		
Neoplasms	Carcinoma of colon Embryonal carcinoma of kidney	Carcinoma of stomach Carcinoma of breast	
Miscellaneous	Treatment of megaloblastic anemia (of pregnancy, pernicious anemia) Acute hemorrhage Acute hemolysis Recovery from agranulocytosis	Dermatitis herpetiformis	
Myeloproliferative diseases			

Increased In

Idiopathic hemochromatosis

Hemosiderosis of excessive iron intake (e.g., repeated blood transfusions, iron therapy, iron-containing vitamins) (may be >300 μg/dL)

Decreased formation of RBCs (e.g., thalassemia, pyridoxine-deficiency anemia, PA in relapse)

Increased destruction of RBCs (e.g., hemolytic anemias)

Acute liver damage (degree of increase parallels the amount of hepatic necrosis) (may be >1,000 μg/dL); some cases of chronic liver disease

Progesteronal birth control pills (may be >200 μg/dL) and pregnancy

Premenstrual elevation by 10% to 30%

Acute iron toxicity; ratio of serum iron:TIBC is not useful for this diagnosis

Decreased In

Iron-deficiency anemia

Normochromic (normocytic or microcytic) anemias of infection and chronic diseases (e.g., neoplasms, active collagen diseases)

Nephrosis (because of loss of iron-binding protein in urine)

PA at onset of remission

Menstruation (decreased by 10% to 30%)

Diurnal variation—normal values in mid-morning, low values in mid-afternoon, very low values (~10 μg/dL) near midnight. Diurnal variation disappears at levels <45 μg/dL.

Iron-Binding Capacity, Total Serum

TIBC (in μmol/L) is obtained by the following equation: transferrin (mg/L) × 0.025.

Unsaturated iron-binding capacity = TIBC minus serum iron (μg/dL).

Use

Differential diagnosis of anemias

Should always be performed whenever serum iron is done to calculate percent saturation (see Fig 11-2) for diagnosis of iron deficiency

Screening for iron overload

Increased In

Iron deficiency

Acute and chronic blood loss

Acute liver damage

Late pregnancy

Progesterone birth control pills

Decreased In

Hemochromatosis

Cirrhosis of the liver

Thalassemia

Anemias of infection and chronic diseases (e.g., uremia, RA, some neoplasms)

Nephrosis

Hyperthyroidism

Transferrin, Serum

Transferrin transports circulating Fe^{3+} molecules. Normally only about 1/3 of iron-binding sites are occupied; the remainder is called unsaturated iron-binding capacity.

Use

Differential diagnosis of anemias

Increased In

Iron-deficiency anemia; is inversely proportional to iron stores

Pregnancy, estrogen therapy, hyperestrogenism

Decreased In

Hypochromic microcytic anemia of chronic disease

Acute inflammation

HEMATOLOGY

Protein deficiency or loss (e.g., burns, chronic infections, chronic diseases [e.g., various liver and kidney diseases, neoplasms]), nephrosis, malnutrition)
Genetic deficiency

Transferrin Saturation, Serum

Serum transferrin saturation is obtained by dividing serum iron by TIBC; normal = 20% to 50%. This figure represents the amount of iron-binding sites that are occupied.

Use
Differential diagnosis of anemias
Screening for hereditary hemochromatosis

Increased In
Hemochromatosis
Hemosiderosis
Thalassemia
Birth control pills (≤75%)
Ingestion of iron (≤100%)
Iron dextran administration causes increase for several weeks (may be >100%)

Decreased In
Iron-deficiency anemia (usually <10% in established deficiency)
Anemias of infection and chronic diseases (e.g., uremia, RA, some neoplasms)

Transferrin Receptor, Soluble, Serum

Soluble transferrin receptors are transmembrane proteins on the surface of most cells. Eighty percent originate from immature RBC progenitors, including reticulocytes, and 20% originate from nonerythroid tissues. This test reflects the degree of iron deficiency in erythroid precursors in marrow. Reference range = 0.57 to 2.8 μg/L; varies with assay system; readings are higher in blacks.

Use
Differential diagnosis of microcytic anemias (increased in IDAs but not increased in anemia of chronic disease [ACD])
Diagnosis of iron deficiency in patients with chronic disease.
Distinguish iron-deficient erythropoiesis (IDA) from physiologic depletion of iron stores (e.g., pregnancy, childhood, adolescence)
>20% increase over baseline within 2 weeks of starting or increasing erythropoietin therapy predicts response to that dosage and indicates that Hb response is likely to follow
Monitor recovery of erythropoietic activity after bone marrow transplantation
Evaluation of anemias when ferritin values may be increased to normal range due to acute-phase reaction if other causes of increased erythropoiesis are ruled out

Increased In
Disorders with hyperplastic erythropoiesis (e.g., IDAs, hemolytic anemias)
Disorders with ineffective erythropoiesis (e.g., myelodysplastic syndromes, megaloblastic anemias)
Residents of high altitude
Erythropoietin therapy

Decreased In
Disorders with reduced erythropoiesis (e.g., aplastic anemia, after bone marrow ablation for stem cell transplantation)
Iron overload disorders for which soluble transferrin receptor (sTfR) reading is not useful.

Anemias

Anemias, Classification by Pathogenesis

Anemias may be classified according to pathogenesis, which is convenient for understanding the mechanism, or according to RBC indices, peripheral blood smear, and reticulocyte count (see Fig. 11-2), which is convenient for workup of a clinical problem.

Marrow hypofunction with decreased RBC production

- Marrow replacement (myelophthisic anemias due to tumor or granulomas [e.g., TB]). *In absence of severe anemia or leukemoid reaction, nucleated RBCs in blood smear suggest miliary TB or marrow metastases.*
- Marrow injury (hypoplastic and aplastic anemias)
- Nutritional deficiency (e.g., megaloblastic anemias caused by lack of vitamin B_{12} or folic acid)
- Endocrine hypofunction (e.g., pituitary, adrenal, thyroid; anemia of chronic renal failure)
- Marrow hypofunction because of decreased Hb production (hypochromic microcytic anemias)

Deficient heme synthesis (IDA, pyridoxine-responsive anemias)
Deficient globin synthesis (thalassemias, hemoglobinopathies)
Excessive loss of RBCs

- Hemolytic anemias caused by genetically defective RBCs

Abnormal shape (e.g., hereditary spherocytosis, hereditary elliptocytosis)
Abnormal Hb (e.g., sickle cell anemia, thalassemias, HbC disease)
Abnormal RBC enzymes (e.g., congenital nonspherocytic hemolytic anemias, G6PD deficiency)

- Hemolysis with acquired defects of RBC and positive Coombs test

Autoantibodies (e.g., autoimmune cold or warm) transfusion reactions, microangio-pathic hemolytic anemia, as in SLE, malignant lymphoma, idiopathic thrombocy-topenic purpura (ITP)
Exogenous allergens, as in penicillin allergy

- Excessive loss of normal RBCs

Hemorrhage
Hypersplenism
Chemical agents (e.g., lead)
Infectious agents (e.g., *Clostridium welchii, Bartonella,* malaria)
Miscellaneous diseases (e.g., uremia, liver disease, cancers)
Physical agents (e.g., burns)
Mechanical trauma (e.g., artificial heart valves, tumor microemboli). *Blood smear shows fragmented, bizarre-shaped RBCs in patients with artificial heart valves.*
Anemias are often multifactorial; the resultant characteristics depend on which factor predominates. The diagnosis must be reevaluated after the apparent causes have been treated.

Chiefly Hypochromic Microcytic Anemias

Earliest change is transient decline in platelets, then an increase (≤ 1 million/μL) within a few hours; coagulation time is decreased.
RBC, Hb, and Hct level are not reliable initially because of compensatory vasocon-striction and hemodilution; they decrease 1 to 3 days after hemorrhage ceases. RBC returns to normal in 4 to 6 weeks; Hb returns to normal in 6 to 8 weeks if no further hemorrhage.
Anemia is normochromic, normocytic (normal MCV, MCHC). *(If hypochromic or micro-cytic, rule out iron deficiency caused by prior hemorrhages.)*
Reticulocyte count increases after 3 to 5 days and reaches a peak in 7 to 10 days ($\leq 15\%$). Persistent increase suggests continuing hemorrhage.
Blood smear shows no poikilocytes. Polychromasia and increased number of nucleated RBCs (up to 5:100 WBCs) may be found.
Increased WBC count (usually $\leq 20,000/\mu$L), reaching peak in 2 to 5 hours and becoming normal in 2 to 4 days. Persistent increase suggests continuing hemor-rhage, bleeding into a body cavity, or infection. Differential count shows shift to the left.
Blood urea nitrogen (BUN) is increased if hemorrhage into lumen of gastrointestinal (GI) tract occurs.
Serum indirect bilirubin is increased if hemorrhage into a body cavity or cystic struc-ture occurs.

HEMATOLOGY

Table 11-5.	Comparison of Neonatal Acute and Chronic Blood Loss in Fetal-Maternal Hemorrhage	
	Acute	Chronic
Hemoglobin	May be normal at first, then rapid drop during first 24 h	Low at birth
RBC morphology	Normochromic, normocytic	Hypochromic, microcytic Anisocytosis, poikilocytosis
Serum iron	Normal at birth	Low at birth

Both types show negative direct Coombs test, low serum bilirubin levels, demonstrable fetal RBCs in maternal blood.

Laboratory findings due to causative disease (e.g., peptic ulcer, esophageal varices, leukemia).

Hemorrhage, Neonatal

See Table 11-5.

Internal Hemorrhage

(e.g., intracranial, large cephalohematoma, rupture of liver or spleen, retroperitoneal hemorrhage)
Anemia without associated jaundice in first 1 to 3 days.
Indirect hyperbilirubinemia appears after third day.

Twin-to-Twin Transfusion

Twin-to-twin transfusion occurs in ~15% of monochorionic twin pregnancies.

♦ Hb difference >5 g/dL in identical twins
♦ Recipient twin shows:

• Erythrocytosis with Hb ≤30 g/dL and Hct up to 82%
• Increased indirect bilirubin
• Laboratory findings due to congestive heart failure, venous thrombosis, respiratory distress, kernicterus

♦ Donor twin shows anemia with Hb as low as 4 g/dL, increased reticulocyte count, and increased number of nucleated RBCs.

Fetal-Maternal Hemorrhage

Anemia varies from mild to severe
Polychromatophilia, increased reticulocyte count, increased number of nucleated RBCs
Serum bilirubin is not increased
Coombs test is negative
If chronic, then findings due to iron deficiency may occur
♦ Diagnosis is established only by demonstrating fetal RBCs in maternal blood (e.g., Kleihauer-Betke test, flow cytometry)
This can be found in ~50% of mothers, but in only 1% of pregnancies is it infant anemic.
May not be found if there is major group incompatibility between mother and infant, in which case buffy coat smears of maternal blood may show erythrophagocytosis; or do serial anti-A or anti-B titers in mother's blood for several weeks after birth.
Concurrent hemolytic disease of the newborn and intraplacental hemorrhage should also be ruled out.
In maternal-to-fetal transfusion, infant may show same findings as in recipient twin.

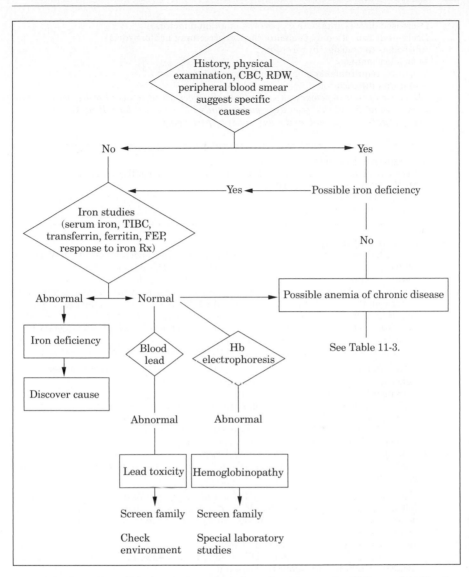

Fig. 11-3. Algorithm for workup for microcytic hypochromic anemia. CBC, complete blood count; RDW, red cell distribution width; TIBC, total iron-binding capacity; FEP, free erythrocyte protoporphyrin; Rx, therapy.

Chiefly Normochromic Normocytic Anemias

Anemia, Iron-Deficiency

See Tables 11-2 to 11-4 and Figures 11-2 and 11-3.
Due To
Usually a combination of factors:

Chronic blood loss (e.g., menometrorrhagia; bleeding from GI tract, especially from carcinoma of colon, hiatus hernia, peptic ulcer, intestinal parasites; marathon runners).

Decreased dietary intake (e.g., poverty, emotional factors)
Decreased absorption (e.g., steatorrhea, gastrectomy, achlorhydria)
Antibodies to transferrin receptor
Atransferrinemia
Increased requirements (e.g., pregnancy, lactation)
Aluminum intoxication
The cause of iron deficiency should always be ascertained to avoid overlooking occult carcinoma. In adults, iron deficiency usually means blood loss. If no GI or gynecologic cause is apparent, endoscopy must be performed.

Diagnostic Criteria
Decreased Hb (<10.5 g/dL in children or women; <13.5 g/dL in men) **and**
MCV <80 fL and serum ferritin <15 ng/mL **or**
Serum sTfR >28 nM **or**
Absence of stainable iron in bone marrow

Laboratory Findings

♦ Decreased serum ferritin is the most sensitive and specific test if MCV is not increased (e.g., pregnancy, infancy, polycythemia) or there is no vitamin C deficiency. Serum ferritin is the first test to reflect iron deficiency; it is *decreased prior to anemia* but may be increased when there is coexisting liver disease, inflammation, or other conditions that increase ferritin, which is an acute-phase reactant. *No other condition causes a low level. Returns to normal range within few days after onset of oral iron therapy; failure to produce serum ferritin level >50 ng/mL suggests noncompliance, malabsorption, or continued iron loss.*
Usually distinguishes iron deficiency from thalassemia in uncomplicated cases.

- <15 ng/mL always indicates iron deficiency and no longer corresponds to severity of deficiency because iron stores are essentially exhausted.
- <18 ng/mL is associated with absent stainable iron in marrow.
- <25 ng/mL in a patient with inflammation suggests iron deficiency
- <30 ng/mL has positive predictive value (PPV) $>92\%$ for IDA
- <50 ng/mL in a transferrin patient suggests iron deficiency
- <100 ng/mL in liver disease suggests iron deficiency
- >80 ng/mL essentially excludes iron deficiency
- >200 ng/mL generally indicates adequate iron stores regardless of underlying conditions

♦ Hb is decreased (usually 6 to 10 g/dL) out of proportion to decrease in RBC (3.5 to 5.0 million/μL); thus, decreased MCV (<80 fL) is a sensitive indicator; MCH is decreased (<30 pg). MCHC (25 to 30 g/dL) is a poor indicator, as is usually normal until anemia is severe.

♦ Increased RDW is first indication of iron deficiency; S/S = $89\%/45\%$; negative predictive value (NPV) of normal RDW = 93%, PPV = 45%. Helps to distinguish iron deficiency from heterozygous thalassemia.

♦ Hypochromia and microcytosis parallel severity of anemia. Polychromatophilia and nucleated RBCs are less common than in PA or thalassemia. Diagnosis from a peripheral blood smear is difficult and unreliable. Target cells may be present but are more common in thalassemias; basophilic stippling and polychromasia also favor thalassemia, although they are absent in 50% of cases. Anisocytosis is less marked in thalassemia.

♦ Ratio of microcytic to hypochromic RBCs (automated hematology analyzer) <0.9 in iron deficiency but >0.9 in β-thalassemia.

♦ Serum iron is decreased (usually 40 μg/dL), TIBC increased (usually 350 to 460 μg/dL), and transferrin saturation decreased ($<15\%$). TIBC may be normal or moderately increased in many patients with uncomplicated iron deficiency. Serum transferrin may be normal or increased (calculated transferrin = TIBC $\times$ 0.7). These have limited value in differential diagnosis, since they are often normal in iron deficiency and abnormal in ACD and may be affected by recent iron therapy.

♦ As iron deficiency progresses, decreased serum ferritin is followed in order by anisocytosis, microcytosis, elliptocytosis, hypochromia, decreases in Hb, decreases in serum iron, decreases in transferrin saturation. See Table 11-6.

Table 11-6. Comparison of Sample Values in Iron-Deficiency States

	Normal	Early Deficiency	Early Anemia	Moderate Anemia	Moderate to Severe Anemia	Severe Anemia
MCV (fL)	82–92	N	N	D	D	D
MCH(pg)	27–31	N	N	Gradually decreases (95→80 fL) →		D
Hb (g/dL)	12–14 M / 14–16 F	N	Gradually decreases to ~10	Usually 7–10 →		
RDW	11.5–14.5	N	N	Gradually increases →		
Blood smear	N	N	Only mild microcytosis	Moderate microcytosis; ovalocytes, target cells, leptocytes	Poikilocytes, severe microcytosis, ovalocytes, elliptocytes	Schistocytes
% Cells hypochromic	N	N		Gradually increases →		
Serum iron (μg/dL)	65–165	N (115)	D (<60)	D (<40)	D (<40)	D (<40)
TIBC (μg/dL)	250–450			Increases to ~480 →		
Transferrin saturation	20–50%	N (30%)	D (<15%)	D (<10%)	D (<10%)	D (<10%)
Serum ferritin (μg/L)	40–160	40–160; decreases to 20	D	<10	<10	<10
RE marrow iron	2–3+	0–1+	0–1+	0	0	0
sTfR	a	N/I	I	I	I	I
Free RBC Protoporphyrin	<100 (μg/dL)	N	I	Gradually increasing to ~200 μg/dL →		
RBC life span	N	N	100 μg/dL	Gradually decreases →		

D, decreased; F, females; I, increased; M, males; N, normal; MCV, mean corpuscular volume; MCH, mean corpuscular hemoglobin; Hb, hemoglobin; TIBC, total iron-binding capacity; RDW, red cell distribution width; RE, reticuloendothelial; sTfR, serum transferrin receptor.

a Depends on method.

Source: Some data from Crosby WH. Iron deficiency anemia: signpost to blood loss. *Emerg Med* Sep 30, 1991:73–83.

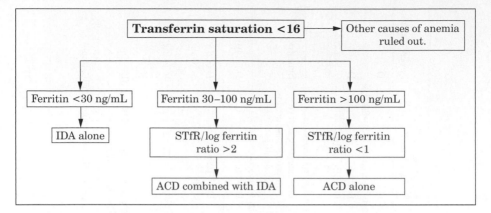

Fig. 11-4. Sequence of laboratory tests to distinguish iron-deficiency anemia (IDA) from anemia of chronic disease (ACD) and ACD combined with IDA. sTfR, soluble transferrin receptor.

◆ sTfR increases only after iron stores are depleted (i.e., decline in serum ferritin below reference range and compensatory erythropoiesis begins) but before changes in other markers of tissue iron deficiency (e.g., transferrin saturation, MCV, erythrocyte protoporphyrin). May be useful in differentiating IDA (increased sTfR) from ACD (normal sTfR) and in diagnosing IDA in patients with chronic disease. Increased S/S when combined with ferritin. sTfR/log serum ferritin (sTfR-F index) has been useful to distinguish IDA coexisting with ACD (>2) from ACD alone (<1) in some reports. See Figure 11-4.

◆ Bone marrow shows normoblastic hyperplasia with decreased hemosiderin, later absent, and decreased percentage of sideroblasts. Decreased to absent iron is the "gold standard" test for diagnosis of iron deficiency.

◆ Free erythrocyte protoporphyrin is increased and is useful screening test since it can be done on fingerstick sample. Is *increased prior to anemia*. Also increased in lead poisoning, ACD, and most sideroblastic anemias but is normal in thalassemias.

WBC is normal or may be slightly decreased in 10% of cases; may be increased with fresh hemorrhage.

Serum bilirubin and lactate dehydrogenase (LD) are not increased.

Platelet count is usually normal but may be slightly increased or decreased; often increased in children.

Coagulation studies are normal.

RBC fragility is normal or (often) increased to 0.21%.

RBC life span is normal.

Reticulocytes are normal or decreased, unless there is recent hemorrhage or administration of iron.

◆ Response to oral iron therapy is the final proof of diagnosis of iron deficiency, *but primary cause of anemia must first be determined; response to iron therapy does not rule out underlying cause.*

• Increased reticulocytes within 3 to 7 days with peak of 8% to 10% (2×–4× above baseline) on fifth to tenth day; is proportional to degree of anemia.

• Followed by increasing Hb (average 0.25–0.4 g/dL/day) and Hct (average = 1%/d) during first 7 to 10 days; thereafter Hb increases 0.1 g/dL/day to level ≥11 g/dL (or 2 g/dL) in 3 to 4 weeks. Should be about half corrected in 3 weeks and fully corrected by 8 weeks. In elderly, increase of 1 g/dL may take 1 month, while younger patients' increases will be Hb 3 g/dL and Hct 10%.

• Failure to respond suggests incorrect diagnosis, coexisting deficiencies (folic acid, vitamin B$_{12}$, thyroid), associated conditions (e.g., lead poisoning, bleeding, transferrin, liver or kidney disease).

Clinical utility is not yet established for RBC ferritin (also decreased in ACD).

Most difficult differential diagnosis is thalassemias and ACD. See Tables 11-7 to 11-8 for additional laboratory findings.

Table 11-7. Laboratory Tests in Differential Diagnosis of Microcytic (MCV <80 fL) and Hypochromic (MCHC <30 g/dL) Anemias

Type of Anemia	Serum Iron	TIBC	Transferrin Saturation	Serum Ferritin	FEP[a]	Marrow Hemosiderin	Sidero-blasts	Type of Hb	Anemia	RBC Count	RDW
Normal values	80–160 µg/dL in men / 50–150 µg/dL in women	250–410 µg/dL	20%–55%	20–150 ng/dL			30%–50%	AA			11.5–14.5
Iron deficiency	D	I	D	D	I	0	D	AA	Hypochromic, normocytic, or microcytic	D	I
Normochromic, normocytic, or microcytic, of chronic disease	D	D or N	D or N	N or slightly I	I	N or I	D	AA	Normochromic, normocytic, or microcytic	D	N
Thalassemia											
Major	I	D	I	I	N	I	I	20%–90% F	Hypochromic	I	N
Minor	N or I	N	N or I	I	N	N or I	I	2%–8% F; A_2 is I	Microcytic	I	N
Sideroblastic	N or I	D or N	I	I	D	I	I	AA	Hypochromic and/or microcytic with normocytic or macrocytic changes, dimorphic RBC population	D	I

0, absent; F, decreased; FEP, free erythrocyte protoporphyrin; I, increased; N, normal.

MCV, mean corpuscular volume; MCHC, mean corpuscular hemoglobin concentration; TIBC, total iron-binding content; RDW, red blood cell distribution width.

Notes: (1) Determine serum iron and TIBC (and also perhaps do iron stain on bone marrow smear—the most reliable index of iron deficiency). (2) If serum iron and TIBC are both normal, Hb electrophoresis will establish the diagnosis of thalassemia. If serum iron is abnormal, the cause may be iron deficiency (e.g., blood loss, dietary deficiency) or normochromic microcytic anemia of chronic disease.

[a]FEP is useful to distinguish between iron deficiency and beta thalassemia.

Iron depletion: Early—serum iron is normal; TIBC may be increased. Later—serum iron decreases; anemia is often normocytic when mild or of rapid onset; anemia first becomes microcytic, then hypochromic.

Iron deficiency may occur without anemia (transferrin saturation <15%; decreased marrow iron and sideroblasts).

HEMATOLOGY

| Table 11-8. | Comparison of Iron-Deficiency Anemia (IDA) Alone and Combined with Thalassemia Minor or Anemia of Chronic Disease (ACD) |

	IDA Alone	ACD Alone	IDA + ACD	Thalassemia Minor Alone	IDA + Thalas. Minor
MCV	D	N or D	D	**Very D**	Very D
RDW	I	I or N	I	D	I
RBC count	V	D	D	**N or I**	N or D
Serum iron	**D**	**D**	D	**N**	D
Serum ferritin	**D**	**N or I**	N or D	N	D
Marrow iron	**D to 0**	N to I	**D to 0**	N	D to 0
TIBC	**I**	**D**	I or N	**N**	I
sTfR	**I**	**N**	**I**	**N**	I
Hb electrophoresis	N	N	N	**Ab**	**Ab**

0, absent; Ab, abnormal; D, decreased; I, increased; N, normal; V, varies.
MCV, mean corpuscular volume; RDW, red blood cell distribution width; TIBC, total iron-binding capacity; sTfR, serum soluble transferrin receptor. Bold type and larger font indicate most useful differences.
Hb electrophoresis is abnormal in β-thalassemia but not in α-thalassemia.
Measurement of globin chain synthesis ratios for confirmation of α- and β-thalassemias.
DNA analysis can detect gene deletions and point mutations, which detect most types of α- and β-thalassemia.

> *In the United States, median Hb is about 1 g/dL lower in blacks without iron deficiency than in whites.*
> Laboratory finding may disclose causative factors (e.g., GI bleeding).

Chiefly Macrocytic/Megaloblastic Anemias[6]

Macrocytic/megaloblastic anemias are possibly caused by blunted erythropoietin (Ep) response by RBC precursors, decreased RBC survival, defective iron absorption, or cytokines blockading iron release from RE system to developing RBCs.

| Table 11-9. | Comparison of Anemia of Chronic Disease (ACD) Alone, Iron-Deficiency Anemia (IDA) Alone, and Combined IDA + ACD |

	ACD Alone	IDA Alone	IDA + ACD
MCV	N or D	D	D (tends to be lower)
RDW	I or N	I	I
RBC count	D	V	D (tends to be lower)
Serum iron	D	D	D
Serum ferritin	N or I	D	N or D
Transferrin	I	D or N	D
Transferrin saturation	D	D	D
Marrow iron	N to I	D to 0	D to 0
TIBC	D	I	I or N
sTfR	N	I	I or N
Ratio sTfR to log ferritin	<1	>2	>2

0, absent; Ab, abnormal; D, decreased; I, increased; N, normal; V, varies.
MCV, mean corpuscular volume; RDW, red blood cell distribution width; TIBC, total iron-binding capacity; sTfR, serum soluble transferrin receptor. Bold type and larger font indicate most useful differences.

[6]Weiss G, Goodnough LT. Anemia of chronic disease. *N Engl J Med* 2005;352:1011–1023.

See Tables 11-3 and 11-4 and Fig. 11-3.
Due To
Chronic kidney disease (BUN >70 mg/dL) and inflammation
Autoimmune disorders

- RA (anemia parallels activity of arthritis)
- SLE, connective tissue diseases
- Sarcoidosis
- Inflammatory bowel disease
- Vasculitis

Neoplasms (solid tumors, leukemias)
Subacute or chronic infections

- Bacterial (especially TB, bronchiectasis, lung abscess, empyema, infective endocarditis, brucellosis, osteomyelitis)
- Viral
- Parasitic
- Fungal

Others (e.g., chronic liver diseases, chronic adrenal insufficiency, hypothyroidism, rheumatic fever)

Laboratory Findings

♦ Anemia is usually mild (Hb 8–9 g/dL) but may be as low as 5 g/dL in uremia when other factors are present. Is insidious over a 3- to 4-week period, then *not progressive*. May be caused by multiple mechanisms (e.g., failure of erythropoiesis, decreased RBC survival, iron deficiency, etc).

♦ Anemia is normocytic, normochromic in 60% to 70% of cases. RDW and indices are usually normal. Anemia is hypochromic and/or microcytic in 30% to 40% of these patients, in which case it is always less marked than in IDA.
Moderate anisocytosis and slight poikilocytosis are present.
Low reticulocyte count.
Polychromatophilia, and nucleated RBCs are absent (may be present with severe anemia or uremia).

♦ Serum iron is decreased. TIBC is decreased or normal; if TIBC is elevated, presence of iron deficiency must be ruled out, but TIBC is not sufficiently sensitive or specific to distinguish ACD from IDA. Transferrin saturation is usually normal; >10% if decreased; <10% implies iron deficiency. IDA may be caused by GI blood loss due to treatment with nonsteroidal anti-inflammatory drugs (NSAIDs) for RA.

♦ Serum ferritin is increased or normal in contrast to iron deficiency. *In RA, liver disease, or neoplasms, normal serum ferritin does not exclude concomitant iron deficiency, but serum ferritin <40 ng/mL indicates iron depletion.*

♦ sTfR is normal. Used to help differentiate from IDA.
Free erythrocyte protoporphyrin is increased.

♦ Hemosiderin is increased or normal; sideroblasts are decreased in bone marrow; cellular elements are generally morphologically normal. Myeloid:erythroid ratio is usually normal.

Platelet count is normal.
Increased WBC, C-reactive protein (CRP), erythrocyte sedimentation rate (ESR), and other acute phase reactants (e.g., fibrinogen, ceruloplasmin) are disproportionate to anemia, and may be a useful clue to distinguish this from IDA.
RBC survival is slightly decreased in patient (80–90 days) but not in normal recipient.

Chronic Renal Disease

Blood smear frequently shows burr cells or schistocytes.
Usually normochromic, normocytic; hypochromic microcytosis may be caused by chronic disease.
Severity of anemia roughly parallels severity of renal disease, but when dialysis is required, anemia is almost always severe.
Decreased serum iron and transferrin. Serum iron, TIBC, and ferritin are often not helpful, and bone marrow stained for iron may be necessary for diagnosis of iron deficiency.

HEMATOLOGY

Concurrent iron deficiency caused by GI tract blood loss may be present.
Bone marrow usually shows erythroid hypoplasia.
Decreased serum erythropoietin. Anemia responds to erythropoietin therapy.
Decreased RBC survival by ^{59}Cr studies.

Hypothyroidism

♦ Occurs in 1/3 to 2/3 of patients with hypothyroidism; usually mild (Hct >35%). May
be secondary to hypopituitarism.
Normochromic normocytic or macrocytic (if hypochromic, rule out associated iron defi-
ciency). No anisocytosis or poikilocytosis.
Reticulocyte count is not increased.
Serum iron is usually decreased and responds only to treatment of hypothyroidism,
unless there is concomitant iron deficiency.
Decreased total blood volume and plasma volume.
Normal RBC survival.
Concurrent iron deficiency or PA may be present.

Hypogonadism

Normochromic, normocytic; only occurs in men.

Hypoadrenalism

Hct is pseudo-normal at presentation due to plasma volume depletion; corticosteroid
therapy unmasks anemia. Is corrected by 1 to 2 months of therapy.

Chronic Liver Disease

○ Increased MCV (100–125 fL) in 1/3 to 2/3 of patients. Indices resemble those in other
megaloblastic anemias. Low MCHC may indicate associated iron deficiency.
♦ *Uniform round macrocytosis* is the cardinal finding. Target cells and stomatocytes
may be present. The presence of hypochromic macrocytes or microcytes may suggest
misleading diagnosis of iron deficiency. Spur cell (acanthocyte) hemolysis may be
caused by abnormal lipid metabolism.
Hemolytic anemia or true folate deficiency is frequent in alcoholic liver disease.
Reticulocyte count is usually increased.
Serum iron, TIBC, and ferritin are often not helpful, and bone marrow stained for iron
may be necessary for diagnosis of iron deficiency.
Decreased RBC survival by ^{59}Cr studies.

Atransferrinemia

**Atransferrinemia is a very rare autosomal recessive congenital isolated absence
of transferrin.**

Can be diagnosed when severe hypochromic, microcytic, iron-deficiency anemia is
unresponsive to iron therapy. TIBC is low (<85 μg/dL).
♦ Bone marrow shows erythroid hyperplasia, which distinguishes it from IDA.
♦ Absence of transferrin (normal = 200–400 mg/dL) is demonstrated by nephelometry
or immunoelectrophoresis (see Serum Transferrin).
♦ Serum protein electrophoresis shows marked decrease in β-globulins and absence of
transferrin band.
Increased iron stores with hemosiderosis of nonhematopoietic tissues with involvement of adrenals, heart, etc. is present.

Disorders of Hemoglobin

**There are >800 Hb variants.[7] However, only nine Hb variants and thalassemia
syndromes have important clinical significance.**

[7]Hardison RC, Chui DH, Riemer C, et al. Databases of human hemoglobin variants and thalassemia
mutations at the globin gene server. *Hum Mutat* 2002;19:225–233.

Table 11-10. Representative Laboratory Values of Some Common Hemoglobinopathies

Laboratory Test	Hemoglobinopathy				
	AS	SS	SC[a]	S-beta$^+$	S-beta^0
Hb (g/dL)	N	7.5	11	11	8
Range		(6–9)	(9–14)	(8–13)	(7–10)
Hct(%)	N	22	30	32	25
Range		(18–30)	(26–40)	(25–40)	(20–36)
MCV (fL)	N	93	80	76	69
Reticulocyte count (%)	N	11	3	3	8
Range		(4–30)	(1.5–6.0)	(1.5–6.0)	(3–18)
RBC morphology	N				
Sickle cells		Many	Rare	Rare	Varies
Target-cells		Many	Many		Many
Microcytosis				Mild	Marked
Hypochromia				Mild	Marked
Nucleated RBC		Many			
Hb electrophoresis (%)	N				
S	38–45	80–95	45–55	55–75	50–85
F	N	2–20	<8	1–20	2–30
A$_2$	1–3	<3.6	<3.6	3–6	3–6
A	55–60	0	0	15–30	0
C	0	0	45–55	0	0
Clinical severity	No symptoms	Moderate/ severe	Mild/ moderate	Mild/ moderate	Mild/ severe
Presence in U.S. blacks	10%	1:625	1:833	1:1667	1:1667

MCV, mean corpuscular volume; MCHC, mean corpuscular hemoglobin concentration; N, normal.
[a]Blood smear shows tetragonal crystals within RBC in 70% of patients; RBCs tend to be microcytic with low or low/normal MCV but high MCHC; typical distorted RBCs in which Hb is concentrated more in one area of cell than another.

Sickle Cell Disease[8]

Sickle cell disease occurs with autosomal recessive inheritance of abnormal Hb β chain (glutamic acid replaced by valine). This results in the precipitation and polymerization of Hb under conditions of deoxygenation and hypertonicity, causing rigid crystals that deform RBCs (sickling), resulting in microvascular occlusions and hemolysis.
See Tables 11-10 and 11-11.

Sickling of RBCs

Tube test (Sickledex) and metabisulfite slide test. Sickling should be confirmed with Hb electrophoresis or equivalent (e.g., high-pressure liquid chromatography [HPLC], isoelectric focusing, DNA analysis) and genetic studies.

Occurs In

- Sickle cell disease
- Sickle cell trait
- Non-S sickling hemoglobins (e.g., HbC$_{Harlem}$, HbC$_{Georgetown}$, HbI)
- Double heterozygosity of certain variants (e.g., HbS/HbD$_{Los Angeles}$, Hb$_{Montgomery}$/HbS, which also occurs in same populations)

[8]Steinberg MH. Management of sickle cell disease. *New Engl J Med* 1999;340:1021–1030.

HEMATOLOGY

Table 11-11.   Hb Percentage in Various Hemoglobinopathies

	B1	B2	Hb Fractions		
Normal	β^A	β^A	HbA = 97%		HbA$_2$ = 3%
β-thalassemia trait	β^0/β^+	β^A	HbA = 95%		HbA$_2$ = 5%^{a}
HbS trait	β^S	β^A	HbA = 60%	HbS = 36%	HbA$_2$ = 4%
Homozygous HbS	β^S	β^S		HbS = 89%	HbA$_2$ = 6% HbF = 5%
HbS/β^+–thalassemia^{b,c}	β^S	β^+	HbA = 30%	HbS = 62%	HbA$_2$ = 5% HbF = 3%
HbS/β^0–thalassemia^d	β^S	β^0		HbS = 88%	HbA$_2$ = 7% HbF = 5%

^{a}HbA$_2$ can be increased in presence of HbS without presence of β-thalassemia.
^{b}Decreased production of HbA from affected β globin gene.
^{c}No production of HbA from affected β globin gene.
^{d}Only situation where HbS >HbA, except for recent transfusion of HbS/S or HbS/β^0–thalassemia patient; is spurious because part of HbS elutes with HbA$_2$.

False-Positive Results In

- First 4 months after transfusion with RBCs having sickle cell trait
- Mixture on slide with fibrinogen, thrombin, gelatin (glue)
- Excessive concentration of sodium metabisulfite (e.g., ≥4% instead of 2%)
- Drying of wet coverslip preparation
- Poikilocytosis

False-Negative Results In

- First 4 months after transfusion with normal RBCs
- Heating, bacterial contamination, or prolonged washing with saline of RBCs
- Newborn because HbF is high during first months of life
- Low % of HbS
- Outdated reagents

Sickle Solubility Test

Inadequate because does not detect carriers of HbC and β-thalassemia and does not differentiate between sickle cell anemia, trait, and other HbS genetic variants. Sodium dithionite is added to lysed RBCs to reduce the Hb. Solution is turbid when HbS is present but remains clear with other Hb. Useful for screening large numbers of people.

False-Negative Results May Occur With

- Patient's Hb <7 g/dL
- Phenothiazine drugs
- Unreliable for newborn screening because of high HbF
- Low % of HbS (e.g., very young infants)

False-Positive Results May Occur With

- Increased turbidity (e.g., lipemic specimens)
- Abnormal γ globulins
- Polycythemia
- Increased number of Heinz bodies (e.g., postsplenectomy)
- Increased number of nucleated RBCs

Sickle Cell Trait

Sickle cell trait is a heterozygous sickle cell (HbAS) disease that occurs in ≤10% of African Americans; it is asymptomatic.

- ◆ Hb electrophoresis: HbS is 20% to 40% and Hb A is 60% to 80%; normal amounts of HbA$_2$ and HbF (≤(≤2%) may be present.
- ◆ Sickle cell preparation is positive.

Blood smear shows only a few target cells; sickle RBCs are not seen but ≤4% may have abnormal shape.

Complete blood count (CBC) and indices are normal; no anemia, hemolysis, or jaundice is present.

Anoxia may cause systemic sickling (see "Sickle Cell Anemia"). HbS concentration is too low for sickling to occur under most conditions, but of *beware anesthesia, airplane flights, etc.*

Hematuria without any other demonstrable cause may be found.

Hyposthenuria may occur.

Postmortem sickle cells are found regardless of cause of death.

Sickle Cell Anemia[7]

In sickle cell anemia, HbS agglutinates with deoxygenation and hypertonicity. In homozygous (HbSS) disease, sickling occurs at physiologic O_2 tensions. Occurs in 1 in 625 African Americans.

♦ Hb electrophoresis: HbS is 80% to 100%, and HbF comprises the rest (see Fetal Hemoglobin); HbA is absent. Because other Hb variants migrate with HbS on electrophoresis, it is important to confirm Hb as a sickle type.

♦ Sickle cell preparation is positive; sickle solubility test is positive but does not differentiate anemia from other HbS genetic variants and may be falsely negative if Hb <5 g/dL.

♦ Blood smear shows a variable number of RBCs with target cells (especially in HbS/HbC disease), abnormal shapes, nucleated RBCs, Howell-Jolly bodies, spherical cells, polychromasia. Sickle cells in smear when RBCs contain >60% Hb S (except in HbS-persistent HbF). After autosplenectomy, basophilic stippling, Pappenheimer bodies, and nucleated RBCs are also present.

Chronic hemolytic normocytic normochromic anemia (Hb = 5–10 g/dL; normal MCV).

Reticulocyte count is increased (5%–30%); may cause slight increase in MCV. Failure of reticulocyte count and indices to show responses.

WBC count is increased (10,000–30,000/μL) during sickling crises, with normal differential or shift to the left. Infection may be indicated by intracellular bacteria (best seen on buffy coat preparations), Döhle bodies, toxic granules and vacuoles of WBCs, Westergren ESR >20 mm/h.

Platelet count is increased (300,000–500,000/μL), with abnormal forms.

Bone marrow shows hyperplasia of all elements, causing bone changes on radiographs.

○ Decreased ESR becomes normal after blood is aerated. An ESR in the normal range may indicate intercurrent illness or crisis.

Osmotic fragility is decreased (more resistant RBCs).

Mechanical fragility of RBCs is increased.

RBC survival time is decreased (17 days in HbSS, 28 days in HbS/HbC).

Laboratory findings of hemolysis (e.g., increased indirect serum bilirubin increased (≤(≤6 mg/dL), increased urobilinogen in urine and stool, but urine is negative for bile).

• Hemosiderin appears in urine sediment.
• Hematuria is frequent.
• Serum uric acid may be increased.
• Serum alkaline phosphatase (ALP) is increased during crisis, representing vaso-occlusive bone injury as well as liver damage.
• Leukocyte ALP activity is decreased.

Laboratory findings due to complications

• Infections due to immunocompromised status (functional asplenia); e.g., *Salmonella* osteomyelitis occurs virtually only in sickle cell syndromes; marked increase in susceptibility to pneumococcal and *Haemophilus influenzae* sepsis and meningitis, *Escherichia coli* and meningococci infections, staphylococcal osteomyelitis, *Mycoplasma pneumoniae*.

• Vaso-occlusive crisis, e.g., infarction of lungs, brain, bowel; spleen is completed infarcted by middle age causing Howell-Jolly bodies, target cells. Bone marrow necrosis causing fat emboli syndrome; bone (e.g., avascular necrosis of hip; dactylitis).

[7]Hardison RC, Chui DH, Riemer C, et al. Databases of human hemoglobin variants and thalassemia mutations at the globin gene server. *Hum Mutat* 2002;19:225–233.

HEMATOLOGY

- Hyperhemolytic crisis—superimposed further hemolysis caused by bacterial or viral infections; Hb falls from usual 6 to 10 g/dL to ≤5 g/dL in a few days with increasing reticulocyte count. When there is hemolysis, G6PD deficiency should be ruled out, as this is also common in blacks.
- Aplastic crisis—acute, self-limited episode of erythroid aplasia lasting 5 to 10 days due to parvovirus B19; falling Hct and reticulocyte count may require prompt transfusion. Recovery is marked by return of reticulocytosis, usually with resolution of infection.
- Hypoplastic crisis—infection or inflammation causes brief suppression of bone marrow with accentuated brief drop in Hct and reticulocyte count.
- Splenic sequestration crisis—seen mostly in children age 5 months to 5 years (before fibrosis of spleen has occurred); enormous enlargement of spleen associated with precipitous drop in Hct and hypovolemic shock. Over age 2 years, occurs more often with other HbS syndromes.
- Megaloblastic crisis—rare occurrence of sudden cessation of erythropoiesis due to folate depletion in persons with inadequate folate (e.g., pregnancy, alcoholism, poor diet).
- Renal concentrating ability is decreased, leading to a fixed specific gravity in virtually all patients after the first few years of life. Microalbuminuria is a preclinical indicator of glomerular damage and predictor or renal failure. (See Sickle Cell Nephropathy, Chapter 14)
- Stasis and necrosis of liver—increased direct serum bilirubin ≤40 mg/dL, bile in urine, other findings of obstructive type of jaundice.
- Bilirubin gall stones in 30% of patients by age 18 and 70% by age 30, may cause cholecystitis or biliary obstruction.
- ♦ *Anemia and hemolytic jaundice are present throughout life after age 3 to 6 months; hemolysis and anemia are increased only during hematologic crises.*
- ♦ Newborn screening by Hb electrophoresis on cord blood or filter paper spot.
- In newborns with HbSS, anemia is rarely present. May cause unexplained prolonged jaundice. May be difficult to distinguish HbSS from HbAS in neonates because of large amount of HbF, which may obscure the HbA. HbA is also not produced in HbS-β^0 thalassemia, so an FS pattern on electrophoresis may indicate either. HbS-β^+ thalassemia usually has an FSA phenotype requiring careful differentiation from sickle cell trait (phenotype FAS). Percent of RBCs that will sickle is much lower in newborn (as low as 0.5%) than in older children. Diagnosis of HbSS is excluded by HbA on Hb electrophoresis of infant's blood or if mother has negative sickle cell prep. *In newborn, cellulose agar electrophoresis is useless to detect HbS because of the small amount present; acidic citrate agar gel is needed. For exchange transfusion, sickle cell test must be performed on donor blood from blacks since these RBCs may sickle in presence of hypoxia as in respiratory distress syndrome. Hb solubility tests (e.g., Sickledex) are usually not suitable on cord blood because a positive result may be easily obscured by a large amount of HbF.* Most children are anemic and symptomatic by age of 1 year; anemia and hemolysis are present throughout life.
- ♦ Antenatal diagnosis is possible as early as 7 to 10 weeks' gestation by gene analysis of fetal DNA on amniotic fluid cells or chorionic villi. Also detects HbS/HbC disease. Diagnosis can also be made by fetal blood sampling.

Hydroxyurea therapy causes these changes after 6 to 8 years:

- Hb increases 1.2 g/dL
- MCV increases 23 fL
- HbF increases >11%
- Reticulocyte count decreases 158,000/μL
- WBC count decreases 5,000/μL
- Platelet count decreases 83,000/μL
- Total bilirubin decreases 2 mg/dL

HbS/HbC Disease

HbS/HbC disease occurs in 1 of 833 African Americans. This is a severe sickling disease intermediate between sickle cell disease and sickle cell trait.

- ♦ Hb electrophoresis: HbA is absent; HbS and HbC are present in approximately equal amounts (30%–60%); HbF is ≤7%.

♦ Blood smear shows tetragonal crystals within RBC in 70% of patients; MCV is usually low or low/normal but MCHC is high; plump and angulated rather than typical sickle cells in which Hb is concentrated more in one area of the cell than another; ≤85% target cells.

Sickling test is positive.

Variable mild to moderate normochromic, normocytic anemia.

○ A valuable diagnostic aid is the presence of target cells with normal MCV.

♦ Other findings are the same as for sickle cell anemia, but there is less marked destruction of RBCs, anemia, etc., and the disease is less severe clinically. *Hematologic crises may cause a more marked fall in RBC than occurs in HbSS disease.*

Sickle Cell-Alpha Thalassemia Disease

Sickle cell α-thalassemia modifies the severity of sickle cell disease. It is usually clinically insignificant.

Sickle Cell-Beta Thalassemia Disease

Sickle cell β-thalassemia occurs in 1 of every 1,667 African Americans.

♦ Hb electrophoresis: HbS is 20% to 90%; HbF is 2% to 20%.

In one syndrome, HbS may be very high and HbA synthesis is suppressed, causing a more severe disease. In the other (milder) syndrome, HbA is 25% to 50%; HbA_2 is increased.

Anemia is hypochromic and microcytic, with decreased MCV; target cells are prominent; serum iron is normal.

Other findings resemble those of sickle cell anemia.

♦ Valuable diagnostic aids are: the presence of target cells with normal MCV, microcytosis or splenomegaly in patients with mild to moderate sickle cell syndrome, apparent increase in HbA_2 (HbC migrates in HbA_2 position on gel electrophoresis), microcytosis in one parent.

Sickle Cell-Persistent High Fetal Hemoglobin

This type of sickle cell disease occurs in 1 in 25,000 African Americans.

Hb electrophoresis: HbF is 20% to 40%; HbA and A_2 are absent; HbS is ~65%.

Findings are intermediate between those of sickle cell anemia and of sickle cell trait, but sickle cells do not form.

Normally, HbF is evenly distributed among RBCs on Kleihauer stain. In contrast, sickle cell-thalassemia patients may have high HbF values, but HbF is seen in only relatively few RBCs.

Sickle Cell-HbD Disease

HbS/HbD disease occurs in 1 in 20,000 African Americans. It resembles HbSC disease, but is less severe than sickle cell anemia.

Findings are intermediate between those of sickle cell anemia and of sickle cell trait. Clinically mild syndrome.

♦ Hb electrophoresis cannot distinguish HbS and HbD at alkaline pH. HbS and HbD can be separated at acid pH 6.2 and distinguished by solubility studies (HbD is more soluble).

○ One parent may have a negative sickling test but with abnormal Hb showing HbS mobility.

Hemoglobin C Disease

In hemoglobin C (HbC) disease, HbC agglutinates and crystallizes with deoxygenation.

HbC Trait

HbAC occurs in 2% of African Americans, less frequently in other Americans; it is prevalent in West Africa. The disease is asymptomatic.

HEMATOLOGY

♦ Hb electrophoresis: HbA = 50% to 60%; HbC = 30% to 40%. Lesser amounts of HbC with microcytosis usually means coexisting α-thalassemia.
○ Blood smear shows variable numbers (≤40%) of target cells and hypochromia.

No other abnormalities are seen.

HbC Disease

♦ HPLC and Hb electrophoresis demonstrate the abnormal hemoglobin.
Mild normochromic, normocytic to microcytic, hemolytic anemia is present.
Blood smear shows many target cells, a variable number of microspherocytes, occasional nucleated RBCs, and a few tetragonal crystals within RBCs that increase following splenectomy.
Reticulocyte count is slightly increased (2%–10%).
Osmotic fragility is decreased.
Mechanical fragility is increased.
RBC survival time is decreased.
HbF is slightly increased.
Increase in serum bilirubin is minimal.
Normoblastic hyperplasia of bone marrow is present.

HbC-Beta-Thalassemia

HbC-β-thalassemia resembles HbC/HbC but a different concentration of HbC is present on electrophoresis and HPLC.
Usually asymptomatic but moderate hemolysis may occur if HbA is absent, in which case family studies may be needed to differentiate from HbC/HbC.

HbSC Disease

See later in this chapter.

Hemoglobin D Disease

Homozygous HbD Disease

♦ HPLC and Hb electrophoresis demonstrate the abnormal Hb at acid pH.
Mild microcytic anemia.
Target cells and spherocytes.
Decreased RBC survival time.

Heterozygous HbD Trait

♦ HPLC and Hb electrophoresis demonstrate the abnormal hemoglobin at acid pH.
There are no other laboratory findings.

Hemoglobin E Disease

HbE disease occurs almost exclusively in Southeast Asia. It is found in 3% of the population in Vietnam and up to 35% of the population in Laos; migrates like HbA$_2$ on electrophoresis.

Homozygous HbE Disease

Mild hypochromic hemolytic anemia or no anemia
○ Marked microcytosis (MCV 55–70 fL) and erythrocytosis (~5,500,000/μL)
○ Smear shows predominant target cells (25%–60%), which differentiates this from HbE trait and microcytes.
♦ HPLC and Hb electrophoresis shows 95% to 97% HbE, and the rest is HbF. Electrophoretic mobility same as HbA$_2$ but concentration is higher (15%–30%).

Heterozygous HbE Trait

Asymptomatic persons found during family studies or screening programs
Phenotype similar to mild form of β-thalassemia
Normal Hb concentration

Slight to moderate microcytosis (MCV 65–80 fL)
Erythrocytosis (RBC = 5.0–5.34 million/μL)
♦ HPLC and electrophoresis show 30% to 35% HbE.

HbE-Beta-Thalassemia

HbE-β-thalassemia is the most common symptomatic thalassemia in Southeast Asia.
○ Hemolytic anemia varies from moderate to marked severity (thalassemia major or
  intermedia phenotype).
○ Smear shows severe hypochromia and microcytosis, marked anisopoikilocytosis
  with many teardrop and target forms. Nucleated RBCs and basophilic stippling may
  be present.

HbE-Alpha-Thalassemia

Analogous to α-thalassemia-1 and 2 and HbH
*In African Americans, 28% have mild α-thalassemia without microcytosis, 3% are
homozygous α-thalassemia with microcytosis, and 1% have microcytosis due to
β-thalassemia. Median Hb is ~1 g/dL lower in blacks without iron deficiency than in
whites.*
α- or β-thalassemia or HbE occur in ~50% of Southeast Asians and cause microcytosis.

Hemoglobin F

**HbF has two alpha and two gamma chains. Normal: >50% at birth; gradual
decrease to ~5% by age 5 months. <2% when older than age 2 years.**

Detected By

• Flow cytometry.
• Hb electrophoresis.
• Kleihauer-Betke stain of peripheral blood smear. Now measured more accurately by
  flow cytometry with anti-HbF antibodies.

Use

Quantitates amount (milliliters) of fetal RBCs in maternal circulation. Normal
<1%. In rhesus-factor (Rh) –negative women with Rh-positive fetuses, to deter-
mine need/dose of RhIg especially in presence of blunt abdominal trauma, invasive procedures (e.g., chorionic villus biopsy), placenta previa, abruptio placenta.
(See Hemolytic Diseases of Newborn.) HbF increases in pregnancy in ≤25% of
women.

Interferences
False-positive result in hemoglobinopathies (SS, SA, hereditary persistence HbF)

Increased In
Various hemoglobinopathies (see Tables 11-10 and 11-12). About 50% of patients with
β-thalassemia minor have high levels of HbF; even higher levels are found in virtually all patients with β-thalassemia major. In sickle cell disease, HbF >30% protects
the cell from sickling; therefore, even infants with homozygous S have few problems
before age 3 months.
Hereditary persistence of HbF: Inherited persistence of increased HbF in adult without clinical manifestations due to many different genetic lesions (probably autosomal dominant). Incidence <0.2%. Hb electrophoresis shows HbF = ≤30% and HbA
= 60% to 70%. May be pancellular or heterocellular (HbF is increased only in some
RBCs) as seen by Kleihauer-Betke stain of peripheral blood smear. Decreased MCV
and MCHC.
Nonhereditary refractory normoblastic anemia (1/3 of patients).
PA (50% of untreated patients); increases after treatment and then gradually decreases
during next 6 months; some patients still have slight elevation thereafter. Minimal
elevation occurs in ~5% of patients with other types of megaloblastic anemia.
Some patients with leukemia, especially juvenile myeloid leukemia with HbF of 30% to
60%, absence of Ph[1], rapid fatal course, more pronounced thrombocytopenia, and
lower total WBC count.
Multiple myeloma.
Molar pregnancy.
Patients with Trisomy 13 or Trisomy 21 (Down syndrome).

HEMATOLOGY

Table 11-12. Classification of Beta-Thalassemia Syndromes

Genotype	Anemia	Microcytosis	Hb Electrophoresis
Normal			
Beta/beta	None	None	HbA_2 <3.5%, HbF <1%
Thalassemia minima			
Beta/beta$^+$ (mild)	None	None	HbA_2 = N or slightly I HbF = I
Thalassemia minor			
Beta/beta$^+$ (severe)	Mild	Mild to moderate	HbA_2 = 3.5%–7.5% HbF = N or slightly I
Beta/beta^0	Mild	Mild to moderate	HbA_2 = 3.5%–7.5% HbF = N or slightly I
Beta/delta beta^0	Mild	Mild to moderate	HbA_2 = N or D HbF = 5%–20%
Beta/beta Lepore	Mild	Mild to moderate	HbA_2 = N or D HbF = I Hb Lepore up to 8%
Thalassemia intermedia			
Beta$^+$ (mild)/beta$^+$ (severe)	Moderate to severe	Moderate to severe	HbA_2 = 6%–8% HbF = 20%–50% HbA = remainder
Delta beta^0/delta beta^0	Moderate to severe	Moderate to severe	HbF only
Thalassemia major			
Beta^0/beta^0	Severe	Severe	HbA_2 = 3%–11% HbA = 0 HbF = remainder
Beta$^+$ (severe)/beta$^+$ (severe)	Severe	Severe	HbA_2 = 3%–11% HbF = 10%–90% HbA = remainder
Beta^0/beta$^+$ (severe)	Severe	Severe	HbA_2 = 3%–11% HbF = 10%–90% HbA = remainder
Beta^0/beta Lepore	Severe	Severe	HbF >80% Hb Lepore = remainder

D, decreased; I, increased; N, normal.

Acquired aplastic anemia (due to drugs, toxic chemicals, or infections, or idiopathic); returns to normal only after complete remission and therefore is reliable indicator of complete recovery. Better prognosis in patients with higher initial level.

Some chronic viral infections (e.g., cytomegalovirus [CMV], Epstein-Barr virus [EBV]).

Decreased In

A rare case of multiple chromosome abnormalities (probably C/D translocation)

Thalassemias

The thalassemias are a heterogeneous group of inherited disorders of impaired rate of Hb polypeptide chain synthesis but usually structurally normal; they occur predominantly in Mediterranean, African, and Asian persons. β-thalassemia is caused by mutations in one or both genes encoding β-globin chains. Shows precipitation of α-globin chains causing premature apoptosis of erythroid precursors and increased production of δ-globin chains, which join with α-globin chains forming HbA_2.

Table 11-13. Comparison of β-Thalassemias

| Phenotype | Genotype | Hb Electrophoresis | | Blood Smear |
		At Birth	Adulthood	
β-thalassemia major	$(\beta^0/\beta^0\beta^0/\beta^0)$, (β^0/β^+)	No HbA	HbF = 70%–100%	Severe hypochromic microcytic anemia. Marked thalassemia picture. Transfusion dependent.
β-intermediate	(β^+/β^+), $(\beta^+/\beta^0)+$ $(-/\alpha\alpha)$	Normal (β^+/β^+) 4%–10% Bart $(--/\alpha\alpha)$	HbA = 0%–80% HbA$_2$ = 2%–7% HbF = 20%–100%	Severe hypochromic microcytic anemia. Nucleated, teardrop, and target RBCs Severe symptoms. Needs occ. transfusions.
β-thalassemia minor	$(\beta^0\beta^0/\beta)$, (β^+/β)	Normal (β^+/β^+)	HbA$_2$ = >3.5% HbF = 2%–5%	Thalassemia picture, few elliptocytes. Slight ↑RDW. Asymptomatic.
HbE/β^0-thalassemia	$(HbE/\beta^0\beta^0)$	No HbA	HbE = 50%–70% HbF = 30%–50%	Severe anemia. Nucleated RBCs. Transfusion dependent.
Triplicate α-globin	$(\beta^0/\beta)+$ $(\alpha\alpha\alpha/\alpha\alpha)$	Normal	HbA$_2$ = >3.5% HbF = 2%–5%	Moderate anemia. Hypo-chromia. ↑RDW. Nucleated RBCs, prominent stippling. Intermediate severity.

Occ., occasional; ↑ increased; ↓ decreased.

- See Tables 11-2, 11-7, and 11-12 to 11-14. In α-thalassemias, β- and γ-globin chains are produced in excess. In β-thalassemias, α-globin chains are produced in excess. β^4 = HbH; γ^4 = HbBart.
- β-thalassemia is confirmed by Hb electrophoresis. α-thalassemia is confirmed by Southern blot, which detects one or both of the two α-globin genes on chromosome 16. HPLC is the method of choice.
- β-chain synthesis is normally low at birth because HbA becomes predominant only after the first few months. Clinical and laboratory findings correspond to this; thus neonatal anemia occurs only with α-thalassemia, not with β-thalassemia.

Beta-Thalassemia Minima

Silent carrier of β-thalassemia trait
Normal RBC morphology and Hb electrophoresis
♦ Demonstrated by reduced rate of β-globin synthesis with increased α:β-globin chain ratio.

Beta-Thalassemia Trait

♦ In uncomplicated cases, Hb is normal or only slightly decreased (11–12 g/dL), while the RBC count is increased (5–7 million/μL). Most nonanemic patients with microcytosis have thalassemia minor.
♦ Microcytic anemia with Hb <9.3 g/dL is unlikely to be thalassemia minor. MCV <75 fL while Hct is >30; may be as low as 55 fL. Microcytosis may be difficult to detect morphologically.
♦ Ratio of microcytic to hypochromic RBCs is >0.9 but <0.9 in iron-deficiency. MCHC >31%.
Blood smear changes are less than in thalassemia major.
Anisocytosis is less marked than in IDA.

HEMATOLOGY

Table 11-14. Comparison of Delta-Beta Thalassemias

Phenotype	Genotype[a]	Hb Electrophoresis		Blood Smear
		At Birth	Adulthood	
δ-β trait	$(\gamma\text{--}/\gamma\delta\beta)$	Normal	HbA$_2$ is N HbF = 5%–20%	Thalassemia picture. Asymptomatic.
Hb Lepore trait	$(\gamma x/\gamma\delta\beta)^a$	Normal	HbF = 1%–6% Hb Lepore = 10%	Thalassemia picture. Asymptomatic.
Homozygous Lepore	$(\gamma x/\gamma x)^a$	Normal	HbF = 75% Hb Lepore = 25%	Severe hypochromic microcytic anemia. Target, teardrop, nucleated RBCs. Severe symptoms. Needs occasional transfusions.
γ-δ-β trait	$(\text{---}/\gamma\delta\beta)$	Normal	Normal	Thalassemia picture in adults. Hypochromic microcytic anemia in neonate with hemolysis that spontaneously resolves.
γ-thalassemia minor	$(\gamma\text{-}/\gamma\gamma)$, $(\text{--}/\gamma\gamma)$	HbF = $\downarrow$/N	Normal	Mild hypochromic microcytic anemia in neonate with hemolysis that spontaneously resolves.

N, normal; $\downarrow$ decreased.
[a]x = β-δ indicates delta-beta fusion gene.

Poikilocytosis is mild to moderate; more striking than IDA,IDA with Hb = 10 to 12 g/dL. Target cells and oval forms may be numerous.

Occasional RBCs show basophilic stippling in β-thalassemia minor (rare in blacks but common in Mediterranean patients).

Reticulocyte count is increased (2%–10%).

Serum iron is normal or slightly increased; transferrin saturation may be increased. TIBC and serum ferritin are normal.

Cellular marrow contains stainable iron.

Osmotic fragility is decreased.

♦ Hb electrophoresis shows increased HbA$_2$ (>4%); a normal value does not rule out this diagnosis.

Definitions:

• HbA$_2$ has two α and two δ chains.
• HbF has two α and two γ chains.
• HbH has four β chains.
• Bart Hb has four γ chains.
• Hb Lepore has two α and two β-δ chains fused.
• HbE is abnormal Hb with altered β chain. HbE disease mimics thalassemia.
• β^0 = absent Hb.
• β^+ = deficient Hb.

Beta-Thalassemia Minor

More than 50 forms of β-thalassemia minor are recognized by gene cloning.

See Table 11-12.

○ Slight or mild anemia. Most important differential diagnosis is iron deficiency (see Anemia, Iron-Deficiency).

MCV usually <75 and Hct >30; RBC count is often increased. *Microcytosis with RBC >4.5 million/mL^3 is said to be diagnostic for thalassemia and to rule out iron deficiency.*
♦ Normal iron, TIBC, serum ferritin
♦ Increased HbA$_2$ (3%–6%) on Hb electrophoresis and a slight increase in HbF (2%–10%). HbA$_2$ is often decreased in iron deficiency; thus A$_2$ level may be normal in concomitant iron deficiency and β-thalassemia minor and the diagnosis of β-thalassemia trait cannot be made until iron deficiency has been treated. HbA$_2$ and F are absent in α-thalassemia. *Thus, normal Hb electrophoresis and England-Fraser <–6 in the absence of iron deficiency implies α-thalassemia minor.*

Thalassemia Intermedia

Two percent to 10% of thalassemics have thalassemia intermedia; they may be homozygous δ–β, β^0, or β$^+$, with or without an α gene, or double heterozygous with an abnormal Hb such as S or E.

Less severe clinical and laboratory findings than major, which occur at later age.
Hb is usually >6.5 g/dL.
Combination of HbE and β-thalassemia results in wide spectrum of clinical disorders, varying from thalassemia to much milder forms that do not require transfusions.

Thalassemia Major (Cooley Anemia, Mediterranean Anemia)

Several Hb electrophoretic patterns are characteristic (see Table 11-12).
♦ Classification of β-thalassemia syndromes):

• Homozygous β^0: HbA is absent; HbF and HbA$_2$ are present.
• Homozygous β$^+$: HbA, HbA$_2$ and HbF are all detected.
• HbF = 10% to 90%; HbA is decreased; HbA$_2$ may be normal, low, or high.

♦ Marked hypochromic microcytic regenerative hemolytic anemia. Often Hb = 2.0 to 6.5 g/dL, Hct = 10% to 24%, RBC count = 2 to 3 million, indices are decreased.
♦ Blood smear shows marked anisocytosis, poikilocytosis, target cells, spherocytes, and hypochromic, fragmented, and bizarre RBCs; also many nucleated RBCs—basophilic stippling, Cabot rings, siderocytes.
Reticulocyte count is increased.
WBCs are often increased, with normal differential or marked shift to left.
Platelets are normal.
Bone marrow is cellular and shows erythroid hyperplasia and increased iron.
Serum iron and TIBC are increased. After age 5 years, iron-binding capacity is usually saturated.
Laboratory findings of hemolysis and liver dysfunction (e.g., increased serum LD, aspartate aminotransferase [AST], ALT, and indirect bilirubin [1–3 mg/dL], urine and stool urobilinogen; serum haptoglobin and hemopexin [normal = 0.5–2 mg/dL] are very decreased or absent).

• Liver dysfunction causing disturbance of factors V, VII, IX, XI, prothrombin.

RBC survival time is decreased.
Osmotic fragility is decreased.
Mechanical fragility is increased.
Laboratory findings due to complications, e.g.,

• Secondary hypersplenism (usually occurs between age 5 and 10 years, detected when transfusion requirement >200–250 mg/kg body weight, at which time splenectomy is indicated).
○• Hemosiderosis (hepatic fibrosis and cirrhosis; endocrinopathies with hypofunction of pituitary, thyroid, etc.)
○• Bone disease (e.g., skull changes, rickets, osteoporosis)
• Cardiac

Proteinuria, hyposthenuria, failure to acidify urine, increased urobilin and urobilinogen with dark color may be present.
β-thalassemia trait demonstrated in both parents.
♦ Prenatal diagnosis is possible at 16 weeks' gestation in 85% of cases by DNA analysis of amniotic cells; the rest can be diagnosed by α:β chain ratios of fetal blood (obtained by fetoscopy).

HEMATOLOGY

Table 11-15. Differentiation of Microcytic Anemias of Iron Deficiency and Thalassemia Minor

	Iron Deficiency	No Differentiation	Thalassemia Minor	Sensitivity (%)[a]	Accuracy (%)[a]
Hb (g/L)	<9.3 M or F	9.3–13.5 M 9.3–12.5 F	>13.5 M >12.5 F	100	65
MCV (fL)		>68	<68		
MCHC (g/dL)	<30	>30			
RBC (per μL)	<4.2	4.2–5.5	>5.5		
Erythrocytosis				68	90
Mentzer formula[b] (MCV/RBC)	>13		<13	95	65
England-Fraser formula[b] (MCV − [5 × Hb + RBC + K, if K = 3.4])	Positive number		Negative number	69	77
Shine-Lal formula[b] (MCV^2 × MCH)			<1,530	100	86
MCV of 1 parent <79				86	86
Free erythrocyte protoporphyrin = 25				60	67
HbA$_2$ >3.5%				85	90
Microcytic/hypochromic ratio[c]	<0.9		>0.9		

F, females; M, males; MCV, mean corpuscular volume; MCHC, mean corpuscular hemoglobin concentration.

[a]Accuracy in distinguishing anemias of thalassemia minor and iron deficiency (%).

[b]In patients with polycythemia vera who develop iron deficiency with microcytosis, a negative number results. These formulas do not account for the indeterminate zone of no differentiation.

[c]Using Technicon H-1 hematology analyzer (Technicon, Tarrytown, NY).

Source: d'Onofrio G, et al. Arch Pathol Lab Med 1992;116:84.

Table 11-16. Classification of Alpha-Thalassemia Syndromes

	Number of Gene Deletions	Anemia	Microcytosis	Hb Electrophoresis	
				At birth	Adulthoed
α-thal trait 2 (silent carrier)	1	0	0	1%–2% Bart	N
α-thal trait 1 (heterozygous; or homozygous)	2	Mild	Mild	5%–10% Bart	N HbA$_2$ not I
HbH disease (α-thal 2 + α-thal 1)	3	Moderate	Marked	20%–40% Bart	HbH Small amount of HbA
Hydrops fetalis (homozygous)	4	Fatal at/before birth		>50% Bart	Hb Bart

α-thal, α thalassemia; I, increased; N, normal.
α-thalassemias are characterized by decreased or absent synthesis of globin chains; very common in African, Asian, and Mediterranean populations. Most prevalent genetic trait in the world.
Hb Bart disappears by age 3–6 mos. Hb Bart acts like very-high-affinity Hb with marked left-shifted oxygen dissociation curve resembling CO poisoning.
Normal Hb electrophoresis and England-Fraser of < −6 in the absence of iron deficiency implies α-thalassemia minor. Screening can be done for most common deletions of α thalassemia using PCR amplification of specific DNA sequences.

Alpha-Thalassemias

α-thalassemias are caused by mutations in one or more of four genes encoding α-globin chains. α-thalassemias are characterized by decreased or absent synthesis of α-globin chains. It is the most prevalent genetic trait in the world and is very common in Asian, African, and Mediterranean populations.

See Tables 11-16 and 11-17.
♦ Isoelectric focusing is more sensitive than Hb gel electrophoresis for variants present in small amounts. HPLC is the current method of choice.
♦ DNA screening can be done for most common deletions of α-thalassemia.
Deletion of one α allele causes asymptomatic but transmissible trait. Occurs in ≤30% of black populations. Coincident with sickle cell or HbC trait, reduces the proportion of HbS or HbC below the usual 35% to 40% (also slightly decreasing the clinical severity); thus <35% variant Hb is good evidence for coexisting α-thalassemia in such patients. No clinical or hematologic findings.
There are two different functional α-globin genes: α-1 and α-2.
Both α-globin genes may be deleted from same chromosome, or one α-globin gene can be deleted from each chromosome; these have different inheritance risks. Most cases are caused by gene deletions.

• Anemia (minimal hypochromic, microcytic) may or may not be present; may show increased target cells, anisocytosis, and erythrocytosis; may resemble β-thalassemia trait but without increased HbA$_2$.

Hypochromic, microcytic hemolytic anemia is moderate to mild (Hb = 7–11 g/dL), with many target or deformed RBCs, and is accentuated by infection, drugs, pregnancy, etc.
♦ Characteristic patterns appear on RBC and platelet histograms due to very small RBCs; may cause inaccurate platelet count.
○ Supravital stain shows granular inclusions (precipitated β-chains), which are very marked after splenectomy.

HbH Disease

HbH disease occurs when three of four α-globin alleles are absent and an excess of β-globins exists.

Table 11-17. Comparison of Alpha-Thalassemias

| Phenotype | Number of α-globin genes | Hb Electrophoresis | | Blood Smear | MCV (fl) | MCH (pg) |
		At Birth	Adult			
Normal	4	N	N Asymptomatic	Normal	85–95	28–32
α-thalassemia minor (mild) (silent carrier)	3 (-α/αα)	Bart Hb = 1%–3%	N Asymptomatic	Normal or mild thalassemia picture	74–88	24–28
α-thalassemia minor (severe)	2 (-α/αα) (-α/-α) (--/αα)	Bart Hb = 4%–10%	HbA$_2$ = ↓/N	Mild hypochromic microcytic anemia	65–73	20–24
HbH disease	1 (--/-α)	Bart Hb = 10%–25% Trace of HbH	HbH = 10%–25%	Moderate-to-severe hypochromic microcytic anemia	59–72	17–21
α-thalassemia major, lethal hydrops fetalis	0 (--/--)	Bart Hb = 75%. Stillbirth			110–120	Greatly decreased

MCH, mean corpuscular hemoglobin; MCV, mean corpuscular volume; N, normal; ↓ decreased.

Inherited α-thalassemia 1 from one parent and α-thalassemia 2 from other. May also be
due to deletion of two α-globin genes and presence of α-chain variant Hb Constant
Spring. May present with neonatal jaundice. Acquired form may occur during course
of myeloproliferative disorders due to relative suppression of α-chain gene.
Laboratory findings of anemia, jaundice, gallstones, iron overload.

Hb Bart

**Hb Bart occurs when all four α-globin genes are deleted (four γ-globin chains are
substituted) with no normal Hb; may cause stillbirth or early postnatal death due
to severe hypoxia and hydrops fetalis.**

Hb Bart disappears by age 3 to 6 months.
Hb Bart acts like very-high-affinity Hb with a marked left-shifted O_2 dissociation curve
resembling CO poisoning.
♦ Prenatal diagnosis by Southern blot of amniotic fluid DNA or chorionic villus or
using PCR techniques or HPLC.

Aplasias and Pancytopenias

Anemia, Aplastic[9]

♦ Aplastic anemia is characterized by peripheral blood pancytopenia with variable
bone marrow hypocellularity in the absence of underlying myeloproliferative or
malignant disease.

• Neutropenia (absolute neutrophil count <1,500/μL) is always present; often monocytopenia is present.
• Lymphocyte count is normal; reduced helper/inducer:cytotoxic/suppressor ratio.
• Platelet count <150,000/μL; severity varies.
• Anemia is usually normochromic, normocytic but may be slightly macrocytic; may
be <7.0 g/L with Hct = 20% to 25%. RDW is normal. Poikilocytes are not seen on
peripheral blood smear.
• Bone marrow is hypocellular; aspiration and biopsy should both be performed to
rule out leukemia, myelodysplastic syndrome, granulomas, tumor.

Reticulocyte count corrected for Hct is decreased; usually <25 × 10^9/L.
Serum iron is increased.
Flow cytometry phenotyping shows virtual absence of CD34 stem cells in blood and marrow.
Laboratory findings represent the whole spectrum, from the most severe condition of
the classic type with marked leukopenia, thrombocytopenia, anemia, and acellular
bone marrow, to cases with involvement only of erythroid elements. In some cases,
the marrow may be cellular or hyperplastic. Related to pure RBC aplasia, agranulocytosis, amegakaryocytic thrombocytopenia.

Criteria for *Severe* Aplastic Anemia (International Aplastic Anemia Study Group)
≥2 peripheral blood criteria plus either marrow criteria

• Peripheral blood criteria:
  Neutrophils <500/μL; <200/μL in *very severe* aplastic anemia
  Platelets <20,000/μL
  Reticulocyte count ≤40 × 10^3/μL or ≤60 × 10^3/μL (to reflect changes in
  instrumentation) or <1% (corrected for Hct) (to reflect changes in instru-
  mentation)
• Marrow criteria:
  Severe hypocellularity
  Moderate hypocellularity with <30% of residual cells being hematopoietic

---

HEMATOLOGY

[9]Young NS. Acquired aplastic anemia. *New Engl J Med* 1999;282:271–278.

Due To

Idiopathic in 50% of cases
Chemicals (e.g., benzene family, insecticides) cause varying degrees of severity up to aplastic anemia. Hemolytic anemia is sometimes produced. Chemicals cause, in order of decreasing frequency, anemia, macrocytosis, thrombocytopenia, leukopenia, decreased lymphocytes, increased eosinophils
Cytotoxic and antimetabolite drugs
Other drugs, e.g.:
    Antimicrobials (especially chloramphenicol, quinacrine), anticonvulsants (especially hydantoin), analgesics (especially phenylbutazone), antihistamines, antidiabetic drugs, sedatives, others (especially gold; NSAIDs, sulfonamides, antithyroid drugs)
Immunologic disorders (e.g., graft-versus-host disease [GVHD], thymoma and thymic carcinoma)
Ionizing irradiation (radiographs, radioisotopes)
Malnutrition (e.g., kwashiorkor)
Viral infections in 10% of cases (especially seronegative hepatitis; EBV, CMV, HIV, parvovirus)
Constitutional, inherited (e.g., Fanconi anemia [see next section]; Down syndrome)
Leukemia is the underlying disease in 1% to 5% of patients who present with aplastic anemia. Fifteen percent of aplastic anemia patients develop myelodysplasia and leukemia.
Paroxysmal nocturnal hemoglobinuria (PNH) develops in 5% to 10% of patients with aplastic anemia, and aplastic anemia develops in 25% of patients with PNH.

Pancytopenia

Pancytopenia is a descriptive term referring to reduced number of all three blood lines: Anemia *plus* leukopenia (absolute myeloid decrease may be associated with relative lymphocytosis or with lymphocytopenia) *plus* thrombocytopenia.

Due To

Hypersplenism
Diseases of marrow (e.g., metastatic carcinoma, multiple myeloma, aleukemic leukemia osteopetrosis, myelosclerosis, myelofibrosis, etc.)
Aplastic anemias (see previous)
Infections
Autoimmune diseases
Megaloblastic anemias (e.g., PA)

Anemia, Fanconi

Fanconi anemia is a simple autosomal recessive syndrome of pancytopenia and characteristic congenital anomalies of rudimentary thumbs, hypoplastic radii, short stature, renal anomalies, skin hyperpigmentation, and random chromosomal breaks.

Pancytopenia is usually noted at 4 to 10 years of age but may be present from infancy into a patient's 20s. Anemia, leukopenia, and thrombocytopenia may not all be present at onset.

* Profound anemia may be macrocytic and hyperchromic or normochromic.
* Increased HbF (>28%).
* Decreased granulocytes.
* Atrophic bone marrow.

Causes >20% of childhood cases of aplastic anemia.
Increased incidence of leukemia in patients and relatives.
Cytogenetic studies show normal chromosome numbers but structural instability causing breaks, gaps, constrictions, rearrangements.
Laboratory findings are due to anemia, hemorrhage, infection, renal abnormalities.

Aplasia, Congenital Pure Red Cell (Diamond-Blackfan Anemia)

Congenital pure red cell aplasia (PRCA) is a rare (usually sporadic but may be familial autosomal dominant) anemia associated with congenital anomalies of

the kidneys, eyes, skeleton, and heart. The usual onset is before age 12 months; it is present at birth in 25% of patients. Spontaneous remissions occur in ~20% of patients after months or years. May be related to human papilloma virus (HPV) B19 infection.

○ Severe normochromic, often macrocytic, anemia that is refractory to all treatment except transfusion and sometimes prednisone. Reticulocytes are <1%.

WBC count, differential blood count, and platelet counts are normal.

○ Bone marrow usually shows marked decrease in erythroid precursors. Myeloid cells and megakaryocytes are normal.

○ Increased erythropoietin level.

○ Increased fetal Hb; adenosine deaminase activity in RBCs is characteristically increased.

There is no evidence of hemolysis.

Normal serum folic acid, vitamin B_{12}, liver function tests, RBC life span, negative Coombs test.

Normal serum iron with increased saturation level.

Laboratory changes caused by effects of therapy, e.g.:

• Hemosiderosis
• Steroids (e.g., infections, diabetes mellitus, gastric ulcer)

Irradiation, Hematologic Effects

The hematologic effects of irradiation depend on the amount of irradiation received.

Severe

• Severe leukopenia with infection
• Thrombocytopenia and increased vascular fragility, causing hemorrhage; begins in 4 to 7 days, with peak severity in 16 to 22 days
• Aplastic anemia if patient survives 3 to 6 weeks; laboratory findings due to complications, such as hemorrhage, infection, dehydration

Mild (<300 R)

• Increased neutrophils within a few hours, with onset of irradiation sickness
• Decreased lymphocytes after 24 hours, causing decrease in total WBC count
• No anemia unless dose of radiation is greater; may appear in 4 to 8 weeks (*Early appearance of anemia with greater irradiation is caused by hemorrhage and changes in fluid homeostasis rather than marrow injury.*)
• Platelets slightly decreased (some patients)

Chronic (Occupational)

• Decreased granulocytes
• Increased lymphocytes, relative or absolute
• Varying degrees of leukocytosis and leukemoid reactions
• Varying degrees of anemia, normocytic or macrocytic; erythrocytosis
• Thrombocytopenia

Late

• Increased incidence of leukemia (e.g., in survivors of atomic bomb explosions)
• Increased incidence of visceral malignancy (e.g., liver cancer caused by Thorotrast, bone cancer caused by radium)

Tests for Hemolysis

Laboratory Tests for Hemolysis

♦ Evidence of hemolysis, e.g. (but may also be altered in other conditions):

(1) Serum haptoglobin <6 mg/dL (is most sensitive) and hemopexin are decreased or absent during an episode.

HEMATOLOGY

(2) Increased serum LD >220 U/L (best analyte for quantitating)

Increased serum indirect bilirubin >1.5 mg/dL; lacks sensitivity. Not >4 mg/dL unless liver disease is also present, except in neonates. Normal in 25% of patients with hereditary spherocytosis and <50% with immunohemolytic anemia. Increased serum potassium.

(3) Hemoglobinemia is present; increases during sleep.

Visual inspection of serum[10]

Red: moderate (≤100 mg/dL) or severe (≥100 mg/dL)

Pink: mild (20–30 mg/dL)

(4) Hemoglobinuria (cola-colored urine)

- Urine may contain hemosiderin (in WBCs and epithelial cells of sediment); because it may last for months, is particularly useful in cases of intermittent hemolysis (e.g., PNH). Also occurs in hemosiderosis and hemochromatosis.
- Increased urobilinogen in urine.
- Stool urobilinogen is usually increased; is rarely used.

(5) Decreased RBC ⁵¹Cr lifespan is gold standard, but this test is expensive and time-consuming; is rarely needed.

- RBC creatine correlates closely with RBC ⁵¹Cr lifespan, even with mild hemolysis.

○ Evidence of antibodies

(6) Coombs test

○ Evidence of increased RBC production

- Increased reticulocyte count >2.06% and possibly nucleated RBCs
- Erythroid hyperplasia may be seen on bone marrow

Haptoglobins, Serum

Haptoglobin is a glycoprotein synthesized mainly in liver. It sequesters free Hb released from hemolyzed RBCs, which is transported by macrophages to liver where the heme is broken down to bilirubin. The normal adult value is between 40 and 180 mg/dL. The same function is served by hemopexin and especially albumin.

Use

Most sensitive test for RBC destruction; absent when rate of destruction is double that of normal.

Indicator of chronic hemolysis (e.g., hereditary spherocytosis, pyruvate kinase [PK] deficiency, sickle cell disease, thalassemia major, untreated PA). Such patients should not have splenectomy if serum haptoglobin is >40 mg/dL if infection and inflammation have been ruled out. Following splenectomy, increased haptoglobin level indicates success of surgery for these conditions (e.g., haptoglobin reappears at 24 hours and becomes normal in 4 to 6 days in hereditary spherocytosis treated with splenectomy).

In diagnosis of transfusion reaction by comparison of concentrations in pretransfusion and posttransfusion samples. In a posttransfusion reaction, the serum haptoglobin level decreases in 6 to 8 hours; at 24 hours it is <40 mg/dL or <40% of pretransfusion level.

In paternity studies, may aid by determination of haptoglobin phenotypes.

Increased In

Conditions associated with increased ESR and α-2 globulin (haptoglobin is also an acute-phase reactant) (infections, inflammation, trauma, necrosis of tissue, hepatitis, scurvy, amyloidosis, nephrotic syndrome, disseminated neoplasms such as lymphomas and leukemias, collagen diseases such as rheumatic fever, RA, and dermatomyositis). *Thus these conditions may mask presence of concomitant hemolysis.*

One third of patients with obstructive biliary disease

Therapy with steroids or androgens

---

[10]Alter D, et al. Q&A: Does the CAP have definitions for marked, moderate, and slight hemolysis? *CAP Today* 2000;7:111.

Aplastic anemia (normal to very high)
Diabetes mellitus
Smoking
Aging
Decreased or Absent In
Hemoglobinemia (related to the duration and severity of hemolysis) due to:
Intravascular hemolysis (e.g., hereditary spherocytosis with marked hemolysis, PK deficiency, autoimmune hemolytic anemia, some transfusion reactions)
Extravascular hemolysis (e.g., large retroperitoneal hemorrhage)
Intramedullary hemolysis (e.g., thalassemia, megaloblastic anemias, sideroblastic anemias)
Genetically absent in 1% of white population and 4% to 10% of US blacks.
Parenchymatous liver disease (especially cirrhosis)
Protein loss via kidney, GI tract, skin
Infancy, pregnancy
Malnutrition

Lactate Dehydrogenase
See Chapter 3.

Hemoglobin, Serum
Hemoglobin is normally <5 mg/dL; it is easily visible at ~50 mg/dL; levels of about 100 to 150 mg/dL cause hemoglobinuria; >200 mg/dL causes clear cherry red color to serum.

Use
Increase indicates intravascular hemolysis
Slight Increase In
Sickle cell thalassemia
HbC disease
Moderate Increase In
Sickle cell HbC disease
Sickle cell anemia
Thalassemia major
Acquired (autoimmune) hemolytic anemia
Marked Increase In
Any rapid intravascular hemolysis

Red Blood Cell Survival (Chromium-51)
Normal RBC survival is 28 to 38 days, not 60 days because ^{51}Cr is eluted from Hb at rate of ~1%/d.

Use
Confirm decreased RBC survival in various disorders affecting RBCs.
If RBC production = RBC destruction, is also a measure of effective erythropoiesis.
Increased In
Thalassemia minor
In pure red cell anemia, half of the plasma radioactivity may not disappear for 7 to 8 hours. In the normal person, half of the radioactivity of plasma disappears in 1 to 2 hours.
Decreased In
Idiopathic acquired hemolytic anemia
PNH
Association with chronic lymphatic leukemia
Association with uremia
Congenital nonspherocytic hemolytic anemia
Hereditary spherocytosis
Elliptocytosis with hemolysis
HbC disease
Sickle cell HbC disease

Sickle cell anemia
PA
Megaloblastic anemia of pregnancy
Normal In
Sickle cell trait
HbC trait
Elliptocytosis without hemolysis or anemia

Coombs (Antiglobulin) Test

Positive Direct Coombs (Antiglobulin) Test

See Figure 11-5.
Use
Detects immunoglobulin antibodies and/or complement (C3) on patient's RBC membrane (e.g., autoimmune hemolysis, hemolytic disease of newborn, drug-induced hemolysis, transfusion reactions)
Interferences
False-positive result may occur in multiple myeloma and Waldenström macroglobulinemia
Positive In
Erythroblastosis fetalis
Most cases of autoimmune hemolytic anemia, including ≤15% of certain systemic diseases, especially acute and chronic leukemias, malignant lymphomas, and collagen diseases
Strength of reaction may be of prognostic value in patients with lymphoproliferative disorders
Delayed hemolytic transfusion reaction
Drug-induced reactions, e.g.:

* Alpha methyldopa (occurs in ≤30% of patients on continued therapy but <1% show hemolysis); rarely in first 6 months of treatment. If not found within 12 months, is unlikely to occur. Is dose-related, with lowest incidence in patients receiving ≤1 g daily. Reversal may take weeks to months after the drug is discontinued.
* L-Dopa
* Others (e.g., acetophenetidin, ethosuximide, cephalosporins [most common with cephalothin; less frequent with cefazolin and cephapirin; reported in 3%–50% of patients]), mefenamic acid, penicillin (with daily IV dose of 20 million units/d for several weeks), procainamide, quinidine, quinine, others.

Healthy blood donors (1:4,000–1:8,000 persons)
May be *weakly* positive in renal disease, epithelial malignancies, RA, inflammatory bowel diseases. Weakly positive reactions are not usually clinically significant.
Negative In
Hemolytic anemias caused by intrinsic defect in RBC (e.g., G6PD deficiency, hemoglobinopathies)
2% to 9% of patients with hemolytic anemia (due to smaller amount of IgG bound to RBCs but similar response to splenectomy or steroid therapy or to IgM, IgA, or IgD rather than IgG). This is a diagnosis of exclusion.

Positive Indirect Coombs Test

The positive indirect Coombs test uses the patient's serum, which contains antibody.

Use
Cross matching for blood transfusion
Detect and identify antibodies

* Specific antibody—usually isoimmunization from previous transfusion
* "Nonspecific" autoantibody in acquired hemolytic anemia

RBC phenotyping

* In genetic and forensic medicine
* To identify syngeneic twins for bone marrow transplantation

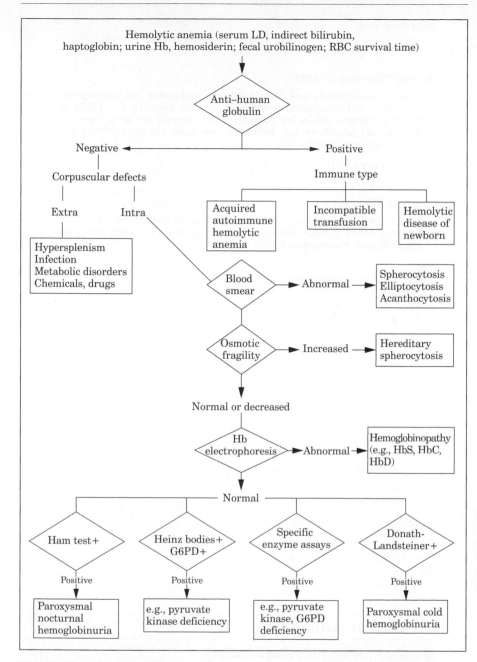

Fig. 11-5. Sequence of laboratory tests in macrocytic anemia. LD, lactase dehydrogenase; G6PD, glucose-6-phosphate dehydrogenase.

Interferences
Beware of false-positive and false-negative results caused by poor-quality test serum, not using fresh blood (must have complement), etc.

Autoantibodies, Warm

The warm autoantibody test detects immune responses that show greatest reactivity at 37°C. The autoantibodies react with the patient's own RBCs as well as donor or reagent RBCs but sometimes are specific for an antigen (especially Rh). Usually polyclonal IgG antibodies are used, but occasionally IgA or IgM; may be accompanied by C3.

♦ Demonstrated by positive DAT (Coombs) test.
See also "Cryoglobulinemia."

Osmotic Fragility

Tests of osmotic fragility use RBCs suspended in buffered solutions of various concentrations of NaCl. Spherocytes and stomatocytes hemolyze at lower NaCl concentration than normal RBCs.

Use
Diagnosis of hereditary spherocytic anemia

Increased In
Hereditary spherocytic anemia (can be ruled out if there is a normal fragility after 24-hour sterile incubation)
Hereditary nonspherocytic hemolytic anemia
Acquired hemolytic anemia (usually normal in PNH)
Hemolytic disease of newborn due to ABO incompatibility
Some cases of secondary hemolytic anemia (usually normal)
After thermal injury
Symptomatic hemolytic anemia in some cases of:

* Malignant lymphoma
* Leukemia
* Carcinoma
* Pregnancy
* Cirrhosis
* Infection (e.g., TB, malaria, syphilis)

Decreased In
Early infancy
IDA
Thalassemia
Sickle cell anemia
Homozygous HbC disease
Nutritional megaloblastic anemia
Postsplenectomy
Liver disease
Jaundice

Hemolytic Anemias

Anemias (Hemolytic), Classification
See Figures 11-1 and 11-5.

Hemoglobin Disorders
Intrinsic
Autosomal

Sickle cell (SS) disease	Common.
Thalassemias	Common.
HbC, HbD, HbE disease	Common.
Unstable hemoglobins	Very rare.

Membrane Disorders

Intrinsic

Congenital or familial (usually autosomal dominant)

Hereditary spherocytosis	Common (~0.02% of Northern European population.
Hereditary elliptocytosis	1:1,000–1:5,000.
Hereditary pyropoikilocytosis	Very rare.
Hereditary stomatocytosis	Very rare.
Acanthocytosis (abetalipoproteinemia)	Very rare.
Rh_{null} disease	Extremely rare.
Acquired—PNH (clonal stem cell disorder)	Rare.

Extrinsic

Acquired

Isoimmune (blood transfusion reaction, HDN)

Autoimmune (AIHA) (Coombs test is usually   Rare
  positive; spherocytes may be present)

Warm antibody 70% of AIHA

Idiopathic

Secondary to disease (e.g., lymphomas,
  leukemia, infectious mononucleosis, SLE)

Cold agglutinin syndrome

Secondary (e.g., *Mycoplasma pneumoniae*
  infection, infectious mononucleosis, viral
  infection, lymphoreticular neoplasms)

Paroxysmal cold hemoglobinuria   Rare.

Idiopathic

Atypical AIHA

Coombs test negative

Combined cold and warm AIHA

Drug induced (e.g., penicillin, methyldopa)   Common.

Nonimmune (*usually Coombs test negative and
  morphologic changes in blood smear*)

Physical or mechanical (e.g., prosthetic
  heart valves)

Microangiopathic hemolytic disease including DIC,
  TTP, HUS, etc.

March hemoglobinuria

Severe burns

Snakebite   See Chapter 17.

Osmotic—distilled water used in prostate resection

Infectious   See Chapter 15.

Protozoan (e.g., malaria, toxoplasmosis,
  leishmaniasis)

Bacterial (e.g., sepsis, clostridial toxins, bartonellosis)

Viral (e.g., echovirus)

PNH, paroxysmal nocturnal hemoglobinuria; HDN, hemolytic disease of newborn; AIHA,
acquired immune hemolytic anemia; SLE, systemic lupus erythematosus; DIC, disseminated
intravascular coagulation; TTP, thrombotic thrombocytopenic purpura; HUS, hemolytic uremic
syndrome.

Metabolic Disorders

Intrinsic

G6PD deficiency	Common.
Pyruvate kinase deficiency	Rare.

Phosphofructokinase deficiency

Hexokinase deficiency

Aldolase deficiency

Defects in nucleotide metabolism

Pyrimidine 5'-nucleotidase

Erythropoietic porphyria

HEMATOLOGY

Extrinsic
Drugs in normal RBCs or in G6PD deficiency
Marked hypophosphatemia (<1 mg/dL) may
  predispose to hemolysis
Others (e.g., lead poisoning, Wilson disease)

G6PD, glucose-6-phosphate dehydrogenase.

A useful approach to the diagnosis of hemolytic anemias may be based on:

- Site of RBC destruction (intravascular or extravascular)
- Site of etiologic defect (intracellular RBC or extracellular)
- Nature of defect (acquired or hereditary)

Hemolytic Anemias, Acquired or Hereditary

See Figure 11-2.
♦ Fifteen percent to 20% of acquired immune hemolytic anemias (AIHA) are related to
  drug therapy.
  - Some 3% of patients taking penicillins and cephalosporins develop a positive
    direct Coombs test; hemolysis is infrequent and usually extravascular.
  - About 10% of patients taking methyldopa develop a positive direct Coombs test
    after 3 to 6 months, but <1% develop hemolysis.
  - Serologic findings cannot be distinguished from idiopathic warm antibody AIHA.

Laboratory findings due to increased destruction of RBCs:

- RBC survival time differentiates intrinsic defect from factor outside RBC.
- Blood smear often shows marked spherocytosis. Anisocytosis, poikilocytosis, and
  polychromasia are seen.
- Slight abnormality of osmotic fragility occurs.
- Increased indirect serum bilirubin (<6 mg/dL because of compensatory excretory
  capacity of liver).
- Urine urobilinogen is increased (may vary with liver function; may be obscured by
  antibiotic therapy altering intestinal flora). Bile is absent.
- Hemoglobinemia and hemoglobinuria are present when hemolysis is very rapid.
- Haptoglobins are decreased or absent in chronic hemolytic diseases (removed fol-
  lowing combination with free Hb in serum).
- WBC count is usually elevated.

Laboratory findings due to compensatory increased production of RBCs:

- Normochromic, normocytic anemia. MCV reflects immaturity of circulating RBCs.
- Polychromatophilia is present.
- Reticulocyte count is increased.
- Erythroid hyperplasia of bone marrow is evident.

Laboratory findings due to mechanism of RBC destruction, e.g.:

- Positive direct Coombs test.
- Warm antibodies are found.
- Cold agglutinins are found.
- Biologic false-positive test for syphilis may occur.

Laboratory findings caused by underlying conditions:

- Malignant lymphoma
- Collagen diseases (e.g., SLE)
- Disseminated intravascular coagulation (DIC)
- Idiopathic pulmonary hemosiderosis
- Infections, especially mycoplasma infection; infectious mononucleosis, cholera
- RBC parasites (e.g., malaria, babesiosis)
- PNH
- Physical/chemical (e.g., burns, drugs, toxins [e.g., phenylhydrazine, benzene])

Antibody-induced:

- Drug-induced (e.g., quinidine, quinine, penicillins, cephalothin, alpha methyldopa)
- Autoantibody (warm, cold)

- Alloantibody (erythroblastosis fetalis, incompatible transfusion)
- Paroxysmal cold hemoglobinuria

Hemolytic Microangiopathic Anemias

Hemolytic microangiopathic anemias are characterized by traumatic intravascular hemolysis due to fibrin strands in vessel lumens.

See Tables 11-2, 11-4, and 11-7, and Figure 11-3.
◆ Peripheral blood smear establishes the diagnosis by characteristic burr cells, schistocytes, helmet cells, microspherocytes.
Nonimmune hemolytic anemia varies in severity depending on underlying condition.
Laboratory findings of hemolysis, e.g., increased serum LD, decreased haptoglobin, hemosiderinuria; hemoglobinemia and hemoglobinuria are less common.
Iron deficiency due to urinary loss of iron.
Direct Coombs test is usually negative.
Laboratory findings towing to causative disease.

Caused By
Renal disease (e.g., malignant hypertension, renal graft rejection)
Cardiac valvular disease (e.g., intracardiac valve prostheses, bacterial endocarditis, severe valvular heart disease)
Severe liver disease (e.g., cirrhosis, eclampsia)
DIC
Autoimmune disorders (e.g., periarteritis nodosa, SLE)
Thrombotic thrombocytopenic purpura (TTP), hemolytic uremic syndrome (HUS)
Snakebite (See Chapter 17.)
Some disseminated neoplasms

Runner's Anemia (March Hemoglobinuria)

Runner's anemia is caused by traumatic hemolysis from the pounding of the feet on the ground. GI blood loss may also contribute in long-distance runners.

Evidence of acute intravascular hemolysis (See "Tests for Hemolysis").
Significant anemia is uncommon.
Indirect bilirubin rarely exceeds 2 mg/dL.

HELLP Syndrome

HELLP syndrome is characterized by: *H* = hemolysis, *EL* = elevated liver enzymes, *LP* = low platelets. It is a DIC-like complication of toxemia of pregnancy or within 48 hours of delivery.

◆ **Diagnostic Criteria**

- Hemolysis (increased serum bilirubin >1.2 mg/dL, LD >600 IU/L, abnormal peripheral blood smear, decreased haptoglobin)
- Abnormal liver enzymes (serum ALT >79 IU/L)
- Platelet count <100,000/μL

Hemolysis and thrombocytopenia are typically milder than in TTP/HUS. Bone marrow shows excessive megakaryocytes.
Normal prothrombin time (PT), activated partial prothrombin time (aPTT), fibrinogen, fibrin degradation products (FDP).

Paroxysmal Cold Hemoglobinuria

In paroxysmal cold hemoglobinuria, microorganism antigens induce antibodies (Donath-Landsteiner) that cross-react with P blood group on RBC membrane, causing osmotic lysis.

HEMATOLOGY

Due To
May be associated with convalescence from an acute viral illness (e.g., mumps, measles, infectious mononucleosis), idiopathic, or caused by syphilis.
♦ Laboratory findings of acute, transient, nonrecurring hemolytic anemia follow exposure to cold environment with sudden hemoglobinuria, hemoglobinemia, spherocytosis, anisocytosis, poikilocytosis, nucleated RBCs, or other laboratory evidence of hemolysis.
○ Erythrophagocytosis is suggestive if present; rarely seen in other AIHAs.
♦ Cold autohemolysin (polyclonal IgG antibodies cross-react with P blood group system) is present (Donath-Landsteiner test—only if blood is chilled and then brought to 37°C in presence of complement and type O RBCs).
Direct Coombs test may be only weakly positive during the attack due only to complement as IgG readily elutes from RBCs.

Cold Agglutinin Disease
Cold agglutinin disease is a group of disorders caused by IgM autoantibodies against RBC (cold agglutinins).

Due To
Chronic
Many have underlying B-lymphocyte neoplasm (e.g., chronic lymphocytic leukemia [CLL], lymphoma, macroglobulinemia)
Acute
Self-limited rare complication of infectious diseases (especially *Mycoplasma pneumoniae [anti-I]* infectious mononucleosis [anti-I]).
Laboratory findings of mild, stable hemolytic anemia.
♦ Cold agglutinin test confirms the diagnosis and determines autoantibody titer.
○ Coombs test is positive only for C3 complement.
Laboratory findings due to underlying disease.

Hemoglobinuria, Paroxysmal Nocturnal[11]
PNH is an acquired clonal stem cell disorder caused by RBC-deficient synthesis of glycosylphosphatidylinositol (GPI)-anchoring proteins, causing increased sensitivity to complement-mediated lysis. The gene is mapped to the short arm of the X chromosome (Xp22.1) with many somatic mutations. PNH is characterized by a clinical triad of intravascular hemolysis, venous thrombosis, and bone marrow failure. PNH Type II RBCs have partial absence or deficiency of GPI, and Type III PNH RBCs completely lack GPI.

○ Insidious slowly progressive hemolytic anemia (mild to moderate, often macrocytic) and cytopenia.
○ Evidence of hemolysis, e.g.:

• Hemoglobinuria (black urine) is evident on arising.
• Urine contains Hb, hemosiderin (in WBCs and epithelial cells of sediment), and increased urobilinogen.
• Hemoglobinemia is present; increases during sleep.
• Methemalbuminemia.
• Increased serum LD and indirect bilirubin.
• Serum haptoglobin is absent during an episode.
• Stool urobilinogen is usually increased.

Severity of hemolysis depends on size of clone (number of affected RBCs), which may vary with time and which coexist with normal cells:

• Mild hemolysis with <20% complement-sensitive RBCs
• Sleep-related hemolysis with 20% to 50% affected RBCs
• Continuous hemolysis with >50% affected RBCs

[11]Brodsky RA, Mukhina GL, Li S, et al. Improved detection and characterization of paroxysmal nocturnal hemoglobinuria using fluorescent aerolysin. *Am J Clin Pathol* 2000;114:459–466.

♦ Flow cytometry is gold standard for diagnosis; has replaced Ham and sugar water tests.

• Demonstrates deficiency of GPI-anchored proteins on RBCs (CD59), granulocytes (CD55 and CD59), and monocytes.

• Permits concomitant diagnosis of PNH in ~20% of patients with myelodysplasia.

♦ Resistance of PNH RBCs, lymphocytes, granulocytes to aerolysin (toxin secreted by bacteria *Aeromonas hydrophila)* compared to normal cells.

Demonstration of increased RBC sensitivity to complement:

• Ham test (RBC fragility is increased in acid medium and in hydrogen peroxide); amount of change is related to clinical severity.

• Sucrose hemolysis test is said to be more sensitive but less specific than Ham test.

Autohemolysis is increased.

Negative direct Coombs test.

Osmotic fragility is normal.

Serum iron may be decreased.

Platelet count usually shows mild to moderate decrease.

WBC count is usually decreased.

Blood smear is not characteristic and often shows hypochromasia and polychromatophilic macrocytes (reticulocytes).

Bone marrow is not diagnostic; most often shows normoblastic hyperplasia with adequate myeloid and megakaryocytic cells, but cellularity may be decreased or aplasia may be present. Stainable iron is often absent.

Leukocyte ALP activity is decreased (as in other marrow stem cell disorders, e.g., CML and myelodysplastic syndromes).

RBC acetylcholinesterase activity is decreased.

Develops in 5% to 10% of patients with aplastic anemia, and aplastic anemia develops in 25% of patients with PNH.

Laboratory findings due to

○• Recurrent arterial and venous thromboses in unusual sites, especially of GI tract, in ~30% of patients (e.g., hepatic, portal, splenic); cerebral, skin and resistance to therapy are major causes of death in Western patients.

• Pancytopenia is major manifestation in younger and Asian patents.

• Hemorrhage.

• Infection—causes death in ~10% of patients.

○• Renal findings similar to those in sickle cell disease (e.g., papillary necrosis, multiple infarcts).

• Spontaneous clinical remission in ~15%, including negative Ham test.

○ Diagnosis should be considered in any patient with Coombs negative–acquired chronic hemolysis, especially if hemoglobinuria, pancytopenia, or thrombosis is present.

Bone marrow transplantation is definitive therapy.

Hemolytic Disease of the Newborn (Erythroblastosis Fetalis)

The probability of isoimmunization of Rh-negative woman by a single Rh-incompatible pregnancy is ~17%. If mother and fetus are ABO incompatible, a protective effect on Rh isoimmunization occurs (due to immediate destruction of fetal RBCs by maternal AB antibodies). An Rh-positive infant occurs in ~10% of Rh-negative white women, 5% of black women, and 1% of Asian women.

Prevalence has been markedly reduced due to prompt therapy with Rh immune globulin after abortion or delivery.

Prenatal Screening and Diagnosis

♦ Blood ABO and Rh type should be done at the first prenatal visit early in pregnancy. Indirect Coombs test should always be performed, regardless of Rh type, because of ABO or irregular antigens.

♦ Fetal RhD genotyping can be determined in DNA by reverse transcriptase PCR (RT-PCR) from maternal serum of RhD-negative pregnant women; is reported to have S/S = 100%. (Substitute for footnote #6: *Am J Obstet Gynecol* 2005;192:666.)[12]

---

[12]Lo YMD, Hjelm NM, Fidler C, et al. Prenatal diagnosis of fetal RhD status by molecular analysis of maternal plasma. *New Engl J Med* 1998;339:1734–1738.

Rh-negative women should be given anti-D immunoglobulin (RhIg) at end of second trimester and again within 72 hours of delivery of Rh-positive baby. RhIg is also given when fetal RBCs can enter maternal circulation. Prevalence of HDN has been markedly reduced by prompt RhIg therapy.

♦ Monitor anti-D titer in maternal serum periodically to detect sensitization (titer >1:8). Severity of anemia typically correlates with antibody titer. If titer ≥1:32, serial amniotic fluid indirect bilirubin is performed every 2 to 3 weeks to determine infant's risk in severe cases, and lung maturity is determined by lecithin/sphingomyelin (L/S) ratio and other studies.

♦ Amniocentesis in sensitized mothers is more reliable than anti-D titer to assess severity of disease. Measure indirect bilirubin (reflects hemolysis) using spectrophotometer at ΔOD_{450}; repeat amniocentesis at appropriate intervals according to values on Lilly Graph and deliver when L/S ratio indicates lung maturity. DNA analysis of amniotic fluid by PCR can also determine D antigen status of fetus.

♦ Can also monitor degree of fetal anemia by umbilical cordocentesis; if Hct <18%, transfuse type O, Rh-negative RBCs in utero (which may cause infant to be typed as Rh-negative). Transfuse infant with CMV-negative, irradiated, antigen-negative (for any fetal antibodies) RBCs every 7 to 21 days; can use maternal RBCs if ABO compatible.

♦ At birth, determine cord blood Hb, bilirubin, and Coombs test (DAT) on infant's RBCs. Positive DAT means probable later exchange transfusions. If test results indicate fetomaternal hemorrhage >30 mL of fetal whole blood (see HbF), additional RhIg should be given.

♦ Fetomaternal hemorrhage (FMH) may be indicated by:

♦ Flow cytometry detects 0.1% Rh-positive RBCs equivalent to FMH of 15 mL whole blood.

• Kleihauer-Betke test detects HbF; is least sensitive.

• Enzyme-linked antiglobulin test (ELAT) detects <12.5 mL (and as little as 3 mL) of Rh-positive whole blood).

• Rosette test: antibody binds to fetal Rh-positive RBCs forming rosette detects 5 mL Rh-positive fetal RBCs (10 mL Rh-positive whole blood); negative with <2.5 mL Rh-positive fetal RBCs.

Postnatal Diagnosis and Therapy

♦ Serum indirect bilirubin shows rapid rise to high levels. May rise 0.3 to 1.0 mg/h to level of 30 mg/dL in untreated infants to its maximum in 3 to 5 days unless they die. Increased urobilinogen in the urine and feces parallels serum levels.

♦ Direct Coombs test is strongly positive on cord blood RBCs when due to Rh, Kell, Kidd, or Duffy antibodies but is usually negative or weakly positive when due to anti-A antibodies. It becomes negative within a few days of effective exchange transfusion but may remain positive for weeks in untreated infants. Indirect Coombs test on cord blood may be positive because of "free" immune antibody.

At birth there is little or no anemia. Anemia may develop rapidly (RBCs may decrease by 1 million/μL/d) in severe cases to maximum by third or fourth day.

MCV and MCH are increased; MCHC is normal.

○ Nucleated RBCs in peripheral blood are markedly increased (10,000 to 100,000/μL) during first 2 days (normal = 200 to 2,000/μL) and are very large. They tend to decrease and may be absent by third or fourth day. Normoblastosis is mild or absent when due to other antigens than Rh_0.

Peripheral smear shows marked polychromatophilia and anisocytosis, macrocytic RBCs, increased reticulocyte count (>6% and up to 30%–40%). In ABO incompatibility, spherocytosis may be marked with associated increased osmotic fragility; *spherocytosis is slight or absent in Rh incompatibility.*

HbF is decreased and adult Hb is increased.

WBC count is increased (usually 15,000–30,000/μL).

Platelet count is usually normal; may be decreased in severe cases but returns to normal after 1 week. With decreased platelets, one may find increased bleeding time, poor clot retraction, and purpura. Prothrombin and fibrinogen deficiencies may occur.

Disease terminates in 3 to 6 weeks after elimination of maternal antibodies from infant's serum.

Table 11-18.   Criteria for Performing Exchange Transfusion

Criteria	Continue to Follow Patient	Consider Exchange	Perform Exchange
Rh antibody titer in mother	<1:64	>1:64	
Cord hemoglobin	>14 g/dL	12–14 g/dL	<12 g/dL
Cord bilirubin	<4 mg/dL	4–5 mg/dL	>5 mg/dL
Capillary blood hemoglobin	>12 g/dL	<12 g/dL	<12 g/dL and decreasing in first 24 h.
Serum bilirubin	<18 mg/dL	18–20 mg/dL	20 mg/dL in first 24 h; after 48 h, 22 mg/dL on two tests 6–8 h apart. In sick premature infants, 15 mg/dL is upper limit of normal to indicate exchange transfusion.

Late anemia occurs during second to fourth week of life in 5% of those receiving exchange transfusion. Reticulocyte count is low, and marrow may not show erythroid hyperplasia.

Hypoglycemia occurs in >15% of infants with cord Hb <10 g/dL; often asymptomatic.

Exchange Transfusion

Use mother's serum for crossmatch.

Use indirect Coombs test for crossmatch.

Use Rh-negative donor unless both mother and baby are Rh positive.

For subsequent transfusions, use blood compatible with that of mother and infant.

Monitor infant's glucose level during exchange with heparinized blood and after exchange with citrated blood, as high glucose content of citrated blood may cause infant hypoglycemia 1 to 2 hours later.

Monitor infant's blood pH, because pH of donor is low; therefore prefer fresh heparinized blood.

In infants, Hb of 15 g/dL corresponds to RBC volume of 30 mL/kg body weight. Transfusion of 6 mL of whole blood equals 2 mL of packed RBCs. Destruction of 1 g of Hb produces 35 mg of bilirubin. Infant with blood volume of 300 mL can have decrease in Hb of 1 g/dL that may be undetected but produces 105 mg of bilirubin.

♦Indications for Exchange Transfusion

See Table 11-18.

If Birth Weight Is (g)	Serum Bilirubin Is (mg/dL)
<1,000	10.0
1,001–1,250	13.0
1,251–1,500	15.0
1,501–2,000	17.0
2,001–2,500	18.0
>2,500	20.0

Transfuse at one step earlier in presence of:

• Serum protein <5 g/dL
• Metabolic acidosis (pH <7.25)
• Respiratory distress (with O_2 <50 mm Hg)
• Certain clinical findings (e.g., hypothermia, central nervous system [CNS] or other clinical deterioration, sepsis, hemolysis)

Other criteria for exchange transfusion are suddenness and rate of bilirubin increase and when it occurs; e.g., an increase of 3 mg/dL in 12 hours, especially after bilirubin has already leveled off, must be followed with frequent serial determinations, especially if it occurs on the first or the seventh day rather than on the third day.

HEMATOLOGY

Beware of rate of bilirubin increase >1 mg/dL during first day. Serum bilirubin = 10 mg/dL after 24 hours or 15 mg/dL after 48 hours in spite of phototherapy usually indicates that serum bilirubin will reach 20 mg/dL. In ABO hemolytic disease, the rate of bilirubin increase is not as great as in Rh disease; if the danger level for exchange transfusion is not reached by the third day, it is unlikely that it will be reached.

Laboratory Complications of Exchange Transfusion

Electrolytes—hyperkalemia, hypernatremia, hypocalcemia, acidosis
Clotting—overheparinization, thrombocytopenia
Infection—bacteremia, serum hepatitis
Other—hypoglycemia
Phototherapy of Coombs-positive infants decreases exchange transfusions (from 25% to 10% of these infants); follow effect of therapy with serum bilirubin every 4 to 8 hours.
Phototherapy is usually not begun until serum bilirubin is 10 mg/dL. Skin color is disguised by phototherapy, so serum bilirubin determination is even more important.
Beware of untreated anemia in these infants occurring in 1 to 8 weeks due to short survival time of Coombs-positive RBCs.
♦ Phototherapy is contraindicated in congenital erythropoietic porphyria and when there is significant direct-reacting bilirubinemia to avoid bronze baby syndrome.

• Serum, urine, and skin become bronze (bronze-black) because of some unknown pigment.
• Onset several hours or more after phototherapy, usually recover without sequelae.
• Most patients have some preexisting liver disease.

Amniocentesis, Indications

Prior immunized pregnancy with maternal antibody titer >1:8 in albumin. History of hemolytic disease of newborn.
After the first amniocentesis at the 24th week, repeat every 2 to 3 weeks to measure presence and increase in bilirubin pigments; the rise in these pigments according to age of fetus correlates with severity of the disease and is an indication for intrauterine transfusion, repeat examination, or immediate delivery. L:S ratio should also be measured to determine pulmonary maturity (see Chapter 14).
ABO hemolytic disease alone does not cause fetal loss and therefore is not an indication for amniocentesis.

Indications for Selection of Patients for Immunosuppression of Rh Sensitization[13]

Passive immunization using RhIg anti-D, which should be administered within hours. Less protective for ≤13 days)

Nonimmunized mother must be Rho (D) negative and weak D expression (formerly D^u), regardless of ABO blood group. Late in pregnancy, 1.8% of Rh-negative mothers become sensitized.
Weak D expression women are classified as Rh positive and not considered at risk for Rh immunization.
Other indications (unless the father or fetus is *known and documented* to be Rh negative (because of prenatal typing errors ≤3%) include:

• Abortion (spontaneous, therapeutic, threatened)
• Abruptio placenta
• Abdominal trauma during pregnancy
• Administration of whole blood, RBCs, granulocytes, or platelet concentrates from Rh-positive donors to Rh-negative patients of childbearing age
• Amniocentesis
• Ectopic pregnancy
• External cephalic version

[13]Hartwell EA. Use of RH immune globulin. ASCP practice parameter. *Am J Clin Pathol* 1998; 1210:281–292.

- Chorionic villus sampling
- Death in utero
- Manual removal of placenta
- Percutaneous umbilical blood sampling
- Placenta previa
- Trophoblastic disease or neoplasm (not complete hydatiform mole)
- Tubal ligation
- Immune thrombocytopenic purpura

Whenever a positive D+W test is found in a woman known to be D+W negative before delivery, the postpartum blood should be tested to confirm fetal-maternal hemorrhage and to quantify the volume of fetal cells in maternal circulation.

The maternal serum must have no Rh antibodies. If antenatal RhIg has been administered, the mother's postpartum serum will contain anti-D (usually weakly reactive [DAT] low titer [≤4]), which does not indicate existing immunization, and she should receive postpartum immunoprophylaxis.

Baby must be Rho (D) positive or D+W positive and have negative direct Coombs test (cord blood).

Protocol to determine postpartum candidacy for RhIg administration:

- Test mother to determine if she is Rh negative; do not perform D+W test.
- If mother is Rh negative, test cord RBCs; if these are Rh positive or D+W positive, the mother is a candidate. Even if baby (cord RBCs) is Rh negative, D+W typing is still necessary, as D+W positive cord RBCs can cause Rh sensitization.
- Quantitate fetal-maternal hemorrhage to determine dose of RhIg. Microscopic D+W test should be performed for routine screening to detect Rh-positive fetal cells; will detect fetal-maternal hemorrhage of ~35 mL of fetal blood in a woman of average size. This is often omitted due to difficulty in reading test and low predictive value of positive test.

The half-life of RhIg is 21 to 30 days (standard dose). Thus most women will have a positive antibody screen. Records must be kept of antenatal RhIg to avoid classifying this as active immunization.

Erythroblastosis, ABO

ABO incompatibility causes approximately 2/3 of cases; Rh incompatibility causes <1/3 of cases, and the latter are more severe. Minor blood factors (e.g., c, E, Kell) cause 2% of cases.

♦ Mother is Group O with Group A_1 or B infant; rarely is mother Group A_2 with Group A_1 or B infant.

♦ Infant's serum shows positive indirect Coombs test with adult RBCs of same group varying up to moderately positive, but positive test is not dependable.

Infant's RBCs show a negative direct Coombs test (by standard methods) due to antibody derived from the mother that has crossed the placenta.

Both Coombs reactions have disappeared after the fourth day.

Marked microspherocytosis is present.

Osmotic fragility is increased.

Anti-A or anti-B titer in mother's serum is not useful, since there is no correlation between the occurrence of hemolytic disease and the presence or height of the titer. If the mother's serum does not hemolyze RBCs of the same type as the infant's, the diagnosis should be questioned.

Rapidly developing anemia is rare; serial bilirubin determinations are indicators for exchange transfusion to prevent a level of 20 mg/dL. Infants may show jaundice in their first 24 hours but rarely require exchange transfusion for anemia or hyperbilirubinemia.

For exchange transfusion, use Group O, Rh type–specific blood or Group O, Rh-negative blood.

Infants born subsequently to the same parents do not have more serious disease, and they may have less serious disease.

Hereditary Hemolytic Nonspherocytic Anemias

This heterogeneous group may be caused by PK deficiency, variants of G6PD deficiency, Hb Zurich, or other rare congenital enzyme defects (e.g., glutathione).

HEMATOLOGY

♦ Hereditary hemolytic nonspherocytic anemias are characterized by persistent hemolysis without demonstrable autoantibodies, abnormal hemoglobins, altered RBC morphology, or other obvious findings indicating etiology. Hemolytic anemia may be severe; may begin in newborn; may be precipitated by certain drugs.

RBCs show Howell-Jolly bodies, Pappenheimer bodies, Heinz bodies, and basophilic stippling; there may be slight macrocytosis.

Increase in renormal.

Autohemolysis is present in some cases but not in others; reduction by glucose is less than in normal blood.

Glucose-6-Phosphate Dehydrogenase Deficiency in Red Blood Cells

G6PD deficiency is an inherited X-linked disorder. It is the most frequent inherited RBC enzyme disorder; there are more than 400 variants.

May be associated with several different clinical syndromes. Classes 2 and 3 represent 90% of cases. Classes 4 and 5 show no clinical findings.

* Class 1 (<5% of normal RBC enzyme activity): Rare, chronic, congenital, nonspherocytic hemolytic anemia worsened by oxidant drugs or febrile illness. Not improved by splenectomy.
* Class 2 (<10% of normal RBC enzyme activity): Episodic acute hemolytic crises induced by some oxidant drugs (e.g., primaquine, sulfonamides, acetanilid) or acidosis. Splenectomy is not helpful.
* Class 3 (10%–60% of normal RBC enzyme activity): Oxidant drugs or infection (e.g., pneumonia, infectious hepatitis) induce acute self-limiting (2–3 days) hemolysis in persons without previously recognized hematologic disease. Also reported in hepatic coma, hyperthyroidism, myocardial infarction (after first week), megaloblastic anemias, and chronic blood loss.
* Many other genetic and clinical variants.

♦ After standard dose of primaquine in adult, intravascular hemolysis is evidenced by:

* Decreasing Hct, usually beginning in 2 to 4 days; reaches nadir by 8 to 12 days.
* Heinz bodies and increased serum bilirubin occur during first few days of hemolysis.
* Reticulocytosis begins at about the fifth day; reaches maximum in 10 to 20 days.
* Hemolysis subsides spontaneously even if primaquine is continued.

♦ In vitro tests of Heinz body formation when patient's RBCs are exposed to acetylphenylhydrazine.

Hb varies from 7 g/dL to normal; is lower when due to exogenous agent; is usually normochromic, normocytic.

Peripheral smear shows varying degree of nucleated RBCs, spherocytes, poikilocytes, crenated and fragmented RBCs, and Heinz bodies, but is not distinctive.

♦ Diagnosis is established by RBC assay for G6PD (using fluorescence); heterozygotes have two RBC populations, and the proportion of each determines the degree of deficiency detected.

○ Screening tests are available.

In Newborn

Five percent develop neonatal jaundice after the first 24 hours (in contrast to erythroblastosis fetalis). Serum indirect bilirubin usually reaches a peak at third to fifth day (often >20 mg/dL). When jaundice appears late in the first week, the peak serum level may occur during the second week of life.

* In Asian and Mediterranean infants, neonatal jaundice and kernicterus are more common. Significant portions of the bilirubin may be conjugated.
* In African American infants at term, incidence of neonatal jaundice is not increased; occurs after exposure to certain drugs (e.g., synthetic vitamin K, naphthalene).

G6PD Is Decreased In

African American males (13%)

African American females (3%; 20% are carriers)

Some other ethnic groups (e.g., Greeks, Sardinians, Sephardic Jews)

All persons with favism (but not all persons with decreased G6PD have favism)

G6PD Is Increased In

PA, to three times normal level; remains elevated for several months, even after administration of vitamin B_{12}.

ITP (Werlhof disease); becomes normal soon after splenectomy.

Erythrocyte Pyruvate Kinase Deficiency

Erythrocyte PK deficiency is a congenital autosomal recessive nonspherocytic hemolytic anemia with splenomegaly showing a wide range of clinical and laboratory findings, from severe neonatal anemia requiring transfusion to a fully compensated hemolytic process in healthy adults, due to a deficiency of PK (10%–25% of normal) in the RBCs.

♦ Assay of RBC PK activity will demonstrate a heterozygous carrier state in persons who are hematologically normal.

○ Laboratory findings due to mild to severe chronic hemolysis that may be exacerbated by pregnancy or viral infections.

* Beyond early childhood, Hb is usually 7 to 10 g/dL.
* Peripheral smear shows no characteristic changes (i.e., few or no spherocytes, occasional tailed poikilocytes, macrocytosis, reticulocytosis).

Abnormal autohemolysis test is variably corrected by glucose.

Normal osmotic fragility.

If an infant has been transfused, the assay should be performed 3 to 4 months later.

○ Diagnosis is difficult to make. *May be suggested by increased P_{50} due to elevated 2,3-diphosphoglycerate (DPG).*

Laboratory findings due to complications (e.g., cholelithiasis, hemosiderosis).

Other rare deficiencies of RBC enzymes also exist.

Hereditary Elliptocytosis[14]

Hereditary elliptocytosis is an autosomal dominant congenital disorder of the RBC membrane affecting 1:2,500 persons in the United States. More than 10 variants are known. More than 90% of RBC cytoskeletal protein spectrin exists in dimeric form. This disease may also be acquired or autosomal recessive.

♦ Blood smear shows 25% to 100% elliptical RBCs; in normal individuals, ≤10% of RBCs may be elliptical. Also seen frequently in thalassemias, hemoglobinopathies, iron deficiency, myelophthisic anemias, megaloblastic anemia; these must be ruled out to establish the diagnosis in a congenital hemolytic anemia with marked elliptocytosis. Only a few abnormal RBCs are present at birth, with a gradual increase to stable value after ~3 months old. Hemolysis is rare in newborns. Splenectomy does not relieve elliptocytosis, despite clinical improvement.

♦ Elliptocytes are found in at least one parent and may be present in siblings.

The severity of disease varies, from severe hemolytic disease to asymptomatic carrier. The degree of hemolysis does not correlate with proportion of abnormal RBCs.

* Elliptocytes are the only hematologic abnormality seen in ~85% of patients; they are asymptomatic with fully compensated hemolysis with no anemia or splenomegaly. Spherocytes are present in some forms.
* Mild normocytic normochromic anemia (Hb 10–12 g/dL) is present in 10% to 20% of patients.
* About 12% of patients show a chronic congenital hemolytic anemia (Hb <9 g/dL) with decreased RBC survival time, moderate anemia, increased serum bilirubin, increased reticulocyte count, increased osmotic fragility, and autohemolysis.
* Severe in ~5% of patients (homozygous)—transfusion-dependent anemia with misshapen RBCs resembling hereditary pyropoikilocytosis.

Mild anemia and reticulocytosis.

Decreased MCV, MCH, MCHC; increased RDW.

Mechanical fragility is increased.

Osmotic fragility and autohemolysis are normal in patients without hemolytic anemia.

Hb electrophoresis is normal.

[14]Kakkar N, et al. Abnormal red blood cell morphology in an elderly male. *Lab Med* 2004;35:534.

HEMATOLOGY

Laboratory findings due to crises (usually precipitated by infection or stress) or complications (e.g., gallstones, hypersplenism).

Hereditary Stomatocytosis

Hereditary stomatocytosis is an uncommon autosomal dominant disease showing defective RBC permeability to sodium and potassium ions, especially at or below room temperature.

Morphologic abnormality of >35% of RBCs in which one or more slitlike areas of central pallor produce a mouthlike appearance.

- Normally <5% of RBCs are stomacytic.
- ≤20% of RBCs are stomacytic in many acquired disorders (e.g., alcoholism, drug-induced hemolytic anemia, various neoplasms, hepatobiliary disease).

Laboratory findings resemble those of hereditary spherocytosis with variable degree of hemolytic anemia, but splenectomy may cause partial or no remission.

Hereditary Spherocytosis

Hereditary spherocytosis is a rare autosomal hereditary morphologic abnormality of the RBCs. Defective RBC membrane is caused by a cytoskeleton protein (e.g., spectrin or ankyrin) deficiency; this ranges from about 30% of normal in severe cases to 80% of normal in the mildest cases. The autosomal dominant form in ~70% of cases shows moderately severe hemolysis in which one parent and half the siblings are affected; ~20% of cases have mild compensated hemolysis. About 10% have severe debilitating disease with severe anemia that makes them transfusion-dependent and causes gallstones in childhood and bone changes. The disease may also be inherited recessively and occur without a family history or may be sporadic.

♦ >35% of RBCs in which one or more slitlike areas of central pallor produce a mouthlike appearance.

- Normally <5% of RBCs are stomacytic.
- ≤20% of RBCs are stomacytic in many acquired disorders (e.g., alcoholism, drug-induced hemolytic anemia, various neoplasms, hepatobiliary disease).
- Heterozygotes show ≤25% of RBC stomatocytes with no anemia.
- Homozygotes show ~1/3 of RBC stomatocytes with mild to moderate hemolytic anemia.
- Macrocytic RBCs with MCV ≤150.
- Osmotic fragility and autohemolysis are increased due to an unknown membrane defect.

♦ Abnormal peripheral blood smear is the most suggestive finding. Many microspherocytes are present. Anisocytosis may be marked; poikilocytosis is slight. RBCs show Howell-Jolly bodies, Pappenheimer bodies, and Heinz bodies. Polychromatophilic reticulocytes and microspherocytes are present.

♦ Coombs-negative hemolytic anemia is moderate (RBC = 3–4 million/μL), microcytic (MCV = 70–80 fL), and hyperchromic (increased MCHC = 36–40 g/dL). *MCHC >36% indicates congenital spherocytic anemia if cold agglutinins and hypertriglyceridemia have been excluded. An isolated increase in MCHC or hyperchromasia may indicate recessive disease.*

♦ Evidence of hemolysis:

- Degree of reticulocytosis (usually 5%–15%) is greater than in other hemolytic anemias with similar degrees of anemia.
- Bone marrow shows marked erythroid hyperplasia except during aplastic crisis; moderate hemosiderin is present.
- Increased serum LD and indirect bilirubin.
- Haptoglobins are decreased or absent.
- Hemolytic crises, usually precipitated by infection (especially parvovirus), cause more profound anemia despite reticulocytosis and increased jaundice and splenomegaly.
- Hemoglobinemia and hemoglobinuria only during hemolytic crises.
- Stool urobilinogen is usually increased.

♦ Osmotic fragility is increased; the increase generally reflects the clinical severity of disease; when normal in some patients, the incubated fragility test shows increased hemolysis. Diagnosis is not established without abnormal osmotic fragility. Increased osmotic fragility does not distinguish hereditary spherocytosis from autoimmune hemolytic disease with spherocytosis, but the latter shows much less increased fragility with incubation.

Autohemolysis (sterile defibrinated blood incubated for 48 hours) is increased (10%–50% of cells, compared to normal reading of <4% of cells); very nonspecific test. May sometimes be found also in nonspherocytic hemolytic anemias.

Abnormal osmotic fragility and autohemolysis are reduced by 10% glucose; false-negative test may occur with concomitant diabetes mellitus.

♦ Direct Coombs test must be negative (in contrast to immune hemolytic conditions, in which spherocytosis is common and direct Coombs test is positive).

Mechanical fragility is increased.

WBC and platelet counts are usually normal; may be increased during hemolysis.

Laboratory findings due to complications (e.g., gallstones, aplastic crises).

Findings resemble hereditary spherocytosis but splenectomy may cause partial or no remission.

Splenectomy should cause a complete response in hemolysis but not in spherocytosis.

Age at diagnosis is related to severity of hemolysis; more severe forms are diagnosed early in life.

In neonates, is associated with jaundice in about 50% of cases. Serum indirect bilirubin may be >20 mg/dL. Anemia is usually mild (Hb ≥10 g/dL) during the first week of life.

Spherocytes are present in infant and one parent and may be present in siblings.

Reticulocyte count is usually 5% to 15%.

May interfere with glycosylated Hb measurement.

Hereditary Pyropoikilocytosis

Hereditary pyropoikilocytosis is a rare autosomal recessive homozygous subset of hereditary elliptocytosis that begins at an early age; it occurs primarily in blacks.

Congenital severe hemolytic anemia with virtually all RBCs markedly misshapen (especially fragments, microspherocytes, elliptocytes, pyknotic forms).

MCV is low (55–74 fL).

Increased fragility of cells is particularly marked when incubated at 37°C to 48°C.

Increased autohemolysis with or without glucose.

Bone marrow shows marked ineffective erythroid hyperplasia.

Splenectomy greatly lessens hemolysis.

Rhesus Factor Null Phenotype

The Rh$_{null}$ phenotype is an extremely rare condition in which RBCs lack all Rh antigens due to absent RhD and RhCcEe proteins; Fy^5 and LW are also lacking, and patients may have markedly decreased S/s and U antigens.

Mild to moderate chronic hemolytic anemia with characteristic stomatocytes and spherocytes.

♦ Absence of all Rh antigens on RBCs.

Shortened RBC life span.

Increased osmotic fragility.

Can become sensitized to multiple Rh antigens.

Disorders of Erythrocytosis

Erythrocytosis, Classification

Polycythemia vera

Hereditary erythrocytosis (rare conditions)

• High-affinity hemoglobinopathies
• Decreased RBC 2,3-DPG (due to high RBC adenosine triphosphate or autosomal recessive DPG mutase deficiency)
• Increased production of erythropoietin (autosomal recessive)
• Erythropoietin-receptor mutations (autosomal dominant)
• Unknown causes

Secondary polycythemia

Relative polycythemia

Neonatal thick blood syndrome

Factitious polycythemia (due to blood doping or ingestion of steroids by athletes)

HEMATOLOGY

Table 11-19.	Comparison of Polycythemia Vera, Secondary Polycythemia, and Relative Polycythemia		
Test	Polycythemia Vera	Secondary Polycythemia[a]	Relative Polycythemia[b]
Hct	I	I	I
Blood volume	I	I	D or N
Red cell mass	I	I	D or N
Plasma volume	I or N	N or I	D
Platelet count	I	N	N
WBC with shift to left	I	N	N
Nucleated RBC, abnormal RBC	I	N	N
Serum uric acid	I	I	N
Serum vitamin B_{12}	I	N	N
Leukocyte alkaline phosphatase	I	N	N
Oxygen saturation of arterial blood	N	D	N
Bone marrow	Hyperplasia of all elements	Erythroid hyperplasia	N
Erythropoietin level	D	I	N

D, decreased; I, increased; N, normal.
[a]Diagnosis of secondary polycythemia is suggested by erythrocytosis without increased WBC, platelets or splenomegaly; causes should be sought.
[b]Relative polycythemia is not secondary to hypoxia but results from decreased volume owing to unknown mechanism or to decreased fluid intake and/or excess loss of body fluids (e.g., diuretics, dehydration, burns) with high normal RBC mass.

Polycythemia Vera

Polycythemia vera (PV) is a clonal disorder of the erythroid cells.

See Table 11-19 and Figure 11-6.

♦ **Diagnostic Criteria**[15]
A1 + A2 + A3; if A3 is absent, then two of four criteria from B must be present.
A1: Increased RBC mass ($\geq$25% above normal predicted value) or Hb >18.5 g/dL in men, >16.5 in women)
A2: No cause for secondary erythrocytosis including
Absence of familial erythrocytosis
No increase of Ep owing to
Hypoxia (arterial PO_2 $\geq$92%)
High oxygen activity Hb
Truncated Ep receptor
Inappropriate Ep by tumor
A3: Splenomegaly (occurs in ~75% of cases)
A4: Clonal genetic abnormality other than Ph^1 or *BCR-ABL* gene in marrow cells
A5: Endogenous erythroid colony formation in vitro
B1: WBC count >12,000/μL (occurs in ~60% of cases) in absence of fever or infection
B2: Platelet count >400,000/μL (occurs in >60% of cases)
B3: Bone marrow biopsy panmyelosis, principally erythroid and megakaryocytic proliferation
B4: Low serum Ep level

---

[15]Jaffe ES, ed. *Pathology and Genetics of Tumours of Haematopoietic and Lymphoid Tissues.* World Health Organisation Classification of Tumors, vol. 3. Lyon: IARC Press; 2001:32.

RBC is increased; often = 7 to 12 million; may increase to >15 million/μL. Increased Hb = 18 to 24 g/dL in males and >16 g/dL in females residing at altitude <2,000 feet, in 71% of cases.

Increased Hct >55% in 83% of cases; >60% indicates increased RBC mass, but <60% may be associated with normal RBC mass.

MCV, MCH, and MCHC are normal or decreased.

Increased ^{51}Cr RBC mass is reported essential for diagnosis; blood volume is increased (using albumin tagged with iodine-125 or ^{131}I); plasma volume is variably normal or slightly increased. RBC mass may be difficult to assess reliably if not done frequently, and some experts omit this test when other criteria are present, especially if serum Ep is decreased and marrow erythroid colony growth occurs in absence of exogenous Ep.

In the presence of active hemorrhage, the isotope is lost via the bleeding site and false values will be produced. *Radioisotopes should not be administered to children or pregnant women.*

Increased platelet count >400,000/μL in 62% of cases; often >1 million/μL.

Increased polymorphonuclear leukocytes (PMNs) >12,000/μL in ~60% of cases; usually >15,000 μL; sometimes there is a leukemoid reaction). Mild basophilia in ~60% of cases.

Oxygen saturation of arterial blood is normal in 84% of cases.

Increased leukocyte ALP score >100 (occurs in ~70% of cases) in absence of fever or infection.

Increased serum vitamin B$_{12}$ >900 pg/mL in ~30% of cases.

Increased unsaturated vitamin B$_{12}$–binding capacity >2,200 pg/mL in ~75% of cases. (Normal range = 870–1,800 ng/L.) Also increased in myeloproliferative diseases (e.g., CML), pregnancy, and oral contraceptive drugs and decreased in hepatitis and cirrhosis.

♦ Ep in plasma or serum is usually decreased (but occasionally normal). Normal level (3.7–16.0 IU/L) is not helpful, but increased level rules out PV and requires search for cause of secondary *erythrocytosis*. Usually increased (but may be normal) in secondary polycythemia; there is overlap between these. Increases may be intermittent; therefore a single normal level is unreliable. Usually normal in relative polycythemia. Usually remains normal during phlebotomy therapy.

Use

• Differential diagnosis of PV.
• Indicator of need for Ep therapy in patients with renal failure.
• Detection of forbidden use of Ep for athletic performance enhancement.

Interferences

• Decreased by high plasma viscosity, estrogens, β-adrenergic blockers, agents that increase renal blood flow (e.g., enalapril, an inhibitor of angiotensin-converting enzyme).
• Circadian rhythm in hospitalized adults with lowest values between 8 AM and 12 PM and 40% higher values in late evening.

Ep Increased *Appropriately**

• Extremely high: Usually transfusion-dependent anemia with Hct = 10% to 25% and Hb = 3 to 7 g/dL (e.g., aplastic anemia, severe hemolytic anemia, hematologic cancers)
• Very high: Patients have mild to moderate anemia with Hct = 25% to 40% or Hb = 7 to 12 g/dL
• High: Patients are more anemic (e.g., hemolytic anemia, myelodysplasia, exposure to chemotherapeutic or immunosuppressive drugs, AIDS)

Ep Increased *Inappropriately**

• Some renal disorders (e.g., renal cysts, postrenal transplant)
• Malignant neoplasms (e.g., renal adenocarcinoma [1%–5% of cases], juxtaglomerular cell tumor, Wilms tumor, hepatocellular carcinoma or hemangiosarcoma, testicular carcinoma, malignant pheochromocytoma, breast carcinoma)

(*Ep is normally inversely related to RBC volume, Hb, or Hct.)

HEMATOLOGY

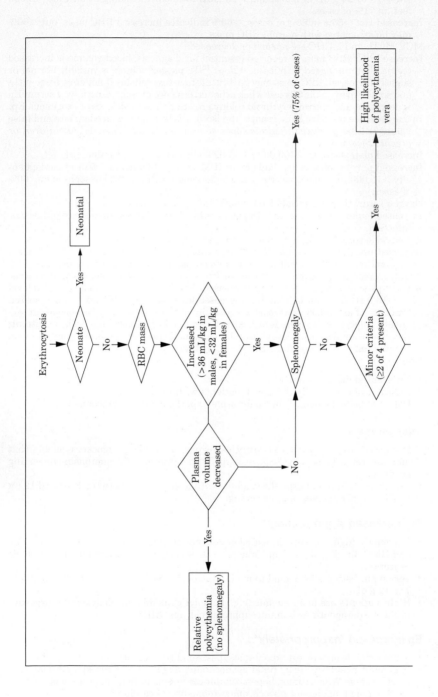

442

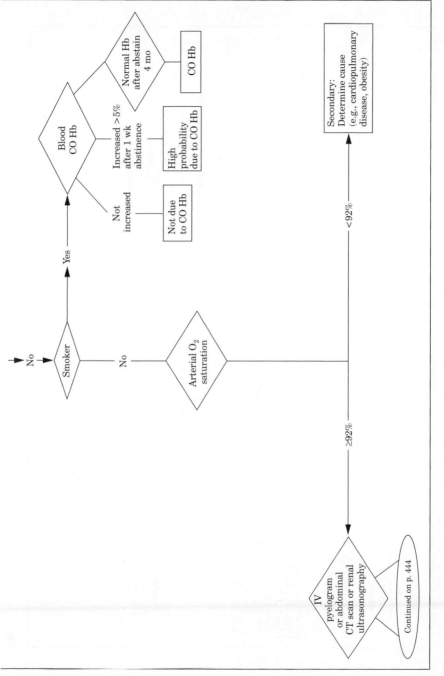

Fig. 11-6. Sequence of laboratory tests in the diagnosis of erythrocytosis. 2,3-DPG, 2,3-diphosphoglycerate.

Continued on p. 444

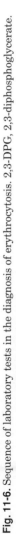

HEMATOLOGY

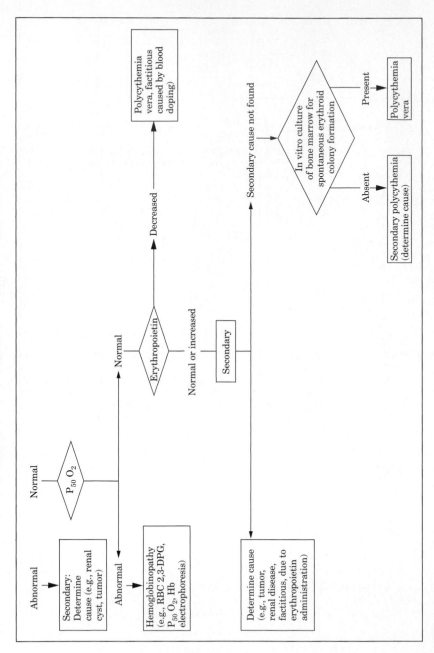

Fig. 11-6. (*continued*)

- Nonmalignant neoplasms (e.g., meningioma, hemangioblastoma of brain [20% of cases], liver, or adrenal, leiomyoma of uterus)

Ep Decreased Inappropriately*

- PV
- Renal failure
- Autonomic neuropathy
- AIDS before zidovudine therapy
- Weeks 3 and 4 after bone marrow transplant

Decreased Appropriately*

- Renal failure, RA, multiple myeloma, cancer

ESR is decreased.
Blood viscosity is increased.
Osmotic fragility is decreased (increased resistance).
Peripheral blood smear may show macrocytes, microcytes, polychromatophilic RBCs, normoblasts, large masses of platelets, neutrophilic shift to the left.
Reticulocyte count >1.5% in 44% of cases.
○ Bone marrow shows general hyperplasia of all elements. Cellularity >75%, especially with megakaryocytic hyperplasia in presence of erythrocytosis, is strong evidence for PV. (Mean cellularity <48% in normal persons and 48%–55% in secondary cases.) Mild myelofibrosis may be present; iron may be decreased or absent.
♦ Spontaneous erythroid colony formation occurs in in vitro culture of marrow erythroid progenitors in PV without addition of exogenous Ep (seen less commonly in other myeloproliferative disorders) but not in secondary polycythemia or normal persons; only available in special laboratories.
Serum uric acid increased in ~50% of cases.
Serum total bilirubin may be slightly increased in ~50% of cases.
Serum iron may be decreased in ~50% of cases.
Serum potassium may be increased (artifactual due to thrombocytosis).
Bleeding time and coagulation time are normal, but clot retraction may be poor.
Urine may contain increased urobilinogen, and occasionally albumin is present.
○ Laboratory findings of associated diseases (e.g., gout, duodenal ulcer, cirrhosis, hypertension).
○ Laboratory findings due to complications such as thromboses (e.g., cerebral, portal vein), intercurrent infection, peptic ulcer, hemorrhage, myelofibrosis, myeloid metaplasia (develops in 3%–10% of patients), CML (develops in 20% of patients), acute leukemia (develops in 1% of patients).

Polycythemia, Secondary

○ Diagnosis is suggested by erythrocytosis without increased WBC count or platelets or splenomegaly; causes listed below should be sought.
Hct is slightly increased.
Leukocyte ALP score is normal or slightly increased.
Serum Ep is usually increased or normal.
Increased plasma cholesterol is frequent.

Due To

Physiologically Appropriate
Arterial hypoxemia, e.g.,

- Decreased atmospheric pressure (e.g., high altitudes)
- Chronic heart disease

Congenital (e.g., pulmonary stenosis, septal defect, patent ductus arteriosus)

- Acquired (e.g., chronic rheumatic mitral disease)
- Arteriovenous aneurysm
- Impaired pulmonary ventilation
- Alveolar-capillary block (e.g., Hamman-Rich syndrome, sarcoidosis, lymphangitic cancer)
- Alveolar hypoventilation (e.g., bronchial asthma, kyphoscoliosis)

(*Ep is normally inversely related to RBC volume, Hb, or Hct.)

HEMATOLOGY

- Restriction of pulmonary vascular bed (e.g., primary pulmonary hypertension, mitral stenosis, chronic pulmonary emboli, emphysema)

Hypoxemia due to intrinsic RBC changes

- Abnormal hemoglobin pigments (methemoglobinemia or sulfhemoglobinemia caused by chemicals, such as aniline and coal tar derivatives)
- High oxygen-affinity hemoglobinopathies
- Carboxyhemoglobinemia ("smoker's erythrocytosis") can be detected by oximetry but not from P_{50}

Physiologically Inappropriate
Increased Ep secretion, e.g.,

- Associated with tumors and miscellaneous conditions (may be first sign of an occult curable tumor)
- Renal disease (hypernephroma, benign tumors, hydronephrosis, cysts, renal artery stenosis, long-term hemodialysis; occurs in up to 5% of renal cell carcinomas; occurs in ≤17% of kidney transplant recipients)
- Hemangioblastoma of cerebellum (occurs in 15%–20% of cases)
- Uterine fibromyoma
- Hepatocellular carcinoma (5% –10% of cases)
- Abnormality in Ep receptor

Increased androgen

- Pheochromocytoma
- Cushing syndrome (adrenocortical hyperplasia or tumor)
- Masculinizing ovarian tumor (e.g., arrhenoblastoma)
- Factitious (use of androgens by athletes)

Polycythemia, Relative (Stress Erythrocytosis)

Recent literature questions the existence of this entity.[16]

Relative polycythemia is not secondary to hypoxia but results from decreased plasma volume due to an unknown mechanism or to decreased fluid intake and/or excess loss of body fluids (e.g., diuretics, dehydration, burns) with normal RBC mass.
Increased RBC (usually <6,000,000/μL), Hb, and Hct.
Normal WBC, platelet, and reticulocyte counts.
Findings of secondary polycythemia (e.g., decreased O_2 saturation) are not present.
Serum Ep is normal.
Leukocyte ALP score is normal or mildly increased.
Bone marrow shows normal cellularity and megakaryocyte count; no myelofibrosis; iron may be absent.
Hypercholesterolemia is frequent.
Laboratory findings due to complications (e.g., thromboembolism).

Polycythemia, Factitious

See Chapter 16.
Due To
Use of androgens by athletes to increase muscle mass and strength.
Intentional blood doping (athlete is phlebotomized and later transfused with own stored blood prior to competitive event to improve performance).
Administration of recombinant human erythropoietin (rHuEPO). For several weeks thereafter, Hb is increased and reticulocyte count is suppressed.[17]
Normal oxygen saturation.
Serum EPO is low in autotransfusion but increased by exogenous rHuEPO.

[16]Fairbanks VF, Klee GG, Wiseman GA, et al. Measurement of blood volume and red cell mass: re-examination of ^{51}Cr and ^{125}I methods. *Blood Cells Mol Dis* 1996;22:169–186.
[17]Ashenden MJ, Sharpe K, Damsgaard R, et al. Standardization of reticulocyte values in an anti-doping context. *Am J Clin Pathol* 2004;121:816–825.

♦ Absolute and percent of reticulocyte count. rHuEPO can be detected in urine.[18]
♦ Use of Hemopure (a glutaraldehyde-polymerized bovine oxygen carrying Hb) is detected by electrophoresis.[19]

Thick Blood Syndrome, Neonatal

Caused By

Transfusion (e.g., maternofetal, twin-to-twin)
Hypoxemia (e.g., postmaturity, small-for-gestational-age neonates)
Decreased deformability of RBC membranes (e.g., sickle cell anemia, spherocytosis)
♦ Hct >64% in a heparinized sample or >67% in an unheparinized sample.
♦ When Hct is 60% to 64%, diagnosis must be made with a microviscometer. If <60%, hyperviscosity is not found.
Hyperbilirubinemia, hypoglycemia, platelet count <130,000/μL, or abnormal blood smear (burr cells, fragmented RBCs, increased erythroid elements) are found in ~50% of cases.
Therapeutic replacement of blood with plasma exchange transfusion aims to reduce Hct to the 50% to 60% range.

Tests for Disorders of White Blood Cells

White Blood Cell Count

Use

Diagnosis of myeloproliferative disorders, myelodysplasias, various other hematologic disorders
Support diagnosis of various infections and inflammation.
Is often ordered inappropriately and has almost no value as a *screening* test. The neutrophil and band counts may be useful in acute appendicitis and neonatal sepsis, with moderate sensitivity and specificity.

Interferences

Associated with automated WBC counters (artifact is corrected when manual WBC counts are performed)

• Leukocyte fragility due to immunosuppressive and antineoplastic drugs
• Lymphocyte fragility in lymphocytic leukemia
• Excessive clumping of leukocytes in monoclonal gammopathies, cryofibrinogenemia, cold agglutinins
• Platelet agglutination (e.g., due to ethylenediaminetetraacetic acid [EDTA]) may cause clumps of platelets to be counted as WBCs.

Causes of Neutropenia/Leukopenia (Figure 11-7)

Neutropenia/leukopenia is diagnosed with an absolute neutrophil count (total WBC × % segmented neutrophils and bands) is <1,800/μL or <1,000 in black persons.

Decreased/ineffective production

• Infections, especially:

Bacterial (e.g., overwhelming bacterial infection, septicemia, miliary TB, typhoid, paratyphoid, brucellosis, tularemia)
Viral (e.g., infectious mononucleosis, hepatitis, influenza, measles, rubella, psittacosis)
Rickettsial (e.g., scrub typhus, sandfly fever)
Other (e.g., malaria, kala-azar)

HEMATOLOGY

[18]Lasne F, Crepin N, Ashenden M, et al. Detection of hemoglobin-based oxygen carriers in human serum for doping analysis: screening by electrophoresis. *Clin Chem* 2004;50:410–415.

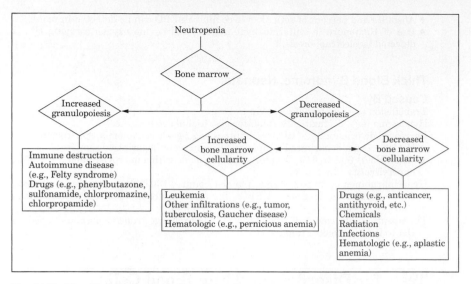

Fig. 11-7. Algorithm for workup of neutropenia.

- Drugs and chemicals (especially sulfonamides, antibiotics, analgesics, marrow depressants, arsenicals, antithyroid drugs, many others)
- Ionizing radiation
- Hematopoietic diseases (e.g., folic acid and vitamin B_{12} deficiency, aleukemic leukemia, aplastic anemia, myelophthisis)

Decreased survival (e.g., Felty syndrome, SLE, autoimmune and isoimmune neutropenias, splenic sequestration, drugs)
Abnormal distribution, e.g., hypersplenism
Miscellaneous, e.g., severe renal injury

Neonatal and Infantile Causes of Neutropenia/Leukopenia

Neutropenia/leukopenia is diagnosed with a neutrophil count <5,000/μL during an infant's first few days or <1,000/μL by the end of the first week of life.

Maternal causes

- Associated with maternal neutropenia (e.g., SLE)
- Maternal drug ingestion, and often associated with thrombocytopenia (e.g., sulfas, thiazides, propylthiouracil, phenothiazines, trimethadione, amidopyrine)
- Associated with maternal isoimmunization to fetal leukocytes

Inborn errors of metabolism (e.g., chronic tyrosinosis, maple syrup urine disease, ketotic hyperglycinemia, methylmalonic acidemia, isovaleric acidemia, propionic acidemia)

Immune defects (e.g., X-linked agammaglobulinemia, dysgammaglobulinemia)

- Associated with phenotypic abnormalities (e.g., cartilage hair dysplasia, dyskeratosis congenita, Shwachman-Diamond syndrome [chronic hypoplastic neutropenia associated with pancreatic insufficiency])
- Infantile genetic agranulocytosis
- Disorders of uncommitted stem cell proliferation
- Cyclic neutropenia
- Reticular dysgenesis (granulocytes and lymphocytes do not develop normally, absent thymus, low immunoglobulin concentrations, platelets and RBCs are unaffected)

Disorders of Myeloid Stem Cell Proliferation

- Kostmann agranulocytosis (moderate to severe neutropenia that may be associated with dysgammaglobulinemia, frequent chromosomal abnormalities, normal granulocytic maturation up to promyelocyte or myelocyte stage)
- Benign chronic granulocytopenia of childhood
- In children:
  Adult-type PA
  Defective secretion or type of gastric intrinsic factor (normal gastric mucosa and acid secretion, no antibodies to intrinsic factor or parietal cells, no associated endocrine deficiency)
  Imerslund-Gräsbeck syndrome
- Pregnancy—progressive decrease in granulocyte count during pregnancy. *Serum B_{12} is normal in megaloblastic anemia of pregnancy.*

Causes of Neutrophilia

Neutrophilia is defined as an absolute neutrophil count >8,000/μL.

See Tables 11-4 and 11-5.
Acute infections

- Localized (e.g., pneumonia, meningitis, tonsillitis, abscess)
- Generalized (e.g., acute rheumatic fever, septicemia, cholera)

Inflammation (e.g., vasculitis)
Intoxications

- Metabolic (uremia, acidosis, eclampsia, acute gout)
- Poisoning by chemicals, drugs, venoms, etc. (e.g., mercury, epinephrine, black widow spider)
- Parenteral (foreign protein and vaccines)

Acute hemorrhage
Acute hemolysis of red blood cells
Myeloproliferative diseases
Tissue necrosis, e.g.:

- Acute myocardial infarction
- Necrosis of tumors
- Burns
- Gangrene
- Bacterial necrosis

Physiologic conditions (e.g., exercise, emotional stress, menstruation, obstetric labor)
Steroid administration (e.g., prednisone 40 mg orally) causes increased neutrophil leukocytes of 1,700 to 7,500 (peak in 4–6 hours and return to normal in 24 hours); no definite shift to left. Lymphocytes decrease 70% and monocytes decrease 90%.
May be accompanied by shift to left of granulocytes, toxic granulation, Döhle bodies, and cytoplasmic vacuolization.

Causes of Lymphocytosis

Lymphocytosis is defined as counts >4,000/μL in adults, >7,200/μL in adolescents, >9,000/μL in young children and infants.

See Figure 11-8.
Infections (e.g., pertussis, infectious lymphocytosis, infectious mononucleosis, infectious hepatitis, CMV, mumps, German measles, chickenpox, toxoplasmosis, chronic TB, undulant fever, convalescence from acute infection)
Thyrotoxicosis (relative)
Addison disease
Neutropenia with relative lymphocytosis
Lymphatic leukemia
Crohn disease
Ulcerative colitis

HEMATOLOGY

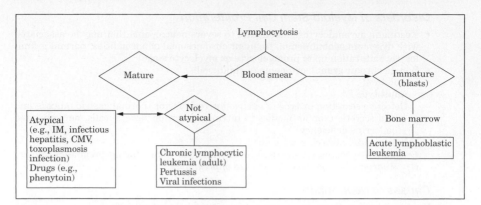

Fig. 11-8. Algorithm for workup of lymphocytosis. IM, infectious mononucleosis; CMV, cytomegalovirus.

Serum sickness
Drug hypersensitivity
Vasculitis

Causes of Lymphocytopenia

Lymphocytopenia is defined as a count of <1,500 in adults, <3,000 in children.

Increased destruction

- Chemotherapy or radiation treatment
- Corticosteroids (Cushing syndrome, stress)

Increased loss via GI tract

- Intestinal lymphectasia
- Thoracic duct drainage
- Obstruction to intestinal lymphatic drainage (e.g., tumor, Whipple disease, intestinal lymphangiectasia)
- Congestive heart failure

Decreased production

- Aplastic anemia
- Malignancy, especially Hodgkin disease
- Inherited immunoglobulin disorders (e.g., Wiskott-Aldrich, combined immunodeficiency, ataxia-telangiectasia)
- Infection (e.g., AIDS)

Others (e.g., SLE, renal failure, miliary tuberculosis, myasthenia gravis, aplastic anemia)

CD4 Lymphocytes

CD4 lymphocyte count is determined by flow cytometry; it is calculated as: total WBC × % lymphocytes × % of lymphocytes stained with CD4.

Use

Diagnosis of immune dysfunction, especially AIDS, in which a severely depressed count is the single best predictor of imminent opportunistic infection and an increase is associated with therapeutic effect of drugs. May also be expressed as CD4:CD8 lymphocyte ratio, but CD8 count is more labile and may diminish the value of the CD4 counts.

Decreased In
Acute minor viral infections. Should recheck in 3 months.
Also diurnal variation, with peak evening values that may be twice morning values. Imprecision in total WBC and differential may cause 25% variability in CD4 values.

Causes of Atypical Lymphocytes
Lymphatic leukemia
Viral infections (e.g., infectious lymphocytosis, infectious mononucleosis, infectious hepatitis, viral pneumonia and other exanthems of childhood, mumps, chickenpox, CMV)
Pertussis
Brucellosis
Syphilis (in some phases)
Toxoplasmosis
Drug reactions and serum sickness
Normal persons may show up to 6% atypical lymphocytes.
"Heterophile-negative" infectious mononucleosis syndrome is most often seen in:

- Early stage of infectious mononucleosis
- Toxoplasmosis
- CMV
- Infectious hepatitis

Basophilic Leukocytes

Use
May be first sign of blast crisis or accelerated phase of CML.
Persistent basophilia may indicate unsuspected myeloproliferative disease.
Diagnosis of basophilic leukemia.

Increased In (>50/μL or >1%)
Lymphoproliferative disorders (e.g., Waldenström macroglobulinemia, CML, basophilic leukemia, PV, myeloid metaplasia, Hodgkin disease)
Postsplenectomy
Chronic hemolytic anemia (some patients)
Chronic sinusitis
Chickenpox
Smallpox
Myxedema
Nephrosis (some patients)
Foreign protein injection
Ionizing radiation

Decreased In
Hyperthyroidism
Pregnancy
Period following irradiation, chemotherapy, and glucocorticoids
Acute phase of infection

Causes of Monocytosis

Monocytosis is defined as >10% of differential count or an absolute count >500/μL.

Monocytic leukemia, other leukemias
Other myeloproliferative disorders (myeloid metaplasia, PV)
Hodgkin disease and other malignant lymphomas, multiple myeloma, carcinomas
Lipid storage diseases (e.g., Gaucher disease)
Postsplenectomy
Tetrachloroethane poisoning
Recovery from agranulocytosis and subsidence of acute infection
Many protozoan infections (e.g., malaria, kala-azar, trypanosomiasis)
Some rickettsial infections (e.g., Rocky Mountain spotted fever, typhus)
Certain bacterial infections (e.g., subacute bacterial endocarditis, TB, brucellosis)
Chronic ulcerative colitis, regional enteritis, and sprue

HEMATOLOGY

Sarcoidosis
Collagen diseases (e.g., RA, SLE)
Most common causes are indolent infections (e.g., mycobacteria, subacute bacterial
    endocarditis) and recovery phase of neutropenia
*Monocyte phagocytosis of RBCs in peripheral smears from earlobe is said to occur often
    in subacute bacterial endocarditis.*

Monocytes Decreased In
Hairy cell leukemia

Plasma Cells

Increased In
Hematologic neoplasms (e.g., plasma cell leukemia, multiple myeloma, Hodgkin dis-
    ease, chronic lymphocytic leukemia [CLL])
Other neoplasias (cancer of liver, kidney, breast, prostate)
Cirrhosis
Collagen diseases (e.g., RA, SLE)
Serum reaction
Bacterial infections (e.g., syphilis, TB)
Parasitic infections (e.g., malaria, trichinosis)
Viral infections (e.g., infectious mononucleosis, rubella, measles, chickenpox, benign
    lymphocytic meningitis)

Decreased In
Not clinically significant

Causes of Eosinophilia

**Eosinophilia is defined as a eosinophil count >250/μL; there is diurnal variation,
with highest levels in morning. Normal = 1 circulating eosinophil for every 100 in
tissues.**

Atopic/allergic diseases (e.g., asthma, hayfever, urticaria, drug therapy, allergic rhinitis,
    eczema)
Parasitic infestation, especially with tissue invasion (e.g., trichinosis, hookworms,
    Ascaris lumbricoides, schistosomiasis, filariasis, fascioliasis)
Mycoses (e.g., coccidioidomycosis following primary infection, allergic bronchopul-
    monary aspergillosis)
Some infectious diseases (e.g., scarlet fever, erythema multiforme, *Chlamydia* infec-
    tion, cat scratch disease, brucellosis)
Collagen-vascular diseases (e.g., periarteritis nodosa, SLE, RA, Churg-Strauss syndrome)
Some diffuse skin diseases (e.g., pemphigus, scabies, dermatitis herpetiformis)
Some hematopoietic diseases (e.g., PA, CML, acute myelomonocytic leukemia, poly-
    cythemia, Hodgkin disease, T-cell lymphomas, eosinophilic leukemia); postsplenectomy
Some immunodeficiency disorders (e.g., Wiskott-Aldrich syndrome, GVHD, cyclic neu-
    tropenia, IgA deficiency)
Some GI diseases (e.g., eosinophilic gastroenteritis, inflammatory bowel diseases)
Some endocrine diseases (e.g., hypopituitarism, Addison disease)
Postirradiation
Miscellaneous conditions

- Certain tumors (ovary, involvement of bone or serosal surfaces)
- Sarcoidosis
- Löffler parietal fibroplastic endocarditis
- Familial conditions
- Poisoning (e.g., phosphorus, black widow spider bite)

Drugs (e.g., aspirin sensitivity)
Idiopathic hypereosinophilic syndrome
Eosinophilic leukemia
Eosinophilia-myalgia syndrome (see Chapter 10)
Eosinophilic fascitis
Toxic oil syndrome (possibly due to rapeseed oil): Eosinophilia, pleural effusion,
    hypoxia, neuritis, vasculitis.
Highest levels occur in trichinosis, *Clonorchis sinensis* infection, and dermatitis her-
    petiformis.

Neutrophil Function Tests

Morphology: Light, Phase, and Electron Microscopy
(e.g., Chédiak-Higashi)

Adherence

- To glass or spreading
- Aggregometer
- Flow cytometry—anti-CD18 and anti–sialyl-Lewis X positive

Locomotion

- Random
- Chemotaxis

Serum deficiencies (e.g., complement, immunoglobulins)
Cell defects (e.g., hyperimmunoglobulinemia E, Chédiak-Higashi syndrome, Kartagener syndrome, drugs, diabetes mellitus, uremia, etc.)

Phagocytosis

- Uptake of latex beads, microorganisms
- Assay hexose monophosphate shunt

Secretion: Assay Lysosome Enzymes, Lactoferrin B_{12}-binding Protein

Bactericidal Activity

- Nitroblue tetrazolium test (see next)
- Killing of bacteria (e.g., *Staphylococcus aureus*)
- Oxygen radical production (e.g., chronic granulomatous disease, G6PD deficiency)

Nitroblue Tetrazolium Reduction In Neutrophils

Usual normal values reported are <10%, but there is considerable variation, and each laboratory should establish its own normal range.

Use

Diagnosis of poor neutrophilic function (failure of nitroblue tetrazolium [NBT] reduction), particularly in chronic granulomatous disease; now replaced by flow cytometry.
Differentiating untreated bacterial infection from other conditions; rarely used.

Increased In

Bacterial infections, including miliary TB and TB meningitis
Nocardia and other systemic fungal infections
Various parasitic infections (e.g., malaria)
Chédiak-Higashi syndrome
Idiopathic myelofibrosis
Normal infants up to age 2 months
Pregnancy
Patients taking birth control pills
Some patients with lymphoma suppressed by chemotherapy

Decreased or Normal In Absence of Bacterial Infection

Chronic granulomatous disease
Normal persons
Postpartum state
Postoperative state (after 7–10 days)
Cancer
Tissue transplantation
Other conditions with fever or leukocytosis not caused by bacterial infection (e.g., RA)

Decreased or Normal In Presence of Bacterial Infection

Antibiotic therapy—effectiveness of treatment indicated by reduction of previous elevation, sometimes in <6 hours
Localized infection
Administration of corticosteroids and immunosuppressive drugs (although contrary findings with corticosteroids have also been reported)

HEMATOLOGY

Miscellaneous conditions, probably involving metabolic defects of neutrophil function:

- Chronic granulomatous disease
- Neutrophilic deficiency of G6PD or myeloperoxidase
- SLE
- Sickle cell disease
- CML
- Lipochrome histiocytosis
- Congenital and acquired agammaglobulinemia
- Other

Increased (from Previously Determined Normal Level) In
Has been used to monitor development of infection in chronically ill patients; may occur before other clinical parameters

- Development of wound sepsis in burn patients
- Development of infection in uremic patients on chronic hemodialysis

Leukocyte Alkaline Phosphatase Staining Reaction
Leukocyte ALP staining reaction is a stain of enzyme present in granules in myelocytes and more mature myeloid cells.

Use
Differentiating CML from leukemoid reaction; now replaced by PCR
Evaluation of PNH; now replaced by flow cytometry

Usually Increased In
Leukemoid reaction
PV
Essential thrombocythemia (may be normal)
Lymphoma (including Hodgkin, reticulum cell sarcoma)
Acute and chronic lymphocytic leukemia
Multiple myeloma
Myeloid metaplasia
Aplastic anemia
Agranulocytosis
Bacterial infections
Cirrhosis
Obstructive jaundice
Pregnancy and immediate postpartum period
Administration of Enovid
Trisomy 21
Klinefelter syndrome (XXY)

Usually Decreased In
CML
PNH
Hereditary hypophosphatasia
Nephrotic syndrome
Progressive muscular dystrophy
Refractory anemia (siderotic)
Sickle cell anemia

Usually Normal In
Secondary polycythemia
Hemolytic anemia
Infectious mononucleosis
Viral hepatitis
Lymphosarcoma

Variable In
PA
ITP
IDA
Acute myelogenous leukemia and idiopathic myelofibrosis
Acute undifferentiated leukemia

Table 11-20.	White Blood Cell Inclusions in Peripheral Blood
Organisms (especially in *Neisseria meningitidis, Staphylococcus aureus*) *Ehrlichia chaffeensis* morulae *Cryptococcus neoformans*	Usually means overwhelming sepsis, with grave prognosis.
Histoplasma capsulatum, Candida organisms	Within histiocytes.
Cytomegalovirus	Within circulating endothelial cells.
Auer rods (linear azurophilic granules)	Pathognomonic for myeloid origin. Occur in blasts and promyelocytes.
Howell-Jolly bodies	Nuclear fragments seen within granulocyte cell series (neutrophils, bands, myelocytes, metamyelocytes) in immunosuppression (e.g., drugs, AIDS, *Mycobacterium avium-intracellulare* infection).
Döhle bodies	Remnants of ribosomes or endoplasmic reticulum (RNA). Seen in many infectious diseases, burns, aplastic anemia, following administration of toxic agents. May resemble inclusions of May-Hegglin anomaly.
Alder-Reilly bodies	Dense azurophilic granulation in all WBCs and marrow macrophages; occurs in genetic mucopolysaccharidoses.
Chédiak-Higashi syndrome	Neutrophils contain coarse, deeply staining, peroxidase-positive, fused large granulations in cytoplasm and are present less frequently in other WBCs.
Batten (Batten-Spielmeyer-Vogt) disease (autosomal recessive type of juvenile amaurotic idiocy)	Azurophilic hypergranulation of leukocytes occurs in patients and in heterozygous and homozygous members of their families. In Giemsa and Wright stained smears, it resembles toxic granulation but differs by the absence of supravital staining in Batten disease and by normal leukocyte alkaline phosphatase activity (markedly increased in toxic granulation). This granulation occurs in ≥15% of neutrophils.

White Blood Cell Inclusions

See Table 11-20.

Disorders of White Blood Cells

Agranulocytosis

Agranulocytosis is characterized by a decreased number of granulocytes in the blood and bone marrow.

See Aplastic Anemia.
♦ In acute fulminant form, WBC count is decreased to ≤2,000/μL, sometimes as low as 50/μL. Granulocytes are 0% to 2%. Granulocytes may show pyknosis or vacuolization.

♦ In chronic or recurrent form, WBC count is decreased to 2,000/μL, with less marked granulocytopenia.
There is relative lymphocytosis and sometimes monocytosis.
♦ Bone marrow shows an absence of cells in granulocytic series but normal erythroid and megakaryocytic series.
ESR is increased.
Hb, RBC count and morphology, platelet count, and coagulation tests are normal.
Laboratory findings due to infection.

Due To
Peripheral destruction of PMNs (often drug related)
Overwhelming sepsis
More generalized bone marrow failure (see Aplastic Anemia)

Alder-Reilly Anomaly

♦ In Alder-Reilly anomaly, heavy, dense, metachromatic-staining cytoplasmic granules (mucopolysaccharides in lysosomes) of neutrophils and some lymphocytes and monocytes are seen. Inconstant in blood but always present in marrow cells. Associated with mucopolysaccharidoses (see Chapter 12). May also be seen in otherwise healthy persons.

Jordan Anomaly

♦ Jordan anomaly is a harmless rare anomaly of fatty inclusions in the cytoplasm of all neutrophils, most monocytes, some basophils and eosinophils, occasional lymphocytes.
♦ Three to 10 vacuoles per neutrophil stain with Sudan III. Fewer vacuoles are found in marrow myeloid cells beginning with promyelocytes.

Langerhans Cell Histiocytosis

This disorder was formerly called Histiocytosis X. It displays rare proliferative abnormalities of macrophages.

Eosinophilic Granuloma

Eosinophilic granuloma is manifested in single or multiple bone lesions.

♦ Biopsy of bone is diagnostic.
May have increased ESR and mild leukocytosis. No specific laboratory findings.

Letter-Siwe Disease

Letter-Siwe disease is a rapidly progressive, frequently fatal disease, primarily of children.

• Laboratory findings due to infiltration of skin and various organs, e.g.:
• Bone marrow: Progressive normocytic normochromic anemia. Hemorrhagic manifestations due to thrombocytopenia.
• Hypersplenism, infections, liver involvement
• Diagnostic biopsy (e.g., bone, skin, lymph nodes) shows characteristic lesions.

Hand-Schüller-Christian Disease

Hand-Schüller-Christian disease is the reactive proliferation of macrophages of uncertain etiology, causing a triad of skull defects, exophthalmos, and diabetes insipidus.

♦ Diagnosis is made by histologic examination of involved tissues (especially bone).
Anemia, leukopenia, and thrombocytopenia may be present.
Diabetes insipidus may occur in ≤50% of patients.

Lymphocytosis (Infectious), acute

Acute infectious lymphocytosis may be associated with coxsackievirus, echovirus, and adenovirus infections.

Markedly increased WBC count (usually 20,000–50,000/μL) is caused by lymphocytosis (60%–90%); normal appearing, small lymphocytes. Eosinophilia is frequent. Heterophil agglutination is negative.

Neutropenia, Periodic (Cyclic)

This rare autosomal dominant condition is caused by the accelerated apoptosis of developing neutrophils. Periodic neutropenia also occurs as an acquired disorder with clonal proliferation of large granular lymphocytes.

◆ Regular periodic occurrence of neutropenia every 10 to 35 days, lasting 3 to 6 days. WBC count is 1,000 to 1,500/μL, and granulocytes are as low as 0%. Diagnosis is made by serial counts two to three times per week for at least six weeks.
Oscillations of monocytes, platelets, reticulocytes may also occur.
Laboratory findings due to bacteremias (usually *Clostridium* species) during neutropenic periods.

Neutrophilia, Hereditary Giant

Hereditary giant neutrophilia is a very rare but innocuous autosomal dominant anomaly.

◆ One percent to 2% of neutrophils are ≤2× normal size and contain 6 to 10 nuclear lobes. In females, drumstick appendages are often duplicated. There are no associated anomalies.
Acquired form may occur in myeloproliferative disease, acute myelogenous leukemia (AML), treatment with alkylating agents.

Neutrophils, Hereditary Hypersegmentation

Hereditary hypersegmentation of neutrophils is a very rare harmless autosomal dominant condition. Must be differentiated from folate and B$_{12}$ deficiency.

◆ Hypersegmentation of neutrophils resembles that seen in PA, but it is a permanent abnormality. Most neutrophils have four or more lobes. There are ≥5 lobes in >10% of heterozygotes and 30% of homozygotes. Number of drumsticks in females may also be increased.
A similar harmless condition exists that affects only the eosinophilic granulocytes (hereditary hypersegmentation of eosinophils).
Hypersegmentation is also found in almost every patient with chronic renal disease with BUN >30 mg/dL for more than 3 months.

Pelger-Huët Anomaly

Pelger-Huët anomaly is caused by an autosomal dominant mutation at chromosome 1q42.1. This usually heterozygous anomaly of WBCs is of no clinical significance.

◆ Nuclei of >80% of granulocytes show hyposegmentation; are shaped like pince-nez eyeglasses, rods, dumbbells, or peanuts; present in peripheral blood and bone marrow. Condensed (mature) pyknotic chromatin is evident in nuclei of granulocytes, lymphocytes, eosinophils, basophils, and monocytes and in marrow metamyelocytes and bands. Heterozygotes have one or two lobed nuclei; homozygotes are uniformly unsegmented.
Cytoplasmic maturation is normal.
Sex chromatin body is not found in these women.
Acquired pseudo–Pelger-Huët changes is dysplastic maturation of nucleus and cytoplasm; are less predominant and nuclear chromatin is immature. May occur in:

• Acute and chronic myeloproliferative disorders (may be a premonitory feature), NHL, myelodysplastic syndrome (predicts poor prognosis), Hodgkin disease, others. Not found in acute lymphocytic leukemia (ALL) and rarely in CLL.
• May be transient in various acute infections (e.g., leukemoid reactions, granulocytosis, TB, HIV, *Mycoplasma* pneumonia, influenza, malaria).
• Due to certain drugs (e.g., colchicine, sulfonamides, ibuprofen, valproic acid, alkylating agents).
• Nonhematologic disorders (e.g., SLE, myxedema)

Disorders of Spleen and Thymus

Spleen, Decreased Function (Hyposplenism)

Caused By

Congenital absence

Splenectomy or autoinfarction (e.g., sickle cell anemia)

Infiltration (e.g., amyloidosis, lymphoma) is rare cause.

Nontropical sprue, dermatitis herpetiformis, ulcerative colitis, regional ileitis (30% of patients), but overwhelming sepsis is rare.

Irradiation

GVHD

♦ Howell-Jolly bodies (is the most consistent abnormality; good indicator of asplenic state), pocked cells, and target cells are seen in peripheral blood smears; also Pappenheimer bodies, Cabot rings, few acanthocytes, nucleated RBCs. Some Heinz bodies can be seen with special stains.

Decreased osmotic fragility may be found.

Increased risk of overwhelming infection by encapsulated bacteria (50% are caused by *Streptococcus pneumoniae;* another 25% are brought on by *Haemophilus influenzae, Neisseria meningitidis,* and group A streptococcus; *Staphylococcus, Pseudomonas,* and other Gram-negative organisms are rarer). High mortality with massive bacteremia. Risk of infection is greater in infants younger than 2 years old, within 2 years of splenectomy, or if underlying disorder is primary hematologic or splenic disease.

Postsplenectomy

Absence of RBC changes may suggest an accessory spleen in postsplenectomy patients.

Increased WBC count (granulocytosis) for several weeks in 75% of patients and indefinitely in 25%. Lymphocytosis and monocytosis occur in several weeks in 50% of patients; some of these may show increased eosinophils or basophils. Platelet, WBC, and reticulocyte counts may increase to a peak in 5 to 14 days in the postoperative period, and then become high-normal.

Spleen, Increased Function (Hypersplenism)

♦ Diagnosis is made by exclusion.

♦ There are various combinations of anemia, leukopenia, and thrombocytopenia associated with bone marrow showing normal or increased cellularity of affected elements (includes primary splenic pancytopenia and primary splenic neutropenia).

* Decreased platelet count is moderate to severe (100,000–30,000/μL).
* Normochromic anemia (Hb = 9.0–11.0 g/dL) may occur.
* WBCs may be decreased with a normal differential count.
* Bone marrow is normal or shows increased cellularity of all lines with normal maturation.

Peripheral blood smear may reflect the underlying cause:

* Spherocytes in hereditary spherocytosis
* Target cells in liver disease
* Atypical lymphocytes in infectious mononucleosis or chronic infection
* Leukoerythroblastosis, nucleated RBCs, and immature granulocytes in myeloid metaplasia with extramedullary hematopoiesis
* Teardrop and hand mirror RBCs in myelofibrosis

Direct Coombs test is negative.

[51]Cr-tagged RBCs from a normal person or from the patient are rapidly destroyed after transfusion, and radioactivity accumulates in spleen. (Normal spleen:liver ratio = 1.0; in hypersplenism it is 1.5–2.0; in hemolysis, the ratio is >3.0.)

Laboratory findings because of underlying disease that can cause splenomegaly:

* Congestion (e.g., cirrhosis with portal hypertension)
* Hematologic disorders (e.g., lymphoma/leukemia)
* Infiltration (e.g., histiocytoses, lipid storage disease)

- Inflammation and infections (e.g., subacute bacterial endocarditis, TB, kala-azar, sarcoidosis, collagen diseases, Felty syndrome)
- Splenic tumors and cysts
- Primary splenic pancytopenia

Thymic Hypoplasia (Digeorge Syndrome)

Hypoplasia or aplasia of thymus and parathyroid and anomalies of other structures formed at same time (e.g., cardiac defects, renal abnormalities, facial abnormalities such as cleft palate, etc.) are caused by chromosome 22q11 deletions.

See Tables 11-33 and 11-34.

♦ **Diagnostic Criteria**
Involvement of ≥2 of the following organ systems:

- Thymus
- Parathyroid
- Cardiovascular

Hypocalcemia may be transient; may cause neonatal seizures.

Serum immunoglobulins are usually near normal for age but may be decreased, especially IgA. IgE may be increased.

Decreased T cells and relative increase in B-cell percentage. Normal ratio of helper and suppressor types.

With complete syndrome, patient is susceptible to opportunistic infection (*Pneumocystis jiroveci [carinii]*, fungi, viruses) and to lethal GVHD from blood transfusion. In partial syndrome (with variable amount of hypoplasia), growth and response to infection may be normal.

Thymus is often absent; when ectopic thymus is found, histology appears normal.

Lymph node follicles appear normal, but paracortical areas and thymus-dependent areas of spleen show variable amount of depletion. Incidence of cancer and of autoimmune disease is not increased.

Thymus Tumors

More than 40% of thymic tumors have parathymic syndromes noted in the following, which are multiple in 1/3 of cases.

○ Associated With

Myasthenia gravis in about 35% of cases. May appear up to 6 years after excision of thymoma in 5% of cases. Thymoma develops in 15% of patients with myasthenia gravis.

Acquired hypogammaglobulinemia. Seven percent to 13% of adults with this condition have an associated thymoma; this does not respond to thymectomy.

Pure red cell aplasia (PRCA) is found in approximately 5% of thymoma patients. Fifty percent of cases of PRCA have thymoma, 25% of whom benefit from thymectomy; onset followed thymectomy in 10% of cases. May be accompanied or followed, but not preceded, by granulocytopenia or thrombocytopenia or both in 1/3 of cases; thymectomy is not useful therapy. PRCA occurs in 1/3 of patients with hypogammaglobulinemia and thymoma.

Autoimmune hemolytic anemia with positive Coombs test and increased reticulocyte count

Cushing syndrome

Multiple endocrine neoplasia (usually type 1)

SLE

Miscellaneous disorders (e.g., giant cell myocarditis, nephrotic syndrome)

Cutaneous disorders (e.g., mucocutaneous candidiasis, pemphigus)

HEMATOLOGY

Myeloproloferative Disorders (Leukemias/Lymphomas)[19,20]

Classification of Lymphoid Neoplasms by Cell of Origin

Eighty-five percent or fewer of lymphoid neoplasms are of B-cell origin, rarely of natural killer (NK) origin; the rest are of T-cell origin.

Immature precursor B-cell neoplasms (precursor B-cell acute lymphoblastic leukemia/lymphoma).

Mature B-cell neoplasms (e.g., CLL/chronic lymphocytic lymphoma, follicular lymphoma, Burkitt lymphoma, multiple myeloma, hairy cell leukemia)

Precursor T-cell neoplasms (precursor-T ALL/acute lymphoblastic lymphoma)

Mature precursor T-cell and NK-cell neoplasms (e.g., mycosis fungoides/Sézary syndrome, adult T-cell leukemia/lymphoma, angioimmunoblastic T-cell lymphoma)

Hodgkin lymphoma

Gene Rearrangement *(bcr)* Assay

♦ **PCR or FISH** have replaced Southern blot as preferred methods to demonstrate Ph[1]. For diagnosis in Ph[1]-negative cases (by cytogenetics, 5% of CML patients) or to confirm Ph[1]-positive CML.

To diagnose CML patients who present in blast crisis or are in blast transformation.

To detect CML in myeloproliferative disorders with similar morphologic features.

To monitor CML patients treated with marrow transplant, chemotherapy, or interferon.

Detection of minimal residual disease or confirm complete remission.

Monitoring for early detection of relapse.

Purging of *bcr*-positive cells from autologous bone marrow before infusion.

Positive *bcr* gene rearrangement in acute leukemia indicates poor prognosis, especially in ALL.

Finding of same gene rearrangement in lymphocytes in a distant site biopsy is proof of metastasis.

Also used for diagnosis of many other genetic disorders (e.g., HbS, HbC, β-thalassemia).

Interferences

False-negative PCR in Ph[1]-positive patients may occur because of therapy with α-interferon or, less commonly, hydroxyurea.

Contamination of PCR material.

Interpretation

♦ Philadelphia chromosome t(9;22) (q34q11.2) (Ph[1]) due to chimeric *BCR-ABL* fusion gene on chromosome 22 is found in 95% of early chronic phase cases; persists in chronic stable phase when marrow and blood appear normal. Causes increased dysregulated tyrosine kinase activity that regulates apoptosis and maturation (specifically inhibited by STI-571, an adenosine triphosphate analogue currently used for treatment).

Presence of Ph[1] affects response to therapy and survival. Persists during blast phase when additional abnormalities may appear in ≤8% of cases (e.g., chronic myelomonocytic leukemias). Other cytogenic abnormalities occur in 1/3 of the 5% of cases who are Ph[1] negative. The Ph[1] chromosome is also found in ≤30% of adults with ALL, 2% of adults with AML, and 5% of children with ALL. The Ph[1] chromosome in acute leukemia indicates a poor prognosis. Ph[1] is present in granulomonocytic, erythroid, and megakaryocytic lines as well as some B-lymphocytes. If karyotyping is negative, Ph[1] may be revealed by FISH or RT-PCR, which are more sensitive. Treatment with imatinib (tyrosine kinase inhibitor) results in cytogenetic hematologic remission in >75% of early chronic phase cases and >40% of late cases; in 50% of these, Ph[1] is no longer detectable but still detectable by RT-PCR in >95% of patients.

[19]Crisan D, ed. Acute leukemias. *Clin Lab Med* 2000;20:1–227.
[20]Schumacher HR, Alvares CJ, Blough RI, et al. Acute leukemia. *Clin Lab Med* 2002;22:153–192.

Hodgkin Disease And Other Malignant Lymphomas

♦ Diagnosis is established by histologic findings of biopsied lymph node.
Blood findings may vary from completely normal to markedly abnormal.
Moderate normochromic normocytic anemia occurs, occasionally of the hemolytic type;
may become severe.
♦ Cytopenias occur commonly due to hypersplenism, immune effect, or lymphoma
effect on marrow.
♦ Bone marrow involvement is found at time of diagnosis in <10% of patients with
Hodgkin disease; in 50% of patients with diffuse, small cleaved lymphoma and mixed
cell type; and 70% to 80% of patients with follicular, small cleaved cell lymphoma;
this is less frequent in large cell lymphomas.
Large intermediate-grade lymphoma with serum LD >500 IU/L is less likely to be cured.
Serum protein electrophoresis: Albumin is frequently decreased. Increased α-1 and
α-2 globulins suggest disease activity. Decreased γ globulin is less frequent in Hodgkin
disease than in lymphosarcoma. γ globulins may be increased, with macroglobulins
present and evidence of autoimmune process (e.g., hemolytic anemia, cold agglutinins). Monoclonal gammopathy in ~20% of small lymphocytic lymphomas.
ESR and CRP are increased during active stages in ~50% of cases; may be normal during remission. ESR >30 after radiotherapy may predict relapse.
Hypercalcemia may be present.

Hodgkin Disease

**Hodgkin disease is a neoplasm of transformed terminal center B-lymphocytes. The
EBV genome is identified in Reed-Sternberg cells in ≤70% of cases.**

• Peripheral blood changes are common (~25% of cases at time of diagnosis) but not
specific. WBC count may be normal, decreased, or slightly or markedly increased
(25,000/μL). Leukopenia, marked leukocytosis, and anemia are bad prognostic
signs. Eosinophilia occurs in ~20% of patients. Relative and absolute lymphopenia
may occur. If lymphocytosis is present, look for another disease. Neutrophilia may
be found. Monocytosis may be found. These changes may all be absent or may even
be present simultaneously or in various combinations. Rarely, Reed-Sternberg cells
are found in marrow or peripheral blood smears in advanced disease. Platelets may
be decreased or increased.
• Patients commonly have abnormal T-cell function with deficiencies of cell-mediated
immunity, with increased susceptibility to bacterial, fungal, and viral (especially
herpes zoster and varicella) infections; these persist even after cure. Serum
immunoglobulins are usually normal.
• More than 50% of cases show evidence of EBV in Reed-Sternberg cells.
• No specific chromosomal abnormalities

Subtype*	~ %	Comment
Lymphocyte predominance	7%	Most frequently in young males. Tend to localize in cervical lymph nodes. Best prognosis, indolent. Not associated with EBV. Lymphocyte-rich is 40% associated with EBV.
Nodular sclerosis	68%	Most frequently in young females presenting as mediastinal mass. Rarely associated with EBV.
Mixed cellularity	23%	70% associated with EBV.
Lymphocyte depletion	2%	Most frequently in older age and in HIV-positive patients. Paucity of peripheral lymphadenopathy. Bone marrow involvement is common. Over 70% associated with EBV.

EBV, Epstein Barr virus.
*Classification is based on histologic findings, usually in a lymph node.

Non-Hodgkin Lymphoma

• Ninety percent or fewer of cases of NHL are derived from B cells. Their immunopheno-
typic abnormalities can be used to distinguish them from benign reactions in lymph nodes.

- Patients often have abnormalities of humoral immunity; hypogammaglobulinemia in 50% of cases and monoclonal gammopathy in ~10% of small lymphocytic lymphomas.
- Autoimmune hemolytic anemia and thrombocytopenia may occur.
- Increased serum cancer antigen 125 in ~40% of cases indicates pleuropericardial or peritoneal involvement; may be useful for staging. Return of increased value to normal indicates therapeutic response, with S/S of 100%/>87%.
- Laboratory findings due to involvement of other organ systems (e.g., liver, kidney, CNS).
- Testicular NHL is often aggressive and associated with CNS and bone marrow disease.
- Laboratory findings due to effects of treatment (e.g., radiation, chemotherapy, splenectomy), including acute and long-term toxicity, gonadal dysfunction, peripheral neuropathy, and second neoplasms (especially AML).
- Occurs frequently in AIDS patients and shows rapid course, poor prognosis, and frequent extranodal and CNS involvement.

Post–organ transplantation malignant lymphomas in ~2% of cases; median time to recurrence ~6 months and two thirds within 10 months. Occurs in 0.8% of recipients of renal allografts, 1.6% of liver allografts, 5.9% of heart allografts. Compared to spontaneous lymphomas, these tend to be more aggressive, frequently large-cell type in extranodal sites, especially CNS; many are immunoglobulin negative.

◆ Gene Rearrangement

Use

Monitor for residual lymphoma during chemotherapy, confirm remission, detect minimal residual disease, detect marrow or distant site involvement, monitor patients undergoing marrow transplantation, diagnose relapse earlier.
In B-cell diffuse lymphoma, *bcl*-2–positive patients are less likely to have complete remission. Detection by PCR after bone marrow has been purged prior to marrow transplant is indicator to predict relapse.

Burkitt Lymphoma

Burkitt lymphoma is a distinctive type of aggressive non-Hodgkin lymphoma with characteristic morphology. It is usually extranodal.

Distinctive neoplastic blast cells in marrow are mature B cells expressing B-cell antigens (CD10) and monotypic surface immunoglobulins.
Leukemic phase has predominantly peripheral blood and marrow involvement.
Cytogenic and molecular studies show one of three characteristic translocations: t(8:14)(q24;q32), t(8;22)(q24;q11), or t(2;8)(p11;q24).
Related to EBV infection.

Diffuse Large B-Cell Lymphoma

Diffuse large B-cell lymphoma appears in 20% of non-Hodgkin lymphoma cases with heterogeneous pathogenesis and typical single nodal or extranodal (e.g., GI tract, brain, bone, skin, viscera) site.

Various chromosomal abnormalities (e.g., t(14;18) of follicular lymphoma)

Follicular Lymphoma

Follicular lymphoma is the most common type of non-Hodgkin lymphoma in the United States. It follows an indolent waxing and waning course.

≤50% transform, especially to diffuse large B-cell lymphoma.
bcl-2 gene rearrangement is molecular counterpart of t(14;18)(q32:q21) reciprocal translocation; found in >80% by cytogenic analysis and virtually all by molecular testing and differentiates this from reactive lymph nodes.

Mantle Cell Lymphoma

Mantle cell lymphoma comprises ~3% of non-Hodgkin lymphoma due to translocation of *BCL1* locus on chromosome 11 to Ig heavy chain locus on chromosome 14, causing overexpression of cyclin D1 protein, resulting in unregulated proliferation of affected B cells.

♦ Microscopic examination of tumor.
♦ Immunohistochemistry to detect cyclin D1 overexpression.
♦ FISH detects the t(11;14)(q13;q32).
♦ PCR is positive in only 30% to 40% of these lymphomas.

Cutaneous T-Cell Lymphoma[21]

Cutaneous T-cell lymphoma is characterized by tumors of the CD4+ helper T cells.

Mycosis Fungoides

♦ Biopsy of lesion (usually skin) shows microscopic findings that parallel clinical findings. Repeated periodic biopsies may be needed before diagnosis is established.
♦ Mycosis fungoides cells in peripheral blood or marrow suggest extensive disease.
Laboratory findings are generally not helpful.
Peripheral blood may occasionally show increased eosinophils, monocytes, and lymphocytes.
Bone marrow may show increase in reticuloendothelial cells, monoblasts, lymphocytes, and plasma cells.
Laboratory findings due to involvement of virtually any other organ.

Sézary Syndrome

♦ Sézary syndrome is a more aggressive form of skin lesions caused by infiltration of Sézary cells associated with >1,000/μL of these cells in peripheral blood
♦ Increased peripheral blood lymphocyte count, >15% of which are atypical lymphocytes (Sézary cells).
Total WBC count is often increased
ESR, Hb, and platelet counts are usually normal.
Bone marrow, lymph nodes, and liver biopsies are usually normal.
Increased serum IgA, IgE, and eosinophilia appear in advanced cases.

Leukemic Involvement

Circulating monoclonal tumor cells >5% to 10% of total WBC or >20% of total lymphocytes or absolute cell count >1,000/mm³.
CD4/CD8 ratio <10

Lymphadenopathy, Angioimmunoblastic

Angioimmunoblastic lymphadenopathy is a rare lymphoproliferative disorder arising from mature postthymic T-lymphocytes with sudden onset of constitutional symptoms and lymphadenopathy. It carries a very poor prognosis.

♦ Diagnosis requires a lymph node biopsy, which shows characteristic changes, but these alone do not permit diagnosis and the clinical findings are required.
Nonspecific polyclonal hypergammaglobulinemia in 75% of cases.
Coombs-positive hemolytic anemia in 50% of cases.
Leukocytosis with lymphopenia.
Thrombocytopenia.
High frequency of autoantibodies and association with other autoimmune syndromes, especially SLE.
Death usually caused by infection associated with T-cell immune deficiency (e.g., CMV, EBV, herpes simplex, *Pneumocystis jiroveci (carinii)*, mycobacteria, opportunistic fungi).
Lymphomas (B- or T-cell type or, rarely, Hodgkin disease) develop in 5% to 20% of cases.
Serologic tests for HIV are negative.

HEMATOLOGY

[21]Girardi M, Heald PW, Wilson LD. The pathogenesis of mycosis fungoides. *N Engl J Med* 2004; 350:1978–1988.

Myelodysplastic (Preleukemic) Syndromes

♦ Myelodysplastic syndromes are clonal proliferative disorders of bone marrow that show peripheral blood cytopenias; disordered, ineffective myelopoiesis; and myeloblasts <20%; 30% to 40% progress to acute nonlymphocytic leukemia, 60% to 80% of patients die of complications (e.g., acute infection, hemorrhage) or associated diseases, and 10% to 20% remain stable and die of unrelated causes. There is no detectable cause, but prior chemotherapy (especially with alkylating agents) or radiation may contribute in some. Partial or complete loss of chromosomes 5 and/or 7 and trisomy 8 is seen in ≤70% of cases. Occurs eventually in some aplastic anemia patients.

World Health Organization Classification of Myelodysplastic Syndromes

♦ Refractory anemia with ringed sideroblasts (RARS) (same as acquired idiopathic sideroblastic anemia):

• Refractory anemia (see above); RBCs may be dimorphic—oval macrocytes and hypochromic microcytes; many siderocytes
• >15% ringed sideroblasts
• Normal megakaryocytes and granulocytes
• <1% blasts in peripheral blood
• <5% blasts in marrow
• ≤10% develop acute myelocytic leukemia

♦ Refractory anemia without ringed sideroblasts:

• Persistent anemia refractory to treatment with vitamin B$_{12}$, folate, or pyridoxine, with decreased reticulocytes and variable dyserythropoiesis. Anemia may be macrocytic, normocytic, or dimorphic with hypochromasia, with changes in size and shape of RBCs.
• <1% blasts in peripheral blood
• <5% blasts in marrow
• <15% ringed sideroblasts in marrow (bone marrow normoblasts)
• Hypercellular marrow with erythroid hyperplasia and/or dyserythropoiesis
• Normal megakaryocytes and granulocytes
• Dysgranulopoiesis is infrequent
• 5% of patients present with these findings but without anemia

♦ Refractory anemia with excess blasts (RAEB) (poor prognosis; usually progresses to acute leukemia within a year):

• Cytopenia affecting ≥2 cell lines
• <5% blasts in peripheral blood and 5% to 20% blasts in marrow; granulocytic maturation is present
• Divided into RAEB-1 (5% to 10% blasts in peripheral blood and marrow) and RAEB-2 (11%–19% blasts in marrow and peripheral blood or blasts with Auer rods)
• <1% marrow sideroblasts
• Variably cellular marrow with granulocytic or erythroid hyperplasia
• Dysgranulopoiesis, dyserythropoiesis, and/or dysmegakaryocytopoiesis

♦ Refractory cytopenia with multilineage dysplasia (RCMD):

• Cytopenia affecting ≥2 cell lines
• Little or no increase in blasts (<5%) in marrow; no increase in monocytes.
• Usually no blasts in peripheral blood. No Auer rods.
• Dysplasia ≥2 myeloid lines. Type and degree of dysplasia vary greatly.

♦ Myelodysplastic syndrome, unclassified (MDS-U):

• Usually no blasts in peripheral blood
• Slight or no increased blasts in marrow
• Dysplasia affects only a single line; slight or marked
• Does not fit other categories

♦ 5q⁻ syndrome:

• Macrocytic anemia, severe to moderate.
• WBC and platelets normal or slightly increased.

- Peripheral blood and marrow as in refractory anemia, RAEB, or RCMD. Numerous small megakaryocytes with hypolobulated (≤3 lobes) nuclei.
- Prolonged course; may become acute leukemia with additional chromosomal abnormalities.

Myelodysplastic/Myeloproliferative Diseases

- Chronic myelomonocytic leukemia
- Atypical CML
- Juvenile myelomonocytic leukemia

French, American, British (FAB) Classification of Myelodysplastic Syndromes

Myelodysplastic Syndromes	Blasts		Other Features
	Peripheral Blood	Bone Marrow	
Refractory anemia	<1%	<5%	Same as WHO classification
Refractory anemia with ringed sideroblasts (RARS)	<1%	<5%	Same as WHO classification. Same as acquired idiopathic sideroblastic anemia.
Refractory anemia with excess blasts (RAEB)	<5%	5%–20%. • Granulocytic maturation is present. • <1% marrow sideroblasts.	Poor prognosis; usually progresses to acute leukemia within a year. • Cytopenia affecting ≥2 cell lines. • Divided into RAEB-1 and RAEB-2 according to % blasts in marrow and peripheral blood. • Variably cellular marrow with granulocytic or erythroid hyperplasia. • Dysgranulopoiesis, dyserythropoiesis, and/or dysmegakaryocytopoiesis
Refractory anemia with excess blasts in transformation (RAEB-T) (from myelodysplasia to overt acute nonlymphocytic leukemia)	>5%	21%–30% (>30% blasts constitutes acute nonlymphocytic leukemia)	• <1% marrow sideroblasts. • Auer rods are present in myeloid precursors. • Do not fit into FAB M1-M7 categories. • 75% develop acute myelocytic leukemia.
Chronic myelomonocytic leukemia	<5%	≤20%. • <1% marrow sideroblasts.	Same as refractory anemia with excess blasts but with:

HEMATOLOGY

- Increased monocytes
  $>100/\mu L$ ($>10\%$)
  in peripheral blood.
- Neutrophilia in
  50% of cases;
  mature granulocytes
  may be increased.
- Increased monocyte
  precursors in
  marrow (may need
  special stains).
- Absent *BCR-ABL*
  gene fusion and
  increased basophils.

WHO, World Health Organization; FAB, French, American, British.

Abnormal and asynchronous maturation of different cell series is defined as:
♦ • Dyserythropoiesis

Anisocytosis, poikilocytosis, oval macrocytes, nucleated RBCs, and normochromia are the most common changes in RBCs on peripheral smear. The RBC population may be dimorphic.

Erythroid maturation defects with bizarre (e.g., multinucleated) forms and megaloblastic features unresponsive to folic acid, vitamin B_{12}, and iron.

♦ • Dysgranulomonopoiesis

Increased or decreased numbers or abnormal nuclei or granulation in blood, acquired Pelger-Huet anomaly.

Variable increase in mature granulocyte precursors (usually myelocytes) and monocytosis occur frequently in marrow.

♦ • Dysmegakaryocytopoiesis

Increased or decreased number.

Atypical, bizarre, or giant platelets, often with giant abnormal granules, are seen in most cases. Marrow megakaryocytes are often atypical or bizarre.

Platelet function defects with prolonged bleeding time and aggregation abnormalities are very common.

Other clinicopathologic forms include refractory anemias of various types, PRCA, PNH, chronic idiopathic neutropenia, chronic idiopathic thrombocytopenia, etc.

Low granulocyte or platelet count or elevated bone marrow blast count are independent indicators of poor outcome. The 5q⁻ karyotype is often found in refractory anemia and carries a relatively good prognosis. Monosomy 7 and trisomy 8 are frequently found in other subclasses of myelodysplasia and are associated with a poor prognosis.

Poor prognosis is indicated by (in decreasing order of importance): >5% blasts in marrow, circulating blasts, abnormal karyotypes, granulocytopenia ($<1,000/\mu L$), monocytopenia, thrombocytopenia ($<140,000/\mu L$), ineffective erythropoiesis, presenting Hb <9.0 g/dL, hemolysis, <20% ringed sideroblasts in marrow, abnormal localization of blasts in center of marrow rather than subendosteal areas, and circulating CD34+ cells.

Leukemias

Acute

Risk Factors

Ionizing radiation, smoking

Chemical agents (e.g., benzene compounds, pesticides) and drugs (e.g., chlorambucil, cyclophosphamide)

Genetic disorders (e.g., trisomy 21, Fanconi syndrome, Klinefelter syndrome, Fanconi anemia, Bloom syndrome, ataxia-telangiectasia, xeroderma pigmentosum)

Oncogenic viruses (e.g., human T-cell lymphotropic virus; EBV)

♦ Diagnosis and prognosis are based on a combination of diagnostic methods:

(1) Microscopic examination of blood, bone marrow, and/or lymph nodes; electron microscopy (EM) (e.g., for myeloperoxidase, platelet peroxidase)

(2) Cytochemical (e.g., myeloperoxidase, chloracetic [specific] esterase, periodic acid–Schiff [PAS]) and immunohistochemical staining
(3) Immunophenotyping by flow cytometry is indispensable to distinguish T-cell, B-cell, and non-T, non-B cell types of ALL, which is important because of different prognoses and relapse patterns in the three types.
(4) Cytogenetics (see Chromosome Abnormalities in the following section)
(5) Molecular methods
(6) Clinical features

♦ **(1) (2) (3) Microscopic examination of blood and bone marrow:**

- WBC count is rarely >100,000/μL. It may be normal and is commonly less than normal.
- Peripheral smear shows many cells that resemble lymphocytes; it may not be possible to differentiate the very young forms as lymphoblasts or myeloblasts, and special cytochemical stains may be used (blast cells are positive for peroxidase, Sudan black B and nonspecific esterase are positive in AML but negative in ALL; cytoplasmic acid phosphatase may be positive in T-cell ALL).
- Auer rods are diagnostic of AML; seen in 10% to 20% of cases.
- Prognosis is poorer in: older children and adults >35 years, those with high initial WBC count, and those with chromosome translocations (e.g., 9,22 in Ph^1 chromosome and 4,11 positive ALL). A favorable response to treatment is more likely if B-cell lymphoblasts are CALLA-positive (common ALL antigen) but cytoplasmic μ-chain-negative. The presence of leukemic lymphoblasts that express myeloid antigens is associated with an unfavorable prognosis.

Anemia is almost always present at clinical onset. Usually normocytic and sometimes macrocytic, it is progressive and may become severe. Normoblasts and polychromatophilia are common.

Platelet count is usually decreased at clinical onset and becomes progressively severe. May show poor clot retraction, increased bleeding time, positive tourniquet test, etc.

♦ Bone marrow:

- Blast cells are present even when none are found in peripheral blood. (This finding is useful to differentiate from other causes of pancytopenia.) There is progressively increasing infiltration with earlier cell types (e.g., blasts, myelocytes).
- The myeloid:erythroid ratio is increased.
- Erythroid and megakaryocyte elements are replaced.
- Cultures (bacterial, fungal, viral) should be done routinely, as they may be the first clue to occult infection.

(4) Chromosome Abnormalities (see Table 11-21)
At initial diagnosis, routine cytogenetic studies show chromosomal abnormality in >50% of cases:

(A) Structural abnormalities, including translocations, deletions, isochromosomes, inversions, and duplications, and
(B) Numeric anomalies (e.g., trisomies, monosomies).

In contrast, molecular tests may detect only one or few specific translocations.
If an abnormal chromosome clone is not observed, the analysis is considered not diagnostic.

Risk assessment in ALL patients:

- Among children <1 year old in whom prognosis is poor, 70% to 80% have MLL gene rearrangements. In adolescents and adult patients, high frequency of MLL rearrangements and BCR-ABL fusion are associated with poor prognosis.
- Favorable genetic abnormalities are hyperdiploidy (>50 chromosomes/cell), which is also associated with low WBC count and ETV6-CBFA2 (TEL-AML1) fusion, which occur mainly at age 1 to 9 years.
- Markedly hypodiploid or near-haploid leukemic cells usually indicate a poor prognosis, regardless of age of WBC count.
- Leukemic cells with BCR-ABL fusion usually indicates high risk. In adults, 20% of acute leukemias are lymphocytic (ALL) and 80% are nonlymphocytic (AML),

♦ In children, 75% of cases are ALL and 25% are AML or chronic; >80% show clonal chromosomal abnormalities. With specific genetic abnormalities, PCR can identify as few as 1 malignant cell per 10^6 normal cells and minimal residual leukemia in >90% of childhood ALL.

Table 11-21. Chromosomal Translocations in Hematologic Malignancies

Hematologic Disorder	Chromosomal Translocation	Gene Rearrangement (Break Points)	Clinical Utility
CML	Ph¹ t(9;22) and variants	BCR/ABL (bcr break point)	D, P, M
B-cell ALL	Ph¹ t(9;22)	BCR/ABL (bcr and BCR break points)	D, P, M
	t(8;14), t(2;8) t(8;22)	IgH, Ig κ Ig λ, and MYC	D, M
	t(1;19)	PBX/TCF (E2A)	D, P
	t(4;11), t(11;19) and variants	MLL/different loci	D, P
	t(5;14)	IL3/IgH	Being evaluated
T-cell ALL	t(1;14) and variants	TAL1/TCR δ, α, SIL	D
B- or T-cell ALL	t(7q35), t(14q11), t (14q32)	Antigen receptor genes	D
AML-M2	t(8;21)	AML1/ETO	D, P, M
AML-M3	t(15;17)	PML/RARA	D, P, M
AML-M4 Eo	inv(16), t(16;16)	CBFB/MYHII	D, P
AML-M5	t(11q23), various partner chromosomes	MLL/different loci	D, P
AML with basophilia	t(6;9)	DEK/CAN	D, P
AML with thrombocytosis	t(3;3), inv(3)	EVII/?	P
Follicular, and subsets of diffuse lymphomas	t(14;18)	BCL-2/IgH	D, M
Burkitt lymphoma	t(8;14), t(2;8), t(8;22)	IgH, Ig κ, Ig λ, and MYC	D, M
Mantle zone lymphoma, rare CLL cases	t(11;14)	BCL-1 (cyclin D or PRAD1)/IgH	D, M

D, diagnosis; M, monitor therapy; P, prognosis; CML, chronic myelogenous leukemia; ALL, acute lymphocytic leukemia; AML, acute myelogenous leukemia; CLL, chronic lymphocytic leukemia. Source: Crisan D. Molecular diagnostics in hematology. *Advance/Laboratory*. Nov 1997:45–48. Adapted from Crisan D, et al. Hematology. *Oncol Clin North Am* 1994;8(9):725–750.

♦ Gene rearrangement assays allows classification of almost all cases of ALL as T, B, or pre-B types. Confirm pathologic-immunologic diagnoses of T-cell and B-cell lymphomas that are difficult to classify. Virtually all cases of non-T, non-B leukemias are recognized as pre-B types.

♦ **(5) Molecular quantification of leukemic cells** (e.g., PCR or antibody detection) in minimal residual disease ALL.[22–24]

• Combinations of surface antigens semispecific for leukemic clone detect level of 10^{-4} cells.
• Various PCR techniques have limit of detection of 10^{-2} to 10^{-6} leukemic cells.
• After end of induction chemotherapy, level of minimal residual disease is useful for prognosis. $>10^{-2}$ cells (which is below detection limit with conventional microscopic examination of bone marrow) or $>10^{-3}$ cells at later time is associated with a very

[22]Cave H, van der Werff ten Bosch J, Suciu S, et al. Clinical significance of minimal residual disease in childhood acute lymphoblastic leukemia. European Organization for Research and Treatment of Cancer—Childhood Leukemia Cooperative Group. *N Engl J Med* 1998;339:591–598.
[23]Pui CH, Evans WE. Acute lymphoblastic leukemia. *N Engl J Med* 1998;339:605–615.
[24]Morley A. Quantifying leukemia. *N Engl J Med* 1998;339:627–629.

high probability of relapse; $<10^{-5}$ ($<.01\%$ nucleated cells) is associated with a very low probability of relapse.
- If $<10^{-3}$ cells in bone marrow, sampling error may be significant because of multifocal clones; therefore use peripheral blood or multiple marrow samples.
- Considered in remission after cytotoxic therapy, $<10^{10}$ cells and leukemic cells cannot be identified by conventional techniques.
- With 10^{11} to 10^{12} leukemic cells, clinical symptoms are present.
- With 10^{13} leukemic cells, death results.

(6) Clinical features

- DIC may be present (especially with M3; also M4 and M5; less commonly with other forms) at onset.
- Tumor lysis syndrome may cause hyperphosphatemia, hypokalemia, hypocalcemia, hypomagnesemia, etc. (see Chapter 17).
- Increased serum creatinine and BUN reflect infiltration of kidneys impairing renal function.
- In AML, serum LD is frequently but inconstantly increased; there is normal to slight increase in serum AST, ALT. LD >400 IU/L predicts shorter survival in elderly patients.
- Urine lysozyme may be increased in acute nonlymphocytic leukemia (M4 and M5).

♦ Laboratory findings due to complications:

- Meningeal leukemia occurs in 25% to 50% of children and 10% to 20% of adults with acute leukemia; the CSF shows pleocytosis and increased pressure and LD. CSF should be examined routinely as "sanctuary" for leukemic cells during chemotherapy and to rule out occult infection. Cranial irradiation may be indicated if leukemic cells are present in CSF, WBC count $\geq 100,000/\mu$L, or Ph^1 chromosome is present.
- Serum uric acid is frequently increased. With large leukemic cell burden: hyperuricemia (may have urate nephropathy), hyperkalemia, and hyperphosphatemia with secondary hypocalcemia are common.
- Infection causes 90% of deaths. The most important pathogens are enteric Gram-negative rods (especially *Pseudomonas aeruginosa*, *Escherichia coli*) and *Staphylococcus aureus*. With cumulative immunosuppression, fungi (especially *Candida albicans*), viruses (especially varicella-zoster and other herpesviruses), and *Pneumocystis jiroveci (carinii)* are common.
- Hemolytic anemia.

Laboratory findings caused by predisposing conditions:

- Genetic (e.g., Down syndrome, Bloom syndrome, Klinefelter syndrome, Fanconi anemia)
- Immunodeficiency (e.g., ataxia telangiectasia, common variable immunodeficiency, severe combined immunodeficiency, Wiskott-Aldrich syndrome)
- Ionizing radiation (therapeutic or accidental)
- Chemotherapeutic drugs (e.g., alkylating agents)
- Toxins (e.g., benzene)

Complete remission is possible with drug therapy (e.g., prednisone in ALL).

- WBC count falls (or rises) to normal in 1 to 2 weeks, with replacement of lymphoblasts by normal PMNs and return of RBC and platelet counts to normal; bone marrow may become normal. Maximum improvement is seen in 6 to 8 weeks.

Laboratory findings caused by toxic effect of therapeutic agents:
- Amethopterin toxicity causes a macrocytic type of anemia, with megaloblasts in marrow, compared to leukemic normocytic anemia, with blast cells in marrow.
- Cyclophosphamide can cause hematuria.
- L-asparaginase can cause coagulopathies, hyperglycemia, etc.
- Daunorubicin can cause cardiac toxicity with fibrosis.
- In childhood ALL, therapeutic agents cause 7× increase in all cancers and 22× increase in CNS tumors.

Leukemia, Lymphoblastic, Acute

ALL primarily affects children; comprises >85% of childhood leukemias. About 90% of patients have chromosomal changes. Children with Down syndrome have a 15× higher incidence of leukemia (especially ALL). An increased incidence is

HEMATOLOGY

seen also in immunodeficiency syndromes (e.g., ataxia-telangiectasia), osteogenesis imperfecta, Poland syndrome, and siblings of ALL patients. There is a high relapse rate. In adults, 80% of ALL are B-cell lineage and 20% are T-cell lineage.

♦ Diagnosis is based on morphology, cytochemistry, immunophenotyping, and genetic analysis. FAB terms L-1, L-2, L-3 are no longer used.
♦ WBC count increased; may be >100,000/μL but normal or low in some patients. Moderate to severe thrombocytopenia.
Variable degree of anemia.
♦ Marrow usually shows >50% lymphoblasts.
♦ High incidence of meningeal involvement; CSF may show increased protein and cells (some recognized as leukemic), where they find sanctuary.
♦ Ph^1 chromosome is present in ≤25% of adults and 3% of children; it is a uniformly poor prognostic sign. Most commonly in non-T, non-B cell ALL; never in T-cell ALL.
Serum LD, uric acid, ESR often increased.
Poor prognostic signs: platelet count <50,000/μL, WBC count >100,000/μL, CD10-negative serotype, cytogenic abnormalities, pre-B phenotype.
ALLs are categorized by immunophenotyping patterns (e.g., CD19, CD20, CD10, TdT)*

Leukemia, Lymphocytic, Chronic

CLL comprises 30% of all leukemias in the United States; <5% are T-cell type. Most are B-cell type. Progression to more aggressive cancers occurs in ~10% of cases (e.g., large B-cell lymphoma, prolymphocytic leukemia, ALL, multiple myeloma).

See Table 11-22.

Diagnostic Criteria
♦ Lymphocyte count >15,000/μL in absence of other causes and marrow infiltration >30% for >6 months. Have characteristic immunophenotype.
♦ Demonstration of monoclonality in the proper clinical context confirms the diagnosis regardless of absolute lymphocyte count. Monoclonality is determined by demonstration of light chain restriction in B-cell lymphocytosis and rearranged T-cell receptor genes in T-cell lymphocytosis; NK cells do not rearrange T-cell receptor genes.

♦ Peripheral blood:

• WBC count is increased (usually 50,000 to 250,000/μL) with 90% lymphocytes, which are uniformly similar, producing a monotonous blood picture of small mature-looking lymphocytes with minimal cytoplasm indistinguishable from normal. Frequent smudge cells. Blast cells are uncommon. Granulocytopenia. Neutropenia is a late occurrence.
• Autoimmune hemolytic anemia and thrombocytopenia occur in 25% of patients. Hb <11 g/dL and/or thrombocytopenia (<100/000/μL), diffuse bone marrow infiltration, and lymphocyte doubling time <1 year correlate with marked decrease in sur­vival time. Progress occurs with rising WBC count but may be absent with WBC count >50,000/μL.
• Platelet count is less likely to increase with therapy than in myelogenous leukemia.

♦ Bone marrow

• Infiltration with earlier lymphocytic cell types is progressively increased.
• There is replacement of erythroid, myeloid, and megakaryocyte series, which show normal morphology and maturation.

♦ Lymph node biopsy shows pattern of diffuse lymphoma with well-differentiated, small, noncleaved cells; aspirate or imprint shows increased number of immature leukocytes, predominantly blast cells.
Serum enzyme levels are less frequently increased and show a lesser increase than in CML. Even serum LD is frequently normal.

(*TdT = terminal deoxynucleotidyltransferase, a specialized DNA polymerase expressed only by pre-T and pre-B lymphoblasts positive in >95% of cases.)

Table 11-22.	Comparison of Chronic Lymphocytic Leukemias (CLLs)

B-lymphocytes

CLL	Autoimmune hemolytic anemia, hypogammaglobulinemia
Prolymphocytic leukemia (not a variant of CLL but a separate entity)	B-type lymphocytes derived from medullary cords of lymph nodes show less mature forms than in CLL extreme leukocytosis with >54% prolymphocytes with a typical phenotype, very high blast counts, prominent splenomegaly often without much lymphadenopathy
Waldenström macro-globulinemia	Increased serum IgM
Leukemic phase of poorly differentiated lymphoma	Usually is leukemic phase of lymphoma, but ≤50% have marrow involvement lymphoma when first seen; occasionally may present without node involvement
Hairy cell leukemia	Pancytopenia and prominent splenomegaly; usually leukopenia with many hairy cells showing characteristic tartrate-resistant acid phosphatase

T-lymphocytes

CLL	Causes <5% of cases of CLL
Adult T-cell leukemia/lymphoma	Hypercalcemia, lytic bone lesions; WRC usually >50,000/μL; due to HTLV-1 infection
Prolymphocytic	Morphologically identical to B-cell type, but lymph-adenopathy is more frequent in T-cell type leukemia
T-γ—chronic lympho-proliferative disease	Severe granulocytopenia; moderate increase in WBC; recurrent infections are common; usually no lymphadenopathy or skin involvement
Cutaneous T-cell lymphoma	Sézary syndrome refers to both skin and systemic involvement; mycosis fungoides is cutaneous form, which may be present for years before clinical systemic involvement

Direct Coombs test is positive in up to 1/3 of patients.

Hypogammaglobulinemia occurs in two thirds of cases, depending on duration of disease; monoclonal gammopathy (most often IgM) is found in <1% of cases.

Uric acid levels are not increased but may increase during therapy.

Chromosomal abnormalities appear in ~50% of patients, most often chromosomes 12 (especially trisomy 12) and 14 (especially 14q+). Ph[1] chromosome is not found. Translocations are rare.

More favorable prognosis is in patients with normal karyotype or with single abnormalities compared to complex abnormalities or with 13q14 deletions. Poorer prognosis with trisomy 12, 11q deletions, or 17p deletions. Chromosomal abnormalities develop over time.

Distinctive immunophenotype on tumor cells (CD19, CD20, CD23, CD5)

○ Leukemic B cells that express IgV$_\text{H}$ (immunoglobulin variable region) gene with somatic mutations confer better prognosis (median survival of >24 years compared to 6–8 years in patients without such mutations).[25] *ZAP-70* expression by flow cytometry (>20%) is surrogate for these gene mutations.

Laboratory findings due to secondary infection (e.g., encapsulated bacteria, herpes zoster, opportunistic organisms).

Leukemia, Myelogenous, Chronic

CML is a malignant clonal disorder of the stem cells and accounts for 20% of all leukemias in the United States; 90% of cases occur in adults, 10% in children.

See Table 11-23 and Figures 11-9 and 11-10.

Types of chronic myeloid leukemias

[25]Shah J, et al. Clinical significance of cytogenetics in multiple myeloma and chronic lymphocytic leukemia. *Lab Med* 2004;35:685.

HEMATOLOGY

Table 11-23.   Differential Diagnosis of Chronic Myelogenous Leukemia

	Chronic Myelogenous Leukemia	Acute Myeloblastic Leukemia	Granulocytic Leukemoid Reaction	Myelo-fibrosis
WBC >100,000/μL	Yes	Rare	No	No
Whole spectrum of immature granulocytes	Yes	No (leukemic hiatus)	No	Yes
Myeloblasts and pro-myelocytes in blood or marrow	>30%	>30%	0	<30%
Leukocyte ALP scores	Usually <10	30–150	>150	Variable
Bone marrow	Granulocytic hyperplasia	>30% myelo-blasts	Granulocytic hyperplasia	Fibrosis
Philadelphia chromosome	Yes	No	No	No

ALP, alkaline phosphatase.

- CML
- Chronic myelomonocytic leukemia
- Mast cell leukemia (rare)
- Chronic monocytic leukemia (rare)
- Chronic eosinophilic leukemia (rare)
- Classified into chronic, accelerated, and blast crisis phases.

Chronic Phase

♦ WBC count is usually 50,000 to 300,000/μL when disease is discovered, predominantly neutrophils and myelocytes with no leukemic hiatus. In earlier stages the

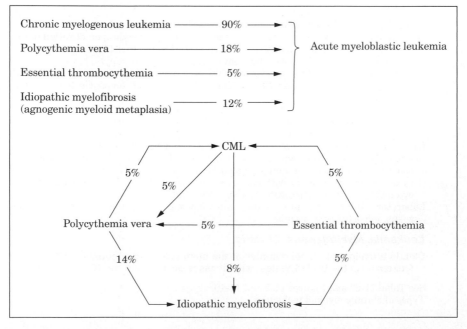

Fig. 11-9. Transformation of myeloproliferative syndromes. CML, chronic myelogenous leukemia.

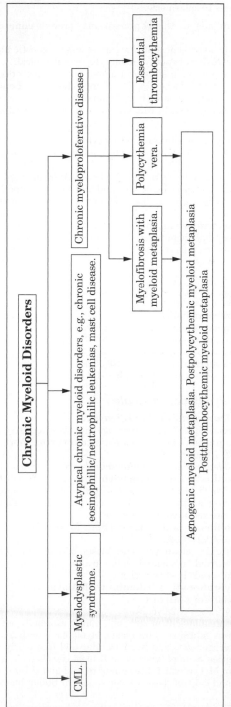

Chronic Myeloid Disorders

- CML.
- Myelodysplastic syndrome.
- Atypical chronic myeloid disorders, e.g., chronic eosinophillic/neutrophilic leukenias, mast cell disease.
- Chronic myeloproliferative disease
  - Myelofibrosis with myeloid metaplasia.
  - Polycythemia vera.
  - Essential thrombocythemia

Agnogenic myeloid metaplasia. Postpolycythemic myeloid metaplasia Postthrombocythemic myeloid metaplasia

Fig. 11-10. Classification of chronic myeloid disorders. CML, chronic myelogenous leukemia.

more mature forms predominate, with sequentially fewer younger forms, and only an occasional blast cell may be seen; later, the younger cells predominate. WBC count corresponds to spleen size.

- Absolute basophilia is invariably present; may precede clinical symptoms by many years.
- Eosinophilia may be present, but this carries less diagnostic utility than basophilia.
- Absolute monocytosis but relative monocytopenia is typical.
- Lymphocytes are normal in absolute number but relatively decreased.
- Decreased leukocyte ALP score in 95% of untreated cases. Leukocyte ALP score can rise to normal or high levels with infection, inflammation, or secondary malignant disease; after splenectomy; in remission due to chemotherapy; or at onset of blast crisis.

○ Anemia is usually normochromic, normocytic; absent in early stage and severe in late stage. Blood smear shows few normoblasts, slight polychromatophilia, occasional stippling.
Reticulocyte count is usually <3%. Anemia is caused by myelophthisis; also caused by bleeding (skin and GI tract), hemolysis, and insufficient compensatory hematopoiesis. Degree of anemia is a good index of extent of leukemic process and therefore of prognosis.
○ Platelet count is increased in ≤50% of cases; decreased in terminal stages with findings of thrombocytopenic purpura. Low count may increase with therapy. Bleeding manifestations are usually caused by thrombocytopenia. Megakaryocytes in blood in ~25% of cases.
♦ Bone marrow

- Hyperplasia of granulocytic elements occurs, with increase in myeloid:erythroid ratio. Myeloblasts <5% of all cells initially.
- Granulocytes are more immature than in the peripheral blood.
- Number of eosinophils and basophils is increased.
- Megakaryocytes may be increased.
- Hemosiderin deposits are increased.
- Focal or diffuse reticulin fibrosis in ~1/3 of cases.
- Macrophages (pseudo-Gaucher cells) in ~1/3 of cases.

Leukemias, Nonlymphocytic, Acute[26]

♦ *French, American, British Classification*
Has 85% concordance. Based on morphology and cytochemistry. Immunophenotyping and cytogenetics provide additional essential information. World Health Organization criteria uses ≥20% blasts.
M-1, M-2, and M-3 leukemias are predominantly granulocytic.
M0: Acute Myeloblastic Leukemia with Minimal Differentiation
Marrow contains ≥30% blasts that do not fulfill FAB morphologic and cytochemical classification criteria. Not included in current FAB classification. Immunologic markers or EM are required for diagnosis.
M1: Acute Myeloblastic Leukemia without Maturation
Incidence: ≤20% of AML cases.
>90% of nonerythroid nucleated cells are blasts, predominantly type 1.
<10% of nonerythroid nucleated cells are of maturing granulocytic lineage. Occasionally, Auer rods may be present.
M2: Acute Nonlymphocytic Leukemia with Maturation
Incidence: 25% to 30% of AML cases.
Patient age: young (mean = 28 years).
Clinical findings: splenomegaly in 28%; chloromas, especially of face area, in 20%.
Morphology: Marrow contains >30% blasts. Myeloblasts with Auer rods in 60% to 70% of cells are heterogeneous and hypogranular and frequently show pseudo–Pelger-Huët abnormalities. Sum of types I and II blast cells is 30% to 89% of nonerythroid cells (differ from M-1 in which the sum of types I and II blast cells is >90% of nonerythroid cells and ≥3% of these are peroxidase or Sudan black positive); monocytic

[26]Lauglin WR, Bick RL. Acute leukemias: FAB classification and clinical correlates. *Lab Med* 1994; 25:11.

cells are <20%; granulocytes from promyelocytes to polynuclear types are >10%. Maturation towards granulocytes is often abnormal; eosinophil precursors are frequently increased and may contain Auer rods.

Histochemistry: cells contain granulocyte but not monocyte enzymes; Sudan black and myeloperoxidase are abnormal (punctate rather than diffuse).

Karyotype: t(8;21)(q22;q22); critical region 21q translocated to 8q; frequent loss of sex chromosome. Increased predilection for M2 leukemia in Down syndrome (trisomy 21).

Oncogenes: c-ets-2 translocates from 21q to 8q, but expression data for the gene are unknown; c-mos remains at 8q and c-myc translocates to 21q, but both are probably not important.

Prognosis: 75% to 85% complete remission rate after chemotherapy, but median survival (9.5 months) is of average duration.

M3: Acute Promyelocytic Leukemia

Incidence: 5% to 10% of AML cases.

Patient age: Median of 31 years.

Clinical findings: Typically present with bleeding diathesis; ≤47% die of early fatal hemorrhage. DIC in ≤80% of cases.

Morphology: <30% blasts in most cases. Predominantly neoplastic promyelocytes with coarse azurophilic granules and multiple Auer rods; a variant (**M3v** is ~30% of M3 cases) shows hypogranular/microgranular promyelocytes on EM. Leukemic cell count in peripheral blood is usually not high (5,000–15,000/μL).

Unusual feature: Blast cells occasionally can be induced to differentiate into mature granulocytes or macrophages by various agents.

Karyotype: t(15;17)(q22;q12) occurs frequently; is diagnostic for M3.

Oncogene: None known.

M3v: Microgranular Variant

Incidence: 20% of AML cases.

Increased WBC count (50,000 to 200,000/μL) with small, difficult to see azurophilic granules. Morphology may vary between marrow (more like M3 AML) and peripheral blood.

M4: Acute Myelomonocytic Leukemia

Incidence: 20% to 25% of AML cases.

Marrow morphology: ≥30% of nonerythroid nucleated cells are myelomonocytic blasts; 2% to 80% of these are of granulocytic lineage and 20% to 80% are of monocytic lineage (demonstrated with combined esterase stain). Peripheral blood typically shows myelomonocytic blasts and >500/μL monocytes; serum lysozyme is often elevated.

- A variant (**M4Eo**) shows 5% to 30% abnormal eosinophils in marrow. Better prognosis and longer remission than for M4.

Cytochemistry is needed for reliable diagnosis; very weak staining for nonspecific esterase; can be distinguished from granulocytic types by monoclonal antibodies demonstrating specific antigens.

Karyotype: Almost all patients show inversion or deletion of chromosome 16 [inv(16)(p13;q22)]; <10% show balanced translocation between short arm of one chromosome 16 and long arm of other chromosome 16 [t(16;16)(p13.1;q22)].

Oncogene: Unknown.

Molecular oncology: Disruption of metallothionein genes by the chromosomal abnormality.

Prognosis: 70% to 90% complete remission rate probably with prolonged median duration (>18 months). >1/3 have relapse in the CNS, including myeloblastomas (compared to 5% of all acute nonlymphocytic leukemia patients, who rarely show CNS myeloblastomas).

M5: Acute Monocytic Leukemia with t(9;11)

Incidence: 10% of AML patients.

Patient age: Often children and young adults.

Clinical findings: Leukemic cells may infiltrate skin or gums, involve CNS; serum lysozyme is often elevated. DIC is frequent. Poor survival rates and shorter remissions.

Morphology: >30% of nonerythroid nucleated cells are blasts; >80% are of monocytic lineage.

Can be distinguished from granulocytic types by monoclonal antibodies demonstrating specific antigens.

M-5a: Acute Monoblastic Leukemia: Poorly differentiated variant comprises 4% of AML cases; >80% of monocytic cells are blasts.

HEMATOLOGY

M-5b: Acute Monocytic Leukemia: A well differentiated variant is 6% of AML cases; <80% of monocytic cells are blasts.
Karyotype: t(9;11)(p22;q23).
Oncogene: c-ets-1 translocated to 9p22 in region of α-interferon gene; expression data not known.

M6: Erythroleukemia
Incidence: 4% to 5% of AML cases.
Marrow morphology: ≥50% of all nucleated cells are erythroblasts. Thirty percent or more of nonerythroid nucleated cells are myeloblasts (if <30%, the diagnosis is myelodysplastic syndrome). Erythroid hyperplasia and marked dyserythropoiesis (e.g., megaloblasts, ringed sideroblasts, Howell-Jolly bodies) are common.
Nucleated RBCs in peripheral blood smear and anemia are common.
Immunologic abnormalities are more frequent in this form (e.g., positive Coombs test, antinuclear antibodies, positive rheumatoid factor (RF), increased serum γ globulins, hemolytic anemia).
Now further divided into **M6a** (acute erythroleukemia; age >50 years), **M6b** (Di Guglielmo syndrome), and **M6c,** which behave differently and require different therapy.

M7: Acute Megakaryocytic Leukemia
Incidence: 1% to 2% of AML cases.
Clinical: Is most common type in Down syndrome between infancy and age 3 years.
Marrow morphology: Myelofibrosis present in almost all patients; 20% to 40% present with acute myelofibrosis, making blast count impossible. Blast cells are highly polymorphic and are often classified as undifferentiated. Megakaryoblasts ≥30% of all cells.
Increased numbers of maturing megakaryocytes may be present. Megakaryocyte fragments, micromegakaryocytes, and blasts are frequently present in peripheral blood.
Cytochemistry is nonspecific: No myeloperoxidase or nonspecific esterase reaction. Unlike all other FAB subtypes except M0, diagnosis is based on EM identification of platelet peroxidase or on specific monoclonal antibodies to megakaryocyte antigens.
Karyotype: Abnormalities of chromosome 21 have been reported but specificity is still uncertain.
High serum LD.
Prognosis: Preliminary reports of poor response to conventional thracycline-cytarabine based therapy

Acute Undifferentiated Leukemia

No evidence of either myeloid or lymphoid lineage. Accounts for <1% of all acute leukemia cases. Not included in current FAB classification.

Acute Mixed-Lineage Leukemia

Myeloid and lymphoid lineages in same clone. Accounts for 10% to 15% of all acute leukemia cases.
Five percent to 10% of acute leukemias convert from one lineage to another.
Not included in current FAB classification.

Therapy-Related Leukemia

Clinical findings: >70% have a preleukemic phase lasting about 11 months; occurs several years (median = 4 years) after chemotherapy (most frequently an alkylating agent, especially melphalan, chlorambucil, or cyclophosphamide) or radiation for another disease such as Hodgkin disease (compared to about 20% of all acute non-lymphocytic leukemias that have a preleukemic phase). Risk is 3% to 10% 10 years after therapy but may be greater after age 40.
Highest risk after combined radiation and alkylating therapy; develop AML. Risk rises 5× to 20× following exposure to nontherapeutic compounds (e.g., benzene).
Unexplained pancytopenia; infection and hemorrhage.
Karyotype: >75% show deletion of chromosome 5/5q⁻ and/or 7/7q⁻.
Prognosis: Shorter survival compared to de novo leukemias; often refractory to therapy.

Table 11-24. Comparison of Types of Adult Human T-Cell Leukemia

Type	% of Cases	Lymphocytes	Hypercalcemia	Median Survival	Organ Involvement
Acute	60	High number	Common	6 mo	LNN, lytic bone, CNS
Lymphomatous	20	<1% abnormal	Less common	6 mo–2 y	LNN
Chronic[a]	15	>4,000/μL. >10% abnormal	Absent $\uparrow$LD >2× ULN	2 y	LNN, skin, liver, spleen, lung in some cases
Smoldering[a]	5	~5% abnormal	Absent	5 y	No LNN; skin, lung in some cases

LNN, lymph node; CNS, central nervous system; LD, lactate dehydrogenase; $\uparrow$, increased; ULN, upper limit of normal.
[a]Chronic and smoldering forms may become acute type.

Leukemia, Hairy Cell (Formerly Leukemic Reticuloendotheliosis)

Hairy cell leukemia is a rare condition of splenomegaly and infrequent lymphadenopathy with characteristic pathologic changes in marrow and spleen.

♦ Diagnosis is established by finding the characteristic mononuclear cells (which show long, delicate cytoplasmic projections) in the peripheral blood (vary from 0%–90%) or bone marrow, which show a characteristic diffuse *intense* histochemical reaction of tartrate-resistant acid phosphatase (isoenzyme-5) activity (mild to moderate staining of leukocytes may be seen in Sézary syndrome, CLL, and infectious mononucleosis, and in various histiocytes). Cells bear B-lymphocyte markers. Isoenzyme-5 may also be increased in the serum. Hairy cells are increased to frankly leukemic levels in ≤20% of cases.
Hypersplenism with pancytopenia is seen in >50% of cases.

• Thrombocytopenia (in 75% of cases), usually <80,000/μL
• Anemia (usually normochromic), usually 7 to 10 g/dL
• Leukopenia (in >60% of cases), usually <4,000/μL

Abnormal platelet function may be found.
Increased ESR may be present.
♦ Bone marrow reticulin fibrosis causes dry tap, requiring core biopsy; hairy cells are readily seen.
Leukocyte ALP activity is markedly increased in some patients.
Laboratory findings due to infection (e.g., pyogenic bacteria, opportunistic organisms).

Leukemia/Lymphoma Syndrome, Adult Human T-Cell[27]

This disease is caused by infection of CD4+ T cells with a retrovirus (human T-cell lymphotropic virus [HTLV-1]) that is endemic in Japan, Caribbean, and southeast United States. See Table 11-24.

♦ Increased antibody titers to HTLV-1 (see Chapter 15).
In Japan, ~25% of healthy persons are antibody positive. HTLV-1 can be isolated from malignant lymphoma or leukemia cells.
♦ Leukemic phase with WBC count ≤190,000/μL is characteristic (but not pathognomonic).
T cells with flowerlike nuclei in peripheral blood. Infrequent anemia and thrombocytopenia. Bone marrow involvement in 50% of patients correlates poorly with extent of peripheral blood involvement.
♦ Hypercalcemia in about 75% of patients is characteristic; may occur without bone involvement. May be very high.

[27]Foss FM, Aquino SL, Ferry JA. Case records of the Massachusetts General Hospital. Case 10-2003. A 72-year-old man with rapidly progressive leukemia, rash, and multiorgan failure. *N Engl J Med* 2003;348:1267–1275.

HEMATOLOGY

♦ Biopsy shows lymphomatous involvement of affected sites (e.g., lymph nodes, liver, spleen, bone, skin, etc.).

Laboratory findings due to involvement of various organs (e.g., liver, CNS)

Marked immunosuppression with opportunistic infections (e.g., cryptococcal meningitis, *Pneumocystis jiroveci [carinii]* pneumonia)

Hypereosinophilic Syndrome

♦ **Diagnostic Criteria**

- Eosinophilia >1,500/μL for >6 months
- No other cause for eosinophilia
- Organ dysfunction:
  Cardiovascular in ~50%–75% of cases (e.g., valve insufficiency, heart failure, mural thrombi cause systemic embolization in 5% of cases)
  Pulmonary in 1/3 of cases (e.g., pleural effusion, diffuse interstitial infiltrates)
  Neurologic in 35%–75% of patients
  Cutaneous in 50% of patients
  Liver function abnormalities in 15% of cases
  Abnormal urine sediment in 20% of patients

~50% of cases have FIP1L1-PDGFRA fusion gene generated by a cryptic interstitial chromosomal deletion, del(4)(q12q12), indicating these are clonal hematologic neoplasms (eosinophilic leukemia).[28]

Total WBC count is usually <25,000/μL but may be >90,000/μL with 30% to 70% eosinophils. Rare immature forms. Abnormalities in morphology of WBCs are frequent.

Mild anemia in ~50% of cases.

Thrombocytopenia in 1/3 of cases.

Hypercellular bone marrow with 25% to 75% eosinophils.

Absence of Ph[1], BCR-ABL gene fusion, clonal proliferation, blasts >2% distinguishes this from eosinophilic leukemia.

Detection of Minimal Residual Disease

Method	Target	Detection Sensitivity
Morphology	Blood/marrow cells	
Cytogenetics	Ph[1] chromosome	1:20
FISH	BCR-ABL fusion gene	1:200–1:500
RT-PCR	Quantify BCR-ABL RNA	1:100,000–1:1,000,000

FISH, fluorescence in situ hybridization; RT-PCR, reverse transcriptase polymerase chain reaction.

Needle aspiration of spleen reveals:
- Number of immature leukocytes is increased.
- Normoblastosis is present.
- Megakaryopoiesis is increased.

Serum and urine uric acid are increased, especially with high WBC count and antileukemic therapy.

Urinary obstruction may develop because of intrarenal and extrarenal uric acid crystallization.

Serum LD is increased; rises several weeks prior to relapse and falls several weeks prior to remission. LD is useful for following course of therapy.

Increased serum AST, ALT, and aldolase show less increase than in acute leukemia; are normal in half the patients.

Serum protein electrophoresis shows decreased albumin with increased α and γ globulins.

Direct Coombs test is positive in ≤20% of patients at some time in course of disease; overt hemolysis in ~25% of these patients.

[28]Cools J, Stover EH, Wlodarska I, et al. The FIP1L1-PDGFRα kinase in hypereosinophilic syndrome and chronic eosinophilic leukemia. *Curr Opin Hematol* 2003;11:51–57.

Laboratory findings due to leukemic infiltration of organs (e.g., kidney [hematuria common; uremia rare], heart, liver). With increasing survival in blast crisis, meningeal leukemia has become more frequent (up to 40%), with leukemic cells in CSF indicative of need for intrathecal chemotherapy.

Serum vitamin B_{12} level is increased (often >1,000 μg/mL); B_{12} binding capacity is increased.

Partial peripheral blood remission caused by drugs—decreased WBC count to nearly normal levels (decrease in spleen size is usually parallel) with only rare immature cells, correction of anemia, platelet count >450,000/μL, and leukocyte ALP may occasionally rise to normal; Ph^1 chromosome. May occur in <90% of cases. Complete cytogenetic response in >60% of cases. Complete molecular response in <5% of cases.

Accelerated phase is experienced by ~50% of patients before a blast crisis

♦ Combination of various criteria described in literature:

* Rapidly increasing WBC count (>50,000/μL) (doubling time <5 days) showing increasing immaturity and increased number of blasts (>5%–15% in marrow, >15% in blood), basophilia (>10% in marrow; >20% in blood)
* Increasing anemia (Hb <7.0 g/dL not caused by therapy) and thrombocytopenia (platelets <100,000/μL not because of therapy or >1,000,000/μL despite therapy)
* Increased leukocyte ALP
* New karyotypic abnormalities (e.g., trisomy 8, trisomy 18, additional Ph^1 chromosomes)
* Myelofibrosis in some cases
* Associated with clinical symptoms
* Increasing doses of drugs are needed to lower neutrophil count

Blast crisis occurs abruptly without an accelerated phase in 50% of cases

♦ Diagnosed by >20% blasts in marrow or peripheral blood or extramedullary proliferation of blasts (chloroma), or large foci of blasts in bone marrow biopsy. About 1/3 of patients with CML in blast crisis have lymphoid transformation (cells show morphologic, antigenic, enzymatic [TdT], and other lymphoid characteristics). The disease is increasingly refractory to therapy in blast phase, and many patients die of acute leukemia or complications in 3 to 6 months.

Platelet count <15,000 or >1,000,000/μL, blasts in peripheral blood, absence of Ph^1, moderate to marked myelofibrosis at time of diagnosis are poor prognostic signs. WBC count <25,000/μL or Hb >14 g/dL are good prognostic signs.

Juvenile Chronic Myelogenous Leukemia[29]

Juvenile CML (JCML) differs from adult CML in several ways:

* Aggressive disease
* 95% of patients are <4 years old
* Leukocytosis (usually <100,000/μL) with absolute monocytosis (>450/μL)
* Immature myeloid cells in peripheral blood in >70% of cases
* <25% marrow blasts
* Absent Ph^1
* Increased HbF (typically 20%–80%); JCML is the only leukemia with this increase
* Lymphadenopathy in 20% of cases
* Skin involvement with monocytic infiltrate is very common; may be preceded by neurofibromatosis
* Viral studies (CMV, EBV, rubella) are usually negative
* Leukocyte ALP is not useful; may be normal, low, or increased

Myeloid Metaplasia, Primary (Idiopathic Myelofibrosis)[30]

Primary myeloid metaplasia is a myeloproliferative clonal stem cell disease stimulating marrow fibroblasts. It is termed idiopathic (agnogenic) if other clonal/nonclonal causes of marrow fibrosis are excluded.

See Figure 11-9.

HEMATOLOGY

[29]Hess JL, Zutter MM, Castleberry RP, et al. Juvenile chronic myelogenous leukemia. *Am J Clin Pathol* 1996;105:238–248.
[30]Tefferi A. Myelofibrosis with myeloid metaplasia. *N Engl J Med* 2000;342:1255–1265.

♦ **Diagnostic Criteria**

Peripheral smear shows characteristic anisocytosis and marked poikilocytosis with teardrop RBCs (dacrocytes); polychromatophilia and occasional nucleated RBCs are found. Rarely seen in other hematologic conditions. Leukoerythroblastosis (granulocytic and RBC and precursors present).

Bone marrow shows fibrosis without apparent cause. Repeated bone marrow aspirations often produce no marrow elements. Biopsy of bone for histologic examination shows fibrosis of marrow that is usually hypocellular.

Progressive splenomegaly caused by disordered, ineffective extramedullary hematopoiesis and osteosclerosis.

Normochromic normocytic anemia caused by hemolysis and decreased production. Reticulocyte count is increased ($\leq$10%) with leukoerythroblastosis.

Hypersplenism may cause thrombocytopenia and leukopenia.

WBC count may be normal (50% of patients) or increased (usually $\leq$30,000/μL), and abnormal forms may occur. Immature cells ($\leq$15%) are usual. Blast cells <5%. Basophils and eosinophils may be increased.

Platelets may be normal, increased, decreased, or abnormal, and large forms may occur. Deficient platelet aggregation after collagen or epinephrine may occur.

♦ Needle puncture of spleen and a lymph node shows extramedullary hematopoiesis involving all three cell lines.

Prolonged PT is found in 75% of patients.

Serum uric acid is often increased.

Leukocyte ALP is usually increased (in contrast to CML); may be marked.

Serum vitamin B_{12} is often increased.

Some patients have trisomies of 8, 9, and 21 (appearance during treatment is a poor prognostic sign), but Ph^1 is rare.

Laboratory findings due to complications (hemorrhage, hemolytic anemia, infection):

* DIC occurs in 20% of patients.

Rule out other myeloproliferative diseases, especially CML.

Disorders of Plasma Cells and of Plasma Proteins

Monoclonal Gammopathies, Classification

Monoclonal gammopathies are clonal disorders of atypical cells of B-lymphocytes. Each is a homogeneous product of a single clone of proliferating cells that secrete a single homogeneous Ig or its fragment; expressed as a monoclonal gammopathy.

Monoclonal proteins each consists of two heavy polypeptide chains of the same class (e.g., γ, α, μ) and subclass and two light polypeptide chains of the same type (either κ or λ); may be present in serum, urine, and CSF. Heavy-chain disease is production of only heavy chains without accompanying light chains; light-chain disease is the reverse. Identified by protein electrophoresis, immunoelectrophoresis, immunofixation, capillary zone electrophoresis, etc.

Idiopathic monoclonal gammopathy of unknown significance (MGUS)

* Benign (IgG, IgA, IgD, IgM; rarely free light chains)
* Associated with neoplasms of cells now known to produce M-proteins
* Biclonal gammopathies
* Only two thirds of patients with monoclonal gammopathy are symptomatic

Malignant

* Multiple myeloma (IgG, IgA, IgD, and Bence-Jones [BJ] gammopathies are associated with classic picture)

Symptomatic
Smoldering (asymptomatic and indolent)

Plasma cell leukemia
Nonsecretory (1%–5% of cases)
Osteosclerotic

- Plasmacytoma (solitary of bone, extramedullary)
- Malignant lymphoproliferative diseases

Waldenström macroglobulinemia
Malignant lymphoma

- Heavy-chain diseases (γ, α, μ, δ [very rare])
- Amyloidosis

Secondary to multiple myeloma (no monoclonal protein in other secondary types)
Primary

- Unknown significance

Idiopathic
Others (e.g., ~10% of patients with chronic hepatitis C virus liver disease)

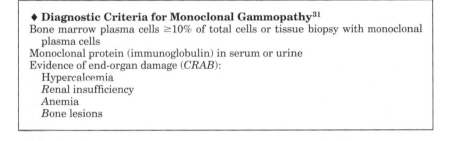

> ◆ **Diagnostic Criteria for Monoclonal Gammopathy**[31]
> Bone marrow plasma cells ≥10% of total cells or tissue biopsy with monoclonal
>   plasma cells
> Monoclonal protein (immunoglobulin) in serum or urine
> Evidence of end-organ damage (*CRAB*):
>   *H*ypercalcemia
>   *R*enal insufficiency
>   *A*nemia
>   *B*one lesions

Myeloma, Multiple

Multiple myeloma is a B-cell neoplasm characterized by skeletal lesions, renal failure, anemia, and hypercalcemia that secretes one homogeneous IgG or its fragments. Secretes excess light or heavy chains along with complete IgG.

See Tables 11-25, 11-26, 11-27.

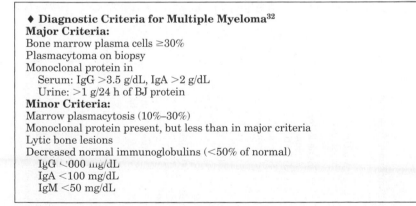

> ◆ **Diagnostic Criteria for Multiple Myeloma**[32]
> **Major Criteria:**
> Bone marrow plasma cells ≥30%
> Plasmacytoma on biopsy
> Monoclonal protein in
>   Serum: IgG >3.5 g/dL, IgA >2 g/dL
>   Urine: >1 g/24 h of BJ protein
> **Minor Criteria:**
> Marrow plasmacytosis (10%–30%)
> Monoclonal protein present, but less than in major criteria
> Lytic bone lesions
> Decreased normal immunoglobulins (<50% of normal)
>   IgG <000 mg/dL
>   IgA <100 mg/dL
>   IgM <50 mg/dL

HEMATOLOGY

[31]International Myeloma Working Group. Criteria for the classification of monoclonal gammopathies, multiple myeloma and related disorders: a report of the International Myeloma Working Group. *Br J Haematol* 2003;121:749–757.
[32]Richardson PG, Kassarjian A, Jing W. Case records of the Massachusetts General Hospital. Case 38-2004: A 40-year-old man with a large tumor of the skull. *N Engl J Med* 2004;351:2637–2745.

Table 11-25. Comparison of Diseases with Monoclonal Immunoglobulins

	Multiple Myeloma	Macroglobulinemia	Benign Monoclonal Gammopathy	Heavy-Chain Diseases		
				Gamma	Alpha	Mu
Clinical	Bone lesions Anemia Infections	Enlarged LNN, L, S	None	Enlarged LNN, L, S	Intestinal malabsorption	Enlarged LNN, L, S
Bone marrow	Sheets of plasma cells	Lymphocytosis or lymphocytoid plasma cells	Up to 10% plasma cells	Plasma cells or lymphocytoid plasma cells	—	Lymphocytosis or lymphocytoid plasma cells with vacuoles
Monoclonal Ig in serum (electrophoresis)	80%	Present	Present	Present	Present	Present
Bence-Jones protein in urine (electrophoresis)	70%–80%	80%–95%	Rare	Common	Rare	Common
Serum (immuno-electrophoresis)	1 type of M chain[a] 1 type of L chain[b]	μ chain 1 type of L chain[a]	1 type of M chain[a] 1 type of L chain[b]	γ chain No L	α chain No L	μ chain Free κ or λ in two thirds
Urine (immuno-electrophoresis)	κ or λ	κ or λ	Rare κ or λ	γ chain	—	κ or λ in tow thirds

Ig, immunoglobulin; LNN, lymph nodes; L, liver; S, spleen.

[a] M chain is γ, α, μ, delta or epsilon.

[b] L chain is kappa or lambda.

Paraproteinemia is caused by monoclonal gammopathy of unknown significance (63%), multiple myeloma (14%), primary amyloidosis (9%), indolent non-Hodgkin lymphoma (5%), extramedullary or solitary bone plasmacytoma (4%), chronic lymphocytic leukemia (3%), or Waldenström macroglobulinemia (2%).

Table 11-26.   Immunochemical Frequency of Monoclonal Gammopathies

IgG (with/without BJ)	60%
IgA (with/without BJ)	15%
IgM (with/ without BJ)	10%–15%
Light chain (BJ only)	15%
Rare	
IgD (with/without BJ)	1%
Heavy chain	1%
γ heavy-chain disease	
α heavy-chain disease	
μ heavy-chain disease	
IgE (with/without BJ)	0.1%
Biclonal (IgG + IgM)	
Triclonal	

Ig, immunoglobulin; BJ, Bence-Jones.

Table 11-27.   Comparison of Immunoproliferative Disorders

Disease	Relative Frequency (%)	Ig Heavy Chain	Ig Light Chain	Urine BJ (%)	Complications/Associated Conditions
Myelomas					
IgG	75	γ	κ or λ	60	Infection
IgA	15	α	κ or λ	70	Infection
IgD	<1	δ	Usually λ	100	Amyloidosis
IgE	Very rare	ε	κ or λ	?	Plasma cell leukemia
Light-chain myeloma	10	None	κ or λ	100	Amyloid kidney, hypercalcemia
Macroglo-bulinemia		μ	κ or λ	30–40	Hyperviscosity Hemolytic anemia (cold agglutinin) Bleeding
Heavy-chain disease					
γ		None	γ chain		
α		None	None		GI tract lymphoma Malabsorption
μ		None	κ chain BJ		Amyloidosis Chronic lymphocytic leukemia

Ig, immunoglobulin; BJ, Bence-Jones.

HEMATOLOGY

♦ Clinical Staging

Parameter	Clinical Stage					
	I A	**I B**	**II A**	**II B**	**III A**	**III B**
Serum creatinine (mg/dL)	<2.0	≥2.0	<2.0	≥2.0	<2.0	≥2.0
Hb (g/dL)	>10.0		8.5–10.0		<8.5	
Serum total calcium (mg/dL)	≤12		12		>12	
Serum M-protein						
IgG (g/dL)	<5		5–7		>7	
IgA (g/dL)	<3		3–5		>5	
Urine light chains (g/24 h)	<4		4–12		>12	
Plasma cells in marrow	<20%		20%–50%		>50%	
Extent of lytic bone lesions	Few, small		Many, variable		Extensive; fractures	
Estimated no. tumor cells/m² body surface area	$<0.6 \times 10^{12}$		$0.6–1.2 \times 10^{12}$		$>1.2 \times 10^{12}$	
Tumor burden ($\times 10^{12}/m^2$)	Low, 0.6		Intermediate 0.6–1.2		High >1.2	
Average survival time (mo)	61		55		30	15

% of Patients	Immunoelectrophoresis or Immunofixation Shows:
≤99%	Monoclonal protein in serum or urine
90%	Serum monoclonal spike
20%	Both serum and urine monoclonal protein
20%	Monoclonal light chains in urine only
<2%	Hypogammaglobulinemia only without serum or urine paraprotein
60%	IgG myeloma protein
20%	IgA myeloma protein
10%	Light chain only (BJ proteinemia)[a]
Very rare	IgE myeloma protein[b]
<1%	IgD myeloma protein[a,c]

BJ, Bence-Jones.
[a]Poorer prognosis because of prominent myeloma nephropathy.
[b]Poor prognosis because of high incidence of plasma cell leukemia.
[c]IgD myeloma is difficult to recognize because serum levels are relatively low and specific antiserum is required to demonstrate IgD; on electrophoresis, IgD is often included in β-globulin peak, and clinical features are the same as in other types of myeloma. *BJ proteinuria is almost always present, and total protein is often normal.*

Very increased serum total protein is caused by increase in globulins (with decreased A/G ratio) in one half to two thirds of patients.

Serum protein immunoelectrophoresis or immunofixation characterizes protein as monoclonal (i.e., one light-chain type) and classifies disease by identifying a specific heavy chain. It reveals abnormal immunoglobulins in 80% of patients. A serum or urine monoclonal paraprotein can be identified in ≤99% of patients with multiple myeloma.

♦ BJ proteinuria occurs in 35% to 50% of patients. More than 50% of IgG or IgA myelomas and 100% of light chain myelomas have BJ proteinuria. Dipstick tests for urine protein will miss BJ protein, and heat precipitation is not a reliable test.

♦ Electrophoresis/immunofixation of both serum and urine is abnormal in almost all patients. If only serum electrophoresis is performed, κ and some λ light-chain myelomas will be missed. Immunofixation determines type of immunoglobulin. Ten percent of patients have hypogammaglobulinemia (<0.6 g/dL). Free Ig light chains are rapidly filtered by the glomerulus and found only in urine. Intact monoclonal Ig is identified only in serum.

♦ Bone marrow aspiration shows >10% plasma cells (normal = <5%) or myeloma cells, usually in sheets; anaplastic and abnormal plasma cells may be found (flaming cells, morular cells, Mott cells, thesaurocytes); multiple sites may be required.

Hematologic findings:

• Anemia (normocytic, normochromic; rarely macrocytic) in 60% of patients suggests tumor mass $>10^{12}$ cells. Hb <8 g/dL suggests poor prognosis.

- Usually normal WBC and platelet counts; 40% to 55% lymphocytes frequently present on differential count, with variable number of immature lymphocytic and plasmacytic forms. Decreased WBC and platelet counts are seen in about 20% of patients, usually with extensive marrow replacement. Eosinophilia may be found.

○ • Rouleaux formation (due to serum protein changes) in 85% of patients, occasionally causing difficulty in cross matching blood.
○ • Increased ESR in 90% of patients and other abnormalities due to serum protein changes. May be normal in light-chain myeloma. ESR >100/hour is rare in any condition other than myeloma.
○ • Cold agglutinins or cryoglobulins.

○ Hyperviscosity syndrome is characteristic of IgM and occurs in 4% of IgG and 10% of IgA myeloma and may be the presenting feature. Symptoms are usually present when relative serum viscosity = 6 to 7 centipoises (normal <1.8).
○ Clinical amyloidosis occurs in ≤10% of cases of multiple myeloma, but monoclonal spikes are present in urine in most, if not all, cases of primary amyloidosis. IgD myeloma and light-chain disease are associated with amyloidosis and early renal failure more frequently than other types of myeloma. See Chapter 16.
Serum β_2 microglobulin is increased in proliferative disorders where there is rapid cell multiplication or increased tumor burden. A level >6 μg/mL indicates poor prognosis (normal <2 μg/mL); may also be increased by renal failure.
Chromosome analysis frequently shows translocation t(11;14)(q13;q32).
Laboratory findings of repeated bacterial infections, especially those caused by *Diplococcus pneumoniae*, *Staphylococcus aureus*, and *Escherichia coli*.
See Bone Diseases of Calcium and Phosphorus, Table 13-6.

- Serum calcium is markedly increased in 25% to 50% of cases.
- Corrected calcium (mg/dL) = serum calcium (mg/dL) – serum albumin (g/dL) + 4.0
- Serum phosphorus is usually normal.
- Serum ALP is usually normal or slightly increased. Increase may reflect amyloidosis of liver or bone disease.
- Hypercalciuria causing dehydration and tubular dysfunction.

See Kidney in Multiple Myeloma, Chapter 14.
○ Presymptomatic phase (may last many years) may show only:

- Unexplained persistent proteinuria
- Increased ESR
- Myeloma protein in serum or urine
- Repeated bacterial infections, especially pneumonias (six times greater incidence)
- Amyloidosis

Serial measurement of serum globulins and/or BJ proteinuria are excellent indications of efficacy of chemotherapy; the decrease in BJ proteinuria occurs before the decrease in abnormal serum globulin peak.
Lowered anion gap in IgG myeloma only (due to cationic IgG paraproteins causing retention of excess chloride ion)
Increased incidence of other neoplasms (not known if this is related to chemotherapy)

- Acute myelomonocytic leukemia, often preceded by sideroblastic refractory anemia, is increasingly seen.
- 20% of patients develop adenocarcinoma of GI tract, biliary tree, or breast.

Markers of poor prognosis:
Plasma cells in peripheral blood
Low serum albumin levels
Increased serum β_2-microglobulin
Plasma cells showing blast features in bone marrow
Increased density of bone marrow microvessels
Hypodiploidy responding poorly to chemotherapy (12.5 months versus 44.5 months survival)
Complete deletion of chromosome 13 or its long arm (karyotyping)
Translocation of t(4;14) or t(4;16) or t(14;16)
Increase of plasma cell–labeling index
Better prognosis with t(11;14)(q13;32)

HEMATOLOGY

Table 11-28.	Comparison of Multiple Myeloma and Monoclonal Gammopathy of Unknown Significance (MGUS)		
		Multiple Myeloma	MGUS
Paraprotein level		Higher	Lower (rarely <3 g/dL)
Nonparaprotein immunoglobulins suppressed		96% of cases	12% of cases
Bence-Jones proteinuria		57% of cases	17% of cases
Bone marrow plasmacytosis >20%		100% of cases	4% of cases
Plasma cell labelling index (using monoclonal antibody to 5-bromo-2-deoxyuridine)		>1%	<1%
Renal failure		May be related	Unrelated if present
Hypercalcemia		May be related	Unrelated if present
Anemia, lytic bone changes		Present	Absent
Progression		Yes	No

Monoclonal Gammopathy of Unknown Significance[33,34]

MGUS is also known as idiopathic ("benign" or "asymptomatic") plasma cell dyscrasia. It is asymptomatic, with no evidence of end-organ damage. Found in 0.5% of normal persons older than age 30, 3% of those above age 70, and ≤10% above age 80.

See Table 11-29.

◆ **Diagnostic Criteria**

- These changes are present for a period of >5 years.
- M-component: Serum IgG ≤3.0 g/dL, IgA ≤2 g/dL; urine ≤1 g/24 h of BJ protein.
- Marrow plasmacytosis <10%.
- No lytic bone lesions.
- No myeloma-related symptoms (e.g., anemia, hypercalcemia, renal insufficiency).
- Normal immunoglobulins may be depressed. In contrast, multiple myeloma *always* shows depression of background immunoglobulins.
- May be associated with aging, cholecystitis, neoplasms, many chronic diseases (most often RA) and infections (e.g., TB).

◆ Periodic reexamination is essential because there is a 1% annual risk of progression to myeloma or related malignancy.

~50% have translocations involving immunoglobulin heavy-chain locus on chromosome 14q32 and one of five partner chromosomes.

See Table 11-29.

Plasmacytoma, Solitary

Solitary plasmacytoma is considered to represent the earliest stage of multiple myeloma, and 50% to 60% of cases progress to multiple myeloma within 5 years. Fifteen percent remain solitary; 12% develop local recurrence; 15% develop new distant lesions. About 30% of patients remain free of disease for >10 years; other patients develop multiple myeloma after a median of 3 years. Following local radiotherapy, the level of any myeloma protein is reduced.

[33]Kyle RA, Thernau TM, Rajkumar SV, et al. A long term study of prognosis in monoclonal gammopathy of undetermined significance. *N Engl J Med* 2002;346:564–569.
[34]Kyle RA, Rajkumar SV. Multiple myeloma. *N Engl J Med* 2004;351:1860–1873.

Table 11-29. Comparison of Various Myelomas

	Multiple Myeloma	Non-secretory Multiple Myeloma	Smoldering Myeloma	Indolent Myeloma	Osteosclerotic Myeloma	Plasma Cell Leukemia
% of patients	–	1%–5%	~15%		<3%	2%
M-protein		Absent. Monoclonal M protein can be identified in plasma cells by immuno-fluorescence.	>3 g/dL	M-component: IgG <7 g/dL, IgA <5 g/dL.	Same as MM.	Primary cases have smaller M-protein peak in serum.
Bone marrow plasma cells		Same as MM.	Same as MM.	>10%–30%	Same as MM.	>20% plasma cells or >2,000/μL in peripheral blood.
Bone lesions	Present.	Same as MM.	Absent.	<3; No fractures.	Sclerotic, not lytic lesions.	Occurs.
↑Creatinine	Occurs; see Chapter 14.	Less frequently.	N	N	Same as MM.	Occurs.
Anemia	Occurs.	Same as MM.	N	N	Same as myeloma.	Present.
↑Calcium	Occurs.	Same as MM.	N	N	Same as myeloma.	
Infection	Occurs.	Same as MM.	Absent.	N	Same as myeloma.	
Other			Condition remains stable.		Frequently associated with POEMS.	~60% of cases are primary; have higher platelet count, younger age and longer survival.

N, normal; MM, multiple myeloma; POEMS, polyneuropathy, organomegaly, endocrinopathy, monoclonal gammopathy, and skin changes.

♦ Diagnosis is based on histologic finding of single tumor of plasma cells, which are identical to those of multiple myeloma. No criteria of multiple myeloma are present.

♦ Bone marrow shows no evidence of multiple myeloma.

♦ Radiographs and bone scans are negative for other myeloma bone lesions.

Myeloma proteins are low or normal concentration in serum or concentrated urine by immunofixation.

Nonmyeloma immunoglobulin concentration in serum is generally normal.

Paraprotein is detectable in 80% to 90% of cases of solitary plasmacytoma of bone, often at very low concentrations. IgG κ is most common; IgA and BJ have been described.

CSF total protein, albumin, and IgG may be increased if a vertebral lesion extends into the spinal canal.

Extramedullary plasmacytoma may occur, chiefly (80%) in upper respiratory tract. About 20% have low level of monoclonal immunoglobulin (not IgM) in urine or tract. Diagnosis is based on histologic examination of tumor and same criteria as above. Development of multiple myeloma is infrequent.

Leukemia, Plasma Cell

Plasma cell leukemia is a rare terminal complication of multiple myeloma.

♦ WBC count usually >15,000, with >20% plasma cells or >2,000/μL in peripheral blood, varying from typical plasmacytes to immature and atypical forms. Occasionally, special studies (cytochemical stains, cell surface and cytoplasmic markers, EM) are needed to confirm identity of plasma cells.

♦ Plasma cell monoclonality.

Frequent complication of IgE and IgD myeloma.

About 60% of cases are primary, and the rest occur in 2% of previously diagnosed cases of multiple myeloma. Primary cases have smaller M-protein peak in serum, higher platelet count, younger age, and longer survival.

Macroglobulinemia (Primary; Waldenström)

Waldenström macroglobulinemia is a hyperviscosity syndrome caused by a low-grade small-cell lymphoma that produces excess monoclonal IgM.

♦ Electrophoresis/immunofixation of serum shows an intense sharp peak in globulin fraction, usually in the gamma zone, identified as IgM by immunofixation (75% are κ). The pattern may be indistinguishable from that in multiple myeloma. IgM protein $\geq$3.0 g/dL. Associated decrease in normal immunoglobulins.

♦ Total serum protein and globulin are markedly increased.

○ ESR is very high.

○ Rouleaux formation is marked; positive Coombs reaction; difficulty in cross matching blood.

○ Severe anemia, usually normochromic normocytic; usually caused by hemodilution, occasionally hemolytic. Increased plasma volume may contribute an artifactual component.

WBC count is decreased, with relative lymphocytosis but no evidence of lymphocytic leukemia; monocytes or eosinophils may be increased.

♦ Bone marrow biopsy is always hypercellular and shows >30% involvement by lymphoplasmacytoid infiltrate with atypical "lymphocytes" and also plasma cells. Increased number of mast cells. Similar spleen and liver involvement occurs in ~50% of patients. Marrow aspirate is often hypocellular.

♦ Lymph node may show lymphoplasmacytoid infiltrate.

○ Flow cytometry shows $\leq$50% of patients have circulating monoclonal B-lymphocyte population.

○ 50% of patients with Waldenström macroglobulinemia have hyperviscosity syndrome due to large IgM molecule causing coagulation abnormalities. (Normal serum viscosity = $\leq$1.8 centipoises). Causes persistent oronasal hemorrhage in ~75% of patients, neurologic and visual disturbances, hypervolemia, and congestive heart failure.

IgM may also cause type I or II cryoglobulinemia, resulting in cold-agglutinin hemolytic anemia.

Table 11-30.	Alleles of the AAT Gene		
	Serum AAT	AAT Function	Phenotype
Normal	Normal (150–350 mg/dL)	Normal	Pi MM
Deficient severe	<50 mg/dL	Normal	Pi ZZ (>95% of cases)
			Pi SZ (rare)
			Pi SS
			Pi MZ
Null	Undetectable		Pi null–null
			Pi Z–null
Dysfunctional	Normal	Abnormal	

Z alleles are rare in Asians and blacks.
Threshold protection level for emphysema is 80 mg/dL.

BJ (light chain) proteinuria is found in 10% of cases. Monoclonal light-chain protein-
uria is found in 70% to 80% of cases.
Coagulation abnormalities: There may be decreased platelets, abnormal bleeding time,
coagulation time, PT, prothrombin consumption, etc.
Serum uric acid may be increased.
Impaired renal function is much less common than in myeloma.
Amyloidosis AL (light chain) occurs in ~5% of patients. (See Chapter 16.)
♦ *Differs from multiple myeloma by absence of lytic bone lesions and of hypercalcemia.*
Macroglobulinemia may also be associated with neoplasms, collagen diseases, cirrho-
sis, and chronic infections.

Other Disorders of Plasma Proteins

Alpha$_1$-Antitrypsin Deficiency

**Alpha$_1$-antitrypsin deficiency is an autosomal recessive deficiency of AAT (chro-
mosome 14), a serine protease inhibitor, the principal substrate of which is neutrophil elastase, which when unchecked is associated with familial pulmonary
emphysema and liver disease. The heterozygous state occurs in 10% to 15% of
the general population who have serum levels of AAT ~60% of normal; homozygous state occurs in 1:2,000 persons who have serum levels ~10% of normal;
there are many alleles of the AAT gene.**

See Table 11-30.
♦ Absent α_1 peak on serum protein electrophoresis. Should be confirmed by assay of
serum AAT (electroimmunoassay) and Pi phenotyping (isoelectric focusing on poly-
acrylamide; DNA analysis also permits prenatal diagnosis) and functional analysis
of total trypsin inhibitory capacity (90% is due to AAT activity).
AAT May Be Decreased In
(Typically <50 mg/dL)
Prematurity
Severe liver disease
Malnutrition
Renal losses (e.g., nephrosis)
GI losses (e.g., pancreatitis, protein-losing diseases)
Exudative dermopathies
AAT deficiency should be ruled out in children with neonatal hepatitis, giant cell
hepatitis, chronically abnormal liver chemistries, or juvenile cirrhosis and in
adults with chronic hepatitis without serologic markers, cryptogenic cirrhosis, and
hepatoma.
AAT Increased In
(AAT is an acute-phase reactant)
Acute or chronic infections

Neoplasia (especially cervical cancer and lymphomas)
Pregnancy
Use of birth control pills
○ Liver biopsy supports the diagnosis and helps stage extent of liver damage. Shows characteristic intracytoplasmic inclusions (in both heterozygotes and homozygotes) that may be found in patients with emphysema without liver disease and in asymptomatic heterozygous relatives, but must be searched for and stained specifically, since the rest of the pathology in the liver is not specific. About 9% of adults with nonalcoholic cirrhosis are MZ phenotype. Hepatoma may occur in cirrhotic livers.
Liver disease occurs in 10% to 20% of children with this deficiency. Clinical picture may be neonatal hepatitis (in 15% of those with ZZ phenotype), prolonged obstructive jaundice during infancy, cirrhosis, or asymptomatic. Five percent to 10% of infants with undefined cholestasis have AAT deficiency. In ~25% of these patients, clinical and biochemical abnormalities become normal by age 3 to 10 years; ~25% have abnormal liver function tests with or without clinical cirrhosis; ~25% survive first decade with confirmed cirrhosis; 25% die of cirrhosis between 6 months and 17 years of age.
○ Pulmonary emphysema occurs in heterozygotes and homozygotes; occurs in family of 25% of patients. Causes 2% of cases of emphysema. Secondary bronchitis and bronchiectasis may occur. Associated with phenotypes Pi ZZ and probably Pi SZ but not Pi MZ.
Purified AAT is now available for augmentation therapy:

- Indicated when AAT is severely deficient, abnormal lung function tests shows deterioration
- Not indicated when lung function is normal, even if AAT deficiency coexists with liver disease; or pulmonary emphysema is associated with normal or heterozygous phenotypes.

Analbuminemia, Congenital[35]

Congenital analbuminemia is a rare autosomal recessive disorder with surprisingly few symptoms.

♦ Serum electrophoresis shows complete absence of an albumin band.
Routine chemistry may show falsely increased albumin ≤1.8 g/dL.
May affect analysis of other analytes that are bound to protein.

Bisalbuminemia

Bisalbuminemia consists of hereditary variations of albumin leading to either slower or faster electrophoretic migration.

♦ Two albumin bands (peaks) are present on serum protein electrophoresis in clinically healthy homozygotes or carriers.

Cryofibrinogenemia[36]

♦ Plasma (as compared to serum in cryoglobulinemia) precipitates when oxalated blood is refrigerated at 4°C overnight. Due to fibrinogen-fibrin complexes that show reversible cold precipitability in anticoagulated blood.
May cause erroneous WBC count when performed on electronic cell counter.
May be associated with increased α-1-antitrypsin, haptoglobin, α-2 macroglobulin (by immunodiffusion technique), and with increased plasma fibrinogen. Not associated with cryoglobulins.
Has been reported in association with many conditions, especially:

- Hematologic and solid neoplasms
- Thromboembolic conditions
- Idiopathic
- Transient benign condition associated with infection

[35]Newstead J, et al. Low serum albumin and abnormal body shape. . . *Lab Med* 2004;35:350.
[36]Nash JW, Ross P Jr, Neil Crowson A, et al. The histopathologic spectrum of cryofibrinogenemia in four anatomic sites. Skin, lung, muscle, and kidney. *Am J Clin Pathol* 2003;119:114–122.

Cryoglobulinemia[37,38]

Cryoglobulinemia occurs when proteins that precipitate spontaneously and reversibly in serum (compared to cryofibrinogenemia in plasma) at less than body temperature within 3 days; they are insoluble at 4°C and may aggregate up to 30°C; can fix complement and initiate inflammatory reaction; 500 to 5,000 mg/dL in serum; normal = <80 mg/dL.

Type I (monoclonal immunoglobulin, especially IgM κ type)

* Causes 25% of cases.
* Most commonly associated with multiple myeloma and Waldenström macroglobulinemia; other lymphoproliferative diseases with M components; may be idiopathic.
* Often present in large amounts (>5 mg/dL serum). Blood may gel when drawn.
* Severe symptoms (e.g., Raynaud syndrome, gangrene without other causes).

Type II (monoclonal immunoglobulin mixed with at least one other type of polyclonal immunoglobulin, most commonly IgM and polyclonal IgG; always with RF)

* Causes up to 25% of cases.
* Associated most often with chronic hepatitis C virus (HCV) infection; less often with HBV, EBV, bacterial and parasitic infections, autoimmune disorders, Sjögren syndrome, syndrome of essential mixed cryoglobulinemia, immune-complex nephritis (e.g., membranoproliferative glomerulonephritis, vasculitis).
* High titer RF without definite rheumatic disease.
* C4 levels decreased.

Type III (mixed polyclonal immunoglobulin, most commonly IgM-IgG combinations, usually with RF)

* Causes ~50% of cases
* Usually present in small amounts (<1 mg/dL serum) in normal persons
* Most commonly associated with lymphoproliferative disorders, connective tissue diseases (e.g., SLE), persistent infections (e.g., HCV)

Recurrent purpura may occur.
♦ Hyperviscosity syndrome is likely at IgM >4.0 g/dL; clinically unpredictable at 2.0 to 4.0 g/dL, therefore serum viscosity should be measured. Viscosity increases exponentially with IgM concentration.
○ Cryoprecipitate may be seen in serum.
○ May cause erroneous WBC when performed on electronic cell counter.
○ Rouleaux formation may occur.
ESR may be increased at 37°C but is normal at room temperature.
Laboratory findings of associated conditions:

* Liver disease (e.g., serologic evidence of viral hepatitis).
* Renal disease (e.g., immune glomerular disease). Renal failure develops in ~50%, and marked proteinuria occurs in ~25%.
* Skin biopsy showing cutaneous vasculitis.

Hypoanabolic Hypoalbuminemia

Hypoanabolic hypoalbuminemia is an inherited disorder that is present from birth, without kidney or liver disease. Growth and development are normal. The patient is unaffected except for periodic peripheral edema.

♦ Serum albumin is <0.3 g/dL. Total globulins are 4.5 to 5.5 g/dL.
Albumin synthesis is decreased, with decreased catabolism of IV-injected albumin.
Serum cholesterol is increased.

[37]Kallemuchikkal U, Gorevic PD. Evaluation of cryoglobulins. *Arch Pathol Lab Med* 1999;123:119–125.
[38]Coblyn JS, McCluskey RT. Case records of the Massachusetts General Hospital. Weekly clinicopathological exercises. Case 3-2003: A 36-year-old man with renal failure, hypertension and neurologic abnormalities. *N Engl J Med* 2003;348:333–342.

HEMATOLOGY

Lymphoproliferative (Autoimmune) Syndrome[39,40]

Lymphoproliferative syndrome is a recently defined inherited disorder arising in early childhood that includes massive persistent lymphadenopathy, splenomegaly, and autoimmune features caused by failure of apoptosis of lymphocytes.

♦ Absolute increase of B-cell and T-cell counts with polyclonal expansion of T cells.
♦ Autoimmune disease

- Hemolytic anemia
- Thrombocytopenia
- Autoimmune neutropenia
- Polyclonal hypergammaglobulinemia
- Others (e.g., glomerulonephritis, primary biliary cirrhosis, Guillain-Barré syndrome)

♦ Circulating autoantibodies

- Positive direct Coombs test
- Anticardiolipin antibody
- Others (e.g., antinuclear antibodies, RF)

♦ Biopsy of lymph nodes or spleen shows characteristic benign lymphoid hyperplasia and plasmacytosis.
Laboratory changes due to infection after splenectomy for hypersplenism and of increased risk of lymphoma.

Tests for Immmunodeficiency Disorders

Immunodeficiency, Screening Tests

See Figure 11-11 and Tables 11-31 and 11-32.

Cell-mediated

- Absolute WBC count, differential, morphology
- Neutrophilic function
- Flow cytometry differentiates cells by lineage or stage of development by expression of surface and cytoplasmic proteins referred to as "CD" (cluster of differentiation) (e.g., for expression of β-integrins. For example, CD11 and CD18 antigens are depressed/absent in leukocyte adhesion deficiency 1 (LAD-1).
- Neutrophil oxidative burst (both abnormal in chronic granulomatous disease).
- Chemotaxis using Rebuck skin window and Boyden chamber or soft agar system. Primarily research assays.
- NK count by flow cytometry. Standard assay for in vitro activity.
- HIV serology
- Total lymphocyte count (lymphopenia usually indicates T-cell dysfunction, since most circulating lymphocytes are T cells).
- T-lymphocyte subsets. T-cell–deficient patients tend to have chronic recurrent *Candida* infection of scalp, nails, mucous membranes.
- Anergy skin tests (PPD, *Candida*)
- B-cell deficiency should be suspected with recurrent, complicated, or severe pyogenic infections.

Humoral immunity

- Antibody defects

Serum IgG, IgM, IgA, anti-A, anti-B isohemagglutinins
Serum IgG antibody titers before and after vaccinations (e.g., diphtheria, tetanus, *Pneumococcus*, *Haemophilus influenzae* type b)

- Complement defects

---

[39]Straus SE, Sneller M, Lenardo MJ, et al. An inherited disorder of lymphocyte apoptosis: the autoimmune lymphoproliferative syndrome. *Ann Intern Med* 1999;130:591–601.
[40]Holzelova E, Vonarbourg C, Stolzenburg MC, et al. Autoimmune lymphoproliferative syndrome with somatic *Fas* mutations. *N Engl J Med* 2004;351:1409–1418.

Table 11-31. Some Infectious Agents in Various Immune Deficiency Disorders

Pathogen	T-cell Defect	B-cell Defect (Humoral)	Neutrophil	Complement Defect
Bacteria	*Mycobacterium avium-intracellulare*	Encapsulated bacteria (e.g., *Haemophilus influenzae, Streptococcus pneumoniae,* staphylococci) causing recurrent lung and sinus infections	Recurrent/deep-seated infections (e.g., abscesses, periodontitis, osteomyelitis, pneumonia)	C3: sinopul-monary infection C6–C9: recurrent systemic infection or meningitis with *Neisseria*
Viruses	CMV, EBV, severe vaccinia, chronic respiratory and intestinal viruses	Enteroviral encephalitis	N/A	N/A
Fungi, parasites	*Candida, Pneumocystis jiroveci (carinii)*	Severe giardiasis	*Candida, Nocardia, Aspergillus*	N/A
Comment	Aggressive infection with opportunistic organisms; failure to resolve infection	Recurrent sino-pulmonary infections, sepsis, chronic meningitis	—	—

CMV, cytomegalovirus; EBV, Epstein-Barr virus.

CH50
C1 to C4 deficiencies associated with pyogenic infections and autoimmunity
C3, C5 to C9 deficiencies associated with neisserial infections

• Phagocyte defects

WBC and differential counts
Serum IgE
NBT test now replaced by flow cytometry respiratory burst assay

Table 11-32. Evaluation of Acquired Immunity

Screening Tests		Secondary Tests	
B-cell Function	T-cell Function	B-cell Function	T-cell Function
Quantitative IgG Specific antibody: Circulating specific antibodies. Pre- and post-immunization antibodies (protein and carbohydrate antigens: 4 × titer increase). IgG subclasses. HIV testing.	HIV testing. Lymphocyte count. Delayed type of hypersensitivity skin tests.	B-cell count by flow cytometry. In vitro B-cell function tests.	T-cell count by flow cytometry. T-cell proliferation (mitogen, antigen). T-cell cytokine production. T-cell cytotoxicity.

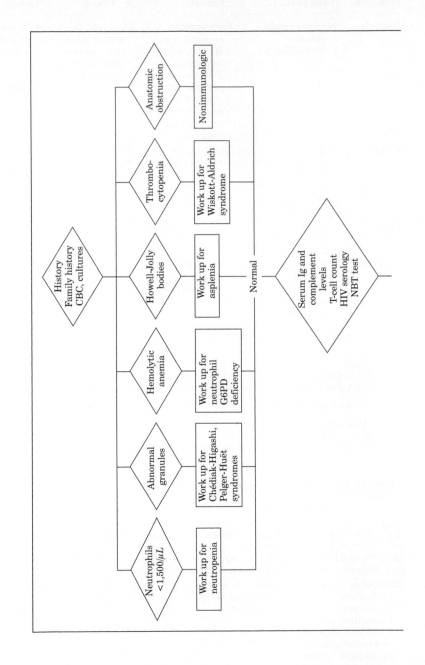

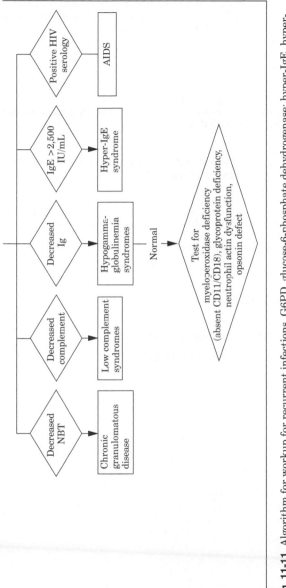

Fig. 11-11. Algorithm for workup for recurrent infections. G6PD, glucose-6-phosphate dehydrogenase; hyper-IgE, hyper-immunoglobulinemia E; Ig, immunoglobulin; NBT, nitroblue tetrazolium.

Immunoglobulin Function

Immunoglobulins are composed of four polypeptide chains—two heavy and two light—linked by disulfide bonds. They differ in their amino acid sequence and in the structure of their heavy chains.

IgG comprises 80% of Ig in blood. Activates complement. Fights infection.
IgA comprises 10% to 15% of Ig in blood. Is first line of defense on mucosal surfaces.
IgM comprises 5% to 10% of Ig in blood. Is first antibody responding to antigen challenge.
IgD is present in trace amounts in blood. Activates some lymphocytes.
IgE mediates allergic or hypersensitivity reactions.

Protein Gammopathies

Use
Identify hereditary and acquired immunodeficiencies.
Identify monoclonal gammopathies (increases) and associated disorders (concomitant hyperproteinemia is very frequent; see Tables 3-4, 3-5)

Monoclonal Increase In
Classification of monoclonal gammopathies
May artifactually increase serum total bilirubin and decrease high-density lipoprotein

Polyclonal Gammopathy with Hyperproteinemia
Collagen diseases (e.g., SLE, RA, scleroderma)
Liver disease (e.g., chronic hepatitis, cirrhosis)
Chronic infection (e.g., chronic bronchitis and bronchiectasis, lung abscess, TB, osteomyelitis, subacute bacterial endocarditis, infectious mononucleosis, malaria, leishmaniasis, trypanosomiasis)
Miscellaneous (e.g., sarcoidosis, malignant lymphoma, acute myeloid and monocytic leukemia, diabetes mellitus)
Idiopathic (family of patients with SLE)

Immunoglobulins A, D, E, G, M

Immunoglobulin A

IgA provides the first line of defense on mucosal surfaces.

Increased In (in Relation to Other Immunoglobulins)
γ-A myeloma (M component)
Cirrhosis of liver
Chronic infections
RA with high titers of RF
SLE (some patients)
Sarcoidosis (some patients)
Wiskott-Aldrich syndrome
Other

Decreased In (Alone) (>7 mg/dL)
Normal persons (1:700)
Hereditary telangiectasia (80% of patients)
Type III dysgammaglobulinemia
Malabsorption (some patients)
SLE (occasionally)
Cirrhosis of liver (occasionally)
Still disease (occasionally)
Recurrent otitis media (occasionally)
Non-IgA myeloma
Waldenström macroglobulinemia
Acquired immunodeficiency

Immunoglobulin D

IgD functions to activate some lymphocytes.

Use
Diagnosis of rare IgD myelomas (greatly increased)

Increased In
Chronic infection (moderately)
Autoimmune disease
Decreased In
Hereditary deficiencies
Acquired immunodeficiency
Non-IgD myeloma
Infancy, early childhood

Immunoglobulin E

IgE mediates allergic and hypersensitivity reactions.

Use
For allergy testing, IgE antibodies and skin tests are essentially interchangeable.[41]
Indicates various parasitic diseases
Diagnosis of E-myeloma
♦ *A normal serum IgE level excludes the diagnosis of bronchopulmonary aspergillosis.*
Increased In
Atopic diseases

• Exogenous asthma in ~60% of patients
• Hay fever in ~30% of patients
• Atopic eczema

Influenced by type of allergen, duration of stimulation, presence of symptoms, hyposensitization treatment
Parasitic diseases (e.g., ascariasis, visceral larva migrans, hookworm disease, *schistosomiasis*, *Echinococcus* infestation)
Normal or Low In
Asthma
Decreased In
Hereditary deficiencies
Acquired immunodeficiency
Ataxia-telangiectasia
Non-IgE myeloma

Immunoglobulin G

IgG activates complement and fights infection.

Use
Diagnosis of IgG myeloma
Diagnosis of hereditary and acquired IgG immunodeficiencies
Serologic diagnosis of infectious diseases and immunity
Increased In
Sarcoidosis
Chronic liver disease (e.g., cirrhosis)
Autoimmune diseases
Parasitic diseases
Chronic infection
Decreased In
Protein-losing syndromes
Pregnancy
Non-IgG myeloma
Waldenström macroglobulinemia
Decreased In (Combined with Other Immunoglobulin Decreases)
Agammaglobulinemia

• Acquired

Primary
Secondary (e.g., multiple myeloma, leukemia, nephrotic syndrome, protein-losing enteropathy)

• Congenital

[41]Homburger HA. Diagnosing allergic diseases in children. *Arch Pathol Lab Med* 2004;128:1028–1031.

Hereditary thymic aplasia
Type I dysgammaglobulinemia (decreased IgG and IgA and increased IgM)
Type II dysgammaglobulinemia (absent IgA and IgM and normal levels of IgG)
Infancy, early childhood

Immunoglobulin M

IgM is the first antibody to appear in response to antigen.

Use

Diagnosis of hereditary and acquired IgM immunodeficiencies
Diagnosis of Waldenström macroglobulinemia
Earliest Ig serologic diagnosis of infectious disease

Increased In

Liver disease
Chronic infections

Decreased In

Protein-losing syndromes
Non-IgM myeloma
Infancy, early childhood
See Neutrophil Function Tests in the section Tests for Disorders of White Blood Cells.

Immunodeficiency Disorders[42]

Immunodeficiency, Classification

Primary (see Tables 11-31, 11-33, and 11-34)

Primary B-cell (antibody) Deficiency Disorders

- X-linked agammaglobulinemia (block in maturation of pre-B cells)
- Common variable immunodeficiency (block in differentiation of B cells to plasma cells)
- Selective IgA deficiency (block in differentiation to a specific isotype)
- Selective IgG subclass deficiency (block in differentiation to a specific isotype)
- Hyper-IgM syndrome

Primary T-cell Deficiency

- DiGeorge syndrome (lack of thymus development causes block in T-cell maturation)
- Chronic mucocutaneous candidiasis (probable absence of T-cell clones that respond to *Candida* infections)
- Hyper-IgE syndrome

Combined T/B Cell Deficiency

- Severe combined immunodeficiency disease (SCID) (defect in adenosine deaminase [ADA] or purine nucleoside phosphorylase [PNP] enzymes)
- Wiskott-Aldrich syndrome
- Ataxia-telangiectasia

Secondary

Associated With

Virus infections (e.g., HIV, CMV, EBV, measles, rubeola)
Metabolic disorders (e.g., uremia, malnutrition, diabetes mellitus)
Protein deficiency (e.g., nephrotic syndrome)
Immunosuppression (e.g., drugs, neoplasms, splenectomy)
Respiratory tract disorders

- Anatomic (e.g., tracheoesophageal fistula, cleft palate, gastroesophageal reflux)
- Other (e.g., cystic fibrosis, immotile cilia, allergy)

Prematurity

[42]Illoh OC. Current applications of flow cytometry in the diagnosis of primary immunodeficiency diseases. *Arch Pathol Lab Med* 2004;128:23–31.

Table 11-33. Comparison of Some Primary Immunodeficiency Diseases

	Name	T cell	B cell	Ig
Combined lymphocyte defects	DiGeorge syndrome	N/D	N/D	N/D
	X linked SCID	D	N/I	D
	X linked hyper-IgM syndrome	N	N	N/I IgM D IgA, IgG
Antibody deficiency	X-linked agammaglobulinemia	N	D/0	D/0
	Common variable immunodeficiency	N	N	D ≥1 subtypes
	Ig deficiency (e.g., IgA, IgG)	N	N	D ≥1 subtypes
	μ heavy-chain deficiency	N	0	0
Phagocyte disorders	Chronic granulomatous disease	N	N	N
	Chédiak-Higashi syndrome	N	N	N
	Leukocyte adhesion deficiency	N	N	N
Complement deficiencies (see Chapter 3)	Individual complement deficiency	N	N	N
Other syndromes	Wiskott-Aldrich syndrome	N	N/D	N (some D IgM)
	Ataxia-telangiectasia	N	N	N
	Hyper-IgE syndrome	N	N	I IgE
	Bloom syndrome	N	N	N
	X linked lymphoproliferative syndrome	N/I	I	I
	Autoimmune lymphoproliferative syndrome	I CD4/ CD8		

0, absent; D, decreased; hyper-IgE, hyperimmunoglobulinemia E; hyper-IgM, hyperimmunoglobulinemia M; I, increased; Ig, immunoglobulin; N, normal; SCID, severe combined immunodeficiency disease.

Acquired Immune Deficiency Syndrome

See Chapter 15.

Ataxia-Telangiectasia

Ataxia-telangiectasia is caused by an autosomal recessive defective gene on chromosome 11. It is a multisystem progressive disorder of humoral and cellular defects. Cerebellar ataxia is apparent when child starts to walk. Oculocutaneous telangiectasias develop between 3 and 6 years of age.

See Table 11-34.
♦ Serum α-fetoprotein is almost always increased.
♦ Selective absence of IgA in 50% to 80% of patients. IgE is usually low. Other immunoglobulins may be abnormal.
Decreased total T cells (CD3) and helper cells (CD4) with normal or increased suppressor cells (CD8).
○ Recurrent infections in 80% of cases, usually bacterial sinopulmonary but not viral.
Delayed cutaneous anergy indicates impaired cell-mediated immunity.
Death is most commonly caused by lymphoid cancers and progressive neurologic disease.

Agammaglobulinemia, X-linked

This type of agammaglobulinemia is an X-linked recessive trait due to deficiency of Bruton tyrosine kinase, causing immunodeficiency.

See Tables 11-33 and 11-34.

HEMATOLOGY

Table 11-34. Classification of Primary Immunologic Defects

	Number of				Lymph Node		
Syndrome	Circulating Lymphocytes	Number of Plasma Cells	Ig Changes	Thymus	Germinal Center	Paracortical Zone	Other Laboratory Findings
X-linked agammaglobulinemia (Bruton disease)	N	O	Markedly D in all	N	O	N	X; increased frequency of malignant lymphoma
Selective inability to produce IgA	N	IgA-producing plasma cells, especially in lamina propria	IgA is O; others are usually N	N	N	N	May have malabsorption syndrome, steatorrhea, bronchitis
Transient hypogammaglobulinemia of infancy	N	D	IgG is D		O or rare		X
Non-sex-linked primary immunoglobulin deficiencies (e.g., dysgammaglobulinemias—acquired, congenital)	N	V (usually D)	Present, but type and amount are V	N	Usually O — Reticulum hyperplasia	Often D	X, Z; increased frequency of malignant lymphoma and autoimmune diseases
Agammaglobulinemia with thymoma (Good syndrome)	Progressively D, often to very low levels	D or O	Markedly D in all	Enlarged (stromal epithelial spindle-cell type)	D or O	May be D	X, Z; thymoma; pure red cell aplasia may occur; eosinophils O or markedly D
Wiskott-Aldrich syndrome (X-linked, recessive immune deficiency with thrombopenia and eczema)	Usually progressively D	N	Usually present, but type and amount are V (frequently IgM is D and IgA is I; IgG usually N)	N	May be D	Progressively D in lymphocytes	X, Z; eczema and thrombocytopenia; increased frequency of malignant lymphoma; serum lacks isohemagglutinins; platelets one-half normal size

Ataxia-telangiectasia (Louis-Bar syndrome), autosomal recessive	V (usually slightly D)	V (usually present)	Usually present, but type and amount are V (frequently IgA and IgE are D or O, and D IgG)	Embryonic type (no Hassall corpuscles or cortical medullary organization)	May be D	Lymphocytes D	Progressive cerebellar ataxia; telangiectasia in tissues; ovarian dysgenesis; increased frequency of malignant lymphoma; frequent pulmonary infections when IgA is D
Primary lymphopenic immunologic deficiency (Gitlin syndrome)	V–D	V	Always present, but type and amount are V	Hypoplastic (Hassall corpuscles and lymphoid cells D)		Marked D in tissue lymphocytes; foci of lymphocytes may be present in spleen and lymph nodes	Z
Autosomal recessive alymphocytotic agammaglobulinemia (Swiss type agammaglobulinemia; Glanzmann and Riniker lymphocytophthisis)	Markedly D	O	Markedly D in all	Hypoplastic (Hassall corpuscles and lymphoid cells O)		Lymphocytes O or markedly D	X, Z; increased frequency of malignant lymphoma
Autosomal recessive lymphopenia with normal immunoglobulins (Neselof syndrome)	D	Present	N	Hypoplastic (Hassall corpuscles and lymphoid cells O)	May be present	Lymphocytes markedly D	Z
DiGeorge syndrome (thymic aplasia)	V (usually N)	Present	N	Absent	Present	Rare paracortical lymphocytes present	Z; absent parathyroids (tetany of the newborn); frequent cardiovascular malformations

N, normal; O, absent; D, decreased; Ig, immunoglobulin; V, variable; X, recurrent infections with pyogenic organisms; Z, frequent virus, fungus, or *Pneumocystis* infection.
Adapted from Seligmann M, Fudenberg HH, Good RA. A proposed classification of primary immunologic deficiencies. *Am J Med* 1968;45:818.

Male patients suffer severe recurrent extracellular pyogenic infections (e.g., streptococci, pneumococci, *Haemophilus influenzae*) after age 4 to 6 months. Often have
persistent viral (e.g., chronic, progressive, fatal CNS infection with echoviruses) or
parasitic infections. *Giardia lamblia* leads to chronic diarrhea. Large-joint arthritis
probably caused by *Ureaplasma urealyticum*. Not unusually susceptible to viral
infections except fulminant hepatitis.
♦ Inability to make functional antibody is the distinguishing feature; antibody
responses to immunization are usually absent. Live virus vaccination may cause
severe disease (e.g., paralytic polio).
♦ Serum levels of IgG, IgA, IgM are very low (<100 mg/dL).
♦ B cells in peripheral blood are absent or found in very low numbers.
♦ T-cell numbers and function are intact.
Natural blood group antibodies are absent. Patients fail to produce antibodies during
immunizations.
Plasma cells in lymph nodes and GI tract are absent or found in very low numbers.
No markers exist for detection of heterozygotes.
Hypoplasia of tonsils, adenoids, lymph nodes with absent germinal centers. Thymus
appears normal, with Hassall corpuscles and abundant lymphoid cells.
Increased frequency of lymphoreticular malignancy (≤6%).
Prone to develop connective tissue diseases (e.g., dermatomyositis, RA-like disorder)
and allergic disorders (e.g., rhinitis, asthma, eczema, drug rash)
Female carriers can be identified by examination of B cells.

Chédiak-Higashi Syndrome

**Chédiak-Higashi syndrome is a rare autosomal recessive mutation in chromosome
1q42 causing fusion of cytoplasmic granules into one large vesicle resulting in
severe immunodeficiency (defective phagocytosis with recurrent bacterial infections); it also causes hypopigmentation of skin, hair, and uvea. The syndrome
can be treated by bone marrow transplant.**

See Table 11-33.
♦ Neutrophils contain coarse, deeply staining, peroxidase-positive, fused, large, dis-
torted granulations in cytoplasm and are present in lymphocytes, monocytes,
platelets, megakaryocytes, Langerhans cells, liver, spleen, Schwann cells. Most
prominent in marrow cells.
♦ Laboratory findings due to frequent severe pyogenic infections and hemorrhage
(which cause death by age 5) or to lymphoreticular malignancy in teens.
Marked deficiency of NK cell function.
♦ Heterozygous carriers are identified by a granulation anomaly in PMNs.
Pancytopenia appears during the (accelerated) "lymphomalike" phase.
Must be differentiated from pseudo–Chédiak-Higashi anomaly, which occurs in rare
cases of AML.

Shwachman-Diamond Syndrome

**Shwachman-Diamond syndrome is a rare autosomal recessive disorder of marrow
failure associated with exocrine pancreatic insufficiency, skeletal abnormalities,
bone marrow dysfunction, and recurrent infections due to defective phagocytosis.**

Neutropenia, cyclic or intermittent; 10% to 25% also have pancytopenia.
Increased risk of marrow aplasia, myelodysplasia, leukemia.

Hyper Immunoglobulin E Syndrome

**This very rare autosomal dominant condition shows severe recurrent staphylococ-
cal infections, chronic candidiasis, and skeletal and dental abnormalities.**

♦ Increased eosinophils in blood (in >90% of cases), sputum, and sections of tissues.
Not correlated with serum IgE.
♦ Very high serum IgE with substantial fluctuations over time. Other immunoglobu-
lins are usually normal.
Normal count of lymphocytes and subsets and phagocytic function.

Hyper Immunoglobulin M Syndrome[43]

Hyper IgM syndrome comprises a heterogeneous group of disorders. Male (X-linked) patients have history of pyogenic infections resembling those in X-linked agammaglobulinemia. The disease confers increased susceptibility to infections, especially *Pneumocystis jiroveci (carinii)*.

♦ Serum usually has decreased concentration of IgG (<150 mg/dL) and undetectable IgA and IgE. Polyclonal IgM is increased and may be $\geq 1,000$ mg/dL.
♦ B-lymphocytes are normal in number but have only surface IgM and IgD; surface IgG and IgA are virtually absent.
Increased frequency of autoimmune disorders; neutropenia is most important and may be recurrent, severe, and prolonged; autoimmune hemolytic anemia, thrombocytopenia. In second decade of life, IgM-producing polyclonal plasma cells may show marked proliferation with extensive invasion of GI tract, liver, gall bladder that may be fatal.
Increased risk of abdominal cancers.

Graft-Versus-Host Disease

GVHD is caused by immunocompetent T-lymphocytes in donor transplant of organs or tissues into a severely immunocompromised host (e.g., bone marrow transplant recipients, congenital immunodeficiency syndromes in infants, but not in patients with AIDS). The transfused T-lymphocytes become functional and recognize host's cells as foreign.

Acute

Acute GVHD occurs within days but <1 to 2 months after transplantation. Cellular cytotoxic response against host in patients receiving hematopoietic cell therapy ($\leq 70\%$ of bone marrow transplants). Most cases are mild but $\leq 20\%$ mortality.

♦ Laboratory findings due to selective epithelial damage involving:

• Positive biopsy of skin, liver, colon, upper GI tract confirms diagnosis
• Liver: Increased serum bilirubin, ALP, ALT, AST; may progress to liver failure with encephalopathy, ascites, coagulation disorders
• Intestine: Bloody diarrhea, paralytic ileus
• Acute form causes persistent severe immunoincompetence with profound immunodeficiency and susceptibility to infection
• Transfusion-associated GVHD in severely immunocompromised patients receiving nonirradiated blood. Rapid onset in <30 days causing bone marrow hypoplasia with pancytopenia; is usually severe in contrast to GVHD after bone marrow transplant. Confirmed by peripheral blood lymphocytes using cytogenetic or HLA studies, engraftment of donor lymphocytes.

Chronic

Chronic GVHD occurs >100 days but as occasionally as early as 40 to 50 days after transplantation in $\leq 40\%$ of long-term survivors. It is caused by a combined cellular and humoral response of transplanted cells against host.

• Biopsy shows changes in affected organs
• Liver: Changes of chronic cholestasis (in 80% of cases) often resembles acute GVHD; rarely progresses to cirrhosis
• Abnormalities of cellular immunity (e.g., decreased B cells, defects in number and function of CD4[+] T cells, increased number of nonspecific suppressor cells, impaired antibody production against specific antigens)
• Thrombocytopenia and/or leukopenia, anemia
• Skin changes resemble Sjögren syndrome and scleroderma

In one report, serum catalase showed S/S = 100%/88% compared to 5′-nucleotidase S/S = 88%/28%.

[43]Winkelstein JA, Marino MC, Ochs H, et al. The X-linked hyper-IgM Syndrome. Clinical and immunologic features of 79 patients. *Medicine (Baltimore)* 2003;82:373–384.

HEMATOLOGY

Granulomatous Disease, Chronic [44,45]

Chronic granulomatous disease is a rare heterogeneous disorder characterized by chronic recurrent suppurative infections by catalase-positive organisms (e.g., *Aspergillus* sp., *Staphylococcus aureus;* also seen frequently are *Burkholderia cepacia, Serratia marcescens, Pseudomonas cepacia, Klebsiella* sp., *E. coli, Nocardia, Chromobacterium violaceum*) that usually have low virulence (e.g., *Salmonella, Candida albicans*). Because of the abnormality of the nicotinamide adenine dinucleotide phosphate (NADPH) oxidase system responsible for generating superoxide, PMNs and monocytes ingest normally but fail to kill certain bacteria and fungi; ~60% are X-linked membrane abnormalities, ~40% due to autosomal recessive inheritance (most are cytosol abnormalities), 5% are membrane abnormalities, and <1% due to autosomal dominant inheritance.

♦ Failure of these cells to reduce NBT to purple formazan on slide test provides a simple, rapid diagnosis in patients and in heterozygotes for the X-linked form (carriers). The NBT test is now replaced by flow cytometry.
♦ Other confirmatory tests in reference laboratory for absent (or severely reduced production of oxygen radicals) include measurement of oxygen consumption, hydrogen peroxide or superoxide production, and chemiluminescence of phagocytes.
♦ Prenatal diagnosis has been established using NBT test on fetal blood leukocytes. Can also analyze fetal DNA from chorionic villus or amniocytes for specific mutation.
WBCs show morphologically normal appearance and granules on routine Wright-Giemsa–stained smears.
Serum complement and immunoglobulin levels are normal.
Laboratory findings due to infection (leukocytosis, anemia, increased ESR, elevated γ globulin levels) are noted.
Laboratory findings due to abscesses of subcutaneous tissue, lung, liver, perirectal area, lymph nodes, bone, brain, others.
Laboratory findings due to granulomas causing obstruction (e.g., GI tract, genitourinary tract).

Immunodeficiency, Cellular, with Normal Immunoglobulins (Nezelof Syndrome)

In Nezelof syndrome, the hypoplastic thymus shows abnormal architecture with no Hassall corpuscles, few lymphocytes, and poor corticomedullary distinction. There is decreased lymphoid tissue with depletion of paracortical lymphocytes. Infants may show recurrent or chronic pulmonary infection, failure to thrive, candidiasis, Gram-negative sepsis, genitourinary tract infection, progressive varicella, etc.

See Table 11-34.
♦ Lymphopenia, neutropenia, eosinophilia.
♦ Marked deficiency of total T cells and T-cell subsets; normal helper:suppressor (CD4:CD8) ratio (in contrast to AIDS patients, who show marked deficiency of CD4 with reverse of ratio).
Normal or increased serum immunoglobulins; some show selective IgA deficiency, increased IgD, and marked increase in IgE.
A few patients have associated enzyme deficiency, causing low or absent serum uric acid.

Severe Combined Immunodeficiency Disorders [46]

SCIDs are rare disorders of many genetic causes that show congenital absence of all immune functions with death due to infection before age 2 years. Failure to thrive is noted. The disease displays diverse immunologic, hematologic, enzymatic, and genetic features. It may be cured with bone marrow transplant.

[44]Winkelstein JA, Marino MC, Johnston RB Jr, et al. Chronic granulomatous disease. Report on a national registry of 368 patients. *Medicine (Baltimore)* 2000;75:155–169.
[45]Segal BH, Leto TL, Gallin JI, et al. Genetic, biochemical, and clinical features of chronic granulomatous disease. *Medicine (Baltimore)* 2000;75:170–200.
[46]McCormack MP, Rabbitts TH. Activation of the T-cell oncogene LMO2 after gene therapy for X-linked severe combined immunodeficiency. *N Engl J Med* 2004;350:91–922.

Autosomal Recessive SCID

♦ Marked lymphopenia (<1,000 lymphocytes/μL) with lack of T- and B-cell function; very low T-cell count but CD4:CD8 ratio is rarely reversed as in AIDS. T- and B-cell counts are very low in most autosomal recessive forms.

Eosinophilia and monocytosis are prominent features.

○ Decreased serum immunoglobulins; no antibody formation after immunization.

○ Delayed cutaneous anergy; cannot reject transplants.

○ Recurrent infections with opportunistic organisms (persistent thrush or diaper monilia rash or *Pneumocystis jiroveci [carinii]* pneumonia; viral infection from varicella, herpes, adenovirus, CMV, measles, progressive vaccinia) finally cause wasting and death. GVHD may develop.

Very small thymus (<1 g) that fails to descend from neck shows few lymphocytes, no corticomedullary distinction, and usually no Hassall corpuscles, but thymic epithelium appears normal.

Lymph nodes show lymphocyte depletion in both follicular and paracortical areas; tonsils, adenoids, and Peyer patches are absent or very underdeveloped.

♦ Enzyme deficiency (e.g., ADA, PNP) occurs in ~40% of autosomal recessive SCID patients. ADA deficiency causes severe depletion of both T cells and B cells and lack of both cell-mediated and humoral immunity. PNP deficiency preferentially affects T cells; severe defect in cell-mediated immunity but humoral immunity is intact. RBCs show ADA deficiency and increased deoxyadenosine triphosphate (deoxy-ATP) and deoxyadenosine diphosphate (deoxy-ADP).

SCID is most commonly X-linked.

Defective Expression of Major Histocompatibility Complex Antigens

Persistent diarrhea in early infancy, often with cryptosporidiosis
Malabsorption
Susceptibility to opportunistic infection
Hypogammaglobulinemia with decreased IgM and IgA
Poor or absent antibody production
Moderate lymphopenia; decreased T-cell function and B-cell percentage
Absent plasma cells in tissues
Severe hypoplasia of thymus and lymphoid tissues

SCID with Leukopenia

SCID with leukopenia is a very rare condition in infants.

Lymphocytes are totally lacking.
A tiny thymus (<1 g) shows no Hassall corpuscles or lymphocytes.

Hypogammaglobulinemia, Common Variable

Common variable hypogammaglobulinemia was formerly known as acquired hypogammaglobulinemia. This is a heterogenous immunodeficiency syndrome; it can result from three different immunologic causes: intrinsic B-cell defects, immunoregulatory T-cell imbalances, or autoantibodies to T or B cells.

See Table 11-33.

Clinically, may resemble X-linked agammaglobulinemia, but infections are less severe and there is equal sex distribution. Patients may have unusual infections (e.g., *P. jiroveci [carinii]*, various fungi); recurrent herpes simplex and herpes zoster viruses in ~20% of patients. Untreated cases present with chronic lung disease and bronchiectasis and infections elsewhere due to other organisms. Many have sprue-like syndrome because of *Giardia lamblia*.

♦ Diagnosis is by exclusion of other causes of humoral immune defects.

Serum IgG is decreased (<250 μg/μL); IgA and IgM are usually decreased.

Associated with increased incidence (~20%) of autoimmune diseases (e.g., PA occurs in ~10% of patients, SLE, RA) and malignancy (especially intestinal lymphomas and gastric adenocarcinoma).

Reactive follicular hyperplasia of lymph nodes, tonsil, spleen, and small bowel (may cause malabsorption) but lack plasma cells.

Sterile noncaseating granulomas can occur in liver, spleen, lung, skin.

HEMATOLOGY

Table 11-35. Comparison of Coagulation Disorders with Platelet or Vascular Disorders

	Coagulation Disorder	Platelet or Vascular Disorder
Hemarthroses and deep hematomas in muscle	Characteristic	Rare
Delayed bleeding	Characteristic	Rare
Bleeding from superficial cuts	Uncommon	Persistent; may be profuse
Petechiae	Rare	Characteristic
Ecchymoses	Common, usually single and large	Characteristic, usually multiple and large
Epistaxis, melena	Seldom predominant	Often causes significant bleeding
Hematuria	Common	Uncommon

T-lymphocyte function may be impaired.
Number of peripheral blood B cells may be low or high but fail to differentiate into immunoglobulin antibody-secreting cells.

Immunoglobulin a Deficiency, Selective

IgA is the first line of defense on mucosal surfaces. Selective IgA deficiency is an immunodeficiency syndrome with lack of IgA-producing cells in the intestinal lamina propria.

See Tables 11-33 and 11-34.
♦ Serum IgA is very low (<5 mg/dL).
♦ Serum IgM and IgG are usually normal.
Serum antibodies to IgA are present in >40% of patients; therefore IV or IM blood products that contain IgA (e.g., immune serum globulin) are contraindicated.
Peripheral blood lymphocytes bearing IgA, IgM, and IgG are normal.
Plasma cells producing IgA are absent in GI and respiratory epithelium.
Clinical features: asymptomatic or recurrent pyogenic respiratory infections; increased incidence of allergic disease (e.g., asthma, eczema), autoimmune diseases (e.g., RA, SLE), and GI complications (e.g., celiac disease, malabsorption, chronic giardiasis). Found in >1:400 persons in general population.

Tests of Coagulation

See Tables 11-35 to 11-37.

Anticoagulants, Circulating

Circulating anticoagulants are usually antibodies that inhibit the function of specific coagulation factors, especially VIII or IX; occasionally V, XI, XIII, von Willebrand factor (vWF). Antibodies may be acquired (e.g., multiple transfusions for congenital deficiency of a coagulation factor) or spontaneous.

Association with Clinical Disorders

Factor	Disorder
VIII and IX	Following replacement therapy for hereditary deficiency
XI	SLE; very rare
IX	SLE; rare
VIII	SLE, RA, drug reaction, asthma, pemphigus, inflammatory bowel disease, postpartum period, advanced age
X	Amyloidosis (tissue binding rather than circulating)
V	Associated with streptomycin administration, idiopathic
X,V	SLE; common
II	Myeloma, SLE
XIII	Associated with isoniazid administration, idiopathic

Table 11-36. Screening Tests for Presumptive Diagnosis of Common Bleeding Disorders[a]

Platelet Count	BT	PT	aPTT[b]	Location of Defect	Most Frequent Causes Acquired	Hereditary
N	N	I	N	Extrinsic pathway[c]	Liver disease, coumarin therapy, vitamin K deficiency, DIC (very rare)	Deficiency of factor VII (very rare)
N	N	N	I	Intrinsic pathway[d]	Heparin therapy, inhibitors	Hemophilia A or B, deficiency of factor XI, XII, prekallikrein, high-molecular-weight kininogen, Passavoy factor
N[e]	N	I	I	Common or multiple pathways	Heparin therapy, liver disease, vitamin K deficiency, DIC, fibrinogenolysis (very common)	Deficiency of factor V, X, prothrombin; dysfibrinogenemias (very rare)
D	I	N	N	Thrombocytopenia	ITP, secondary (e.g., drugs)	Wiskott-Aldrich syndrome, etc.
N or I	I	N	N	Disorder of platelet function	Thrombocythemia, drugs, uremia, dysproteinemias	Thrombasthenia, deficient release reaction
N	I	N	I	von Willebrand disease		
N	I	N	N	Vascular abnormality	Allergic purpura, drugs, scurvy, etc.	Deficiency of factor XIII, telangiectasia

BT, bleeding time; PT, prothrombin time; aPTT, activated partial thromboplastin time; D, decreased; I, increased; N, normal; DIC, disseminated intravascular coagulation; ITP, idiopathic thrombocytopenia purpura.

[a] Screening tests may be normal in mild von Willebrand disease that has borderline or intermittent normal BT, in mild hemophilia, and in factor XIII deficiency.

[b] Concentration of factors must be decreased to ≤30% of normal for these tests to be abnormal.

[c] Extrinsic pathway function depends on factors VII, X, V, II (prothrombin), I (fibrinogen); is assessed by PT.

[d] Intrinsic pathway depends on factors XII, XI, IX, VIII, X, V, II, I; is assessed by aPTT.

[e] May be I in acquired disorders that produce abnormalities of platelets and multiple coagulation factors.

Table 11-37. Summary of Coagulation Studies in Hemorrhagic Conditions

Condition	Screening Tests				Capillary Fragility (Tourniquet Test)	Accessory Tests			Factor Assay
	Platelet Count	BT	PT	aPTT		Coagulation Time	Clot Retraction	Prothrombin Consumption Time	
Thrombocytopenic purpura	D	I	N	N	+	N	Poor	I	
Nonthrombocytopenic purpura	N	N	N	N	V	N	N	N	
Glanzmann thrombasthenia	N^a	N or I	N		+ or N	N	Poor	I Corrected by platelet substitute	
von Willebrand disease	N	I or N	N	N or I	N, + in severe	V	N	I	+
AHF (factor VIII) deficiency (hemophilia)	N	N	N	I	N	I N in mild	N	I	+
PTC (factor IX) deficiency (hemophilia B; Christmas disease)	N	N	N	I^c	N	I N in mild	N		+
Factor X (Stuart) deficiency	N	N	I^b	I^b	N	N or slightly I	N	I	+
PTA (factor XI) deficiency	N I in severe	N	N	I^c	N	I	N	I	+
Factor XII (Hageman) deficiency	N	N	N	I^c	N	I	N	I	+
Factor XIII deficiency	N	N	N	N	N	N	N	N	+
Fibrinogen deficiency	N	N I in severe	I	I	N	I	N	N	+

Hypoprothrombinemia	N	N or I	I	I	N	I	N	N
Excess dicumarol therapy	N	N I in severe	I	I	N + in severe	I N in mild	N	N
Heparin therapy	N	N to I	May be I	I	N	I	N	N
Vascular purpura (e.g., Schönlein-Henoch disease, hereditary hemorrhagic telangiectasia)	N	N	N	N	N	N	N	N
Increased antithromboplastin	N		I	I	N	I		I
Increased antithrombin	N	N	I	N	N	N May be I in severe	N	N[d]
Increased fibrinolysin	N	N or I	N	N	N	N or I	Lysis of clot	N[d]

BT, bleeding time; PT, prothrombin time; aPTT, activated partial thromboplastin time; +, positive; D, decreased; I, increased; N, normal; AHF, antihemophilic factor; PTC, plasma thromboplastin components; PTA, plasma thromboplastin antecedent; V, variable.

[a]Platelets appear abnormal.
[b]Corrected by serum.
[c]Corrected by serum or plasma.
[d]Not useful; may be difficult to do.

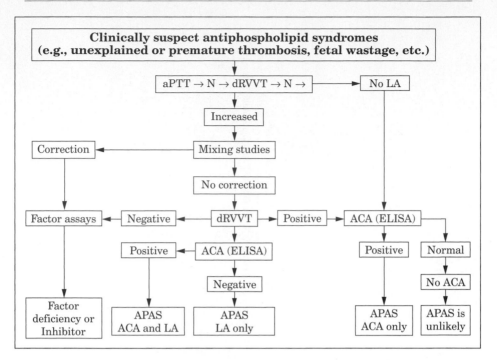

Fig. 11-12. Laboratory diagnosis of antiphospholipid syndromes. APAS, antiphospholipid antibody syndromes; aPTT, activated partial thromboplastin time; LA, lupus anticoagulant; ACA, anticardiolipin antibody; dRVVT, dilute Russell venom viper time; N, normal; ELISA, enzyme-linked immunosorbent assay.

Also associated with pregnancy, lymphoproliferative diseases, certain drugs (e.g., penicillin, sulfonamides, phenytoin)

♦ ***Antiphospholipid-thrombosis syndrome[47]*** defined as ≥1 autoantibodies (anticardiolipin antibodies [ACA], lupus anticoagulant [LA]) and/or biologic false-positive result for syphilis found on ≥2 occasions at least 12 weeks apart associated with thrombocytopenia, recurrent fetal loss, or noninflammatory venous or arterial thrombosis. Most patients have positive assay for both LA and ACA. May be secondary to SLE (in ~50% of SLE patients) or primary (i.e., without signs of autoimmune disease). Clinical syndrome occurs only in those with autoimmune diseases. Directed against phospholipids rather than against a specific factor. (See Figure 11-12.)

Anticardiolipin Antibodies

♦ ACAs can be detected by ELISA against IgG, IgM, and IgA. Requires protein cofactors β-2 glycoprotein (B2GPI) to detect antibodies relevant to thrombosis. Patients with antiphospholipid syndrome are B2GPI-dependent. Patients with infectious diseases and drug reactions are B2GPI-independent.
Can also detect human anti-B2GPI antibodies rather than bovine anti-B2GPI antibodies.
Common in SLE—correlates with lab features (e.g., thrombocytopenia, prolonged aPTT, positive direct and indirect Coombs test); may not correlate with clinical manifestations in contrast to primary syndrome.
ACAs are five times more common than LAs.

Lupus Anticoagulant

Sixty percent of LA-positive patients have ACA.

[47]Levine JS, Branch DW, Rauch J. The antiphospholipid syndrome. *N Engl J Med* 2002;346: 752–763.

◆ **Diagnostic Criteria**

1. Prolonged coagulation in ≥ 1 phospholipid-dependent test using platelet-poor plasma from two different parts of coagulation cascade (e.g., intrinsic pathway—aPTT, kaolin coagulation time [CT]; extrinsic pathway—dilute PT; final common pathway—dilute Russell viper venom time [dRVVT]).
2. Failure to correct CT by mixing patient's plasma with normal plasma demonstrates that abnormality is caused by an inhibitor rather than factor deficiency

   • Rosner index >15 indicates an inhibitor:

   $$\frac{(\text{CT of mixture of patient} + \text{normal plasma}) \text{ minus } (\text{normal plasma CT})}{(\text{normal plasma CT})}$$

   • Prolonged incubation with normal plasma does not increase inhibitor effect.
3. Confirmation of inhibitor specificity for phospholipid. Shorten/correct CT by adding excess phospholipids.
4. No evidence of another coagulopathy to account for abnormal coagulation reaction.

If confirmatory test is negative, rule out other coagulopathies with factor assays.

CT, clotting time.

Dilute Russell Venom Viper Time

dRVV is a serine protease that directly activates factor X in the presence of Ca^{2+}, bypassing intrinsic and extrinsic pathways.

Use
Detection of LA (IgG and IgM autoantibodies that interfere with function of anionic phospholipids and prolong phospholipid-dependent clotting tests [e.g., aPTT, dRVVT]).
dRVVT is more specific than aPTT because dRVVT is not influenced by deficiencies of intrinsic pathway factors or antibodies to factors VIII, IX, or XI.

Antithrombin[48]

Antithrombin is synthesized in the liver and circulates in plasma. It inactivates thrombin, plasmin, and factors IXa, Xa, XIa, and XIIa, helping to regulate the coagulation cascade. Activity level is usually 35% to 70%.

See Figure 11-13.
Use
Assess response to heparin therapy.
To detect hypercoagulable state associated with episodes of venous thrombosis; decreased in ~4.5% of patients with idiopathic venous thrombosis.
Functional tests are required since the antigen level may be normal in ~10% of cases of hereditary qualitative deficiency by immunologic method.
Decreased In
Hereditary deficiency (typically 40%–60% of normal); >80 mutations; autosomal dominant trait
Chronic liver disease (>80% of cases of cirrhosis)
Nephrotic syndrome, other protein-wasting diseases
Heparin therapy for >3 days
L-Asparaginase therapy
Acute-phase reaction (e.g., thrombotic, inflammatory, surgical)
DIC (not diagnostically useful)
Last trimester of pregnancy (rarely <75% of normal)
Newborns (~50% of adult levels, which are attained by age 6 months)
Others (e.g., acute leukemia, carcinoma, Gram-negative septicemia)
Increased In
Patients with increased ESR, hyperglobulinemia
Coumadin anticoagulation

[48]Kottke-Marchant K, Duncan A. Antithrombin deficiency: issues in laboratory diagnosis. *Arch Pathol Lab Med* 2002;126:1326–1336.

HEMATOLOGY

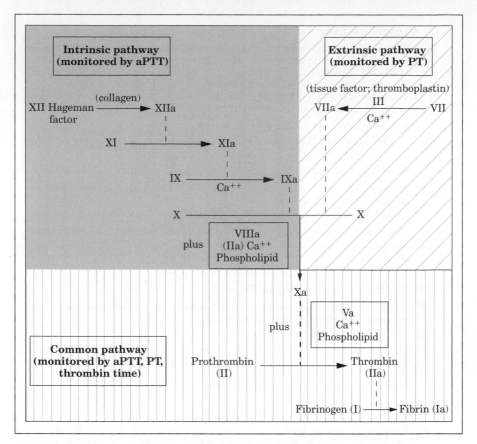

Fig. 11-13. Blood coagulation cascade. ***Shaded Area:*** Monitored by activated partial thromboplastin time (aPTT). Encloses the intrinsic coagulation reactions that occur on the surface membrane of platelets. Hemostasis begins when exposed tissue factor from injured vessel activates factor VII. Platelets collect at site of vascular injury and are acted upon by activated factor VIIa and tissue factor in the presence of calcium. This induces the activation of factors X and IX, leading to thrombin generation. ***Diagonal Lines Area:*** Monitored by prothrombin time (PT). ***Vertical Lines Area:*** Encloses common pathway. Monitored by aPTT, PT, thrombin time. Thrombin cleaves fibrinogen into fibrin and activates XIIIa to crosslink it. Thrombin also mediates formation of activated protein C, which binds to free protein S; this complex inhibits factors VIIIa and Va. Antithrombin also controls thrombin production and activity by acting at different levels of cascade.

Bleeding Time

See Figure 11-14.

To determine bleeding time (BT), use the Mielke modification of Ivy method; should use a standardized technique: blood pressure cuff on upper arm inflated to 40 mm Hg; two small, standardized skin incisions are made on volar surface of forearm using a specially calibrated template. Normal = 4 to 7 minutes. Longer in women than men. Limited precision, accuracy, reproducibility.

Use

BT is functional test of primary hemostasis. Measures platelet response to vessel injury. BT is best single screening test for acquired (e.g., uremia) or congenital functional or structural disorders of platelets. Normal BT without suggestive history usually

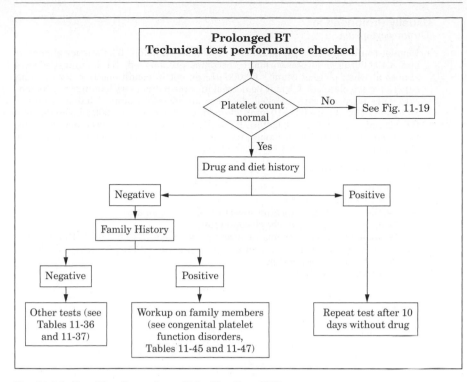

Fig. 11-14. Algorithm for prolonged bleeding time (BT).

excludes platelet dysfunction. However, a normal BT does not rule out a significant defect; with clinical suspicion, platelet aggregation should be performed. Also depends on fibrinogen.

Useful as part of workup for coagulation disorders in patients with history of excess bleeding (e.g., associated with dental extraction, childbirth, circumcision, tonsillectomy), even with a normal platelet count.

Normal in all other disorders of coagulation except vWF deficiency and some cases of very low plasma fibrinogen (because platelets contain fibrinogen).

May be useful to monitor treatment of active hemorrhage in patients with prolonged BT due to uremia, von Willebrand disease (vWD), congenital platelet function abnormalities, or severe anemia.

No value in performing BT if platelet count <100,000/μL, as BT is usually prolonged.

Prolonged BT with platelet count >100,000/μL usually indicates impaired platelet function (e.g., due to aspirin) or vWD.

Not recommended for prediction of bleeding in myeloproliferative diseases or neonates receiving NSAIDs.

S/S and predictive value of BT in perioperative hemorrhage are not known.

Not recommended for routine preoperative screening because:

- General surgery patients without obvious risk factors for bleeding rarely have a clinically significant increase in BT
- Even with a prolonged BT, blood loss does not exceed that of patients with normal BT
- Prolonged BT does not necessarily cause increased bleeding
- Therapeutic decisions are not likely to be changed by results of BT
- Clinical history is the best preoperative screening
- Not recommended for preoperative evaluation of patients receiving aspirin or NSAIDs, patients with liver disease, patients for coronary bypass
- May be useful in preoperative screening of patients for eye, middle ear, brain, or knee surgery

HEMATOLOGY

Usually Prolonged In
Thrombocytopenia

- Platelet count <100,000/μL and usually <80,000/μL before BT becomes abnormal and <40,000/μL before abnormality becomes pronounced. BT is almost always abnormal when platelet count <60,000/μL, except in conditions that have young supereffective platelets. BT may be normal in some patients with immune thrombocytopenic purpura with marked decrease in platelet count. Platelet count = 80,000/μL should have BT ~10 minutes and platelet count = 40,000/μL should have BT ~20 minutes and at <10,000/μL BT will always be >30 minutes if platelet function is normal; beyond these values, the patient may also have a qualitative platelet abnormality.

Platelet Function Disorders

- Hereditary
  Defect in plasma proteins
  vWD (especially 2 hours after ingestion of 300 mg of aspirin)
  Deficient release of platelet glycoproteins
  Glanzmann thrombasthenia (deficient or defective glycoprotein [GP] iib/iiia)
  Bernard-Soulier syndrome (deficient glycoprotein [GPibIX])
  Defective release mechanisms
  Gray platelet syndrome
  Aspirinlike defect
  Storage pool deficiency
  Others, e.g.:
  Wiskott-Aldrich syndrome
  Chédiak-Higashi syndrome
  Oculocutaneous albinism (Hermansky-Pudlak syndrome)
  Hereditary hemorrhagic telangiectasia
  Ehlers-Danlos syndrome
- Acquired
  Abnormal plasma factors
  Drugs
  Aspirin, NSAIDs (indomethacin, ibuprofen, phenylbutazone, etc.). Ingestion ≤7 days is the most common cause of prolonged BT. Aspirin may double the baseline BT, which may still be within normal range. A dose of 325 mg of aspirin will increase BT of most persons.
  Antimicrobials (especially high dose beta-lactam, [e.g., carbenicillin; cephalosporins, nitrofurantoin, hydroxychloroquine])
  Anticoagulants (e.g., heparin, prostacyclin, streptokinase-streptodornase)
  Tricyclic antidepressants (e.g., imipramine, amitriptyline, nortriptyline)
  Phenothiazines (e.g., chlorpromazine, promethazine, trifluoperazine)
  Anesthetic (e.g., halothane, local)
  Methylxanthines (e.g., caffeine, theophylline, aminophylline)
  Others (e.g., dextrans, calcium channel-blocking agents, radiographic contrast agents, β-adrenergic blockers, alcohol, aminocaproic acid, nitroglycerin)
  Uremia (may be corrected with vasopressin or cryoprecipitate)
  Fibrin degradation products (e.g., DIC, liver disease, fibrinolytic therapy)
  Macromolecules (e.g., dextran, paraproteins [e.g., myelomas, Waldenström macroglobulinemia])
  Other immune thrombocytopenias
  Myeloproliferative diseases, including myelodysplastic syndrome, preleukemia, acute leukemia, hairy cell leukemia)
  Vasculitis
  Others (e.g., amyloidosis, viral infections, scurvy, after circulating through an oxygenator during cardiac bypass surgery)
  Vascular disorders
  Increased BT or BT increased out of proportion to platelet count suggests vWD or qualitative platelet defect.

Usually Normal In
Hemophilia
Severe hereditary hypoprothrombinemia
Severe hereditary hypofibrinogenemia

Clot Retraction

Clot retraction is an outmoded test that reflects platelet number and function. It is a poor test of clotting function. It has little value for detection of mild to moderate bleeding disorders. It may be abnormal in various thrombocytopenias and thrombasthenia.

Coagulation (Clotting) Time ("Lee-White Clotting Time")

Coagulation time was formerly a routine method for control of heparin therapy but is now replaced by aPTT. It is not a reliable screening test for bleeding conditions because it is not sensitive enough to detect mild conditions; it will only detect severe ones. Normal clotting time does not rule out a coagulation defect. There are many variables in the technique of performing the test. Routine preoperative BT and clotting time are of little value for routine preoperative screening.

Fibrinogen Degradation Products

The rapid latex agglutination test kit detects increased level (10 μg/mL) of fibrinogen degradation products in serum and parallels results with hemagglutination inhibition (HAI) method. It detects major breakdown products of fibrin or fibrinogen. However, it does not distinguish between fibrinolysis and fibrinogenolysis.

Use
Aid in diagnosis of DIC
Increased In Serum
DIC
In association with fibrinolytic therapy
Thromboembolic events

- Pulmonary embolism—peak values may be transient
- Postoperative deep vein thrombosis
- Acute myocardial infarction during first 24 to 48 hours
- Certain disorders of pregnancy
- Small increases with exercise, anxiety, stress, severe liver disease

Increased In Urine
Kidney disease

- Urinary tract infection—increased in infection of upper tract but not of bladder
- Proliferative GN—level falls during response to drug therapy
- Rejection of renal transplant

Conditions causing increased serum level (see previous paragraph)
Interferences
RF may cause a false-positive result

Heparin, Plasma

Use of Plasma Heparin Assay

Monitor heparin therapy in selected situations:

- Combined heparin and warfarin therapy
- Combined heparin and recombinant tissue plasminogen activator therapy
- Heparin resistance in presence of a circulating anticoagulant
- Altered plasma clotting proteins (e.g., increased factor I or VIII or platelet factor 4 or decreased antithrombin)
- When aPTT appears to be unsatisfactory for heparin therapy control (e.g., overwhelming infections, myocardial infarction, severe liver disease)
- Use of low-molecular-weight heparins (LMWHs)

To prove unrecognized heparin administration (e.g., indwelling catheter)

Partial Thromboplastin Time, Activated

See Table 11-38 and Figures 11-15 to 11-18.

HEMATOLOGY

Table 11-38. Effect of Anticoagulant Drugs on Coagulation Tests

Test	Heparin	Warfarin	Aspirin	Dipyridamole/ Sulfinpyrazone	Urokinase/ Streptokinase
Platelet count	N[a]	N	N	N	N
Inhibition of platelet aggregation	N or I	N	I	N	I
Bleeding time	N or I	N[b]	I	N	I
Clotting time	I	N[b]	N	N	I
Thrombin time	I	N	N	N	I
Prothrombin time	I	I	N[b]	N	I
Partial thrombo-plastin time	I	N[b]	N	N	I
Fibrinogen	N	N	N	N	D

D, decreased; I, increased; N, no change.
[a]Decreased in 25% of cases.
[b]Increased with high drug dosage.

Use

Monitor heparin therapy. Often does not correlate with heparin blood levels. Cannot be used to monitor LMWH or danaparoid and cannot be used in presence of LA and certain factor (e.g., XII) deficiencies; instead, monitor with factor Xa inhibition or protamine neutralization.

Screen for hemophilia A and B.

Detect clotting inhibitors.

aPTT is the *best single screening test* for disorders of coagulation; it is abnormal in 90% of patients with coagulation disorders when properly performed. It screens for all coagulation factors that contribute to thrombin formation except VII and XIII.

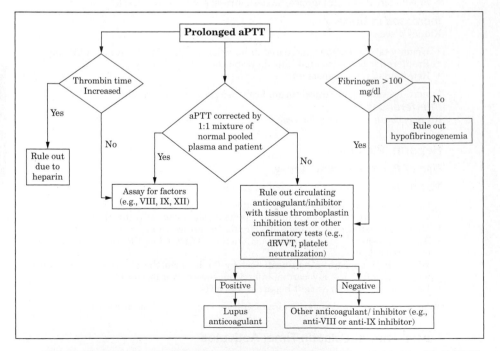

Fig. 11-15. Algorithm for isolated prolonged activated partial thromboplastin time (aPTT). dRVVT, dilute Russell venom viper time.

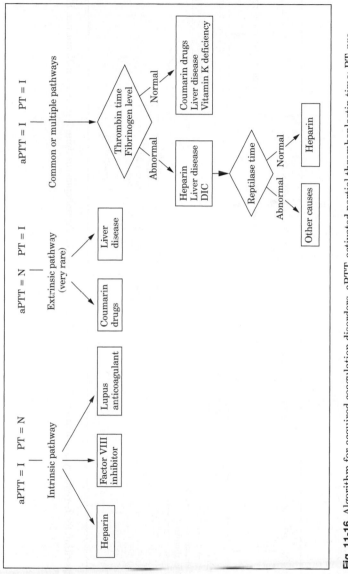

Fig. 11-16. Algorithm for acquired coagulation disorders. aPTT, activated partial thromboplastin time; PT, prothrombin time; I, increased; N, normal; DIC, disseminated intravascular coagulation.

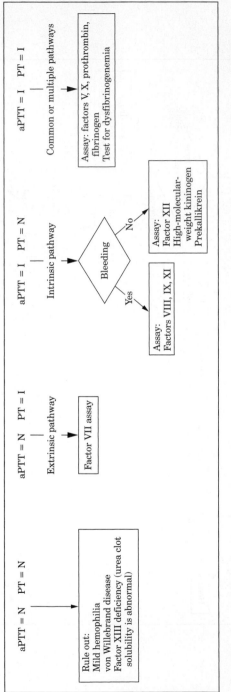

Fig. 11-17. Algorithm for hereditary coagulation disorders. aPTT, activated partial thromboplastin time; I, increased; N, normal; PT, prothrombin time.

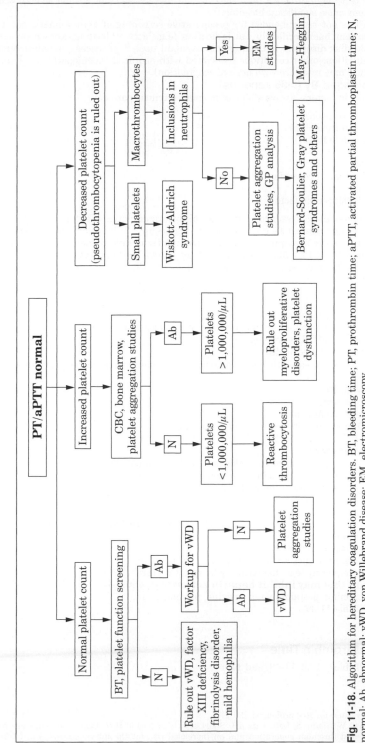

Fig. 11-18. Algorithm for hereditary coagulation disorders. BT, bleeding time; PT, prothrombin time; aPTT, activated partial thromboplastin time; N, normal; Ab, abnormal; vWD, von Willebrand disease; EM, electromicroscopy.

HEMATOLOGY

The test may not detect mild clotting defects (25%–40% of normal levels), which seldom cause significant bleeding.

aPTT is not recommended for preoperative screening of asymptomatic adult unless patient has specific clinical indication (e.g., active bleeding, known or suspected bleeding disorders [including anticoagulant use], liver disease, malabsorption, malnutrition, other conditions associated with acquired coagulopathies, where procedure may interfere with normal coagulation).

Prolonged By (>36 seconds)

Defect in factors (assays <30% of normal; intrinsic pathway)

- I (fibrinogen)
- II (prothrombin)
- V (labile factor)
- VIII*
- IX*
- X (Stuart-Prower factor)
- XI*
- XII (Hageman factor)

Mixing studies: Presence of specific inhibitors of clotting factors* (most frequently antibody against factor VIII, which occurs in ~15% of multitransfused patients with severe hemophilia A and less frequently in mild/moderate hemophilia A; and circulating LA). *Mixing equal parts of patient and normal plasma corrects aPTT (or PT) if caused by a coagulation factor deficiency but not if caused by an inhibitor.*

Heparin

Warfarin

Lupus anticoagulant*

Traumatic venipuncture may prolong (if baseline aPTT is normal) or shorten aPTT (if baseline aPTT is prolonged).

Short (<24 seconds)

Caused by increased thrombin generation, causing increased risk of venous thrombosis.[49]

Normal In

Thrombocytopenia

Platelet dysfunction

vWD (may be prolonged in some patients)

Isolated defects of factor VII

Interferences

Very increased or decreased Hct (e.g., polycythemia) that alters citrate concentration or inadequate citrate in collection tube

Specimen contamination with EDTA

Clots in specimen

Partially filled collection tube

Values may be falsely very high if plasma is very turbid or icteric when photoelectric machines are used

Drugs other than heparin

Hirudin analogues and argatroban, warfarin

Less frequently (e.g., hematin, hydroxy-ethyl starch, suramin)

Drugs that may inhibit heparin action (e.g., antihistamines, digitalis, nicotine, IV penicillin, protamine, tetracycline, phenothiazine)

See Table 11-39.

Prothrombin Time

See Tables 11-38, 11-43, and 11-44

(*May cause isolated prolonged aPTT)

[49]Korte W, Clarke S, Lefkowitz JB. Short activated partial thromboplastin times are related to increased thrombin generation and an increased risk for thromboembolism. *Am J Clin Pathol* 2000;113:123–127.

Table 11-39.	Interaction Between Prothrombin Time and Partial Thromboplastin Time		
		Partial Thromboplastin Time	
		Normal	Prolonged
Prothrombin time	Normal	fXIII, dysfibrinogenemia, vWD; mild fVIII, fIX, fXI	*Intrinsic pathway:* Lupus anticoagulant, fVII, fVIII, fIX, fXI, fXIII
	Prolonged	*Extrinsic pathway:* Liver disease, coumarins, fVII, dysfibrinogenemia, DIC	*Common or multiple pathways:* Liver disease, vitamin K deficiency, coumarin, heparin, fV, fVIII, fX, prothrombin, dysfibrinogenemia, fibrinogen

f, factor deficiencies or inhibitors; coumarin/heparin, effect of drug administration; vWD, von Willebrand disease; DIC, disseminated intravascular anticoagulant.

Use

Primarily for three purposes:

- Monitor long-term oral anticoagulant therapy with coumarins and indanedione derivatives.
- Evaluation of liver function—PT is the most useful test of impaired liver synthesis of prothrombin complex factors (factors II, VII, X; proteins C and S).
- Evaluation of coagulation disorders—Screen for abnormality of factors involved in extrinsic (factors V, VII, X; prothrombin; fibrinogen) and common pathways (i.e., production of fibrin and fibrin formation). Should be used with aPTT.

Prolonged By Defect In

(Assays <30% of normal; extrinsic pathway)
Factor I (fibrinogen)
Factor II (prothrombin)
Factor V (labile factor)
Factor VII (stable factor)
Factor X (Stuart-Prower factor)

Prolonged In

Inadequate vitamin K in diet
Premature infants
Newborn infants of vitamin K-deficient mothers (hemorrhagic disease of the newborn)
Poor fat absorption (e.g., obstructive jaundice, fistulas, sprue, steatorrhea, celiac disease, colitis, chronic diarrhea)
Severe liver damage (e.g., poisoning, hepatitis, cirrhosis)
Drugs (e.g., coumarin-type drugs for anticoagulant therapy, salicylates)
Factitious ingestion of warfarin
Idiopathic familial hypoprothrombinemia
Circulating anticoagulants
Hypofibrinogenemia (acquired or inherited)
Heparin
LA

Reporting

PT should be reported as ratio of patient to control, rather than as %.
PT may also be reported as an international normalized ratio (INR) only in patients on oral anticoagulants for ≥2 weeks who have stable PTs and responded appropriately to the drug.

$$INR = (patient\ PT)^{ISI*} \div (mean\ of\ PT\ reference\ range\ for\ that\ laboratory)$$

where *International Sensitivity Index (ISI) is provided by the thromboplastin manufacturer. Is intended to take into account differences caused by different methods or thromboplastin-instrument combinations in interpretation of results.

HEMATOLOGY

Suggested INR range = 2.0 to 3.0 for standard-dose therapy for treatment or prophylaxis of venous thrombosis or pulmonary or systemic embolus.
Suggested INR range = 2.5 to 3.5 for high-risk patients with mechanical heart valves.
Suggested INR range = 3.0 to 3.5 for patients with LAs.
INR is sensitive to levels of factors II, VII, and X.
NOTE: INR is dependent on instrumentation. Sensitive thromboplastin (low ISI) leads to undertreatment, and insensitive thromboplastin (high ISI) leads to overtreatment.

Plasminogen and Tissue-Type Plasminogen Activator[50]

Tissue-type plasminogen activator (tPA) is an inactive precursor of plasmin released from endothelium, leukocytes, and other tissues, forming plasmin that cleaves fibrin and leading to lysis of fibrin clots. Reference ranges: males = 76% to 124%; females = 65% to 153%; infants = 27% to 59%.

Use
Is one indicator of fibrinolytic activity
Monitor fibrinolytic therapy with streptokinase or urokinase
Not warranted for routine assay of plasminogen and tPA in patients with thrombophilia
May Be Decreased In
Presence of plasminogen-activator inhibitor
Some familial or isolated cases of idiopathic deep venous thrombosis; autosomal deficiency or dysplasminogenemia
Diabetics with thrombosis
DIC and systemic fibrinolysis
Behçet disease
Cirrhosis of the liver

Protein C, Plasma[51]

Protein C is a vitamin K-dependent protease principally produced in liver. It acts as an anticoagulant that inactivates factors Va and VIIIa and enhances fibrinolytic activity in plasma. A normal range is from about 70% to 140%.

Use
Detect hypercoagulable states associated with venous thrombosis, especially in unusual sites (e.g., cerebral, portal, retinal).
Decreased In
Hereditary (autosomal with variable penetrance) deficiency (heterozygote levels are usually 30%–65%; found in screening in 1/500 persons; thrombosis is not usual if level >50%). *Purpura fulminans in homozygous infants* (usually <1% of normal) *establishes the diagnosis*. There are more than 160 unique mutations. Type I deficiency (most common): Decrease of protein C antigen and activity. Type II deficiency: Decreased functional activity with usually normal antigenic levels.
Acquired
• *Warfarin-induced skin necrosis is almost pathognomonic for protein C deficiency.*

High loading dose of warfarin causes transient rapid drop in protein C levels.

• Liver disease
• Vitamin K deficiency
• L-asparaginase therapy
• DIC
• Acute-phase reaction (e.g., thrombotic, inflammatory, surgical)

Decreases with age (~4% per decade)
Increased In
Nephrotic syndrome
Ischemic heart disease
Pregnancy, use of oral contraceptives or hormone replacement

[50]Brandt JT. Plasminogen and tissue-type plasminogen activator deficiency as risk factors for thromboembolic disease. *Arch Pathol Lab Med* 2002;126:1376–1381.
[51]Kottke-Marchant K, Comp P. Laboratory issues in diagnosing abnormalities of protein C, thrombomodulin, and endothelial cell protein C receptor. *Arch Pathol Lab Med* 2002;126:1337–1348.

Activated Protein C Resistance[52]

The activated protein C resistance (APC-R) assay is a modified version of aPTT. Caused by factor V Leiden mutation in >95% of cases found in 5% of persons in the United States. It is the most common recognized familial thrombophilia. APC resistance interferes with the pathway that inhibits fibrin formation.

Use
Common risk factor for venous thrombosis
Interferences
Invalidated by oral anticoagulants within 7 to 14 days, other causes of prolonged clotting times (e.g., factor deficiencies, autoantibodies, or inhibitors), increased factor VIII, presence of platelets in test plasma.

APC protein added to normal plasma prolongs PTT in normal person, but not in patients with APC-R who have ratio <2.0 (normal ratio >2.0); S/S = 50%–86%/75%–98%. Interferences due to any causes of shortened (increased factor VIII) or prolonged PTT (e.g., deficiency of factors VIII, IX, XI, XII).

Modified assay uses patient's plasma diluted with factor V–deficient plasma (but otherwise normal plasma); S/S approaches ≤100%; LA still affects PTT.

♦ DNA testing, usually by PCR, is gold standard.

Protein S, Plasma[53]

Protein S is manufactured mainly in the liver. It acts as a cofactor for protein C. There are acquired and hereditary forms of the protein S deficiency (gene located on chromosome 3); prevalence of the deficiency is 1 in 500. The rare homozygous type may cause severe neonatal purpura fulminans. Protein S deficiency may be responsible for venous but rarely arterial thrombosis.

Use
Detect hypercoagulable states associated with episodes of venous thrombosis.
Should be assayed whenever protein C is assayed; both are vitamin K-dependent inhibitors of coagulation. Heterozygotes with levels of 30% to 60% may have episodes of recurrent thrombosis. Measured by functional (high rate of false-positive results due to many interferences) or ELISA (which is preferred method); the gold standard precipitation method is difficult to reproduce.

Decreased In
Pregnancy, hormone replacement therapy, oral contraceptives
First year of life (adult levels reached by 1 year of age)
Values lower in women than men; increase with age in women but not in men
Oral anticoagulants (vitamin K antagonists)
Acute-phase reaction (e.g., thrombotic, inflammatory, surgical); normal value during such events excludes deficiency
Proteinuria
1% to 3% of patients with deep venous thrombosis
Others

Homocysteine[54]

Use
To exclude or confirm deficiencies of cobalamine or folate (see Chiefly Macrocytic/Megaloblastic Anemias)
Renal failure: >30 μmol/L is prognostic factor for mortality and cardiovascular events
Risk factor for cardiovascular disease
To confirm or exclude diagnosis of homocystinuria, monitor treatment response and compliance

[52]Van Cott EM, Soderberg BL, Laposata M. Activated protein C resistance, the Factor V Leiden mutation, and a laboratory testing algorithm. *Arch Pathol Lab Med* 2002;126.577–582.
[53]Goodwin AJ, Rosendaal FR, Kottke-Marchant K, et al. A review of the technical, diagnostic, and epidemiologic considerations for protein S assays. *Arch Pathol Lab Med* 2002;126:1349–1366.
[54]Refsum H, Smith AD, Ueland PM, et al. Facts and recommendations about total homocysteine determinations: an expert opinion. *Clin Chem* 2004;50:3–32.

HEMATOLOGY

Increased In
Certain drugs (e.g., methotrexate, phenytoin, theophylline)
Pregnancy to screen for folate deficiency
Hypothyroidism

Prothrombin Consumption

Impaired by
Any defect in phase I or phase II of blood coagulation (e.g., thrombocytopathies, thrombocytopenia, hypoprothrombinemia, hemophilias, circulating anticoagulants, etc).

Ristocetin Cofactor Activity

Use
Differential diagnosis of vWD (see Table 11-49)

Thrombin Time[55]

Use
Detects decreased or abnormal fibrinogen
Detects unreported therapeutic heparin
Detects other antithrombins
Increased In
Fibrinogen levels that are very low (<80 mg/dL) or high (>400 mg/dL)
Interference with polymerization of fibrin

- Fibrin degradation products, especially DIC
- High concentrations of monoclonal immunoglobulins (e.g., myeloma, macroglobulinemia, AL-type amyloidosis), which interfere with fibrin monomer polymerization
- Uremia
- Dysfibrinogenemia (abnormal fibrinogen present)

Heparin contamination of specimen is common cause in hospital patients; a reptilase test is normal in presence of heparin but prolonged by other causes listed previously
Various radiocontrast agents (e.g., metrizamide, diatrizoate)

Reptilase Time

Reptilase is a thrombinlike enzyme derived from venom of fer-de-lance (*Bothrops atrox*) that measures the conversion of fibrinogen to fibrin.

Use
Evaluate prolonged aPTT
Exclude dysfibrinogenemia
Increased In
Hypofibrinogenemia
Dysfibrinogenemia
Fibrin degradation products (slight increase)

Tourniquet Test

Use
Differential diagnosis of purpura
Positive In
Thrombocytopenic purpuras
Nonthrombocytopenic purpuras
Thrombocytopathies
Scurvy

[55]Cunningham MT, Brandt JT, Laposata M, et al. Laboratory diagnosis of dysfibrinogenemia. *Arch Pathol Lab Med* 2002;126:499–505.

Vitamin K

Vitamin K is a fat-soluble vitamin that is necessary to synthesize various coagulation factors. Assayed by PT.

Use

Useful as test for severe liver function abnormality by measuring PT before and after administration of vitamin K.

Monitor anticoagulation with Coumadin (e.g., patients with myocardial infarction). Coumadin is a vitamin K antagonist and induces relative vitamin K deficiency.

Decreased In

Hemorrhagic disease of the newborn

Fat malabsorption

Use of drugs that interfere with vitamin K metabolism (e.g., coumarin, phenytoin, some broad-spectrum antibiotics)

Disorders of Coagulation Factors[56]

Fibrinogen (Factor I)

Factor I, or fibrinogen, is an acute-phase reactant. It is a glycoprotein and is synthesized in liver. It is modified by thrombin to produce fibrinogen. A normal level is 200 to 400 mg/dL.

Increased In (May contribute to thrombophilia)

Acute-phase response

Pregnancy

Older age

Atherosclerosis

Smoking

Diabetes mellitus

Myocardial infarction, sudden cardiac death

Decreased In (May increase risk of bleeding; Detected by TT)

DIC

Severe liver disease

Congenital Afibrinogenemia (rare inherited autosomal recessive congenital absence)

♦ Plasma fibrinogen is absent.

BT is increased in 1/3 of patients.

PT, aPTT, and TT are abnormal.

Platelet-to-glass adhesiveness is abnormal unless fibrinogen is added.

Congenital Hypofibrinogenemia (inherited autosomal dominant)

♦ Plasma fibrinogen is moderately decreased (usually <80 mg/dL).

Bleeding and coagulation times are normal.

Blood clots are soft and small.

Dysfibrinogenemia[57,58]

Dysfibrinogenemia is a rare inherited (autosomal dominant) or acquired heterogeneous group of disorders caused by the synthesis of abnormal fibrinogen molecules. Over 50% of cases have no bleeding diathesis; 20% to 25% of cases have mild to moderate bleeding or thrombosis or both.

[56]Chandler WL, Rodgers GL, Sprouse JT, et al. Elevated hemostatic factor levels as potential risk factors for thrombosis. *Arch Pathol Lab Med* 2002;126.1405–1414.

[57]Cunningham MT, Brandt JT, Laposata M, et al. Laboratory diagnosis of dysfibrinogenemia. *Arch Pathol Lab Med* 2002;126:499–505.

[58]Le Groupe de Etudes sur l'Hemostase et la Thromboise (GEHT) website (http://www.geht.org/pages/database_ang.html).

HEMATOLOGY

♦ Fibrin formation is abnormally slow, with prolonged plasma TT and reptilase time used for screening. S/S are not known.
♦ Confirmatory test is fibrinogen clotting activity/antigen ratio. S/S are not known. Excluded by normal TT and fibrinogen level. Prolonged TT and decreased fibrinogen may also occur in DIC, liver disease, recent birth.
♦ Inherited form has normal liver function tests and mutation of one of three fibrinogen genes.
♦ Acquired form is distinguished by abnormal liver function tests and absence of disorder in family members.

Factor II (Prothrombin)

Factor II is synthesized in the liver in the presence of vitamin K; it is converted to thrombin during coagulation.

Factor IIa (Thrombin)

Factor IIa converts fibrinogen into fibrin clot.

Also binds to thrombomodulin on endothelial cell surface to become activated; in this form, converts protein C to activated form.

Factor III (Tissue Thromboplastin)

Factor III is released from damaged tissue in the first phase of extrinsic coagulation cascade. It activates factor IV.

Factor IV (Calcium Ions)

Factor IV activates thromboplastin and the conversion of prothrombin to thrombin.

Factor V (Proaccelerin or Labile Factor)

Factor V is a protein synthesized in the liver. Twenty percent comes from platelets. It helps accelerate the conversion of prothrombin to thrombin.

Decreased In
Congenital Deficiency
Parahemophilia: inherited autosomal recessive deficiency syndrome. Infrequent bleeding occurs only in the homozygote
Acquired Deficiency in association with severe liver disease or DIC.
PT and aPTT are increased but corrected by addition of absorbed plasma.
Variable increase in PT, prothrombin consumption, and coagulation time is not corrected by administration of vitamin K.
♦ Factor V assay

Factor VI

This factor is no longer used. May be identical to factor V.

Factor VII (Proconvertin)

Factor VII is also called stable factor, proconvertin, and serum prothrombin conversion accelerator. It is synthesized by the liver and is a critical part of extrinsic coagulation pathway.

Decreased In
Congenital deficiency (infrequent autosomal recessive trait; bleeding occurs in homozygotes; heterozygotes have few or no manifestations).
Acquired type may be due to liver disease, vitamin K deficiency, or dicumarol therapy.
Only PT is prolonged (normal when viper venom is used as thromboplastin; this does not correct PT in factor X deficiency) and is not corrected by administration of vitamin K; corrected by aged serum.
BT, coagulation time, aPTT, clot retraction, and prothrombin consumption are normal.
♦ Factor VII assay

Increased In
Pregnancy, oral contraceptives, hyperlipidemia, aging, obesity
No decisive links to disease

Factor VIII (Antihemophiliac Globulin or Factor)

Factor VII is an acute-phase reactant. It is synthesized in liver and is required in the first phase of the intrinsic system.

Decreased In
Hemophilia[59] (X-linked recessive deficiency or abnormal synthesis of factor VIII)
♦ Classic (severe) hemophilia (factor VIII assay <1%) shows increased coagulation time, prothrombin consumption time, and aPTT; prolonged BT in ~20% of patients.
♦ Moderate hemophilia (factor VIII assay 1%–5%) shows normal coagulation time and normal prothrombin consumption time but increased aPTT.
♦ In mild hemophilia (factor VIII assay <16%) and "sub-hemophilia" (factor VIII assay 20% to 30%), these laboratory tests may be normal; patients seldom bleed excessively except after surgery.
Screening tests for factor VIII deficiency: Normal PT and platelet count, prolonged aPTT, thrombin time, BT
Secondary tests: Factor VIII:C, factor VIIIR:Ag, platelet aggregation, platelet agglutination, ristocetin cofactor
♦ Specific factor assay is required to differentiate from factor IX deficiency (hemophilia B).
Laboratory findings caused by hemorrhage and anemia.
"Acquired" hemophilia may occur when an inhibitor (autoantibody) is present usually spontaneously but may be associated with autoimmune or lymphoproliferative disorders, pregnancy and postpartum states, and allergy to drugs, especially penicillin. aPTT mixing studies distinguish factor deficiency from antibody: pooled normal plasma supplies missing factor and corrects clotting time in case of deficiency, but antibody inhibits normal plasma, causing incomplete correction of aPTT.
Antibodies develop in ~20% of patients receiving repeated transfusion of factor VIII products, prolonging aPTT and lowering VIII activity of normal plasma.
♦ Prenatal diagnosis during 8th to 10th week of pregnancy by DNA analysis of amniocytes or chorionic villous material or by analysis of fetal blood at 12 to 14 weeks for VIII:C and VIII:Ag.
Carrier status is 95% accurate in ~80% of women by pedigree analysis and laboratory studies.
>75% of patients with severe hemophilia who received multiple doses of factor concentrate before 1985 are HIV positive; many have AIDS. High incidence of viral hepatitis seropositivity.

Increased In
Clotting activity >150% on >1 occasion in absence of acute-phase response, pregnancy, aerobic exercise is risk factor for venous or arterial thrombosis.
Blood types A or B in persons are ~15% higher than in type O persons.

Incidence of Inherited Congenital Coagulation Factors[63]

Autosomal recessive except factors IX and VIII, which are X-linked recessive, and II.

VIII	1:10,000
IX	1:60,000
VII	1:500,000
X	1:1,000,000
V	1:1,000,000
I (fibrinogen)	1:1,000,000
XI	1:1,000,000
XIII	1:1,000,000
II (prothrombin)	1:2,000,000

HEMATOLOGY

[59]Mannucci P, Tuddenham E. The hemophilias—from royal genes to gene therapy. *N Engl J Med* 2001;344:1773–1779.

Factor IX

Factor IX is also known as plasma thromboplastin component. Factor X is a vitamin K–dependent protein made in the liver. It is activated by factors III and VII.

Decreased In
Inherited (recessive X-linked deficiency; Christmas disease, hemophilia B)
Acquired due to vitamin K deficiency, liver disease, warfarin therapy, nephritic syndrome, factor IX Ig inhibitors
In severe cases, coagulation time, BT, prothrombin consumption time, and aPTT are increased
Defect is corrected by frozen plasma just as well as by bank blood
♦ Factor IX assay

Increased By
With age
Use of oral contraceptives
Risk of venous thrombosis if activity >129%

Factor X (Stuart-Prower Factor)

Factor X is also known as Stuart-Prower factor. It is a protein synthesized by the liver in presence of vitamin K. It is activated by factor VII in extrinsic pathway and factor IX in intrinsic coagulation pathways.

Increased In
Use of oral contraceptives
Pregnancy

Decreased In
Inherited deficiency: Rare autosomal recessive defect resembles factor VII deficiency; heterozygotes show mild or no clinical manifestations.
Form may be associated with amyloidosis, coumarin anticoagulant therapy, vitamin K deficiency (e.g., malnutrition, liver disease).
Increased PT (not corrected by use of viper venom as thromboplastin) is not corrected by administration of vitamin K. Heterozygotes may have only slight increase in PT.
♦ Factor X assay

Factor XI (Plasma Thromboplastin Antecedent)

Factor XI is also called plasma thromboplastin antecedent. It is a protein that is synthesized in liver and megakaryocytes. It activates factor IX in intrinsic pathway.

Decreased In
Inherited autosomal recessive deficiency is usually mild; acquired forms are recognized. In mild form, coagulation time may be normal, whereas prothrombin consumption time is slightly increased.
Severe cases display increased coagulation time and increased prothrombin consumption time.
Usually do not bleed spontaneously but may have postoperative bleeding.
♦ Factor XI assay

Factor XII (Hageman Factor) Deficiency

Factor XII is a protein synthesized by the liver. It circulates as inactive form until activated by collagen, basement membrane, or activated platelets; then with a cofactor, it becomes factor XIIa to ultimately form fibrin.

Coagulation time and prothrombin consumption time are increased.
Specific factor assay is needed to distinguish from factor XI deficiency.
No hemorrhagic symptoms occur, but tendency for thrombosis.

Factor XIII (Fibrin-Stabilizing Factor) Deficiency

In presence of calcium, factor XIII stabilizes a polymerized fibrin clot into initial clot. Does not circulate in plasma.

Factor XIII deficiency is an inherited autosomal recessive deficiency with severe coagulation defect.
The acquired type may occur in

- AML
- Liver disease
- Association with hypofibrinogenemia in obstetric complications
- Presence of circulating inhibitors

All standard clotting tests appear normal.
Patient's fibrin clot is soluble in 5M urea.
Whole blood clot is qualitatively friable.

Disorders of Coagulation

Stages of Coagulation

1. Vessel constriction
2. Platelet plug formation (primary hemostasis)
3. Coagulation and fibrin generation
4. Fibrinolysis, healing, repair (see Table 11-45)

Classification of Hemorrhagic Disorders

Vascular abnormalities

- Congenital (e.g., hereditary hemorrhagic telangiectasia [Osler-Weber-Rendu disease]), Marfan syndrome, Ehlers-Danlos syndrome, osteogenesis imperfecta)
- Acquired (see Nonthrombocytopenic Purpura)
    Infection (e.g., bacterial endocarditis, rickettsial infection)
    Immunologic (e.g., Schönlein-Henoch, allergic purpura, drug sensitivity)
    Metabolic (e.g., scurvy, uremia, diabetes mellitus)
    Miscellaneous (e.g., neoplasms, amyloidosis, angioma serpiginosum)

Connective tissue abnormalities

- Congenital (e.g., Ehlers-Danlos syndrome)
- Acquired (e.g., Cushing syndrome)

Platelet abnormalities (see sections on thrombocytopenic purpura, thrombocythemia, thrombocytopathies)
Plasma coagulation defects

- Causing defective thromboplastin formation (deficiency of factors VIII, IX, XI), vWD
- Causing defective rate or amount of thrombin formation
    Vitamin K deficiency (due to liver disease, prolonged bile duct obstruction, malabsorption, hemorrhagic disease of the newborn, anticoagulants)
    Congenital deficiency of factors II, V, VII, X
- Decreased fibrinogen due to intravascular clotting and/or fibrinolysis (e.g., DIC))
    Congenital deficiency of factor XIII, congenital afibrinogenemia and hypofibrinogenemia, etc.)
    Neoplasms (leukemia, carcinoma of prostate, etc.)
    Transfusion reactions
- Circulating anticoagulants
    Heparin therapy
    Dysproteinemias, SLE, postpartum state, some cases of hemophilia, etc.

Coagulation Disorders, Neonatal

Severe forms of factors VIII and IX deficiency cause most hemorrhagic congenital coagulation problems in newborns. Bleeding occurs within the first week in 50% of cases, especially following circumcision.
Congenital deficiency of factor XIII
Hemorrhagic disease of the newborn (due to lack of vitamin K) may be associated with a mother on anticonvulsant drug therapy (e.g., phenytoin, phenobarbital), severe liver disease in the infant, or to a variety of transient defects in clotting; this is more

HEMATOLOGY

Table 11-40. Comparison of Hemorrhagic Diseases of the Newborn

Test	Hemorrhagic Disease of the Newborn caused by Vitamin K Deficiency	Secondary Hemorrhagic Disease of the Newborn
Capillary fragility	Normal	Usually abnormal
Bleeding time	Normal	Often increased
Clotting time	Increased	Variable
One-stage prothrombin	Marked increase ($\leq$5%)	Moderate increase (usually 5%–25%)
Factor V	Normal	Often decreased (<50%)
Fibrinogen	Normal	Occasionally marked decrease
Platelet count	Normal	Occasionally decreased
Response to vitamin K	Improvement in clotting factors appears in 2–4 h; almost complete correction in 24 h	Little or no response

commonly seen in low-birthweight premature infants and anoxic or septic neonates. (See Table 11-40.) *Water-soluble forms of vitamin K may precipitate hemolysis in newborns, especially in presence of G6PD.*

- PT is markedly increased.
- PTT and coagulation time are increased.
- BT is normal or may be slightly increased.
- Capillary fragility, prothrombin consumption, and platelet count are normal.
- Laboratory findings due to blood loss.

DIC
Abnormal hemostasis is rare in the healthy term infant. Most of the bleeding disorders seen by primary care physicians are acquired rather than inherited abnormalities of coagulation and are expressions of underlying disease.
In the sick neonate, thrombocytopenia is the most common cause of abnormal hemostasis; less common are DIC, vitamin K deficiency, and inadequate liver function. The cause of neonatal thrombocytopenia (e.g., sepsis, DIC) is discovered in only 40% of the cases.

Coagulopathy Due to Liver Disease

Screening tests may include any combination of abnormal PTT, aPTT, TT, euglobulin or whole-blood clot lysis times, or increased fibrin degradation products. These will be corrected by an equal mixture of patient and normal plasma except TT in presence of large amounts of fibrin degradation products due to hyperplasminemia or if fibrin polymerization is faulty. Special tests may show decreased antithrombin, decrease in any coagulation factor (except VIII:C, which is normal or increased in liver disease but decreased in DIC), decreased α-2-antiplasmin. PT is corrected by parenteral administration of vitamin K.
Abnormal liver function chemistries.

Disseminated Intravascular Coagulation[60]

DIC is an acquired coagulation disorder caused by excessive overwhelming systemic activation of the coagulation system showing widespread fibrin thrombi in microcirculation with rapid concurrent depletion of platelets and coagulation proteins (causing bleeding) and activation of thrombin, leading to thrombosis of small and midsized vessels; more than one mechanism is often present.

See Tables 11-41 to 11-44.

[60]Levi M, ten Cate H. Disseminated intravascular coagulation. *N Engl J Med* 1999;341:586–592.

Table 11-41. Disseminated Intravascular Coagulation (Consumption Coagulopathy)

Determination	% of Cases Abnormal	Abnormal Level for DIC	Mean Values for DIC	Response to Heparin Therapy	Tests
Decreased platelet count (per µL)	93	<150,000	52,000	None or may take wks[a]	Platelet count, PT, fibrinogen level are performed first as screening tests; if all three are positive, diagnosis is considered established. If only two of these are positive, diagnosis should be confirmed by at least one of the tests for fibrinolysis.
Increased PT (s)	90	>15	18.0	Becomes normal or falls >5 s in few hours to 1 d	
Decreased fibrinogen level (mg/dL)	71	<160	137	Rises significantly (>40 mg) in 1–3 d	
Latex test for fibrinogen degradation products (titer)	92	>1:16	1:52	Begins to fall in 1 d, if very high, may take >1 wk to become normal	
Prolonged thrombin time (s)	59	>25	27		Tests for fibrinolysis.
Euglobulin clot lysis time (min)	42	<120		Returns to normal	

DIC, disseminated intravascular coagulation; PT, prothrombin time.

[a] Platelet count is not a satisfactory indicator of response to heparin therapy.

Adapted from Colman RW, Robboy SJ, Minna JD. Disseminated intravascular coagulation (DIC): an approach. *Am J Med* 1972;52:679.

Table 11-42.	Comparison of Acute Disseminated Intravascular Coagulation (DIC) and Primary Fibrinogenolysis	
	Acute DIC	Fibrinogenolysis
Platelet count	D	Usually N
Fibrinogen	D	D
Fibrin degradation products	O to very marked I	Very marked I
Protamine sulfate test	Positive	Negative
Euglobulin clot lysis time	N	D
Factor V	D	D
Factor VIII	D	N to moderate D

O, absent; D, decreased; I, increased; N, normal.

Causes	Occurs in % of Cases
• Infections	
Sepsis is most common cause (Gram positive and negative)	30%–50%
Meningococcemia	
Rocky Mountain spotted fever	
Viremia (CMV, HIV, hepatitis, varicella)	
• Pregnancy and obstetric complications, e.g.:	50%
Retained dead fetus syndrome (in 50% of cases with fetus retained 5 weeks)	
Eclampsia (fulminant in 10%–15% of patients)	
Amniotic fluid embolism	
Abruptio placentae	
Saline-induced abortion	
• Trauma with extensive tissue injury (e.g., crush injuries, burns, extensive surgery, shock, fat embolism)	50%–70%
• Metastatic neoplasms, especially prostate	10%–15%
Necrosis due to chemotherapy or irradiation	
Acute leukemia, especially acute promyelocytic	15%
• Vascular disorders:	
Giant hemangioma	25%
Large aortic aneurism	<1%
Cardiac, peripheral	
• Connective tissue diseases	
• Toxins (e.g., snake bites, brown recluse spider bite, drugs)	
• Injury to platelets or RBCs (e.g., immunologic hemolytic anemias)	

Table 11-43.	Comparison of Acute and Chronic Disseminated Intravascular Coagulation (DIC)	
	Acute DIC	Chronic DIC
Platelet count	D (moderate/marked)	D (mild/marked)
Prothrombin time	I	N or slight I
Activated partial thromboplastin time	I	N or D
Thrombin time	I	N or moderate I
Fibrinogen	D	I, N, or moderate D
Fibrin degradation products	Present	Present
Protamine sulfate test	Positive	Positive
Factors V and VIII	D	N

D, decreased; I, increased; N, normal.

Table 11-44. Differential Diagnosis of Disseminated Intravascular Coagulation (DIC)

	DIC	Chronic Liver Disease	Primary Fibrinolysis	TTP	Hemolytic Uremic Syndrome	Multiple Transfusion
Platelet count	D	D	N	N–D	D	D
PT	I	I	I	N	N	I
aPTT	I	N–I	I	N	N	I
FDP	I	N–I	I	N–I	N–I	N
D-Dimer assay	I	N	I	N	N	N
Fibrinogen	D	V	D	N	N	I
Schistocytes	+	O	+	+	+	O
BUN	I	N	N	I	I	N
Liver function tests	N	I	N	N	N	N
Protamine sulfate	I	N–I	I	N-I	N	N
Euglobulin clot lysis	N	N	D	N	N	N

I, increased; N, normal; +, present; PT, prothrombin time; aPTT, activated partial thromboplastin time; D, decreased; FDP, fibrin degradation products; BUN, blood urea nitrogen; O, absent; V, variable; TTP, thrombotic thrombocytopenic purpura.

- Prosthetic devices (e.g., aortic balloon, LeVeen shunt)
- Reticuloendothelial system injury—liver disease (e.g., acute hepatic failure, obstructive jaundice, cirrhosis, hepatitis), postsplenectomy

♦ *Criteria for specific diagnosis are not well defined. No single test is diagnostic, and diagnosis usually depends on a combination of findings. A single normal level does not rule out DIC, and a repeat test screen should be done a few hours later for changes in platelet count and fibrinogen.* Some have defined DIC as: systemic bleeding, PT >3 seconds above upper limit of normal, fibrinogen <150 mg/dL, and platelet count <100,000/μL.
♦ In acute cases, repeated aPTT and PT (if initially prolonged), decreased platelet count, and decreased fibrinogen levels are particularly useful for screening. All may be normal in 25% of acute DIC. If any are abnormal, follow with fibrin degradation products (FDP) and D-dimer.
♦ Most sensitive and specific tests:

- Test for FDP in serum >20 μg/mL (may be >100 μg/mL; normal = 0 to 10 μg/mL); S/S = 85% to 100%/~50%.
- D-dimer positive assay is specific for fibrin and is more reliable indicator of DIC (~100% specificity) than FDP assay, since D-dimer is negative in cases of primary fibrinolysis. Thus, the combination of FDP and D-dimer has S/S = 100%.
- Declining serial fibrinogen levels to <150 μg/dL; S/S = ~25%/>95%.
- Antithrombin is useful for diagnosis and to monitor therapy, but immunologic assay should not be used.
- Fibrinopeptide A is increased.
- Protamine sulfate or ethanol gelation (reflect FDP but are less specific). A negative protamine is against ongoing DIC; ethanol test is less sensitive and may produce false-negative results. Less sensitive and specific tests
- PT (should be done serially if prolonged; increased in ~70% of acute DIC)
- aPTT (increased in ~50% of acute DIC)
- Decreased platelet count (in ~90% of acute cases) and abnormal platelet function tests (e.g., BT, platelet aggregation)
- Thrombin time may be increased

Least sensitive and specific tests:

- Euglobulin clot lysis, which measures fibrinolytic activity in plasma
- Peripheral blood smear examination

HEMATOLOGY

Table 11-45. Congenital Functional Platelet Disorders

		Platelet Aggregation			
		ADP or Epinephrine			
Disorder	Platelet Retention in Glass Bead	First Phase	Second Phase	Ristocetin	Collagen
Bernard-Soulier syndrome	D	N	N	D	N
Glanzmann thrombasthenia	D	D	D	N	D
Release defect	N or D	N	D	N	D
Storage pool disease	N or D	N	D	N	D
Von Willebrand disease	D	N	N	D	N

D, depressed; N, normal; ADP, adenosine diphosphate.
Source: Bowie DJW. Recognition of easily missed bleeding mistakes. *Mayo Clin Proc* 1982;57:263.

In addition, the following abnormalities often occur:

- Schistocytes in the peripheral blood smear and other evidence of microangiopathic hemolytic anemia may be present (e.g., increased serum LD, decreased serum haptoglobin).
- Cryofibrinogen may be present.
- Observation of the blood clot may show the clot that forms to be small, friable, and wispy because of the hypofibrinogenemia.
- Plasma factors V, VIII, and XIII are usually significantly decreased, but results are useless for diagnosis.
- Survival time of radioiodine-labeled fibrinogen and rate of incorporation of ^{14}C-labeled glycine ethyl ester into soluble "circulating fibrin" are sensitive indicators of DIC.

Clotting time determinations are used to monitor heparin therapy.

Laboratory findings due to multiorgan failure resulting from microvascular thrombi and ischemia

Chronic DIC is most often caused by a malignancy causing chronic low-grade activation of the coagulation system. PT and aPTT may be shortened because of the increase in activated coagulation factors. Large vessel thrombosis may occur in neoplasia (Trousseau sign).

○ *Suspect clinically in patients with underlying conditions who show bleeding (frequently acute and dramatic), purpura or petechiae, acrocyanosis, arterial or venous thrombosis.*

Tests of Platelet Function

Platelet Aggregation Studies

Platelet aggregation, stimulated by certain agonistic drugs, is measured *in vitro* by a turbidimeter and shown graphically by wave patterns.

See Table 11-45.

Disorder	Aggregation Results
vWD	Ristocetin cofactor assay
Bernard-Soulier syndrome	Ristocetin; ADP, collagen are normal
Thrombasthenia	All agents decreased except ristocetin
Release defects	
Storage pool disease	ADP, epinephrine, ristocetin: no secondary wave; ristocetin may be normal
Idiopathic	ADP, epinephrine, collagen
Abnormal thromboxane A2 synthesis	Arachidonic acid, ADP, epinephrine, collagen
Afibrinogenemia	No primary or secondary waves to ADP

Use

Classification of congenital qualitative platelet functional abnormalities of adhesion, release, or aggregation (e.g., storage pool disease, Glanzmann thrombasthenia, Bernard-Soulier syndrome)

Rarely useful to evaluate acquired bleeding disorders

Interferences

Aspirin and rare aspirin-like defect block arachidonic acid and reduce collagen aggregation

Myeloproliferative diseases and uremia: Abnormal aggregation to epinephrine, ADP and collagen

Aggregation may also be abnormal due to dysproteinemia, lipemia, hemolysis, various drugs (e.g., NSAIDs), and cardiopulmonary bypass

Interpretation

ADP and epinephrine produce primary and secondary waves of aggregation; collagen, arachidonic acid, and ristocetin produce only primary waves

Platelet Aggregation, Ristocetin-Induced

Ristocetin-induced platelet aggregation is not the same as ristocetin cofactor assay.

Increased In

vWD (type IIB)

Platelet-type vWD

Type 1 New York vWD

Decreased In

vWD (type I, IIA, IIC, III)

Idiopathic thrombocytopenic purpura (ITP)

Storage pool disease

Bernard-Soulier syndrome

Acute myeloblastic leukemia

Aspirin ingestion

Infectious mononucleosis

Cirrhosis

Platelet Count

The platelet life span is 8 to 10 days. It takes 5 days for a megakaryocyte to shed a platelet. Seventy percent of platelets are present in blood; 30% are in the spleen. Measured by automated analyzers using electrical impedance or light scattering, accurate to ±5% between 1,000 and 3,000,000/μL. Measures mean platelet volume (MPV) and platelet size distribution curve at same time.

See Tables 11-45 to 11-47 and Figure 11-19.

Increased In

(>400,000/μL; <1,000,000/μL in 97% of patients. Plasma thrombopoietin levels are high.)

Essential thrombocythemia and other clonal myeloproliferative disease (e.g., PV, CML, agnogenic myeloid metaplasia)

Reactive

* Malignancy (especially disseminated, advanced, or inoperable) accounts for ~13% of cases in hospital patients. *About 50% of patients with an "unexpected" increase in platelet count are found to have a (especially visceral) malignancy.*
* Patients recently having surgery, especially splenectomy (accounts for 19% of cases in hospital patients); severe trauma; massive acute hemorrhage; or thrombotic episodes.
* Infections account for ~31% of cases in hospital patients.
* Chronic inflammation (e.g., TB, inflammatory bowel disease, collagen diseases, RA)
* IDA
* Miscellaneous disease states (e.g., cardiac disease, cirrhosis, chronic pancreatitis, neonates with acute respiratory distress syndrome, burns, hypothermia, preeclampsia, ethanol withdrawal, renal failure, splenectomy) and many other causes
* Drug reactions (e.g., vincristine)

HEMATOLOGY

Table 11-46.	Some Congenital Hemorrhagic Diseases Caused by Disorders of Platelet-Vessel Wall

Platelet Defects

Bernard-Soulier syndrome	Moderate thrombocytopenia
	Bleeding time markedly increased
	Large platelets
	Decreased ristocetin-induced agglutination not corrected by vWF
Glanzmann thrombasthenia	Normal platelet count and morphology
	Increased bleeding time
	Clot retraction absent or much decreased
	No platelet aggregation with any agonists
Pseudo-von Willebrand disease	Variable mild thrombocytopenia
	Increased bleeding time
	Increased ristocetin-induced agglutination
	Variable plasma immunoreactive vWF
Gray-platelet syndrome	Moderate thrombocytopenia
	Large platelets
	Bleeding time slightly increased
	Platelets agranular on blood smear
	Abnormal platelet aggregation with collagen or thrombin
Dense-granule deficiency syndrome	Normal platelet count
	Normal platelet morphology on blood smear
	Bleeding time variably increased
	Abnormal aggregation with ADP and collagen
Deficiency of platelet enzyme (cyclo-oxygenase or thromboxane synthetase)	Normal platelet count and morphology
	Abnormal aggregation with ADP collagen, and arachidonic acid
May-Hegglin anomaly	Autosomal dominant trait
	Moderate thrombocytopenia with huge platelets; normal platelet function
	Döhle bodies in granulocytes

Plasma Defects

Von Willebrand disease	Normal platelet count and morphology
	Increased bleeding time
	Abnormal ristocetin-induced agglutination
	Abnormal plasma vWF
Afibrinogenemia	Normal platelet morphology
	Mild thrombocytopenia occasion
	Bleeding time variably increased
	Plasma coagulation abnormalities

Vessel Wall Defects

Genetic disorders of connective tissue	Platelets may be large
	Collagen-induced aggregation may be abnormal

ADP, adenosine diphosphate; vWF, von Willebrand factor.

Table 11-47.   Comparison of Congenital Disorders of Platelet Function

Platelet Disorder	Platelet Count	Bleeding Time	PT/aPTT	Fibrinogen	Aggregation	
					Ristocetin	ADP
Aspirin induced	N	A	N	N	N	A
Bernard-Soulier syndrome	A	A	N	N	A	N
Congenital afibrino-genemia	N	A	A	A	N	A
Glanzmann throm-basthenia	N	A	N	N	N	A
Storage pool deficiency	N	A	N	N	N	A
Von Willebrand disease	N	A	N/A	N	A	N

N, normal; A, abnormal; PT, prothrombin time; aPTT, activated partial thromboplastin time; ADP, adenosine diphosphate.

Decreased In
(thrombocytopenic purpura; <150,000/μL)
Acquired:

- Decreased platelet production (e.g., aplastic anemia, myelophthisis, ionizing radiation, nutritional deficiencies [e.g., folate, vitamin B_{12}], drugs [e.g., alcohol, chemotherapeutic agents])
- Infections (e.g., AIDS, CMV, subacute bacterial endocarditis, septicemia, rubella, infectious mononucleosis, most rickettsial infections) may have several mechanisms
- Hypersplenism
- Increased platelet destruction:

♦ *Antiplatelet antibodies* (IgG and IgM) may be found in plasma and by flow cytometry may be detected on platelets in most patients with drug-induced thrombocytopenia (sensitivity = 90%). Fifteen percent to 29% of patients with autoimmune thrombocytopenia have only platelet-associated IgM. Negative results in plasma and on platelets is strongly against an immune etiology of thrombocytopenia. Platelet-associated IgG may be seen in ITP, sepsis, aplastic anemia, acute leukemia, SLE (see Chapter 17), immune vasculitis, and drugs.
Drug-induced immune thrombocytopenia (e.g., heparin quinidine, quinine, gold, sulfonamides, penicillins; causes thrombocytopenia in ≤10% of patients, usually in 5–10 days).
Neonatal alloimmune thrombocytopenia, an uncommon condition that may cause intracranial hemorrhage in utero or at birth, with death or neurologic impairment. Caused by maternal platelet-specific antibody against infant platelet antigen inherited from father but absent in mother. Unexplained petechiae/purpura at birth, platelet count <100,000/μL.
Lymphoproliferative disorders
Posttransfusion (develops in 5–10 days; complement-fixing antibody for platelet antigen Pl[A1] establishes diagnosis)
Extracorporeal circulation

- Increased platelet consumption:
  TTP/HUS
  DIC
  Septicemia
  Toxemia of pregnancy (≤20% of cases)
  Massive blood loss

Hypersplenism (e.g., cirrhosis)

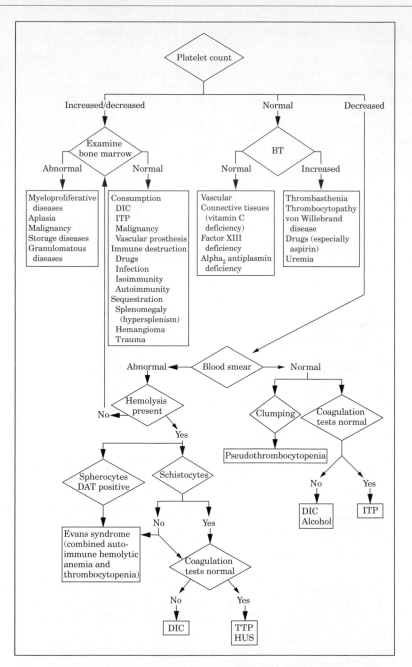

Fig. 11-19. Evaluation of hemostatic abnormalities. (For algorithms of prothrombin time and activated partial thromboplastin time, see Figures 11-16 and 11-17.) BT, bleeding time; DIC, disseminated intravascular coagulation; ITP, idiopathic thrombocytopenic purpura; DAT, direct antiglobulin test (Coombs); TTP, thrombotic thrombocytopenic purpura; HUS, hemolytic uremic syndrome.

- Dilutional (e.g., following massive transfusion)
- Renal insufficiency
- PNH

Inherited:

- Allport syndrome
- Bernard-Soulier syndrome
- Chédiak-Higashi syndrome
- Ehlers-Danlos syndrome
- May-Hegglin anomaly
- vWD type 2B, pseudo-vWD
- Wiskott-Aldrich syndrome
- Glanzmann thrombasthenia
- Hermansky-Pudlak syndrome
- TAR (*t*hrombocytopenia, *a*bsent *r*adius bones) syndrome

When associated with anemia and microangiopathy on peripheral smear, rule out DIC, TTP/HUS, prosthetic valve dysfunction, malignant hypertension, eclampsia, vasculitis, leaking aortic aneurysm, disseminated metastatic cancer.

Interferences
Pseudothrombocytopenia diagnosis by examination of stained blood smear

- Platelet clumping induced by EDTA blood collection tubes is the most common cause. Due to IgG autoantibodies.
- Platelet satellitosis (platelet rosettes around WBCs; rare)
- Platelet cold agglutinins
- Giant platelets
- RBC count >6,500,000/μL

Artifacts (e.g., overfilling vacuum tubes, clot formation)
Pseudothrombocytosis (spurious)

- Cold agglutinins
- Malaria parasites
- Fragments of RBCs or WBCs, or other particles of debris
- Microspherocytes
- Howell-Jolly bodies, nucleated RBCs, Heinz bodies, clumped Pappenheimer bodies

Usual range is 150,000 to 400,000/μL
Between 50,000 and 150,000/μL, there is usually no bleeding
Between 20,000 and 50,000/μL, there is minor spontaneous bleeding; postoperative bleeding
Levels under 20,000/μL denote an increasing risk of more serious bleeding
Those with counts under 5,000/μL frequently have serious bleeding
Platelet transfusions are not used if count is >20,000/μL except preoperatively or if there is a specific bleeding lesion (e.g., peptic ulcer).
One unit of platelet concentrate will increase the platelet count by 15,000/μL in the average 70-kg adult; therefore, the minimal dose to administer is six units. No increment in 60 minutes suggests alloimmunization has occurred (should use single-donor platelets; >5,000/μL increment suggests that alloimmunization has not occurred).
If count is atypical, peripheral smear should always be examined for platelet size, morphology, granularity, associated abnormalities of RBCs and WBCs.
Estimate of platelet count from peripheral smear: = no. of platelets/100× oil immersion field × 10,000.
See Fig 11-20.

Platelet Function Defects

Hereditary:

- Defect in plasma proteins
  - vWD (especially 2 hours after ingestion of 300 mg of aspirin)
- Deficient release of platelet glycoproteins
  - Glanzmann thrombasthenia (deficient or defective glycoprotein IIb/IIIa)
  - Bernard-Soulier syndrome (deficient glycoprotein Ib)
- Defective release mechanisms

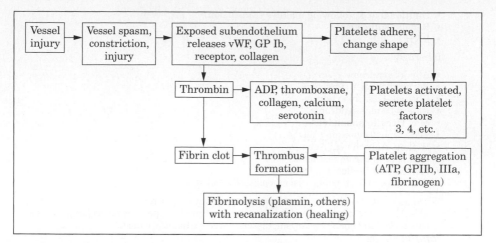

Fig. 11-20. Steps in normal hemostasis. vWF, von Willebrand factor; GPIb, IIB, IIa, glyco-proteins; ADP, adenosine diphosphate; ATP, adenosine triphosphate.

- Gray platelet syndrome (deficient α granules)
- Aspirinlike defect
- Deficient dense bodies (e.g., Wiskott-Aldrich, Chédiak-Higashi, Hermansky-Pudlak [oculocutaneous albinism] syndromes)
- Others (e.g., Ehlers-Danlos, hereditary hemorrhagic telangiectasia)
- Others (e.g., concomitant finding: May-Hegglin anomaly, Down syndrome, congenital heart disease)

Acquired:

- Abnormal plasma factors
- Drugs
  - Aspirin, NSAIDs (indomethacin, ibuprofen, phenylbutazone, etc.) by inhibition of prostaglandin pathways. Ingestion of aspirin ≤7 days is the most common cause of prolonged BT. Aspirin may double the baseline BT, which may still be within normal range. A dose of 325 mg of aspirin will increase the BT of most persons.
- Antiplatelet therapeutic drugs for ischemic heart disease (e.g., clopidogrel) inhibit ADP receptor–mediated platelet activation. Abciximab, eptifibatide, tirofiban inhibit glycoprotein IIb/IIIa.
  - Antimicrobials (especially high dose β-lactam, e.g., carbenicillin; cephalosporins, nitrofurantoin, hydroxychloroquine)
  - Anticoagulants (e.g., heparin, dicumarol, streptokinase-streptodornase)
  - Tricyclic antidepressants (e.g., imipramine, amitriptyline, nortriptyline) by interference with platelet membrane receptors
  - Phenothiazines (e.g., chlorpromazine, promethazine, trifluoperazine)
  - Anesthetic (e.g., halothane, local cocaine, Xylocaine) by interference with platelet membrane receptors
  - Methylxanthines (e.g., caffeine, theophylline, aminophylline) by inhibition of platelet phosphodiesterase activity
  - Others (e.g., dextrans, calcium channel-blocking agents, radiographic contrast agents, β-adrenergic blockers, alcohol, aminocaproic acid, nitroglycerin)
- Uremia (may be corrected with vasopressin or cryoprecipitate)
- Fibrin degradation products (e.g., DIC, liver disease, fibrinolytic therapy)
- Macromolecules (e.g., dextran, paraproteins [e.g., myelomas, Waldenström macroglobulinemia, monoclonal gammopathy]) coat platelet membranes
- Autoimmune diseases (e.g., collagen vascular disease, antiplatelet antibodies, immune thrombocytopenias)
- Myeloproliferative diseases, including myelodysplastic syndrome, preleukemia, acute leukemias, and lymphomas may show any combination of platelet aggregation defects that are not characteristic
- Vasculitis

- Others (e.g., amyloidosis, viral infections, scurvy, after circulating through an oxygenator during cardiac bypass surgery)
- Anemias (e.g., severe deficiency of iron, B_{12}, or folate)

Platelet Volume, Mean

Measurement of mean platelet volume is of limited value when measured by routine automated hematology instruments. Normal is about 7 to 11 fL.

Use
Younger platelets tend to be larger. In study of thrombocytopenic patients:

- Increased MPV with thrombocytopenia indicates that thrombopoiesis is stimulated and platelet production is increased.
- Normal MPV with thrombocytopenia indicates impaired thrombopoiesis.

Increased In
Immune thrombocytopenic purpura
Thrombocytopenia due to sepsis (recovery phase)
Myeloproliferative disorders
Massive hemorrhage
Prosthetic heart valve
Splenectomy
Vasculitis
Bernard-Soulier syndrome
Decreased In
Wiskott-Aldrich syndrome

Disorders of Platelets[61,62]

See Tables 11-45 to 11-47.

Bernard-Soulier Syndrome

Bernard-Soulier syndrome is a rare heterogeneous autosomal recessive condition characterized by the absence or dysfunction of the platelet membrane glycoproteins that enable platelets to bind vWF. An autosomal dominant variant has been described.

○ Mild or moderate thrombocytopenia, with platelet counts usually 50,000 to 80,000/μL. Hemorrhage and increased BT are excessively severe for degree of thrombocytopenia.
○ Giant round platelets on peripheral smear; MPV is increased.
Bone marrow shows increased megakaryocytes with disordered maturation and increased cytoplasmic granularity.
♦ Failure of vWF and ristocetin aggregation; other aggregations normal.
♦ Flow cytometry allows definite diagnosis by demonstration of abnormal expression of GPIb/IX/V.
Normal clot retraction.

Glanzmann Thrombasthenia

Glanzmann thrombasthenia is a rare autosomal recessive absence or dysfunction of the glycoprotein receptors (GPIIb/IIIa) that enable platelets to bind a family of integrins (to generate large platelet aggregates), of which fibrinogen is most important. Variant forms exist.

Prolonged BT.
Impaired clot retraction. Normal in essential athrombia, in which other laboratory abnormalities are the same.

[61]Kottke-Marchant K, Corcoran G. Chasing after the causes of platelet disorders. *CAP Today* 2002;6:20.
[62]Kottke-Marchant K. The laboratory diagnosis of platelet disorders. *Arch Pathol Lab Med* 2002; 126:133–146.

HEMATOLOGY

Normal platelet count and morphology but unusually well dispersed on smear with no clumping.

Normal coagulation time.

♦ Flow cytometry shows abnormal expression of GPIIb/IIIa.

♦ Totally absent primary platelet aggregation with all agonists except ristocetin and vWF.

♦ Prothrombin consumption tests abnormal but corrected by adding platelet substitute.

Gray-Platelet Syndrome

Gray-platelet syndrome is an extremely rare congenital autosomal recessive or dominant disorder; it is characterized by childhood onset of mild-moderate bleeding.

○ Platelet count 20,000/μL up to normal. Median MPV = 13 fL. Shortened life span. BT is prolonged (10 to >30 minutes), related to degree of thrombocytopenia, but is increased even with normal platelet count.

♦ Large agranular gray or gray-blue platelets (Wright-Giemsa stain). Marrow biopsy may show normal number of megakaryocytes and nonprogressive reticulin fibrosis. Neutrophils may be hypogranular.

♦ Absent or very deficient α granules by EM, by ELISA for α granule constituents, or by flow cytometry. Normal number of dense bodies.

Platelet aggregation to ristocetin is reduced or normal; deficient by collagen or thrombin; normal to ADP and arachidonic acid.

Heparin-Induced Thrombocytopenia

Type 1 heparin-induced thrombocytopenia (HIT) (nonimmune) occurs in ≤10% of patients receiving heparin. Platelet count rapidly decreases in first 2 days. Usually is >100,000/μL; returns to normal without therapy.

Type 2 HIT (immune) occurs in ≤10% of patients receiving heparin. Platelet count rapidly decreases within 5 to 14 days. Usually <100,000/μL or <30% from baseline (range 20–150/μL); returns to normal in 4 to 7 days after heparin is stopped; antibodies disappear within 3 months. May produce venous thrombosis (especially in postoperative patients); arterial thrombosis (especially in cardiac patients), often in large vessels (e.g., aorta, femoral); skin necrosis; adrenal infarction. Bleeding is uncommon.

Platelet aggregation has poor sensitivity.

♦ Platelet serotonin release assay has S/S >85%/99%; not widely available. Heparin-induced platelet agglutination assay, flow cytometry, heparin antibodies.

May-Hegglin Anomaly

May-Hegglin anomaly is a rare autosomal dominant abnormality of granulocytes and platelets with mild to severe bleeding symptoms. It is associated with chronic renal disease and neutrophil inclusions but not with deafness or eye findings.

♦ Large, poorly granulated platelets are associated with large abnormal Döhle-like inclusion bodies in cytoplasm of granulocytes in absence of infection (Döhle bodies may also be found in neutrophilic response to infection). In absence of infection, these bodies are pathognomonic.

♦ Diagnosis is confirmed by finding Döhle-like bodies in a parent or sibling.

Thrombocytopenia of 60,000 to 100,000/μL with normal life span and clot retraction may occur. Median MPV = 12.5 fL. Prolonged BT.

Normal platelet aggregation, platelet ultrastructure, granulocyte function.

Purpura, Henoch-Schönlein[63]

See Vasculitis, Chapter 5.

[63]Triplett D. Coagulation and bleeding disorders: review and update. *Clin Chem* 2000;46: 1260–1269.

Table 11-48. Comparison of Acute and Chronic Forms of Immune Thrombocytopenia

	Acute	Chronic
Population	Children aged 2–9 y	Adults; mostly women aged 20–40 y
Onset	Usually follows recent infectious illness	Insidious
Platelet count (per μL)	Often <20,000	Usually 30,000–70,000
CBC	Mild anemia, eosinophilia, and lymphocytosis	Normal
Megakaryocytes	Increased number	Increased number and volume

Purpura, Immune, Thrombocytopenic, Idiopathic (Werlhof Disease)[64]

◆ Diagnosis By

• May be primary or secondary to other causes of thrombocytopenia (e.g., SLE, leukemias, HIV and HCV infections, thyroid disorders, etc.), which must be excluded.
• Isolated low platelet count with quantitatively and qualitatively normal RBCs and WBCs.
• Bone marrow—normal or increased number and volume of megakaryocytes but without marginal platelets.

Decreased platelet count (<100,000/μL) due to markedly diminished half-life; no bleeding until <50,000/μL; postoperative and minor spontaneous bleeding may occur at 20,000 to 50,000/μL. Significant bleeding is unusual until counts are >5,000/μL and even then does not occur in most adults. Routine platelet counts have discovered many asymptomatic patients.

Normal blood count and blood smear except for decreased number of platelets; platelets may appear abnormal (small or large immature or deeply stained). MPV is normal or increased.

Positive tourniquet test
Increased BT
Poor clot retraction
Normal PT, aPTT, and coagulation time
Laboratory findings due to hemorrhage:

• Increased WBC with shift to left
• Anemia proportional to hemorrhage, with compensatory increase in reticulocytes, polychromatophilia, etc.

Platelet IgG and autoantibodies (in ~33% of ITP patients) to specific platelet-membrane glycoproteins are not important for diagnosis or treatment; platelet IgG found in ≤75% of patients with other immune-associated thrombocytopenias.

Thrombopoietin is not increased, reflecting normal megakaryocyte mass.

◆ *A palpable spleen is evidence against ITP.*

In children, 80% to 90% of acute cases remit spontaneously in 6 to 12 months; the rest become chronic; in adults almost all are chronic (see Table 11-48). ≤80% of children have preceding viral infection.

Two thirds of children and 85% of adults with chronic ITP develop normal platelet count after splenectomy.

Platelet transfusions are indicated in ITP if:

• Platelet count <5,000/μL, even if asymptomatic
• Severe mucosal bleeding at any platelet count
• Bleeding after splenectomy

[64]Cines DB, Blanchette VS. Immune thrombocytopenic purpura. *N Engl J Med* 2002;346: 995–1008.

HEMATOLOGY

- Impending/actual CNS hemorrhage at any platelet count
- Before major surgery (other than splenectomy) that requires platelet count >50,000/μL

Purpura, Nonthrombocytopenic

Due To
Abnormal platelets (e.g., thrombocytopathies, thrombasthenia, thrombocythemia)
Abnormal serum globulins (e.g., multiple myeloma, macroglobulinemia, cryoglobulinemia, hyperglobulinemia)
Infections (e.g., meningococcemia, subacute bacterial endocarditis, typhoid, Rocky Mountain spotted fever)
Other diseases (e.g., amyloidosis, Cushing syndrome, PV, hemochromatosis, diabetes mellitus, uremia)
Drugs and chemicals (e.g., mercury, phenacetin, salicylic acid, chloral hydrate)
Allergic reaction (e.g., Schönlein-Henoch purpura, serum sickness)
Diseases of the skin (e.g., Osler-Weber-Rendu disease, Ehlers-Danlos syndrome)
vWD
Avitaminosis (e.g., scurvy)
Miscellaneous (e.g., mechanical, orthostatic)
Blood coagulation factors (e.g., hemophilia)

Purpura, Thrombotic Thrombocytopenic; Hemolytic Uremic Syndrome[65–67]

TTP and HUS are caused by deficiency of a plasma metalloprotease (known as ADAMTS-13) that cleaves the vWF subunit at a specific peptide bond, thereby decreasing the multimer size and biologic activity. ADAMTS-13 prevents inappropriate platelet aggregation.

TTP Due To
Congenital (inherited disorder)
Acquired

- Nondiarrhea-associated form is associated with:
  Complications of pregnancy (e.g., eclampsia, abruptio placenta, amniotic fluid embolism)
  Drugs (e.g., oral contraceptives, phenylbutazone, cyclosporin, 5-fluoruracil, mitomycin C, quinine)
  Underlying systemic diseases (e.g., primary glomerulopathies, rejection of renal transplant, vasculitis, cryoglobulinemia, septicemia, hypertension, adenocarcinoma)
  Nonenteric pathogens
  Idiopathic due to autoantibodies

Closely related HUS showing acute renal failure is associated with other conditions:

- Diarrhea-associated form: related commonly to a verocytotoxin-producing strain of *E. coli O157:H7* and to *Shigella* with gastroenteritis and bloody diarrhea
- 10% of bone marrow transplant patients
- Normal pregnancy (usually postpartum)
- Drugs (e.g., oral contraceptives, mitomycin, immunosuppressive agents)
- Carcinoma (e.g., prostate, pancreas)
- Autoimmune disorders
- Immune deficiency disorders

◆ Classic pentad of consumptive thrombocytopenia, microangiopathic hemolytic anemia, neurologic involvement, fever, and minor renal involvement, or triad of throm-

---

[65]TTP and HUS may be two different syndromes. See Hosler GA, Cusumano AM, Hutchins GM. Thrombotic thrombocytopenic purpura and hemolytic uremic syndrome are distinct pathologic entities. Review of 56 Autopsy Cases. *Arch Pathol Lab Med* 2003;127:834–839.
[66]Noake JL. Thrombotic microangiopathies. *N Engl J Med* 2002;347:589.
[67]Wyrick-Glatzel J. Thrombotic thrombocytopenic purpura and ADAMTS-13: new insights into pathogenesis, diagnosis and therapy. *Lab Med* 2004;35:733.

bocytopenia, schistocytosis, and increased LD. Diagnostic hallmark of TTP is decreased/absent (0%–10%) vWf-cleaving metalloprotease activity (vWF-CP) and by excluding other known causes of these features. vWF-CP is often normal or only moderately decreased in HUS. vWF-CP is decreased to 40% to 50% of normal in decompensated cirrhosis and acute inflammation.

♦ Severe consumptive thrombocytopenic purpura due to platelet thrombi with normal or increased megakaryocytes in bone marrow. Platelet count usually <20,000/μL. Caused by decreased/absent or antibody against vWf-CP.

♦ Multiorgan microvascular platelet thrombi in various organ systems result in clinical manifestations (e.g., brain, heart, kidneys, spleen, GI, adrenals) in ~90% of cases. Presence in gingival biopsy supports the diagnosis but present in <50%. Other sites (skin, liver, lymph nodes, bone marrow) are rarely useful.

♦ Microangiopathic Coombs-negative hemolytic anemia (normochromic, normocytic) is present at onset or within a few days, resulting in:

• Hb usually <10 g/dL; is often <6 g/dL; may fall 50% in 2 days.
• Numerous fragmented and misshapen RBCs (schistocytes, burr cells) on blood smear are virtually required for this diagnosis.
• Increased reticulocytes, nucleated RBCs, basophilic stippling, and polychromatophilia.
• Increased serum Hb, indirect bilirubin, LD, and decreased serum haptoglobin.

♦ In HUS, BUN may rise as much as 50 mg/dL/day; is often >100 mg/dL. Urine may show blood, protein, casts, or anuria. Progressive renal disease or recovery. Oliguria and acute renal failure are uncommon. Renal biopsy shows fibrin thrombi damaging glomerular endothelium primarily (usually in children, associated with gastroenteritis, bloody diarrhea) or primarily arterial changes (associated with scleroderma, malignant hypertension, after mitomycin treatment).

Increased or normal WBCs and neutrophils.

In contrast to DIC, PT and aPTT are usually normal or may be mildly increased; clotting and fibrinogen are normal or only slightly increased; fibrin split products are usually present in low levels.

Bone marrow is hypercellular, with erythroid and megakaryocytic hyperplasia in response to hemolysis and consumptive thrombocytopenia.

Serum AST and ALT may be slightly increased.

High initial BUN and creatinine, decreasing Hb, and failure of platelet count to increase are poor prognostic signs.

Serum complement is normal.

Laboratory findings due to associated diseases (e.g., gastric adenocarcinoma).

Sticky Platelet Syndrome[68]

Diagnostic Criteria:
History of thrombosis plus hyperaggregability to one concentration of ADP and EPI or to two different concentrations of ADP or EPI on >1 occasion.
Type I sticky platelet syndrome (SPS): hyperaggregability to both EPI and ADP.
Type II SPS: hyperaggregability to EPI alone.
Type III SPS: hyperaggregability to ADP alone.

Storage Pool Disorders

Storage pool disorders are congenital or acquired abnormalities of platelet secretion caused by deficiency or defective release of α or dense granules or both. They may be solitary, or they may be part of hereditary disorders (e.g., Chédiak-Higashi, Wiskott-Aldrich syndrome, TAR syndrome, others).

BT is usually abnormal.
Various platelet aggregation abnormalities.

[68]Bick RL, Goeddecke C. Limitations, challenges of SPS testing. ADVANCE/Laboratory. June 2002:100.

HEMATOLOGY

♦ EM shows absence of or improperly formed dense granules.
Dense granules contain serotonin, ADP, ATP.
α granules contain fibrinogen, factors V and VIII, etc.

Thrombocytosis, Primary (Essential Thrombocythemia)

Primary thrombocytosis is classified as a clonal myeloproliferative disorder predominantly involving the megakaryocytes.

See Figure 11-19.

Diagnostic Criteria
Platelet count >600,000/μL on two occasions (>1,000,000/μL in 90% of cases)
Is diagnosis of exclusion; no cause for reactive thrombocytosis

- No iron deficiency (marrow contains stainable iron or <1 g Hb increase after 1 month of iron therapy)
- No evidence of leukemia in peripheral blood or marrow (Ph[1] chromosome; *abl-bcr* rearrangement is not found)
- No evidence of polycythemia (normal Hb, RBC mass)
- Bone marrow

Fibrosis is minimal or absent to rule out agnogenic myeloid metaplasia, or in absence of both splenomegaly and leukoerythroblastosis, it must be <1/3 of area of biopsy specimen
Hypercellular with hyperplasia of all elements, with giant dysplastic megakaryocytes with increased ploidy, associated with large masses of platelet debris; eosinophilia, basophilia; no evidence of masked PV; no ring sideroblasts of myelodysplastic syndrome; normal megakaryocyte morphology in reactive thrombocytosis

---

Platelets appear normal early in disease; later, size and shape are abnormal; changes in structure occur. Aggregation may be abnormal with epinephrine, ADP, thrombin.
Mild anemia (10–13 g/dL) in 1/3 of patients due to blood loss.
WBC count usually >12,000/μL without cells earlier than myelocyte forms in ≤40% of patients; leukocyte ALP is usually normal or may be increased.
Increased serum LD, uric acid.
Artifactual increase in serum potassium, calcium, oxygen.
Thrombohemorrhagic disease (bleeding—skin, GI tract, nose, gums in 35% of patients but normal BT) and thromboses of major vessels (arterial and venous). Hepatic vein thrombosis (Budd-Chiari syndrome) and portal vein thrombosis are characteristic of myeloproliferative diseases.
Terminally, may show marrow fibrosis or transformation to AML.
See Platelet Count.

Von Willebrand Disease[69,70]

vWD is a heterogeneous group of autosomal (>20 subtypes) and acquired disorders of vWF with mucocutaneous bleeding due to abnormal vWF quantity or quality. It is the most common inherited hemostatic abnormality. No single lab test can detect all forms of vWD. vWD is part of a larger complex of hemostatic changes associated with inflammation, atherosclerosis, and arterial thrombosis rather than a solitary risk factor.

See Tables 11-47 and 11-49.

[69]Kujovich J. Approach to a bleeding patient. *Lab Med* 2001;32:250.
[70]Mannucci PM. Treatment of von Willebrand's disease. *N Engl J Med* 2004;351:683–694.

Table 11-49.   Types of von Willebrand Disease[a]

Type	Defect	vWF Antigen	vWF Activity	Factor VIII	Multimer	Genetic Transmission[b] (% of Cases)
1	Normal qualitative vWF. Partial (5%–30% of normal) quantitative deficiency of vWF and fVIII.	D	D	D	N	AD (60%–80%)
2	Qualitative defects of vWF					AD.
2A	Defect in platelet adhesion due to loss of HMWM.	D	DD	D	0	Rarely AR. (10%–30%)
2B	Increased affinity of vWF causes spontaneous binding of HMWM to platelet Gp1b. Associated with lack of larger multimers.	D	DD	D	0	
2M	Defective platelet-dependent vWF functions. Not associated with multimer defects.					
2N	Normal platelet adhesion but defective fVIII binding site.	N	N	DD	N	
3	Complete absence (<1% of normal) of vWF; secondary deficiency (1%–10% of normal) of fVIII.	N	N	DD	0	AR (1%–10%)

D, decreased; DD, markedly decreased; N normal; I, increased; 0, absent; vWF, von Willebrand factor; fVIII, factor VIII; HMWM, high-molecular-weight multimer; AD, autosomal dominant; AR, autosomal recessive.
[a]Kujovich J. Approach to a bleeding patient. *Lab Med* 2001;32:250; Mannucci PM. Treatment of von Willebrand disease. *N Engl J Med* 2004;351:683–694.
[b]www.sheffield.ac.uk/vwf.

A number of clinical variants have been described.

Difficulty in diagnosis arises from temporal variation in clinical and laboratory findings in an individual patient, as well as from patient to patient

All tests have limited S/S and reproducibility; therefore none alone is sufficient for diagnosis.

Can usually diagnose vWD with BT, factor VIII levels, vWF:Ag, and ristocetin cofactor (RCoF) activity. For appropriate therapy, subtypes must be distinguished, for which multimeric analysis and factor VIII binding assay are needed.

Due To

Hereditary deficiency (types 1 and 3) or qualitative defect (type 2) of vWF.[71] All show mild to moderate bleeding, except type 3, which is severe.

[71]von Willebrand factor [vWF] is a high-molecular-weight glycoprotein synthesized in megakaryocytes and endothelial cells, stored in Weibel-Palade bodies, secreted by endothelial cells into extracellular matrix to facilitate platelet adhesion to injured endothelium by binding to platelet surface GPIb/IX/V. vWF circulates complexed to (carrier for) factor VIII:C which also responds as an acute phase protein.

MUSCULOSKEL

- Type 1 (comprises 60%–80% of cases): Decreased amount of vWF without qualitative abnormality.
- Type 2: Qualitative abnormalities of vWF due to loss of various multimers.
- Type 3: vWF completely or almost completely absent from plasma and platelets.
- Pseudo-vWD is a rare platelet disorder in which platelet receptors have marked avidity for vWF that causes spontaneous clumping, depletes the plasma of vWF, and may cause mild to moderate thrombocytopenia.
- Platelet-type vWD is distinguished from type 2B by mixing studies with normal platelets and plasma.

Acquired vWD due to formation of autoantibodies (in association with autoimmune lymphoproliferative disorders or monoclonal paraproteinemias), decreased synthesis or other mechanisms (e.g., in myeloproliferative, vascular, and congenital heart diseases) or idiopathic.

○ BT is prolonged; in a few patients, may only be prolonged after administration of 300 mg of aspirin. Poor S/S for mild vWF deficiency.

aPTT is prolonged.

Platelet adhesiveness to glass beads is decreased. Ristocetin-induced aggregation of platelets is abnormal if RCoF activity <30%; thus may be normal in mild vWD. May not identify some mild cases in which activity is >30% but less than normal of 50% to 150%.

Platelet count is usually normal but may be mildly decreased in type IIB or platelet-type vWD.

PT and clot retraction are normal.

Tourniquet test may be positive.

Factor VIII coagulant activity (VIII:C) may range from normal to severely reduced (assayed directly or with aPTT or thromboplastin generation time tests).

♦ Factor VIII–related antigen (vWF:Ag) measured by special electroimmunoassay is decreased.

May be increased in endothelial cell injury (e.g., trauma, surgery, surgical graft failure, clotting)

♦ Transfusion of normal plasma (or of hemophiliac plasma, cryoprecipitate, serum) causes a rise in factor VIII activity greater than the amount of factor VIII infused, which does not peak until 8 to 10 hours and slowly declines for days; in contrast, hemophilia shows rapid peak and fall after infusion of normal plasma or cryoprecipitate. This response to transfusion is a good diagnostic test in patients in whom diagnosis is equivocal. Factor VIII levels may increase to normal during pregnancy or use of oral contraceptives with subsidence of hemorrhagic episodes, although bleeding time is often unaffected. Therefore diagnostic evaluation should not be done in the presence of these two circumstances.

Screening tests: aPTT, BT, platelet count.

Confirmatory tests:

♦ RCoF assay that measures vWF-mediated agglutination of platelets in presence of ristocetin.

♦ Collagen-binding assay (ELISA) measures interaction of vWF and collagen.

Screening of family members may be useful in difficult diagnostic cases, even if they are asymptomatic and have no history of unusual bleeding.

Laboratory findings due to complications, (e.g., viral infections, development of antibodies to vWF [occurs in severe type 3], atherothrombosis).

Comparison of Hemophilia A and Von Willebrand Disease

	Hemophilia A	von Willebrand Disease
Bleeding time	Normal	Prolonged
Factor VIIIR:Ag	Normal	Low
Factor VIII:C	Low	Prolonged/normal
Platelet adhesion	Normal	Retarded
Platelet aggregation (RIPA)	Normal	Decreased
Ristocetin cofactor	Normal	Deficient
aPTT	Prolonged	Prolonged/normal

Source: Triplett D. Coagulation and bleeding disorders: review and update. *Clin Chem* 2000;46:1260.

Transfusion of Blood and Tissue Products

Adverse effects[72–74]

Adverse effects occur in ~1 in 1,000 components transfused in the United States.
~1 in 12,000 transfusions are given to the wrong person. These are fatal in 1:600,000
  transfusions, which are almost always caused by ABO incompatibility (usually due
  to clerical error).
Most common causes are transfusion-related acute lung injury (TRALI), ABO incompatibility, and bacterial contamination.

Condition	Frequency or Risk/Unit Transfused
Immune-Mediated	
Acute	
Fatal acute hemolysis (ABO) (mortality ~3.3%) (isoimmune). Laboratory findings due to complications of hemolysis (e.g., DIC, acute renal failure, cardiovascular failure).	1:633,000 (fatal). 1:33,000 (nonfatal).
Alloimmune minor transfusion reactions due to sensitization of RBCs against foreign, minor, non-ABO antibodies. Delayed (3–10 d) reaction of extravascular hemolysis produces milder clinical and laboratory findings.	
Febrile nonhemolytic reaction (WBC or cytokine induced), including especially TRALI	1:200
Allergic transfusion reaction	1:333
Acute anaphylaxis	1:20,000–1:50,000
Acute lung injury	>1:5,000
Hemolytic transfusion reaction	1:200
Chronic	
Alloimmunization	
RBC hemolysis	1:1,500
Platelet refractoriness	1:3,300–1:10,000
Delayed hemolysis	1:4,000
Graft-versus-host disease (transfusion associated)	Unknown
Posttransfusion purpura	Rare to very uncommon
NonImmune-Mediated	
Acute (immediate)	
Volume overload	1:100–1:200
Nonimmune hemolysis (e.g., heat, cold, osmotic, mechanical)	Infrequent
Electrolyte imbalance (K^+, Mg^{2+}, Ca^{2+})	Uncommon
Chemical effects (e.g., citrate)	Uncommon
Coagulopathy (e.g., DIC; usually with massive transfusions)	Uncommon
Bacterial contamination	See below
Chronic (delayed)	
Alloimmunization	
RBC hemolysis	1:1,500
Platelet refractoriness	1:3,300–1:10,000
Delayed hemolysis	1:4,000

[72]Simon TI, Alverson DC, AuBuchon J, et al. Practice parameter for the use of red blood cell transfusions. *Arch Pathol Lab Med* 1998;122:130–138.
[73]Practice parameter for the recognition, management, and prevention of adverse consequences of
blood transfusion. College of American Pathologists.
[74]Goodnough LT, Brecher ME, Kanter MH, et al. Transfusion medicine. First of two parts—blood
transfusion. *N Engl J Med* 1999;340:438–447.

HEMATOLOGY

Graft-versus-host disease (transfusion associated)	1:400,000
Posttransfusion purpura	Rare to very uncommon
Transfusional hemosiderosis	Uncommon

Infections[a]

Viruses

Hepatitis A virus	Unknown; presumably 1:<1 million
Hepatitis B virus	1:63,000–1:200,000
Hepatitis C virus[b]	1:1,667,000
HIV I[b] and HIV II	1:2,000,000
Human T-cell lymphotrophic viruses I and II	1:641,000
Cytomegalovirus	3–12/100; infrequent with leukocyte-reduced components
Parvovirus B19. More common with plasma-derived products.	Unknown; presumably 1:<1 million
Epstein-Barr virus	Rare
Human herpes virus 8	3.2% seroprevalence
Severe acute respiratory syndrome	Not known but has been isolated from blood
West Nile, other arboviruses	Regional/seasonal risk; incidence of transmission during 2003 ~1:1 million recipients

Prions

Classic and variant Creutzfeldt-Jakob diseases (CJD)	One probable case reported in United Kingdom. Has eliminated ≤5% of donors. Caused CJD disease in recipients of cadaveric dura mater grafts.[c]

Bacteria

Syphilis	Not reported since 1968; <1,000,000
Malaria	<1,000,000
Bacterial contamination—platelet units (e.g., *Staphylococcus aureus*, *Klebsiella pneumoniae*, *Serratia marcescens*, *S. epidermidis*)	Contamination found in 1:500–1:2,500 units in United States. Mortality rates = 1:20,000–1:85,000
Bacterial contamination—RBCs	7:12,000,000
Chlamydia pneumoniae	Is likely but no definite evidence.
Rocky Mountain spotted fever (*Rickettsia rickettsii*), *Rickettsia* (reclassified as bacterium)	

Parasites

Plasmodium sp.	1:4 million
Babesia sp.	<1:1 million. >20 reported cases.
Trypanosoma cruzi (see Chagas disease)	Unknown; presumably <1:1 million. Seroprevalence 1:7,500 in Los Angeles. Nine reported cases.
Leishmania sp.	<1:20 million
Borrelia burgdorferi (Lyme disease)	No reported cases
Anaplasma phagocytophilum (Human granulocytic ehrlichiosis) and *Ehrlichia chaffeensis* (ehrlichiosis)	One reported case
Toxoplasma gondii	Few or no cases
Wuchereria bancrofti (lymphatic filariasis)	Few or no cases

TRALI, transfusion-related acute lung injury.

[a]Some data from: Pomper GJ. Risks of transfusion-transmitted infections. *Curr Opin Hematol* 2003;10:405; Fiebig EW, Busch MP. Emerging infections in transfusion medicine. *Clin Lab Med* 2004;24:797; Stramer SL, et al. *N Engl J Med* 2004;35 1:760; and Transfusion Medicine. *The ACP Guide for Hospitalists*. March 2006.

[b]New nucleic acid tests may detect ≤5 HIV-1 and ≤100 HCV–infected units/y that were previously seronegative.

[c]*Morbid Mortal Weekly Rep* Dec. 2003;48:1179.

Transfusion-Related Acute Lung Injury

TRALI is a recently recognized cause of immediate transfusion reactions (dyspnea, hypoxemia, fever, and possibly hypotension) possibly caused by the presence of donor leukocyte antibodies or lipids (e.g., endotoxin and platelet activating factor), especially in multiparous women transfused into patients who have had recent surgery, infection, or massive transfusion. Mortality = 5% to 10%; 80% resolve within 4 days.

Adverse Effects of Marrow Transplantation

Acute GVHD develops in 25% to 30% of recipients and is fatal in 8%.
Chronic GVHD develops in 20% to 30% of patients who survive >6 months.
Most infections occur within 6 months. Interstitial pneumonia occurs in 16% of those conditioned by cyclophosphamide and ≤50% of those conditioned with whole-body irradiation: mortality is 40% to 50%; half of cases are caused by CMV and half are of unknown cause. Classic Creutzfeldt-Jakob disease cornea, dura mater, pituitary hormone.

Indications for Red Cell Transfusion

Hb <8 g/dL (Hct <26%) and MCV within normal limits (81–100 fL; 70–125 fL if age 14 years or less)
Hb <8 g/dL (Hct <26%) in patients with acute bleed or high risk*
Hb <11 g/dL (Hct <36%) and clinically symptomatic*†
Hb <11 g/dL (Hct <36%) or bleeding >1 unit/24 h
Any Hb level in high-risk* patients with acute bleed
Any Hb level in symptomatic*† patients with acute bleed
Any Hb level in patients bleeding >2 units/24 h or >15% of blood volume/24 h
Death is unlikely until Hb falls to 3 g/dL or Hct to 10%.
After bleeding has stopped, one unit of packed RBCs typically increases recipient's Hct by 2% to 3% and Hb 1 g/dL; 2 units increases Hct ~6.4% and Hb ~2 g/dL.

Indications for Cryoprecipitate (Cryoprecipitated AHF) Transfusion

Received massive transfusions >8 units/24 h
Received transfusion of >6 RBC units/case (e.g., open heart surgery)
Bleeding or invasive procedure in patients with hypofibrinogenemia or DIC.
Deficient factor VIII or vWD (if desmopressin acetate or factor VIII are not effective or available), or abnormal or markedly decreased fibrinogen in bleeding patients or before surgery or invasive procedure
Typical bag of cryoprecipitate contains 100 units of factor VIII (the amount normally present in 100 mL of plasma)
Risk of viral transmission same as for 1 unit of packed RBCs

Indications for Fresh Frozen Plasma Transfusion

In actively bleeding patients or before surgery or invasive procedures documented by (1) increased PT >1.5 times midnormal range (usually >18 seconds) or (2) increased aPTT >1.5 times upper normal range (usually >55–60 seconds) (normal fibrinogen and no heparin in specimen); and (3) coagulation assay <25% activity:

- After massive blood transfusion (>1 blood volume within several hours with evidence of coagulation deficiency)
- Deficient various coagulation factors or vWD (if desmopressin acetate or factor VIII are not effective or available)
- Reverse warfarin effect for immediate hemostasis when PT >18 seconds; INR >1.6

---

*High risk: Coronary artery disease, chronic pulmonary disease, cerebrovascular disease, or known anemia.
†Symptomatic: Patients with signs or symptoms of anemia (such as tachycardia, angina, electrocardiographic changes) or of respiratory distress; known hemoglobinopathy, etc.

• Deficiency of antithrombin (when concentrate is not available), protein C, protein S, heparin cofactor II

Hypoglobulinemia (rarely).
Plasma exchange for TTP or HUS
Contraindicated as volume expander
Each unit increases any clotting factor by 2% to 3% in average adult

Indications for Platelet Transfusion

Unit of platelets = $5.5 \times 10^{10}/\mu L$.
Platelet count >50,000/μL: unlikely to be needed; bleeding unlikely due to low count
Platelet count <5,000/μL

• Spontaneous bleeding is likely except in platelet destruction disorders; prophylactic use is indicated.

Platelet count <10,000/μL

• Prophylactic with minor hemorrhage; fever

Platelet count <20,000 in patients

• Without TTP, ITP, posttransfusion purpura, or HUS
• Prophylactic in leukemia in presence of coagulation disorders, during induction therapy
• Before minor surgical procedures

Platelet count <50,000 in patients with

• Minor bleeding
• Preoperatively for a minor procedure
• Prematurity
• High blast count

Platelet count <90,000 in patients with

• Bleed requiring RBC transfusion
• Preoperatively for a major procedure

Received massive RBC transfusion (>8 units/24 h)
BT >10 minutes
Received transfusion of >6 RBC units/case (e.g., open heart surgery)
Platelets are used only in first 5 days because of contamination
Incidence of bacterial contamination: ~1:500 to 1:2,000
Each platelet transfusion is accompanied by 200 to 400 mL of donor plasma

12

Metabolic and Hereditary Disorders

METAB/HERED

METAB/HERED

METAB/HERED

Acid-Base Disorders

See Tables 12-1 to 12-4.

pH represents the negative logarithm of H^+ concentration; changes nonlinearly masking magnitude of acid-base disorders.

In analyzing acid-base disorders, several points should be kept in mind:

- Determination of pH and blood gases should preferentially be performed on arterial blood. Venous blood is useless for judging oxygenation or if perfusion is not adequate, but it offers an estimate of acid-base status. Venous pH is ~0.03 to 0.04 lower than in arterial blood, and CO_2 pressure (pCO_2) is normally ~3 to 4 mm higher.
- Blood specimens should be packed in ice immediately; a delay of even a few minutes will cause erroneous results, especially if the white blood cell (WBC) count is high.
- Determination of electrolytes, pH, and blood gases should be performed on blood specimens obtained simultaneously, since the acid-base situation may be very labile.
- Repeated determinations are often indicated because of the development of complications, the effect of therapy, and other factors.
- Acid-base disorders are often mixed rather than in the pure form. These mixed disorders may represent simultaneously occurring diseases, complications superimposed on the primary condition, or the effect of treatment.
- Changes in chronic forms may be notably different from those in the acute forms.
- For judging hypoxemia, it is also necessary to know the patient's hemoglobin (Hb) or hematocrit (Hct) and whether the patient was breathing room air or oxygen when the specimen was drawn.
- Arterial blood gases cannot be interpreted without clinical information about the patient.

Renal compensation for a respiratory disturbance is slower (3 to 7 days) but more successful than respiratory compensation for a metabolic disturbance but cannot completely compensate for arterial CO_2 pressure ($PaCO_2$) >65 mm Hg, unless another stimulus for HCO_3 retention is present. The respiratory mechanism responds quickly but can only eliminate sufficient CO_2 to balance the most mild metabolic acidosis.

See Figures 12-1 and 12-2 and Table 12-5.

Most laboratories measure pH and pCO_2 directly and calculate HCO_3 using the Henderson-Hasselbalch equation:

$$\text{Arterial pH} = 6.1 + \log [(HCO_3) + (0.03 \times pCO_2)]$$

where 6.1 is the dissociation constant for CO_2 in aqueous solution and 0.03 is a constant for the solubility of CO_2 in plasma at 37°C.

Table 12-1.   Metabolic and Respiratory Acid-Base Changes in Blood

	pH	pCO_2	HCO_3^-
Acidosis			
Acute metabolic	D	N	D
Compensated metabolic	N	D	D
Acute respiratory	D	I	N
Compensated respiratory	N	I	I
Alkalosis			
Acute metabolic	I	N	I
Chronic metabolic	I	I	I
Acute respiratory	I	D	N
Compensated respiratory	N	D	D

D = decreased; I = increased; N = normal.

METAB/HERED

Table 12-2.   Illustrative Serum Electrolyte Values in Various Conditions

Condition	pH	HCO_3^-	Potassium	Sodium	Chloride
Normal	7.35–7.45	24–26	3.5–5.0	136–145	100–106
Metabolic acidosis					
Diabetic acidosis	7.2	10	5.6	122	80
Fasting	7.2	16	5.2	142	100
Severe diarrhea	7.2	12	3.2	128	96
Hyperchloremic acidosis	7.2	12	5.2	142	116
Addison's disease	7.2	22	6.5	111	72
Nephritis	7.2	8	4.0	129	90
Nephrosis	7.2	20	5.5	138	113
Metabolic alkalosis					
Vomiting	7.6	38	3.2	150	94
Pyloric obstruction	7.6	58	3.2	132	42
Duodenal obstruction	7.6	42	3.2	138	49
Respiratory acidosis	7.1	30	5.5	142	80
Respiratory alkalosis	7.6	14	5.5	136	112

A normal pH does not ensure the absence of an acid-base disturbance if the pCO_2 is not known.
An abnormal HCO_3 indicates a metabolic rather than a respiratory problem;

- Decreased HCO_3^- indicates metabolic acidosis.
- Increased HCO_3^- indicates metabolic alkalosis.
- Respiratory acidosis is associated with a pCO_2 >45 mm Hg.
- Respiratory alkalosis is associated with a pCO_2 <35 mm Hg.
- Thus, mixed metabolic and respiratory acidosis is characterized by low pH, low HCO_3^-, and high pCO_2.
- Mixed metabolic and respiratory alkalosis is characterized by high pH, high HCO_3^-, and low pCO_2.

In severe metabolic acidosis, respiratory compensation is limited by inability to hyperventilate pCO_2 to $<\sim 15$ mmHg; beyond that, small increments of the H^+ ion produce disastrous changes in pH and prognosis; thus patients with lung disorders (e.g., chronic obstructive pulmonary disease [COPD], neuromuscular weakness) are very

Table 12-3.   Upper Limits of Arterial Blood pH and HCO_3^- Concentrations (Expected for Blood pCO_2 Values)

	Arterial Blood	
pCO_2 (mm Hg)	pH	HCO_3^- (mEq/ L)
20	7.66	22.8
30	7.53	25.6
40	7.57	27.3
60	7.29	27.9
80	7.18	28.9

Values shown are the upper limits of the 95% confidence bands.
Source: Coe FL. Metabolic alkalosis. *JAMA* 1977;238:2288.

Table 12-4. Summary of Pure and Mixed Acid-Base Disorders

	Decreased pH	Normal pH	Increased pH
Increased pCO_2	Respiratory acidosis with or without incompletely compensated metabolic alkalosis or coexisting metabolic acidosis	Respiratory acidosis and compensated metabolic alkalosis	Metabolic alkalosis with incompletely compensated respiratory acidosis or coexisting respiratory acidosis
Normal pCO_2	Metabolic acidosis	Normal	Metabolic alkalosis
Decreased pCO_2	Metabolic acidosis with incompletely compensated respiratory alkalosis or coexisting respiratory alkalosis	Respiratory alkalosis and compensated metabolic acidosis	Respiratory alkalosis with or without incompletely compensated metabolic acidosis or coexisting metabolic alkalosis

Source: Adapted from Friedman HH. *Problem-oriented medical diagnosis*, 3rd ed. Boston: Little, Brown, 1983.

vulnerable because they cannot compensate by hyperventilation. In metabolic alkalosis, respiratory compensation is limited by CO_2 retention, which rarely causes pCO_2 >50 to 60 mm Hg (because increased CO_2 and hypoxemia stimulate respiration very strongly); thus, pH is not returned to normal.

Base excess (BE) is a number that hypothetically "corrects" pH to 7.40 by first "adjusting" pCO_2 to 40 mmHg, thereby allowing comparison of resultant HCO_3^- with normal value at that pH (24 mEq/L). Normal $= -2$ to $+2$ mEq/L.

BE can be calculated from by determined values for pH and HCO_3^- by this formula:

$$BE \ (mEq/L) = HCO_3^- + 10(7.40 - pH) - 24$$

Negative BE indicates depletion of HCO_3^-. It does not distinguish primary from compensatory derangement.

See Table 12-6.

(1) Respiratory Alkalosis

Respiratory alkalosis is defined as a decreased pCO_2 of <38 mm Hg.

Caused By
Hyperventilation

- Central nervous system (CNS) disorders (e.g., infection, tumor, trauma, cerebrovascular accident, anxiety-hyperventilation)
- Hypoxia (e.g., high altitudes, ventilation-perfusion imbalance)
  - Cardiovascular (e.g. congestive heart failure, hypotension)
  - Pulmonary disease (e.g., pneumonia, pulmonary emboli, asthma, pneumothorax)
- Drugs (e.g., salicylate intoxication, methylxanthines, β-adrenergic agonists)
- Metabolic (e.g., acidosis [diabetic, renal, lactic], liver failure)
- Others (e.g., fever, pregnancy, Gram-negative sepsis, pain)
- Mechanical overventilation, cardiopulmonary bypass

Laboratory Findings
Acute hypocapnia—usually only a modest decrease in plasma HCO_3^- concentrations and marked alkalosis
Chronic hypocapnia—usually only a slight alkaline pH (not usually >7.55)

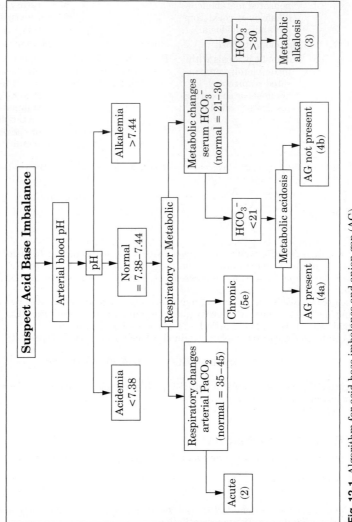

Fig. 12-1. Algorithm for acid-base imbalance and anion gap (AG).

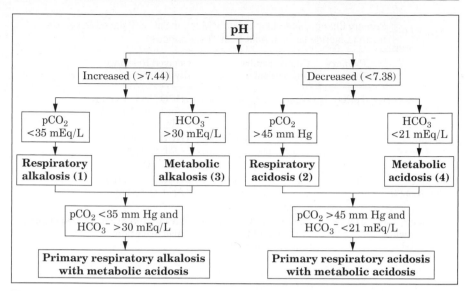

Fig. 12-2. Algorithm illustrating effects of metabolic and respiratory acid-base changes in blood.

(2) Respiratory Acidosis

Laboratory findings differ in acute and chronic conditions.

(2a) Acute

Caused by decreased alveolar ventilation impairing CO_2 excretion:

- Cardiopulmonary (e.g., pneumonia, pneumothorax, pulmonary edema, foreign body aspiration, laryngospasm, bronchospasm, mechanical ventilation, cardiac arrest)
- CNS depression (e.g., general anesthesia, drugs, brain injury, infection)
- Neuromuscular (e.g., Guillain-Barré syndrome, hypokalemia, myasthenic crisis)

Acidosis is severe (pH 7.05–7.10), but HCO_3^- concentration is only 29 to 30 mEq/L. Severe mixed acidosis is common in cardiac arrest, when respiratory and circulatory failure causes marked respiratory acidosis and severe lactic acidosis.

Table 12-5. Immediate and Delayed Compensatory Response to Acid-Base Disturbances

Acid-Base Abnormality	Immediate Response (By Lungs)	Delayed Response (By Kidneys)
Respiratory alkalosis (1)	↑pCO_2 by decreasing ventilation	↓HCO_3^- excretion. ↓Acid excretion
Respiratory acidosis (2)	↓pCO_2 by increasing ventilation	↑HCO_3^- retention. ↑Acid excretion
Metabolic alkalosis (3)	↑pCO_2 by decreasing ventilation	↓HCO_3^- excretion. ↓Acid excretion
Metabolic acidosis (4)	↓pCO_2 by increasing ventilation	↑HCO_3^- retention. ↑Acid excretion

↑, increases;   ↓, decreases.

METAB/HERED

Table 12-6.	Primary Change, and Compensatory Mechanisms in Delayed Response to, and Chloride Level in Acid-Base Disturbances			
	Primary Change	Compensatory Mechanism	Delayed Response (By Kidneys)	Cl^-
Respiratory alkalosis (1)	$\downarrow pCO_2$	None.	$\downarrow HCO_3^-$ 3–5 mmol/L for every 10 mm Hg $\uparrow pCO_2$	$\uparrow$
Respiratory acidosis (2)	$\uparrow pCO_2$	$\uparrow HCO_3^-$ 1 mmol/L for every 10 mm Hg$\uparrow pCO_2$.	$\uparrow HCO_3^-$ 3–5 mmol/L for every 10 mm Hg $\uparrow pCO_2$.	$\downarrow$
Metabolic alkalosis (3)	$\uparrow HCO_3^-$	$\uparrow pCO_2$ 3–5 mm Hg for every 10 mmol/L $\uparrow HCO_3^-$	$\downarrow HCO_3^-$ excretion. $\downarrow$ Acid excretion	$\downarrow$
Metabolic acidosis with increased anion gap (4a)	$\downarrow HCO_3^-$	$\downarrow pCO_2$ 1.0–1.3 mm Hg mmol/L for every 1 mmol/L $\uparrow HCO_3^-$	$\uparrow HCO_3^-$ retention $\uparrow$ Acid excretion	No change
Metabolic acidosis normal anion gap (4b)	$\downarrow HCO_3^-$	pCO_2 changes 2 for every pH change after decimal (e.g., if pH = 7.25, $pCO_2 = 25 \pm 2$).		$\uparrow$
Respiratory alkalosis (1)	$\downarrow pCO_2$	*Acute:* none *Chronic:* $\downarrow HCO_3^-$ 3–5 mmol/L for every 10 mm Hg $\uparrow pCO_2$.		$\uparrow$
Respiratory acidosis (2)	$\uparrow pCO_2$	*Acute:* $\uparrow HCO_3^-$ 1 mmol/L for every 10 mm Hg $\uparrow pCO_2$ *Chronic:* $\uparrow HCO_3^-$ 3–5 mmol/L for every 10 mm Hg $\uparrow pCO_2$		$\downarrow$
Metabolic alkalosis (3)	$\uparrow HCO_3^-$	$\uparrow pCO_2$ 3 to 5 mm Hg for every 10 mmol/L $\uparrow HCO_3^-$		$\downarrow$
Metabolic acidosis with increased anion gap (4a)	$\downarrow HCO_3^-$	$\downarrow pCO_2$ 1.0–1.3 mm Hg for every 1 mmol/L $\downarrow HCO_3^-$		No change
Metabolic acidosis with normal anion gap (4b)	$\downarrow HCO_3^-$	pCO_2 changes 2 for every pH change after decimal (e.g., if pH = 7.25, $pCO_2 = 25 \pm 2$)	Hyperchloremic metabolic acidosis	$\uparrow$

$\uparrow$, increased; $\downarrow$, decreased.

(2b) Chronic

Due to chronic obstructive or restrictive conditions

- Nerve disease (e.g., poliomyelitis)
- Muscle disease (e.g., myopathy)
- CNS disorder (e.g., brain tumor)

- Restriction of thorax (e.g., musculoskeletal, scleroderma, Pickwickian syndrome)
- Pulmonary disease (e.g., prolonged pneumonia, primary alveolar hypoventilation)

Acidosis is not usually severe.

Beware of commonly occurring mixed acid-base disturbances (e.g., chronic respiratory acidosis with superimposed acute hypercapnia resulting from acute infection, such as bronchitis or pneumonia).

Superimposed metabolic alkalosis (e.g., due to diuretics or vomiting) may exacerbate the hypercapnia.

(3) Metabolic Alkalosis

Caused By

Loss of acid:

- Vomiting, gastric suction, gastrocolic fistula
- Diarrhea in mucoviscidosis (rarely)
- Villous adenoma of colon
- Aciduria secondary to potassium depletion

Excess of base caused by administration of:

- Absorbable antacids (e.g., sodium bicarbonate; milk-alkali syndrome)
- Salts of weak acids (e.g., sodium lactate, sodium or potassium citrate)
- Some vegetarian diets
- Citrate due to massive blood transfusions

Potassium depletion (causing sodium and H^+ to enter the cells):

- Gastrointestinal (GI) loss (e.g., chronic diarrhea)
- Lack of potassium intake (e.g., anorexia nervosa, intravenous fluids without potassium supplements for treatment of vomiting or postoperatively)
- Diuresis (e.g., mercurials, thiazides, osmotic diuresis)
- Extracellular volume depletion and chloride depletion
- Dehydration reducing intracellular volume, thereby stimulating aldosterone, causing excretion of potassium and H^+
- All forms of mineralocorticoid excess (e.g., primary aldosteronism, Cushing syndrome, administration of steroids, large amounts of licorice) causing excretion of potassium and H^+
- Glycogen deposition
- Chronic alkalosis
- Potassium-losing nephropathy

Hypoproteinemia per se may cause a nonrespiratory alkalosis. Decreased albumin of 1g/dL causes an average increase in standard bicarbonate of 3.4 mmol/L, an apparent base excess of $+3.7$ mEq/L, and a decrease in anion gap (AG) of ~ 3 mEq/L.

Laboratory Findings

Serum pH is increased (>7.60 in severe alkalemia).

Total plasma CO_2 is increased (bicarbonate >30 mEq/L).

pCO_2 is normal or slightly increased.

Serum pH and bicarbonate above those predicted by the pCO_2 (by nomogram or Table 12-3).

Hypokalemia is an almost constant feature and is the chief danger in metabolic alkalosis.

Decreased serum chloride is relatively lower than sodium.

Blood urea nitrogen (BUN) may be increased.

Urine pH is >7.0 (≤ 7.9) if potassium depletion is not severe and concomitant sodium deficiency (e.g., vomiting) is not present. With severe hypokalemia (<2.0 mEq/L), urine may be acid in presence of systemic alkalosis.

○ Metabolic alkalosis patients may be volume depleted and chloride responsive or have volume expansion and be chloride resistant. When the urine chloride is low (<10 mEq/L) and the patient responds to chloride treatment, the cause is more likely loss of gastric juice, diuretic therapy, or rapid relief of chronic hypercapnia. Chloride replacement is completed when urine chloride remains >40 mEq/L. When the urine chloride is high (>20 mEq/L) and the patient does not respond to NaCl treatment, the cause is more likely hyperadrenalism or severe potassium deficiency.

METAE/HERED

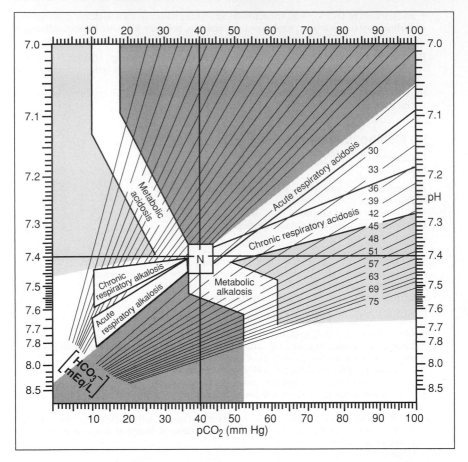

Fig. 12-3. Acid-base map. The values demarcated for each disorder represent a 95% probability range for each *pure* disorder. Coordinates lying outside these zones suggest mixed acid-base disorders. N, normal. (Adapted from Goldberg M, Green SB, Moss ML, et al. Computer-based instruction and diagnosis of acid-base disorders. *JAMA* 1973;223:269.)

Acid-base maps (see Figure 12-3) are a graphic solution of the Henderson-Hasselbalch equation, which predicts the HCO_3^- value for each set of pH/pCO_2 coordinates. They also allow a check of the consistency of arterial blood gas and automated analyzer determinations, since these may determine the total CO_2 content, of which 95% is HCO_3^-. These maps contain bands that show the 95% probability range of values for each disorder. If the pH/pCO_2 coordinate is outside the 95% confidence band, then the patient has at least two acid-base disturbances. These maps are of particular use when one of the acid-base disturbances is not suspected clinically. If the coordinates lie within a band, it is not a guarantee of a simple acid-base disturbance.

Anion Gap Classification

AG is arithmetic approximation of difference between routinely measured serum anions and cations = 23 mEq/L minus 11 mEq/L = 12 mEq/L.
Unmeasured ions include proteins (mostly albumin) = 15 mEq/L, organic acids = 5 mEq/L, phosphates = 2 mEq/L, sulfates = 1 mEq/L; total = 23 mEq/L.
Unmeasured cations include calcium = 5 mEq/L, potassium = 4.5 mEq/L, magnesium = 1.5 mEq/L; total = 11 mEq/L.

Calculated as $Na^+ - (Cl^- + HCO_3^-)$; typical normal values = 8 to 16 mEq/L; if K^+ is included, normal = 10 to 20 mEq/L; reference interval varies considerably depending on instrumentation and between individuals. Increased AG reflects amount of organic (e.g., lactic acid, ketoacids) and fixed acids present.

AG initially began as a measure of quality assurance.

Use

Identify cause of a metabolic acidosis

Supplement to laboratory quality control, along with its components

Increased AG In

○ Increased "unmeasured" anions
- Organic (e.g., lactic acidosis, ketoacidosis)
- Inorganic (e.g., administration of phosphate, sulfate)
- Protein (e.g., hyperalbuminemia, transient)
- Exogenous (e.g., salicylate, formate, paraldehyde, nitrate, penicillin, carbenicillin)
- Not completely identified (e.g., hyperosmolar hyperglycemic nonketotic coma, uremia, poisoning by ethylene glycol, methanol)
- Artifactual
  Falsely increased serum sodium
  Falsely decreased serum chloride or bicarbonate

○ *When AG >12 to 14 mEq/L, diabetic ketoacidosis is the most common cause, uremic acidosis is the second most common cause, and drug ingestion (e.g., salicylates, methyl alcohol, ethylene glycol, ethyl alcohol) is the third most common cause; lactic acidosis should always be considered when these three causes are ruled out. In small children, rule out inborn errors of metabolism.*

♦ Mnemonic for AG acidosis: *A MUDPIE*: A, aspirin; M, methyl alcohol; U, uremia; D, diabetic acidosis; P, propyl alcohol or paraldehyde administration; I, isopropyl alcohol or idiopathic lactic acidosis; E, ethylene glycol.

Decreased AG (<6 mEq/L) In

○ Decreased unmeasured anion (e.g., hypoalbuminemia is probably commonest cause of decreased AG); also hypocalcemia, hypomagnesemia.

○ Artifactual
- "Hyperchloremia" in bromide intoxication (if chloride determination by colorimetric method)
- False increase in serum chloride or HCO_3^-
- False decrease in serum sodium (e.g., hyperlipidemia, hyperviscosity)

○ Increased unmeasured cations
- Hyperkalemia, hypercalcemia, hypermagnesemia
- Increased proteins in multiple myeloma, paraproteinemias, polyclonal gammopathies (these abnormal proteins are positively charged and lower the AG)
- Increased lithium, tris buffer (tromethamine)

○ *AG >30 mEq/L almost always indicates organic acidosis, even in presence of uremia.*

AG = 20 to 29 mEq/L occurs in absence of identified organic acidosis in 25% of patients.

AG is rarely >23 mEq/L in chronic renal failure.

Simultaneous changes in ions may cancel each other out, leaving AG unchanged (e.g., increased Cl and decreased HCO_3^-).

Change in AG should equal change in HCO_3^-; otherwise a mixed rather than simple acid-base disturbance is present.

(4) Metabolic Acidosis

(4a) With Increased Anion Gap (AG >15 mEq/L)

Lactic acidosis—commonest cause of metabolic acidosis with increased AG (frequently >25 mEq/L) (see following section)

Renal failure (AG <25 mEq/L)

Ketoacidosis

- Diabetes mellitus (AG frequently >25 mEq/L)
- Associated with alcohol abuse (AG frequently 20 to 25 mEq/L)
- Starvation (AG usually 5 to 10 mEq/L)

Drugs

- Salicylate poisoning (AG frequently 5 to 10 mEq/L; higher in children)
- Methanol poisoning (AG frequently >20 mEq/L)

METAB/HERED

- Ethylene glycol poisoning (AG frequently >20 mEq/L)
- Paraldehyde (AG frequently >20 mEq/L)

(4b) With Normal Anion Gap (AG)
Hyperchloremic metabolic acidosis

Decreased serum potassium

- Renal tubular acidosis (RTA)
  Acquired (e.g., drugs, hypercalcemia)
  Inherited (e.g., cystinosis, Wilson disease)
  Carbonic anhydrase inhibitors (e.g., acetazolamide, mafenide)
- Increased loss of alkaline body fluids (e.g., diarrhea, loss of pancreatic or biliary fluids)
- Ureteral diversion (e.g., ileal bladder or ureter, ureterosigmoidostomy)

Normal or increased serum potassium

- Hydronephrosis
- Early renal failure
- Administration of HCl (e.g., ammonium chloride)
- Hypoadrenalism (diffuse, zona glomerulosa, or hyporeninemia)
- Renal aldosterone resistance
- Sulfur toxicity

In lactic acidosis, the increase in AG is usually greater than the decrease in HCO_3^-, in contrast to diabetic ketoacidosis, in which the increase in AG is identical to the decrease in HCO_3^-.

Laboratory Findings
Serum pH is decreased (<7.3).
Total plasma CO_2 content is decreased; <15 mEq/L almost certainly rules out respiratory alkalosis.
Serum potassium is frequently increased; it is decreased in RTA, diarrhea, or carbonic anhydrase inhibition. Increased serum chloride.
Azotemia suggests metabolic acidosis due to renal failure.
Urine is strongly acid (pH = 4.5–5.2) if renal function is normal.
In evaluating acid-base disorders, calculate the AG (see previous).

Lactic Acidosis
Indicates acute hypoperfusion and tissue hypoxia.
Should be considered in any metabolic acidosis with increased AG (>15 mEq/L).
Diagnosis is confirmed by exclusion of other causes of metabolic acidosis and serum lactate ≥5 mEq/L (upper limit of normal = 1.6 for plasma and 1.4 for whole blood). There is considerable variation in the literature in limits of serum lactate and pH to define lactic acidosis.
Exclusion of other causes by

- Normal serum creatinine and BUN *(increased acetoacetic acid [but not beta-hydroxybutyric acid] will cause false increase of creatinine by colorimetric assay)*
- Osmolar gap <10 mOsm/L
- Negative nitroprusside reaction *(nitroprusside test for keto-acidosis measures acetoacetic acid but not β-hydroxybutyric acid; thus blood ketone test may be negative in diabetic ketoacidosis)*
- Urine negative for calcium oxalate crystals
- No known ingestion of toxic substances

Laboratory findings due to underlying diseases (e.g., diabetes mellitus, renal insufficiency, etc.)
Laboratory tests for monitoring therapy:

- Arterial pH, pCO_2, HCO_3^-, serum electrolytes every 1 to 2 hours until patient is stable
- Urine electrolytes every 6 hours

Associated or compensatory metabolic or respiratory disturbances (e.g., hyperventilation or respiratory alkalosis may result in normal pH)

Caused By

Type A due to tissue hypoxia (e.g., acute hemorrhage, severe anemia, shock, asphyxia), marathon running, seizures
Type B without tissue hypoxia caused by:

- Common disorders (e.g., diabetes mellitus, uremia, liver disease, infections, malignancies, alkaloses)
- Drugs and toxins (e.g., ethanol, methanol, ethylene glycol, salicylates, metformin)
- Hereditary enzyme defects (e.g., methylmalonic acidemia, propionic aciduria, defects of fatty acid oxidation, pyruvate-dehydrogenase deficiency, pyruvate-carboxylase deficiency, multiple carboxylase deficiency, glycogen storage disease [GSD] type I).
- Others (e.g., starvation, short-bowel syndrome)

With a typical clinical picture (acute onset following nausea and vomiting, altered state of consciousness, hyperventilation, high mortality)

- Decreased serum bicarbonate
- Low serum pH, usually 6.98 to 7.25
- Increased serum potassium, often 6 to 7 mEq/L
- Serum chloride normal or low with increased AG
- ○ • Increased serum phosphorus. Phosphorus:creatinine ratio >3 indicates lactic acidosis either alone or as a component of other metabolic acidosis.
- WBC count is increased (occasionally to leukemoid levels).
- Increased serum uric acid is frequent (up to 25 mg/dL in lactic acidosis)
- Increased serum aspartate aminotransferase (AST), lactase dehydrogenase (LD), and phosphorus

See Table 12-3.

(5) Mixed Acid-Base Disturbances

Mixed acid-base disturbances must always be interpreted with clinical data and other laboratory findings.

See Table 12-7.

(5a) Respiratory Acidosis with Metabolic Acidosis

Examples: Acute pulmonary edema, cardiopulmonary arrest (lactic acidosis due to tissue anoxia and CO_2 retention due to alveolar hypoventilation)
Acidemia may be extreme with

- pH <7.0 (H^+ >100 mEq/L)
- HCO_3^- <26 mEq/L. Failure of HCO_3^- to increase ≥3 mEq/L for each 10 mm Hg rise in pCO_2 suggests metabolic acidosis with respiratory acidosis.

Mild metabolic acidosis superimposed on chronic hypercapnia causing partial suppression of HCO_3^- may be indistinguishable from adaptation to hypercapnia alone.

(5b) Respiratory Acidosis with Metabolic Alkalosis

Examples: Chronic pulmonary disease with CO_2 retention developing metabolic alkalosis due to administration of diuretics, severe vomiting, or sudden improvement in ventilation ("posthypercapnic" metabolic alkalosis)
○ Decreased or absent urine chloride indicates that chloride-responsive metabolic alkalosis is a part of the picture.
○ In clinical setting of respiratory acidosis but with normal blood pH and/or HCO_3 higher than predicted, complicating metabolic alkalosis may be present.

(5c) Metabolic Acidosis with Respiratory Alkalosis

Examples: Rapid correction of severe metabolic acidosis, salicylate intoxication, Gram-negative septicemia, initial respiratory alkalosis with subsequent development of metabolic acidosis. *Primary metabolic acidosis with primary respiratory alkalosis with an increased AG is characteristic of salicylate intoxication in absence of uremia and diabetic ketoacidosis.*

METAB/HERED

Table 12-7. Illustrative Serum Values in Acid-Base Disturbances

Condition	Sodium (mEq/L)	Chloride (mEq/L)	HCO$_3$$^-$ (mEq/L)	pCO$_2$ (mm Hg)	pH
Normal	140	105	25	40	7.40
Metabolic acidosis	140	115	15	31	7.30
Chronic respiratory alkalosis	136	102	25	40	7.44
Mixed metabolic acidosis and chronic respiratory alkalosis (e.g., sepsis: addition of respiratory alkalosis to metabolic acidosis further decreases HCO$_3$$^-$ but pH may remain normal; lactic acidosis plus respiratory alkalosis due to severe liver disease, pulmonary emboli, or sepsis)	136	108	14	24	7.39
Metabolic alkalosis	140	92	36	48	7.49
Chronic respiratory acidosis	140	100–102	28	50	7.37
Mixed metabolic alkalosis and chronic respiratory acidosis (e.g., patient with COPD receiving glucocorticoids or diuretics; pCO$_2$ and HCO$_3$$^-$ are increased by both conditions, but pH is neutralized)	140	90	40	67	7.40
Metabolic alkalosis	139	89	35	47	7.49
Respiratory alkalosis	136	102	20	30	7.44
Mixed alkalosis, mild	139	92	32	39	7.53

Mixed alkalosis, severe (e.g., postoperative patient with severe hemorrhage stimulating hyperventilation [respiratory alkalosis] plus massive transfusion and nasogastric drainage [metabolic alkalosis])	139	92	32	30	7.63
Mixed chronic respiratory acidosis and acute metabolic acidosis (e.g., COPD [chronic respiratory acidosis] with severe diarrhea [metabolic acidosis]; pH is too low for pCO_2 of 55 mm Hg in chronic respiratory acidosis, indicating low pH due to mixed acidosis, but HCO_3^- effect is offset.)	136	102	22	55	7.22
Mixed metabolic acidosis and metabolic alkalosis (e.g., gastroenteritis with vomiting [metabolic alkalosis] and diarrhea [metabolic acidosis due to loss of HCO_3^-]; surprisingly normal findings with marked volume depletion)	140	103	25	40	7.40

METAB/HERED

571

pH may be normal or decreased.

Hypocapnia remains inappropriate to decreased HCO_3^- for several hours or more.

(5d) Metabolic Alkalosis with Respiratory Alkalosis

Examples: Hepatic insufficiency with hyperventilation plus administration of diuretics or severe vomiting; metabolic alkalosis with stimulation of ventilation (e.g., sepsis, pulmonary embolism, mechanical ventilation), which causes respiratory alkalosis

Marked alkalemia with decreased pCO_2 and increased HCO_3^- is diagnostic.

(5e) Acute and Chronic Respiratory Acidosis

Examples: Chronic hypercapnia with acute deterioration of pulmonary function causing further rise of pCO_2.

May be suspected when HCO_3^- is in intermediate range between acute and chronic respiratory acidosis (similar findings in chronic respiratory acidosis with superimposed metabolic acidosis or acute respiratory acidosis with superimposed metabolic alkalosis)

(5f) Coexistence of Metabolic Acidosis of Hyperchloremic Type and Increased AG

Examples: uremia and proximal RTA, lactic acidosis with diarrhea, excessive administration of NaCl to patient with organic acidosis

May be suspected by plasma HCO_3^- that is lower than is explained by the increase in anions (e.g., AG = 16 mEq/L and HCO_3^- = 5 mEq/L)

(5g) Coexistence of Metabolic Alkalosis and Metabolic Acidosis

Examples: Vomiting causing alkalosis plus bicarbonate-losing diarrhea causing acidosis

May be suspected by acid-base values that are too normal for clinical picture

Pearls

Pulmonary embolus: Mild to moderate respiratory alkalosis is present unless sudden death occurs. The degree of hypoxia often correlates with the size and extent of the pulmonary embolus. pO_2 >90 mm Hg when breathing room air virtually excludes a lung problem.

Acute pulmonary edema: Hypoxemia is usual. CO_2 is not increased unless the situation is grave.

Asthma: Hypoxia occurs even during a mild episode and increases as the attack becomes worse. As hyperventilation occurs, the pCO_2 falls (usually <35 mm Hg); a normal pCO_2 (>40 mm Hg) implies impending respiratory failure; increased pCO_2 in a true asthmatic (not bronchitis or emphysema) indicates impending disaster and the need to consider intubation and ventilation assistance.

COPD (bronchitis and emphysema) may show two patterns—"pink puffers," with mild hypoxia and normal pH and pCO_2, and "blue bloaters," with hypoxia and increased pCO_2; normal pH suggests compensation and decreased pH suggests decompensation.

Neurologic and neuromuscular disorders (e.g., drug overdose, Guillain-Barré syndrome, myasthenia gravis, trauma, succinylcholine): Acute alveolar hypoventilation causes uncompensated respiratory acidosis with high pCO_2, low pH, and normal HCO_3^-. Acidosis appears before significant hypoxemia, and rising CO_2 indicates rapid deterioration and need for mechanical assistance.

Sepsis: Unexplained respiratory alkalosis may be the earliest sign of sepsis. It may progress to cause metabolic acidosis, and the mixed picture may produce a normal pH; low HCO_3^- is useful to recognize this. With deterioration and worsening of metabolic acidosis, the pH falls.

Salicylate poisoning characteristically shows poor correlation between serum salicylate level and presence or degree of acidemia (because as pH drops from 7.4 to 7.2, the proportion of nonionized to ionized salicylate doubles and the nonionized form leaves the serum and is sequestered in the brain and other organs, where it interferes with function at a cellular level without changing blood levels of glucose, etc.). Salicylate poisoning in adults typically causes respiratory alkalosis, but in children this progresses rapidly to mixed respiratory alkalosis/metabolic acidosis and then to metabolic acidosis (in adults, metabolic acidosis is said to be rare and a near-terminal event).

Isopropyl (rubbing) alcohol poisoning produces enough circulating acetone to produce a positive nitroprusside test (it therefore may be mistaken for diabetic ketoacidosis; thus insulin should not be given until the blood glucose is known). In the absence of a history, positive serum ketone test associated with normal anion gap, normal serum HCO_3^-, and normal blood glucose suggests rubbing alcohol intoxication.

A change in chloride concentration independent of, or out of proportion to, changes in sodium usually indicates an acid-base disorder.

Nutritional Deficiencies

Copper Deficiency

Copper is a metal component of various enzymes (e.g., cytochrome oxidase, superoxide dismutase, tyrosinase) involved in Hb synthesis, bone and elastic tissue development, and CNS function.

Nutritional Copper Deficiency

Found in patients on parenteral nutrition and in neonates and premature infants and children recovering from severe protein/calorie malnutrition fed iron-fortified milk formula with cane sugar and cottonseed oil.
Anemia not responsive to iron and vitamins
Leukopenia with WBC <5,000/μL and neutropenia (<1,500/μL)
♦ Copper administration corrects neutropenia in 3 weeks and anemia responds with reticulocytosis.
Decreased copper and ceruloplasmin in plasma and decreased hepatic copper confirm diagnosis.

"Kinky Hair" (Menkes) Syndrome

Menkes syndrome is an X-linked recessive error of copper metabolism caused by gene mutations that block copper transport from intestinal mucosa cells to blood, causing copper deficiency. It is a syndrome of neonatal hypothermia, feeding difficulties, and sometimes prolonged jaundice; at 2 to 3 months, seizures and progressive hair depigmentation and twisting take place. The syndrome also includes a striking facial appearance, increasing mental deterioration, infections, failure to thrive, death in early infancy and changes in the elastica interna of arteries.

♦ Decreased copper in serum and liver; normal in red blood cells (RBCs).
Increased copper in amniotic fluid, cultured fibroblasts, and amniotic cells
Decreased serum ceruloplasmin

Serum Copper Also Decreased In

Wilson disease (total copper is decreased; see Chapter 8): mutation interferes with copper transport from intestinal mucosal cytoplasm to Golgi apparatus, where it becomes bound to protein.
Nephrosis (ceruloplasmin lost in urine)
Acute leukemia in remission
Some iron-deficiency anemias of childhood (that require copper as well as iron therapy)
Kwashiorkor, chronic diarrhea
Adrenocorticotropic hormone and corticosteroids

METAB/HERED

Serum Copper Increased In

Wilson disease (free copper is increased; see Chapter 8)

Anemias

- Pernicious anemia
- Megaloblastic anemia of pregnancy
- Iron-deficiency anemia
- Aplastic anemia

Leukemia and lymphoma

Infection, acute and chronic

Biliary cirrhosis

Hemochromatosis

Collagen diseases (including systemic lupus erythematosus [SLE], rheumatoid arthritis, acute rheumatic fever, glomerulonephritis)

Hypothyroidism

Hyperthyroidism

Frequently associated with increased c-reactive protein (CRP)

Ingestion of oral contraceptives and estrogens

Pregnancy

Zinc Deficiency or Toxicity

Zinc is required for production of functionally mature T cells and for activation of T cells. It is a component of many enzymes, including DNA and RNA polymerases.

Deficiency Caused By

Acrodermatitis enteropathica (rare autosomal recessive disease of infancy due to block in intestinal absorption of zinc)

Inadequate nutrition (e.g., parenteral alimentation)

Excessive requirements

Decreased absorption or availability

Increased losses

Iatrogenic

Plasma concentrations

- Normal range = 70 to 120 μg/dL
- Moderate depletion = 40 to 60 μg/dL
- Severe depletion = 20 μg/dL

No accurate indicators of zinc status. Zinc levels in plasma, RBC, and hair are frequently misleading.

Decreased or very excessive urinary zinc excretion may be helpful.

Toxicity Caused By

Acute: ingestion of >200 mg/d

Chronic: ingestion of >25 mg/d may cause copper deficiency. Ingestion of >150 mg/d may decrease high-density lipoprotein cholesterol (HDL-C).

Failure to Thrive[1]

In evaluations for failure to thrive, premature infants (shortened gestation period) should be differentiated from infants with weight below that expected for gestational age.

Intrauterine Growth Retardation

Intrauterine growth retardation refers to low-birth-weight infants who are mature by gestational age.

---

[1]Stoler JM, Leach NT, Donahoe PK. Case records of the Massachusetts General Hospital. Case 36-2004: A 23-day-old infant with hypospadias and failure to thrive. *N Engl J Med* 2004;351:2319–2326.

Due To
Maternal factors

- Chronic hypertension, especially with renal involvement and proteinuria
- Chronic renal disease
- Severe, long-standing diabetes mellitus
- Preeclampsia and eclampsia with underlying chronic vascular disease
- Maternal protein-calorie malnutrition
- Hypoxia, e.g., cyanotic heart disease, pregnancy at high altitudes, hemoglobinopathies, especially sickle cell disease
- Alcohol and other drug abuse

Placental conditions

- Extensive infarction
- Parabiotic transfusion syndrome
- Hemangioma of placenta or cord
- Abnormal cord insertion

Fetal factors

- Chromosomal abnormalities, especially trisomies of D group and chromosome 18
- Malformations of GI tract that interfere with swallowing
- Chronic intrauterine infections (e.g., rubella, cytomegalovirus [CMV], herpes simplex virus, syphilis, toxoplasmosis)

Unexplained

Postnatal Failure to Thrive

Due To

Cause	% of Cases
Inadequate caloric intake	87
Maternal (e.g., caloric restriction, child abuse, emotional disorders)	
Congenital abnormalities (e.g., cleft lip or palate, tracheoesophageal fistula, esophageal webs, macroglossia, achalasia)	
Acquired abnormalities (e.g., esophageal stricture, subdural hematoma, hypoxia, diabetes insipidus)	
Decreased intestinal function	
Abnormal digestion, e.g.:	
Cystic fibrosis	3.0
Trypsin deficiency	
Monosaccharidase and disaccharidase deficiencies	
Abnormal absorption, e.g.:	
Celiac syndrome	0.5
Gastroenteritis	
Biliary atresia	
Megacolon	
Giardiasis	
Protein-losing enteropathy	
Increased utilization of calories	
Infant of narcotic-addicted mother	
Prolonged fever (e.g., chronic infections)	
Excessive crying	
Congenital heart disease	
Renal loss of calories	
Aminoaciduria, e.g.:	
Maple syrup urine disease	0.5
Methylmalonic academia	0.5
Chronic renal disease, e.g., renal tubular acidosis, pyelonephritis, polycystic disease, congenital/acquired nephritis, congenital nephrosis, nephrogenic diabetes insipidus	
Other	
Anemias, e.g., fetal-maternal transfusion, hemoglobinopathies, iron deficiency	

> Hypercalcemia, e.g., hyperparathyroidism, vitamin A or D
> intoxication, idiopathic
> Endocrine
> Hypothyroidism   2.5
> Hypoadrenalism
> Hyposomatotropism
> Congenital hyperthyroidism
> Metabolic
> Glycogen storage disease   0.5
> Galactosemia
> Hypophosphatasia
> Mucopolysaccharidosis
> Rickets
> CNS lesions
> Subdural hematoma   2.5
> Intracerebral hemorrhage
> Tumors
> Unknown
> CNS, central nervous system.

Laboratory Evaluation
Initial

- Pathologic examination of placenta
- Complete blood count (CBC) (anemia, hemoglobinopathy)
- Urine—reducing substances, ferric chloride test, pH, specific gravity, microscopic examination, colony count and culture
- Stool—occult blood, ova and parasites, pH
- Serum—sodium, potassium, chloride, bicarbonate, creatinine, calcium, albumin, protein
- State newborn screening

More detailed tests

- Sweat chloride and sodium (see section on cystic fibrosis)
- Serum thyroid-stimulating hormone and T_4 (hypothyroidism)
- Serum and urine amino acids (aminoacidurias) and organic acids
- Rectal biopsy
- Serologic tests for congenital infection (HIV, rubella, CMV, toxoplasmosis, syphilis)
- Duodenal enzyme measurements
- Chromosome studies (trisomy D, E)

Imaging studies (e.g., GI series, renal ultrasound, brain MRI or CT scan, echocardiography)

Adult Malnutrition and Kwashiorkor

Adult malnutrition and kwashiorkor occur in patients with inadequate protein intake in presence of low caloric intake or normal caloric intake and increased catabolism (e.g., trauma, severe burns, respiratory or renal failure, nonmalignant GI tract disease); they may develop quickly. A major loss of protein from visceral compartments may impair organ function.

○ These laboratory tests all have low sensitivity/specificity (S/S) or may not be easily available.
Decreased serum proteins

- Albumin has half-life of 21 days (2.8–3.4 mg/dL in mild deficiencies, 2.1–3.0 mg/dL in moderate deficiencies, <2.1 mg/dL in severe deficiencies) is a poor marker for early malnutrition.
- Prealbumin (transthyretin) is more sensitive than albumin because of its shorter half-life of 1.9 days. Normal range = 18 to 36 mg/dL: severe malnutrition <10.7 mg/dL; moderate malnutrition = 10.7 to 16 mg/dL; is likely to benefit from early therapy. With therapy, increases >1 mg/dL daily. Decreased in renal failure.
- Retinol-binding protein (carrier for vitamin A) has a half-life of 12 hours; is effective monitor of growth rate in preterm infants. Also decreased in impaired liver function (e.g., hepatitis, cirrhosis, obstructive jaundice), vitamin A deficiency, hyperthyroidism, and some types of amyloidosis. Increased in renal failure.

- Transferrin (150–200 mg/dL in mild, 100–150 mg/dL in moderate, <100 mg/dL in severe deficiencies) or total iron-binding capacity. Increase in transferrin caused by inflammation decreases diagnostic utility. Direct measurement is preferred because calculation is affected by iron metabolism and laboratory variability. Poor sensitivity in this condition.
- CRP rises rapidly during catabolism and declines during anabolism.
- Other protein markers with short-lives have been suggested, such as fibronectin.

Other chemistry values

- BUN is decreased.
- Fluid and electrolyte disorders are common, e.g., hyperchloremic metabolic acidosis, decreased potassium, and decreased phosphate.

Hematologic values

- Decreased total lymphocyte count evidencing diminished immunologic resistance (normal = 2,000–3,500/μL; <1,500/μL is indication for further assessment; moderate = 800–1,200/μL; severe <800/μL); should always be interpreted with total WBC count.
- Mild normochromic, normocytic anemia is common.
- All serum complement components except C4 and sometimes C5 are decreased.

Marasmus

Marasmus is a chronic deficiency in total energy intake, as in wasting illnesses (e.g., cancer) with protein loss from somatic compartment without necessary losses in visceral component.

Serum protein levels are usually normal.
Mild anemia is common.
Immune function is impaired.
Clinically, show severe wasting of skeletal muscle and fat; edema is distinctively absent. May progress to marasmic kwashiorkor.
Laboratory findings due to underlying diseases (e.g., cancer) or complications (e.g., infection).

Monitor Nutritional Therapy

Weekly 24-hour urine nitrogen excretion 1×/week reflects degree of hypermetabolism and correction of deficits.
Increase of serum prealbumin and retinol-binding proteins by 1 mg/dL/day indicates good response. Measure two to three times per week. May precede improvement in albumin levels by 7 to 10 days.
Somatomedin C has also been suggested for monitoring.
Fluid and electrolyte levels should be corrected.

Nutritional Factors in Young Children, Laboratory Indicators

BUN <6 mg/dL or urine <8 mg/g of creatinine suggests recent low protein intake.
Serum albumin <3.2 g/dL suggests low protein intake, but this is a rather insensitive nonspecific indicator of protein status.
Iron—see Chapter 11.
Vitamin A—serum carotene <40 μg/dL suggests low intake of carotene. Serum vitamin A <20 μg/dL, suggests low stores of vitamin A or may indicate failure of retinol transport out of liver into circulation.
Ascorbic acid—serum ascorbate <0.3 mg/dL suggests recent low intake. Whole blood ascorbate <0.3 mg/dL indicates low intake and reduction in body pool of ascorbic acid. Leukocyte ascorbic acid <20 mg/dL suggests poor nutritional status.
Riboflavin—<250 μg/g of creatinine in urine suggests low recent intake of riboflavin. Glutathione reductase-flavin adenine dinucleotide effect, expressed as ratio >1.2:1, suggests poor nutritional status.
Thiamine—<125 μg/g of creatinine in urine suggests low intake of thiamine. Transketolase–thiamine pyrophosphate effect, expressed as a ratio >1.5:1, suggests poor nutritional status.

Folate—serum folate <6 μg/dL suggests low intake. RBC folate <20 μg/dL or increased excretion of formiminoglutamic acid (FIGLU) in urine following histidine load suggests poor nutritional status.

Iodine—<50 μg/g of creatinine in urine suggests recent low intake of iodine.

Calcium, phosphorus, alkaline phosphatase (ALP)—rickets (see Chapter 10).

Total Parenteral Nutrition, Metabolic Complications

Decreasing serum prealbumin (transthyretin) level after 2 weeks of total parenteral nutrition (TPN) indicates poor prognosis, but increasing or unchanged level indicates anabolism and protein replenishment and suggests probable survival.

Serum cholesterol decreases rapidly during first 2 days, then remains at low level. Apolipoprotein A (Apo A) decreases 30% to 50% after long-term TPN, but Apo B is usually unchanged.

Hyperglycemia (which may cause osmotic diuresis and hyperosmolarity) or hypoglycemia.

Serum electrolytes are usually unchanged, but sodium may decrease slightly and potassium may increase slightly after fifth day. Changes depend on solution composition and infusion rate. Frequent monitoring is indicated.

Ketosis develops if insufficient calories or low glucose concentration; may indicate onset of infection.

Hyperosmolarity due to TPN infusion.

Lactic or hyperchloremic metabolic acidosis develops in some patients.

Serum creatinine and creatinine clearance are not significantly changed.

Serum uric acid decreases markedly by second to 17th day of TPN and returns to pretreatment level 3 to 7 days after cessation of TPN.

Transiently increased serum AST ($3\times$ to $4\times$), alanine aminotransferase (ALT) ($3\times$ to $7\times$), ALP ($2\times$), and γ-glutamyltransferase (GGT). Direct bilirubin and LD normal or slightly increased. Levels improve 1 week after cessation of TPN and return to normal in 1 to 4 months.

Serum folate falls 50% if not supplemented.

67% of children show eosinophilia ($>140/\mu$L) after 9 days of TPN.

Abnormal plasma amino acid levels.

Deficiency of essential fatty acids (on fat-free TPN), zinc, or copper

Laboratory findings of sepsis (e.g., *Candida*) due to infection of catheter

Some Guidelines for Monitoring Patients on TPN

Twice weekly: chemistry profile, electrolytes, transthyretin

Weekly: CBC, urinalysis, chemistry and acid-base profiles, iron, zinc, copper, magnesium, triglycerides (TG), ammonia

Every 2 weeks: Folate, vitamin B_{12}

Baseline: All of the above tests

Patient with an unstable clinical condition may require testing daily or more often. Fever must always be explained.

Vitamins

Vitamins are essential chemical micronutrients that cannot be synthesized. Fat-soluble vitamins are A, D, E, and K; water-soluble vitamins are C (ascorbic acid) and the B vitamins (see following).

Vitamin A Deficiency

♦ Decreased plasma level of retinol vitamin A.

Elevated carotenoids may cause false low values for vitamin A.

Laboratory findings due to preceding conditions (e.g., malabsorption, alcoholism, restricted diet).

Toxicity caused by daily ingestion of $>33,000$ IU (chronic) or $>500,000$ IU (acute) may cause hepatocellular necrosis, intracranial hypertension.

Vitamin B$_1$ (Thiamine) Deficiency (Beriberi)

Thiamine deficiency causes inadequate adenosine triphosphate (ATP) synthesis and abnormal carbohydrate metabolism.

Increased blood pyruvic acid level
♦ ○ Decreased thiamine levels in blood and urine; become normal within 24 hours after therapy begins (thus, baseline levels should be established first).
RBC transketolase <8 IU (baseline), and addition of thiamine pyrophosphate causes >20% increase.
Laboratory findings due to complications (e.g., heart failure)
○ Laboratory findings due to underlying conditions (e.g., renal dialysis, chronic diarrhea, inadequate intake [polished rice], alcoholism)

Vitamin B₂ (Riboflavin) Deficiency

Riboflavin is a coenzyme for various biochemical reactions.

♦ Decreased riboflavin level in plasma, RBCs, WBCs
○ RBC glutathionine reductase activity decreased in RBCs; not useful in persons with glucose-6-phosphate dehydrogenase (G6PD) deficiency.

Vitamin B₃ (Niacin) Deficiency

A deficiency of niacin causes pellagra—dermatitis, dementia, and diarrhea (the "three D's").

○ Decreased excretion of niacin metabolites (nicotinamide) in urine
○ Blood niacin level <24 μmol/L is not reliable.
○ Plasma tryptophan level is markedly decreased; also occurs in carcinoid syndrome.

Vitamin B₆ (Pyridoxine) Deficiency

♦ Decreased serum or RBC levels of vitamin B₆.
♦ Decreased pyridoxic acid in urine.
♦ Measure xanthurenic acid after oral tryptophan load.

Vitamin B₁₂ and Folic Acid Deficiency

See Chapter 11 and Table 11-13.

Vitamin C Deficiency (Scurvy)

The vitamin C level is measured as the sum of ascorbic and dehydroascorbic acid concentrations.

♦ Plasma level of ascorbic acid is decreased; <0.2 mg/dL suggests vitamin C deficiency; usually 0 in frank scurvy. Reflects recent dietary intake. (Normal = 0.5–1.5 mg/dL, but lower level does not prove diagnosis.) Decreased by smoking. Levels are 20% higher in women.
♦ Ascorbic acid in buffy coat (WBC) reflects tissue stores, is decreased—usually absent in clinical scurvy. (Normal is 30 mg/dL.) Decreased by smoking.
Ascorbic acid is measured in two 24-hour urine samples; one at baseline and the other 2 days after oral ascorbic acid administration. Vitamin C deficiency is indicated by <50 mg/dL in second specimen.
After protein meal or administration of tyrosine, tyrosyl compounds are present in urine (detected by Millon's reagent) in patients with scurvy but are absent in normal persons.
Serum ALP is decreased; serum calcium and phosphorus are normal.
Rumpel-Leede test is positive.
Microscopic hematuria is present in one third of patients.
Stool may be positive for occult blood.
Laboratory findings due to associated deficiencies (e.g., anemia caused by folic acid deficiency) are present.

Vitamin D Deficiency or Excess

See Rickets, Chapter 10, and discussion of excess vitamin D in Chapter 13.

METAB:HERED

Vitamin E Deficiency

Vitamin E acts as an antioxidant and free radical scavenger, especially in cell membranes.

♦ Plasma α-tocopherol <0.4 mg/dL in adults; <0.15 mg/dL in infants age 1 month
Laboratory findings due to underlying conditions (e.g., malabsorption in adults; diet high in polyunsaturated fatty acids in premature infants)

Vitamin K Deficiency

See Chapter 11.

Vitamins, Reference Ranges (Blood)

Reference ranges for vitamins* have limited utility because blood levels may not reflect tissue stores.

Vitamin A	
Retinol	360–1,200 μg/L
	<20 μg/dL indicates low intake and tissue stores
	20–36 μg/dL is indeterminate
Retinyl esters	≤1.0 μg/dL
Carotene	48–200 μg/dL
Vitamin C (ascorbic acid)	0.2–2.0 mg/dL
	<0.2 mg/dL represents deficiency
Vitamin D	Indirect estimate by measuring serum ALP, calcium, and phosphorus
Total 25-hydroxy vitamin D	14–42 ng/mL (winter)
	15–80 ng/mL (summer)
1,25-dihydroxy vitamin D	15–60 pg/mL
Vitamin E (alpha-tocopherol)	
Children	3.0–15.0 μg/mL
Adults	5.5–17.0 μg/mL
Deficiency	<3.0 μg/mL
Excess	>40 μg/mL
Vitamin B_1 (thiamine)	5.3–7.9 μg/dL
Vitamin B_2 (riboflavin)	3.7–13.7 μg/dL
Vitamin B_{12} (cobalamin)	
Low	<150 pg/mL
Normal	190–900 pg/mL
Unsaturated vitamin B_{12}-binding capacity	870–1,800 pg/mL
Folate	
Serum	Usual normal range is 5–15 ng/mL; is associated with normal hematologic findings.
	3–5 ng/mL is borderline; is associated with variable hematologic findings.
	<3 ng/mL is associated with positive hematologic findings.
RBC	
<1 y old	74–995 ng/mL
1–11 y old	96–362 ng/mL
≥12 y old	180–600 ng/mL

ALP, alkaline phosphatase.
*Values are for serum unless otherwise indicated.

Table 12-8.   Serum Markers in Detection of Various Prenatal Conditions

Condition	AFP	hCG	Unconjugated Estriol	Detection Rate
Anencephaly	4+	—	—	95%
Open spina bifida	3+	—	—	80%
Abdominal wall defects	3+	—	—	75%
Trisomy 21 (Down syndrome)	D	I	D	60%
Trisomy 18	DD	DD	DD	60%
Other chromosomal abnormalities	I/D	I/D	I/D	50%

D = decreased; DD = strongly decreased; I = increased; I/D = increased or decreased.
Source: Wasserman ER. Preventing problem pregnancies. *Advance/Laboratory* Nov 1997:53.

Inherited Metabolic Disorders

Laboratory Tests For Prenatal Screening and Diagnosis[2]

See also Obstetric Monitoring of Fetus and Placenta, Chapter 14.
Use
General Risk Factors:

- Maternal age ≥35 years at delivery
- Abnormal maternal serum α-fetoprotein (AFP), human chorionic gonadotropin (hCG), or unconjugated estriol

Ethnic Risk Factors:

- Sickle cell anemia (presence of sickling; confirmed by Hb electrophoresis)
- Tay-Sachs disease (decreased serum hexosaminidase A)
- α- and β-thalassemia (decreased mean corpuscular volume; confirmed by Hb electrophoresis)

Specific Risk Factors:

- Rubella, toxoplasmosis, or CMV infection
- Maternal disorder (e.g., diabetes mellitus, phenylketonuria [PKU])
- Teratogen exposure (e.g., radiation, alcohol, isotretinoin, anticonvulsants, lithium)
- Previous stillbirth or neonatal death
- Previous child with chromosomal abnormality or structural defect
- Inherited disorders (e.g., cystic fibrosis, metabolic disorders, sex-linked recessive disorders)
- Either parent with balanced translocation or structural abnormality

Maternal Serum Sampling

See Table 12-8 and Figure 12-4.
See AFP in open neural tube, anencephaly, ventral wall defects, etc.
See trisomy 21 (Down syndrome) and trisomy 18.
Fetal DNA in maternal serum has been reported for diagnosis of fetal Rh(D) status, β-thalassemia, myotonic dystrophy, achondrodysplasia, trisomy 21, and preeclampsia.[3]

[2]Donnenfeld AE, Lamb AN. Cytogenetics and molecular cytogenetics in prenatal diagnosis. *Clin Lab Med* 2003;23:457–480.
[3]Lo YM, Tein MS, Lau TK, et al. Quantitative analysis of fetal DNA in maternal plasma and serum: implications for noninvasive prenatal diagnosis. *Am J Hum Genet* 1998;62:768–775.

METAB/HERED

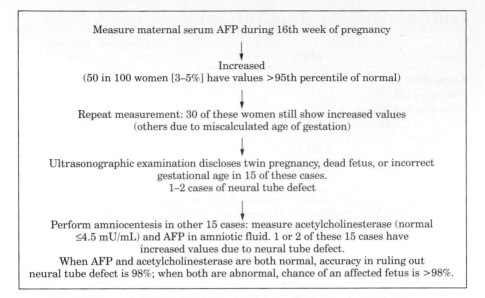

Measure maternal serum AFP during 16th week of pregnancy

↓

Increased
(50 in 100 women [3–5%] have values >95th percentile of normal)

↓

Repeat measurement: 30 of these women still show increased values
(others due to miscalculated age of gestation)

↓

Ultrasonographic examination discloses twin pregnancy, dead fetus, or incorrect
gestational age in 15 of these cases.
1–2 cases of neural tube defect

↓

Perform amniocentesis in other 15 cases: measure acetylcholinesterase (normal
≤4.5 mU/mL) and AFP in amniotic fluid. 1 or 2 of these 15 cases have
increased values due to neural tube defect.
When AFP and acetylcholinesterase are both normal, accuracy in ruling out
neural tube defect is 98%; when both are abnormal, chance of an affected fetus is >98%.

Fig. 12-4. Algorithm for α-fetoprotein (AFP) testing in pregnancy (detects virtually all cases of anencephaly and 80% of cases of open spina bifida, with very few false-positive results).

Amniocentesis

Generally not done before 14 weeks of gestation. Risk of fetal loss ~0.5%.
Cell culture takes 5 to 7 days; activity similar to that in fibroblasts.
Use
In women >35 years old to detect various chromosomal abnormalities.
Can detect intermediary metabolites of some inborn errors, especially organic acid disorders.
Confirm abnormal maternal serum findings, e.g., AFP, hCG.

Chorionic Villus Sampling[4]

Generally done between 10 to 13 weeks of gestation; sometimes as early as 6 to 7
weeks. Risk of fetal loss is ≤2%. Failure to obtain results = 2%.
Contamination with maternal decidua must be avoided for accurate diagnosis based on
fetal chromosomes, enzyme assay, or DNA analysis.
In some patient populations, a negative culture for *Neisseria gonorrhoeae* or herpes
simplex virus may be required.
Associated with ~7% fetal loss similar to amniocentesis (spontaneous rate ~4.5%).
False-positive result in 2% of cases compared with 0.3% of cases using amniocentesis.
Most prenatal diagnoses of enzyme defects are now made with this assay.
Does not include biochemical analysis of amniotic fluid (AF) (e.g., AFP, others).
Therefore cannot test for neural tube defects.
Primary advantage is to provide earlier results than AF, allowing pregnancy termination in first trimester or relieving anxiety.
Both parents carry recessive gene (e.g., sickle cell anemia, cystic fibrosis, Tay-Sachs).
X-linked recessive gene (e.g., hemophilia, Duchenne muscular dystrophy).
Not reliable for diagnosis of Fragile X syndrome.

[4]Cole HM (Ed.) Chorionic villus sampling: a reassessment. Diagnostic and therapeutic technology assessment. *JAMA* 1990;263:305.

Indications

Chromosomal examination:

- 80% for trisomies 21, 18, 13; aneuploidies or mosaicism involving sex chromosomes
- 20% unbalanced translocations or deletions, others.
- Previous child with chromosomal trisomy
- Mother carrier of X-linked disorder (to determine fetal sex)
- Parent carrier of chromosomal translocation
- Maternal age >35

Restriction enzyme assay:

- Hemoglobinopathy (e.g., thalassemia)
- Lesch-Nyhan syndrome
- α_1-antitrypsin deficiency
- PKU

Metabolic assay:

- Adenosine deaminase deficiency
- Adrenoleukodystrophy
- Argininosuccinic aciduria
- Citrullinemia
- Cystinosis
- Fabry disease
- Fanconi anemia
- Farber disease
- Gaucher disease
- Gm_1 gangliosidosis
- Gm_2 gangliosidosis (Tay-Sachs disease)
- Homocystinuria
- Krabbe disease
- Lesch-Nyhan syndrome
- Maple syrup urine disease
- Menkes syndrome
- Metachromatic leukodystrophy
- Methylmalonic acidemia
- Mucolipidosis II (I-cell disease)
- Mucopolysaccharidosis (Ia, II, III, IV)
- Multiple sulfatase deficiency
- Niemann-Pick disease
- Pompe disease
- Wolman disease
- Zellweger syndrome

Fetal Blood Sampling

Generally done ~15th week but usually also successful between 18 and 23 weeks. Check for maternal serum contamination by determining hCG concentration. Additional risk to fetus of 2%.

Use

Prenatal diagnosis of

- RBC isoimmunization, e.g., rhesus factor, minor antigens
- Alloimmune or autoimmune thrombocytopenia
- Hemoglobinopathies (e.g., thalassemias, sickle cell disorders, spherocytosis, enzyme deficiencies [e.g., G6PD])
- Coagulation defects (e.g., Factor VIII and IX hemophilias and fetal sex, other factor deficiencies, von Willebrand disease)
- Immune-deficiency disorders (e.g., severe combined immunodeficiency, Wiskott-Aldrich syndrome, ataxia telangiectasia, chronic granulomatous disease, homozygous C3 deficiency, Chédiak-Higashi syndrome)
- Intrauterine infections (e.g., rubella, toxoplasmosis, varicella, CMV, parvovirus B19) to determine specific IgM and increased total IgM, increased WBC and eosinophil count, decreased platelet count, various blood chemistries
- Chromosomal disorders (e.g., mosaicism, Fragile X)

METAB/HERED

- Metabolic and cytogenetic disorders (e.g., phenylketonuria, α_1-antitrypsin deficiency, cystic fibrosis, Duchenne muscular dystrophy)
- Others (e.g., familial hypercholesterolemia, hyperphenylalaninemia, adrenoleukodystrophy)
- Fetal acid-base balance and metabolic state
- Fetal drug administration

Fetal Biopsy
Use
Liver biopsy for diagnosis of deficiency of long chain 3-hydroxyacyl-CoA dehydrogenase, ornithine transcarbamylase deficiency, atypical PKU due to deficiency of glutamyl transpeptidase cyclohydrolase I, type I hyperoxaluria, GSD type I.
Skin biopsy, e.g., certain severe genetic disorders such as epidermolysis bullosa
Muscle biopsy for Duchenne muscular dystrophy

Fetal Urine
Use
In cases of oligohydramnios when AF cannot be obtained.
To diagnose and treat fetal obstructive uropathy.

Cystic Hygroma Fluid
Use
To diagnose associated chromosomal abnormalities (e.g., 45 X, trisomy 21, trisomy 18).

Genetic Testing
Use
Carrier identification (e.g., Tay-Sachs disease, sickle cell trait)
Prenatal diagnosis (e.g., Down syndrome)
Newborn screening (e.g., PKU, congenital hypothyroidism)

Ultrasound and Echocardiography
Use
To guide sampling techniques.
To verify gestational age.
Karyotyping is done if malformations are found, since one third of these fetuses will have a chromosomal disorder.
Nuchal thickness and nasal bone absence for prenatal diagnosis of trisomy 21.
May be abnormal in trisomy 13, 18, 21, and 45X and triploidy.
Detection of ~50% of major heart, kidney, and bladder abnormalities, which are not detected by maternal serum AFP screening.

Karyotype Analysis
Use
Determine status of chromosomes X, Y, 21, 18, and 13.

Molecular Diagnosis
Use
Direct detection of gene deletions and mutations and linkage analysis using cultured amniocytes or chorionic villi can make some diagnoses, even when gene products are not present (e.g., adult polycystic kidney disease, sickle cell disease, α-thalassemia, cystic fibrosis, Gaucher disease, Duchenne muscular dystrophy, fragile X syndrome, factor deficiencies).

Isolation of Fetal Cells in Maternal Blood or Fetal DNA
Usual ratio of fetal cells to maternal cells = 1:1,000 to 1:5,000.
Use
Allows diagnosis by flow cytometry and polymerase chain reaction (PCR). PCR can demonstrate a Y chromosome in women carrying male fetuses.

Laboratory Tests For Newborn Screening[5]

Nuclear Sexing (Sex Chromatin; Barr Bodies)

In nuclear sexing, epithelial cells from a buccal smear (or vaginal smear, etc.) are stained with cresyl violet and examined microscopically. A dense body (Barr body) on the nuclear membrane represents one of the X chromosomes and occurs in 30% to 60% of female somatic cells. The maximum number of Barr bodies is 1 less than the number of X chromosomes.

Largely replaced by chromosome analysis. A normal count does not rule out chromosomal abnormalities.

If there are <10% of cells containing Barr bodies in a patient with female genitalia, karyotyping should be done to delineate probable chromosomal abnormalities.

No Barr bodies in:

• Normal males
• Turner syndrome (ovarian dysgenesis)

Two Barr bodies may be found in:

• 47 XXX female
• 48 XXXY male (Klinefelter syndrome)
• 49 XXXYY male (Klinefelter syndrome)

Three Barr bodies may be found in:

• 49 XXXXY male (Klinefelter syndrome)

Are same as drumstick nuclear appendages in 2% to 3% of leukocytes in normal females and indicate the presence of two X chromosomes in the karyotype. It is not found in males. There is a lower incidence of drumsticks in Klinefelter syndrome (XXY) as opposed to the extra Barr body. (*Mean lobe counts of neutrophils are also decreased.*)

Incidence of drumsticks is decreased and mean lobe counts are lower also in trisomy 21.

Double drumsticks are exceedingly rare and diagnostically impractical.

Chromosome Analysis (Karyotyping)

Every nucleated human cell contains a complete genome of 6×10^9 base pairs of DNA packed into 46 chromosomes consisting of 22 pairs of autosomes and one pair of sex chromosomes (XX in females, XY in males). Cytogenic disorders are present in ≤1% of live births, <50% of spontaneous fetal losses.

Use

Suspected autosomal syndromes:
    Down (trisomy 21), trisomy 18, trisomy 13, Cri du chat syndrome
Suspected sex-chromosome syndromes:
Klinefelter XXY, XXXY
    Turner XO
    "Superfemale" XXX, XXXX
    "Supermale" XYY
    "Funny-looking kid" syndromes, especially with multiple anomalies, including mental retardation and low birth weight
    Possible myelogenous leukemia to demonstrate Philadelphia chromosome
    Ambiguous genitalia
    Infertility (some patients)
    Repeated miscarriages
    Primary amenorrhea or oligomenorrhea
    Mental retardation with sex anomalies
    Hypogonadism
    Delayed puberty or abnormal development at puberty
    Disturbances of somatic growth

[5]Waisbren SE. Newborn screening for metabolic disorders. *JAMA* 2006;296:993.

Newborn Screening[6-8]

Use

Genetic tests are available for >940 diseases, of which 400 are only research tests.

The most current methodology employs tandem mass spectrometry (MS/MS), which can detect >50 genetic disorders.

Amino acids that can be measured include glycine, alanine, histidine, glutamic acid, glutamine, arginine, and ornithine.

Can also detect carnitine, acylcarnitines, fatty acids, methylmalonic academia, propionic acidemia, various cobalamin defects, and vitamin B_{12} deficiency.

Patterns rather than only single metabolites are significant.

Ideally, to screen for disorders that are asymptomatic, can cause irreversible damage, and for which there is effective treatment.

Population prevalence sufficient to limit false-positive and false-negative results.

High cost:benefit ratio.

Adequate follow-up to assure appropriate treatment.

Neonatal Screening, Disorders and Incidence

Disorder	Incidence
Phenylketonuria and its milder variations	Among Caucasians, between 1:10,000 and 1:25,000; 1 in 50 persons is a carrier
Iminoglycinuria	1:10,000
Cystinuria	1:7,000
Histidinemia	1:14,000–1:20,000 live births in United States and 1:8,000 in Japan
Hartnup disease	1:30,000
Genetic mucopolysaccharidoses	1:25,000
Galactosemia	
Galactokinase deficiency	1:150,000
Classic galactose-1-phosphate uridyltransferase	1:60,000
Uridinediphosphate-galactose-4- epimerase	<1:50,000
Argininosuccinic acidemia	1:100,000
Cystathioninemia	1:100,000
Hyperglycinemia (nonketotic)	1:150,000
Fanconi syndrome (renal)	1:150,000
Propionic acidemia	1:50,000
Hyperlysinemia	<1:300,000
Hyperornithinemia	<1:300,000
Hyperprolinemia	<1:300,000
Maple syrup urine disease	1:250,000–1:400,000
Homocystinuria	1:50,000–1:150,000
Tyrosinemia	1:40,000–1:50,000
Hypothyroidism	1:3,600–1:4,800
Cystic fibrosis of pancreas	1:2,400 in United States and Western Europe; 1:90,000 in native Hawaiians
Congenital adrenal hyperplasia (90% are of 21-hydroxylase type)	1:67,000 in Maryland; 1:490 in Ypik Eskimos of Alaska

Some Laboratory Clues to Metabolic Diseases in Infants and Children

Various genetic metabolic diseases are so often associated with certain laboratory findings that such clues should alert the physician to rule them out.

[6]Chace DH, Kalas TA, Naylor EW. Use of tandem mass spectrometry for multianalyte screening of dried blood specimens from newborns. *Clin Chem* 2003;49:1797–1817.
[7]www.cdc.gov/nceh/dls/newborn_screening.htm; www.savebabies.org.
[8]http://www.ncbi.nlm.nih.gov/omim/.

Hypoglycemia:

- Galactosemia
- GSDs (IA, IB, III, VI, IX A, B, C)
- Hereditary fructose intolerance
- Organic acidemias (e.g., maple syrup urine disease, propionic acidemia, methyl-malonic acidemia, isovaleric acidemia, glutaric acidemia, etc.)
- Tyrosinemia
- Biotinidase deficiency
- Endocrine disorders (e.g., adrenal insufficiency, diabetic mother, hypopituitarism.)
- Others (e.g., Reye syndrome, sepsis, liver disease, drugs.)

Ketosis (massive ketosis, especially in the presence of severe vomiting, is otherwise rare in neonates, even in juvenile diabetes):

- Galactosemia
- Hereditary fructose intolerance
- Maple syrup urine disease
- Organic acidemias

Acidosis

Amino acid disorders:

- Maple sugar urine disease
- Hypervalinemia
- Hyperleucine-isoleucinemia

Organic acid defects:

- Isovaleric acidemia
- Propionic acidemia
- Methylmalonic acidemia
- Glutaric acidemia
- Combined carboxylase deficiency
- 3-Hydroxy-3-methylglutaric acidemia
- 2-Methyl-3-hydroxybutyric acidemia
- Acyl CoA dehydrogenase deficiencies

Glycogen storage diseases:

- Type Ia
- Type III

Hyperammonemia

(May be associated with failure to thrive, low birth weight, strong body odor, decreased albumin and calcium, etc.). (*Plasma ammonia should be determined in any neonate with unexplained neurologic deterioration or any patient with unexplained encephalopathy or episodic lethargy and vomiting.*) Marked hyperammonemia without significant acidosis suggests a urea cycle disorder; should perform serum amino acid assay by High-performance liquid chromatography (HPLC) and urine organic acid assay by GC/MS.

Defects in urea cycle: severe hyperammonemia with respiratory alkalosis:

- Arginosuccinate synthetase deficiency
- Arginosuccinate lyases deficiency
- Arginase deficiency
- Ornithine transcarbamylase deficiency
- N-Acetylglutamate synthetase deficiency
- Carbamyl phosphate synthetase deficiency

Organic acid defects: mild to moderate hyperammonemia (≤500 mg/dL):

- Methylmalonic acidemia
- Isovaleric acidemia*

METAB.HERED

- Multiple carboxylase deficiency*
- Propionic acidemia*
- Glutaric acidemia type I and II
- Ketothiolase deficiency

Disorders of dibasic amino acid transport (e.g., hyperornithinemia)

Fatty acid oxidation defects

Transient hyperammonemia of newborn

Reye syndrome

Hepatic failure

Drugs (e.g., valproate)

Increased serum indirect bilirubin:

- Inborn errors of RBC metabolism (e.g., pyruvate-kinase deficiency or G6PD deficiency)
- Crigler-Najjar syndrome
- Gilbert syndrome
- Hypothyroidism

Increased serum direct bilirubin:

- Rotor syndrome
- Dubin-Johnson syndrome
- Galactosemia
- Hereditary fructose intolerance
- α_1-antitrypsin deficiency

Hepatomegaly is prominent in:

- Lysosomal storage diseases, (e.g., mucopolysaccharidoses, mucolipidoses, glycoprotein storage diseases, gangliosidosis)
- Lipidoses (e.g., Gaucher disease, Niemann-Pick disease, Wolman disease)
- Disorders of carbohydrate metabolism (e.g., galactosemia, hereditary fructose intolerance, GSDs)
- Tyrosinemia
- α_1-antitrypsin deficiency

Feeding difficulties or vomiting are associated with many metabolic diseases but are most prominent with:

- Protein intolerance (e.g., organic acidemias or hyperammonemia syndromes)
- Carbohydrate intolerance (e.g., hereditary fructose intolerance)
- Adrenogenital syndrome

Seizures:

- Glycogen storage disease (hypoglycemia)
- Galactosemia
- Fructose intolerance
- Maple syrup urine disease
- Congenital lactic acidosis
- Vitamin D–resistant rickets
- Organic acidemias
- Urea cycle disorders
- Hyperglycemia
- Pyridoxine dependency

Some Laboratory Clues to Acute Neonatal Illness

Thrombocytopenia
Anemia

*Also characterized by lactic acidosis.

Hypoglycemia
Metabolic acidosis
Hyperammonemia

Classification of Inherited Metabolic Conditions (Abbreviated)

Inherited metabolic conditions are classified according to involved metabolic pathway (e.g., carbohydrate, amino acid, fatty acids), involved cell organelles (e.g., lysosomes, mitochondria), and/or phenotypes.

Disorder	Deficiency	Substances Detected
Disorders of carbohydrate metabolism		
Diabetes mellitus	See Chapter 13	Glucose
Pentosuria		L-xylulose
Fructose		Fructose
Fructosuria	Fructose 1–6 phosphate aldolase B deficiency (hereditary fructose intolerance)	
	Fructose 1–6 diphosphatase deficiency	
	Essential fructosuria (hepatic fructokinase deficiency)	
Lactose	Familial lactose intolerance	Lactose
Galactose		Galactose
Galactosemia	Galactose-1-phosphate uridyltransferase	
	Galactokinase deficiency	
	Galactose-4-epimase deficiency	
Glycogen storage diseases		
Disorders of amino acid and organic acid metabolism[a]		
Hyperphenylalaninemia	Phenylalanine hydroxylase	Phenylalanine (B) and its metabolites (phenylpyruvic acid, ortho-hydroxyphenylacetic acid) in blood, urine and CSF; tyrosine and the derivative catecholamines are deficient.
	Type I (phenylketonuria)	Mental retardation
	Type II	Milder form of type I
	Type III	Transient
Tyrosinemia I	Fumarylacetoacetate and maleylacetoacetate hydrolases	Succinylacetone, tyrosine (U)
Tyrosinemia II	Tyrosine aminotransferase	Tyrosine (B, U)
Alkaptonuria	Homogentisic acid oxidase	Homogentisic acid (U)
Histidinemia	Histidase	
Homocystinuria	Cystathionine synthase	Homocystine and methionine (B, U); D cysteine (B)
	Cobalamin metabolism (see "Megaloblastic Anemia," Chapter 11)	Homocystine and methylmalonic acid (B, U), cystathionine (U)

METAB-HERED

	Methylenetetra-hydrofolate reductase	Homocystine (B, U), cystathionine (U)
Hyperlysinemia		
Persistent	Lysine ketoglutarate reductase	Lysine (B,U)
Periodic	Lysine dehydrogenase	Lysine (B) ammonia (B)
Citrullinemia	Argininosuccinate synthetase	Argininosuccinic acid
Hyperargininemia	Arginase	
Argininosuccinic aciduria	Argininosuccinate (B, U)	Citrulline
Hyperammonemias		
Ornithine carbamoylsynthase deficiency	Ammonia (B), orotic acid (U); D citrulline	
Carbamyl phosphate synthetase deficiency	Ammonia (B), orotic acid (U); citrulline (B)	
N-acetylglutamate synthetase deficiency	Ammonia (B)	
Maple syrup urine disease (branched-chain ketoaciduria)	Branched-chain ketoacid dehydrogenase	Leucine, isoleucine, valine, branched-chain ketoacids (B, U)
Isovaleric acidemia	Isovaleryl-CoA dehydrogenase	Isovaleric acid (B), hydroxyisovaleric acid (U), isovalerylglycine (U)
Glutaric aciduria	Glutaryl-CoA dehydrogenase	Accumulation of glutaric acid and its metabolites (glutaconic acid and 3-hydroxyglutaric acid)
Nonketotic hyperglycinemia	Glycine cleavage system	Glycine (B, U, CSF)
Propionic acidemia	Propionyl-CoA carboxylase	
Methylmalonic acidemia	Methylmalonyl-CoA mutase, adenosyl-cobalamin synthesis	
Imino acids		
Hyperprolinemia	Proline oxidase	Proline (B, U), glycine (U), hydroxyproline (U)
Hyperhydroxyprolinemia	Pyrroline-5-carboxylate dehydrogenase	Proline (B, U), glycine (U), hydroxyproline (U), pyrroline-5-carboxylate (U)
Hyperimidodipeptiduria	Prolidase (peptidase)	Imidodipeptides (U)
Urea cycle disorders		
Phenylketonuria	Phenylalanine hydroxylase	Phenylalanine and its metabolites (phenylpyruvic acid, ortho-hydroxyphenylacetic acid) in B, U, CSF; tyrosine and the derivative catecholamines are deficient
Citrullinemia	Argininosuccinic acid synthetase	Argininosuccinic acid
Argininemia	Arginase	
Argininosuccinic aciduria	Argininosuccinate lyase	Citrulline
		Ornithine carbamoyl-transferase deficiency
		N-acetylglutamate synthetase deficiency
		Carbamyl phosphate synthetase deficiency

Disorders of proline and hydroxyproline metabolism

Hyperprolinemia I	Proline oxidase	Proline
Hyperprolinemia II	Pyrroline-5-carbgoxylate dehydrogenase	Proline
Hyperimidodipeptiduria	Prolidase	
HHH syndrome	*H*yperornithinemia, *H*yperammonemia, *H*omocitrullinuria)	

Organic acid disorders/organic acidurias

Biotinidase deficiency (one cause of multiple carboxylase deficiency)		
Cobalamin C defect		
Pyruvate and lactate metabolism	Lactate dehydrogenase deficiency	
	Pyruvate dehydrogenase deficiency	
	Pyruvate carboxylase deficiency	
	Phospho*enol*pyruvate carboxykinase deficiency	

Branched-chain organic acidemias

Isovaleric acidemia	Isovaleryl-CoA dehydrogenase	Isovaleric acid (B), hydroxyisovaleric acid (U), isovalerylglycine (U)
Mevalonic acidemia	Mevalonate	Leucine, isoleucine, valine,
Maple syrup urine disease (branched-chain ketoaciduria)	Branched-chain ketoacid dehydrogenase	branched chain ketoacids (B, U)

Organic acid disorders

Propionate and methylmalonate metabolism

Propionic acidemia	Propionyl-CoA carboxylase
Methylmalonic acidemia	Methylmalonyl-CoA mutase, adenosyl-cobalamin synthesis
Multiple carboxylase deficiency	Holocarboxylase synthetase, biotinidase

Other organic acid disorders

Alkaptonuria (see Chapter 8)	Homogentisic acid oxidase	
Hyperoxaluria type I (glycolic aciduria)	Alanine:glyoxylate aminotransferase	Glycolic and oxalic acid
Hyperoxaluria type II (glyceric aciduria)	Glyceric dehydrogenase	
	Glycerol kinase deficiency	
Canavan disease	Aspartoacylase	

Lysosomal storage disorders

Metachromatic leukodystrophy	Arylsulfatase A
Multiple sulfatase deficiency	Multiple lysosomal sulfatases
Niemann-Pick disease	Sphingomyelinase
Farber disease	Ceramidase
Gaucher disease	Glucocerebrosidase
Pompe disease (GSD II)	α-1,4-glucosidase deficiency

METAB/HERED

Krabbe disease   Galactocerebrosidase
Fabry disease α-galactosidase
Gm$_1$ gangliosidosis β-galactosidase
Wolman disease   Acid lipase
Cholesteryl ester   Acid lipase
  storage disease
Mucolipidosis type IV

Acylcarnitine Disorders

Fatty acid oxidation   e.g., Carnitine   Various
  disorders   transporter defects;
                                 medium, short, long,
                                 and very-long-chain
                                 Acyl-CoA dehydroge-
                                 nase deficiencies;
                                 others

Peroxisomal disorders

Acatalasia   Catalase
Refsum disease   Phytanic acid   Various, e.g., very-long-chain
                                 hydroxylase   fatty acids
Zellweger syndrome   Peroxisome biogenesis

Purine and pyrimidine metabolism disorders

Lesch-Nyhan syndrome   Hypoxanthine   Increased uric acid (B)
                                 phosphoribosyl-
                                 transferase
Orotic aciduria   Uridine-5'-monophos-   Increased orotic acid (B)
  (see Chapter 11)   phate synthase
Xanthinuria   Xanthine oxidase   Decreased uric acid (B, U)

Disorders of metal metabolism

Wilson disease (see Chapter 8)
Hemochromatosis
Menkes syndrome

Disorders of lipid metabolism (see Table 12-9)

Disorders of heme proteins
Porphyrinurias
Bilirubin metabolism   See Chapter 8
  Crigler-Najjar
    syndromes I, II
  Gilbert's disease
  Dubin-Johnson syndrome
  Rotor syndrome

Membrane transport disorders

Cystinuria
Hartnup disease
Iminoglycinuria   Proline, hydroxyproline,
                                                              glycine (all N or D)

Disorders of serum enzymes

Hypophosphatasia   Alkaline phosphatase   Alkaline phosphatase (D)
Hyperphosphatasia
α_1-antitrypsin deficiency

Disorders of plasma proteins

Analbuminemia
Agammaglobulinemia
Atransferrinemia

Disorders of blood

Coagulation diseases (e.g., hemophilias)	See Chapter 11
RBC G6PD deficiency	See Chapter 11
Hemoglobinopathies (including sickle cell disease and α- and β- thalassemias)	See Chapter 11
Hereditary spherocytosis	See Chapter 11
Hereditary nonsphero-cytic hemolytic anemia	See Chapter 11

Endocrine disorders

Neonatal hypothyroidism	See Fig 13-7
Congenital adrenal hyperplasia	See Chapter 13

Infectious diseases, (transmitted) e.g.:

HIV, toxoplasmosis	See Chapter 15
Hepatitis B, C	See Chapter 8

Others

Cystic fibrosis	See Chapter 8
Duchenne muscular dystrophy	See Chapter 10

D, decreased; I, increased; N, normal; B, blood; U, urine; CSF, cerebrospinal fluid; GSD, glycogen storage disease; G6PD, glucose-6-phosphate dehydrogenase.
[a]Stern HJ, Finkelstein JD. Heritable diseases of amino-acid metabolism. In: Becker KL, ed. *Principles and Practice of Endocrinology and Metabolism.* 3rd ed. Philadelphia: Lippincott Williams & Wilkins; 2001; also Wapner RS. In McMillan J, Feigin RD, DeAngelis C, Jones DJ, eds. Inborn Errors of Metabolism; *Oski's Pediatrics.* 4th ed. Philadelphia: Lippincott Williams & Wilkins; 2006.

Tests of Lipid Metabolism

See Chapter 5.

Disorders of Lipid Metabolism

Acid Lipase Deficiencies

Acid lipase deficiencies are characterized by the inability to hydrolyze lysosomal TG and cholesteryl esters.

◆ Decreased acid lipase in lymphocytes or fibroblasts. Increased serum TG, LDL-C, and cholesterol esters.

Wolman Disease

Wolman disease is a rare autosomal recessive absence of enzyme A of lysosomal acid lipase activity, causing accumulation of total cholesterol (TC) and TG throughout body tissues; death occurs within the first 6 months of life.

Prominent anemia develops by 6 weeks of age.
Peripheral blood smear shows prominent vacuolation (in nucleus and cytoplasm) of leukocytes.
◯ Characteristic foam cells in bone marrow resemble those in Niemann-Pick disease.
◆ Abnormal accumulation of cholesterol esters and TGs in tissue biopsy (e.g., liver) establishes the diagnosis.
◆ Assay shows absent acid lipase activity in many tissues, including leukocytes and cultured fibroblasts. Heterozygotes have enzyme activity of ~50% of normal in leukocytes or cultured fibroblasts.

METAB/HERED

♦ Prenatal diagnosis by demonstrating enzyme deficiency in cultured amniocytes.
Laboratory findings due organ involvement:

• Abnormal liver function tests (caused by lipid accumulation)
• Malabsorption
• Decreased adrenal cortical function (diffuse calcification on CT scan).

Cholesteryl Ester Storage Disease

This is a rare, inherited, marked deficiency of isoenzyme A of lysosomal acid lipase activity, causing accumulation of cholesterol ester.

Similar to Wolman disease but is less severe, lacks intestinal malabsorption, and deposits are predominantly cholesterol esters in lysosomes.

Metabolic Syndrome (Syndrome X)[9]

Metabolic syndrome is a recently recognized constellation of findings, possibly caused by insulin resistance, including hypertension, abdominal obesity, and prothrombotic and proinflammatory states.

Glucose intolerance with fasting blood glucose 110 to 125 mg/dL
Atherogenic dyslipidemia (TG >150 mg/dL, HDL-C <40 mg/dL in men and <50 mg/dL in women, small dense LDL particles
Abnormalities in fibrinolysis and coagulation
Exclusion of other causes of dyslipidemia (e.g., cholestasis, hypothyroidism, chronic renal failure, nephrotic syndrome)

Hyperlipidemias, Primary

See Table 12-9. See also Chapter 5.

Hyperalphalipoproteinemia (HDL-C Excess)

Hyperalphalipoproteinemia is inherited as a simple autosomal dominant trait in families with longevity, or it may be caused by alcoholism, extensive exposure to chlorinated hydrocarbon pesticides, or exogenous estrogen supplementation.

Occurs in 1 in 20 adults with mildly increased TC levels (240–300 mg/dL) secondary to increased HDL-C (>70 mg/dL). LDL-C is not increased, TG is normal.

• Hyperalphalipoproteinemia (HDL-C excess)

  1 in 20 adults with mild increased TC levels (240–300 mg/dL) secondary to increased HDL-C (>70 mg/dL)
  LDL-C is not increased
  TG is normal

• Hypobetalipoproteinemia (see Table 13-6)

Severe Hypertriglyceridemia (Type I) (Familial Hyperchylomicronemia Syndrome)

Hypertriglyceridemia is a rare autosomal recessive trait due to deficiency of lipoprotein lipase (LPL) or Apo C-II or circulating inhibitor of LPL. There is marked heterogeneity in causative molecular defects.

Persistent very high TG (>1,000 mg/dL) with marked increase in very-low-density lipoprotein (VLDL) and chylomicrons.
Responds to marked dietary fat restriction.
Patients with Apo C-II deficiency cannot activate LPL in vitro. Deficiency of Apo C-II is shown by isoelectric focusing or two-dimensional gel electrophoresis of plasma.
Associated with recurrent pancreatitis rather than coronary artery disease (CAD).
Laboratory changes due to fatty liver (increased serum transaminase).

[9]Reaven GM. The metabolic syndrome: requiescat in pace. *Clin Chem* 2005;51:931.

Familial Hypercholesterolemia (Type II)

Familial hypercholesterolemia is inherited as an autosomal dominant disorder.

♦ LDL receptors in fibroblasts or mononuclear blood cells are <25% in homozygous and 50% of normal levels in heterozygous patients (performed at specialized labs).

Homozygous—very rare condition (1 per million) in which serum TC is very high (600–1,000 mg/dL) with corresponding increase in LDL. Both parents are heterozygous. Clinical manifestations of increased TC (xanthomata, corneal arcus, CAD that causes death usually before age 30 years).

♦ • Neonatal diagnosis requires finding increased LDL-C in cord blood; serum TC is unreliable. Because of marked variation in serum TC levels during the first year of life, diagnosis should be deferred until 1 year of age.

♦ • Prenatal diagnosis of homozygous fetus can be made by estimation of binding sites on fibroblasts cultured from amniotic fluids; useful when both parents are heterozygous.

Heterozygous—increased serum TC (300–500 mg/dL) and LDL (two to three times normal) with similar change in a parent or first-degree relative; serum TG and VLDL are normal in 90% and slightly increased in 10% of these cases. Gene frequency occurs 1 in 500 in the general population, but 5% in survivors of acute myocardial infarction (AMI) <60 years old. Premature CAD, tendinous xanthomas, and corneal arcus are often present.

Plasma TG is normal in type II-A but increased in type II-B. This is not the most common cause of phenotype II-A.

Polygenic Hypercholesterolemia (Type IIA)

Polygenic hypercholesterolemia can be diagnosed only after secondary causes of hypercholesterolemia and autosomal dominant traits have been excluded.

Persistent TC elevation (>240 mg/dL) and increased LDL without familial hypercholesterolemia or familial combined hypercholesterolemia. In Type IIB, both LDL and VLDL are increased.

Premature CAD occurs later in life than with familial combined hyperlipidemia.

Xanthomas are rare.

Familial Combined Hyperlipidemia (Types IIB, IV, V)

Familial combined hyperlipidemia occurs in 0.5% of general population and 15% of survivors of AMI <60 years old.

There may be any combination of increased LDL-C and VLDL and chylomicrons; HDL-C is often low; different family members may have increased serum TC or TG or both.

Premature CAD occurs later in life (after age 30 years) than with familial hypercholesterolemia.

Xanthomas are rare.

Patients are often overweight.

Familial Dysbetalipoproteinemia (Type III)

Familial dysbetalipoproteinemia occurs in 1 per 5,000 to 10,000 persons.

Abnormality of apoprotein E with excess of abnormal lipoprotein (beta mobility-VLDL); TC >300 mg/dL plus TG >400 mg/dL should suggest this diagnosis.

VLDL cholesterol:TG ratio = 0.3 (normal ratio = 0.2).

Diagnosis by combination of ultracentrifugation and isoelectric focusing that shows abnormal apoprotein E pattern.

Tuberous and tendinous xanthomas and palmar and plantar xanthomatous streaks are present.

Atherosclerosis is more common in peripheral than coronary arteries.

Familial Hypertriglyceridemia (Type IV)

Familial hypertriglyceridemia is an autosomal dominant condition present in 1% of general population and 5% of survivors of AMI <age 60 years.

Elevated TG (usually 200–500 mg/dL) and VLDL with normal LDL-C and decreased HDL-C.

METAB/HERED

Table 12-9.	Comparison of Classic Types of Hyperlipoproteinemia	

Point of Comparison	Type I (Rarest)	Type II-a (Relatively Common)
Origin	Exogenous hyperlipidemia due to deficient lipoprotein lipase	
Definition	Familial fat-induced hyperglyceridemia	Hyperbetalipoproteinemia (hypercholesterolemia)
Age	Usually younger than age 10 yrs	
Gross appearance of plasma	On standing: supernatant creamy, infranatant clear	Clear (no cream layer on top)
Serum cholesterol	N or slightly I	Markedly I (300–600 mg/dL)
LDL cholesterol	N	I
HDL cholesterol	N to D	N to D
Apolipoprotein (apo)	I (B-48) I (A-IV) V (C-II)	I (B-100)
Increased lipoprotein	Chylomicrons	LDL
Serum triglycerides	Markedly I (usually >2,000 mg/dL)	N
Appearance of lipoprotein components visualized by electrophoresis		
Chylomicron[a]	Marked I	0
Beta-lipoprotein[b]	N or D	I
Pre–beta-lipoprotein[c]	N or D	N
Alpha-lipoprotein[d]		
Other laboratory abnormalities	Glucose tolerance usually	N
Triglyceridecholesterol ratio	8	1
Lipid changes resembling primary hyperlipidemias		
Diet		
Drugs		Triglyceride-lowering drugs in types III and IV

Type II-b (Relatively Common)	Type III (Relatively Uncommon)	Type IV (Most Common)	Type V (Uncommon)
Overindulgence lipidemia		Endogenous hyperlipidemia	Mixed endogenous and exogenous hyperlipidemia (combined types I and IV)
Combined hyperlipidemia (mixed hyperlipidemia)	Carbohydrate-induced hyperglyceridemia with hypercholesterolemia	Carbohydrate-induced hyperglyceridemia without hypercholesterolemia	Combined fat- and carbohydrate-induced hyperglyceridemia
	Not known younger than age 25 yrs	Only occasionally seen in children	
No cream layer on top; clear to turbid infranatant	Clear, cloudy, or milky	Slightly turbid to cloudy On standing: unchanged	Markedly turbid On standing: supernatant, creamy, infranatant milky
Markedly I (300–600 mg/dL)	Markedly I (300–600 mg/dL)	N or slightly I	I (250–500 mg/dL)
I	I	N	N
N to D	N to D	N to D	N to D
I(B-100)	I(E-II) D(E-III) D(E-IV)	V(C-II) I(B-100)	V(C-II) I(B-48) I(B-100)
LDL, VLDL	IDL	VLDL	VLDL, chylomicrons
1 ≤ 400 mg/dL	Markedly I (200–1,000 mg/dL)	Markedly I (500–1,500 mg/dL)	Markedly I (500–1,500 mg/dL)
0	0	0	
I	I, floating beta	N or I	I
I	I	I	N or I
			I
	Hyperglycemia; glucose tolerance often abnormal; serum uric acid I	Glucose tolerance often abnormal; serum uric acid often I	Glucose tolerance usually abnormal; serum uric acid usually I
Variable	<2	1–5	>5
Very high cholesterol diet	Same as for type II-a	Caffeine or alcohol before testing	
Same as for type II-a	Triglyceride-lowering drugs in type IV	Cholesterol-lowering drugs, chlorothiazide, birth control pills, or estrogens	

METAB/HERED

(continued)

| Table 12-9. | *(continued)* |

Point of Comparison	Type I (Rarest)	Type II-a (Relatively Common)
Primary disease		Myxedema, nephrosis, obstructive liver disease, stress, porphyria, anorexia nervosa, idiopathic hyper-calcemia
Origin	[a]Chylomicrons Gut	[c]VLDL Liver
Function	Transport dietary triglycerides	Transport endogenous triglycerides
Electrophoretic mobility	Origin	Pre-beta
Major apolipoproteins	B-48, A-1, C, E	B-100, C, E
Protein	1%	10%
Triglyceride	90%	60%
Cholesterol	5%	15%
Phospholipid	4%	15%

0 = absent; D = decreased; I = increased; N = normal; HDL = high-density lipoprotein; IDL = intermediate density; LDL = low-density lipoprotein; VLDL = very low density lipoprotein.
Since apo B is the only protein in LDL and apo A-I is the major protein constituent of HDL and VLDL, the ratio of apo-B to apo A-I reflects the ratio of LDL to HDL and may be a better discriminator of coronary artery disease than the individual components; however, data on apolipoproteins are still limited. Obtain blood only after at least 12–14 hrs' fasting and when patient has been on usual diet for at least 2 wks.
Rule out diabetes, pancreatitis, and hypothyroidism in all groups.
Increased susceptibility to coronary artery disease occurs in types II, III, and IV; accelerated peripheral vascular disease in type III.

Distinction from familial combined hyperlipidemia is made only by extensive family screening.

Abetalipoproteinemia (Bassen-Kornzweig Syndrome)

Abetalipoproteinemia is a rare autosomal recessive disorder in which the liver and intestine cannot secrete Apo B; should be ruled out in children with fat malabsorption, steatorrhea, failure to thrive, neurologic symptoms, pigmented retinopathy, acanthocytosis.

○ Abnormal RBCs (acanthocytes) are present in the peripheral blood smear; may be 50% to 90% of RBCs and are characteristic (see Chapter 11).
Decreased RBC life span may vary from severe hemolytic anemia to mild compensated anemia.
○ Erythrocyte sedimentation rate (ESR) is markedly decreased (e.g., 1 mm/h).
○ There may be
  • Marked decrease of serum beta-lipoprotein and cholesterol.
  • Marked decrease in serum TG (<30 mg/dL) with little increase after ingestion of fat, and in TC (20–50 mg/dL).
  • Chylomicrons, LDL-C, VLDL, Apo B-48, and Apo B-100 are absent; HDL-C may be lower than in normal persons.
  • Marked impairment of GI fat absorption.
  • Low serum carotene levels.
  • Abnormal pattern of RBC phospholipids.
Plasma lipids are normal in heterozygotes.
Malabsorption causes low serum fat-soluble vitamin (A, K, E) levels.
○ Biopsy of small intestine shows characteristic lipid vacuolization, but this is not pathognomonic (occasionally seen in celiac disease, tropical sprue, juvenile nutritional megaloblastic anemia).

Type II-b (Relatively Common)	Type III (Relatively Uncommon)	Type IV (Common)	Type V (Uncommon)
Same as for type II-a	Myxedema, dysgam-maglobulinemia, liver disease	Nephrotic syndrome, hypothyroidism, pregnancy, glycogen storage disease	Myeloma, macro-globulinemia, nephrosis
IDL	bLDL		dHDL
VLDL	VLDL and IDL		Liver, gut, intravascular metabolism
Transport cholesteryl esters; LDL precursor	Transport cholesteryl esters		Reverse cholesterol transport
Beta, pre-beta	Beta		Alpha
B-100, E	B-100		A-I, A-II, C, E
15%	20%		50%
	5%		5%
35%	50%		20%
	25%		25%

Xanthomas appear in types I, II, and III.
Abdominal pain occurs in types I and V.
If dietary or drug treatment has begun, it may not be possible to classify the lipoproteinemia or the classification may be erroneous.
Type II-b is overindulgence hyperlipidemia; shows increased cholesterol and triglycerides, with increased beta and pre-beta; can be distinguished from type III only by detection of abnormal beta-migrating lipoprotein in serum fraction with density >1.006.
Source: Office of Medical Application of Research. National Institutes of Health. Treatment of hypertriglyceridemia. *JAMA* 1984;251:1196.

Negative sweat test distinguishes this from cystic fibrosis.
Arteriosclerosis is absent.
A variant is normotriglyceridemic abetalipoproteinemia in which patient can secrete Apo B-48 but not Apo B-100, resulting in normal postprandial TG values but marked hypocholesterolemia; associated with mental retardation and vitamin E deficiency.

Hypobetalipoproteinemia

Hypobetalipoproteinemia is an autosomal dominant disorder with increased longevity and lower incidence of atherosclerosis; at least one parent will show decreased β-lipoprotein.

Marked decrease in LDL-C and LDL-C/HDL-C ratio.
Homozygous patients have decreased serum TC (<50 mg/dL) and TG and unde-tectable or trace amounts of chylomicrons, VLDL, and LDL.
Heterozygotes are asymptomatic and have serum TC, LDL-C, and Apo B values that are 50% of normal (consistent with codominant disorder). May also be caused by malabsorption of fats, infection, anemia, hepatic necrosis, hyperthyroidism, AMI, acute trauma.

Tangier Disease

Tangier disease is a rare autosomal recessive disorder caused by mutations at chromosome 9q31 causing a defect in the metabolism of Apo A, In which there is a marked decrease (heterozygous) or absence (homozygous) of HDL.

♦ Plasma levels of Apo A-I and A-II are extremely low. In homozygotes, HDL-C is usu-ally <10 mg/dL and Apo A-I is usually <5 mg/dL. In heterozygotes, HDL-C and Apo A-I are ~50% of normal.

Pre-beta lipoprotein is absent.

Serum TC (<100 mg/dL), LDL-C, and phospholipids are decreased; TG = 100 to 250 mg/dL.

Deposits of cholesterol esters in reticuloendothelial cells cause enlarged liver, spleen, and lymph nodes; enlarged orange tonsils; and small orange-brown spots in rectal mucosa. Patients may have premature CAD, mild corneal opacification, and neuropathy in homozygous type.

Lecithin-Cholesterol Acyltransferase Deficiency (Familial)

Lecithin-cholesterol acyltransferase (LCAT) deficiency is a very rare autosomal recessive disorder of adults. It is associated with premature CAD, corneal opacities, glomerulosclerosis.

Serum TC is normal but cholesterol esters are virtually absent. Plasma free cholesterol is extremely increased. HDL-Cs low.

Normochromic anemia with large RBCs that are frequently target cells.

Proteinuria.

Isolated Lipidemias

High HDL-C

High HDL-C is a rare autosomal recessive disorder causing cholesteryl ester transfer protein gene defects.

Due To

Active life style (physical exercise)

Drugs (e.g., estrogens, alcohol, phenytoin, phenobarbital, rifampicin, griseofulvin)

Low HDL-C

Due To

Sedentary life style (physical inactivity)

Drugs (isotretinoin, anabolic steroids)

Familial hypoalphalipoproteinemia (autosomal dominant disorder with HDL-C)

Deficiency of Apo A-I and Apo C-III

Abetalipoproteinemia, hypobetalipoproteinemia (<30 mg/dL in women and <40 mg/dL in men)

Hyperlipidemias, Secondary

Due To

(Many are combined hyperlipidemias)

- Diabetes mellitus*
  Increased VLDL with increased serum TG, low HDL-C; LDL-C may be normal or mildly increased.
- Hypothyroidism[†]
  Increased LDL-C and TC. *Test for hypothyroidism whenever LDL-C >190 mg/dL.*
  Rapidly becomes normal with treatment.
  Serum TC is not always increased.
- Nephrotic syndrome*
  Increased serum TC and LDL-C is usual.
  Increased VLDL and therefore increased serum TG may also occur.
- Other renal disorders (chronic uremia, hemodialysis, following transplantation)[†]
  Increased TG and TC and low HDL-C may occur.
- Hepatic glycogenoses
  Increased serum lipoprotein is common in any of the forms, but the pattern cannot be used to differentiate the type of GSD.
  Predominant increase in VLDL in G6PD deficiency.
  Predominant increase in LDL-C in debrancher and phosphorylase deficiencies.
- Obstructive liver disease*
  Increased serum TC is common until liver failure develops.
  Resistant to conventional drug therapy. The type of lipoproteinemia is variable.

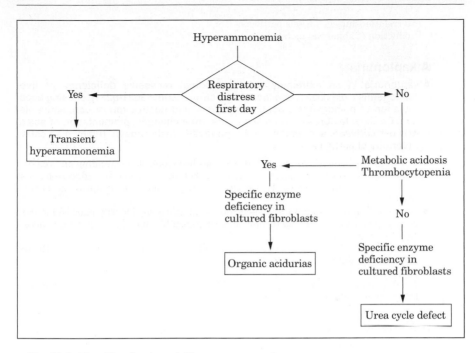

Fig. 12-5. Algorithm for neonatal hyperammonemia.

In intrahepatic biliary atresia, there is often an increase in lipoprotein X, with a marked increase in serum TC and even more marked increase in serum phospholipids.
- Chronic alcoholism[†]
  Marked increase in VLDL, producing type IV or V patterns.
  - Hyperlipoproteinemia of "affluence" (dietary)[*]
  - Pregnancy[*]
  - Drugs (e.g., estrogens[*], steroids[*], beta blockers[*], diuretics[†], cyclosporine[†])

[*]Predominantly hypertriglyceridemia
[†]Predominantly hypercholesterolemia

Disorders of Amino Acid Metabolism

See Figure 12-5.
Genetic disorders of amino acid metabolism may be caused by:

- Enzyme defects
- Membrane transport defects
- Miscellaneous (including storage diseases)

Enzyme deficiency may be caused by:

- Defective synthesis rate
- Synthesis of abnormal protein
- Multiple abnormal alleles may affect the same enzyme protein

Clinical findings depend on:

- Location of block (deficiency distal to block or toxic increase proximal to block)
- Degree of abnormality

METAB/HERED

- Interrelationships of various pathways
- Production of abnormal metabolites

Alkaptonuria

Alkaptonuria is an extremely rare autosomal recessive deficiency of liver homogentisic oxydase (gene located on chromosome 3q21-q231), causing accumulation of homogentisic acid, ochronosis, and destruction of connective tissue. Cardinal features of the disease are urine changes, pigmentation of sclera and ear cartilage, and lumbosacral spondylitis (ochronosis). It may also cause deformity of aortic valve cusps.

♦ Presumptive diagnosis by urine that becomes brown-black on standing and reduces Benedict solution (urine turns brown) and Fehling solution, but glucose-oxidase reagent strips are negative. Ferric chloride test is positive (urine turns purple-black).

♦ Thin-layer chromatography and spectrophotometric assay identify marked increase in urinary homogentisic acid (is normally undetectable) but are not generally necessary for diagnosis.

♦ An oral dose of homogentisic acid is largely recovered in the urine of affected patients but not in normal persons.

Kidney stones occur with increased frequency.

Urine may contain increased osteocalcin (due to new bone formation) and collagen N-telopeptide (because of bone resorption).

Aminoaciduria, Secondary

See Tables 12-10 and 12-11.

Occurs in
- Severe liver disease
- Renal tubular damage caused by:
  Lysol
  Heavy metals
  Maleic acid
  Burns
  Galactosemia
  Wilson disease
  Scurvy
  Rickets
  Fanconi syndrome (e.g., outdated tetracycline, multiple myeloma, inherited)
- Neoplasms:
  Cystathionine excretion in neuroblastoma of adrenal gland
  Ethanolamine excretion in primary hepatoma

Argininosuccinic Aciduria

Argininosuccinic aciduria is an autosomal recessive deficiency of argininosuccinase that may cause brittle hair, neurologic changes, and absence of metabolic acidosis. More than 12 mutations are located on chromosome 7cen-q11.2.

○ Fasting blood ammonia is normal but may be markedly increased after eating.

♦ Argininosuccinic acid is markedly increased in plasma and urine; it may also be increased in cerebrospinal fluid (CSF).

Because of block in urea cycle, plasma arginine is markedly decreased, and glutamine and alanine are increased.

Urine orotic acid is increased.

Serum ALP may be increased.

♦ Heterozygous carriers show increased argininosuccinic acid in urine and decreased argininosuccinase in RBCs, liver biopsy, and cultured skin fibroblasts.

♦ Prenatal diagnosis by assay of enzyme in cultured amniocytes (*Mycoplasma* contamination may cause a false-negative result) or assay of amniotic fluid for argininosuccinic acid.

Neonatal type is usually fatal in infancy. Late-onset type may present at any age triggered by intercurrent infection or stress.

Table 12-10. Summary of Primary Overflow Aminoacidurias (Increased Blood Concentration with Overflow into Urine)

Disease	Increased Blood Amino Acids	Urine Abnormalities*	Other Laboratory Findings
Phenylketonuria	Phenylalanine	Orthohydroxyphenylacetic acid; phenylpyruvic, acetic, and lactic acids	Blood tyrosine does not rise after phenylalanine load
Maple syrup urine disease			
Severe infantile form	Valine, leucine, isoleucine, alloisoleucine	Branched-chain ketoacids in great excess: urine has odor of maple syrup	
Intermittent form	Same	Ketoaciduria and urine odor present only during attacks	
Hypervalinemia	Valine		
Homocystinuria	Methionine; homocystine	Homocystine in great excess in urine	Vascular accidents, Marfan-like syndrome, osteoporosis
Tryptophanemia	Tryptophan	Decreased excretion of kynurenine after tryptophan load	
Hyperlysinemia	Lysine	Ornithine, gamma-aminobutyric acid, and ethanolamine in excess	
Congenital lysine intolerance	Lysine, arginine		Ammonia intoxication
Tyrosinosis	Tyrosine; methionine may be markedly increased	p-Hydroxyphenylpyruvic, acetic, and lactic acids; methionine may be prominent	Generalized aminoaciduria, renal glycosuria, renal rickets, cirrhosis, Fanconi's syndrome
Cystathioninuria	Cystathionine slightly increased	Cystathionine (may be >1 gm/day)	Congenital acidosis, thrombocytopenia, pituitary gland abnormalities
Hyperglycinemia			
Severe infantile	Glycine (other amino acids may be elevated)	Acetone	May have ammonia intoxication, ketosis, neutropenia, and osteoporosis
With hypo-oxalusia	Glycine	Decreased oxalate excretion	

(continued)

METAB·HERED

Table 12-10. (continued)

Disease	Increased Blood Amino Acids	Urine Abnormalities*	Other Laboratory Findings
Argininosuccinicaciduria	Argininosuccinic acid (~4 mg/dL); Citrulline	Argininosuccinic acid (2.5–9.0 gm/day); Citrulline	Ammonia intoxication
Citrullinemia	Citrulline; alanine	Citrulline; glutamine	Liver disease, ammonia intoxication; BUN may be low
Ornithinemia	Ornithine	Ornithine may be normal	Ammonia intoxication
Histidinemia	Histidine (alanine may also be increased)	Alanine may be increased; imidazolepyruvic, acetic, and lactic acids	Urocanic acid absent in sweat and urine after oral histidine load
Carnosinuria		Carnosine (20–100 mg/day)	
Hyper-beta-alaninemia	Beta-alanine, GABA	Beta-aminoisobutyric acid, GABA, and taurine in excess	Beta-alanine and GABA increased in CSF
Hyperprolinemia			
Type I	Proline	Hydroxyproline, glycine elevated	Patient may have hereditary nephritis
Type II	Proline	Delta^1-pyrroline 5-carboxylate, hydroxyproline, glycine elevated	No nephritis
Hydroxyprolinemia	Hydroxyproline	No excretion of delta^1-pyrroline 3-hydroxy-5-carboxylate or gamma-hydroxyglutamic acid after hydroxyproline load	
Hypophosphatasia	Phosphoethanolamine slightly elevated (≈0.4 mg/dL)	Phosphoethanolamine (≧ 150 mg/day)	Bone disease

GABA = gamma-aminobutyric acid.
*In addition to overflow aminoaciduria:
Mental retardation is often present in these patients.
For proper interpretation of aminoaciduria, avoid all drugs and medications for 3–4 days (unless immediate diagnosis is required), since they may cause renal tubular damage with aminoaciduria or may produce confusing spots on chromatograms. Use fresh urine specimens without urinary tract infection or else amino acid pattern may be abnormal. Since aminoaciduria may occur with various acute illnesses, repeat amino acid chromatogram after recovery from acute illness to avoid misdiagnosis. Some aminoacidurias may not be clinically significant (e.g., newborn aminoaciduria, glycinuria, beta-aminoisobutyricaciduria).
Source: Efron MD, Ampola MG. The aminoacidurias *Pediatr Clin North Am* 1967;14:881.

Table 12-11.	Summary of Renal or Gut Transport Aminoacidurias (Blood Amino Acids Are Normal or Low)
Disease	Amino Acids Increased in Urine
Oasthouse urine disease	Methionine (may not be much increased on normal diet but is on high-methionine diet); smaller amounts of valine, leucine, isoleucine, tryosine, and phenylalanine
Hartnup disease	Neutral amino acids (monoamine, monocarboxylic acid) and basic amino acids (methionine, proline, hydroxyproline, and glycine) normal or only slightly increased
Glycinuria (may be harmless; patient may be heterozygous for benign prolinuria; may be associated with many conditions)	Glycine
Severe prolinuria (Joseph's syndrome)	Proline, hydroxyproline, and glycine in great excess ($\leq$3 gm/day of proline)
Benign prolinuria	Proline, hydroxyproline, and glycine ($\leq$600 mg/day of proline)
Cystine-lysinuria Type I (renal calculi) Type II Type III	Cystine and dibasic amino acids
Isolated cystinuria (familial hypoparathyroidism, ? incidental)	Cystine

Source: Efron MD, Ampola MG. The aminoacidurias. *Pediatr Clin North Am* 1967;14:881.

Beta-Aminoisobutyricaciduria

Beta-aminoisobutyricaciduria is a familial disorder of thymine metabolism. It is a benign metabolic polymorphic trait.

♦ Increased beta-aminoisobutyric acid in urine (50–200 mg/24 h)
May also occur in leukemia because of increased breakdown of nucleic acids.

Carnitine Deficiency

Carnitine deficiency is a very rare autosomal recessive disorder of mitochondrial fatty acid metabolism caused by impaired carnitine transport in muscle, heart, fibroblasts, and renal and intestinal epithelia.

Two types

• Myopathic: Deficiency limited to muscle; normal levels in plasma and other tissues. Myoglobinuria in older children or young adults. Biopsy shows lipid deposits. Tissue homogenates do not support normal rates of beta-oxidation of long-chain fatty acids unless carnitine is added. Serum carnitine is normal or slightly decreased.
• Systemic: More acute clinical picture, presents earlier in life; may mimic Reye syndrome.

Carnitine depleted in blood and all tissues.
Tissue contains marked decreased activity of medium-chain acyl coenzyme A (CoA) dehydrogenase.
Hepatic encephalopathy
Hypoglycemia without ketosis
Hyperammonemia may be present
Increased serum uric acid may be present
Laboratory findings due to cardiomyopathy

METAB/HERED

Due To
- Dietary deficiency
- Low renal reabsorption (e.g., Fanconi syndrome)
- Inborn deficiency of medium-chain acyl CoA dehydrogenase
- Valproic acid therapy (inducing excretion of valprolycarnitine in urine)
- Excessive loss of free carnitine in urine because of failure of carnitine transport across cells of renal tubule, muscle, and fibroblasts
- Organic acidurias (e.g., methylmalonic aciduria, propionic acidemia)
- Others (e.g., maternal deficiency, prematurity)

Citrullinemia

Citrullinemia is a rare autosomal recessive deficiency of argininosuccinate synthetase with metabolic block in citrulline utilization and associated mental retardation. It is genetically heterogeneous (like other disorders of the urea cycle), with various clinical pictures and onset from neonatal to adult period. Many mutations are identified, located at chromosome 9q34.

See Table 12-10.
○ Massive hyperammonemia (>1,000 mg/dL) in neonatal form.
♦ Markedly increased citrulline levels in blood, CSF, and urine in acute neonatal citrullinemia. May also be mildly to moderately increased in argininosuccinic aciduria.
♦ Blood argininosuccinic acid is absent.
○ Serum levels of glutamine and alanine are usually increased.
○ Urine orotic acid is increased.
Laboratory findings due to liver disease.
♦ Deficient enzyme activity can be demonstrated in liver biopsy and cultured skin fibroblasts.
♦ Prenatal diagnosis by assay of citrulline in amniotic fluid or of enzyme in cultured amniocytes. Carrier detection is available.

Cystathioninuria

Cystathioninuria is a rare autosomal recessive deficiency of cystathionine γ-lyase, probably a benign trait, that is corrected by vitamin B_6.

Increased cystathionine in urine

Glutaric Acidemia (Type I)[10]

Glutaric acidemia is an autosomal recessive inborn error of metabolism caused by a deficiency of glutaryl-CoA dehydrogenase, resulting in progressive neurodegenerative disease. Glutaryl-CoA dehydrogenase is a mitochondrial matrix enzyme encoded by nuclear gene on chromosome 19p13.2.

♦ Deficiency of this enzyme causes accumulation of glutaric acid and its metabolites (glutaconic acid and 3-hydroxyglutaric acid) which can be detected in urine by gas chromatographic (GC) MS and is diagnostic.
♦ Deficiency of this enzyme occurs in cultured skin fibroblasts.
♦ Prenatal diagnosis and carrier detection are available
○ Can also use dried blood spots for newborn screening (increased glutarylcarnitine) by MS/MS. May be negative in asymptomatic persons.

Histidinemia

Histidinemia is a rare autosomal recessive deficiency of histidase in liver and skin (converts histidine to urocanic acid). It results from mutations at 12q22-q23.

♦ Plasma histidine is increased to 500 to 1,000 μmol/L (normal = 85–120 μmol/L).
♦ Urine histidine is increased to 0.5 to 4.0 g/d (normal <0.5 g/d). Histidine metabolites (imidazole acetic, imidazole lactic, and imidazole pyruvic acids) are also increased in urine; alanine may be increased.

---

[10]Rakheja D, et al. *Lab Med* 2005;36:174.

Urine may show green color with Phenistix or ferric chloride test because of imidazole pyruvic acid.

With oral histidine load, no FIGLU appears in urine.

Most children show no sequelae; therefore neonatal screening is not performed.

Heterozygote detection is not established yet.

Homocystinuria/Homocysteinemia

Homocystinuria/homocysteinemia are caused by a genetic deficiency of methionine synthase on chromosome 1q43. Homocysteine is the reduced (sulfhydryl) form and homocystine is the oxidized (disulfide) form of homologues cysteine and cystine. The term refers to the combined pool of homocystine and homocysteine and their mixed disulfides. May also be caused by inherited disorders in folate or cobalamin metabolism.

Use

Unexplained thromboembolic disease. Homocysteinemia is independent risk factor for premature arteriosclerosis (e.g., coronary, cerebral, and peripheral vessels) and venous thromboembolic disease. Gradient response to risk of thrombosis: <7.0 μmol/L = no risk; 9.0 μmol/L = low risk; 14.0 μmol/L = moderate risk; >14.0 μmol/L = high risk.

Early diagnosis of cobalamin deficiency.

Due To

Autosomal recessive error of methionine metabolism with deficient methionine synthase in liver and brain, with inability to catalyze homocysteine to methionine. Incidence of mild form = 5% to 7% of general population; severe form is rare.

May also be caused by other rare genetic disorders, e.g., cobalamin C disease.

Increased In

Deranged vitamin B_{12} metabolism, block in folate metabolism, or deficiency of vitamin B_{12}, folate, or vitamin B_6

Chronic renal or liver failure, postmenopausal state, drugs (e.g., methotrexate, phenytoin, theophylline, cigarette smoking)

Various neoplastic diseases (e.g., acute lymphoblastic leukemia, cancers of breast, ovary, pancreas)

Preanalytic factors, e.g., nonfasting sample, delay in separating plasma from cells

♦ Urine excretion of homocysteine is increased (positive nitroprusside screening test). May also contain increased methionine and other amino acids.

♦ Increased serum homocysteine (up to 250 mg/d; normal = trace or not detected) and methionine (up to 2,000 mg/d; normal up to 30 mg/d); also increased in CSF.

♦ Abnormal homocysteine metabolism may only be shown after methionine-loading test. Blood samples before and at 4- to 8-hour intervals after 100 mg/kg methionine oral load. Normal = transient increase free and protein-bound homocysteine peaking between 4 and 8 hours. Abnormal = plasma homocysteine >2 SD greater than normal controls.

In homozygous form, laboratory findings due to associated clinical conditions:

• Mild variable hepatocellular dysfunction
• Mental retardation, Marfan syndrome, osteoporosis, etc.

Serum methionine levels should be kept at 20 to 150 μmol/L by a low-methionine diet and pyridoxine therapy.

♦ Patients have enzyme activity levels of 0% to 10% in fibroblasts and lymphocytes; heterozygotes (their parents) have levels <50% of normal.

♦ For neonatal detection, measure methionine in filter paper specimen of blood; confirm by measuring blood and urine amino acids. Methionine tends to be very low in newborns.

♦ Can also measure specific enzyme in cultured fibroblasts.

Hydroxyprolinemia

Hydroxyprolinemia is a very rare autosomal recessive benign trait.

♦ Increased hydroxyproline in blood

METAB/HERED

Hyperglycinemia

Hyperglycinemia is a rare autosomal recessive disease with ketotic and long-chain ketotic forms (without hypoglycemia) and ketonuria accentuated by leucine ingestion.

Same findings (neutropenia, thrombocytopenia, hypogammaglobulinemia, increased glycine in blood and urine, osteoporosis, hypoglycemia) may occur in propionic acidemia, methylmalonic acidemia, isovaleric acidemia, and 3-keto-thiolase deficiency.

Hyperoxaluria

Hyperoxaluria is a rare autosomal recessive organic acid disorder.

Type I (glycolic aciduria) is caused by deficiency of alanine:glyoxylate aminotransferase (converts glycolic acid to glycine). In absence, glycolic acid is converted to oxalic acid.
♦ Early childhood calcium oxalate renal calculi and nephrocalcinosis with extrarenal deposition of calcium oxalate in eye, heart, skin, other sites. Uremia causes death.
♦ Increased glycolic and oxalic acid in urine in large amounts.
Type II (glyceric aciduria), caused by deficiency of glyceric dehydrogenase or glycerol kinase, is milder and may be asymptomatic.
♦ Increased serum and urinary oxalic acid
Increased urinary glycolic and glyoxylic acid
Must be distinguished from secondary increased absorption from bowel (e.g., inflammatory bowel disease, fat malabsorption)

Hyperprolinemia

There are two types of hyperprolinemia, caused by rare autosomal recessive traits. Type I is benign and due to decreased activity of proline oxidase encoded on chromosome 22q11.2. Type II may have seizures; due to deficient activity of delta-1-pyrroline-5-carboxylate-dehydrogenase encoded on chromosome 1p36.)

Type II shows
♦ Increased proline in blood and urine
Increased glycine and hydroxyproline in urine
Severe prolinuria (Joseph syndrome)
♦ Urine shows marked increase in proline, hydroxyproline, and glycine.
Heterozygotes may show mild prolinuria.
Type II shows same findings as Type I, along with:
♦ Increased blood and urine levels of pyrroline-5-carboxylate and increased urine level of pyrroline-3-hydroxy-5 carboxylate.
♦ Deficient enzyme activity in WBCs and cultured skin fibroblasts.

Maple Syrup Urine Disease[11]

Maple syrup urine disease (MSUD) is caused by an autosomal recessive deficiency of mitochondrial multienzyme complex branched-chain α-keto acid-dehydrogenase; the incidence is about 1 in 200,000 live births. There is a characteristic maple syrup odor in urine, sweat, hair, and cerumen. Genes are encoded at chromosomes 19q13.1-q13.2, 6p22-p21, and 1p31.

♦ Blood shows greatly increased branched-chain amino acids (leucine, isoleucine, and valine) and their ketoacids. Presence of alloisoleucine (stereoisomeric metabolite of isoleucine) is characteristic.
○ Metabolic ketoacidosis occurs, often with hyperammonemia and hypoglycemia.
○ Ferric chloride test of urine produces green-gray color.
○ Newborn screening testing for leucine may be available.

---

[11]www.msud-support.org.

♦ MSUD is divided into six severity classes (Ia, Ib, II, III, IV, V) depending on which enzyme has been mutated and identifying that enzyme.

Loading tests with isoleucine and measuring increased alloisoleucine in blood may be performed for variant MSUD.[12]

Patient must be monitored to avoid ketoacidosis.

♦ Prenatal diagnosis can be performed by measuring enzyme concentration in cells cultured from amniotic fluid.

Methylmalonic Acidemia

Methylmalonic acidemia is a very rare autosomal recessive error of metabolism, with neonatal metabolic acidosis and mental and somatic retardation. There are at least four distinct forms; the screening incidence is 1 in 48,000 in infants 3 to 4 weeks old.

○ Metabolic acidosis
○ Increased methylmalonic acid in urine and plasma
Long-chain ketonuria
Intermittent hyperglycinemia
○ All findings accentuated by high-protein diet or supplemental ingestion of valine or isoleucine
Hypoglycemia, neutropenia, thrombocytopenia may occur
Heterozygote detection is not reliable
♦ Prenatal diagnosis by assay of methylmalonyl CoA mutase in cultured amniocytes, increased methylcitric or methylmalonic acids in amniotic fluid, or (late in pregnancy) increased methylmalonic acid in maternal urine
♦ Identify by MS/MS spectrometry

Methylmalonic acidemia and aciduria are direct measures of tissue vitamin B_{12} deficiency. (See Chapter 11.)

Nephron Transport Defects, Classification

Proximal Tubule

Selective transport defects

(A) Renal glycosuria (primary; combined)
(B) Renal aminoaciduria
  • 1. Basic aminoacidurias
      ○ (a) General cystinuria (cystine, lysine, arginine, ornithine)
      ○ (b) Specific hypercystinuria, dibasic aminoaciduria, lysinuria
  • 2. Neutral aminoacidurias
      ○ (a) General (Hartnup disease)
      ○ (b) Specific (methioninuria, tryptophanuria, histidinuria)
  • 3. Dicarboxylic aminoaciduria
      ○ (a) General (glutamic, aspartic acids)
  • 4. Iminoglycinuria
      ○ (a) General (proline, hydroxyproline, glycine)
      ○ (b) Specific (glycinuria)
(C) Proximal RTA (primary or due to carbonic anhydrase change)
(D) Uric acid disorders
(E) Calcium and phosphate disorders

Nonselective (Fanconi syndrome)

(A) Genetic (e.g., cystinosis, tyrosinemia, Wilson disease)
(B) Tubulointerstitial (e.g., Sjögren syndrome, medullary cystic disease, renal transplant)
(C) Heavy metals (lead, cadmium, mercury)
(D) Drugs, toxins (e.g., outdated tetracycline, gentamicin)
(E) Monoclonal gammopathies (see Chapter 11)

[12]Schadewaldt P, Bodner-Leidecker A, Hammen HW, Wendel U. Significance of L-alloisoleucine in plasma for diagnosis of maple syrup urine disease. *Clin Chem* 1999;45:1734–1740.

METAB/HERED

(F) Secondary hyperparathyroidism
(G) Others (e.g., nephrotic syndrome, amyloidosis, paroxysmal nocturnal hemoglobinuria)

Loop of Henle

Bartter syndrome
Drugs (e.g., ethacrynic acid, furosemide)

Distal Tubule

I. Selective transport defects

(A) Distal RTA
- 1. Genetic disorders (e.g., medullary cystic disease **[see Chapter 14]**, sickle cell anemia, elliptocytosis **[see Chapter 11]**)
- 2. Nephrocalcinosis (e.g., hyperparathyroidism, hyperthyroidism, medullary sponge kidney, Wilson disease, Fabry disease)
- 3. Tubulointerstitial (e.g., chronic pyelonephritis, obstructive uropathy, renal transplant) **(see Chapter 14)**
- 4. Autoimmune disorders (e.g., Sjögren syndrome, SLE, primary biliary cirrhosis)
- 5. Drugs (e.g., analgesics, amphotericin B)
(B) Renal tubular acidosis of glomerular insufficiency **(see Chapter 14)**
(C) Potassium secretory disorders

II. Nonselective transport defects (distal RTA, hyperkalemia, renal salt wasting) (see Chapter 13)

(A) Primary mineralocorticoid deficiency
(B) Hypoangiotensinemia drugs (e.g., captopril, angiotensin receptor blockers)
(C) Hyporeninemic hypoaldosteronism (e.g., diabetic nephropathy, tubulointerstitial nephropathies, nephrosclerosis, AIDS, nonsteroidal anti-inflammatory drugs)
(D) Mineralocorticoid-resistant hyperkalemia with or without salt wasting

Medullary Collecting Ducts (see Chapter 13)

Disorders of concentration and dilution (e.g., diabetes insipidus, syndrome of inappropriate excretion of antidiuretic hormone, others)

Oasthouse Urine Disease

Oasthouse urine disease is an autosomal recessive disorder of methionine malabsorption in GI tract with diarrhea, failure to thrive, mental retardation, and white hair.

♦ Distinctive odor of urine
Increase of various amino acids in blood and also in urine (e.g., phenylalanine, tyrosine, methionine, valine, leucine, isoleucine)

Ornithine Transcarbamoylase Deficiency

This is caused by an X-linked recessive deficiency of ornithine transcarbamoylase (OTC), a mitochondrial enzyme in the urea cycle that converts ornithine to citrulline. This disorder may cause seizures, cerebral palsy, mental retardation, hyperammonemic encephalopathy, and death.

○ Increased blood ammonia, usually $2\times$ to $10\times$ normal; glutamine, glycine, alanine are increased.
○ Markedly decreased citrulline and decreased arginine in blood.
○ Markedly increased orotic acid in blood and urine. May also be increased in lysinuric protein intolerance.
♦ Decreased OTC in biopsy of liver.
♦ To detect asymptomatic carriers, female heterozygotes may require measurement of urine orotic acid before and 6 hours after an oral protein loading test. Can also be

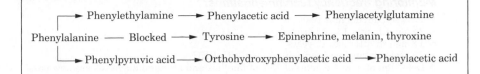

Fig. 12-6. Pathways of phenylalanine metabolism.

detected by a cDNA probe for the ornithine transcarbamylase gene using restriction fragment length polymorphism analysis (RFLP).
♦ Prenatal diagnosis using RFLP for chorionic villus DNA analysis.
OTC deficiency can occur after a bacterial or viral infection, causing confusion with Reye syndrome.

Phenylketonuria

PKU is an inherited autosomal recessive disorder caused by a variety of mutations on chromosome 12. The absence of phenylalanine hydroxylase activity in liver causes increased phenylalanine and its metabolites (phenylpyruvic acid, ortho-hydroxyphenylacetic acid) in blood, urine, and CSF; tyrosine and the derivative catecholamines are deficient. The condition results in mental retardation. Among Caucasians, 1 in 50 persons is a carrier and ~1 in 12,000 in the United States is affected with PKU. See Figure 12-6.

Unrestricted protein diet:

• Normal blood phenylalanine = 2 mg/dL.
♦ • Classic PKU patients: high blood phenylalanine (usually >30 mg/dL and always >20 mg/dL in infancy) with phenylalanine and its metabolites in urine; normal or decreased tyrosine concentration.
♦ • Less severe variant forms of PKU: blood phenylalanine levels are 15 to 30 mg/dL and metabolites may appear in urine (incidence = 1:15,000).
♦ • Mild persistent hyperphenylalaninemia: blood phenylalanine may be 2 to 12 mg/dL and metabolites are not found in urine (incidence 1:30,000).
♦ For screening of newborns, urine amounts of phenylpyruvic acid may be insufficient for detection by colorimetric methods when blood level is <15 mg/dL. May not appear in urine until 2 to 3 weeks of age. False-negative results on the Guthrie bacteria inhibition test may also occur if capillary tubes and venipuncture specimens are used for blood collection rather than direct application to filter paper, especially if level is within 0.2 mg of cutoff value. Preliminary blood screening tests detects >4 mg/dL. Screening should be performed after protein-containing feedings have begun.
♦ When repeat screening test is positive, quantitative blood phenylalanine and tyrosine are performed to confirm phenylalaninemia and exclude transient tyrosinemia of newborn, which is the most common cause of a positive screening. Tandem mass spectrometry or fluorometry confirms the increased level and also measures tyrosine levels.
♦ Serial determinations should be performed on untreated borderline cases, because blood levels may change markedly with time or stress and infection.
♦ Diagnosis of PKU may be confirmed by giving 100 mg of ascorbic acid and collecting blood and urine 24 hours later.

Adjust diet throughout life by monitoring blood phenylalanine:

• Up to 12 years old: 2 to 6 mg/dL.
• After age 12: 2 to 10 mg/dL.
• After adolescence: 2 to 15 mg/dL.
• During pregnancy: 2 to 5 mg/dL, because with increased serum phenylalanine there is greatly increased frequency of mental retardation, microcephaly, and congenital heart disease in offspring.

META3/HERED

Monitoring frequency recommendations:

- 1×/week during first year
- 2×/month ages 1 to 12 years
- 1×/month after age 12 years
- 2×/week during pregnancy in women with PKU
- ◆ Detection of heterozygotes of 75% of families and prenatal diagnosis are now possible using cDNA probe.

Laboratory findings due to congenital heart disease in ≤15% of PKU patients.

Urine $FeCl_3$ dipstick test is positive because of phenylpyruvic acid.

Comparison of PKU and Transient Tyrosinemia

Substance	PKU	Transient Tyrosinemia
Serum phenylalanine	>15 mg/dL	>4 mg/dL (15–20 mg/dL)
Serum tyrosine	<5 mg/dL (is never increased)	>4 mg/dL (5–20 mg/dL)
Urine o-hydroxyphenylacetic acid	Present	Absent
Urine	Phenylalanine is >100 µg/mL	Large amounts of tyrosine and its metabolites

Propionic Acidemia

Propionic acidemia is characterized by an autosomal recessive deficiency of propionyl CoA carboxylase, which prevents degradation and therefore results in intolerance of isoleucine, valine, threonine, and methionine. Incidence in the United States = ~1:50,000 live births.

○ Recurrent episodes (often following infections) of massive ketosis, metabolic acidosis, vomiting, and dehydration progressing to coma.

Same picture as hyperglycinemia (see previous).

○ Increase plasma and urine glycine.

Urine is tested (daily in infants) for ketones (e.g., Acetest reagent strips or tablets) and blood for propionic acid to monitor treatment.

Laboratory findings of complications (e.g., sepsis, ventricular hemorrhage)

- ◆ Prenatal diagnosis is available.
- ◆ Positive assay of enzyme in cultured fibroblasts can indicate heterozygosity, but negative assay may not be reliable to indicate absence.

Renal Amino Acid Transport Disorders

Cystinuria

Cystinuria is an autosomal recessive failure of amino acid transport, resulting in renal tubular reabsorption and intestinal uptake of cystine, ornithine, lysine, arginine.

- ◆ Markedly increased cystine in urine (20×−30× normal). May also be increased in organic acidemias, hyperuricemia, trisomy 21, hereditary pancreatitis, muscular dystrophy, hemophilia, retinitis pigmentosa.
- ◆ Presence of characteristic hexagonal crystals in urine is diagnostic.
- ◆ Confirm diagnosis by identifying increased urinary arginine, lysine, and ornithine in urine. Homozygotes excrete >800 mg/24 h of cystine.
- ◆ Cystine renal and bladder stones make up ≤8% of stones in children, 1% in adults.

Laboratory findings due to genitourinary (GU) tract infections. *Bacteria can degrade cystine.*

Hartnup Disease

Hartnup disease is a rare autosomal recessive defect in transport in GI tract and renal tubules of "neutral" amino acids, which causes nicotinamide deficiency (due to faulty metabolism of tryptophan) and may lead to pellagra. Incidence = 1:26,000 births.

♦ Urine contains increased (5×−1×) amounts of alanine, threonine, valine, leucine, isoleucine, phenylalanine, tyrosine, tryptamine, histidine.

Iminoglycinuria

Iminoglycinuria is a rare benign inherited autosomal recessive defect of renal tubule amino acid transport.

♦ Increased urine glycine, imino acids (proline, hydroxyproline) but normal or low in blood.

Tyrosinemia

Occurs as both persistent hereditary and transient forms.

Tyrosinemia I (Hepatorenal) (Tyrosinosis) Persistent Hereditary Form

Type I tyrosinemia is a rare autosomal recessive condition caused by deficiency of fumaryl acetoacetase, with an incidence of 1 per 50,000 live births; it is usually fatal in the first year.

♦ Increased blood and urine tyrosine; methionine may also be markedly increased; increased blood phenylalanine may cause positive test when screening for PKU.
○ Urinary excretion of tyrosine metabolites p-hydroxyphenylpyruvic and p-hydroxyphenylacetic acids is increased. *May also be increased in myasthenia gravis, liver disease, ascorbic acid deficiency, and malignancies.*
♦ Detection of succinylacetone in urine is virtually diagnostic.
Acetic and lactic acids may be increased in urine.
Anemia, thrombocytopenia, and leukopenia are common.
Urine δ-aminolevulinic acid (δ-ALA) may be increased.
Laboratory findings due to Fanconi syndrome, hepatic cirrhosis, and liver carcinoma are noted.
Dietary restriction of tyrosine, phenylalanine, and methionine can correct biochemical and renal abnormalities but does not reverse or prevent progression of liver disease. A liver transplant can correct biochemical abnormalities.
♦ Prenatal diagnosis by measurement of succinylacetone in amniotic fluid has been used.

Tyrosinemia II (Oculocutaneous)

Type II tyrosinemia is a rare condition caused by a deficiency of tyrosine aminotransferase.

♦ Plasma tyrosine markedly increased (30–50 mg/dL)
Tyrosine is found in urine
No findings of liver or kidney disease

Tyrosinemia III

Type III tyrosinemia is caused by a deficiency of 4-hydroxyphenylpyruvic acid oxidase.

Transient Tyrosinemia

Transient tyrosinemia may occur in incomplete development of tyrosine oxidizing system, especially in premature or low-birth-weight infants.

♦ Serum phenylalanine is >4 mg/dL (5–20 mg/dL).
♦ Serum tyrosine is between 10 and 75 mg/dL.
♦ Tyrosine metabolites in urine are ≤1 mg/mL (parahydroxyphenyl-lactic and parahydroxyphenylacetic acids can be distinguished from o-hydroxyphenylacetic acid by paper chromatography).
♦ O-hydroxyphenylacetic acid is absent from urine.
Without administration of ascorbic acid, 25% of premature infants may have increased serum phenylalanine and tyrosine for several weeks (but reversed in 24 hours after ascorbic acid administration) and increased urine tyrosine and tyrosine derivatives.

METAB/HERED

Similar blood and urine findings that are not reversed by administration of ascorbic acid may occur in untreated galactosemia, tyrosinemia, congenital cirrhosis, and giant-cell hepatitis; jaundice occurs frequently.

Serum serotonin (5-hydroxytryptophan) is decreased.

Urine 5'-hydroxyindoleacetic acid excretion is decreased.

Blood levels of phenylalanine deficiency should be monitored frequently during treatment (e.g., 2×/week during first 6 months, 1×/week during next 6 months, 2×/month up to age 18 months, 1×/month thereafter).

Adjust diet by monitoring blood phenylalanine (e.g., 10 mg/dL with consistently negative $FeCl_3$ urine test.)

In women with untreated PKU and increased serum phenylalanine, there is a greatly increased frequency of mental retardation, microcephaly, and congenital heart disease in offspring.

♦ Detection of heterozygotes in 75% of families and prenatal diagnosis are now possible using cDNA probe.

Xanthinuria

Xanthinuria is a rare autosomal recessive deficiency of xanthine oxidase in tissues, which catalyzes conversion of hypoxanthine to xanthine and xanthine to uric acid.

♦ Enzyme activity <10% of normal in biopsy of liver and jejunal mucosa.

♦ Decreased serum uric acid; <1 mg/dL strongly suggests this diagnosis.

Decreased urine uric acid (usually <30 mg/24 h; normal up to 500 mg/24 h).

Increased urine and serum levels of xanthine and hypoxanthine.

○ Laboratory findings due to urinary xanthine calculi.

Disorders of Carbohydrate Metabolism

Fructosuria, Essential

Fructosuria is a benign asymptomatic autosomal recessive disorder caused by a deficiency of hepatic fructokinase, which metabolizes fructose to fructose-1-phosphate. The gene is encoded at chromosome 2p23.3-p23.2.

○ Large amount of fructose in urine gives a positive test for reducing substances (Benedict reagent, Clinitest) but not with glucose-oxidase methods (Clinistix, Tes-Tape).

♦ Fructose is identified by paper chromatography.

♦ Fructose tolerance test shows that blood fructose increases to 4× more than in normal persons, blood glucose increases only slightly, and serum phosphorus does not change.

Fructose Intolerance, Hereditary

Hereditary fructose intolerance is a severe autosomal recessive disease of infancy caused by a virtual absence of fructose-1-phosphate aldolase, causing fructose-1-phosphate accumulation in liver; clinically, it resembles galactosemia.

○ Fructose in urine of 100 to 300 mg/dL gives a positive test for reducing substances (Benedict reagent, Clinitest) but not with glucose oxidase methods (Clinistix, Tes-Tape).

♦ Fructose is identified by chromatography.

♦ Fructose tolerance test shows prolonged elevation of blood fructose and marked decrease in serum glucose, which may cause convulsions and coma. Serum phosphorus shows rapid prolonged decrease. Aminoaciduria and proteinuria may occur during test.

○ Fructosemia, fructosuria, hypoglycemia, and lactic acidosis are present, with increased blood potassium, magnesium, and uric acid and decreased phosphate.

Increased serum ALT, AST, and bilirubin; cirrhosis may occur.

♦ Carriers and prenatal testing by molecular genetic techniques.

♦ Aldolase B assay in liver biopsy confirms diagnosis.

Fructose-1,6-Diphosphatase Deficiency

Fructose-1,6-diphosphatase deficiency is a rare severe autosomal recessive disease of infancy due to deficiency of enzyme in liver, kidney, and jejunum. It is caused by a mutation at chromosome 9q22.2-q22.3.

Episodes of hypoglycemia, lactic acidosis, increased pyruvate, alanine, uric acid, usually without fructosuria.
♦ Deficient fructose-1,6-diphosphatase in WBCs and liver and jejunal biopsies.
♦ Prenatal diagnosis and carrier testing are available.

Galactosemia, Classic

Classic galactosemia is an autosomal recessive inherited defect in liver and RBCs of galactose-1-phosphate uridyltransferase, which converts galactose to glucose; the deficiency causes accumulation of galactose-1-phosphate located on chromosome 9p13. Rarer variant forms are caused by galactokinase deficiency and uridinediphosphate-galactose-4-epimerase deficiency.)

♦ Increased blood galactose ≤300 mg/dL (normal <5 mg/dL).
♦ Increased urine galactose of 500 to 2,000 mg/dL (normal <5 mg/dL). Positive urine reaction with Clinitest but negative with Clinistix and Tes-Tape may be useful for pediatric screening up to 1 year of age.
♦ Reduced RBC galactose-1-phosphate uridyltransferase establishes diagnosis.
Serum glucose may appear to be elevated in fasting state but falls as galactose increases; hypoglycemia is usual.
Galactose tolerance test is positive but not necessary for diagnosis and may be hazardous because of induced hypoglycemia and hypokalemia.

* Use an oral dose of 35 g of galactose/m^2 body area.
* Normal: Serum galactose increases to 30 to 50 mg/dL and returns to normal within 3 hours.
* Galactosemia: Serum increase is greater, and return to baseline level is delayed.
* Heterozygous carrier: Response is intermediate.
* The test is not specific or sensitive enough for genetic studies.

Albuminuria
General aminoaciduria is identified by chromatography.
Laboratory findings due to complications:

* Jaundice (onset at age 4–10 days)
* Liver biopsy—dilated canaliculus filled with bile pigment with surrounding rosette of liver cells, leading to cirrhosis
* Severe hemolysis
* Coagulation abnormalities
* Vomiting, diarrhea, failure to thrive
* Hyperchloremic metabolic acidosis
* Cataracts
* Mental and physical retardation
* Decreased immunity (~25% of infants develop Gram-negative [especially *Escherichia coli*] sepsis, which may cause death). *Newborns with positive screening should be worked up for sepsis.*

Findings disappear (but are not reversed) when galactose is eliminated from diet (e.g., milk). Efficacy of diet is monitored by RBC level of galactose-1-phosphate (desired range <4 mg/dL or <180 μg/g Hb).
Screening incidence = 1:7,500 live births. Cord blood is preferred, but this prevents simultaneous screening for PKU, which is normal in neonatal cord blood. Filter paper blood may show false-positive test for PKU, tyrosinemia, and homocystinuria. Test is invalidated by exchange transfusion. One in 40 persons is a carrier.
♦ Prenatal diagnosis is done by measurement of galactose-1-phosphate uridyltransferase in cell culture from amniotic fluid. Parents show <50% enzyme activity in RBCs.
In galactokinase deficiency (gene located on chromosome 17q21-q25), the accumulation of galactose is reduced by alternate pathway to galactitol, causing osmotic damage to lens fibers (cataracts in childhood).

METAB/HERED

♦ • RBCs show absent galactokinase and presence of galactose-1-phosphate uridyl-transferase.

• No liver, kidney, or CNS sequelae.

Lactase Deficiency; Intestinal Deficiency of Sugar-Splitting Enzymes (Milk Allergy; Milk Intolerance; Congenital Familial Lactose Intolerance; Disaccharidase Deficiency)

Lactase deficiency is a familial disease with failure of lactose to be hydrolyzed to glucose and galactose that often begins in infancy with diarrhea, malabsorption, etc. Patients become asymptomatic when lactose is removed from the diet.

Oral lactose tolerance test shows a rise in blood sugar <20 mg/dL in blood drawn at 15, 30, 60, and 90 minutes (usual dose = 50 g). *In diabetics, blood sugar may increase >20 mg/dL despite impaired lactose absorption. Test may also be influenced by impaired gastric emptying or small bowel transit.*

If test is positive, repeat using glucose and galactose (usually 25 g each) instead of lactose; subnormal rise indicates a mucosal absorptive defect; normal increase (>25 g/dL) indicates lactase deficiency only.

♦ Biopsy of small intestine mucosa shows low level of lactase in homogenized tissue. Is used to assess other diagnostic tests but is seldom required, except to exclude secondary lactase deficiency with histologic studies.

♦ Hydrogen breath test (measured by gas chromatography) is noninvasive, rapid, simple, sensitive, and quantitative. Patient expires into a breath-collecting apparatus; complete absorption causes no increase of H_2 formed in colon to be excreted in breath. Malabsorption causes H_2 production by fermentation in colon that is proportional to the amount of test dose not absorbed. False-negative test in ~20% of patients due to absence of H_2-producing bacteria in colon or prior antibiotic therapy.

○ Lactose in urine amounts to 100 to 2,000 mg/dL. It produces a positive test for reducing sugars (Benedict reagent, Clinitest) but a negative test with glucose-oxidase methods (Tes-Tape, Clinistix).

After ingestion of milk or 50 to 100 g of lactose, stools have a pH of 4.5 to 6.0 (normal pH is >7.0) and are sour and frothy. Fecal studies are of limited value in adults.

Pentosuria

Pentosuria is a benign autosomal recessive deficiency in L-xylitol dehydrogenase, which catalyzes the reduction of L-xylulose to xylitol in the metabolism of glucuronic acid.

♦ Urinary excretion of L-xylulose is increased (1–4 g/d), and the increase is accentuated by administration of glucuronic acid and glucuronigenic drugs (e.g., aminopyrine, antipyrine, menthol).

○ Urine positive for reducing substances but negative for glucose using glucose-oxidase enzymatic strips.

♦ Heterozygotes can be detected by glucuronic acid loading, followed by measuring serum xylulose or assay nicotinamide adenine dinucleotide phosphate–L-xylulose dehydrogenase in RBCs.

Differential Diagnosis

Alimentary pentosuria—arabinose or xylose excreted after ingestion of large amount of certain fruits (e.g., plums, cherries, grapes)

Healthy normal persons—small amounts of d-ribose or trace amounts of ribulose in urine

Muscular dystrophy—small amounts of d-ribose in urine (some patients)

Sucrosuria

Sucrosuria is caused by a deficiency of sucrase.

Urine specific gravity is very high (≤1.07).
Urine tests for reducing substances are negative.
Sucrosuria may follow intravenous administration of sucrose or the factitious addition of cane sugar to urine.

Glycogen Storage Diseases

GSDs are inherited autosomal recessive disorders (except for type IXb, which is X-linked) with abnormal concentrations or structure of glycogen molecule due to deficient activity of various enzymes in different organs. GSDs are characterized by an abnormally increased concentration of glycogen in the liver (>70 mg/g of liver) or muscle (>15 mg/g of muscle) or abnormal glycogen molecule structure. See Table 12-12.

Type IA GSD (Glucose-6-Phosphatase Deficiency; Von Gierke Disease)

Type IA GSD is caused by a lack of glucose-6-phosphatase (G6P) in liver, kidney, and intestine, with an incidence of 1:200,000 births. It may appear in the first days or weeks of life.

○ Blood glucose is markedly decreased.
○ After overnight fast, marked hypoglycemia, increased blood lactate, and occasionally pyruvate with severe metabolic acidosis, ketonemia, and ketonuria. *(Recurrent acidosis is most common cause for hospital admission.)*
Blood TGs are very high, cholesterol is moderately increased, and serum free fatty acids are increased. Results in xanthomas and lipid-laden cells in bone marrow.
Mild anemia is present.
Impaired platelet adhesiveness may cause bleeding tendency.
Increased serum uric acid may cause clinical gout, nephrocalcinosis, proteinuria.
Serum phosphorus and ALP are decreased.
Urinary nonspecific amino acids are increased, without increase in blood amino acids.
Other renal function tests are relatively normal despite kidney enlargement; Fanconi syndrome is rare.
Liver function tests (other than those related to carbohydrate metabolism) are relatively normal, but serum GGT, AST, and ALT may be slightly increased.
Glucose tolerance may be normal or diabetic type; diabetic type is more frequent in older children and adults.
○ Functional tests
  • Administer 1 mg of glucagon intravenously or intramuscularly after an 8-hour fast. Blood glucose increases 50% to 60% in 10 to 20 minutes in a healthy person. Little or no increase occurs in infants or young children with von Gierke disease; delayed response may occur in older children and adults.
  • Intravenous administration of glucose precursors (e.g., galactose or fructose) causes no rise in blood glucose in von Gierke disease (demonstrating block in gluconeogenesis), but normal rise occurs in limit dextrinosis (type III GSD).
♦ Biopsy of liver shows absent or markedly decreased G6P on assay of frozen liver provides definitive diagnosis. Other enzymes (other GSDs) are present in normal amounts. Increased glycogen content (>4% by weight), but normal biochemically and structurally. Histologic findings are not diagnostic; show vacuolization of hepatic cells and abundant glycogen granules confirmed with Best stain.
♦ Biopsy of jejunum shows intestinal glucose-6-phosphatase is decreased or absent.
Biopsy of muscle shows no abnormality of enzyme activity or glycogen content.
Can be cured by liver transplant.
Late complications include liver adenomas that tend to become malignant and progressive glomerulosclerosis with renal failure.

Type IB GSD

Type IB GSD shows all the clinical and biochemical features of von Gierke disease, except that liver biopsy does not show deficiency of G6P. It is caused by defective transport of G6P across microsomal membrane of liver cells and granulocytes.

○ May have maturation arrest neutropenia; varies from mild to agranulocytosis; usually constant but may be cyclic. Associated increased frequency of staphylococcal and *Candida* infections and Crohn disease.

Table 12-12. Comparison of Glycogen Storage Diseases

Type	Gene Location	Frequency (%)	Deficient Enzyme	Principal Organ Involved	Usual Age at Onset	Laboratory Findings
O	12p12.2		Glycogen synthetase	No glycogen synthesis in liver	First year	Hypoglycemia, ketosis
I von Gierke disease		20			Newborn or 3–4 mo	
Ia	17q21		Glucose-6-phosphatase	Normal glycogen accumulates in liver, kidney		↓↓↓glucose, ↑uric acid, ↑lipids, lactic acidosis, platelet dysfunction
Ib	11q23		Microsomal transport of glucose-6-phosphatase	Liver, WBCs		Similar to Ia but less severe. ↓↓↓WBCs. Recurrent bacterial infections, Crohn disease
Ic	11q23	Rare	Deficient microsomal transport of phosphate	Liver, kidney		Similar to Ia
II Pompe disease	12q25.2–q25.3	20	Lysosomal α-glucosidase			
IIa				↔Heart, MM	Infancy	Normal glycogen in lysosomes of all organs
IIb				Heart, MM	Juvenile	Normal glycogen in lysosomes of MM
IIc				MM	Adult	Little/no glycogen

IIIa to **IIIf** Forbes or Cori disease	1p21	20	Amylo-1,6-glucosidase (debrancher enzyme)	Accumulation of highly branched, short-chain abnormal glycogen in liver. In some subtypes, also in MM and heart	Infancy	↓↓Glucose
IV Andersen syndrome	3p12	<1	Amylo-1,4→1,6 transglucosidase (brancher enzyme)	Accumulation of abnormally structured glycogen in liver, MM	Severe; death in <48 mo	Cirrhosis, late-onset myopathy
V McArdle syndrome	11q13	5	Muscle phosphorylase	Moderate accumulation of normal structure MM		Cramps on exercise → no ↑blood lactate; myoglobinuria
VI Hers disease	14q21-q22	Rare	Liver phosphorylase	Accumulation of normal glycogen in liver		↓Glucose; may be asymptomatic
VII Tarui disease	12q13.3	25 for VI and VII	Phosphofructokinase	Enzyme ↓↓↓ in MM; ↓50% in RBCs; Accumulation of normal glycogen in MM	Adult	Hemolysis; cramps on exercise; causes no ↑blood lactate
VIII Hug, Huijing	?	Very rare	Inactive liver phosphorylase	Accumulation of glycogen in liver, CNS	Death in childhood	
IXa	Xp22.2–p22.1	25	Deficient phosphorylase kinase in liver	Glycogen accumulates in liver, RBCs, WBCs		
IXb	16q12–q13			Glycogen accumulates in liver, MM, RBCs, WBCs		

(continued)

Table 12-12. *(continued)*

Type	Gene Location	Frequency (%)	Deficient Enzyme	Principal Organ Involved	Usual Age at Onset	Laboratory Findings
IXc	16p12.1–p11.2		Deficient phosphorylase kinase in liver, testis	Glycogen accumulates in liver, RBCs, WBCs		
IXd	Xq12–q13		Deficient phosphorylase kinase in muscle	Glycogen accumulates in MM		
X	?		cAMP-dependent kinase	Glycogen accumulates in liver, MM		Mild hypoglycemia
XI Fanconi-Bickel syndrome	3q26.1–26.3		Microsomal transport of glucose	Glycogen accumulates in liver, proximal renal tubules	Galactose intolerance, mild fasting hypoglycemia	Proximal renal tubular wasting of PO_4, HCO_3^-

MM, skeletal muscle; CNS, central nervous system; cAMP, cyclic adenosine monophosphate; ↔, variable; ↓ to ↓↓↓↓, degree of decrease.

♦ Establish diagnosis by impaired function of G6P activity in granulocytes and impaired transport protein in liver biopsy.

Type II GSD (Pompe Disease; Generalized Glycogenosis; A-Glucosidase Deficiency)

Type II GSD is an autosomal recessive disease showing absence in infantile onset, or marked reduction in juvenile/adult onset, of lysosomal α-glucosidase (acid maltase) activity. The classic infantile form (type IIA) shows neurologic, cardiac, and muscle involvement; frequent liver enlargement; and death within the first year. The juvenile form (type IIB) displays muscle disease resembling pseudohypertrophic dystrophy, and in the adult form (type IIC), there is progressive myopathy.

Fasting blood sugar, glucose tolerance test, glucagon responses, and rises in blood glucose after fructose infusion are normal. No acetonuria is present.
General hematologic findings are normal.
♦ Staining of circulating leukocytes for glycogen shows massive deposition.
♦ Confirm diagnosis by absence of α-glucosidase in muscle or liver biopsy or cultured fibroblasts or leukocytes. Assay of amniotic cells or chorionic villus biopsy allows prenatal diagnosis. Neonatal diagnosis may also be possible using dried blood spots.

Type III GSD (Cori-Forbes Disease; Debrancher Deficiency; Limit Dextrinosis)

Type III GSD is an autosomal recessive (gene on chromosome 1p21) disease with enlarged liver, retarded growth, chemical changes, and benign course caused by a deficiency of amylo-1,6-glucosidase (debrancher enzyme). About 80% of those affected lack enzyme in liver and muscle (IIIa), ~15% lack enzyme only in liver (IIIb); IIIc lacks only enzyme glucosidase and type IIId lacks transferase enzyme only.

Serum creatine kinase (CK) may be markedly increased.
Mild increases in cholesterol and TG are less marked than in type I.
Marked fasting acetonuria (as in starvation).
Fasting hypoglycemia is less severe than in type I.
Normal blood lactate; uric acid is usually normal.
Serum AST and ALT are increased in children but normal in adults.
Diabetic type of glucose tolerance curve, with associated glucosuria.
Infusions of gluconeogenic precursors (e.g., galactose, fructose) causes a normal hyperglycemic response, in contrast to type I.
○ Low fasting blood sugar does not show expected rise after administration of subcutaneous glucagon or epinephrine but does increase 2 hours after high-carbohydrate meal.
♦ Confirm diagnosis by deficient debrancher activity in liver and muscle biopsy, WBCs, RBCs, cultured skin fibroblasts. Biochemical findings of increased glycogen, abnormal glycogen structure. Normal phosphorylase and G6P activity.
♦ Assay of amniotic cells or chorionic villus biopsy allows prenatal diagnosis.
♦ DNA-based diagnosis is available.

Type IV GSD (Andersen Disease; Brancher Deficiency; Amylopectinosis)

Type IV GSD is an extremely rare fatal condition caused by the absence of amylo-(1,4-1,6)-transglucosylase.

Hypoglycemia is not present.
Liver function tests may be altered as in other types of cirrhosis (e.g., slight increase in serum bilirubin, reversed albumin/globulin ratio, increased AST, decreased cholesterol). There may be a flat blood glucose response to epinephrine and glucagon.
♦ Biopsy of liver may show a cirrhotic reaction to the presence of glycogen of abnormal structure, which stains with Best carmine and periodic acid–Schiff stain but normal glycogen concentration.
♦ Enzyme defect shows in liver, WBCs, cultured fibroblasts.
♦ Assay of amniotic cells or chorionic villus biopsy allows prenatal diagnosis.

METAB/HERED

Type V GSD (Mcardle Disease; Myophosphorylase Deficiency)

Type V GSD is caused by absent myophosphorylase in skeletal muscle; affected persons show very limited ischemic muscle exercise tolerance in the presence of normal appearance of muscle.

Epinephrine or glucagon causes a normal hyperglycemic response.
Biopsy of muscle is microscopically normal in young; vacuolation and necrosis are seen in later years. Increased glycogen is present.
♦ Definitive diagnosis is made by absence of phosphorylase.
○ After exercise that quickly causes muscle cramping and weakness, the regional blood lactate and pyruvate do not increase (in a normal person they increase two to five times). A similar abnormal response occurs in type III involving muscle and in types VII, VIII, and X.
Myoglobulinuria may occur after strenuous exercise.
○ Increased serum muscle enzymes (e.g., LD, CK, aldolase) for several hours after strenuous exercise.

Type VI GSD (Hers Disease; Hepatic Phosphorylase Deficiency)

Type VI GSD is a rare disorder caused by a deficiency of hepatic phosphorylase.

Enlarged liver, present from birth, is associated with hypoglycemia.
Serum cholesterol and TGs are mildly increased.
Serum uric acid and lactic acid are normal.
Liver function tests are normal.
Fructose tolerance is normal.
Response to glucagon and epinephrine is variable but tends to be poor.
♦ Diagnosis is based on decreased phosphorylase activity in liver, but muscle phosphorylase is normal.

Type VII GSD (Muscle Phosphofructokinase Deficiency; Tarui Disease)

Type VII GSD is caused by a deficiency of muscle phosphofructokinase, which regulates glycolysis in muscle.

Fasting hypoglycemia is marked.
Other members of family may have reduced tolerance to glucose.
♦ RBCs show 50% decrease in phosphofructokinase activity.
♦ Biopsy of muscle shows marked decrease (1%–3% of normal) in phosphofructokinase activity and increased glycogen and abnormal morphology. Increased glycogen is found in the brain. Clinically identical to type V.

Type VIII GSD

Type VIII GSD is a very rare X-linked recessive deficiency of phosphorylase kinase with progressive CNS degeneration and enlarged liver.

Blood glucose is markedly decreased, causing hypoglycemic seizures and mental retardation.
Glucagon administration causes no increase in blood glucose (see von Gierke disease), but ingestion of food causes a rise in 2 to 3 hours.
♦ Biopsy of liver shows marked decrease in glycogen synthetase.

Type IX GSD

Type IX GSD is usually mild and is caused by a liver phosphorylase kinase deficiency.

May have fasting hypoglycemia that is unusual.
Mild increase in serum AST, ALT, cholesterol, TGs may be present.
Normal uric acid and blood lactate.
Functional tests are not usually useful.
With increasing age, the enzyme deficiency persists, but chemical and clinical abnormalities gradually disappear.

Porphyrias[13]

The porphyrias are a group of inherited metabolic disorders caused by enzyme defects in heme synthesis (porphyria cutanea tarda, however, is mainly acquired). Diagnosis is made by patterns of porphyrins and metabolites in urine, stool, RBCs, and plasma; by plasma fluorescence screening; by measuring deficient enzyme; and by genetic testing. More than 80% of heterozygotes are asymptomatic.

See Figures 12-7 and 12-8 and Table 12-13.

Acute episodes (may include abdominal pain and psychiatric symptoms; hypertension, paresthesias, fever, and seizures less frequently; neuromuscular weakness, hyponatremia) are characteristic of acute intermittent porphyria, coproporphyria, and variegate porphyria; may be precipitated by certain drugs (especially barbiturates, alcohol, and sulfonamides; also diphenylhydantoin, chlordiazepoxide, ergots, certain steroids, etc.), infection, starvation. Can be rapidly confirmed by markedly increased urine porphobilinogen (PBG) in single void specimen.

Asymptomatic carriers of acute porphyrias may have few acute attacks throughout life, and levels of ALA, PBG, and porphyrins in urine, serum, and feces are normal in most.

♦ Laboratory confirmation may include: 24-hour urine for quantitative 5-aminolevulinic acid, PBG, uroporphyrin, and coproporphyrin (urine should be kept refrigerated, as porphyrins quickly deteriorate, especially at room temperature); plasma porphyrin; free RBC protoporphyrin; spot stool quantitative coproporphyrin and protoporphyrin; Watson-Schwartz test to demonstrate porphyrin precursors in urine (Ehrlich reagent and sodium acetate added to urine; positive turns cherry red with addition of chloroform) is qualitative and lacks sensitivity; evidence of hemolytic anemia or liver disease; fluorescence of appropriate tissues; and enzyme activity assay of RBCs, liver tissue or cultured fibroblasts. Urine δ-ALA and PBG should be measured during episodes. Some drugs may precipitate acute porphyria (stimulate heme synthesis by induction of δ-ALA synthase), e.g., alcohol, antipyretics, barbiturates, estrogens, phenylhydrazine, phenytoin, and sulfonamides.

♦ Measurement of enzyme activity and DNA testing help confirm type of porphyria. See Table 12-13.

Porphyrin Tests of Urine (Fluorometric Methods)

Some drugs that produce fluorescence, e.g., acriflavine, ethoxazene, phenazopyridine, sulfamethoxazole, tetracycline

Classification

Erythropoietic

- Congenital erythropoietic porphyria (CEP)
- Erythropoietic protoporphyria
- Erythropoietic coproporphyria

Hepatic

- Acute intermittent porphyria (AIP)
- Variegate porphyria (VP)
- Hereditary coproporphyria (HC)
- ALA dehydrase deficiency porphyria
- Porphyria cutanea tarda (PCT)

Hepatoerythropoietic

- Hepatoerythropoieic porphyria

(1) Ala Dehydratase Deficiency Porphyria (Porphobilinogen Synthase Deficiency)

ALA dehydrase deficiency porphyria is a very rare autosomal recessive condition with 98% deficiency of enzyme; parents had 50% of normal activity. Acute porphyria-type symptoms are present.

[13]Anderson KE, Bloomer JR, Bonkovsky HL, et al. Recommendations for the diagnosis and treatment of the acute porphyrias. *Ann Intern Med* 2005;142:439–450 [erratum 2005;143(4):316].

METAB/HERED

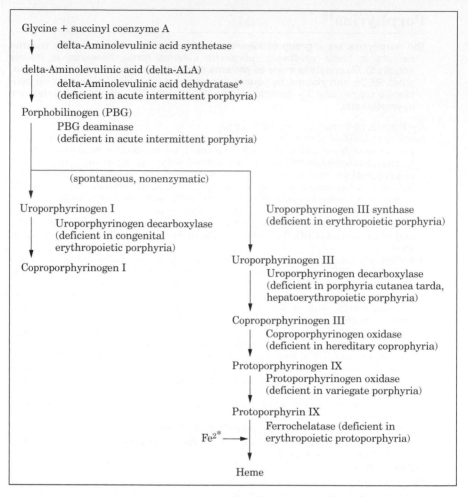

Glycine + succinyl coenzyme A

↓   delta-Aminolevulinic acid synthetase

delta-Aminolevulinic acid (delta-ALA)

↓   delta-Aminolevulinic acid dehydratase*
(deficient in acute intermittent porphyria)

Porphobilinogen (PBG)

PBG deaminase
(deficient in acute intermittent porphyria)

(spontaneous, nonenzymatic)

Uroporphyrinogen I

Uroporphyrinogen decarboxylase
(deficient in congenital
erythropoietic porphyria)

Coproporphyrinogen I

Uroporphyrinogen III synthase
(deficient in erythropoietic porphyria)

Uroporphyrinogen III

Uroporphyrinogen decarboxylase
(deficient in porphyria cutanea tarda,
hepatoerythropoietic porphyria)

Coproporphyrinogen III

Coproporphyrinogen oxidase
(deficient in hereditary coprophyria)

Protoporphyrinogen IX

Protoporphyrinogen oxidase
(deficient in variegate porphyria)

Protoporphyrin IX

Fe^{2*} →

Ferrochelatase (deficient in
erythropoietic protoporphyria)

Heme

Fig. 12-7. Heme biosynthesis pathway showing site of enzyme action and disease caused by enzyme deficiency. Accumulation of porphyrins and their precursors preceding the enzyme block are responsible for the clinical and laboratory findings of each syndrome. PBG and ALA are increased in all hepatic porphyrias. ALA and PBG cause abdominal pain and neuropsychiatric symptoms. Increased porphyrins (with or without increased PBG or ALA) cause photosensitivity. Thus, deficiencies near the end of the metabolic path cause more photosensitivity and fewer neuropsychiatric findings.

◆ Urine—marked increase in ALA, increased coproporphyrin III (resembles lead intoxication), and uroporphyrin; normal PBG.
◆ RBC—ALA dehydrase <5% of normal. Protoporphyrins are increased.
RBC, but not plasma, protoporphyrins are also increased in iron-deficiency anemia and lead intoxication. Screening tests using fluorescence microscopy of RBCs or Wood lamp viewing of treated whole blood may also be positive in iron-deficiency anemia, lead intoxication, and other dyserythropoietic states. In congenital erythropoietic porphyria, 5% to 20% of RBCs show fluorescence that lasts up to a minute or more, in contrast to erythropoietic protoporphyria, where fluorescence is half that and lasts about 30 seconds, and in lead poisoning, where almost all RBCs fluoresce for only a few seconds. Fluorescence of hepatocytes occurs in erythropoietic protoporphyria, PCT, VP, HC.

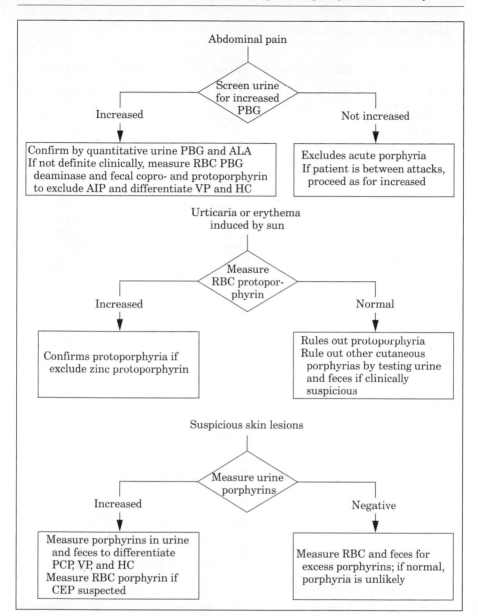

Fig. 12-8. Diagnostic strategy (algorithm) for suspected porphyria according to symptoms. Excess production of porphyrins is associated with cutaneous photosensitivity. Excess production of only porphyrin precursors is associated with neurologic symptoms. Excess production of both is associated with both types of clinical symptoms. PBG, porphobilinogens; ALA, aminolevulinic acid; RBC, red blood cells; AIP, acute intermittent porphyria; VP, variegate porphyria; HC, hereditary coproporphyria; PCP, porphyria cutanea tarda; CEP congenital erythropoietic porphyria.

Table 12-13a.   Comparison of Porphyrias

	Enzyme Defect	Inheritance, Location[a]	Usual age at onset	Frequency
1. ALA Dehydratase Deficiency Porphyria	ALA dehydratase, ~5% of normal	AR 9q34 7 mutations	Variable	Extremely rare; few reported cases
2. Acute Intermittent Porphyria	Porphobilinogen deaminase, 50% of normal	AD 11q23.3 >227 mutations	Rare before puberty	Lapland, 1:1,000; elsewhere, 1.5:100,000
3. Congenital Erythropoietic Porphyria	Uroporphyrinogen III cosynthase	AR 10q25.2–26.3	Fetal life At birth	Very rare; <200 reported cases
4. Porphyria Cutanea Tarda	Uroporphyrinogen decarboxylase	Mostly acquired Also AD 1p34	30s–40s	Most common type in United States and Europe
5. Hepatoerythropoietic Porphyria	Uroporphyrinogen decarboxylase	AR	Before age 2 y	Extremely rare; <20 reported cases
6. Hereditary Coproporphyria	Coproporphyrinogen oxidase, 50% of normal	AD 3q12 36 mutations	Any age	Very rare. <50 reported cases
7. Variegate Porphyria	Protoporphyrinogen oxidase, 50% of normal	AD 1q22 120 mutations	Usually 15–30 y	South Africa, 3:1,000; rare elsewhere
8. Erythropoietic Protoporphyria	Ferrochelatase	AD 18q21.3	1–4 y	Very rare; <50 reported cases

ALA, aminolevulinic acid; PBG, porphobilinogen; AD, autosomal dominant; AR, autosomal recessive.
[a]Number of known mutations.

(2) Acute Intermittent Porphyria[14]

AIP is the most frequent and severe form of porphyria seen in the United States. It comprises an autosomal dominant (>200 mutations) deficiency of PBG deaminase. Adult onset is usual, with acute attacks of various neuropsychiatric and abdominal symptoms. Patients do not exhibit photosensitivity. It is often precipitated by drugs or hormones.

♦ Diagnosed in acute or latent states by finding decreased δ-ALA dehydratase PBG deaminase (~50% of normal) activity in RBCs and in liver samples, fibroblasts, and lymphocytes; normal in other porphyrias. RBCs may be used to confirm diagnosis, since urine findings may occur during acute attacks of VP and HC.
○ Urine may be of normal color when fresh and becomes red/brown on exposure to sunlight.
♦ Urine—Diagnostic finding is marked increase of PBG and, to a lesser extent, of δ-ALA; these decrease during remission but are rarely normal; not increased in silent carriers; also increased in plasma. Watson-Schwartz screening test for PBG should be confirmed by quantitative test. Coproporphyrin and uroporphyrin may be increased.

[14]von und zu Fraunberg N, Pischik E, Udd L, et al. Clinical and biochemical characteristics and genotype-phenotype correlation in 143 Finnish and Russian patients with acute intermittent porphyria. *Medicine (Baltimore)* 2005;84:35–47.

Table 12-13b.   Comparison of Porphyrias *(continued)*

	Chief Site of Porphyrin Overproduction	Chief Laboratory Findings			
		Urine	Feces	RBCs	Plasma
1. ALA Dehydratase Deficiency Porphyria	Liver	↑**ALA,** ↑**copropor-phyrin,** ↑uroporphyrin	0	ALA <5% of normal; ↑protopor-phyrin	
2. Acute Intermittent Porphyria	Liver	**Watson-Schwartz positive;** darkens on exposure to sunlight; ↑**ALA**[b], ↑**uropor-phyrin I,** ↑**PBG constant**	Porphyrins normal or may be slightly ↑	Porphyrins normal; ↓porphobili-nogen deaminase activity by 50% in 90% of cases	Normal or slightly ↑; ↑ porphyrins during attacks
3. Congenital Erythropoietic Porphyria	Bone marrow	Watson-Schwartz negative[a] ↑**uropor-phyrin I** >copropor-phyrin	↑copropor-phyrin	↑uropor-phyrin I and/or zinc porphyrin	↑ uropor-phyrin I, copropor-phyrin I
4. Porphyria Cutanea Tarda	Liver	↑**uropor-phyrin I** >**III;** pink fluorescence	↑copropor-phyrin	Porphyrins normal	↑ carboxyl-porphyrins
5. Hepatoery-thropoietic Porphyria	Bone marrow, Liver	Pink urine; ↑carboxyl-porphyrins, ↑porphobili-nogen	↑copropor-phyrins, ↑uroporphyrino-gen	↑**protopor-phyrin (zinc)**	Normal serum iron
6. Hereditary Copropor-phyria	Liver	↑copropor-phyrin III; ↑PBG and ↑ALA during attacks	**Marked** ↑**copropor-phyrin III,** >↑**proto-porphyrin;** ↑**PBG and** ↑**ALA during attacks**	Normal	Usually normal
7. Variegate Porphyria	Liver	↑copropor-phyrin ↑PBG and ↑ALA during attacks; normal otherwise	↑**Protopor-phyrin,** >↑**copropor-phyrin constant**	Normal	**Plasma fluoresence scanning distinguishes it from other porphyrias**
8. Erythro-poietic Protopor-phyria	Bone marrow; liver variable	Normal porphyrins	↑**Protopor-phyrin**	↑**protopor-phyrin,** Red fluorescence	↑Protopor-phyrin

0, absent; ↑, increased; ↑, decreased; >, more than.
[a]Present during acute attack; may be absent during remission.
[b]ALA may be increased even more in chronic lead poisoning. Boldface type indicates body material used for diagnosis.

METAB/HERED

Table 12-13c.	Comparison of Porphyrias *(continued)*					
	Clinical Manifestations					
	Skin	Neuro	Liver	RBCs	Precipitated by	Comment
1. ALA Dehydratase Deficiency Porphyria	0	4+			Alcohol, stress	
2. Acute Intermittent Porphyria	0	4+	0		Drugs, hormones	
3. Congenital Erythropoietic porphyria	4+	0	0	Fluorescent RBCs and normoblasts		Erythrodontia, hemolytic anemia
4. Porphyria Cutanea Tarda	1+	0	Cirrhosis, hepatitis; ↑iron		Chemicals, iron, alcohol, estrogens. Photosensitivity to sunlight.	Diabetes mellitus. 50% have HCV, hepatoma, cirrhosis
5. Hepatoerythropoietic porphyria	4+	0	1+		Photosensitivity to sunlight	Erythrodontia, normochromic anemia.
6. Hereditary Coproporphyria	1+	1+	↑ALA synthase		Drugs, especially barbiturates. Photosensitivity to sunlight.	
7. Variegate Porphyria	3+	4+	0		Estrogens, barbiturates. Photosensitivity to sunlight.	
8. Erythropoietic Protoporphyria	3+	0	1+	1+		Anemia is unusual

0, absent; 1+ to 4+, degree of severity; HCV, hepatitis C virus.

Stool—protoporphyrin and coproporphyrin are usually normal; may be slightly increased. During acute attack, there may be decreased serum sodium (may be marked), chloride, and magnesium, increased BUN, and slight leukocytosis.

Liver function tests are normal.

Other frequent laboratory abnormalities are increased serum cholesterol, hyperbetalipoproteinemia (type IIa), increased serum iron, abnormal glucose tolerance, and increased T-4 and thyroxine-binding globulin without hyperthyroidism.

(3) Congenital Erythropoietic PORPHYRIA

CEP is an extremely rare, autosomal recessive disorder caused by decreased activity of uroporphyrinogen III cosynthase in RBCs, causing overproduction of uroporphyrinogen I and coproporphyrinogen, which have no role in heme synthesis, but their oxidation causes findings listed in the following. The usual onset of CEP is in infancy; patients exhibit extreme cutaneous photosensitivity with mutilation and red urine and teeth.

♦ Ultraviolet fluorescence of variable number of RBCs and normoblasts; also urine, teeth, and bones.
Normocytic, normochromic, anicteric hemolytic anemia that tends to be mild; may be associated with hypersplenism and increased reticulocytes and normoblasts.
♦ Urine—marked increase of uroporphyrin I is characteristic; coproporphyrin shows lesser increase. Excretion of PBG and δ-ALA is normal. Watson-Schwartz test is negative.
♦ RBCs—increased uroporphyrins I and/or zinc protoporphyrins.
♦ Plasma—marked increase of uroporphyrins; increased coproporphyrin.
♦ Stool—marked increase of coproporphyrins.

(4) Porphyria Cutanea Tarda

PCT is the most common porphyrin disorder. It is caused by a deficiency (~50%) of uroporphyrinogen decarboxylase. It is basically an acquired disorder (inhibitor of uroporphyrinogen decarboxylase may be generated in liver) that may be caused by hepatoma, cirrhosis, or chemicals (e.g., an epidemic in Turkey was caused by contamination of wheat by hexachlorobenzene). The disease may be activated by increased ingestion of iron, alcohol, or estrogens.

The inherited form (autosomal dominant) is expressed in ~20% of patients with this gene and is caused by a deficiency of uroporphyrinogen decarboxylase in liver in toxic/sporadic forms (type I) and in all tissues in familial form (type II). Associated with alcoholic liver disease and hepatic siderosis.

♦ Urine—marked increase of uroporphyrin (frequently up to 1,000 to 3,000 µg/24 h [normal <300 µg]) with only slight increase of coproporphyrin and ratio of uroporphyrin/coproporphyrin >7.5 (ratio <1 in VP). In biochemical remission, 24-hour uroporphyrin is <400 µg.
Stool—isocoproporphyrins are present.
Plasma—increased protoporphyrin.
RBC porphyrins are normal.
♦ Distinguished from VP, in which there is increased fecal protoporphyrins and urine coproporphyrins exceed uroporphyrins during cutaneous symptoms.
Serum ferritin, iron, and transferrin saturation are increased in ~50% of cases.
Laboratory findings of underlying liver disease; ~50% have hepatitis C. Liver biopsy shows morphologic changes of underlying disease and fluorescence under ultraviolet light; usually shows iron overload.
Diabetes mellitus in ≤33% of patients due to associated hemochromatosis.
Phlebotomy therapy to remove iron is monitored by decreased urinary excretion of uroporphyrins.

(5) Hepatoerythropoietic Porphyria

Hepatoerythropoietic porphyria is an extremely rare (few reported cases) autosomal recessive severe deficiency of uroporphyrinogen decarboxylase. Onset occurs before age 2 years.

♦ Marked deficiency of uroporphyrinogen decarboxylase (5%–10% of normal; 50% of normal in parents).
♦ Pink urine, increased uroporphyrinogens I, III.
♦ RBCs contain increased zinc protoporphyrin.
Plasma contains increased uroporphyrin.
♦ Porphyrin abnormalities resemble porphyria cutanea tarda but additionally zinc protoporphyrin is increased in RBCs.
Mild normochromic anemia; fluorescent normoblasts in bone marrow. Normal serum iron.
Increased serum GGT and transaminase may occur. Liver disease may progress to cirrhosis.
Severe skin involvement. Pink teeth.

(6) Hereditary Coproporphyria

HC is a very rare autosomal dominant deficiency of coproporphyrinogen oxidase. Two-thirds of patients are latent. It is precipitated by the same factors as is AIP.

META3/HERED

♦ Stool—coproporphyrin III is always increased—very markedly during an acute attack; coproporphyrin III is also increased in plasma. Protoporphyrin is normal or only slightly increased.

Urine—coproporphyrin III may be increased or not; is usually normal during remission. Isolated increase may be secondary to liver, hematologic, neoplastic, and toxic conditions. Increased PBG and to a lesser extent ALA during acute attacks.

♦ RBCs—diminished coproporphyrinogen oxidase is strongly indicative.

♦ Liver—diminished coproporphyrinogen oxidase is diagnostic; increased ALA synthase.

(7) Variegate Porphyria[15]

VP is an autosomal dominant condition caused by a deficiency of protoporphyrinogen oxidase (by ~50%), which can also be found in cultured fibroblasts, liver tissue, and peripheral blood lymphocytes. Skin or neurologic manifestations may occur. VP is precipitated by the same factors as is AIP.

♦ Plasma fluorescence scanning at 625 nm efficiently distinguishes VP from other porphyrias. Plasma scanning is more sensitive and specific than fecal testing, but neither is sensitive in children and both are less sensitive in asymptomatic carriers.

♦ Stool chromatography—characteristic change is marked increase of protoporphyrin, which is found during attack, remission, or only with skin manifestations. When stool is normal or borderline or in asymptomatic patients, can demonstrate increased porphyrins in bile.

Urine—marked increase of δ-ALA and PBG during an acute attack; levels are usually normal after acute episode, in contrast to AIP and HC.

Blood—porphyrin levels are not increased.

♦ DNA analysis for the appropriate gene mutation is preferred to identify carriers, especially children.

(8) Erythropoietic Protoporphyria

Erythropoietic protoporphyria is a relatively common type of porphyria caused by an autosomal dominant deficiency of ferrochelatase activity in bone marrow, reticulocytes, liver, and other cells.

Mild microcytic hypochromic anemia in 20% to 30% of patients.

Laboratory findings due to liver disease (severe in 10% of cases) with increased serum direct bilirubin, AST, and ALP (due to intrahepatic cholestasis), and gallstones containing porphyrins may be found.

Urine—porphyrins within normal limits.

♦ RBCs—marked increase of free protoporphyrin in symptomatic patients (zinc-chelated form may also be increased in iron-deficiency anemia and lead poisoning, but nonchelated form is present in protoporphyria). May be normal or slightly increased in asymptomatic carriers. Examination of dilute blood by fluorescent microscopy may show rapidly fading fluorescence in variable part of RBCs.

♦ Stool—protoporphyrin is usually increased in symptomatic patients and in some carriers, even when carrier RBC porphyrins are normal.

♦ Three chemical patterns consist of increased free RBC and stool protoporphyrin alone or with each other.

Lysosomal Storage Disorders

Lysosomes are acidic organelles containing hydrolases that normally degrade larger molecules. Lysosomal storage diseases are a group of >50 inherited diseases due to deficient activity of these enzymes causing abnormal accumulation of substrates. Clinical syndromes depend on different organ accumulations and lysosome-associated protein, neonatal, juvenile, and adult onsets.

---

[15]Hift RJ, Davidson BP, van der Hooft C, et al. Plasma fluorescence scanning and fecal porphyrin analysis for the diagnosis of variegate porphyria: precise determination of sensitivity and specificity with detection of protoporphyrinogen oxidase mutations as a reference standard. *Clin Chem* 2004;50:915–923.

Lysosomal Storage Disorder	Deficient Enzyme	Stored Material	Chief Sites of Involvement
Sphingolipidoses			
GM_1 and GM_2	β-galactosidase	GM_1 ganglioside	CNS
Tay-Sachs	Hexosaminidase A	GM_2 ganglioside, other metabolites	CNS
Sandhoff	Hexosaminidase B	GM_2 ganglioside, other metabolites	CNS
Gaucher types	Glucocerebrosidase (acidic β-glucosidase	Glucocerebroside	CNS, spleen, liver, bones
Niemann-Pick types A, B	Sphingomyelinase	Sphingomyelin	CNS, liver, spleen, lungs; no CNS in type A
Niemann-Pick type C, D	Mutant protein leading to block in cholesterol esterification. Sphingomyelinase not deficient.	?	CNS, liver, spleen
Krabbe (globoid cell leukodystrophy)	β-galactosylceramidase		CNS, peripheral NS
Metachromatic leukodystrophy	Arylsulfatase A	Cerebroside sulfate	CNS, peripheral NS
Multiple sulfatase deficiency	Various sulfatases	Sulfate-containing glycolipids, MPS, steroids	CNS, spleen, liver, bones
Fabry disease	α-galactosidase A	Ceramide trihexoside	Skin, peripheral NS, kidney, eye, heart and brain vessels
Mucopolysaccharidoses see Table 12-14			
MPS IH (Hurler syndrome)	α-L-iduronidase	Dermatan sulfate, heparan sulfate	CNS, bone liver, heart
MPS IS (Scheie syndrome)	α-L-iduronidase	Dermatan sulfate, heparan sulfate	Eye, bone, heart
MPS IH/IS (Hurler/Scheie)	α-L-iduronidase		
MPS II (Hunter syndrome)	Iduronate sulfatase	Dermatan sulfate, heparan sulfate	CNS, bone liver, heart
MPS III, Sanfilippo type A	Heparan N-sulfatase	Heparan sulfate	CNS, bone
MPS III, Sanfilippo type B	N-acetyl-α-D-glucosaminidase		
MPS III, Sanfilippo type C	Acetyl-CoA: α-glucosaminide-N-acetyltransferase		
MPS III, Sanfilippo type D	N-acetylglucosamine-6-sulfatase		
MPS IV, types A, B (Morquio syndrome)	Type A: N-acetyl-galactosamine-6-sulfate sulfatase	Keratan sulfate	Bone

META/HERED

	Type B: β-galactosidase (specific for keratan sulfate)		
MPS VI (Maroteaux-Lamy)	Arylsulfatase B	Dermatan sulfate	Bone
MPS VII (Sly syndrome)	β-glucuronidase	Dermatan sulfate, heparan sulfate	Bone, liver, CNS
MPS IX hyaluronidase deficiency	Hyaluronidase		
Sphingolipidoses Mucopolysaccha-ridoses			
Mucolipi-doses (Oligosacchari-doses)			
Sialidosis type I and II	α-neuroaminidase	Sialooligosaccharides	CNS, peripheral NS, eye, skin
Mannosidosis	Mannosidase	Oligosaccharides	CNS, mild bone changes, hepatosple-nomegaly
Fucosidosis types I, II	Fucosidase	Oligosaccharides, sphingolipids	CNS, high sweat electrolytes
Aspartylglycosa-minuria	Aspartyl-glucosa-minidase	Glycoasparagines	
Mucolipidosis II (I-cell disease) (formerly MPS VII)	N-acetylglucosamine-1-P-transferase		CNS, bone, connective tissue
Mucolipidosis III (Pseudo-Hurler polydystrophy)	N-acetylglucosamine-1-P-transferase		Predominant-ly joint and connective tissue
Mucolipidosis IV (ML IV)		Gangliosides, glycosaminoglycans	CNS, eye
Lysosomal Efflux			
Cystinosis	?		Kidney
Salla disease	?		CNS
Chédiak-Higashi syndrome (see Chapter 11)			

GM$_1$, GM$_2$, gangliosides 1 and 2; CNS, central nervous system; MPS, mucopolysaccharidosis.

Cystinosis[16]

Cystinosis is an autosomal recessive lysosomal storage disease caused by impaired transport of cystine from lysosomes to cytoplasm; this causes abnormal accumulation of soluble and crystalline cystine amino acid in various organs. It is mapped to chromosome 17p13; there are >50 mutations.

[16]Gahl WA, Thoene JG, Schneider JA. Cystinosis. *N Engl J Med* 2002;347:111–121.

Table 12-14. Classification of Mucopolysaccharidoses

Type of Mucopolysaccharidosis (clinical name)	Deficient Enzyme	Mucopolysaccharide Excreted in Urine	Signs/Symptoms
IH (Hurler's syndrome)	Alpha-L-iduronidase	Dermatan sulfate and heparan sulfate in 7:3 ratio	Progressive mental/physical disability from 1 yr of age; hyperplastic gums; coarse face; stiff joints (clawhands); organomegaly; dwarfing; dysostosis multiplex
IS (Scheie's syndrome)	Alpha-L-iduronidase	Dermatan sulfate and heparan sulfate	Mild form of MPS I; mild or no mental retardation; clawhands; aortic stenosis
IH/S (Hurler-Scheie syndrome)	Aplha-L-iduronidase		Features intermediate between Hurler's and Scheie's syndromes
II (Hunter's syndrome)	Iduronate sulfatase	Dermatan sulfate and heparan sulfate	Dysostosis multiplex; mild to severe mental retardation; no corneal opacity; longer life compared with MPS I
IIIA (Sanfilippo's syndrome, type A)	Heparan N-sulfatase (sulfamidase)	Heparan sulfate	Mild or no connective tissue abnormalities; marked hirsutism; behaviorism progresses to severe mental retardation; no corneal opacity
IIIB (Sanfilippo's syndrome, type B)	Alpha-N-acetylglu-cosaminidase (alpha-hexosaminidase)	Heparan sulfate	Same as in MPS IIIa
IIIC (Sanfilippo's syndrome, type C)	Acetyl CoA: alpha-glucosaminide N-acetyltransferase	Heparan sulfate	Same as in MPS IIIa
IIID (Sanfilippo's syndrome, type D)	N-Acetylglucosamine-6-sulfatase	Heparan sulfate	Same as in MPS IIIa
IVA (Morquio's syndrome, type A)	N-Acetylgalactosamine-6-sulfatase	Keratan sulfate	Marked skeletal abnormalities; small stature; short neck; prominent lower ribs; normal intellect; coma

(continued)

Table 12-14. Classification of Mucopolysaccharidoses

Type of Mucopolysaccharidosis (clinical name)	Deficient Enzyme	Mucopolysaccharide Excreted in Urine	Signs/Symptoms
IVB (Morquio's syndrome, type B)	Beta-galactosidase	Keratan sulfate	
V	This class is vacant now (formerly was Scheie's syndrome)		
VI (Maroteaux-Lamy syndrome)	N-Acetylgalactosamine-4-sulfatase (arylsulfatase B)	Dermatan sulfate	Severe dysostosis multiplex and corneal opacity; retarded growth; normal intellect; cardiac abnormalities; a mild form also occurs
VII (Sly's syndrome)	Beta-glucuronidase	Dermatan sulfate, heparan sulfate, chondroitin 4, 6-sulfate	Mild mental retardation; organomegaly; corneal opacity may occur; coarse facies; gingivitis; very heterogeneous clinical appearance

CoA = coenzyme A; MPS = mucopolysaccharidosis.
Inheritance in Hunter's syndrome is X-linked recessive; others are autosomal recessive.
Cloudy cornea in IH, IS, IVA, IVB, VI, VII.
Mental retardation in IH, II, IIIA, IIIB, IIIC, IIID, VII.
Hepatosplenomegaly in IH, II, IIIA, IIIB, IIIC. IIID, IVB, VI, VII.
Skeletal defects in all.

Infantile (acute nephropathic form)

Renal Fanconi syndrome (aminoaciduria, glycosuria, proteinuria, renal tubular acidosis, phosphaturia, hypophosphatemic rickets) and also glomerular disease, leading to end-stage renal disease by age 10 years.

Polyuria: 2 to 6 L/d (<300 mOsm/L) may cause dehydration with loss of electrolytes.

♦ Prenatal diagnosis by testing cultured amniocytes or chorionic villus.

♦ Neonatal diagnosis is performed by measuring cystine in leukocytes or placenta.

Crystalline inclusions in conjunctiva, cornea (slit lamp examination confirms diagnosis after 1 year of age) and leukocytes, bone marrow, rectal mucosa. Biopsy is not required for diagnosis.

Late manifestations: type 1 diabetes mellitus, pancreatic insufficiency, primary testicular failure, hypothyroidism, myopathy, etc.

Juvenile (late onset) has much lower progression of nephropathic disease.

Adults/benign disease may show

Only cystine crystals in cornea
Urinary tract calculi
Cystinuria (cystine crystals in urine; >200 mg of cystine in 24-hour urine)
Asymptomatic

Sphingolipidoses

See Table 12-15.

Tay-Sachs Disease (GM₂ Gangliosidosis, Type I)

Tay-Sachs disease is an autosomal recessive (chromosome 15) lysosomal storage disease found predominantly in Ashkenazi Jews, French Canadians, and Cajuns, characterized by appearance in infantile form by psychomotor deterioration, blindness, cherry-red spot in the macula, and an exaggerated extension response to sound, with death by age 4; juvenile form (with death by age 15), and chronic form in adults. Macula spots appear only in the infantile form.

♦ Diagnosis is established by absence of hexosaminidase A activity in serum, plasma, leukocytes, and cultured skin fibroblasts (also absent in all tissues of body and tears). Accumulation of ganglioside 2 (GM₂) in the brain is caused by a deficiency or absence of hexosaminidase A.

♦ Heterozygotes can be identified by plasma assay showing 50% decrease in activity of hexosaminidase A; screening should be done before pregnancy, which may cause false-positive results; oral contraceptives, diabetes mellitus, and liver disease may also cause false-positive results; in these cases, WBCs are used for hexosaminidase A assay.

♦ Prenatal diagnosis using cultured amniotic cells is superior to that done using amniotic fluid or uncultured amniotic cells; false-negative results can occur because of contamination with maternal blood or tissue or bacteria.

♦ PCR for specific DNA mutations in WBCs or fibroblasts is more specific than enzyme assay, can detect various mutations, and can predict severity of disease in affected child.

There is early marked increase of serum LD and AST, which return to normal if patient survives 3 to 4 years.

Decrease in serum fructose-1-phosphate aldolase; also decreased in *heterozygotes*.

CSF AST parallels serum AST.

Occasional vacuolated lymphocytes are seen.

Liver function tests are normal.

Serum acid phosphatase is normal.

♦ Electron microscopy shows characteristic cytoplasmic bodies in brain. (In Sandhoff disease [similar to Tay-Sachs disease] total deficiency of β-hexosaminidase, glycolipids, and other substances accumulate in brain as well as other tissues.)

METAB/HERED

Table 12-15. Classification of Sphingolipidosis

Clinical Name	Enzyme Defect Specimen for Assay	Major Lipid Accumulation	Signs/Symptoms
Gaucher's disease	Cerebroside beta-glucosidase in L, F	Glucosyl ceramide	Enlarged spleen and liver; erosion of long bones and pelvis; mental retardation only in infantile form
Niemann-Pick disease	Sphingomyelinase in F, U, S	Sphingomyelin	Enlarged liver and spleen; mental retardation; ~30% have cherry-red spot in retina
Krabbe's disease (globoid cell leukodystrophy)	Cerebroside beta-glucosidase in F, L, A, S	Galactosyl ceramide	X-linked; mental retardation; almost total absence of myelin; globoid bodies in brain white matter; increased CSF protein
Metachromatic leukodystrophy	Arylsulfatase A in L, U, F, S	Sulfatide	Mental retardation; psychological disturbances in adult form
Multiple, sulfatase deficiencies	Arylsulfatase A, B, C in F, L	Sulfatide	Resembles metachromatic leukodystrophy; dermatan sulfate and heparan sulfate increased in urine
Ceramide lactoside lipidosis	Beta-galactosidase in L, S	Ceramide lactoside	Slowly progressive brain damage; enlarged liver and spleen

Disease	Enzyme deficiency and source	Accumulated substance	Clinical features
Fabry's disease (angio-keratoum corporis diffusum universale)	Alpha-galactosidase in S, L, F, U, T	Trihexosyl ceramide	Skin lesions; loss of renal function; involvement of heart, and brain vessels; pain in lower limbs; cherry-red spot in retina
GM_2 gangliosidosis Tay-Sachs disease	Hexosaminidase A in S, L, A, F, U, T	Gangliositle GM_2	Mental retardation; cherry-red spot in retina; blindness; muscle weakness
Sandhoff's disease	Hexosaminiriase A, B in S, T, A, F, U, T	Ganglioside GM_3 and globoside	Clinical picture same as in Tay-Sachs disease but mild peripheral neuropathy and organomegaly
Landing's disease (GM_1 gangliosidosis)	Lysosomal acid-beta-galactosidase in L, F, U	Ganglioside GM_1	Psychomotor deterioration; cherry-red spot in retina; enlarged liver and spleen; dysostosis multiplex
Farber's lipogranu-lomatosis*	Acid ceramidase in L, F	Ceramide	Granulomas of dermis and viscera; joint disease in infancy
Fucosidcsis	Alpha-fucosidase in L	H-isoantigen	
Lactosyl ceramidosis	Neutral beta-galactosidase in F	Lactosyl ceramide	

A = amniocytes; F = fibroblasts; L = leukocytes; S = serum; U = urine; T = tears; CSF = cerebrospinal fluid.
Note: Molecular techniques are now available for diagnosis of Gaucher's, Niemann-Pick, Tay-Sachs, Sandhoff's, Fabry's, and Wolman's diseases and for generalized gangliosicosis.
*Diagnosis confirmed by biopsy of subcutaneous nodules rather than by determination of enzyme activity.

Fabry Disease (α-Galactosidase A Deficiency)[17]

Fabry disease is a rare X-linked recessive lysosomal storage disease caused by a deficiency of α-galactosidase A (α-gal A) that results in progressive accumulation of globotriaosylceramide (Gb_2) and related glycosphingolipids in plasma and vascular endothelium, leading to ischemia and infarction in various organs (e.g., kidney, heart, brain, eye, nerves) and characteristic angiokeratomas of skin. Carrier females may have mild or severe disease. The gene for the disease is located on chromosome Xq22.

♦ Absent ($<$1%) α-gal A in plasma and leukocytes in classical form and $<$10% of normal in cardiac variant in males. In female carriers, may be very low or normal; therefore must demonstrate the specific family genetic mutation (of $>$300 mutations).
♦ Heterozygote detection by enzyme assay of cultured cells or by assay of Gb_2 content of 24-hour urine sediment.
♦ Urine lipid profiles by MS/MS (including various ceramides) may be useful for identifying hemizygotes and heterozygotes.[18]
♦ Prenatal diagnosis by demonstration of XY karyotype and enzyme deficiency in cultured amniotic fluid cells or chorionic villi. If family mutation is known, molecular studies can replace or confirm enzymatic diagnosis.
○ Laboratory findings due to Gb_2 accumulation in vascular endothelium and organs, especially of kidneys (e.g., renal failure), heart (e.g., mitral valve disease left ventricular hypertrophy), and brain (e.g., stroke).
Patients with blood group B antigen (a glycosphingolipid) may have a more severe prognosis.

Gaucher Disease

Gaucher disease is an autosomal recessive deficiency of glucocerebrosidase (glucosylceramidase), which causes deposition of glucocerebroside in cells of macrophage-monocyte system. It is the most frequent lipid storage disease and may be present in 10,000 to 20,000 Americans, with the highest prevalence of type 1 in Ashkenazi Jews. The gene is located on chromosome 1q21.

♦ Decreased β-glucocerebrosidase activity in leukocytes or fibroblasts is reliable diagnostic method; substantial overlap between heterozygotes and normal persons. Confirmed by DNA testing.
♦ Diagnostic Gaucher cells are seen in bone marrow aspiration or in needle biopsy or aspiration of spleen, liver, or lymph nodes examined for thrombocytopenia or unrelated disorder and cause the nonneurologic manifestations.
○ Serum acid phosphatase is increased in most patients (substrate for test is different from that for prostatic acid phosphatase; i.e., uses phenyl phosphate or p-nitrophenylphosphate instead of glycerophosphate). It may return to normal following splenectomy.
Serum angiotensin-converting enzyme is increased in most patients.
Serum cholesterol and total fats are normal.
Laboratory findings due to involvement of specific organs

• Spleen—hypersplenism occurs with anemia (normocytic normochromic), leukopenia (with relative lymphocytosis; monocytes may be increased), thrombocytopenia without bleeding.
• Bone—serum ALP may be increased; osteopenia.
• Liver—serum AST may be increased.
• Lung infiltrates
• CNS involvement only in types 2 and 3; AST may be increased in CSF.

Laboratory findings due to increased incidence of lymphoproliferative disorders (e.g., multiple myeloma, chronic lymphocytic leukemia).

---

[17]Desnick RJ, Brady R, Barranger J, et al. Fabry disease, an under-recognized multisystemic disorder: expert recommendations for diagnosis, management, and enzyme replacement therapy. *Ann Intern Med* 2003;138:338.
[18]Fuller M, Sharp PC, Rozaklis T, et al. Urinary lipid profiling for the identification of Fabry hemizygotes and heterozygotes. *Clin Chem* 2005;51:688–694.

♦ Prenatal diagnosis by enzymatic determination of cultured amniotic fluid cells. If both parental mutations have been identified by DNA, chorionic villus sampling for fetal DNA can be done.

♦ Carrier identification by enzymatic methods are confirmed by DNA.

♦ Phenotype cannot be predicted from genotype. Common mutations can be detected using PCR and aid in genetic counseling for general risk of transmitting the gene but not specific prognosis for future affected children.

Type 1 (99% of patients): adult; no neurologic involvement.

Type 2: fulminating disorder with severe neurologic involvement and death within first 18 months.

Type 3: juvenile form with later onset of neurologic symptoms and milder course, with death in early childhood.

Bone marrow transplantation is effective therapy but has associated morbidity and mortality. Enzyme replacement therapy usually obviates need for splenectomy.

Niemann-Pick Disease

Niemann-Pick disease is a syndrome of autosomal recessive traits causing accumulation of sphingomyelin and cholesterol in lysosomes of macrophage-monocyte system. There are four major subtypes.

♦ Diagnosis by demonstrating sphingomyelinase deficiency in cultured fibroblasts or circulating leukocytes: 1% to 10% of normal in types A and B; 50% to 75% of normal in types C and D.

♦ Diagnosis of types C and D by showing biochemical defect in cholesterol transport in cultured fibroblasts.

♦ Heterozygote identification of types A and B by DNA analysis. Heterozygote identification of types C and D not available.

○ Foamy histiocytes (Niemann-Pick [NP] cells) may be found in bone marrow aspiration and in liver, spleen, skin, skeletal muscle, and eye, and may appear in peripheral blood terminally; not pathognomic.

Peripheral blood lymphocytes and monocytes may be vacuolated (2%–20% of cells).

WBC count is variable.

Rectal biopsy may show changes in ganglion cells of myenteric plexus.

Laboratory findings due to involvement of specific organs:

• Anemia is caused by hypersplenism or microcytic anemia associated with anisocytosis, poikilocytosis, and elliptocytosis.

• AST may be increased in serum and CSF.

• Enzyme changes in CSF are same as in Tay-Sachs disease, except that LD is normal.

Acid phosphatase is increased (same as in Gaucher disease).

LD is normal in serum and CSF.

Different enzyme activities result in different clinical forms.

• Type A: acute progressive neuropathic loss of motor and intellectual function early in life, with death common in infancy. Cherry-red macula is often present. Enlarged liver and spleen.

• Type B similar to type A but later onset and not neuropathic.

• Type C may have prolonged neonatal jaundice; variable CNS; less severe liver and spleen enlargement.

• Type D: not neuropathic; later onset.

♦ Prenatal diagnosis of types A and B by measuring acid sphingomyelinase activity in cultured amnoicytes or chorionic villi.

GM$_1$ Gangliosidosis (Landing Disease; Systemic Late Infantile Lipidosis)

GM$_1$ gangliosidosis is a rare autosomal recessive deficiency of acid β-galactosidase with no racial predilection characterized by psychomotor deterioration, enlargement of liver and/or spleen, cherry-red macular spots, and dysostosis multiplex. There are infantile, juvenile, and adult forms.

METAB/HERED

♦ Diagnosis by absence of lysosomal acid β-galactosidase enzyme in leukocytes, cultured fibroblasts, or brain. Tissue biopsy or culture of marrow or skin fibroblasts shows accumulation of ganglioside GM_1; also can demonstrate GM_1 in brain and viscera and mucopolysaccharides in viscera.

♦ Heterozygote carriers can be detected by enzyme assay in leukocytes.

○ Abnormal leukocytic granulations (Alder-Reilly bodies) may be present. Vacuolated lymphocytes may be found.

○ Foam cell histiocytes (resembling Niemann-Pick cells) may be seen in biopsy from bone marrow, liver, or rectum.

♦ Prenatal diagnosis by enzyme assay in cultured amniotic fluid cells or by HPLC analysis of galactosyl oligosaccharides in amniotic fluid.

Serum LD, AST, and fructose-1-phosphate aldolase are normal.

Mucolipidoses

I-Cell Disease (Mucolipidosis II)

I-cell disease is an autosomal recessive deficient activity of N-acetylglucosamine 1-phosphotransferase, which causes deficiency of multiple lysosomal enzymes. Clinical features resemble Hurler syndrome, but without corneal changes or increased mucopolysaccharides in urine.

♦ Deficiency of N-acetylglucosaminylphosphotransferase in cultured fibroblasts establishes the diagnosis.

♦ Vacuolation (cytoplasmic inclusions on phase contrast microscopy) in lymphocytes, fibroblasts, liver and kidney cells, which are positive for Sudan and acid phosphatase. Lysosomal enzyme activity (hexosaminidase A and B and α-galactosidase) is low in these cells but high in serum or culture medium.

♦ Prenatal diagnosis by high levels of multiple acid hydrolases in amniotic fluid or deficiency of them in cultured amniocytes.

Some heterozygotes have abnormal inclusions in fibroblasts. Some heterozygotes may have intermediate enzyme levels in leukocytes and cultured fibroblasts.

Urine mucopolysaccharides are not increased.

Mucolipidosis III (*N*-Acetylglucosaminylphosphotransferase Deficiency; Pseudo-Hurler Dystrophy)

The clinical features of type III mucolipidosis resemble those of Hurler syndrome but without increased mucopolysaccharides in urine.

♦ Autosomal recessive transmission of fundamental defect in recognition or catalysis and uptake of certain lysosomal enzymes due to deficient activity of N-acetylglucosamine-1-transferase.

♦ Heterozygotes may have intermediate enzyme levels in leukocytes and cultured fibroblasts.

Mucopolysaccharidoses, Genetic

The mucopolysaccharidoses (MPSs) are chronically progressive, clinically heterogeneous diseases resulting from defects in stepwise degradation of mucopolysaccharides caused by enzyme blocks in catabolism of keratin, heparin, or dermatan. See Table 12-14.

♦ All MPSs show metachromatically staining inclusions of mucopolysaccharides in circulating polynuclear leukocytes (Reilly granulations) or lymphocytes, cells of inflammatory exudate, and bone marrow cells (most consistently in clasmatocytes). Mucopolysaccharide is also deposited in various parenchymal cells. Detection of deficiency of lysosomal enzyme in cultured fibroblasts establishes the diagnosis and makes prenatal diagnosis possible. Serum can be used for diagnosis in MPS II, IIIB, and VI. Leukocytes can be used for diagnosis in MPS IH, IS, IIIA, and IIIC. RBCs can be used for diagnosis in III, IV, and VI. Enzyme deficiency is demonstrable in liver in all except V and VII; demonstrable in muscle in all except IH and II. Increased glycogen in affected organs except in IV; glycogen structure is normal except in III and IV. Carrier state detection of IH, III, IV, and VI is not reliable because of overlapping with normal persons of enzymatic activity values.

Inheritance in Hunter syndrome is X-linked recessive; all others are autosomal recessive.
Cloudy cornea in IH, IS, IVA, IVB, VI, and VII.
Mental retardation in IH, II, IIIA, IIIB, IIIC, IIID, and VII.
Hepatosplenomegaly in IH, II, IIIA, IIIB, IIIC, IIID, IVB, VI, and VII.
Skeletal defects in all.

Hurler Syndrome (Mucopolysaccharidosis IH)

Hurler syndrome is a lysosomal disorder caused by deficient activity of α-L-iduronidase Most with the disorder die by age 10 years.

♦ Initial diagnosis by quantitative increase of mucopolysaccharides in urine; confirmed by assay of α-L-iduronidase in cultured fibroblasts or leukocytes.
Similar enzyme assay detects carriers who have ~50% activity, but the wide range with overlap between normal and carriers may make the diagnosis difficult in individual cases.
♦ Prenatal diagnosis by assay of enzyme or mucopolysaccharides in amniocytes or chorionic villi sampling.

Hunter Syndrome (Mucopolysaccharidosis II)

Hunter syndrome is clinically similar to Hurler syndrome but milder, with no corneal opacity.

♦ Initial diagnosis by quantitation of total glucosaminoglycans in urine and accumulation of keratan sulfate in tissues is confirmed by enzyme assay in fibroblasts.
♦ Heterozygous female carriers recognized by MPS in fibroblasts or enzyme assay in individual hair roots.
♦ Prenatal diagnosis by enzyme assay of amniotic fluid should be confirmed by assay of cultured cells.
♦ Maternal serum shows increased activity of iduronate sulfate sulfatase with a normal or heterozygous fetus but no increase if fetus has Hunter syndrome.
Mild and severe subtypes

Sanfilippo Type A Syndrome (Mucopolysaccharidosis III)

The four types of Sanfilippo syndrome cannot be distinguished clinically.

♦ Only MPS in which heparan sulfate is found in urine, which confirms diagnosis.
♦ Assay of fibroblasts shows deficiency of enzyme in patient and decrease of normal activity in carrier who also show mucopolysaccharide accumulation.
○ Metachromatic inclusion bodies in lymphocytes are coarser and sparser than in Hurler syndrome and may be seen in bone marrow cells. Severe cerebral changes with relatively mild changes in other body tissues.

Morquio Syndrome (Mucopolysaccharidosis IV)

♦ Keratan sulfate is increased in urine (often 2×–3× normal).
○ Metachromatic granules may be seen in polymorphonuclear leukocytes.
♦ Diagnosis by enzyme assay in fibroblasts and leukocytes.
♦ Prenatal diagnosis by assay of enzymes in cultured amniocytes.

Maroteaux-Lamy Syndrome (Mucopolysaccharidosis VI)

○ Metachromatic cytoplasmic inclusions (Alder granules) may be seen in 50% of lymphocytes and 100% of granulocytes are more marked than in other MPSs.
♦ Large amount of dermatan sulfate occurs in urine.
♦ Diagnosis is established by deficiency of specific enzyme in cultured fibroblasts.
♦ Enzyme assay also allows diagnosis of heterozygotes and prenatal diagnosis.
Other rare diseases due to enzyme deficiencies that resemble these conditions include I-cell disease (mucolipidosis I) and mucolipidosis III and related disorders.

Leukodystrophies

The leukodystrophies are autosomal or x-linked inherited disorders of myelination that cause destruction or abnormal formation of nervous system white

matter. This category also includes Canavan disease, adrenoleukodystrophy, and others.

Metachromatic Leukodystrophy

Metachromic leukodystrophy is a rare autosomal recessive lipidosis caused by a deficiency of arylsulfatase A. There are infantile and adult forms with inability to degrade sphingolipid, sulfatide, or galactosylceramide, causing accumulation of sulfatide.

♦ Urine sediment may contain metachromatic lipids (from breakdown of myelin products).
CSF protein may be normal or increased ≤200 mg/dL.
♦ Biopsy of dental or sural nerve stained with cresyl violet showing accumulation of metachromatic sulfatide is diagnostic. Also increased in brain, kidney, liver.
♦ Conjunctival biopsy shows metachromatic inclusions within Schwann cells.

Krabbe Disease (Globoid Cell Leukodystrophy)

Krabbe disease is an autosomal recessive deficiency of galactosylceramidase mapped to chromosome 14, which causes progressive disease of CNS myelination from ~3 months of age, ending in death by ~2 years.

♦ Diagnosis by deficiency of this enzyme (5%–10% of normal) in leukocytes or cultured fibroblasts.
♦ Conjunctival biopsy shows characteristic ballooned Schwann cells.
♦ Brain biopsy (massive infiltration of unique multinucleated inclusion-containing globoid cells in white matter due to accumulation of galactosylceramide; also diffuse loss of myelin, severe astrocytic gliosis).
CSF protein electrophoresis shows increased albumin and α-globulin and decreased β- and γ-globulin (same as in metachromatic leukodystrophy).
♦ Prenatal diagnosis by measuring enzyme activity in cultured amniotic fluid cells.

Other Genetic Disorders

See Table 12-16. See Chapter 13.

Batten Disease (Batten-Spielmeyer-Vogt Disease)

See Chapter 11, Table 11-20.

Down Syndrome (Trisomy 21; Mongolism)

Down syndrome is the most common autosomal trisomy.

See Table 12-16.
♦ Karyotyping shows 47 chromosomes with trisomy 21 in most patients; caused by translocation, usually to chromosome 14 or to other D group chromosome in <5% of cases. Two percent of patients have mosaicism, with one cell population trisomic.
Leukocytes show decreased incidence of drumsticks (see Chapter 4) and mean lobe counts.
Increased leukocyte alkaline phosphatase staining reaction.
Serum acid phosphatase may be decreased.
Risk of developing acute lymphocytic or nonlymphocytic leukemia is increased. Incidence is 10 to 20× greater than in the general population.
Congenital acute myelogenous leukemia may occur within several months of birth; it is always fatal.
Transient leukemoid reaction (WBC count ≤400,000/μL) with many blasts without anemia, thrombocytopenia, or neutropenia; becomes normal within 3 months. Occurs only with trisomy 21; differentiated from congenital leukemia by bone marrow biopsy, including cytogenetic and immunohistochemical studies. Twenty-five percent or fewer of these Down syndrome infants develop acute leukemia within 3 years.
Increased susceptibility to infection (e.g., hepatitis).

Table 12-16. Chromosome Number and Karyotype in Various Clinical Conditions

	Chromosome Number and Karyotype	Incidence
Normal male	46 XY	
Normal female	46 XX	
Suspected autosomal syndromes		
Down syndrome (mongolism; trisomy 21)	47 XX, G+, or 47 XY, G+	1 in 700 live births (2% are 46 count due to translocation and have 10% risk of Down syndrome in subsequent pregnancies; 2% are 46/47 mosaics)
Trisomy D 1	47 XX, D+, or 47 XY, D+	1 in 5,000 live births
	Translocations	Rare
	Mosaics	Rare
Trisomy E 18	47 XX, E+, or 47 XY, E+	1 in 3,000 live births
	Translocations	Rare
	Mosaics	Rare
Trisomy D 13		
Trisomy 8, 9, 4p, 9p		Rare
Cri du chat syndrome	46 with partial B deletion	1 in 30,000 births
Others (e.g., 4p-, 5p-, 9p-, 13q-)		
Suspected sex chromosome syndromes		
Klinefelter's syndrome	47 XXY	1 in 600 live male births
	48 XXXY	Rare
	48 XXYY	Rare
	49 XXXXY	Rare
	49 XXXYY	Rare
	Mosaics	Infrequent
Turner's syndrome	45 XO	1 in 3,000 live female births
	46 XX	Rare
	Mosaics	Infrequent
"Superfemale"	47 XXX	1 in 1,000–2,000 live female births
	48 XXXX	Rare
	49 XXXXX	Rare
	Mosaics	Rare
"Supermale"	47 XXY	1 in 1,000 live male births

METAB/HERED

Laboratory findings due to associated congenital abnormalities (e.g., GI, GU, cardiovascular systems).

Prenatal Screening and Diagnosis [19,20]

See Table 12-8 and Figure 12-4.

Optimum first-trimester screening (10–13 weeks) combines maternal age >35 years with 2 analytes: Free β-hCG (increased average of ≤2×) and pregnancy-associated plasma protein A (PAPP-A) (decreased average of 2.5×) combined with ultrasound nuchal translucency thickness. Detects ~85% of cases, with 5% false-positive rate. There should be a 2- to 6-week interval between first and second screenings.

Optimum second-trimester screening (at 15–22 weeks) combines maternal age >35 years with four analytes in maternal serum: β-hCG (increased average of 2×), AFP, unconjugated estriol levels (decreased average of 30%), and inhibin A (increased average of 2×). Detects ≤80% of cases, with 5% false-positive rate, using ultrasound to date fetal age.

Ultrasound may also detect major malformations associated with fetal Down syndrome (e.g., nonimmune hydrops, thickened nuchal fold, cystic hygroma, especially absent nasal bone).

Combination of first- and second-trimester screenings detects ~90% of cases, with <2% false-positive rate. In first trimester, nuchal translucency thickness and serum PAPP-A; wait for second-trimester tests; in second trimester AFP, hCG, urine estriol are performed.

	Normal Average Change	Average Value Change in Down Syndrome	Average Value Change in Trisomy 18
Maternal serum AFP[a]	15%/week during second trimester.	25%–30% lower	40% lower
Unconjugated estriol[a]	25%/week	25%–30% lower	60% lower
hCG[a]		2× higher	70% lower
Maternal serum Inhibin A[a]		2× higher	
PAPP-A[b]	50%/week	2.5× lower	Lower
Free β-hCG[b]	Increased	Increased	Lower
Nuchal translucency thickness[b] (typically 0.5–1.5 mm)	20%/week	2× higher	Higher

PAPP-A, pregnancy-associated plasma protein A; β-HcG, β-human chorionic gonadotropin.
[a]Optimum time for screening = 15 to 22 weeks.
[b]Optimum time for screening = 10 to 13 weeks.
Use of Inhibin is moot. Ultrasound nuchal translucency thickness interpretation requires special training.

Maternal Serum AFP

AFP is a glycoprotein produced first by the yolk sac, then by the fetal liver. It reaches its maximum at 10 to 13 weeks of gestation, then declines to <100 μg/L by term. By age 2 years, reaches adult levels <5 μg/L.

See "Obstetric Monitoring of the Fetus and Newborn," Chapter 14.

Interpretation

- Use of maternal serum AFP alone detects ≤25% of cases but should be combined (see previous). Ultrasound is used to verify gestational age, which has a profound effect on the calculated risk of Down syndrome.

[19]Canick JA, Saller DN Jr, Lambert-Messerlian GM. Prenatal screening for Down syndrome. Current and future methods. *Clin Lab Med* 2003;23:395–411.
[20]Wapner R, Thom E, Simpson JL, et al. First-trimester screening for trisomies 21 and 18. *N Engl J Med* 2003;349:1405–1413.

◆ • *Decreased maternal blood level of AFP in pregnancy is a valuable screening test, but diagnosis should be confirmed by finding increased levels in amniotic fluid and sonography* (to rule out missed abortion, molar pregnancy, absent pregnancy), and by chromosomal studies to confirm or refute the diagnosis. Average AFP is 25% to 30% lower in Down syndrome.

• In midtrimester, usual range is 10 to 150 ng/mL; is usually reported as multiple of median (MoM) (normal 0.4–2.5 MoM) to minimize interlaboratory variability and adjust for patient's race, gestational age, diabetes mellitus, twin pregnancy, and patient weight. MoM relates specific patient to entire screened population. 1.0 MoM is central value of a normal pregnancy. 2.0 MoM = 2× central value; 0.5 MoM = half central value.

• MoM = measured AFP (μg/L) ÷ median AFP for gestational age (μg/L) × adjustments (especially for gestational age and race).

Decreased In
Down syndrome (trisomy 21; average value is 2× higher) and trisomy 18
Long-standing death of fetus
Overestimation of gestational age (underestimation of age in amniotic fluid sample)
Choriocarcinoma, hydatidiform mole
Increased maternal weight (does not affect amniotic fluid concentration)
Pseudopregnancy, nonpregnancy
Various drugs (therefore no medications for at least 12 hours before test)
Other unknown factors
Women with diabetes mellitus have values 20% to 40% lower than nondiabetic women.

Increased In
(Should confirm by increase in amniotic fluid)
  Multiple pregnancy (>4.5 MoM)
  Gestational age (for which values must be adjusted)
  Race (10%–15% higher in blacks) (for which values must be adjusted)
Open neural tube defects (e.g., open spina bifida, anencephaly, encephalocele, myelocele); 80% of severe cases will be detected by AFP; hydrocephaly and microcephaly
Ventral wall defects associated with exposed fetal membrane and blood vessel surfaces, e.g., omphalocele, gastroschisis
Hydrops fetalis
Intrauterine death
Fetal-maternal hemorrhage
Esophageal or duodenal atresia
Cystic hygroma
Renal disorders (e.g., polycystic kidneys, renal agenesis, urethral obstruction)
Aplasia cutis
Sacrococcygeal teratoma
Tetralogy of Fallot
Turner syndrome
Oligohydramnios
Maternal causes (e.g., neoplasm that produces AFP, hepatitis)
Placental causes (e.g., infarction, thrombosis, inflammation, cystic changes, very large placenta)
Very rare benign hereditary familial elevation of serum AFP

Maternal Serum Human Chorionic Gonadotropin
hCG appears in maternal serum soon after pregnancy and reaches a peak by 8 to 10 weeks of gestation, then decreases to nadir at 18 weeks and then remains constant to end of pregnancy.

Use
Best *single* marker for Down syndrome screening but usually done as part of a three- or four-test analyte screen. Average value is 2× higher in Down syndrome.
Diagnosis of early pregnancy (see Pregnancy Test)
Diagnosis and effectiveness of therapy of germ cell tumors (see Chapter 14)

METAB/HERED

Maternal Serum Unconjugated Estriol

Estriol originates from fetal adrenal, liver, and placenta. It begins to appear by the seventh to the ninth week of gestation.

See Chapter 4.

Decreased In

Average value is 25% to 30% lower in Down syndrome.

Low values at 35 to 36 weeks of gestation will identify one third or fewer of "light for dates" infants.

Interpretation

Level >12 ng/mL rules out postmaturity in cases of prolonged gestation if there are no other diseases (e.g., diabetes mellitus, isoimmunization).

≤0.6 MoM in 5% of unaffected pregnancies and 26% of Down syndrome.

Safe levels indicate fetal well-being.

Increasing serial values rule out prolonged pregnancy and postmaturity.

Constant normal values are consistent with 40 to 41 weeks of gestation.

Declining values are consistent with prolonged gestation.

Low or significantly falling values are seen in fetal distress and postmaturity.

Pregnancy-Associated Plasma Protein A

PAPP-A is a high-molecular-weight glycoprotein of uncertain function. Levels normally increase 50%/week during the first trimester.

≤2.5× lower in Down syndrome pregnancy in second trimester.

After 14 weeks, PAPP loses its effectiveness; similar in affected and unaffected pregnancies.

Chromosomal Analysis of Amniotic Fluid

Can detect ~20% of cases.

Trisomy 18 (Edward Syndrome)

Trisomy 18 is the second most common autosomal trisomy. Occurrence is usually sporadic; due to nondisjunction; increased maternal age. Seventy percent of pregnancies miscarry. Ninety percent of newborns die in the first year.

♦ Screening in second trimester: maternal age>35combined with decreased AFP (average 40%), hCG (average 70%), and unconjugated estriol (average 60%) in maternal serum detects ~70% of cases, with 0.4% false-positive rate.

♦ Screening in first trimester: maternal age>35, decreased PAPP-A and free β-hCG with ultrasound. Inhibin A use is moot.

Triple screen of AFP, total hCG, unconjugated estriol has reported detection rate of 60%, with <0.7% false positives.

♦ Karyotyping shows 47 chromosomes, with trisomy 18 in most patients or mosaicism or translocations.

Laboratory findings due to congenital abnormalities (e.g., cardiovascular, GU, GI systems).

Trisomy 13 (D₁ Trisomy; Patau Syndrome)[21]

Trisomy 13 is the third most common autosomal trisomy, usually caused by chromosomal nondisjunction (>75% of cases). It may also be caused by translocation (10% of cases; parental carrier) or mosaicism (5% of cases). Over 80% of patients die in the first month; the 6-month survival rate is 5%.)

See Table 12-8.

○ In peripheral blood smears, ≤80% of polymorphonuclear leukocytes (neutrophils and eosinophils) show an increased number of anomalous nuclear projections (tags,

[21]Baty BJ, Blackburn BL, Carey JC. Natural history of trisomy 18 and trisomy 13. I. Growth, physical assessment, medical histories, survival, and recurrence risk. *Am J Med Genet.* 1994;49: 175–188.

threads, drumsticks, clubs); the nuclear lobulation may appear abnormal (nucleus may look twisted without clear separation of individual lobes, coarse lumpy chromatin, etc.). Present in almost all complete trisomic cases. Nuclear coils of chromatin by electron microscopy.

Fetal hemoglobins may persist longer than normal (i.e., be increased); these include HbF, Bart, Gower 2.

O Decreased AFP in maternal serum and amniotic fluid. Has no *pattern* of diagnostic markers for prenatal screening.

Laboratory findings due to multiple congenital abnormalities (including almost pathognomonic tetrad of narrow palpebral fissures, microphthalmos, cleft palate, parieto-occipital scalp defect, and polydactyly).

♦ Karyotyping shows numeric abnormality in 80% of cases: 47 XX, +13 or 47 XY, +13. Mosaicism is rare.

Dysautonomia, Familial (Riley-Day Syndrome)

Dysautonomia is an autosomal recessive disorder (localized to chromosome 9 at 9q31-q33) of autonomic dysfunction occurring in Ashkenazi Jews; patients show difficulty in swallowing, corneal ulcerations, insensitivity to pain, motor incoordination, excessive sweating, diminished gag reflex, lack of tongue papillae, progressive kyphoscoliosis, pulmonary infections, etc.

Urine vanillylmandelic acid (VMA) (3-methoxy-4-hydroxymandelic acid) may be low, and homovanillic acid is increased.

In asymptomatic carriers, urine VMA may be lower than in healthy adults.

Decreased plasma dopamine β-hydroxylase (converts dopamine to norepinephrine).

Fragile X Syndrome of Mental Retardation

Fragile X syndrome is the most common form of inherited mental retardation. It is caused by mutations that increase the size of a specific DNA fragment of the X chromosome (in Xq27.3).

♦ Direct diagnosis by DNA analysis using Southern blotting and PCR. Can also be used for prenatal diagnosis and to detect asymptomatic carriers. Can distinguish between full mutation, in which 100% of males and about 50% of females will be mentally impaired, and permutation, in which only ~3% will be impaired.

Lesch-Nyhan Syndrome

Lesch-Nyhan syndrome is an X-linked recessive trait of complete absence of hypoxanthine-guanine phosphoribosyl transferase (HGPRT) that catalyzes hypoxanthine and guanine to their nucleotides, causing an accumulation of purines. The syndrome appears in male children, with choreoathetosis, mental retardation, and tendency to self-mutilation, biting, and scratching.

♦ Increased serum uric acid levels (9–12 mg/dL).
♦ Hyperuricuria
  • 3 to 4 mg of uric acid/mg creatinine
  • 40 to 70 mg of uric acid/kg body weight
  • 600 to 1,000 mg/24 h in patients weighing ≥15 kg
  • Marked variation in purine diet causes very little change
  • Orange crystals or sand in infants' diapers
♦ Deficiency of HGPRT activity detected in cultured fibroblasts (<1.2% of normal), RBC hemolysates (0%) establishes the diagnosis; in amniotic cells allows diagnosis in utero. DNA probes allow prenatal diagnosis.
♦ Heterozygotes can be detected by study of individual hair follicles.
♦ Variants with partial deficiency of HGPRT show 0% to 50% of normal activity in RBC hemolysates and >1.2% in fibroblasts; accumulate purines but no orange sand in diapers; no abnormality of CNS or behavior.

Laboratory findings due to secondary gout (tophi after 10 years, crystalluria, hematuria, urinary calculi, urinary tract infection, gouty arthritis, response to colchicine); patients die of renal failure by age 10 years unless treated.

METAB/HERED

Table 12-17.   Comparison of Some Periodic Fever Syndromes[24]

	Familial Mediterranean Fever	Hyper-IgD Syndrome	TNF-Receptor-Associated Periodic Syndrome
Ancestry	Sephardic Jews, Arabs, Turks, Armenians	Western European (60% are Dutch, French)	Scottish, Irish; now reported in others
Usual age at onset	<20 y	<1 y	<20 y
Usual duration of attack	<2 d	4–6 d	>14 d
Inheritance	Autosomal recessive	Autosomal recessive	Autosomal dominant
Chromosome	16 short arm	12 long arm	12 short arm
Gene	*MEFV* encodes protein pyrin or marenostrin; five mutations are most frequent	Mevalonate kinase gene; V377I mutation in >80% of patients	Type 1 TNF receptor gene
AA amyloidosis	Nephropathy develops in ≤60% of patients	Not reported	In 25% of affected families
Laboratory findings	Decreased C5a inhibitor in serosal fluids	Increased serum IgD (>100 IU/mL); associated increased IgA in 80% of cases	Soluble type 1 TNF receptor is usually <1 ng/mL and mevalonate kinase activity is 5%–15% of normal in serum
Clinical symptoms of abdominal pain, skin lesions, arthralgia			
Other findings	Myalgia is uncommon	Cervical lymphadenopathy, enlarged liver, spleen	Variable; conjunctivitis, localized myalgia

TNF, tumor necrosis factor.

Periodic Fever Syndromes[22]

The periodic fever syndromes are inherited disorders with limited periods of fever and serositis that recur for years in otherwise healthy persons; the fever is accompanied by an increase in acute inflammatory reactants (e.g., ESR, CRP, WBC, fibrinogen, A amyloid, etc.) and different fever patterns.

See Table 12-17.

Mediterranean Fever, Familial (Familial Paroxysmal Peritonitis)[23]

Familial Mediterranean fever is an autosomal recessive disorder caused by a defect on chromosome 16; it results from a lack of a specific protease in serosal fluids with recurrent polyserositis (peritonitis 93%, arthritis 47%, pleuritis 31%) and fever (92%) and myalgia (39%) lasting ≤96 hours, predominantly in Sephardic Jews, Arabs, Turks, and Armenians.

[22]Drenth JPH, van der Meer JWM. Hereditary periodic fever. *N Engl J Med* 2001;345:1748.
[23]Tunca M, Akar S, Onen F, Turkish FMV Study Group, et al. Familial Mediterranean fever (FMF) in Turkey. *Medicine (Baltimore)* 2005;84(1):1–11.

Diagnostic Criteria
Major
  AA amyloidosis without predisposing disease
  Recurrent febrile episodes of peritonitis, pleuritis, synovitis
  Favorable response to colchicine
Minor
  Recurrent febrile episodes
  Erysipelas-like erythema
  Positive history in first-degree relative
  Definite: 2 major criteria or 1 major and 2 minor criteria
  Probable: 1 major and 1 minor criteria

○ AA amyloidosis nephropathy develops in ≤60% of patients (arrested by colchicine prophylaxis); is usually fatal. Is not related to frequency or severity of clinical attacks; also involves GI, liver, spleen, skin, other sites.
♦ Genetic labs usually screen for five most common mutations, which cause >70% of deleterious alleles.

Hyper-IgD Syndrome

♦ Increased IgD (>100 IU/mL on more than one occasion) is constant. Associated with increased IgA in 80% of cases.
Mevalonate kinase activity = 5% to 15% of normal; complete deficiency in <1% of patients, causing mevalonic aciduria.
Variant form is also recognized.

Tumor Necrosis Factor Receptor-Associated Periodic Syndrome

♦ Serum level of soluble type 1 tumor necrosis factor receptor is low (usually <1 ng/mL; increased in renal insufficiency, e.g., amyloidosis).
♦ DNA gene sequencing detects mutations.

Other Periodic Syndromes include familial cold urticaria, Muckle-Wells syndrome, and aphthous stomatitis.

METAB/HERED

13 Endocrine Diseases

ENDOCRINE

General Principles in Diagnosis of Endocrine Diseases

Perform stimulatory tests if hypofunction is suspected and suppression tests if hyperfunction is suspected.

Suppression tests will suppress normal glands but not autonomous secretion (e.g., functioning neoplasm).

Multiple or pooled samples of baseline specimens and drawing specimens from indwelling lines are often required to obtain optimal specimens.

Patient preparation is particularly important for hormone studies, results of which may be markedly affected by many factors such as stress, position, fasting state, time of day, preceding diet, drug therapy, all of which should be recorded on the lab test requisition form and discussed with the laboratory prior to test ordering.

Appropriate (e.g., frozen) and timely transportation to laboratory and preparation of specimen (e.g., separation of serum may be vital for some tests).

No single test adequately reflects the endocrine status in all conditions.

Multiple gland hypofunction should evaluate pituitary.

Tests of Thyroid Function

Thyroid function hormone tests are not indicated for *screening* programs without suspicion of thyroid disease (overall yield ~0.5% and varies from 0% in young men to 1% in women >40 years).

May be useful for selective screening in certain populations such as newborns (mandatory), strong family history of thyroid disease, elderly, 4 to 8 weeks postpartum women, patients with autoimmune diseases (e.g., Addison disease, type 1 diabetes mellitus). May be useful in some women >40 years with nonspecific complaints.

Calcitonin

Secreted by parafollicular C cells of thyroid; acts directly on osteoclasts to decrease bone-resorbing activity and causing decreased serum calcium

Use

To diagnose recurrence of medullary carcinoma or metastases after the primary tumor has been removed or to confirm complete removal of the tumor if basal calcitonin has been previously increased.

Basal fasting level may be increased in patients with medullary carcinoma of the thyroid even when there is no palpable mass in the thyroid. Circadian rhythm with rise to peak after lunchtime. Basal level is normal in approximately one third of medullary carcinoma cases.

Normal basal calcitonin levels: Males, <12 pg/mL; females, <5 pg/mL; children <6 months, <40 pg/mL; children 6 months to 3 years, <15 pg/mL[1]

- Levels of >2,000 pg/mL are almost always associated with medullary carcinoma of thyroid with rare cases due to obvious renal failure or ectopic production of calcitonin.
- Levels of 500 to 2,000 pg/mL generally indicate medullary carcinoma, renal failure, or ectopic production of calcitonin.
- Levels of 100 to 500 pg/mL should be interpreted cautiously with repeat assays and provocative tests; if repeat tests in 1 to 2 months are still abnormal, some authors recommend total thyroidectomy.

Calcium infusion and/or pentagastrin injection are used as provocative tests in patients with normal calcium basal levels in whom there is a high index of suspicion, e.g., family history of thyroid carcinoma, a calcified thyroid mass, pheochromocytoma, hyperparathyroidism, hypercalcemia, amyloid-containing metastatic carcinoma of unknown origin, or facial characteristics of the mucosal neuroma syndrome. Normally should not rise above 0.2 ng/mL. Peak values >1 ng/mL are indicative of C-cell malignancy. Pentagastrin is more sensitive than calcium stimulation.

[1]Basuyau JP, et al. Reference intervals for serum calcitonin in men, women, and children. *Clin Chem* 2004;50:1828.

Increased In Some Patients
Carcinoma of lung, breast, islet cell, or ovary and carcinoid due to ectopic production
and in myeloproliferative disorders.
Hypercalcemia of any etiology stimulating calcitonin production
Zollinger-Ellison syndrome
C-cell hyperplasia
Pernicious anemia
Acute or chronic thyroiditis
Chronic renal failure

Thyrotropin (TSH)

Secreted by anterior pituitary.

Use
Assess true metabolic status.
Screening for euthyroidism—normal level in stable ambulatory patient not on inter-
fering drugs excludes thyroid hormone excess or deficiency. Recommended as the
initial test rather than T_4.
Screening is not recommended for asymptomatic persons without suspicion of thyroid
disease or for hospital patients with acute medical or psychiatric illness.
Initial screening and diagnosis for hyperthyroidism (decreased to undetectable levels
except in rare TSH-secreting pituitary adenoma) and hypothyroidism.
Especially useful in early or subclinical hypothyroidism before the patient develops
clinical findings, goiter, or abnormalities of other thyroid tests.
In very early cases with only marginal elevation, the TRH stimulation test may be preferred.
Differentiation of primary (increased levels) from central [pituitary or hypothalamic]
hypothyroidism (decreased levels).
Monitor adequate thyroid hormone replacement therapy in primary hypothyroidism
although T_4 may be mildly increased; up to 6 to 8 weeks before TSH becomes normal. Serum TSH suppressed to normal level is the best monitor of dosage of thyroid
hormone for treatment of hypothyroidism.
Monitor adequate thyroid hormone therapy to suppress thyroid carcinoma (should
suppress to <0.1 mU/L) or goiter or nodules (should suppress to subnormal levels)
with third- or fourth-generation assays.
Replace TRH stimulation test in hyperthyroidism since most patients with euthyroid
TSH level will have a normal TSH response and patients with undetectable TSH
level almost never respond to TRH stimulation.
May Not Be Useful
To evaluate thyroid status of hospitalized ill patients (see Nonthyroidal Illness [NTI])
First, ~3 months of treatment of hypo- or hyperthyroidism; free T_4 (FT_4) is test of
choice.
Lag time of 6 to 8 weeks required for normalization of TSH after initiation of thyroid
hormone replacement therapy.
Interferences
Dopamine or high doses of glucocorticoids may cause false normal values in primary
hypothyroidism and may suppress TSH in nonthyroid illness.
Rheumatoid factor, human anti-mouse antibodies, and thyroid hormone autoantibod-
ies may produce spurious results especially in patients with autoimmune disorders
(≤10%).
Heterophile antibodies
Amiodarone
Not affected by variation in thyroid binding proteins
Increased In
Primary untreated hypothyroidism. Increase is proportionate to the degree of hypo-
function, varying from 3× normal in mild cases to 100× normal in severe myxedema.
A single determination is usually sufficient to establish the diagnosis.
Patients with hypothyroidism receiving insufficient thyroid hormone replacement
therapy
Patients with Hashimoto thyroiditis, including those with clinical hypothyroidism and
about one-third of those patients who are clinically euthyroid

Table 13-1.   Free Thyroxine (FT$_4$) and Thyroid-Stimulating Hormone (TSH) Levels in Various Conditions

		Sensitive TSH		
		Normal	Low	High
T_4	**Normal**	Euthyroid	Subclinical/early hyperthyroidism* NTI Drug effects (e.g., L-dopa, glucocorticoids) Replacement therapy or excess T$_4$ therapy for hypothyroidism Rule out thyrotoxicosis	Subclinical/early hypothyroidism† NTI Drug effects (e.g., iodine, lithium, antithyroid drugs, amiodarone, interferon alfa) Insufficient T$_4$ therapy for hypothyroidism First 4–6 wks of therapy for hypothyroidism
	Low	Secondary hypothyroidism Drug effects (e.g., T$_3$, phenytoin, androgens, salicylates, carbamazepine, rifampin)	Secondary hypothyroidism NTI Drug effects (e.g., dopamine, T$_3$, corticosteroids) T3 hyperthyroidism (e.g., Graves disease, toxic goiter, thyroiditis, factitious/iatrogenic, hyperthyroidism, struma ovarii, thyroid carcinoma)	Primary hypothyroidism Drug effects (e.g., iodine, lithium, antithyroid drugs, amiodarone) Insufficient T$_4$ therapy for hypothyroidism
	High	NTI (e.g., psychiatric and acute illness) Abnormal binding (excess TBG, familial dysalbuminemic hyperthyroxemia, some monoclonal proteins) Thyroid hormone resistance Drug effects (e.g., estrogen, iodine drugs or contrast media, thyroxine [factitious])	NTI (e.g., psychiatric and acute illness) Primary hyperthyroidism‡	TSH-secreting tumor Thyroid hormone resistance

T$_3$, triiodothyronine; T$_4$, thyroxine; NTI, nonthyroid illness.
*Low TSH with normal T$_4$.
†High TSH with normal T$_4$.
‡In 95% of cases of thyrotoxicosis. Serum T$_3$ is needed for diagnosis of T$_3$-thyrotoxicosis in the other 5% of cases of thyrotoxicosis.

Use of various drugs

- Amphetamine abuse
- Iodine-containing (e.g., iopanoic acid, ipodate, amiodarone)
- Dopamine antagonists (e.g., metoclopramide, domperidone, chlorpromazine, haloperidol)

Other conditions (test is not clinically useful)

- Iodide deficiency goiter
- Iodide-induced goiter or lithium treatment
- External neck irradiation
- Post-subtotal thyroidectomy
- Neonatal period

Thyrotoxicosis due to pituitary thyrotroph adenoma or pituitary resistance to thyroid hormone
Euthyroid sick syndrome, recovery phase
TSH antibodies
Increased in first 2 to 3 days of life due to postnatal TSH surge.

Decreased In
Hyperthyroidism due to

- Toxic multinodular goiter
- Autonomously functioning thyroid adenoma
- Ophthalmopathy of euthyroid Graves disease
- Treated Graves disease
- Thyroiditis
- Extrathyroidal thyroid hormone source
- Factitious

Overreplacement of thyroid hormone in treatment of hypothyroidism
Secondary pituitary or hypothalamic hypothyroidism (e.g., tumor, infiltrates)
Euthyroid sick patients (some patients)
Acute psychiatric illness
Severe dehydration
Drug effect, especially large doses—use FT_4 for evaluation

- Glucocorticoids, dopamine, dopamine agonists (bromocriptine), levodopa, T_4 replacement therapy, apomorphine, pyridoxine; T_4 may be normal or low
- Antithyroid drug for thyrotoxicosis, especially early in treatment; T_4 may be normal or low
- Assay interference, e.g., antibodies to mouse IgG, autoimmune disease

First trimester of pregnancy
Isolated deficiency (very rare)

May Be Normal In
Central hypothyroidism
Recent rapid correction of hyperthyroidism or hypothyroidism
Pregnancy
Phenytoin therapy
In absence of hypothalamic or pituitary disease, normal TSH excludes primary hypothyroidism.

Thyroglobulin (Tg)

Glycoprotein secreted only by thyroid follicular cells. Involved in iodination and synthesis of thyroid hormones. Proportional to thyroid mass.

See Table 13-2.

Use
To assess the presence and possibly the extent of residual or recurrent or metastatic follicular or papillary thyroid carcinoma after therapy. In patients with these carcinomas treated with total thyroidectomy or radioiodine and taking thyroid hormone therapy, Tg is undetectable if functional tumor is absent, but is detected by sensitive immunoassay if functional tumor is present. Tg correlates with tumor mass with highest values in patients with metastases to bones and lungs.
Diagnosis of factitious hyperthyroidism: Tg is very low or not detectable in factitious hyperthyroidism and is high in all other types of hyperthyroidism (e.g., thyroiditis, Graves disease).
Not recommended for initial diagnosis of thyroid carcinomas. Not a tumor marker.
Do not use in patients with preexisting thyroid disorders.
Predict outcome of therapy for hyperthyroidism; higher remission rates in patients with lower Tg values. Failure to become normal after drug-induced remission suggests relapse after drugs are discontinued.

Table 13-2. Thyroid Function Tests in Various Conditions

Condition	TSH	TT$_4$	FT$_4$	T$_3$	Tg	RAIU	Comment
Hypothyroidism							
Primary							
Clinical	<u>I</u>	<u>D</u>	<u>D</u>	D	N/I	D	Increased response to TRH administration
Subclinical	<u>I</u>	N	N	N	N	NA	
Secondary	<u>N/D</u>	D	D	<u>D</u>			No response to TRH administration
Tertiary	<u>N/D</u>	D	D	D			
Nonthyroidal* illness	<u>V</u>	N/D	N/D	<u>D</u>	D		
Hyperthyroidism							
Primary							
Clinical	<u>D</u>	<u>I</u>	<u>I</u>	I	N	I	
Subclinical	<u>D</u>	N	N	N	N	NA	
T$_3$ thyrotoxicosis	<u>D</u>	N	N	<u>I</u>	N	NA	
TSH-secreting tumor	I	I	I	I	N	NA	
TRH-secreting tumor	I	I	I	I	N	NA	
Factitious							
T$_4$ ingestion	<u>D</u>	<u>I</u>	<u>I</u>	I	<u>D/N</u>	D	Augmented RAIU response to TSH administration
T$_3$ ingestion	D	N	N	<u>I</u>	D/N		
Pregnancy	N	I	N	I	I	X	
With hyperthyroidism	N	I	I	I	I	X	
With hypothyroidism	I	I	D	I	I	X	I T$_4$ and T$_3$ to normal range
Hereditary increased TBG					<u>I</u>		
Hereditary decreased TBG	N	D	N		<u>D</u>		
Hashimoto's thyroiditis	V	V	V	V		V	Thyroid antibodies; biopsy
Goiter	N	N	N	N	N	A	Biopsy
Thyroid carcinoma	N	N	N	N	I	N	Serum calcitonin I in medullary CA; Tg I in differentiated
Nephrosis	N	D	D		D	VI	
Drug effects							
Thyroxine	D	I					
Inorganic iodine	I						
Radiopaque contrast media		I	I				
Estrogen; birth control pills		I	N		I		
Testosterone	N	D	N	D	D		D TBH
ACTH and cortico-steroids	N	D	N	D	D		D TBH
Dilantin	V/I	D	N	N	D		Tissue resistance to T$_4$
Pituitary only	I	I	I				T$_4$ administration does not suppress TSH
Generalized tissue	V/I	V/I	V/I				

0 = absent; A = abnormal; D = decreased; I = increased; N = normal; NA = not useful; TT$_4$ = total thyroxine; V = variable; VD = variable decrease; VI = variable increase; X = contraindicated. Underlined test indicates most useful diagnostic change.
* Forms of nonthyroidal illness (euthyroid sick syndrome).

Diagnosis of thyroid agenesis in newborn.
Presence in pleural effusions indicates metastatic differentiated thyroid cancer.

Interferences

Tg autoantibodies: patients' serum must always first be screened for these antibodies (present in <10% of persons). In such cases, can measure Tg mRNA using RT-PCR.

Increased In

Most patients with differentiated thyroid carcinoma but not with undifferentiated or medullary thyroid carcinomas
Patients with hyperthyroidism—rapid decline after surgical treatment; gradual decline after radioactive iodine (RAI) treatment
Silent (painless) thyroiditis
Some patients with endemic goiter
Marked liver insufficiency

Decreased In

Thyroid agenesis in newborn
Total thyroidectomy or destruction by radiation

Thyroid-Stimulating Hormone; Thyrotropin, Sensitive (sTSH)

Hormone secreted by anterior pituitary; third- and fourth-generation assay detection limits are 0.01/mIU/L and 0.001/mIU/L, respectively.

See Tables 13-1, 13-2, and Fig. 13-1.
Euthyroid: 0.3–5.0 mIU/L
Possible hypothyroid: >5.0 mIU/L
Possible hyperthyroid: <0.10 mIU/L
Borderline: 0.10–0.29 mIU/L

Thyroid Autoantibody Tests

Antithyroid peroxidase antibodies are replacing antimicrosomal antibodies and antithyroglobulin antibodies.

Use

Positive in ~95% of cases of Hashimoto disease and ~85% of Graves disease. Very high titer is suggestive of Hashimoto thyroiditis but absence does not exclude Hashimoto thyroiditis. >1:1,000 occurs virtually only in Graves disease or Hashimoto thyroiditis.
Significant titer of microsome antibodies indicates Hashimoto thyroiditis or postpartum thyroiditis.
To distinguish subacute thyroiditis from Hashimoto thyroiditis, as antibodies are more common in the latter
Hashimoto thyroiditis is very unlikely cause of hypothyroidism in the absence of antibodies.
Significant titer of antibodies in euthyroid patient with unilateral exophthalmos suggests the diagnosis of euthyroid Graves disease.
Occasionally useful to distinguish Graves disease from toxic multinodular goiter when physical findings are not diagnostic
Graves disease with elevated antibody titer should direct surgeon to perform a more limited thyroidectomy to avoid late post-thyroidectomy hypothyroidism.
Tg antibodies may interfere with assay for serum Tg.
Thyroid receptor antibodies mainly used in Graves disease, especially as a predictor of relapse of hyperthyroidism

Increased In

Occasionally positive in papillary-follicular carcinoma of thyroid, subacute thyroiditis (briefly), lymphocytic (painless) thyroiditis (in ~60% of patients)
Primary thyroid lymphoma often shows very high titers; should suggest need for biopsy in elderly patient with a firm enlarging thyroid.
Low titers are present in >10% of normal population, increasing with age.
Other autoimmune diseases (e.g., PA, RA, SLE, myasthenia gravis)

Thyroid Uptake of Radioactive Iodine (RAIU)

See Table 13-2.

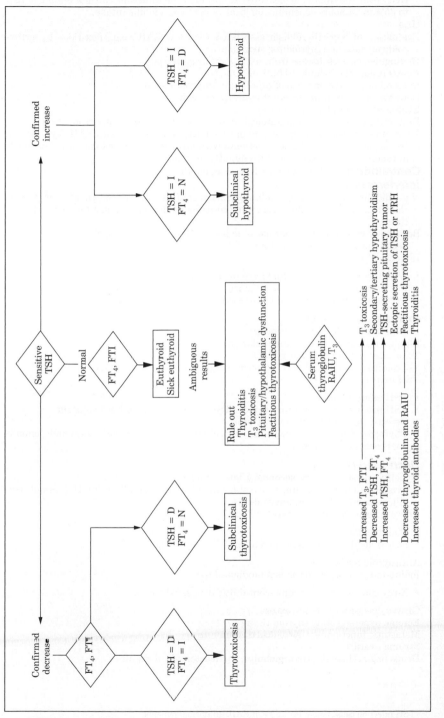

Fig. 13-1. Algorithm for thyroid function testing. (D, decreased; I, increased; N, normal.)

A tracer dose of radioactive iodine (^{131}I or ^{123}I) is administered orally, and the radioactivity over the thyroid is measured at specific time intervals. Normal uptake is 10% to 35% in 24 hours depending on local variations in iodine intake.

Use
Evaluation of hyperthyroidism associated with low RAIU, e.g., factitious hyperthyroidism, subacute thyroiditis, struma ovarii

Distinguish Graves disease from toxic nodular goiter

Assess function of nodules ("hot" or "cold")

Determine location and size of functioning thyroid tissue

Detect metastases from differentiated thyroid cancers

Evaluate use of radioiodine therapy

Determine presence of an organification defect in thyroid hormone production

T_3 suppression test. Administration of triiodothyronine suppresses RAIU by >50% in the normal person but not in patients with Graves disease or toxic nodules; shows autonomy of TSH secretion. Infrequently used now.

Contraindications: Pregnancy, lactation, childhood

Interferences
Not valid for 2 to 4 weeks after administration of antithyroid drugs, thyroid, or iodides; the effect of organic iodine (e.g., x-ray contrast media) may persist for a much longer time.

Because of widespread dietary use of iodine in the United States, RAIU should not be used to evaluate euthyroid state.

Increased by

* Withdrawal rebound (thyroid hormones, propylthiouracil)
* Increased iodine excretion (e.g., diuretics, nephrotic syndrome, chronic diarrhea)
* Decreased iodine intake (salt restriction, iodine deficiency)

Increased (>12%) In
Graves disease (diffuse toxic goiter)

Plummer disease (toxic multinodular goiter)

Toxic adenoma (uninodular goiter)

Thyroiditis (early Hashimoto; recovery stage of subacute thyroiditis)

TSH excess

* TSH administration
* TSH production by pituitary tumor (TSH >4 μU/mL) or other neoplasm
* Defective thyroid hormone synthesis
* Thyrotropin-producing neoplasms (e.g., choriocarcinoma, hydatidiform mole, embryonal carcinoma of testis)

Decreased (<3%) In
Hypothyroidism (tertiary, secondary, late primary)

Thyroiditis (late Hashimoto; active stage of subacute thyroiditis; RAIU does not usually respond to TSH administration)

Thyroid hormone administration (T_3 or T_4)

* Therapeutic
* Factitious (RAIU is augmented after TSH administration*)

Antithyroid medication

Iodine-induced hyperthyroidism (Jodbasedow)[†‡],

* X-ray contrast media, iodine-containing drugs, iodized salt

Graves disease with iodine excess

Ectopic hypersecreting thyroid tissue

Metastatic functioning thyroid carcinoma*

Struma ovarii*

Drugs (e.g., calcitonin, thyroglobulin, corticosteroids, dopamine)

---

*TSH injection causes increase ≥50% of RAIU in normal persons.

[†]TSH injection does not cause a normal increase ≥50% of RAIU.

[‡]Urinary iodine >2,000 g/24 hrs.

Triiodothyronine (T$_3$)

T$_4$ (thyroxine) is converted to T$_3$ in peripheral tissues; ~20% is synthesized by follicular cells. Most T$_3$ is transported bound to protein; only 0.3% is in free unbound state.

See Table 13-2 and Fig. 13-1.

Use

Diagnosis of T$_3$ thyrotoxicosis (when TSH is suppressed but T$_4$ is normal) or cases in which FT$_4$ is normal in presence of symptoms of hyperthyroidism

Evaluating cases in which FT$_4$ is borderline elevated

Evaluating cases in which overlooking diagnosis of hyperthyroidism is very undesirable (e.g., unexplained atrial fibrillation)

Monitoring the course of hyperthyroidism

Monitoring T$_4$ replacement therapy—is better than T$_4$ or FT$_4$ but TSH is preferred to both

Predicting outcome of antithyroid drug therapy in patients with Graves disease

Evaluation of amiodarone-induced thyrotoxicosis

Serum T$_3$ parallels FT$_4$; is early indicator of hyperthyroidism but TSH is better

Good biochemical indicator of severity of thyrotoxicity in hyperthyroidism

Not recommended for diagnosis of hypothyroidism; decreased values have minimal clinical significance

May decrease by ≤25% in healthy older persons while FT$_4$ remains normal

FT$_3$ gives corrected values in patients in whom the total T$_3$ (TT$_3$) is altered on account of changes in serum proteins or in binding sites e.g., pregnancy, drugs (e.g., androgens, estrogens, birth control pills, phenytoin [Dilantin]), altered levels of serum proteins (e.g., nephrosis)

Reverse T$_3$ (rT$_3$)

Hormonally inactive isomer of T$_3$.

Use

To distinguish low T$_3$ "sick thyroid" patients (usually increased) from true hypothyroidism

In severe NTI is increased except in some liver disorders, HIV, renal failure

Usually increased in hyperthyroidism and increased serum TBG; often decreased in hypothyroidism but overlaps with normal range

Thyroxine, Total (T$_4$)

T$_4$ is major secretion of thyroid. Bound to TBG, prealbumin, and albumin in blood. In tissues, is deiodinated to T$_3$ which causes hormonal action. Is responsible for hormonal action.

See Tables 13-1, 13-2, and Fig. 13-1.

Use

Reflects secretory activity; diagnosis of hyper- and hypothyroidism especially when overt or due to pituitary or hypothalamic disease

Increased In

Hyperthyroidism

Pregnancy

Drugs (e.g., estrogens, birth control pills, d-thyroxine, thyroid extract, TSH, amiodarone, heroin, methadone, amphetamines, some radiopaque substances for x-ray studies [ipodate, iopanoic acid])

Euthyroid sick syndrome

Increase in TBG or abnormal thyroxine-binding prealbumin (TBPA)

- Familial dysalbuminemic hyperthyroxinemia—albumin binds T$_4$ but not T$_3$ more avidly than normal, causing changes similar to thyrotoxicosis (TT$_4$ ~20 μg/dL, normal thyroid-hormone-binding ratio, increased FT$_4$I) but patient is not clinically thyrotoxic.
- Serum T$_4$ >20 μg/dL usually indicates true hyperthyroidism rather than increased TBG.
- May be found in euthyroid patients with increased serum TBG.
- Much higher in first 2 months of life than in normal adults.

Decreased In
Hypothyroidism
Hypoproteinemia (e.g., nephrosis, cirrhosis)
Certain drugs (phenytoin, triiodothyronine, testosterone, ACTH, corticosteroids)
Euthyroid sick syndrome
Decrease in TBG

Normal Levels May Be Found in Hyperthyroid Patients With
T_3 thyrotoxicosis
Factitious hyperthyroidism owning to T_3 (Cytomel)
Decreased binding capacity due to hypoproteinemia or ingestion of certain drugs (e.g., phenytoin, salicylates)

Interferences
Various drugs.

Not Affected By
Mercurial diuretics
Nonthyroidal iodine

Thyroxine, Free (FT$_4$)
See Table 13-2.

Use
Gives corrected values in patients in whom the TT_4 is altered on account of changes in serum proteins or in binding sites, e.g., pregnancy, drugs (such as androgens, estrogens, birth control pills, phenytoin), altered levels of serum proteins (e.g., nephrosis)
Monitoring restoration to normal range is only laboratory criterion to estimate appropriate replacement dose of levothyroxine because 6–8 wks are required before TSH reflects these changes.
Not generally helpful unless pituitary/hypothalamic disease is suspected.

Increased In
Hyperthyroidism
Hypothyroidism treated with thyroxine
Euthyroid sick syndrome
Occasional patients with hydatidiform mole or choriocarcinoma with marked hCG elevations may show increased FT_4, suppressed TSH, and blunted TSH response to TRH stimulation. Return to normal with effective treatment of trophoblastic disease. Severe dehydration (may be >6.0 ng/dL).

Decreased In
Hypothyroidism
Hypothyroidism treated with triiodothyronine
Euthyroid sick syndrome

Thyroxine-Binding Globulin (TBG)
Binds and transports most T$_4$ and T$_3$.

Use
Diagnosis of genetic or idiopathic excess TBG
Sometimes used to detect recurrent or metastatic differentiated thyroid carcinoma, especially follicular type and where patient has had an increased level due to carcinoma.
To distinguish increased/decreased TT_3 or TT_4 concentrations due to changes in TBG. Same purpose as T_3 resin uptake and free thyroxine index (see below).

Increased In
Pregnancy
Certain drugs (e.g., estrogens, birth control pills, perphenazine, clofibrate, heroin, methadone)
Estrogen-producing tumors
Systemic illness is increased early
Acute intermittent porphyria
Acute or chronic active hepatitis
Lymphocytic painless subacute thyroiditis.
Neonates
Inherited
Idiopathic

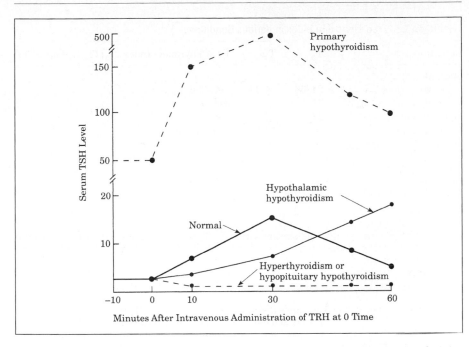

Fig. 13-2. Sample curves of serum thyroid-stimulating hormone (TSH) response to administration of thyrotropin-releasing hormone (TRH) in various conditions.

An increased TBG is associated with increased serum T_4 and decreased T_3 resin uptake; a converse association exists for decreased TBG.

Decreased In
Nephrosis and other causes of marked hypoproteinemia such as liver disease, severe illness (late), stress (thyroxine-binding-prealbumin [TBPA] also decreased)
Deficiency of TBG, genetic or idiopathic
Acromegaly (TBPA also decreased)
Severe acidosis
Certain drugs (e.g., androgens, anabolic steroids; glucocorticoids [TBPA is increased])
Testosterone-producing tumors

Decreased Binding of T_3 and T_4 Due to Drugs
Salicylates, phenytoin, Orinase, diabinase, penicillin, heparin, barbital

Thyrotropin-Releasing Hormone (TRH) Stimulation Test
See Fig. 13-2.
TSH high-sensitivity <0.1 mU/L, obviates need for TRH, except for TSH-secreting tumor and thyroid hormone resistance (in which case TSH thyroxine is high.)
Contraindicated in pregnancy. No T_4 or T_3 for 3 wks prior to test.
TRH can cause smooth muscle spasm; use with caution in asthma and ischemic heart disease.
Serum TSH is measured before, and 15 and 30 minutes after IV administration of TRH (200–500 μg).
Normal response: a significant rise from a basal level of 2 to 3 μU/mL that returns to normal by 120 minutes. Response is usually greater in women than in men.
Hyperthyroidism is ruled out by a normal increase of >2 to 3 μU/mL after TRH administration. A blunted response indicates hyperthyroidism but may occur in other conditions (e.g., uremia, Cushing syndrome, starvation, elevated levels of glucocorticoids, depression, some elderly patients). Largely replaced by sensitive TSH assays.
Primary hypothyroidism: an exaggerated prolonged rise of an already increased TSH level
Secondary (pituitary) hypothyroidism: no rise in the decreased TSH level

Table 13-3.	Free Thyroxine Index in Various Conditions		
Condition	T_3	T_4	Free Thyroxine Index (T_7) (T_3 Uptake $\times$ T_4)
Normal			
Range	24–36	4–11	96–396
Mean	31	7	217
Hypothyroid	22	3	66
Hyperthyroid	38	12	456
Pregnancy, estrogen use (especially birth control pills)	20	12	240*

*Normal even though T_3 and T_4 alone are abnormal.

Hypothalamic hypothyroidism: low serum T_3, T_4 and TSH levels, with a TRH response that may be exaggerated or normal or (most characteristically) with a peak delay 45 to 60 minutes.

Use

Interpretation must be based on clinical studies that exclude the pituitary gland as the site of the disease.

Lack of response shows adequate therapy in patients receiving thyroid hormones to shrink thyroid nodules and goiters and during long term treatment of thyroid carcinoma.

Differentiate two forms (whether or not owning to tumor) of thyrotropin-induced hyperthyroidism

May be particularly useful in T_3 toxicosis in which the other tests are normal or in patients clinically suspicious for hyperthyroidism with borderline serum T_3 levels. TRH stimulation test is superior to the T_3 suppression test of RAIU. Abnormal TSH response to TRH administration does not definitely establish the diagnosis of hyperthyroidism (because autonomous production of normal or slightly increased amounts of thyroid hormones causes pituitary suppression). TRH test may remain abnormal even after successful therapy of Graves disease.

Hyperthyroid patients in whom associated nonthyroid conditions result in only slight elevation of serum T_4 and T_3.

Euthyroid Graves disease presenting with only exophthalmos (unilateral or bilateral). *TRH stimulation test may sometimes be normal in these patients, and T_3 suppression test may be required.*

Elderly patients with or without symptoms of hyperthyroidism may have serum T_4 and T_3 in upper normal range.

Euthyroid sick syndrome—generally serum TSH is normal with a relatively normal TSH response to TRH.

May help differentiate hypothalamic from pituitary hypothyroidism (see above)

Interference

The TSH response to TRH is modified by thyroxine, antithyroid drugs, corticosteroids, estrogens, large amounts of salicylates, and levodopa. Response is increased during pregnancy.

Triiodothyronine (T_3) Resin Uptake (RUR)

Measures unoccupied binding sites on TBG. Now replaced by FT$_4$. Is not a measure of T_3 concentration, which is assayed by other methods for diagnosis of T_3 thyrotoxicosis.

See Table 13-3.

Use

Only with simultaneous measurement of serum T_4 to calculate T_7 in order to exclude the possibility that an increased TT_4 is due to an increase in TBG.

- RUR is inversely proportional unsaturated hormone binding sites.
- RUR decreases when binding protein increases (pregnancy).
- RUR increases when binding protein decreases (hyperthyroidism).

- In some cases of severe NTI, RUR does not fully compensate and does not adjust the T_4 into the normal range.
- $T\hat{T}_4 \times$ RUR is proportional to FT_4 and inversely proportional to TSH.

Increased In
See causes of *decreased* serum TBG.

Decreased In
See causes of *increased* serum TBG.

Normal In
Pregnancy with hyperthyroidism
Nontoxic goiter
Use of certain drugs (e.g., mercurials, iodine)

Free Thyroxine Index (FT$_4$ I)

American Thyroid Association now recommends term *thyroid hormone-binding ratios* (THBR) = T$_3$ resin uptake divided by mean of a reference population. FT$_4$ I = THBR × TT$_4$.)

See Table 13-3.

Use
This calculated product permits correction of misleading results of T_3 and T_4 determinations caused by conditions that alter the thyroxine-binding protein concentration (e.g., pregnancy, estrogens, birth control pills).

Free Triiodothyronine Index (FT$_3$ I)

$FT_3 I = TT_3 \times T_3$ uptake. Provides an estimate of serum free T_3. May aid in diagnosis of T_3 toxicosis when serum T_4 is normal.

Disorders of the Thyroid

See Table 13-2.

Thyroid Masses (Goiter, Carcinoma)

Goiter[2]
Diffuse toxic—Graves disease; most common cause of endogenous hyperthyroidism
Toxic adenoma (uninodular goiter)
Diffuse nontoxic (simple) (colloid)—relative deficiency of thyroid hormone
Endemic—iodine-deficient area
Sporadic—high incidence at puberty
Multinodular goiter—often food or drug induced (goitrogens: Cabbage, cauliflower, Brussels sprouts, turnips); Plummer disease is toxic multinodular goiter.
Hyperplastic nodule of a multinodular goiter (most common)
Clinical "solitary" follicular lesion, mimics adenoma
Neonatal, due to

- Maternal ingestion of iodine (e.g., for thyroid disease, for asthma), propylthiouracil
- Inherited hypothyroidism (diminished ability to synthesize thyroid hormone)
- Neonatal hyperthyroidism
- Dyshormonogenesis
- Hemangioma, lymphangioma

Medullary Carcinoma (MCT)
Arises from calcitonin-secreting C cells

- Sporadic (noninherited): accounts for 80% of cases; usually unilateral
- Familial: accounts for 20% of cases; usually bilateral, multicentric (multiple endocrine neoplasia [MEN] types 1 and 2 and familial non-MEN)

[2]Hegedüs L. The thyroid nodule. *N Engl J Med* 2004;351:1764.

◆ Basal serum calcitonin may be increased in patients with C-cell hyperplasia and MCT and correlates with tumor mass. Stimulation with calcium and pentagastrin will increase 3 to 5× in C-cell hyperplasia and MCT but not in other conditions.

◆ Serum Tg levels are increased in most patients with differentiated thyroid carcinoma but not in undifferentiated or MCT. May not be increased with small occult differentiated carcinoma. May be useful to detect presence and possibly the extent of residual, recurrent, or metastatic differentiated carcinoma. *Increased levels may be found in patients with nontoxic nodular goiter; presence of autoantibodies interferes with the test.*

◆ Serum T_3, T_4, TSH are almost always normal in untreated patients. Rarely, evidence of hyperthyroidism may be found with large masses of follicular carcinoma.

◆ Genetic screening makes diagnosis of familial cases possible before clinical changes or increased calcitonin.

Serum CEA may be increased in MCT and may correlate with tumor size or extent of disease.

Laboratory findings owning to associated lesions (e.g., pheochromocytoma and parathyroid tumors) *(10%–20% of cases of MCT occur as part of MEN)* and owning to production of additional substances (e.g., ACTH, serotonin) by MCT

RAIU is almost always normal.

Papillary/Follicular Carcinoma

Serum LD, CEA, and Tg may be increased in advanced follicular carcinoma.

See Fig. 13-3.

◆ FNA biopsy will produce a definitive diagnosis in 80% of cases of thyroid nodules. Radioactive iodine scan of thyroid. Functioning nodule is almost always benign; nonfunctioning nodule is malignant in 5% of cases.

◆ Isotope scanning of thyroid may show decreased ("cold") or increased ("hot") uptake. 10% of functioning solitary adenoma have suppressed TSH indicating hyperfunction.

Should do antithyroid peroxidase antibodies to detect Hashimoto thyroiditis.

In multinodular goiter, TSH usually is in normal or low-normal range; is rarely increased. T_4, T_3, TBG, Tg do not differ in benign and malignant cyst fluid.

Euthyroid Sick Syndrome (Nonthyroidal Illness [NTI])

Wide variety of nonthyroidal acute and chronic conditions such as infection, liver disease, cancer, starvation, renal failure, heart failure, severe burns, trauma, surgery may be associated with abnormal thyroid function tests in euthyroid patients, especially in aged; artifactual changes in thyroid tests are not included in euthyroid sick syndrome.

See Table 13-4.

	T_4	T_3	rT_3	TSH
Moderate illness	N	D	I	N
Severe illness	D	D	I	D

N, normal; D, decreased; I, increased.

Initial change in all NTI patients is decreased T_3 with increased rT_3. With increasing severity, serum T_4 declines producing low T_3–low T_4 state.

Low T_3 syndrome is the most common NTI. Occurs in most illnesses, starvation, after surgery or trauma. T3 is decreased in ~70% of hospitalized patients without intrinsic thyroid disease and is normal in 20% to 30% of hypothyroid patients; therefore T_3 should not be ordered. In AMI T_3 falls by ~20%and FT_3 by ~40% to nadir on 4th day.

• Increased rT_3.
• Serum TSH is typically normal or slightly increased; TSH response to TRH is usually normal.

Increased T_4 syndrome is most common (≤20%) in acute psychiatric admissions, especially in the presence of certain drugs (e.g., amphetamines, phencyclidine) and old

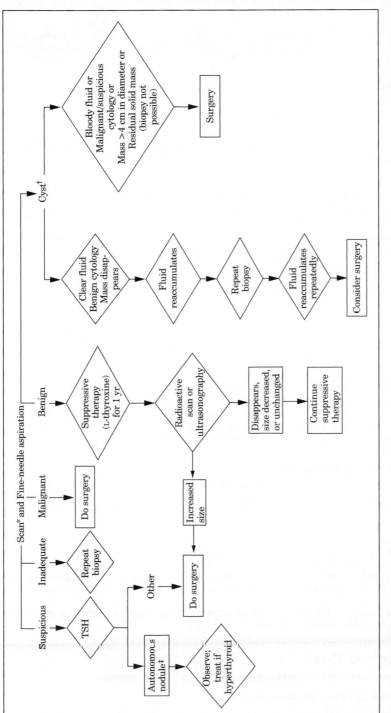

Fig. 13-3. Algorithm for tests for solitary nodule of thyroid. TSH, thyroid-stimulating hormone. *Scan refers to ultrasound, CT scan, and MRI, which may identify nodules associated with increased risk of cancer but cannot reliably distinguish benign lesions from cancer. †Contrary to common belief, cystic lesions may be malignant; thus a "hot" nodule on scan may not require surgery. ‡Autonomous nodules are rarely malignant. (Modified from RH Caplan, et al. Fine-needle aspiration biopsy of thyroid nodules. *Postgrad Med* 1991;90:183.)

Table 13-4.   Differential Diagnosis of Euthyroid Sick Syndrome

	Euthyroid Sick Syndrome	Primary Hypothyroidism	Primary Hypothyroidism with Concomitant Illness
Serum T_4	N or D	D	D
Serum T_3 uptake	I	D	
Serum T_3	D	N or D	D
T_7 (FTI)	I, N, or D	D	D
Reverse T_3	I	D	D, N, or I
Serum TSH	N	I	I, occasionally N
TSH response to TRH	N or D	I	I

D = decreased; I = increased; N = normal.
Definitely increased T_3 uptake associated with decreased serum T_4 strongly indicates euthyroid sick syndrome, whereas in hypothyroidism T_3 uptake tends to be decreased.
In hypothyroidism with concomitant illness, T_3 uptake tends to increase into normal range but not above normal.
Serum TSH is increased in primary hypothyroidism as the earliest and most specific test; in contrast, basal and TRH-stimulated TSH are typically normal in euthyroid sick syndrome.
Reverse T_3 may be a useful discriminator in many euthyroid sick patients without renal failure, but it is not as useful as serum TSH.
Pituitary hypothyroidism may be difficult to distinguish, since serum TSH is low and not responsive to TRH, which is a common pattern in euthyroid sick patients.

age ($\leq$15% of elderly patients); increased values tend to decrease during first 2 weeks after admission as patient improves. Rarely occurs in acutely ill medical patients (e.g., those with acute hepatitis).

- Increased serum T_4, and T_3
- TSH is usually normal in mild to moderate illness.
- TRH test is often not useful due to flat TSH response.
- 50% of patients with hyperemesis gravidarum show elevated TT_4 and sometimes FT_4 that persists until hyperemesis abates. Patients with symptomatic hyponatremia show transient increase until low sodium is corrected.

Decreased T₄ syndrome

- Occurs in >50% of severe or chronic illness.
- TT_4 is decreased; FT_4 may be normal or low.
- TSH is normal; becomes transiently (few days or wks) increased during recovery.

No single test is clearly diagnostic, especially in elderly and acutely or severely ill patients.
Ideally, thyroid status should be deferred until this illness is resolved.
Use TSH with broader reference values (e.g., .05–10 mIU/L) and FT_4. If FT_4 is abnormal, confirm with TT_4. If results are discordant, thyroid disease is unlikely; if abnormal values are concordant, thyroid disease may be present. FT_4 by equilibrium dialysis may be useful.
Repeat tests in ~8 weeks: Normal or increased TSH suggests recovery from NTI or hypothyroid phase of thyroiditis.

Hyperthyroidism

Hypermetabolic state due to excess circulating thyroid hormone.

See Table 13-2 and Figs. 13-4 and 13-5.

Thyrotoxicosis with Hyperthyroidism

Many authors, especially clinical, consider hyperthyroidism and thyrotoxicosis synonymous.

Due To

Thyroid-stimulating immunoglobulins (TSIs)

> Diffuse toxic goiter (Graves disease—autoimmune disorder due to TSH receptor antibody that stimulate excess secretion of T_4, T_3, or both; absent in 5% to 20% of these patients depending on the assay used)

Autonomous nodules in thyroid (**serum TSH is low**)

> Toxic adenoma
> Toxic multinodular goiter

Neonatal thyrotoxicosis associated with maternal Graves disease

Thyrotropin-induced (TRH) hyperthyroidism (**serum TSH is increased**)

- With pituitary tumor
- Without pituitary tumor

Secretion of nonpituitary TSH

> Trophoblastic tissues (neoplasms that secrete hCG that binds to TSH receptors), e.g., choriocarcinoma, hydatidiform mole, embryonal carcinoma of testis

Thyrotoxicosis without Hyperthyroidism

Increased release of thyroid hormone after cell injury is early and transient.

Thyroiditis

- Hashimoto
- Lymphocytic (painless)
- Subacute granulomatous

Iodide-induced (Jod-Basedow)
Metastatic functioning thyroid carcinoma
Struma ovarii with hyperthyroidism
Ectopic thyroid tissue
Factitious
Drugs (e.g., ≤23% of persons receiving amiodarone)
In neonate, is usually due to transplacental maternal TSH receptor-stimulating antibodies that mimic TSH action. May persist for several months.

2% of hospitalized elderly patients have unsuspected hyperthyroidism.

- ♦ Decreased serum TSH will detect virtually all hyperthyroid patients except the very rare cases of pituitary neoplasms that secrete TSH, ectopic secretion of TSH, or TRH, resistance to thyroid hormone (pituitary, generalized), artifact (e.g., autoantibodies to TSH, human antimouse antibodies).
- ♦ Serum TT_4 and FT_4 are increased. With an atypical clinical picture of hyperthyroidism, serum $T_4 > 16$ μg/dL confirms the diagnosis. Normal T_4 (usually in upper range) with low TSH suggests subclinical hyperthyroidism. Severity of hyperthyroidism does not correlate with T_4 levels.
- ♦ Serum T_3 concentration and T_3 resin uptake are increased in ≤85% of patients. T_3 is usually elevated to a greater degree than T_4. $T_3:T_4$ ratio >20:1 occurs in T_3 dependent type of Graves disease.

TRH stimulation test
Serum TBG is normal.
RAIU is increased. It is relatively more affected at 1, 2, or 6 hours than at 24 hours. It may be normal with recent iodine ingestion. May be used to differentiate this from thyroiditis or factitious thyrotoxicosis. Is no longer used for diagnosis of hyperthyroidism but should be performed prior to administration of therapeutic dose of [131]I.

- ○ 99m Technetium pertechnetate uptake parallels hormone production and may be useful when T_4 and TSH results are discordant.
- ○ 24-hour urinary iodide excretion is increased in hyperthyroidism with low RAIU owing to exogenous iodide ingestion.
- ○ Microsomal antibodies are found in moderate to high titers in most patients with Graves disease; may be helpful in confirming diagnosis in a hyperthyroid patient without ocular findings or a euthyroid patient with eye findings.
- ○ Other thyroid autoantibodies are thyroid stimulating immunoglobulins (TSI) and TSH-binding inhibitory immunoglobulins (TBII) found only with Graves disease; sometimes helpful in diagnosis and management. TSH receptor antibody (formerly called LATS or long-acting thyroid stimulator) is present in 80% to 100% of untreated Graves disease patients.

Thyroid suppression test: T_3 administration decreases RAIU in normal persons but not in hyperthyroid persons. Now replaced by TRH stimulation test.

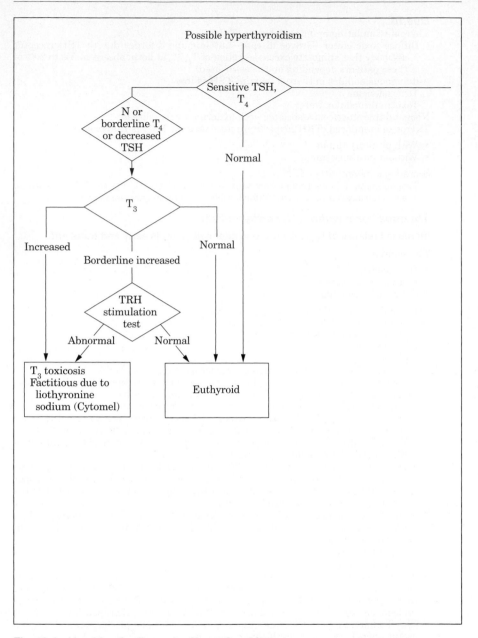

Fig. 13-4. Algorithm for diagnosis of hyperthyroidism.

Serum cholesterol is decreased, and total lipids are usually decreased.
Hyperglycemia and glycosuria are present.
Liver function tests show impairment.
Normal serum creatine almost excludes hyperthyroidism.
Serum total and ionized calcium are increased in 5% to 10% of patients. Serum phosphorus is high-normal or increased. Serum PTH and 1,25-dihydroxyvitamin D are decreased. Increased serum ALP in 75% of patients (liver and bone origin; only liver ALP in 7%; only bone ALP in 15%). After successful treatment, may continue to increase and not become normal for up to 18 months. More common in children and young adults.
Serum ferritin is increased.

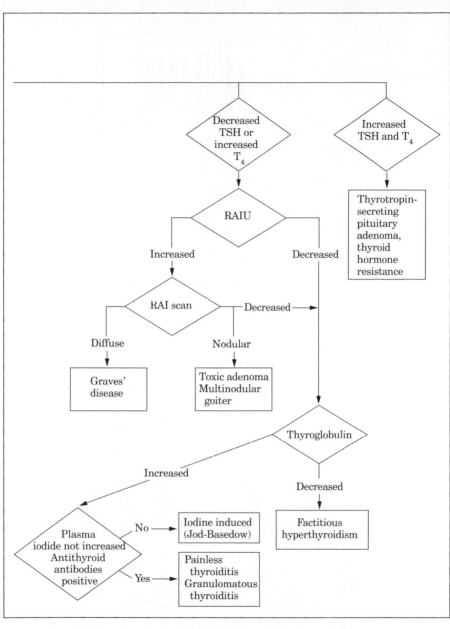

Normochromic anemia in long-standing Graves disease
Unusual laboratory manifestations of hyperthyroidism include hypoproteinemia, mal-
    absorption.
Serum angiotensin-converting enzyme is increased.
Laboratory findings owning to complications of treatment

- Surgery—hypothyroidism (30%–50% of cases), hypoparathyroidism (3% of cases)
- Drugs—agranulocytosis, hepatitis, vasculitis, drug-induced lupus
    Laboratory findings due to associated autoimmune diseases, e.g., type 1 diabetes
mellitus, pernicious anemia, myasthenia gravis, Addison disease

Subclinical Hyperthyroidism

♦ TSH is increased with normal FT_4.

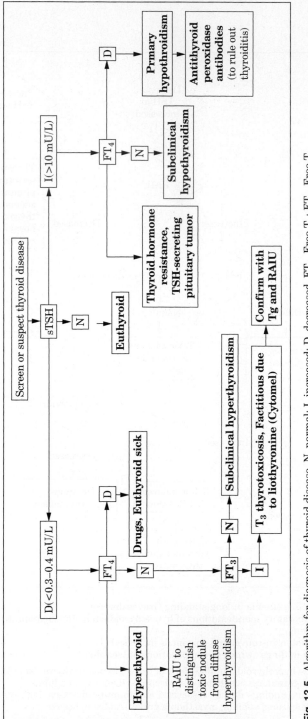

Fig. 13.5. Algorithm for diagnosis of thyroid disease. N, normal; I, increased; D, decreased. FT_3, Free T_3; FT_4, Free T_4.

T_3 Toxicosis Causes 5% of Cases of Hyperthyroidism.

◆ Should be suspected in patients with clinical thyrotoxicosis in whom usual laboratory tests are normal (serum T_4, 24-hour RAIU, TBG, and thyroxine-binding albumin [TBPA]), but serum T_3 is increased

RAIU is autonomous (not suppressed by T_3 administration).

TSH may be increased.

Abnormal TRH test (lack of TSH response to TRH)

Factitious Hyperthyroidism

Self-induced hyperthyroidism by ingestion of thyroxine (T_4) or Cytomel (T_3).

◆ Increased total and free serum T_4 or T_3, depending on which drug is ingested. T_4 may be absent if T_3 is ingested.

◆ Serum thyroglobulin is depressed to low-normal level or undetectable unless patient is taking desiccated thyroid extract of thyroglobulin.

◆ RAIU is low when all other thyroid function tests indicate hyperthyroidism. RAIU is augmented after TSH administration whereas patients with subacute and painless thyroiditis usually do not have any response to TSH administration.

Thyroid Storm

Occurs in operative/perioperative period; fever, symptoms of CNS, GI, and cardiovascular systems

Thyroid function test values may be somewhat higher than in uncomplicated thyrotoxicosis but are useless for differentiation.

Transient hyperglycemia is common.

Abnormal liver function tests are common.

Abnormal serum electrolytes (especially decreased potassium, mild to moderate hypercalcemia) and decreased arterial pCO_2 are common.

Laboratory findings due to associated conditions, especially bacterial infection (increased WBC, shift to left; bacteria in urine, sputum, etc.), pulmonary or arterial embolism

Hypothyroidism

See Table 13-6 and Figs. 13-1, 13-4, 13-5.

Due To

Treatment of preceding hyperthyroidism (surgery, drugs, radioiodine)

Radiation (e.g., treatment of head and neck cancer)

Autoimmune disease, thyroiditis

Central hypothyroidism (TSH level may be normal but is not as biologically active)
  Pituitary disease (e.g., tumors, granulomas, cysts, vascular)
  Hypothalamic disease (e.g., granulomas, TRH deficiency, pituitary-stalk section)

Iodine deficiency

Drugs (e.g., iodides, propylthiouracil, methimazole, phenylbutazone, lithium; 5%–25% of persons receiving amiodarone)

Congenital developmental defects

Organification defect (diagnosis by perchlorate washout test)

4.6% of US population has hypothyroidism; 90% are subclinical, especially in elderly and in psychiatric hospital admissions patients.

◆ Serum TSH is increased in proportion to degree of hypofunction; is at least 2× and often 10× normal value; is best test and first to order. A single determination is usually sufficient to establish the diagnosis. Serum TSH should always be measured prior to treatment of all patients with clinical hypothyroidism to distinguish primary from secondary (pituitary) or tertiary (hypothalamic) types, since the latter two are often associated with secondary adrenal insufficiency, which could be lethal if unrecognized.

• Increased serum TSH is earliest evidence of hypothyroidism. Increased TSH (usually 5–10 mU/L) and normal FT_4 indicates subclinical hypothyroidism.

• If TSH >10 mU/L, repeat TSH with FT_4 before starting lifelong therapy.

• Increased TSH and decreased FT_4 establish diagnosis of primary hypothyroidism.

• Normal or decreased TSH and decreased FT_4 suggest hypothyroidism secondary to decreased TSH secretion (hypopituitarism).

• TSH is undetectable or inappropriately low in relation to degree of thyroid hormone deficiency in secondary or tertiary hypothyroidism.

Table 13-5. Comparison of Causes of Thyrotoxicosis

Disorder	FT$_4$	T$_3$	TSH	TBG	RAIU	RAI scan	Comment
Graves disease	I	I <85% of cases	**D**	I			Other autoimmune diseases present
Toxic multinodular or solitary autonomous nodule	I		**D**	I		+	
Thyroiditis	I/D	I/D	I/D	I/D		**Irregular scan**	**High antibody titer**
TSH-secreting pituitary tumors (rare)	I or N		**I**				TSH responds poorly to TRH stimulation or T$_4$ suppression. Other pituitary secretions CT/MRI of sella
Euthyroid sick (increased T$_4$) syndrome	I	I	N				Drugs, acute psychiatric admissions, elderly
Factitious/iatrogenic							
Thyroxine (T$_4$)	**I**		D	D	D		
Cytomel (T$_3$)		**I**	D	D	D		
Iodide/amiodarone	May be I, N, D	D	I	D	D	D	I urinary iodide History
Thyroid hormone resistance	I	I	**Inappropriately N**				No clinical findings of hyper- or hypothyroidism
Struma ovarii	I		D			D in neck	+ pelvic or abdominal RAIU
Trophoblastic tumors	I		D				hCG is I
Metastases from thyroid cancer	I		D	I		+	+ scan over metastases

Most useful diagnostic test in bold type.
I, increased; D, decreased; N, normal; +, positive.

Table 13-6.	Laboratory Tests in Differential Diagnosis of Primary and Secondary Hypothyroidism	

Test	Panhypopituitarism	Primary Myxedema
Serum TSH	Decreased	Increased
Serum TSH response to TRH administration	Absent	Normal or exaggerated
Response to administration of thyrotropic hormone	Responds with increase in RAIU	No response
Urine 17–ketosteroids	Absent	Low
Response to insulin	Prompt decrease in blood sugar; fails to return to normal	Usually delayed fall in blood sugar and sometimes delayed return to normal

♦ Serum T_4 and FT_4 concentration are decreased; $T_4 > 7$ μg/dL almost certainly excludes hypothyroidism.

Serum T_3 concentration is decreased (may be normal in 20%–30% of hypothyroid patients). Serum TT_3 and FT_3 may not fall until disease is far advanced because increased TSH stimulates thyroid to release T_3. Classic findings of hypothyroidism appear when T_3 falls below normal level.

Serum T_3 has little role in this diagnosis.

Serum T_3 resin uptake is decreased (may be normal in ≤50% of hypothyroid patients).

Serum T_3:T_4 ratio is increased.

RAIU is usually decreased; is not helpful in diagnosis. Salivary and urinary excretion of RAI are decreased.

TSH stimulation (20 units/day for 3 days) increases RAIU to ~normal (20%) in secondary but not in primary hypothyroidism. Diagnosis of primary hypothyroidism is unlikely if RAIU increases substantially after administration of TSH. Replaced by serum TSH.

A TRH-provocative test shows a normal or delayed TSH response in tertiary, no response in Secondary, and exaggerated and prolonged response in primary hypothyroidism (see Fig. 13-2).

Serum TBG is normal.

Serum cholesterol is increased (may be useful to follow effect of therapy, especially in children).

Serum myoglobin is significantly increased in 90% of untreated, long-term hypothyroid patients; inversely proportional to serum T_3 and T_4. Gradual decrease after T_4 therapy begins with return to normal before TSH becomes normal.

Serum CK (10–15×), CK-MM, AST (2–6×), LD (2–3×) are increased above upper reference limit in 40% to 90% of cases owing to myopathy of hypothyroidism.

Serum calcium is sometimes increased.

Serum ALP is decreased.

Serum carotene is increased.

Normocytic normochromic anemia is present.

Serum iron and total iron-binding capacity (TIBC) may be decreased.

Serum sodium is decreased in approximately 50% of cases.

CSF protein is elevated (100–340 mg/dL) in 25% of cases of myxedema.

Proteinuria in ~8% of cases.

Adequate levothyroxine treatment results in normal serum T_4 and TSH. When hypothyroidism is due to thyroid failure, the dose is gradually increased, and adequate therapy is indicated when serum T_4 increases to normal and TSH decreases to normal (may take several months). TSH response to TRH also returns to normal if originally abnormal, but this test is generally not necessary. When hypothyroidism is secondary or tertiary, the TSH is not useful and serum T_4 is used to judge adequacy of therapy. When levothyroxine is used for TSH suppression in patients with thyroid cancer, nodular disease, or chronic thyroiditis, the decreased TSH cannot be distinguished from normal levels; therefore levothyroxine dose is increased until serum T_4 is normal and TSH is undetectable, or an abbreviated TRH test is performed with a single TSH measurement 15 minutes after injection of TRH—if TSH is undetectable, then TSH secretion is considered adequately suppressed.

Table 13-7.   Sensitivity and Specificity of Thyroid Function Tests

	Sensitivity			Specificity	
Patients	All	Hyperthyroid	Hypothyroid	All	Nonthyroid Illness
T_4	76	89	61	90	83
Free T_4	82	96	65	94	94
T_3	80	85	74	87	72
Free T_3	73	93	48	90	80
TSH	89–95	86–95	92–94	92–95	85–90

T_3 = triiodothyronine; T_4 = thyroxine; TSH = thyroid-stimulating hormone.
Source: de los Santos ET, Starich GH, Mazzaferri EL. Sensitivity, specificity and cost-effectiveness of the sensitive thyrotropin assay in the diagnosis of thyroid diseases in ambulatory patients. *Arch Intern Med* 1989;149:526.

Laboratory findings indicative of other autoimmune diseases (e.g., pernicious anemia and primary adrenocortical insufficiency occur with increased frequency in primary hypothyroidism)

Thyroid hormone status should be reassessed at least yearly in treatment of hypothyroidism.

Laboratory findings owning to involvement of other organs, e.g., muscle, heart, ileus, CNS, etc.

Myxedema Coma

Hypoglycemia, hyponatremia and changes due to adrenocortical insufficiency may be found.

Serum creatinine may be increased.

Arterial pCO_2 may be increased and pO_2 decreased.

Increased WBC and shift to left may occur.

Hypothyroidism, Neonatal

Approximately 2% to 4% of cases of infantile hypothyroidism are not detected on neonatal screening. Neonatal screening is usually performed on same filter paper specimen of blood used for PKU screening on third to fifth day of life. Cretinism with mental retardation and growth delay is usually not clinically apparent at birth.

*Do **not** do T_4 or TSH during first few days of life when levels may surge* (see Table 13-7). T_3 rises more rapidly. TSH peaks 30 minutes after birth. Changes in T_4, T_3, and TSH are less marked in premature infants.

♦ RAIU (^{123}I) scan should be done on babies with confirmed hypothyroidism to differentiate thyroid agenesis/dysgenesis from dyshormonogenesis.

If mother has autoimmune thyroid disease, baby should be checked for TSH receptor-blocking antibodies since this type of hypothyroidism cannot be distinguished clinically from thyroid agenesis/dysgenesis and RAIU may be absent. Hypothyroidism is transient.

Due To

Primary Hypothyroidism (Incidence, 1:3,600 to 1:4,800)

Aplasia and hypoplasia	63%
Ectopic gland	23%
Inborn errors of thyroid hormone synthesis or metabolism	14%

• Increased serum TSH is most sensitive test for primary hypothyroidism.
• Decreased serum T_4
• Normal or decreased serum T_3
• Normal serum TBG
• Increased serum CK

Deficiency of TBG (Incidence, 1:8,000 to 1:12,000)
Hereditary
Drug effect

Hypoproteinemia

- Decreased serum T_4 (e.g., 3.2 µg/dL), but normal serum TSH

Secondary Hypothyroidism (Incidence, 1:50,000 to 1:70,000)
Pituitary aplasia, septo-optic dysplasia
Idiopathic hypopituitarism
Hypothalamic disease
  Serum TSH is low or not detectable
  Decreased serum T_4
  TSH response to TRH differentiates pituitary from hypothalamic hypothyroidism
  Normal serum TBG
Transient
Prematurity
Euthyroid sick syndrome
Small for gestational age
Maternal ingestion of iodides or antithyroid drugs
Idiopathic
Treatment of neonatal hypothyroidism is based on frequent T_4, TSH tests.

Pregnancy and Thyroid Function Tests

See Tables 13-2, 13-7.
Thyroid function test values are very different in normal pregnancy.

- Serum TBG gradually increases to 2 to 3 × prepregnancy values causing the serum TT_4 to rise from nonpregnant level of 4 to 8 µg/dL to 10 to 12 µg/dL from 12th week of gestation until 6 weeks postpartum.
- Serum FT_4 and FT_3 are normal.
- T_3 uptake is decreased.
- Increased serum T_3, rT_3.
- TSH is slightly increased by 16th week.
- RAIU is increased but is contraindicated.

T_3 uptake gradually decreases (as early as 3–6 weeks after conception) until the end of the first trimester and then remains relatively constant. It returns to normal 12 to 13 weeks postpartum. Failure to decrease by the eighth to tenth week of pregnancy may indicate threatened abortion (the patient's normal nonpregnant level should be established).
Maternal hypothyroidism has adverse effects on the fetus that can be prevented with treatment.
  Screen using sTSH. If increased, treat patient and assess during each trimester (see Table 13-7). Increased serum thyroid peroxidase antibody in first trimester is a risk factor for postpartum thyroiditis.
Maternal hyperthyroidism: Serum T_4 is increased above the normal range for pregnancy (>12 µg/dL) with T_3 uptake increased to normal nonpregnant range. In hyperthyroidism, both serum T_3 uptake and T_4 are increased, but in the pregnant euthyroid patient or euthyroid patient taking birth control pills or estrogens, the T_4 is increased and the T_3 uptake is decreased. Hyperthyroidism may be indicated by the failure of the T_3 uptake to decrease during pregnancy.

Tissue Resistance to Thyroid Hormone

Genetic syndromes with different phenotypes.

- ◆ TSH is inappropriately normal (nonsuppressed) with increased FT_4 and FT_3.
- In generalized resistance: The patient has no clinical signs or symptoms of hypo- or hyperthyroidism.
- In selective pituitary resistance: The patient has signs and symptoms of hyperthyroidism.
- In selective peripheral resistance: The patient has signs and symptoms of hypothyroidism.

Thyroiditis

Hashimoto (Autoimmune; Chronic Lymphocytic) Thyroiditis

Thyroid function may be normal; occasionally a patient passes through a hyperthyroid stage. 15% to 20% of patients develop hypothyroidism, but Hashimoto disease is a

Table 13-8.   Comparison of Laboratory Findings in Types of Thyroiditis

	Hashimoto Thyroiditis	Painless Sporadic/ Postpartum	Painful Subacute	Suppurative	Riedel
Thyroid function	D	V	V	Usually N	Usually N
Thyroid peroxidase antibodies	Persistent high titer	Persistent high titer in 50%	Transient low or O	O	Usually present
24-hr ^{123}I uptake	V	<5%	<5%	N	D/N
ESR	N	N	I	I	N

N, normal; I, increased; D, decreased; V, varies; O, absent.

very unlikely cause of hypothyroidism in the absence of microsomal and thyroglobulin antibodies.

♦ Test for antimicrosomal antibodies is S/S >90%. Test for antithyroglobulin antibodies is S/S = 36%/98% and is seldom positive if microsomal antibodies are negative. Thus, antimicrosomal antibody alone is sufficient for diagnosis. High titers are pathognomonic.

♦ Serum TSH is earliest indicator of hypothyroidism; is increased in one-third of persons who are clinically euthyroid and in those with clinical hypothyroidism, many of whom have normal T_4 and T_3.

♦ Biopsy of thyroid may be diagnostic.

♦ RAI scan may show involvement of only a single lobe (more common in younger patients); "salt and pepper" pattern is classical.

RAIU is usually normal or low.

Silent (Painless) Thyroiditis; Lymphocytic Thyroiditis

This form of hyperthyroidism comprises ≤25% of all cases of hyperthyroidism that resolves spontaneously in several weeks to months and is often followed by a transient hypothyroidism during recovery period; common in postpartum period; multiple episodes may occur. Pathologic changes are less severe than in Hashimoto thyroiditis, but the latter cannot be ruled out in biopsy specimens.

Hyperthyroid phase is briefer in postpartum type (≤3 months) than in sporadic type (≤12 months)

♦ • Increased serum T_4, T_3, and low serum TSH with RAIU that is very low (<5%)

• Antithyroglobulin antibodies are found in most patients in low titers. Titers in the very high ranges of Hashimoto thyroiditis are rare.

• Nonspecific markers of inflammation are generally normal in contrast to granulomatous thyroiditis. ESR is increased in 50% of patients to range of 20 to 40 mm/hour. WBC and serum proteins are normal.

Recovery phase is complete in ~50%; long-term hypothyroidism in ~50%.

• Serum T_4 and T_3 fall into normal range, but RAIU remain suppressed.

Hypothyroid phase occurs in 20% to 30% of patients; lasts 1 to 8 months; most recover completely but few develop permanent hypothyroidism; recurs in >10% of sporadic type and more often in postpartum type. Permanent hypothyroidism in ~25% of postpartum type.

• Antithyroid antibody titers are highest during this phase (especially in postpartum patients). Gradually decrease with time; 50% become negative within 6 months.

• Serum TSH, T_4, and T_3 gradually return to normal.

• RAIU, TRH tests begin to normalize toward the end of this phase, and urinary iodide falls to normal levels (50–200 μg/day).

Subacute (Painful) Thyroiditis; Granulomatous (De Quervain) Thyroiditis

Probably of viral origin.

◆ Biopsy of thyroid confirms diagnosis.
◆ Decreased RAIU is the characteristic finding and differentiates it from acute thyroiditis; may be <5% during thyrotoxic and euthyroid phase.
◆ Serum thyroglobulin is often markedly increased in contrast to factitious hyperthyroidism.

Antithyroglobulin antibodies may be present for up to several months in low titer.
○ ESR is increased; often >55 mm/hour.
WBC is normal or decreased.
Four sequential phases may be identified: hyperthyroid, euthyroid, hypothyroid, recovery.

Hyperthyroid phase lasts 1 to 2 months

• Increased TT_4 and FT_4; T_3 may be only mildly increased; T_3:T_4 ratio <20:1.
• Serum TSH is very low and does not respond to TRH.
• ESR is markedly increased.

Euthyroid phase lasts 1 to 2 weeks.

• RAIU remains low.
• TSH is normal.

Hypothyroid phase lasts 2 to 6 months.

• TSH increases.

Recovery

• Return of radioactive iodine trapping is the first indication.
• 24-hour RAIU may rise above normal.
• Thyroid hormone levels rise to normal.
• TSH falls to normal.

Relapses occur in up to 47% of patients, usually in first year.

Acute Suppurative Thyroiditis

WBC and PMNs are increased in 75% of cases; absence may indicate anaerobic infection.
ESR is increased.
24-hour RAIU is decreased in <50% of cases.
Thyroid function tests are usually normal.
Staphylococcus causes one third of cases; other organisms include *Streptococcus pyogenes*, *S. pneumoniae*, Enterobacteriaceae, *H. influenzae*, *Pseudomonas aeruginosa*, anaerobes. Fungi are rare and principally occur in immunocompromised patients; may also be caused by mycobacteria or parasites.

Riedel Chronic (Fibrous) Thyroiditis

◆ Biopsy of thyroid confirms diagnosis.
Thyroid function tests, ESR, thyroid antibodies may be normal.
RAI scan may be decreased in involved areas.
Hypothyroidism in ~30% of cases when complete thyroid involvement occurs.

Tests of Parathyroid Function and Calcium/Phosphate Metabolism

Alkaline Phosphatase (ALP)

Alkaline phosphatase enzyme in many body tissues. Bone isoenzymes are different from tissue isoenzymes in that heat and urea denature it.

See Chapter 3, 8, and 9.

Calcitonin

Calcitonin has a minor role in calcium homeostasis. Opposes action of PTH inhibits osteoclast bone resorption and decreases tubular resorption of calcium.

Calcitriol (1,25-Dihydroxy-Vitamin D), Serum

Secreted by the kidney.

Interpretation

Suppressed during hypercalcemia unless there is autonomous source of PTH as in hyperparathyroidism (HPT). (Normal range <42 pg/mL in hypercalcemic and <76 pg/mL in normocalcemic patients.) Failure to suppress indicates extrarenal production as it is normally secreted only by kidney.

Increased In

Sarcoidosis (synthesized by macrophages within granulomas)
Non-Hodgkin lymphoma (~15% of cases). Returns to normal after therapy.

Not Increased In

HPT
Humoral hypercalcemia of malignancy (HHM)

Calcium, Ionized and Total, Serum

Ninety-eight percent of calcium is within bones in form of hydroxyapatite. Calcium exists in plasma in three forms: Ionized (free) calcium is physiologically active; 45% to 50% of total plasma calcium is bound to plasma proteins, mostly to albumin; 10% to 15% is complexed to various anions, e.g. calcium phosphate and calcium citrate. In general is affected by changes in plasma protein concentration and pH of extracellular fluid. Ionized calcium increases in acidosis and decreases in alkalosis. Increase in plasma proteins results in increased total serum calcium; decreased plasma proteins results in decreased in total serum calcium. Heparin should be used for anticoagulant because EDTA and calcium chelators [e.g., citrate] lower total and ionized calcium. Serum or plasma calcium >10.3 mg/dL or ionized calcium >1.30 mmol/L characterize hypercalcemia.

See Chapter 3.

Phosphorus, Serum

Metabolism is linked to calcium. Approximately 85% is in bone, part of hydroxyapatite. Organic phosphate (e.g. phospholipids, proteins, carbohydrates, nucleic acids) is not measured in assay of inorganic phosphate.

See Chapter 3.

Parathyroid Hormone (PTH), Serum

Peptide hormone secreted by parathyroid gland chief cells that controls ionized calcium levels in blood and body fluids by increasing 1,25 dihydroxy vitamin D_3 (by kidney), mobilizing calcium from bone [due to increased osteoclast activity], increasing renal tubular resorption of calcium and reducing renal clearance of calcium, increasing intestinal calcium absorption. Half-life is <5 minutes. Reference range = 8–74 pg/mL (0.8–7.8 pmol/L). Ionized calcium in blood inhibits PTH secretion. Biological activity resides in first 34 terminal amino acids. The intact hormone has 84 amino acids, but can be quickly cleaved by proteolysis into smaller less-active fragments. Assay for the intact PTH has largely superseded tests for various PTH fragments. Important that the PTH assay not cross react with PTH (7-84) lacking the 6 N-terminal, shown to be a weak antagonist to PTH activity and may lower serum and plasma calcium levels.

See Fig. 13-7.

Use

Differential diagnosis of HPT and hypoparathyroidism.
Very sensitive in detecting PTH suppression by 1,25-dihydroxyvitamin D; therefore used for monitoring that treatment of chronic renal failure.

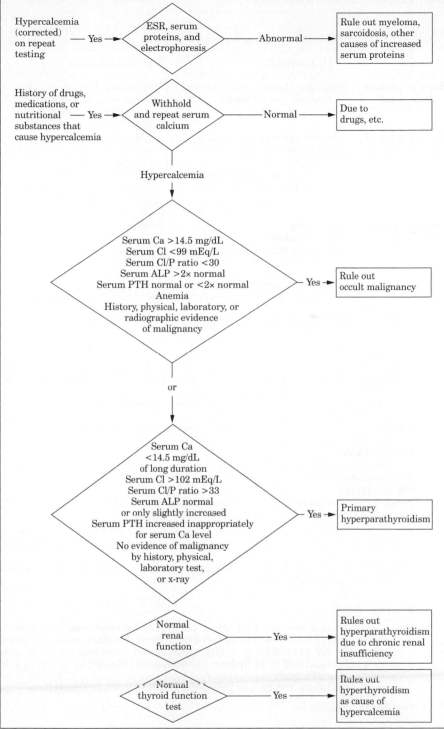

ENDOCRINE

Fig. 13-6. Algorithm for diagnosis of hypercalcemia. (ESR, erythrocyte sedimentation rate; PTH, parathyroid hormone.) (Data from ET Wong, EF Freier. The differential diagnosis of hypercalcemia: an algorithm for more effective use of laboratory tests. *JAMA* 1982;247:75, and KR Johnson, AT Howarth. Differential laboratory diagnosis of hypercalcemia. *CRC Crit Rev Clin La Sci* 1984;21:51.)

Table 13-9.   Serum Calcium and PTH in Various Conditions

	PTH Increased	PTH Not Increased
Serum calcium decreased*	Secondary hyperparathyroidism (chronic renal disease)	Hypoparathyroidism (surgical, autoimmunity, hormone resistance, magnesium deficiency)
Serum calcium increased†	Primary hyperparathyroidism Familial hypocalciuric hypercalcemia Lithium-induced hypercalcemia Tertiary hyperparathyroidism	HHM, milk-alkali syndrome, thiazide diuretics, vitamin D or A intoxication, granulomatous diseases (sarcoidosis, TB), multiple myeloma, thyrotoxicosis, immobilization
Serum calcium normal	Pregnancy Nephrolithiasis Secondary hyperparathyroidism (chronic renal disease)	Normal

HHM, humoral hypercalcemia of malignancy; PTH, parathyroid hormone.
*PTH may be normal or increased in hypocalcemic patients due to renal failure, acute pancreatitis, vitamin D deficiency.
†PTH may be normal or increased in hypercalcemic patients due to acromegaly, vitamin A intoxication, MEN type IIA, renal tubular acidosis, chronic renal failure.

Intraoperative PTH assay to determine removal of abnormally secreting tissue. May replace routine frozen section. Can replace traditional 4-gland explorations and distinguishes single from multiglandular disease.

Preoperative venous catheterization of neck can locate adenoma when prior neck exploration and/or scanning have failed.

♦ Preoperative and 10 to 20 minutess postresection assay of PTH causes 50% to 75% reduction indicating successful resection of parathyroid adenoma.

Interferences

Sedative-hypnotic drug propofol (Diprivan®) may give falsely low PTH values.
Avoid high concentrations of hemolysis, lipemia, bilirubin.

Interpretation

Serum calcium should always be measured at same time as PTH.
Assay of choice detects intact PTH.

- Distinguish HPT from HHM. PTH is suppressed (<1 pmol/L) in 95% of cases of HHM unless there is coexisting parathyroid adenoma, which occurs in 4% of HHM cases.
- RI-PTH that declines ≥50% from the highest baseline in 10 minutes after resection indicates successful total excision.[3]

Vitamin D

Group of fat-soluble vitamins that affect calcium and phosphorus metabolism. Vitamin D_2 = ergosterol. Vitamin D_3 = cholecalciferol is dietary and synthesized in skin under UV irradiation of 7-dihyydrocholesterol. Cholecalciferol to liver where it is hydroxylated to 25-hydroxycholecalciferol (25-[OH]D_3). In kidney it is hydroxylated to dihydroxy metabolite. PTH increases production 1,25-(OH)$_2$ D_3 in renal proximal tubule and causes increased intestinal calcium absorption.

See Chapter 12 and Index.

[3]Guarda LA. Rapid intraoperative parathyroid hormone testing with surgical pathology correlations. *Am J Clin Pathol* 2004;122:704.

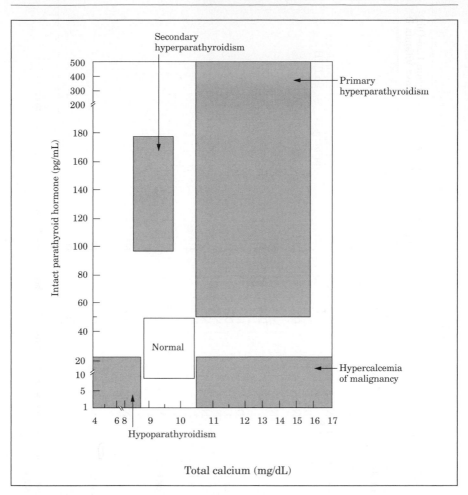

Fig. 13-7. Diagrammatic illustration of distribution of patients according to serum calcium and serum PTH. The values of some patients may lie outside the exact boundaries indicated, and some conditions may overlap. (From *Mayo Laboratories Test Catalog*. Rochester, MN: Mayo Medical Laboratories, 1995.)

Disorders of the Parathyroid Gland and of Calcium, Phosphorus, Alkaline Phosphatase Metabolism

Humoral Hypercalcemia of Malignancy (HHM)

Due to production of parathyroid hormone-related protein (PTHrP) that mediates bone resorption, increases tubular resorption of calcium, decreases tubular resorption of phosphate with phosphaturia and hypophosphatemia, and increases cAMP.

See Tables 13-9, 13-10, and 13-11, and Figs. 13-6 and 13-7.
- ♦ Hypercalcemia occurs in patients with cancer (typically squamous, transitional cell, renal, ovarian), 5% to 20% of whom have no bone metastases compared to patients with widespread bone metastases (myeloma, lymphoma, breast cancer).

- • Occurs in ~20% to 35% of patients with breast cancer, ~10% to 15% of cases of lung cancer, ~70% of cases of multiple myeloma, rare in lymphoma and leukemia.

Table 13-10. Laboratory Findings in Various Diseases of Calcium and Phosphorus Metabolism

Disease	Serum Calcium[a]	Serum Phosphorus	Serum ALP	Urine Calcium[b]	Urine Phosphorus	Serum PTH	Serum 1.25-Dihydroxy-Vitamin D
Primary hyperparathyroidism	I	D (<3 mgdL in 50%)	I slightly in 50% (N if no bone disease)	I in two-thirds	I	I	I
Humoral hypercalcemia of malignancy	I; frequently marked	D in 50%	Frequently I	I	I	D	D
Familial hypocalciuric hypercalcemia	Mild I	N or slightly D	N	D or low N		I or inappropriately N	Proportional to PTH
Hypoparathyroidism	D	I	N	D	D[c]	D	D
Pseudohypoparathyroidism	D	I	N; occasionally D	D	D[c]	N or I	D
Pseudohypoparathyroidism	N	N		N	N	N	
Secondary hyperparathyroidism (renal rickets)	D or N	I	I or N	D or I	I	I	D
Vitamin D excess	I	N	D	I	D	D	I
Rickets and osteomalacia	D or N	D or N	I	D	D		D
Osteoporosis	N	N	N	N or I	N		
Polyostotic fibrous dysplasia	N	N	N or I	N or I	N		
Paget's disease	N or I	N or I	I	N or I	I		
Metastatic neoplasm to bone	N or I	V	N or I	V	I		
Multiple myeloma	N or I	V	N or I	N or I	N or I	I	
Sarcoidosis	N or I	N or I	N or I	I	N		
Fanconi's syndrome or renal loss of fixed base	D or N	D	N or I	I	I		
Histiocytosis X (Letterer-Siwe disease, Hand-Schüller-Christian disease, eosinophilic granuloma)	N	N	N or I	N or I	N		
Hypercalcemia and excess intake of alkali (Burnett's syndrome)	I	I or N	N	N	N		
Solitary bone cyst	N	N	N	N	N		N

D = decreased; I = increased; N = normal; V = variable.

[a] Serum calcium. Repeated determinations may be required to demonstrate abnormalities. Serum total protein level should always be known. See also response to cortisone.

[b] Urine calcium. Patient should be on a low-calcium diet (e.g., Bauer-Aub).

[c] See Ellsworth-Howard Test.

Table 13-11.	Comparison of Primary Hyperparathyroidism (HPT) and Humoral Hypercalcemia of Malignancy (HHM)	
	HHM	HPT
Etiology	Squamous or large cell carcinoma of bronchus, hypernephroma of kidney, cancer of ovary, colon, others	Primary hyperplasia, adenoma, carcinoma of parathyroids
Serum calcium	Very high: >14 mg/dL in 75% of patients	Moderately high: >14 mg/dL in 25% of patients
	Suppressed by cortisone in 25–50% of patients	Suppressed by cortisone in 50% of cases with and 23% of cases without osteitis fibrosa
Serum PTH	Decreased	Increased
Serum PTHRP	Increased	Not increased
Serum chloride	Low: <99 mEq/L	High: >102 mEq/L
Serum chloride phosphorus ratio	<30	>33
Serum bicarbonate	Increased or normal	Normal or low
pH	Alkalosis	Acidosis
Serum ALP	Increased in 50% of patients, even without bone disease	Seldom increased unless bone disease is present
Serum phosphorus	Increased, normal, or low	Normal or low
Urine calcium	Often >400 mg/24 hrs	Usually <400 mg/24 hrs
Serum 1,25-dihydroxy-vitamin D	Decreased	Increased
Urine cAMP	Increased in HHM but not due to bone metastases only	Increased in 90% of cases
ESR	Usually increased	Normal
Anemia	May be present	Absent
Serum albumin	Often decreased	Usually normal
Renal stones	Absent	Common
Pancreatitis	Rare	Occurs
Radiographic changes in hand bones	Absent	May be present

- Patients have increased total and ionized S-calcium and low PTH (which excludes 1° and 2° HPT) and low or normal 1,25 $(OH)_2$ Vit D_3.
- Rarely may occur in association with benign tumors (e.g., pheochromocytoma, dermoid cyst of ovary) ("humoral hypercalcemia of benignancy").

○ • Very high serum calcium (e.g., >14.5 mg/dL) is much more suggestive of HHM than primary HPT; less marked increase with renal tumors. ≤5% of hypercalcemia patients have simultaneous HPT and HHM.

♦ Increased PTHrP in serum (>2.6 pmol/L) can make a positive diagnosis in most of these patients. Approximately 20% of cancers with hypercalcemia have only local osteolytic changes but not increased PTHrP.

PTHrP Is Also Increased In (>2.6 pmol/L)
>80% of hypercalcemic patients with solid tumors with or without bone metastasis
Some patients with hypercalcemia and hematologic cancers
~10% of cancers without hypercalcemia
Becomes normal when hypercalcemia is corrected by treatment of cancer
May be increased in nonmalignant pheochromocytoma

PTHrP Is Not Increased In
Most healthy persons have values <1.0 pmol/L.
Other causes of hypercalcemia (e.g., sarcoidosis, vitamin D intoxication)

♦ Low-normal or suppressed intact PTH (<20 pg/mL) excludes HPT.

○ Serum 1,25-dihydroxy vitamin D is usually decreased or low-normal in HHM but is increased in HPT.

Urinary cAMP is increased in 90% of cases of HHM and of primary HPT; not increased in hypercalcemia due to bone metastases.

Hypercalciuria much greater than in HPT at any serum calcium level.

Decreased serum phosphorus in >50% of patients.

Decreased serum chloride

Alkalosis is present.

Serum ALP is frequently increased.

Decreased serum albumin; serum proteins are not consistently abnormal.

○ Occult cancer should be ruled out as the cause of hypercalcemia in presence of

* Hypercalcemia without increased serum PTH together with increased urinary cAMP
* Serum ALP >2× upper limit of normal
* Increased serum phosphorus
* Serum chloride:phosphorus ratio <30
* Serum calcium >14.5 mg/dL without florid HPT
* Urine calcium >500 mg/24 hours; urine calcium and phosphorus and renal tubular reabsorption of phosphate are not useful in differential diagnosis
* Anemia, increased ESR

Multiple and repeat tests may be necessary in differential diagnosis of some cases of hypercalcemia.

Primary HPT occurs in ≤10% of patients with HHM as well as in those receiving thiazides, or with other causes of hypercalcemia.

Hyperparathyroidism (HPT), Primary

Due to inappropriate secretion of PTH causing efflux of calcium from bone, reabsorption of urine calcium, and promoting absorption of dietary calcium by activating vitamin D. Initially described as a "disease of bones, stones, and groans." Prevalence increases with age.

See Figs. 13-6, 13-7, and Tables 13-9 through 13-11.

Due To

* Parathyroid adenoma (weight >40 mg) in ≤90% of cases; double adenomas are reported in 3% to 12% of cases.
* Hyperplasia of all four glands in ≤15% of cases, sometimes with hereditary syndromes (e.g., MEN-1)
* Parathyroid carcinoma is rare (<1% of cases) or multiple adenomas
* No laboratory test can differentiate these.
* ~15% of these lesions may be ectopic; these must be sought if biochemical changes are not reversed by surgery.

♦ Increased serum calcium is hallmark of HPT and first step in diagnosis.

* Ionized calcium is more sensitive than total calcium and should be assayed whenever serum protein and albumin are abnormal.
* *Serum total protein and albumin must always be measured simultaneously, as marked decrease may cause a decrease in calcium. (Add 0.8 mg/dL to total calcium for every 1.0 g/dL of serum albumin below 3.5 g/dL.)*
* Any increased serum calcium must be confirmed by repeat test in fasting state and discontinuance for 2 to 3 months of drugs that may increase serum calcium (e.g., thiazide diuretics); cessation of thiazides may unmask primary HPT. ≤5% of hypercalcemia patients have simultaneous HPT and HHM.
* Parathyroid carcinoma presents with severe progressive hypercalcemia.
* Normal calcium level may occur in HPT with coexistence of conditions that decrease serum calcium level (e.g., malabsorption, acute pancreatitis, nephrosis, infarction of parathyroid adenoma). High-phosphate intake can abolish increased serum and urine calcium and decreased serum phosphorus; low-phosphate diet unmasks these changes. In these cases, ionized calcium should always be measured.

♦ Serum intact PTH level is increased; a few patients have only high-normal PTH levels. Serum calcium must always be measured concurrently, since PTH is *inappropriately* high in relation to a distinctly increased calcium level, which is consistent with HPT.

Blood should always be drawn after 10 A.M. because of circadian rhythm. PTH $>2\times$ upper limit of normal is almost always due to primary HPT. Nonparathyroid disease causing hypercalcemia (e.g., sarcoidosis, vitamin D intoxication, hyperthyroidism, milk-alkali syndrome, most malignancies) will have a normal or low (suppressed) PTH value (see Serum PTH).

Intraoperative rapid assay of PTH (RI-PTH) in peripheral blood that declines $>50\%$ within 10 minutes after gland resection predicts postoperative return of calcium to normal with 97% accuracy; failure to do this suggests multiglandular disease.[4,5] RI-PTH values can be reported in <30 minutes. After 20 minutes, there may be a 70% decline in RI-PTH. Preoperative [99mTc] scintigraphy imaging gives approximate location of abnormal parathyroid glands with reported sensitivity $= 90\%$; if inconclusive, selective catheterized venous sampling from neck and mediastinum can be done.

Indirect studies of parathyroid function (e.g., cortisone suppression test, decreased tubular reabsorption of phosphate, phosphate deprivation, chloride:phosphorus ratio, calcium infusion, urine cAMP) are no longer used in diagnosis of HPT.

Serum chloride is increased (>102 mEq/L; <99 mEq/L in other types of hypercalcemia). HPT patients tend toward hyperchloremic (nonanion gap) acidosis, whereas other hypercalcemic patients tend toward alkalosis.

Chloride:phosphorus ratio >33 supports the diagnosis of HPT and <30 contradicts this diagnosis.

O Serum phosphorus is decreased (<3 mg/dL) in $\sim 50\%$ of cases. It may be normal in the presence of high-phosphorus intake or renal damage with secondary phosphate retention.

It may be normal in one-half of patients, even without uremia. Low serum phosphorus in hypercalcemic patients suggests the diagnosis of primary HPT, an increased level supports the diagnosis of nonparathyroid hypercalcemia, but a normal level is not useful.

Serum ALP is of limited value. Normal in 50% of patients with primary HPT and only slightly increased in the rest.

Urine calcium is increased (>400 mg on a normal diet; >180 mg on a low-calcium diet) in only 70% of patients with HPT. See Chapter 4.

- Urine calcium excretion is often >500 mg/24 hours in malignancy, sarcoidosis, hyperthyroidism.
- Is <200 mg/24 hours in benign familial hypocalciuric hypercalcemia.
- Lithium-induced hypercalcemia resembles that of familial hypocalciuric hypercalcemia in that both show increased PTH levels and low urine calcium concentrations.

Urine phosphorus is increased unless there is renal insufficiency or phosphate depletion (especially due to commonly used antacids containing aluminum). Phosphate loading unmasks the increased urine phosphorus of HPT.

Polyuria is present, with low specific gravity.

Serum α_2- and β_1-globulins are slightly increased. *Serum protein electrophoresis should be performed in HPT to rule out multiple myeloma and sarcoidosis.*

Serum 1,25-dihydroxy-vitamin D may be increased in primary HPT and in sarcoidosis (and other granulomatous diseases) but not in HMM; serum 25-hydroxy-vitamin D may be useful to establish vitamin D intoxication, especially in factitious cases.

Urinary cAMP (adenosine monophosphate) may be high (>4.0 mmol/L) in $>90\%$ of cases of primary HPT and of HHM but low in vitamin D intoxication and sarcoidosis. Not usually increased in multiple myeloma or other hematologic malignancies; not increased in hypercalcemia owing to osteolytic metastases.

Uric acid is increased in $>15\%$ of patients. Uric acid level is not affected by cure of HPT, but a postoperative gout attack may occur. Increased uric acid level favors hypercalcemia due to thiazides, neoplasm or renal failure rather than HPT.

Increased hydroxyproline in serum and urine may occur with bone disease.

O Increased ESR is infrequent in HPT (may be caused by infection or moderate renal insufficiency).

Marked increase occurs in multiple myeloma.

[4]Sokoll LJ. Measurement of parathyroid hormone and application of parathyroid hormone in intraoperative monitoring. *Clin Lab Med* 2004;24:199.
[5]Strewler GJ. A 64-year-old woman with primary hyperparathyroidism. *JAMA* 2005;293:1772.

○ *HPT must always be ruled out in the presence of*:

- Most HPT patients are now discovered incidentally by routine blood testing (blood calcium within <1 mg/dL of upper limit of normal); PTH usually <2× upper limit of normal.
- Renal stones or calcification (2%–3% have HPT) (see Table 15-7)
- Peptic ulcer (occurs in 15% of patients with HPT)
- Calcific keratitis
- Bone changes (present in 20% of patients with HPT)
- Jaw tumors
- Clinical syndrome of hypercalcemia (nocturia, hyposthenuria, polyuria, abdominal pain, adynamic ileus, constipation, nausea, vomiting) *(present in 20% of patients with HPT; only clue to diagnosis in 10% of patients with HPT)*
- MEN (e.g., islet cell tumor of pancreas, pituitary tumor, pheochromocytoma)
- Relatives of patients with HPT or "asymptomatic" hypercalcemia
- Mental aberrations

Some patients with asymptomatic primary HPT may be followed medically but surgery may be indicated in presence of serum calcium >1 mg/dL above normal range, 24-hr urine calcium >400 mg/24 hours, presence of kidney stones, decreased renal function, decreased bone density, <50 years old, or history of any episode of life-threatening hypercalcemia.

Associated with increased incidence of pseudogout (even after successful removal of parathyroid adenoma) and gout.

Laboratory changes in HPT

- Serum calcium and PTH are stable in most patients.
- 4% have significant worsening of serum calcium.
- 15% develop marked hypercalciuria (>400 mg/24 hours).
- 12% have progressive decline in bone density.
- Most HPT patients remain stable.

Hyperparathyroidism, Secondary

Chronic advanced renal disease causes retention of phosphate, inadequate vitamin D activation, chronic low serum calcium, and therefore compensatory hyperplasia of parathyroid glands with compensatory secretion of PTH.

See Figure 13-7.

Serum PTH should be monitored to identify autonomous (tertiary) hyperparathyroidism.

Laboratory findings owning to underlying causative disease are noted (e.g., renal insufficiency).

♦ Classic findings in renal osteodystrophy are

- Serum phosphorus is increased.
- Serum calcium is low or normal.
- Serum ALP is increased.
- These levels can also be used to monitor response to treatment with calcitriol or alpha-calcidiol.
- Increased serum PTH is suppressed by 1,25-dihydroxyvitamin D which can be used to monitor this treatment of chronic renal failure.

Hyperphosphatasemia

Benign Familial

Rare familial benign persistent increase of serum ALP in the absence of any known disease. Found in Vitamin D hypervitaminosis, hypoparathyroidism, and renal failure.

Serum ALP (usually <5× upper limit of normal). Increase is usually of intestinal or bone (but occasionally of liver) origin.

Mild increase of serum acid phosphatase in some family members does not correlate with increase or type of ALP.

Benign Transient

Incidental discovery in healthy children usually <5 years old, especially after summer months and following recent weight loss.

○ Sudden transient increase in serum ALP, often to very high levels, that return to normal usually within 4 months. Isoenzymes of bone and liver origin are increased without evidence of liver or bone disease.
Plasma 25-hydroxyvitamin D 2× normal for age and time of year.
Occasional slight increase of AST, ALT, and gamma-glutamyl transfera (GGT).
Normal serum ALP in family members.

Hyperphosphatasia

Autosomal recessive syndrome beginning early in life of fragile bones with multiple fractures and deformities, skeletal X-ray changes, increased serum ALP; also referred to as *osteoectasia* and *osteochalasia desmalis familiaris*.

♦ Serum ALP is usually chronically increased, sometimes markedly; electrophoresis indicates bone origin. Serum acid phosphatase is also increased. Indicates increased activity of osteoblasts and osteoclasts.
Serum LAP may also be increased.
Serum calcium is normal or slightly decreased.
Serum phosphorus is normal or increased.
Serum magnesium, proteins and electrolytes are usually normal.
Uric acid is increased in blood and urine.

Hypervitaminosis D

Vitamin D originates in skin by action of UV radiation. Maintains calcium and phosphate concentrations by increasing intestinal absorption and bone mobilization. Excess due to ingestion of >500 μg/day in adults or >50 μg/day in infants.

See Table 13-9.
Serum calcium may be increased; preceded by hypercalciuria.
Serum phosphorus may be increased.
Serum ALP is decreased.
Serum PTH is low or normal.
Urine calcium excretion is increased.
Renal calcinosis may lead to renal insufficiency and uremia.
♦ Serum 25-hydroxyvitamin D is increased. Does not occur until >125 ng/mL.

Hypocalcemia, Neonatal

Since pH affects ionized calcium values, obtain free-flowing sample anaerobically and seal in capillary tube until analysis.
Defined as: From age 1 to 4 weeks, serum calcium <7 mg/dL or ionized calcium <4 mg/dL.
Due To
Early (age 1–3 days)—associated with

• Prematurity and low birth weight (occurs in ≤30% of infants)
• Maternal diabetes (occurs in ≤25% of infants)
• Birth asphyxia (occurs in ≤30% of infants)
• Preclampsia

Late (age 5–10 days)—associated with

• Feeding of cow's milk (increased dietary phosphate causing increased serum phosphate and decreased serum calcium)
• Slight vitamin D insufficiency
• Hypomagnesiumia (<1.4 mg/dL)

"Late-late" (within first 3–4 mos)—rarely associated with

• Maternal hypercalcemia or HPT
• Congenital hypoparathyroidism syndromes (e.g., DiGeorge syndrome)

- Hypoproteinemia (e.g., nephrosis, liver disease)
- Maternal osteomalacia
- Renal disease (primary renal tubular defect; decreased glomerular filtration rate causing phosphate retention)
- Iatrogenic disorders (e.g., exchange transfusions with citrated blood, lipid infusions)

○ *When tetany syndrome is associated with a normal serum calcium or not relieved by administration of calcium, rule out decreased serum magnesium. Hypocalcemia associated with hypomagnesemia will not respond unless hypomagnesemia is treated.*

○ *Serum phosphorus is >8 mg/dL when neonatal hypocalcemia is due to high phosphate feeding. BUN is increased when neonatal hypocalcemia is due to severe renal disease.*

Check serum total calcium for values of <5 to 6 mg/dL or ionized calcium of <2.5 to 3 mg/dL at the following intervals:

- Infants of diabetic mothers: 6, 12, 24, 48 hours
- Infants with intrapartum asphyxia: 1, 3, 6, 12 hours
- Premature infants: 12, 24, 48 hours

Hypercalcemia, Hypocalciuric, Familial (Familial Benign Hypocalciuric Hypercalcemia)[6]

Rare familial autosomal dominant disorder usually due to inactivating mutations of gene for calcium-sensing receptor resulting in inappropriate secretion of PTH. Chronic lifelong, asymptomatic, nonprogressive, mild hypercalcemia; onset before age 10 years without renal stones, kidney damage, peptic ulcer; no response to parathyroidectomy. Parathyroid glands are histologically normal.

◆ Has many of same biochemical findings as primary HPT, including

- Mildly increased serum total and ionized calcium.
- PTH is within normal range but inappropriately increased for level of hypercalcemia.
- Serum phosphorus is slightly decreased or normal.
- Urinary cAMP is increased in about one-third of patients.

◆ Urine calcium excretion is decreased or low-normal despite hypercalcemia.

- ≤200 mg/24 hours in familial hypocalciuric hypercalcemia. Calcium/creatinine clearance ratio is usually <0.01 (but usually >0.02 in primary HPT).
- ≤300 mg/24 hours in normal adult males.
- Increased (often >250 mg/24 hours) in two thirds of patients with HPT.
- Increased (often >500 mg/24 hours) in patients with malignancies.

Serum magnesium is mildly increased in 50% of patients; this is the only condition in which serum magnesium and calcium are both increased. Urine magnesium excretion is decreased also.

Renal function is maintained with normal creatinine clearance.

Serum 25-hydroxyvitamin D is normal and 1,25-dihydroxyvitamin D is proportional to PTH level.

Serum ALP is normal.

No dysfunction of other endocrine glands.

Fifty percent of first-degree relatives have hypercalcemia.

May also be acquired due to autoantibodies against calcium-sensing receptor.[6]

Hypoparathyroidism

Rare disorder often detected in childhood; may be autoimmune disorder associated with Addison disease, diabetes mellitus, hypothyroidism, pernicious anemia, chronic hepatitis, moniliasis, malabsorption, or hypogonadism. May also result from thyroid surgery or idiopathic or familial.

See Table 13-9 and Fig. 13-7.

[6]Pallais JC, et al. Acquired hypocalciuric hypercalcemia due to autoantibodies against calcium-sensing receptor. *N Engl J Med* 2004;351:362.

♦ Serum calcium is decreased (as low as 5 mg/dL) in presence of low or inappropriately low PTH and normal serum Mg which affects PTH secretion and action. Hypocalcemia stimulates PTH secretion in pseudohypoparathyroidism but not in hypoparathyroidism.

○ Serum phosphorus is increased (usually 5–6 mg/dL; as high as 12 mg/dL).

Serum ALP is normal or slightly decreased.

Urine calcium is decreased.

Urine phosphorus is decreased. Phosphate clearance is decreased.

Serum PTH is decreased.

Serum PTHrP is undetectable.

Serum 1,25 $(OH)_2 D_3$ is low.

♦ Renal resistance to PTH is shown by Ellsworth-Howard test

- PTH challenge (IV administration of 200 IU of synthetic PTH) causes increased urine phosphate ($>10\times$) and cAMP in normal persons and in primary hypoparathyroidism but little or no increase in urine phosphorus
- Increased urine phosphate ($<2\times$) and cAMP in classical type I pseudohypoparathyroidism or pseudopseudohypoparathyroidism
- In type II pseudohypoparathyroidism cAMP increases without phosphaturia.
- Decreased response may occur in basal cell nevus syndrome.

Alkalosis is present.

Serum uric acid is increased.

CSF is normal, even with mental or emotional symptoms or with calcification of basal ganglia.

○ Hypoparathyroidism should be ruled out in presence of mental and emotional changes, cataracts, faulty dentition in children, associated changes in skin and nails (e.g., moniliasis is frequent). One third of these patients may present as "epileptics."

Congenital absence may be associated with thymic aplasia (DiGeorge syndrome).

Pseudohypoparathyroidism

Rare heterogeneous group of inherited disorders with renal resistance to PTH action. Patients may be short, stocky with round face, short metacarpals and metatarsals, calvarial thickening, mental retardation.

♦ Serum calcium, phosphorus, and ALP are the same as in hypoparathyroidism but cannot be corrected by (or respond poorly to) administration of PTH.

Lack of response to PTH infusions and renal resistance to PTH is shown by Ellsworth-Howard test.

♦ Serum PTH level is normal or increased in the presence of a low serum calcium, in patients with the signs and symptoms of hypoparathyroidism.

Pseudo-Pseudohypoparathyroidism

Clinical anomalies are the same as in pseudohypoparathyroidism.

Serum and urine calcium, phosphorus, and ALP are normal.

Ellsworth-Howard test (see Hypoparathyroidism, above).

Hypophosphatasia

Rare autosomal recessive disease of impaired bone mineralization with X-ray changes; at least three different clinical syndromes (rickets, hyperparathyroidism, and Fanconi syndrome) are found in infants (most severe), children, and adults (least severe).

♦ Serum ALP is decreased to ~25% of normal (may vary from $0 \leq 40\%$ of normal); is not correlated with severity of disease. Enzymopathy of bone, kidney, liver isoenzymes; normal intestine and placenta isoenzymes. Is decreased in heterozygotes but the level cannot distinguish patients from carriers.

Serum calcium may be increased in severe cases with hypercalciuria, nephrocalcinosis.

Serum phosphorus is normal.

♦ Serum and urine levels of phosphoethanolamine are increased; may also be increased in asymptomatic heterozygotes and useful for detection.

♦ Treatment with corticosteroids usually causes an increase in serum ALP (but it never attains normal level) with a marked fall in serum calcium; phospho-ethanolamine excretion in urine continues high.
♦ Prenatal diagnosis by assay of ALP in amniotic fluid cells but activity in amniotic fluid is unreliable; first trimester diagnosis by assay of ALP in chorionic villus samples.
Urine hydroxyproline is low; in contrast, it is high in vitamin D-resistant rickets or hyperphosphatasia.

Pseudohypophosphatasia

Clinical syndrome and x-ray findings resembling infantile hypophosphatasia.

Serum ALP is normal.

Hypophosphatemia, Primary

Familial but occasionally sporadic condition of intrinsic renal tubular defect in phosphate resorption.

♦ Serum phosphorus is always decreased in the untreated patient.
Serum calcium is usually normal.
Serum ALP is often increased.
Serum PTH is normal.
♦ Bone biopsy shows a characteristic pattern of demineralization around osteocyte lacunae.

Milk-Alkali (Burnett) Syndrome

Due to consumption of large amounts of milk/dairy products and usually >5,000 mg/day of antacids for peptic ulcer or osteoporosis treatment.

○ Increased serum calcium (without hypercalciuria) and serum phosphorus, and mild alkalosis should suggest the diagnosis in a patient with peptic ulcer.
○ Renal insufficiency with increased BUN
Normal serum ALP
Metastatic calcinosis

Tetany Syndrome Due to Magnesium Deficiency

♦ Serum magnesium is decreased (usually <1 mEq/L).
Serum calcium is normal (slightly decreased in some patients).
Blood pH is normal.
♦ Tetany responds to administration of magnesium but not of calcium.

Tetany with Decreased Tissue Calcium

♦ Tetany associated with normal serum calcium, magnesium, potassium, and CO_2 responds to vitamin D therapy.
♦ Special radioactive calcium studies show decreased tissue calcium pool that returns toward normal with therapy.

Tests for Diagnosis of Diabetes Mellitus (DM) and Hypoglycemia

Islet Autoantibodies

Use
Marker for type 1 DM. ≤1 of 4 is positive in 95% of cases of new onset type 1 DM.

Islet Antibody	Frequency at Onset of Type 1 DM
Glutamic acid decarboxylase autoantibodies*	70%–80%
Islet cell cytoplasmic autoantibodies	70%–80%

Insulin autoantibodies	Adults <10%; children ~50%
Insulinoma-2 associated autoantibodies (1A-2A)	~60%

*Recommended because it is most persistent islet autoantibody after onset of autoimmune DM. Glutamic acid decarboxylase is present in pancreatic islet β cells.

C-Peptide, Serum

Formed during conversion of proinsulin to insulin; peptide is released into circulation in equimolar quantities to insulin following conversion of proinsulin to insulin; C-peptide serum levels correlate with insulin levels in blood, except in islet cell tumors and possibly in obese patients.

Use
For estimating insulin levels in the presence of antibodies to exogenous insulin.
Diagnosis of factitious hypoglycemia due to surreptitious administration of insulin in which high serum insulin levels will occur with low C-peptide levels.
Increased In
Insulinoma
Type 2 DM
Decreased In
Exogenous insulin administration (e.g., factitious hypoglycemia)
Type 1 DM

Fructosamine, Serum

Measures concentration of nonlabile glycated serum proteins. Manufacture is now discontinued.

Use
Said to give a reliable estimate of mean blood glucose levels during preceding 1–3 wks.
Allows a shorter time frame than glycohemoglobin (GHb).
When GHb cannot be used due to interferences (e.g., abnormal Hb [see GHb below]), which invalidate HbA_{1c}.
Interpretation
Correlates with HbA_{1c} but is not affected by abnormal hemoglobins, fetal hemoglobin (HbF), increased RBC turnover; shows changed glucose levels earlier than HbA_{1c}.
180 μmol/L increase in fructosamine is related to ~30 mg/dL increase in glucose.
Reference range in nondiabetic persons: Fructosamine = 2.4 to 3.4 μmol/L; fructosamine:albumin ratio = 54 to 86 μmol/g). Should be compared with previous values in same patient rather than reference range.
Reference range = 205–285 μmol/L for second-generation assay.
Interferences
Changes in fructosamine values correlate with significant changes in serum protein concentrations (e.g., liver disease, acute systemic illness). Abnormal values also occur during abnormal protein turnover (e.g., thyroid disease) even though patients are normoglycemic. May be obviated by using fructose:albumin ratio.

Glycated Albumin
Half life ~14 days.

Use
Monitor degree of hyperglycemia during previous 1 to 2 weeks when GHb cannot be used. Not yet shown to be related to risk of progression of diabetic complications. Use is same as for fructosamine.

Glycohemoglobin (Glycated Hemoglobin [GHb])

Glucose combines with Hb continuously and nearly irreversibly during life span of RBC (120 days); thus GHb will be proportional to mean plasma glucose level during previous 6 to 12 weeks.

May be reported as HbA_{1c} or as total of A_{1b}, A_{1a}, A_{1c}.
Values may not be comparable with different methodologies and even different laboratories using same methodology.

Use

Monitor diabetic patients' compliance and long-term blood glucose level control.
Index of diabetic control (direct relationship between poor control and development of complications.)
Predicts development and progression of diabetic microvascular complications.
Utility for diagnosis of DM is still to be determined.

Interpretation

Dietary preparation or fasting not required.

♦ Increase almost certainly means DM if other factors (see below) are absent (>3SD above the mean has S/S = 99%/48%), but a normal value does not rule out impaired glucose tolerance. Values less than the normal mean are not seen in untreated DM.

May rise within one week after rise in blood glucose due to stopping therapy but may not fall for 2 to 4 weeks after blood glucose decrease when therapy is resumed.

Mean blood glucose in first 30 days (days 0–30) before sampling GHb contributes ~50% to final GHb value, whereas days 90 to 120 contribute only ~10%. Time to reach a new steady state is ~30 to 35 days.

When fasting blood glucose is <110 mg/dL, HbA_{1c} is normal in >96% of cases.
When fasting blood glucose is 110–125 mg/dL, HbA_{1c} is normal in >80% of cases.
When fasting blood glucose is >126 mg/dL, HbA_{1c} is normal in >60% of cases.

Normal (A_{1a}, A_{1b}, A_{1c}) = 4%–8%
For level of 4% to 20%, this formula may estimate daily average plasma glucose:

$$\text{Mean daily plasma glucose (mg/dL)} = 10 \times (\text{GHb level} + 4).$$

1% increase in GHb is related to ~30 mg/dL increase in glucose.
In known diabetics:

* <7% indicates good diabetic control
* 10% indicates fair diabetic control
* 13% to 20% indicates poor diabetic control
* When mean annual HbA_{1c} is <1.1 × ULN, renal and retinal complications are rare, but complications occur in >70% of cases when HbA_{1c} is >1.7 × ULN.

Increased In

HbF > normal or 0.5% (e.g., heterozygous or homozygous persistence of HbF, fetomaternal transfusion during pregnancy)
Chronic renal failure with or without hemodialysis
Iron deficiency anemia
Splenectomy
Increased serum triglycerides
Alcohol
Lead and opiate toxicity
Salicylate treatment

Decreased In

Shortened RBC life span (e.g., hemolytic anemias, blood loss)
Following transfusions
Pregnancy
Ingestion of large amounts (>1 g/day) of vitamin C or E
Hemoglobinopathies (e.g., spherocytes) produce variable increase or decrease depending on assay method.

1,5 Anhydroglucitol (1,5 AG; GlycoMark)

1-deoxy form of glucose. Glucose competitively inhibits kidney reabsorption; therefore concentration is inversely related to glucose. Recently approved by the FDA.

Use

Monitor degree of hyperglycemia during previous 1- to 14-day period. Utility still being evaluated.
Reference range: 6.8 to 29.3 μg/mL in women; 10.7–32.0 μg/mL in men.

Insulin, Plasma

Peptide hormone enzymatically processed from proinsulin in pancreatic secretory granules of beta cells. Approximately 50% is removed from blood during initial passage through liver; half-life = 4 to 9 minutes. Secretion is regulated primarily

by blood glucose levels; therefore should always be measured with a concomitant blood glucose. Insulin deficiency is the crucial factor in the pathogenesis of Type 1 DM.)

Use
Diagnosis of insulinoma

Not clinically useful for diagnosis of DM

Increased In
Insulinoma. Fasting blood insulin level >50 μU/mL in presence of low or normal blood glucose level. IV tolbutamide or administration of leucine causes rapid rise of blood insulin to very high levels within a few minutes with rapid return to normal.

Factitious hypoglycemia in presence of normal blood glucose

Insulin autoimmune syndrome

Untreated obese mild DM. The fasting level is often increased.

Cirrhosis due to insufficient clearance from blood

Acromegaly (especially with active disease) after ingestion of glucose

Reactive hypoglycemia after glucose ingestion, particularly when diabetic type of glucose tolerance curve is present

Absent In
Severe DM with ketosis and weight loss. In less severe cases, insulin is frequently present but only at lower glucose concentrations.

Normal In
Hypoglycemia associated with nonpancreatic tumors

Idiopathic hypoglycemia of childhood, except after administration of leucine

Insulin/C-Peptide Ratio

Insulin and C-peptide are secreted into portal vein in equimolar amounts but serum ratio = 1:5 to 1:15 due to removal of ~50% of insulin from blood during initial passage through liver. C-peptide half-life = ~30 minutes.

Use
To differentiate insulinoma from factitious hypoglycemia owning to insulin.

Interpretation
Normal fasting molar ratio C-peptide:insulin = 5.

<1.0 in molarity units (or >47.17 μg/ng in conventional units)

• Increased endogenous insulin secretion (e.g., insulinoma, sulfonylurea administration)
• Renal failure

>1.0 in molarity units (or <47.17 μg/ng in conventional units)

• Exogenous insulin administration
• Cirrhosis

Proinsulin

Enzymatic process forms insulin in pancreatic secretory granules of beta cells. Proinsulin level is normally ≤20% of total insulin. Proinsulin is included in the immunoassay of total insulin and separation requires special technique.

Increased In
Insulinoma tumor may secrete predominantly insulin or proinsulin.

Proinsulin >30% of serum insulin after overnight fast suggests insulinoma.

Factitious hypoglycemia due to sulfonylurea (see Table 13-16)

Familial hyperproinsulinemia—heterozygous mutation affecting cleavage of proinsulin leading to secretion of excess amounts of proinsulin

Non–insulin-dependent DM

Interferences
May also be increased in renal disease

Insulin Tolerance Test

Administer 0.1 unit insulin/kg body weight IV.

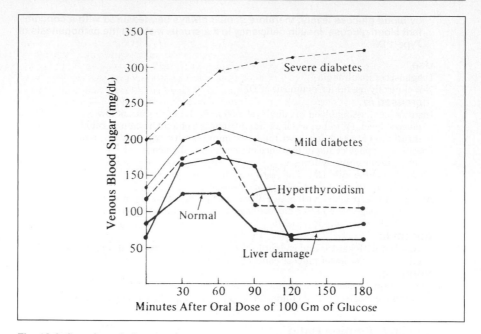

Fig. 13-8. Sample oral glucose tolerance curves in various conditions.

Use smaller dose if hypopituitarism is suspected. Always keep IV glucose available to prevent severe reaction

Use

Assess syndromes of extreme insulin resistance

Crude classification of insulin sensitivity

Assess growth hormone deficiency

Normal

Blood glucose falls to 50% of fasting level within 20 to 30 minutes; returns to fasting level within 90 to 120 minutes.

Increased Tolerance

Blood glucose falls <25% and returns rapidly to fasting level.

• Hypothyroidism
• Acromegaly
• Cushing syndrome (peak cortisol response <18–20 μg/dL and change over baseline <7 μg/dL indicates glucocorticoid deficiency)
• DM (some patients; especially older, obese ones)

Decreased Tolerance

Increased sensitivity to insulin (excessive fall of blood glucose)

Hypoglycemic irresponsiveness (lack of response by glycogenolysis)

• Pancreatic islet cell tumor
• Adrenocortical insufficiency
• Adrenocortical insufficiency secondary to hypopituitarism
• Hypothyroidism
• von Gierke disease (some patients)
• Starvation (depletion of liver glycogen)

Glucose Tolerance Test, Oral (OGTT)[7]

See Fig. 13-8.

[7]American Diabetes Association. Diagnosis and classification of diabetes mellitus. *Diabetes Care* 2005;28:S37–S42.

Standards for OGTT: Prior diet of >150 g of carbohydrate daily, no alcohol, and unrestricted activity for 3 days before test. Test in morning after 10 to 16 hours of fasting. No medication, smoking, or exercise (remain seated) during test. Not to be done during recovery from acute illness, emotional stress, surgery, trauma, pregnancy, inactivity due to chronic illness; therefore is of limited or no value in hospitalized patients. Certain drugs should be stopped several weeks before the test (e.g., oral diuretics, oral contraceptives, phenytoin). Loading dose of glucose consumed within 5 minutes: For adults = 75 g, for children = 1.75 g/kg (of ideal body weight in obese children but never >75 g), for pregnant women = 100 g. Draw blood at fasting, 30, 60, 90, 120 minutes; 30-minute sample offers little additional information but can confirm adequate gastric absorption when patient is nauseous.

Use

OGTT should be reserved principally for patients with "borderline" fasting plasma glucose levels (i.e., fasting range 110–140 mg/dL). Necessary for diagnosis of impaired fasting glucose (IFG) and impaired glucose tolerance (IGT).

All pregnant women should be tested for gestational DM with a 50-g dose at 24 to 28 weeks of pregnancy; if that is abnormal, OGTT should be performed for confirmation. Is gold standard and currently chief use is diagnosis of gestational DM.

OGTT is not indicated in

*   Persistent fasting hyperglycemia (>140 mg/dL)
*   Persistent fasting normoglycemia (<110 mg/dL)
*   Patients with typical clinical findings of DM and random plasma glucose >200 mg/dL
*   Secondary diabetes (e.g., genetic hyperglycemic syndromes, following administration of certain hormones)
*   Should never be done to evaluate reactive hypoglycemia
*   Test is of limited value for diagnosis of DM in children and is rarely indicated for that.

Interpretation

For diagnosis of DM in nonpregnant adults, at least two values of OGTT should be increased (or fasting serum glucose ≥140 mg/dL on more than one occasion) and other causes of transient glucose intolerance must be ruled out.

Diabetes Mellitus (DM) and Other Hyperglycemic and Hypoglycemic Disorders

Diabetes Mellitus (DM)

Chronic metabolic diseases associated with increased blood sugar levels in which the body does not produce, or improperly uses, insulin; associated vascular and neuropathic complications

Types 1 and 2 (see Table 13-12)
Other specific types (represents 1%–2% of diabetic patients), e.g.,
A. Genetic defects of beta cell function (e.g., chromosome 12, 7, 20). Formerly referred to as maturity-onset diabetes of the young. Onset of mild hyperglycemia usually before age 25 years, impaired insulin secretion. Autosomal dominant inheritance.
B. Genetic defects in insulin resistance (e.g., leprechaunism, type A insulin resistance, Rabson-Mendenhall syndrome, lipoatrophic diabetes)
C. Diseases of exocrine pancreas (e.g., pancreatitis, pancreatectomy, neoplasia, cystic fibrosis, hemochromatosis)
D. Endocrine disorders (e.g., Cushing syndrome, acromegaly, pheochromocytoma, aldosteronoma, hyperthyroidism, glucagonoma)
E. Drug/chemical induced (e.g., glucocorticoids, Dilantin, β-adrenergic agonists, pentamidine, thiazides, α-interferon)
F. Infections (e.g., CMV, congenital rubella)
G. Uncommon forms of immune-mediated diabetes (e.g., anti-insulin receptor antibodies, "stiff-man" syndrome)
II. Other genetic syndromes that may be associated with DM (e.g., Down syndrome, Klinefelter syndrome, Turners syndrome, Friedreich ataxia, Huntington chorea, porphyria)
I. Gestational diabetes mellitus (represents 2%–5% of all pregnancies; see below)

Table 13-12. Classification of Diabetes Mellitus (DM) and Other Hyperglycemic Disorders

Type 1 DM	Type 2 DM
Formerly called insulin-dependent (IDDM), juvenile-onset, or brittle DM	Formerly called non–insulin-dependent [NIDDM] or adult-onset DM
Represents 5%–10% of diabetic patients	Represents 90%–95% of diabetic patients
Autoimmune disease in which pancreatic beta islet cell are targets of destruction	Varies from predominantly insulin resistance in muscle and fat with relative deficiency to predominantly insulin secretory defect with insulin resistance
	Relative rather than absolute insulin deficiency
Autoantibodies are present in 85%–90% of cases	Associated with dyslipidemia, obesity (in 80%–90% of cases), increasing age, hypertension, family history
Other autoimmune disorders may be present (e.g., Graves disease, Hashimoto thyroiditis, Addison disease, pernicious anemia)	
Insulin secretion is virtually absent	Plasma insulin may be normal or increased but is expected to be higher relative to blood glucose concentration
Plasma C-peptide is low or undetectable in contrast to Type 2	
Ketosis prone	Ketosis occurs with stress (e.g., infection), but seldom spontaneously

---

♦ **Criteria for Diagnosis in Nonpregnant Adults**
Diabetes Mellitus

- Random plasma glucose >200 mg/dL when there are classical symptoms **or**
- Fasting (>8 hrs) plasma glucose ≥126 mg/dL **or**
- 2-hr plasma glucose >200 mg/dL after 75 g glucose load.
- Any of the above must be confirmed on subsequent day.
- "Acute metabolic decompensation with hyperglycemia" need not be confirmed on a subsequent day.

A suggested alternative criterion:*

- Random plasma glucose >200 mg/dL when there are classical symptoms **or**
- Fasting plasma glucose ≥126 mg/dL confirmed on subsequent day or
- HbA_{1c} >2 SDs the mean for that laboratory or >1% above upper limit of normal should be confirmed by one of the above.

OGTT is not recommended for routine use. Needed to diagnose IFG and IGT.

Impaired Fasting Glucose

- Fasting glucose ≥110 mg/dL but <126 mg/dL **or**

In absence of pregnancy, IGT and IFG are risk factors for future DM and cardiovascular disease; they are not clinical entities.

Impaired Glucose Tolerance

- With OGTT 2-hr value ≥140 and <200 mg/dL in nonpregnant adult

Replaces terms *latent* or *chemical* diabetes.
Other causes of transient glucose intolerance must be ruled out before an unequivocal diagnosis of DM is made.

*Barr RG, et al. Tests of glycemia for the diagnosis of type 2 diabetes mellitus. *Ann Int Med* 2002;137:263.

Test asymptomatic undiagnosed individuals > age 45 every 3 years.
Test at younger age if:

- HDL cholesterol ≤35 mg/dL or triglyceride ≥250 mg/dL
- Previous IGT or IFG
- Obese
- First-degree relative with DM
- High-risk ethnic population (e.g., African American, Native American, Hispanic)
- Delivered baby weighing >9 pounds

Routine screening of DM patients should include: albuminuria (if negative, microalbuminuria), lipid profile, renal function (creatinine, creatinine clearance), Kimmelstiel-Wilson nephropathy, GU tract infection, etc. (see Chapter 14).

Diabetes Mellitus, Gestational

Hyperglycemia that develops for the first time during pregnancy; affects ~4% of pregnant women.

Diagnosis is necessary for short-term identification of increased risk of fetal morbidity. *Screening* of all pregnant women should include:

- Random (need not be fasting) venous blood glucose 1 hourr after ingestion of 50 g of glucose at 24 to 28 weeks' gestation. Values >140 mg/dL are indication for 3-hour 100-g glucose GTT. 1-hour, 50-g test is abnormal in ~15% of pregnant women, ~14% of whom have abnormal 3-hour OGTT. S/S = ~79%/~87%.

◆ **Diagnostic Criteria**
At least two of the following glucose plasma levels are found on OGTT with 100-g glucose loading dose; is gold standard for diagnosis of gestational diabetes.

Fasting	≥95 mg/dL
1 hr	≥180 mg/dL
2 hrs	≥155 mg/dL
3 hrs	≥140 mg/dL

If abnormal results during pregnancy, repeat OGTT at first postpartum visit; if GTT is normal, diagnose as DM only during pregnancy but blood glucose should be tested at every subsequent visit because of increased risk (30% during next 5–10 yrs) of developing diabetes mellitus. If postpartum GTT is abnormal, classify as IGT or IFG (~5%–10%), or DM (10%) using above criteria; remainder appear normal but 30% will develop DM in 5 to 10 years.

GHb and fructosamine are not recommended for detection of gestational DM.

For management of DM during pregnancy, goal is fasting plasma glucose of 60 to 110 mg/dL and postprandial levels <150 mg/dL. Measure serum or 24-hour urine estriol for fetal surveillance.

Test amniotic fluid to evaluate fetal pulmonary maturity.

During labor, keep maternal glucose at 80 to 100 mg/dL; beware of markedly increased insulin sensitivity in immediate postpartum period.

At least 6 weeks postpartum, reclassify as DM, IGF, IGT, or normoglycemic.

Laboratory Evaluation of Fetus

During third trimester, urinary estriol level is used as indicator of fetoplacental integrity.

Placental function is also indicated by hCG, human placental lactogen, estradiol, and progesterone levels. L:S ratio on amniotic fluid is used to predict pulmonary maturity.

At time of cesarean section, before opening amniotic sac, obtain sterile sample of amniotic fluid for culture, Gram stain, L:S ratio.

Infants of Diabetic Mothers

Blood glucose <30 mg/dL in ≤50% of infants of diabetic mothers usually within first hours after birth; usually asymptomatic. Glucose levels should be checked every hour for first hours.

Hypocalcemia is common and occurs 24 to 36 hours after birth.

Diabetes Mellitus, Neonatal

Blood glucose often between 245 and 2,300 mg/dL
Metabolic acidosis of some degree usually present
Variable ketonuria
Laboratory findings owning to dehydration
Laboratory findings owning to infection or CNS lesions, which are present in one third
    of patients
Has been detected as early as fourth day; usually transient

Ketoacidosis, Diabetic (DKA)

**Acute life-threatening metabolic acidosis due to uncontrolled DM (usually type 1;
infrequently type 2) when decompensated by intercurrent illness; owning to
severe insulin deficiency and excess hormone-producing glucose.**

See Table 13-13.

♦ Blood glucose is increased (>250 mg/dL); ranges from slightly increased to very
  high. Very increased glucose (>500–800 mg/dL) suggests nonketotic hyperosmolar
  hyperglycemia (because glucose levels become very high only when extracellular
  fluid volume is markedly decreased). Glucose <200 mg/dL may occur, especially in
  alcoholics or pregnant insulin-dependent diabetics. Glucose concentration is not
  related to severity of DKA.
♦ Plasma acetone is increased (4+ reaction when plasma is diluted 1:1 with water).
  (Acetone is usually 3 to 4× the concentration of acetoacetate but does not contribute
  to acidosis.) Nitroprusside reagent tests (e.g., Acetest, Ketostix, Chemstrip) react
  with acetoacetate, not with β-hydroxybutyrate, weakly with acetone; therefore weak
  positive reaction with ketone does not rule out ketoacidosis. β-hydroxybutyrate:ace-
  toacetate ratio varies from 3:1 in mild up to 15:1 in severe DKA. With correction of
  DKA, conversion of β-hydroxybutyrate to acetoacetate gives a stronger nitroprusside test reaction; this should not be mistaken for worsening of DKA.

Urine ketone tests are not reliable for diagnosing or monitoring DKA.

• May be positive in ≤30% of first morning specimens in pregnancy.
• False-positive results reported in presence of some sulfhydryl drugs (e.g., captopril).
• False-negative results may occur in highly acidic urine, after large doses of ascorbic
  acid, test strips exposed in air for extended time.

♦ Metabolic acidosis (pH <7.3 and/or bicarbonate <15 mEq/L) is mainly due to beta-
  hydroxybutyrate and acetoacetate. Some lactic acidosis may exist, especially if
  shock, sepsis, or tissue necrosis is present; suspect this if pH and anion gap do not
  respond to insulin therapy. Whole spectrum of patterns from pure hyperchloremic
  acidosis to wide-anion-gap acidosis. May be obscured by complicating metabolic
  alkalosis.
♦ Volume and electrolyte depletion (owning to glucose-induced osmotic diuresis)

• Absence of volume depletion should arouse suspicion of other possibilities (e.g.,
  hypoglycemic coma, other causes of coma).
• Very low sodium (120 mEq/L) is usually due to hypertriglyceridemia and hyperosmolality, although occasionally may be dilutional due to vomiting and water intake. Low
  in 67%, normal in 26%, increased in 7% of cases. Depleted body stores are not reflected
  in these initial values, which reflect relative water loss and blood glucose level.
• Serum potassium is normal in 43%, increased in 39% due to potassium exit from
  cells secondary to acidosis; initial low potassium in 18% of cases indicates severe
  depletion.
• Serum phosphate decreased in 10% of cases, normal in 18%, and increased in 71% of
  cases; falls with onset of therapy due to loss by osmotic diuresis and cellular uptake.
  Severe depletion (<0.5 mg/dL may cause muscle weakness, rhabdomyolysis,
  impaired cardiac function, etc.). Excessive replacement may cause hypocalcemia and
  hypomagnesemia.
• Serum magnesium may be decreased in 7% (in prolonged ketoacidosis), normal in
  25%, increased in 68% of cases.

Azotemia is present (BUN is usually 25–30 mg/dL); creatinine may be proportionally
    increased >BUN due to methodologic interference by acetoacetate.
Serum osmolality is slightly increased (≤340 mOsm/L).

Table 13-13.	Comparison of Diabetic Ketoacidosis and Hyperosmolar Hyperglycemic Nonketotic Coma	

	Diabetic Ketoacidosis (DKA)	Hyperosmolar Hyperglycemic Nonketotic Coma (HHS)
Laboratory findings[*]		
Plasma glucose (mg/dL)	250–600	>600; often >1,000
Plasma acetone	+ in diluted plasma	Less + in diluted plasma[†]
Serum sodium (mEq/L)[‡]	Usually low	N, I, or low
Serum potassium (mEq/L)	N, I, or low	N or I
Serum phosphorus (mEq/L)	N or I	N or I
Serum magnesium	N or I	N or I
Serum bicarbonate (mEq/L)	Usually <15	Usually >20
Blood pH	<7.30	>7.30
Anion gap (mEq/L)	>12	10–12
Serum osmolality (mOsm/L)	<320	>330; may reach 380
Serum BUN (mg/dL)	Lesser increase	Greater increase
Serum lactate (mmol/L)	2–3	1–2
Plasma insulin	Low to 0	Some
Clinical findings		
Age	Younger	Usually elderly or middle aged
Type of diabetes	Usually Type 1	Usually Type 2
Previous history of diabetes	Usually	50% of cases
Onset	Acute/subacute	Insidious
Precipitating factors	Infection (30%), noncompliance (20%), new diagnosis (25%), unknown (25%)	Most common: infection MI, CVA; new onset (35%), drugs (e.g., diuretics, glucocorticoids)
Prodrome	<1 day	Several days
Dehydration	Less	More
Acetone breath	Yes	No
Kussmaul respiration	Yes	No
Abdominal pain	Yes	No
Temperature	N or low	N or I
Change in mental status	Moderate	Severe (coma, seizures)
Neurologic findings	Rare	Very Common
Cardiovascular or renal disease	15%	85%
Thrombosis	Rare	Frequent
Mortality	<10%	20%–50%

CVA, cerebrovascular accident (stroke); MI, myocardial infraction; N, normal; I, increased.
[*]Depends on stage of patient's coma and treatment, degree of dehydration, precipitating illness, complications (e.g., vomiting, etc).
[†]Principally beta-hydroxybutyrate that is not detected by nitroprusside reaction.
[‡]Sodium is decreased by 1.6 mEq/L for each 100 mg/dL increment in glucose.
Data from Jabbour SA, Miller JL. Uncontrolled diabetes mellitus. 2001;21:99.

WBC is increased (often >20,000/cu mm) even without infection; associated with decreased lymphocytes and eosinophils.

Hb, Hct, total protein may be increased due to intravascular volume depletion.

Serum amylase may be increased (may originate from salivary glands rather than pancreas) in ≤36% of patients or from both sources in 16% of cases.

Serum AST, ALT, LD, and CK are increased in 20% to 65% of cases partly owing to methodologic interference of acetoacetate in colorimetric methods. CK may be increased due to phosphate depletion and rhabdomyolysis.

Table 13-14.   Differential Diagnosis of Diabetic Coma

Condition	Serum Glucose (mg/dL)	Serum Ketones (undiluted)	Blood pH	Serum Osmolality (mOsm/kg)	Serum Lactate (mmol/L)	Plasma Insulin
Diabetic ketoacidosis	300–1,000	++++	D	300–350	2–3	0–L
Lactic acidosis	100–200	0	D	N–300	≥7	L
Alcoholic ketoacidosis	40–200	++++	D	290–310	2–6	L
Hyperosmolar coma	500–2,000	0/+	N	320–400	1–2	Some
Hypoglycemia	10–40	0	N	285 ± 6	Low	I

0 = none; + = small amount; up to ++++ = large amount; D = decreased; I = increased; L = low; N = normal.
Normal serum lactate = 0.6–1.1 mmol/L.
Lactic acidosis occurs in one-third of patients with diabetic ketoacidosis.
Hypersomolar coma and alcoholic ketoacidosis may occur in diabetic ketoacidosis.

Laboratory findings due to precipitating medical problem (e.g., infection, myocardial infarction, vascular, trauma, pregnancy, emotional, endocrine; not found in 25% of cases); these should always be sought.

Follow-up lab tests every 2 to 4 hours initially and less often with clinical improvement. Bedside fingerstick glucose can be determined initially every 30 to 60 minutes to determine rate of fall of glucose and when to add glucose to IV fluids.

ESR may be increased in diabetic patients even in absence of infection and when serum protein is normal, particularly when glycemic control is poor; does not necessarily indicate underlying infection.

Hyperosmolar Hyperglycemic Nonketotic Coma (HHS)

Acute syndrome due to hyperglycemia, hyperosmolality, and combination of severe dehydration caused by inadequate fluid intake and insulin deficiency; occurs in type 2 diabetes mellitus. Precipitating factors include: Infections and myocardial infarct and both may be complicated by lactic acidosis. Use of corticosteroids and thiazide diuretics have been implicated in the etiology of HHS. As in DKA, there is relative insulin deficiency in the presence of excess catabolic hormone concentrations.

See Tables 13-13 and 13-14.

♦ Blood glucose is very high, often 600 to 1,200 mg/dL, but contrary to expectation in diabetic coma, acidosis and ketosis are minimal and plasma acetone is not found.

♦ Serum osmolality is very high (normal = 280–300 mOsm/L).

• In mildly drowsy patients, mean is 320 mOsm/L.
• At level of 350 mOsm/L, there will be some confusion or some stupor.
• >350 mOsm/L many patients are in coma.
• At 400 mOsm/L, most patients are obtunded.
  State of consciousness does not correlate with height of acidemia.
○ Serum sodium may be increased, normal, or decreased but is disproportionately decreased for degree of dehydration due to marked hyperglycemia (artifactual decrease 1.6 mEq/L for every 100 mg/dL increase of serum glucose).

• Increased sodium with marked hyperglycemia indicates severe dehydration.

Serum potassium may be increased (due to hyperosmolality), low (due to osmotic diuresis with urinary loss), or normal, depending on balance of factors.

BUN is increased (70–90 mg/dL) more than diabetic ketoacidosis.

Laboratory findings owning to complications or precipitating factors

• Renal insufficiency in 90% of cases
• Infection (e.g., pneumonia)

- Drugs (e.g., steroids, phenytoin, potassium-wasting diuretics such as thiazides and furosemide, others [propranolol, diazoxide, azathioprine])
- Other medical conditions (e.g., cerebrovascular or cardiovascular accident, subdural hematoma, severe burns, acute pancreatitis, thyrotoxicosis, Cushing syndrome)
- Glucose overloading or use of concentrated glucose solutions (e.g., hyperalimentation, dialysis, IV infusions in treatment of burns)
- Spontaneous in 5% to 7% of cases
- Preexisting mild DM Type 2
- Dehydration

Clinical picture: A middle-aged or older person with diabetes of recent onset or unrecognized diabetes, who shows neurologic symptoms (e.g., convulsions or hemiplegia) and then becomes stuporous or comatose.

One third of patients admitted for hyperglycemia show characteristics of both DKA and HHS.

Hypoglycemia, Classification

Lowest capillary blood glucose concentrations in normal people has been arbitrarily set at ~2.2 mmol/L (40 mg/dL) in capillary or venous blood, below which is considered hypoglycemic. Systematic studies have shown that the lowest capillary blood glucose concentration is about 2.8 mmol/L in normal elderly patients (>65 years old). The lowest observed random blood glucose concentrations are ~2.5 mmol/L.

See Table 13-15.

◆ Diagnosis requires triad of low blood glucose at the time of spontaneous hypoglycemic symptoms and alleviation by administration of glucose that corrects hypoglycemia.
(Glucose concentration is 15% lower in whole blood than in serum or plasma.)

Reactive (i.e., after eating)

- Alimentary (rapid gastric emptying, e.g., after subtotal gastrectomy, vagotomy)
- Impaired glucose tolerance as in DM (mild maturity-onset)
- Functional (idiopathic)
- Rare conditions (e.g., hereditary fructose intolerance, galactosemia, familial fructose and galactose intolerance)

Fasting (spontaneous)—almost always indicates organic disease

- Liver—severe parenchymal disease (including sepsis, congestive heart failure, Reye syndrome) or enzyme defect (e.g., glycogen storage diseases, galactosemia)
- Chronic renal insufficiency
- Pancreatic
  Insulinoma (pancreatic islet cell tumor)
  MEN-I
  Pancreatic hyperplasia
- Deficiency of hormones that oppose insulin (e.g., decreased function of thyroid, anterior pituitary, or adrenal cortex)
- Postoperative removal of pheochromocytoma
- Large extrapancreatic tumors (65% are intra- or retroperitoneal fibromas or sarcomas)
- Certain epithelial tumors (e.g., hepatoma, carcinoid, Wilms tumor)
- Drugs (including factitious, e.g., insulin, sulfonylureas, alcohol, salicylates, quinine); others may potentiate effect of sulfonylurea (e.g., sulfonamides, butazones, coumarins, clofibrate)
- Artifactual (high WBC or RBC count, e.g., leukemia or polycythemia)
- Starvation, anorexia nervosa, lactic acidosis, intense exercise
- Insulin antibodies or insulin receptor antibodies

Combined reactive and fasting types

- Insulinoma
- Adrenal insufficiency
- Insulin antibodies or insulin receptor antibodies

Table 13-15. Laboratory Interpretation of 72-Hr Fast for Hypoglycemia

	Glucose (mg/dL)	Insulin (μU/mL)	C-Peptide (mmol/L)	Proinsulin (pmol/L)	Beta-hydroxybutyrate (mmol/L)	Change in Glucose (mgd/L)
Normal[a]	≥40	<6	<0.2	<5	>2.7	<25
Insulinoma	≤45	≥6	>0.2	≥5	≤2.7	≥25
Factitious						
Insulin	≤45	≥6	<0.2	<5	≤2.7	≥25
Sulfonylurea[b]	≤45	≥6	≥0.2	≥5	≤2.7	≥25
Insulin-like growth factor	≤45	≤6	<0.2	<5	≤2.7	≥25
Not insulin-mediated hypoglycemia	≤45	<6	<0.2	<5	>2.7	<25
Eating during 72-hr "fast"[a]	≥45	<6	<0.2	<5	≤2.7	≥25
Nonhypoglycemic syndrome	≥40	<6	<0.2	<5	>2.7	<25

[a]Not symptomatic; all others have signs or symptoms.
[b]Sulfonylurea in plasma only if patient has taken this drug. Tolbutamide detection is a separate analysis.
All blood measurements should be performed on the same specimen drawn at start and end of fast and every 6 hrs until plasma glucose is ≤60 mg/dL; then every 1–2 hrs.
Terminate when patient has hypoglycemic signs or symptoms *and* plasma glucose is ≤45 mg/dL.
Draw specimens for cortisol, growth hormone, glucagon at beginning and end of fast if deficiency of these is suspected.
Diagnosis of reactive hypoglycemia is based on decreased blood glucose at time of signs and symptoms with improvement by eating and a repetitive pattern of occurrence.
Diagnosis should not be based on glucose tolerance test, since 25% of healthy young men may have postprandial glucose <50 mg/dL and 2–3% of subjects may have level <40 mg/dL.
Diagnosis of "nonhypoglycemic syndrome"—normal blood glucose associated with symptoms similar to those in hypoglycemia.
Source: Service FJ. Hypoglycemic disorders. *N Engl J Med* 1995;332:1144.

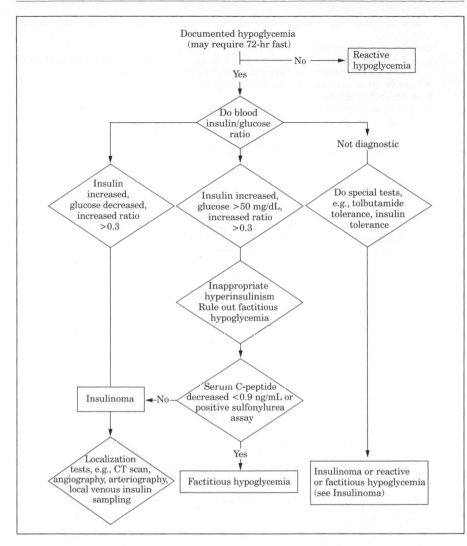

Fig. 13-9. Algorithm for diagnosis of suspected insulinoma. (CT, computed tomography.)

Hypoglycemia, Factitious

See Tables 13-12 and 13-13, Fig. 13-9.

Due To Insulin

♦ During hypoglycemic episode, high insulin and low C-peptide levels in serum confirm diagnosis of exogenous insulin administration (diagnostic triad). (Increased endogenous insulin secretion is always associated with increased C-peptide secretion, which is the part of the proinsulin molecule cleaved off when insulin is secreted and therefore is produced in equimolar amounts with insulin.)

Insulin:glucose ratio >0.3 in serum (normal is <0.3). Increased ratio is also seen in autonomous production due to insulinoma.

♦ Extreme elevations of serum insulin (e.g., >1,000 μU/mL) suggest factitious hypoglycemia (fasting levels in patients with insulinoma rarely >200 μU/mL).

Insulin antibodies appear in 90% of persons injected with beef or pork insulin and 50% of those injected with human insulin for more than a few weeks but are almost never present in persons not taking insulin (rarely occurs on an autoimmune basis), although this may be less useful with the future use of more purified and human insulin.

Due To Sulfonylureas

Biochemically indistinguishable from insulinoma (increased serum C-peptide and insulin levels with insulin: C-peptide molar ratio <1.0).

♦ Specific chemical assay can identify the agent in serum or urine.

Due To Tolbutamide

Acidification of urine causes a white precipitate due to formation of carboxytolbutamide.

Hypoglycemia, Infants and Children

♦ **Diagnostic Criteria**

Plasma glucose <25 mg/dL in low-birth-weight infants

Plasma glucose <35 mg/dL in full-sized-birth-weight infants in first 72 hrs.
    Plasma glucose <45 mg/dL in full-sized-birth-weight infants after 72 hrs.

Make diagnosis on basis of 2 abnormal glucose values, e.g., 2 blood levels, 1 plasma and 1 CSF level.

• Plasma glucose values are 14% higher than whole blood.
• Take capillary blood samples from warm heel, bring to lab on ice (glucose level decreases 18 mg/dL/hr at room temperature).
• Do not be use bedside glucose monitors that are not reliable in low glucose range. Use techniques that measure glucose specifically (e.g., glucose oxidase).

Due To

Transient (<14 days) (symptomatic or asymptomatic); occurs 1 to 3 in 1,000 full-term infants

• Maternal (e.g., diabetes, toxemia, complicated labor or delivery)
• Infant, e.g., Beckwith-Wiedemann syndrome (loss of maternal chromosome 11p15) (children also have Wilms and other embryonal tumors, macroglossia, umbilical hernia, gigantism that may be unilateral, facial changes, etc). Symptomatic hypoglycemia in ≤50% of patients within 1 to 3 days; may be severe, difficult to control, and last for several months.

Prematurity, small size for gestational age
Intrauterine malnutrition
Erythroblastosis
Secondary, e.g., sepsis, asphyxia, anoxia, cerebral or subdural hemorrhage
Congenital anomalies
Iatrogenic, e.g., abrupt cessation of glucose infusion, after exchange transfusion
    Leucine induced (symptoms within 30 minutes of high-protein meal or after prolonged fast). May be neonatal or appear later in first year; symptoms become increasingly severe; tends to improve spontaneously by 4 to 6 years of age. Blood glucose falls >50% within 20 to 45 minutes after oral administration of L-leucine. *Same result in 70% of patients with insulinoma.*

Persistent

Hyperinsulinism

• Focal β-cell hyperplasia
• Diffuse β-cell hyperplasia (nesidioblastosis)
• Islet-cell adenoma
• Teratoma

Endocrine disorders

• Hypothyroidism
• Congenital adrenal hyperplasia
• Anterior pituitary hypofunction
• Decreased glucagons

Hereditary metabolic disorders

* Types I, III, VI, 0 glycogen storage diseases (GSD)
* Fructosemia
* Galactose-1-phosphate deficiency
* Maple syrup urine disease
* Galactosemia
* Propionicacidemia
* Amino acid disorders (e.g., tyrosinemia type I)
* Organic acid disorders (e.g., methylmalonic acidemia, propionic acidemia)
* Carnitine deficiency disorders (e.g., carnitine palmityl transferase deficiency)
* Disorders of fat oxidation (e.g., acyl CoA dehydrogenase deficiencies)
* Disorders of gluconeogenesis (e.g., pyruvate carboxylase deficiency)

Others

Insulin Autoimmune Syndrome

Cause is unknown but patients may be receiving drugs containing a sulfhydryl group (e.g., methimazole, pyritinol). Common in Japan. Appears to be a self-limiting condition usually lasting <1 year.

Spontaneous hypoglycemia, frequently postprandial.
High titers of low-affinity insulin autoantibodies without prior insulin administration.
Elevated serum insulin and C-peptide levels that are discordant (insulin:C-peptide molar ratio >1.0) indicate the possible presence of these antibodies. These elevations are artifactual due to effect of antibody on assay method.
May be difficult to distinguish from factitious hypoglycemia.

Endocrine-Secreting Tumors of Pancreas (Islet Cell)

Cell Type	Hormone Secreted	Tumor	% of Pancreatic Endocrine Tumors	% Malignant	% Part of Familial MEN 1	Usual location
B cell	Insulin	Insulinoma	≤75%	<10%	≤5%	Pancreas, >99%
D cell	Gastrin	Gastrinoma (Z-E syndrome)	≤25%	>50%	≤25%	Pancreas, >25%; duodenum, 75%
A cell	Glucagon	Glucagonoma	≤2%	>70%	≤20%	Pancreas, 100%
H cell	Vasoactive intestinal peptide (VIP)	VIPoma	≤5%	>50%	6%	Pancreas, >90%
D cell	Somatostatin	Somatostatin-oma	<1%	>50%	45%	Pancreas, >55; duodenum, jejunum, 44%
HPP cell	Human pancreatic polypeptide (HPP)	HPP-secreting tumor	<1%			
Argentaffin cell		Carcinoid	<1%	90%	Rare	Foregut, ≤33%; midgut, ≤87%; hindgut, ≤8%; unknown, ≤15%

Other rare (<1% incidence) endocrine-secreting tumors have been identified as causing ectopic ACTH syndrome, atypical carcinoid syndrome, syndrome of inappropriate secretion of antidiuretic hormone (SIADH), ectopic hypercalcemia syndrome, etc.

Table 13-16. Comparison of Laboratory Findings in Causes of Hypoglycemia

	Insulinoma	Factitious — Exogenous Insulin	Factitious — Sulfonylurea	Factitious — Insulin Autoimmune Syndrome
Serum Insulin	High; usually <200 μU/mL Occasionally very low because serum has a very high proinsulin level that interferes with the insulin assay	Very high; often ≤2,000 μU/mL	High	High
Serum C-peptide	Increased endogenous insulin secretion is always associated with increased C-peptide	During hypoglycemic episode, high insulin and low C-peptide levels in serum confirm diagnosis of exogenous insulin administration	N or L	
Serum Insulin/C-peptide ratio			Absent	Very high levels, fall rapidly
Insulin antibodies	Absent	In 90% of persons injected with beef or pork insulin and 50% of those injected with human insulin for more than a few weeks but are almost never present in persons not taking insulin (rarely occurs on an autoimmune basis), although this may be less useful with the future use of more purified and human insulin		
Serum proinsulin*	I in ~95% of cases	N or L	I	
Insulin-glucose ratio	>0.3 in serum (normal is <0.3) Increased ratio is also seen in autonomous production due to insulinoma			
Other	Fasting provokes hypoglycemia Infusion of fish insulin (not measured by assay for human insulin) does not suppress serum insulin in patients with insulinoma but does in normal persons		Demonstration of sulfonylurea or tolbutamide in urine	Other autoimmune syndromes may be present May be receiving drugs containing sulfhydryl groups

N, normal; I, increased; L, low.
*Serum proinsulin is ≤20% of total insulin in normal persons.

Insulinoma

Insulin-secreting tumor of pancreatic islet beta-cell origin; most often benign solitary tumor but ~5% are malignant; 5% to 10% may have MEN I.

See Fig. 13-9, Tables 13-15 and 13-17.

♦ *In patients with fasting hypoglycemia, insulinoma should be considered the cause until another diagnosis can be proved.* No single test is certain to be diagnostic; multiple tests may be required.

♦ Fasting 24 to 36 hours will provoke hypoglycemia in 80% to 90% of these patients; 72 hours of fasting will provoke hypoglycemia in >95% of these patients, especially if punctuated with exercise. Absence of ketonuria implies surreptitious food intake or excess insulin effect (differentiate by blood glucose level). Low serum glucose and high serum insulin establish the diagnosis, i.e., insulin level is inappropriately elevated for the degree of hypoglycemia (in normal persons, insulin level becomes <5 µU/mL or undetectable). *Serum insulin rarely reaches these high levels in patients with reactive hypoglycemia.* Serum C-peptide is similarly inappropriately elevated, in contrast to factitious hypoglycemia. In women, serum glucose during fasting can fall to 20–30 mg/dL and return to normal without treatment; in men, a fall in serum glucose to <50 mg/dL is considered abnormal.

♦ Serum insulin/C-peptide ratio <1.0 in molarity units

♦ Proinsulin level is normally ≤20% of total insulin; increased in insulinoma.

♦ Proinsulin >30% of serum insulin after overnight fast suggests insulinoma. (May also be increased in renal disease.) *(Proinsulin is included in the immunoassay of total insulin and separation requires special technique.)*

♦ Serum insulin:glucose ratio >0.3 when serum glucose >50 mg/dL indicates inappropriate hyperinsulinism, and this usually indicates insulinoma if factitious hypoglycemia is ruled out. Ratio may be slightly higher (e.g., ≤0.35 in obese persons). Has no diagnostic value in insulinoma. Intraoperative immunochemiluminescent assay for insulin can give results within 15 mins; useful for determining completeness of excision since multiple insulinomas occur ≤24% of time and in MEN I, ≤40% are malignant. Insulin:glucose ratio ≤0.4 with normal insulin level predicts successful removal with accuracy = 89%.[8]

♦ Hypoglycemia with markedly increased insulin, C-peptide, and proinsulin strongly indicates insulin-secreting insulinoma.

Serum insulin values are not useful in reactive hypoglycemia but should always be performed in cases of fasting hypoglycemia.

Occasional patients with insulinoma have very low serum insulin levels; their serum shows very high proinsulin level that interferes with the insulin immunoassay giving falsely low values.

Stimulation tests are usually not necessary and may be dangerous if serum glucose <50 mg/dL. Too many false-positive and false-negative results make these tests unreliable.

• Tolbutamide tolerance test
• Glucagon stimulation test: Administer 1 mg of glucagon IV during 1 to 2 minutes; measure serum insulin three times at 5-minute intervals and then twice at 15-minute intervals. Patients with insulinoma show an exaggerated response of serum immunoreactive insulin. Serum insulin >100 µU/mL after glucagon stimulation in a patient with fasting hypoglycemia and inappropriate insulin secretion strongly suggests insulinoma.
• Infusion of exogenous insulin to reduce serum glucose level will also suppress the secretion of insulin and of C-peptide in normal persons but not in patients with insulinoma. C-peptide level usually remains elevated if insulinoma is present (C-peptide is also not suppressed in islet cell hyperplasia and nesidioblastosis) but falls to very low level if beta-cell function is normal.

OGTT is useless for diagnosis; may be normal, flat (in ~20% of normal persons), or show impaired tolerance.

Following overnight fast, reference ranges are

• Serum insulin: 1 to 25 µU/mL
• Serum proinsulin: <20% of total measurable insulin

---

[8]Carneiro DM, et al. Rapid insulin assay for intraoperative confirmation of complete resection of insulinomas. *Surgery* 2002;132:937.

Table 13-17. Comparison of Laboratory Findings in Causes of Hypoglycemia

	Insulinoma	Factitious — Exogenous Insulin	Factitious — Sulfonylurea	Insulin Autoimmune Syndrome
Serum insulin	High; usually <200 μU/mL Occasionally very low because serum has a very high proinsulin level that interferes with the insulin immunoassay	Very high; often up to 2,000 μU/mL	High	High
Serum C-peptide	Inappropriate I; parallels serum insulin Insulin infusion suppresses the C-peptide levels in normal case but not in insulinoma	Not I; does not parallel serum insulin	N or L	Disproportionately not as high as serum insulin indicates the possible presence of these antibodies >1.0 in molarity units
Serum insulin/C-peptide ratio during hypoglycemia	>1.0 in molarity units (or <47.17 μU/ng in conventional units)	<1.0 in molarity units		
Insulin antibodies	Absent	Present after using beef or pork insulin for more than a few weeks Species-specific for beef or pork insulin Present in 50% after using human insulin	Absent	Very high levels, fall rapidly
Serum proinsulin (is ≤20% of total insulin in normal persons)	I in ~95% of cases	N or L	I	
Other	Fasting provokes hypoglycemia Infusion of fish insulin (not measured by assay for human insulin) does not suppress serum insulin in insulinoma but does in normal persons		Demonstration of sulfonylurea or tolbutamide in urine	Other autoimmune syndromes may be present May be receiving drugs containing sulfhydryl groups

- Serum C-peptide: 1 to 2 ng/mL
- Insulin:glucose ratio: <0.3 (up to 0.35 in obese persons). During fasting, ratio decreases in healthy persons and increases in insulinoma patients.

Glucagonoma

Rare tumors that arise from α-cells of pancreatic islets; 60% are malignant. Proglucagon is normally synthesized by α-cells of pancreatic islets and L cells of distal small bowel. Pancreatic glucagon stimulates glucose production; intestinal glucagonlike peptide stimulates insulin production in response to a meal.

Mild DM
Anemia
♦ Increased serum insulin level is characteristic.
♦ Increased serum level of glucagon; is rarely measured clinically. Serum proglucagon is also increased occasionally.
○ Clinical clue is association of dermatitis (necrolytic migratory erythema) with insulin-requiring diabetes.

Glucagon Increased In
Glucagonoma: usually >120 pg/mL but can be 900 to 7,800 pg/mL.
Mild increase in DM, Cushing syndrome, acromegaly, various neuroendocrine tumors, cirrhosis, pancreatitis, renal insufficiency, familial hyperglucagonemia (autosomal dominant disorder with increased glucagon not owning to tumor).

Somatostatinoma

Rare tumors that secrete high levels of somatostatin. Normally somatostatin is secreted by delta-cells of pancreas and inhibits hormone secretion by pituitary (GH and thyrotropin), pancreatic (insulin, glucagon), GI (gastrin, secretin, VIP). Also inhibits gastric emptying and acid secretion and release of pancreatic enzymes.

DM that improves after resection of the tumor
Hypochlorhydria
Steatorrhea
Anemia is occasionally present.

Somatostatin Increased In
Somatostatinoma
Medullary thyroid cancer
Pheochromocytoma
Small-cell cancer of lung

VIPoma (*V*asoactive *I*ntestinal *P*olypeptide-Secreting Tumor)

Secreted by rare tumors of specialized endocrine cells of the amine precursor uptake and decarboxylation (ADUP) system that inhibit gastric acid production and stimulate gastrointestinal secretion of water and electrolytes; most tumors are found in pancreas but ~30% are extrapancreatic (e.g., bronchogenic carcinoma, pheochromocytoma, ganglioneuroblastoma [20%]). Sixty percent are malignant.

♦ Increased plasma vasoactive intestinal polypeptide (VIP), >75 pg/mL. RIA may show cross-reactivity with other gastrointestinal hormones. (Should be collected in special chilled syringe containing EDTA and a plasma protease inhibitor and frozen immediately after centrifugation.) Specificity $>88\%$ and positive predictive value ~86% (varies between laboratories). Increased values may also occur in patients with cutaneous mastocytoma, severe hepatic failure, or portacaval shunts.
♦ Voluminous watery diarrhea (700 mL/day; 70% secrete >3 L/day) with dehydration
Hypokalemia that may be associated with hypokalemic nephropathy
Metabolic acidosis
Hypercalcemia in 50% of cases
Achlorhydria or hypochlorhydria

Table 13-18.	Serum Gastrin Response to Provocative Tests in Hypergastrinemia		
Cause	Secretin Injection	Calcium Infusion	Test Meal
Gastrinoma (Z-E syndrome)	I >200 pg/mL (95 pM) over basal	I >400 pg/mL (190 pM) over basal	I <50% over basal or NC
Hypochlorhydric states	I <200 pg/mL, D, or NC	Small I or NC	I <50% over basal or NC
Antral–G cell hyperplasia	I <200 pg/mL	Small I or NC	I >100% over basal
Ordinary duodenal cancer	I <200 pg/mL	Small I	Moderate I
Others (e.g., excluded gastric antrum, gastric outlet obstruction, small intestine resection, thyrotoxicosis)	1 <200 pg/mL, D or NC	Small I or NC	I >50% over basal

D = decrease; I = increase; NC = no change.

Zollinger-Ellison (Z-E) Syndrome (Gastrinoma)[9]

Disorder of autonomous gastric acid hypersecretion caused by gastrin-secreting tumor (non-β-cell tumors often arising in pancreas).

See Table 13-18.

Due To

- *Tumors are multiple* in 28% of patients and may be ectopic (e.g., ≤40% are in duodenal wall; 9% are extrapancreatic and extraintestinal (bone, liver, ovary, stomach, lymph nodes; selective venous sampling for gastrin may be helpful for localizing tumor).
- *Tumors are malignant* in 50% of patients; 34% of patients have metastases.
- *Diffuse hyperplasia* occurs in 10% of patients.

Condition	Serum Gastrin	Serum Gastrin after Intragastric Administration of 0.1N HCl
Peptic ulcer without Z-E syndrome	Normal range	—
Z-E syndrome	Very high	No change
Pernicious anemia	High level may approach that in Z-E syndrome	Marked decrease

◆ Increased basal serum gastrin; normal levels = 0 to 200 pg/mL serum

- Fasting serum gastrin >1,000 pg/mL and basal acid output >15 mEq/hourr with recurrent peptic ulcer is virtually diagnostic.
- Increased levels >500 pg/mL are highly suggestive for gastrinoma in absence of achlorhydria or renal failure.
- 100 to 500 pg/mL occurs in ~40% of gastrinoma patients and ~10% of ulcer patients without gastrinoma. If fasting serum gastrin is increased, but <1,000 pg/mL, secretin-provocative test and acid secretory rate should be performed.
- <100 pg/mL is unlikely to be gastrinoma.

Provocative Tests:

◆ *Secretin* (2 mg/kg body weight IV) with blood specimens drawn before and at intervals.

---

[9]Jensen RT, Fraker DL. Zollinger-Ellison syndrome. Advances in treatment of gastric hypersecretion and the gastrinoma. *JAMA* 1994;271:1429.

ENDOCRINE

- Is the preferred first provocative test because of greater sensitivity and simplicity. Is most accurate provocative test.
- Patients with Z-E syndrome show 200 pg/mL increased serum gastrin within 15 minutes in 90% of cases, peaks in 45 to 60 minutes (usually >400 pg/mL). With fasting gastrin <1000 pg/mL, sensitivity = 85% for an increased serum gastrin >200 pg/mL.
- Normal persons and patients with duodenal ulcer show no increase in serum gastrin. Serum gastrin decreases in most nongastrinoma patients. Some ulcer patients may increase serum gastrin ≤200 pg/mL.
- With other causes of hypergastrinemia associated with hyperchlorhydria (e.g., retained antrum syndrome, gastric outlet obstruction, small bowel resection, renal insufficiency), serum gastrin is unchanged or decreases.
- Selective injection of secretin into gastroduodenal artery causes serum gastrin to increase >50% in 30 seconds in hepatic or portal vein blood (both should be sampled).
- Postoperative fasting serum gastrin and secretin are both necessary to determine cure.
- Calcium gluconate or a standard test meal is not as sensitive or specific as secretin test.

Calcium gluconate (5 mg/kg body weight/hour IV for 3 hourrs) with preinfusion blood specimen compared to specimens every 30 minutes for up to 4 hours.

- Reserved for when secretin test is negative in patients suspicious for Z-E syndrome.
- Normal patients and those with ordinary duodenal ulcer show minimal serum gastrin response to calcium.
- Z-E syndrome patients show increase in serum gastrin >400 pg/mL in 3 hours in 80% of cases. Many false-positive results; adverse effects due to systemic hypercalcemia. Positive in one third of patients with a negative secretin test.[10]
- Patients with antral G-cell hyperfunction may or may not increase serum gastrin >400 pg/mL.

Insulin Test Meal

Aspirate gastric fluid and measure gastric acid every 15 minutes for 2 hours after IV administration of sufficient insulin (usually 15–20 units) to produce blood sugar <50 mg/dL.

Use
Differentiate causes of hypergastrinemia (see Table 13-17)
Supplanted by other tests; formerly used to
  Aid in distinguishing benign and malignant gastric ulcers
  Aid in diagnosis of pernicious anemia
  Evaluation of patients with ulcer dyspepsia but normal X-rays

Interpretation
Normal: Increased free HCl owning to hypoglycemia
Successful vagotomy produces achlorhydria.
Indications for measurement of serum gastrin and gastric analysis include:

- Atypical peptic ulcer of stomach, duodenum, or proximal jejunum, especially if multiple, unusual location, poorly responsive to therapy, or multiple, rapid, or severe recurrence after adequate therapy
- Unexplained chronic diarrhea or steatorrhea with or without peptic ulcer
- Peptic ulcer disease with associated endocrine conditions, especially hyperthyroidism (see MEN)

Serum gastrin levels are indicated with any of the following:

- Basal acid secretion >10 mEq/hour in patients with intact stomachs
- Ratio of basal to poststimulation output >40% in patients with intact stomachs
- All patients with recurrent ulceration after surgery for duodenal ulcer
- All patients with duodenal ulcer for whom elective gastric surgery is planned
- Patients with peptic ulcer associated with severe esophagitis or prominent gastric or duodenal folds or hypercalcemia or extensive family history of peptic ulcer disease

Measurement for screening of all peptic ulcer patients would not be practical or cost effective.

[10]Frucht H, et al. Secretin and calcium provocative tests in the Zollinger-Ellison syndrome. *Ann Int Med* 1989;111:713.

Increased Serum Gastrin without Gastric Acid Hypersecretion

Atrophic gastritis, especially when associated with circulating parietal cell antibodies
Achlorhydria and hypochlorhydria with or without pernicious anemia
Some patients with carcinoma of body of stomach, a reflection of the atrophic gastritis
that is present
Gastric acid inhibitor therapy
After vagotomy

Increased Serum Gastrin with Gastric Acid Hypersecretion

Z-E syndrome
Hyperplasia of antral gastrin cells
Isolated retained antrum—a condition of gastric acid hypersecretion and recurrent
ulceration following antrectomy and gastrojejunostomy that occurs when the duodenal stump contains antral mucosa

Increased Serum Gastrin with Gastric Acid Normal or Slight Hypersecretion

Rheumatoid arthritis
DM
Pheochromocytoma
Vitiligo
Chronic renal failure with serum creatinine >3 mg/dL; occurs in 50% of patients
Pyloric obstruction with gastric distention
Short-bowel syndrome owning to massive resection or extensive regional enteritis
Incomplete vagotomy
♦ There is a large volume of highly acidic gastric juice in the absence of pyloric
obstruction. (12-hour nocturnal secretion shows acid of >100 mEq/L and volume of
>1,500 mL; baseline secretion is >60% of the secretion caused by histamine or beta-
zole stimulation.) It is refractory to vagotomy and subtotal gastrectomy.
Hypochlorhydria (basal pH >3) or achlorhydria excludes diagnosis of Z-E syndrome
(see Gastric Analysis).
♦ Basal acid output >15 mEq/hour (normal <10 mEq/hour) occurs in 90% of cases
if no previous gastric surgery was done or >5 mEq/hour if previous vagotomy or
gastric resection was done. Ratio of basal acid output:maximal output >0.6
strongly favors gastrinoma, but false-positive and false-negative results are common. If basal acid output determination is not possible, pH >3 excludes Z-E syndrome if patient is not on antisecretory drugs. Fasting serum gastrin >1,000
pg/mL and gastric pH <2.5 almost certainly indicate Z-E syndrome; both should
be measured because there may be a poor correlation between them in individual
patients.
Hypokalemia is frequently associated with chronic severe diarrhea, which may be a
clue to this diagnosis.
Serum albumin may be decreased.
Steatorrhea occurs rarely due to low pH produced in intestine.
High-output secretory diarrhea occurs in ~50% of patients.
Laboratory findings owning to peptic ulcer (present in 70% of patients) of stomach,
duodenum, or proximal jejunum (e.g., perforation, fluid loss, hemorrhage) are noted.
♦ *Clues to Z-E syndrome are ulcers in unusual locations or giant or multiple ulcerations (25% of these patients), rapid or severe recurrence of ulcer after adequate therapy, recurrent ulcer after surgery, prominent gastric folds, gastric acid hypersecretion with hypergastrinemia, family history of peptic ulcer or ulcers with other
endocrine disorders, duodenal ulcers without H. pylori. Also high-output secretory
diarrhea.*
♦ *MEN-I should be ruled out in all patients with Z-E syndrome, which may be the initial manifestation of MEN-I. Twenty-five percent of cases of Z-E syndrome are associated with MEN-I. Forty percent to 60% of cases of MEN-I have Z-E syndrome.
Thirteen percent of patients with Z-E syndrome and MEN-I develop gastric carcinoid
tumors.*
Gastrinomas may produce other peptides (e.g., somatostatin, pancreatic polypeptide,
ACTH, VIP)
Ultrasonography, angiography, CT scan, and MRI are normal in 50% of patients.

Laboratory Tests for Evaluation of Adrenal-Pituitary-Hypothalamus Function

Complete 24-hour urine collections may be difficult to obtain in some patients.

Plasma samples are simple to obtain but are altered by diurnal variation, episodic pulsatile secretion, renal and metabolic clearance, stress, protein binding, and effect of drugs. Therefore abnormal screening tests must be confirmed by tests that stimulate or suppress the pituitary adrenal axis.

Increased function is tested by suppression tests and decreased function is tested by stimulatory tests.

Cortisol measurements have largely replaced other steroid determinations in diagnosis of Cushing syndrome.

ACTH Stimulation (Cosyntropin) Test[11]

Cosyntropin is a potent synthetic rapid stimulator of cortisol and aldosterone secretion.

Use

Initial test to distinguish primary from secondary adrenal insufficiency.
Not helpful in diagnosis of Cushing syndrome.

Rapid Screening Test

Administer 0.25 mg of synthetic ACTH (cosyntropin) IM or IV and measure baseline, 30-min, and 60-min plasma cortisol levels. If response is not normal, perform long test (see below).

Interpretation

Normal: Baseline plasma cortisol >5.0 $\mu g/dL$ with increase to $2\times$ baseline level ≥ 20 $\mu g/dL$ is sufficient single criterion of normal adrenal function to preclude need for further workup; 60 level can be omitted. Less than 5.0 $\mu g/dL$ indicates primary or secondary adrenal insufficiency.

Addison disease: Is ruled out by a positive response

Hypopituitarism: A slight increase is shown the first day and a greater increase the next day

Adrenal carcinoma: Little or no response; marked increase in urine 17-KS

Adrenal hyperplasia increases $3\times$ to $5\times$ baseline level.

Long Test

Daily infusion of ACTH for 5 days, with before and after measurement of serum cortisol, 24-hour urines for cortisol. (Protect possible Addison disease patient against adrenal crisis with 1 mg of dexamethasone.)

Interpretation

Long ACTH stimulation test is necessary for diagnosis of secondary adrenal insufficiency.

Normal: At least $3\times$ increase with maximum above upper reference value

Complete primary adrenal insufficiency (Addison disease): No increase in urine steroids or increase of <2 mg/day

Incomplete primary adrenal insufficiency: Less than normal increases on all 5 days or slight increase on first 3 days that may be followed by decrease on days 4 and 5

Secondary adrenal insufficiency (Owning to pituitary hypofunction): "Staircase" response of progressively higher values each day (delayed but normal response)

♦ Metyrapone inhibition test is performed if ACTH test causes some increase in blood cortisol

Cortisol treatment interferes with all of the above tests and must be discontinued for prior 24 to 48 hours. Dexamethasone will interfere with metyrapone test and plasma ACTH levels.

♦ Antiadrenal antibodies are found in most cases of idiopathic Addison disease and are said to rule out adrenoleukodystrophy and secondary adrenal insufficiency. Said to have very high S/S and is predictive of impending or compensated adrenocortical failure.

---

[11]Dorin RI, et al. Diagnosis of adrenal insufficiency. *Ann Int Med* 2003;139:194.

Idiopathic Addison disease requires ruling out tumor, TB, and other granulomatous diseases of adrenals.

Serum potassium is increased; may be low in secondary adrenal insufficiency.

Serum sodium and chloride are decreased. Sodium:potassium ratio is <30:1.

BUN and creatinine may be moderately increased; may be decreased in secondary adrenal insufficiency.

Fasting hypoglycemia is present.

Neutropenia and relative lymphocytosis are common.

Eosinophilia is present (300/cu mm). *(A total eosinophil count of <50 is evidence against severe adrenocortical hypofunction.)*

Normocytic anemia is slight or moderate but difficult to estimate because of decreased blood volume.

Hct level is increased because of water loss.

Aldosterone, Plasma/Serum

Primary mineralocorticoid secreted by adrenal zona glomerulosa.

Use
Diagnosis of primary hyperaldosteronism
Differential diagnosis of fluid and electrolyte disorders
Assessment of adrenal aldosterone production

Increased In
Primary aldosteronism
Secondary aldosteronism
Barter syndrome
Pregnancy
Very-low-sodium diet
Urine aldosterone is also increased in nephrosis.

Decreased In
Hyporeninemic hypoaldosteronism
Congenital adrenal hyperplasia (CAH)
Congenital deficiency of aldosterone synthetase
Addison disease
Very-high-sodium diet

Androstenedione, Serum

A major adrenal androgen in serum; also produced by testes and ovaries.

Use
Diagnosis of virilism and hirsutism

Increased In
CAH owning to 21-hydroxylase deficiency; marked increase is suppressed to normal levels by adequate glucocorticoid therapy. Suppressed level reflects adequacy of therapeutic control. May be better than 17-hydroxyprogesterone for monitoring therapy because it shows minimal diurnal variation, better correlation with urinary 17-KS excretion, and plasma levels are not immediately affected by a dose of glucocorticoid.
Adrenal tumors
Cushing disease
Polycystic ovarian disease

Decreased In
Addison disease

Dehydroepiandrosterone Sulfate (DHEA-S), Serum

Produced by androgenic zone of adrenal cortex.

Use
Indicator of adrenal cortical function, especially for differential diagnosis of virilization.
Differential diagnosis of Cushing syndrome.
Replaces 17-KS urine excretion with which it correlates; shows no significant diurnal variation, thereby providing rapid test for abnormal androgen secretion.

Increased In

CAH: markedly increased values can be suppressed by dexamethasone. Highest values occur in CAH due to deficiency of 3β-hydroxysteroid dehydrogenase.

Adrenal carcinoma: Markedly increased levels cannot be suppressed by dexamethasone

Cushing syndrome owning to bilateral adrenal hyperplasia shows higher values than Cushing syndrome owning to benign cortical adenoma in which values may be normal or low.

Cushing disease (pituitary etiology): Moderate increase

In hypogonadotropic hypogonadism, DHEA-S is usually normal for chronologic age and high for bone age in contrast to idiopathic delayed puberty in which DHEA-S is low relative to chronologic age and normal relative to bone age.

First few days of life, especially in sick or premature infants

Decreased In

Addison disease

Adrenal hypoplasia

Diseases of Adrenal Gland

Adrenal Adenoma, Nonfunctioning ("Incidentaloma")

Autopsy prevalence of clinically inapparent adenomas ~2.1%. Ultrasound prevalence = 0.1% in asymptomatic persons, 0.42% in nonendocrinologic patients, 4.3% in cancer patients.

To rule out functioning tumor, measure plasma potassium and aldosterone:plasma renin activity (PRA) ratio in hypertensive persons and measure free metanephrines and do 1 mg dexamethasone suppression test in all patients. 21-hydroxylase deficiency should be ruled out in these patients.

Surgery if tumor >4 to 6 cm in size

Adrenal Hyperplasia, Congenital (CAH)[12]

Family of inherited autosomal recessive errors of metabolism due to enzymatic defect in 1 of 5 enzymes responsible for cortisol synthesis. Causes cortisol deficiency and compensatory increased secretion of CRH and ACTH, which causes adrenocortical hyperplasia and hypersecretion of other pathways: mineralocorticoids (17-deoxy pathway), glucocorticoids (17-hydroxy pathway), and sex steroids. Clinical pattern of CAH depends on severity and location of enzyme defect. In United States, occurs 1:80,000 to 100,000 live births.

The most common forms are summarized in Table 13-19. The synthetic pathways are shown schematically in Figure 13-10 to illustrate the altered hormonal levels.

♦ Establish diagnoses by increase in specific precursor steroids in blood or urine that can be suppressed by administration of glucocorticoids.

♦ Finding of increased 17-OHP or androstenedione in amniotic fluid permits prenatal diagnosis.

Increased incidence of adrenal "incidentalomas" and of polycystic ovary syndrome

CAH should always be ruled out in infants with:

• Ambiguous genitalia and presence of nuclear sex chromatin
• Continued vomiting after pyloroplasty
• Siblings affected with CAH
• Salt loss

21-Hydroxylase (P450c21) Deficiency

More than 90% of cases of CAH are owning to deficiency of P450 enzyme (21-hydroxylase deficiency) attributable to mutations in gene *CYP21* and pseudogene *CYP21P* on short arm of chromosome 6; less commonly due to enzyme deficiencies noted in Figure 13-11.

[12]Speiser PW, White PC. Congenital adrenal hyperplasia. *N Engl J Med* 2003;349:776.

Table 13-19. Comparison of Different Forms of Congenital Adrenal Hyperplasia

Enzyme Deficiency	Sexual Ambiguity in Newborn Female	Sexual Ambiguity in Newborn Male	Postnatal Virilization	Hypertension	Salt-Wasting	Urine Hormone Concentrations			Blood Hormone Concentrations					
						17-KS	17-OH	Pregnanetriol	Aldosterone	17-OHP	Delta-4	DHEA	Testosterone	Renin
21-Hydroxylase														
Salt-wasting	+	0	+	0	+	II	D	II	D	II	II	N/I	I	II
Simple virilizing	+	0	+	0	0	II	N/D	II	N/I	II	II	N/I	I	N/I
Late-onset	0	0	+	0	0	I	N	I	N/I	I	I	N/I	N/I	N
11-Beta-hydroxylase[a]	+	0	+	+	0	II	II	I	D	I	II	I	I	DD
3-Beta-HSD														
Salt-wasting	+	+	+	0	+	I	DD	N/D	D	N/I	N/I	III	b	I
Non-salt-wasting	+	+	+	0	0	I	DD	N/D	N	N/I	N/I	III	b	N
Late-onset	0	?	+	0	0	N/I	N	N	N	N/I	N/I	I	N/I	N
17-Alpha-hydroxylase[a]	0	+	0	+	0	DD	DD	N	D	D	D	D	D	D
Cholesterol desmolase	0	+	0	0	+	DD	DD	N	DD	D	D	D	D	I

17-OH = 17-hydroxylase; 17-OHP = 17-hydroxyprogesterone; DHEA = dehydroepiandrosterone; I, II = degrees of increased; D, DD = degrees of decresed; 0 = none, + = present.

[a]Increased 17-deoxycortisol (corticosterone) and 11-deoxycortisol (compound B).

[b]N/D in males; N/I in females.

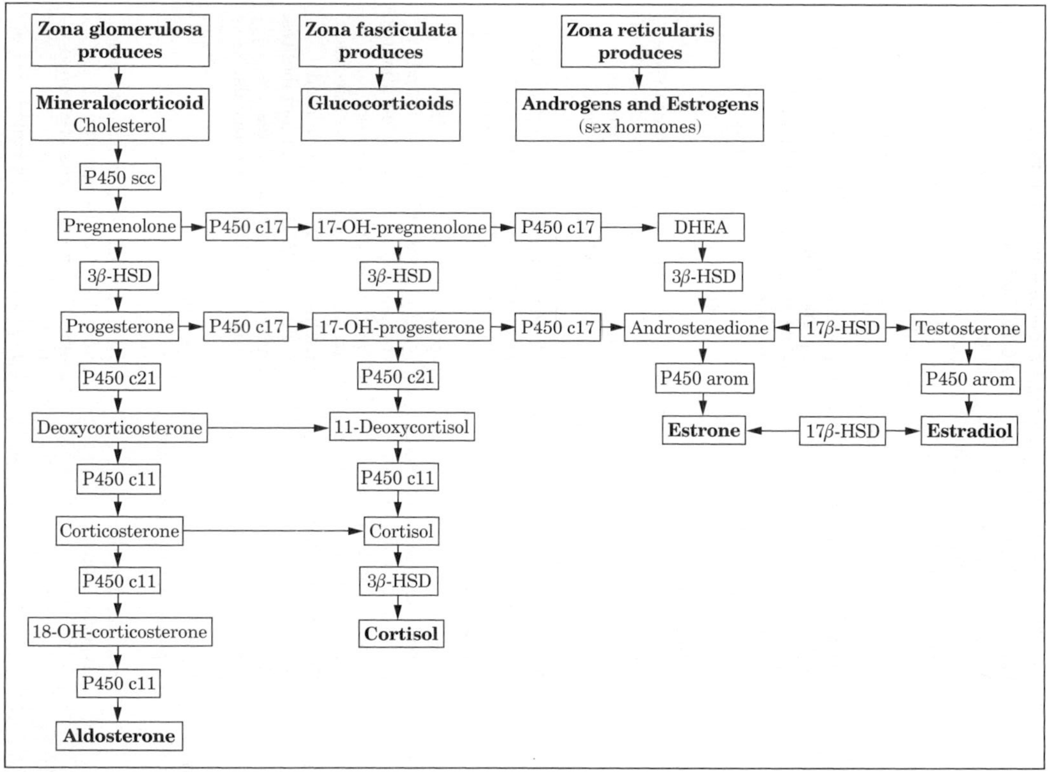

Fig. 13-10. Pathway of adrenal hormone synthesis. Hormones above the level of the deficient enzyme are present in increased amount; those below this level are decreased in amount. Shunting to other pathways may occur. Findings depend on completeness of enzyme deficiency, degree of hormone deficiency, or excessive accumulation. (DHEA, dehydroepiandrosterone; 3β-HSD, 3β-hydroxysteroid dehydrogenase; 17β-HSD, 17β-hydroxysteroid dehydrogenase. P450scc is also termed CYP11A, 20,22-desmolase, 17,20-cholesterol-desmolase. P450c11 is also termed 18-hydroxylase [CYP11B2]. P450c21 is also termed CYP21, CYP21A2, and 21-hydroxylase; is located in endoplasmic reticulum.)

Table 13-20.   Summary of Characteristics of CAH

Deficient Enzyme	Phenotype	Steroid hormones. Response to ACTH. Response to hCG.
Cholesterol desmolase (P450scc) (lipoid CAH)	Salt-wasting crisis Male pseudohermaphroditism	↑ACTH and PRA ↓ all steroid hormones; ↓/0 response to ACTH ↓/0 response to hCG in male pseudohermaphroditism
3β-HSD Classic.	Salt-wasting crisis Male and female pseudohermaphroditism Precocious puberty	↑ACTH and PRA ↑↑I baseline and ACTH-stimulated pregnenolone 17-OH- pregnenolone, DHEA and metabolites I steroids are suppressed by glucocorticoids
3β–HSD Nonclassic.	Precocious puberty Acne Hirsutism Irregular menses Infertility	↑baseline and ACTH-stimulated pregnenolone 17-OH pregnenolone, DHEA and metabolites ↑steroids are suppressed by glucocorticoids
21-OH (P450c21) Classic.	Salt-wasting crisis Female pseudohermaphroditism Postnatal virilization	↑ACTH and PRA ↑↑baseline and ACTH-stimulated 17-OH-progesterone, pregnanetriol ↑↑androgens and metabolites are suppressed by glucocorticoids
21-OH (P450c21) Nonclassic.	Precocious puberty Acne Hirsutism Irregular menses Infertility	↑baseline and ACTH-stimulated 17-OH-progesterone, pregnanetriol ↑androgens and metabolites are suppressed by glucocorticoids
11β-OH (P450c11) Classic.	Female pseudohermaphroditism Postnatal virilization in males and females Hypertension	Hypokalemia. ↑ACTH. ↓PRA. ↑↑baseline and ACTH-stimulated compound S, DOC, and metabolites. ↑↑androgens and metabolites are suppressed by glucocorticoids.
11β-OH (P450c11) Nonclassic.	Precocious puberty Acne Hirsutism Irregular menses Infertility	↑baseline and ACTH-stimulated compound S, DOC, and metabolites. ↑androgens and metabolites are suppressed by glucocorticoids.
17α-OH/17,20 lysase	Male pseudohermaphroditism Sexual infantilism Hypertension	Hypokalemia ↑ACTH D PRA ↑↑DOC, 18-OH DOC, corticosterone, and 18-OH corticosterone ↓some 17 α steroids and ↓response to ACTH ↓/0 response to hCG in male pseudohermaphroditism

↑ = increased; ↑↑ = more increased; ↓ = decreased; 0 = absent. CAH, congenital adrenal hyperplasia

Severe Deficiency, Classic Form

Complete reduction of 21-hydroxylase activity.

♦ Severe enzyme deficiency not compensated for by increased ACTH secretion; and cortisol levels are decreased.
♦ Random specimen showing markedly increased (>20×) 17-hydroxyprogesterone (17-OHP) is a diagnostic indicator (usually 10,000 ng/dL).

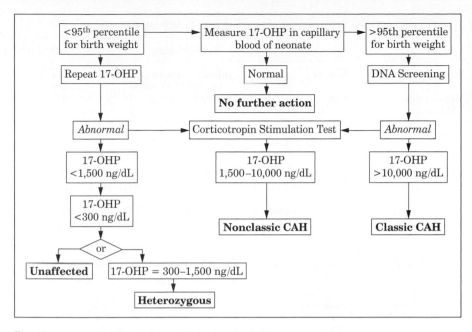

Fig. 13-11. Algorithm for newborn screening for CAH.

♦ Excess production of salt-losing steroids plus inability to secrete aldosterone causes characteristic acute adrenal crisis.
♦ Salt-wasting crisis in ~75% of patients due to inability to synthesize aldosterone; usually occurs 1 to 2 weeks after birth with hyponatremia, hyperkalemia, acidosis, severe dehydration, and shock.
♦ Increased ACTH causes hypersecretion of androgens and virilization of female external (ambiguous) genitalia but usually normal internal genitalia. Males do not show abnormal genitals at birth but may show precocious puberty at 2 to 4 years of age. Both show rapid early growth but premature closure of epiphyses causes shorter stature.
Adrenal medullary function is impaired; plasma epinephrine and metanephrine and urine epinephrine values are 40% to 80% lower.
♦ DNA analysis on fetal cells from amniotic fluid or chorionic villus detects 95% of all abnormal genes for CAH and some with nonclassical CAH.
♦ Analysis of dried blood spot samples for 17-OHP obtained at 48 to 72 hours of age is usual method for neonatal screening (normal newborns <100 ng/dL). False-negative results due to early sampling. False-positive results in sick or premature infants. Positive test requires confirmation with urine steroids or mutation analysis of *CYP21* gene.
CYP21 heterozygotes may have only slight increased 17-OHP levels after adrenal stimulation.

Moderate Deficiency (Simple Virilizing) Form
Approximately 2% reduction of 21-hydroxylase activity.

Salt wasting is mild or absent.
♦ Moderate enzyme deficiency compensated by increased ACTH secretion causing cortisol secretion close to normal and marked increase in androgens (characteristic *increase in androstenedione* and, to a lesser extent, testosterone) and cortisol precursors, some of which (progesterone, 17-OHP) cause some salt wasting; the latter causes compensatory increase in PRA and increased aldosterone secretion.
♦ Androgen ratio in urine of 11-desoxy to 11-oxy-17-KS is ~1:1 (normal adult ratio = 1:4).

Table 13-21.   Different Phenotypes of 21-Hydroxylase (P450c21) Deficiency

	Salt wasting	Simple virilizing	Nonclassic form
Age at onset	Infants	Infants (females) or children (males)	Children or adults
Aldosterone	Low	Normal	Normal
Virilization	++ to ++++	++ to ++++	0 to +

+ to ++++ = degree of severity

Urinary excretion of 17-KS and blood steroid secretion can be suppressed by dexamethasone (1.25 mg/m²/d for 7 days) which differentiates CAH from virilizing adrenal tumors.

Normal or low cortisol levels show little or no response to ACTH administration.

Karyotype should be done to establish genetic sex whenever ambiguous external genitalia are present.

Mild Deficiency (Attenuated; Late Onset) (Nonclassic) Form

At puberty, females show hirsutism and oligomenorrhea; must be differentiated from polycystic ovary syndrome.

♦ Increased 17-OHP: Extreme increase in salt-wasting form of 21-hydroxylase deficiency (20–500× normal; often >25,000 ng/dL) is usually diagnostic; 24-hr urinary metabolite (pregnanetriol) is also increased. Not as increased in simple virilizing form. In mild deficiency, enzyme block is evident only after ACTH stimulation: Excessive rise (5–10×) of 17-OHP 30 or 60 minutes after administration of ACTH (cosyntropin) 0.25–1.0 mg IV or 6 hrs after 0.40 mg IV; (normal <900 ng/dL; late-onset form >2,000 ng/dL; severe form >16,000 ng/dL). Response of exaggerated increase of 17-OHP is used to identify carriers.

♦ Cortisol levels are usually fixed and unresponsive.

♦ Excess adrenal androgen production (e.g., androstenedione, DHEA, testosterone, urinary 17-KS), which is suppressed by glucocorticoids

Aldosterone deficiency is also present in salt-wasting form, but not in simple virilizing form; increased in both forms.

In nonclassical forms (10%–75% reduction of 21-hydroxylase activity) same biochemical pattern occurs (with lower levels) but symptoms of virilization, abnormal growth and puberty, infertility, etc., may be slight or absent.

17-OHP and Δ⁴ levels are used to monitor glucocorticoid therapy by reduction to normal.

♦ Genetic testing and prenatal diagnosis is available.

♦ Neonatal screening shows increased 17-OHP in dried filter paper blood spot. False-positive results may occur due to prematurity and low birth weight, illness, <24 hours old.

11-β-Hydroxylase Deficiency

Causes <3% of cases CAH; excess mineralocorticoids cause hypertension, which may not appear until adulthood; excess androgen causes female pseudohermaphrodites at birth, postnatal virilism in males and females; males with mild form may have only hypertension or gynecomastia.

♦ Increased serum deoxycorticosterone (DOC) causing hypokalemia and suppression of rennin and aldosterone.

♦ Increased 11-deoxycortisol and 17-OHP and increase of their metabolites in urine: tetrahydrodeoxycorticosterone and tetrahydro-11-deoxycortisol.

PRA levels can be used to monitor therapy.

Glucocorticoid therapy returns DOC to normal.

3-β-Hydroxysteroid Dehydrogenase (3-β-HSD) Deficiency

Rare autosomal recessive; complete deficiency causes death.

♦ Impaired secretion with decrease of cortisol, aldosterone, androstenedione, and sex steroids

ENDOCRINE

♦ Increased plasma 17-hydroxypregnenolone, pregnenolone, dehydroepiandrosterone (DHEA), increased ratio of Δ^5 (pregnenolone, 17-hydroxypregnenolone, DHEA) to Δ^4 (progesterone, 17-OHP, Δ^4-androstenedione) causing mild virilization

17-α-Hydroxylase Deficiency

♦ Decreased serum 17-hydroxylated steroids and androgens
♦ Increased serum corticosterone and deoxycorticosterone and their urinary metabolites in urine, causing hypertension, hypokalemia
♦ Decreased aldosterone and PRA; PRA levels can be used to monitor therapy

Cholesterol Desmolase (P450 scc) Deficiency

Due to defective regulatory protein. Complete deficiency incompatible with life. Mild condition in females may cause short stature, virilization, irregular menses, infertility. Males may show short stature, infertility. Early diagnosis and therapy may prevent this. Ambiguous or female genitalia in male children.

♦ Virtually no steroids (cortisol, aldosterone, androgens) are produced.
♦ Very low urine cortisol is not increased by ACTH stimulation.
♦ Aldosterone is very low in plasma and urine.
♦ Hyponatremia, hyperkalemia, rapid dehydration, shock, and early death if not recognized at birth.

Corticosterone Methyloxidase (P450 c18) Deficiency

Type I

• Hyponatremia and hyperkalemia
• Decreased aldosterone and 18-hydroxycorticosterone (18-OHB)
• Increased corticosterone

Type II

• Ratio of urinary metabolites of 18-OHB to aldosterone is markedly increased (normal is <3.0); is a better marker than 18-OHB levels.

17-β-HSD (P450c11) Deficiency

♦ Increased Δ^4-testosterone ratios in peripheral and spermatic blood is diagnostic.
During First Week of Life

• Urine total 17-KS in normal infants may be as high as in CAH due to maternal steroids. Normally falls to <1 mg/24 hours during second week of life; therefore should do serial determinations in suspected cases. Level <1 mg/24 hours rules out CAH; an increasing level suggests CAH but a decreasing level does not rule out CAH. Is increased in all virilizing forms except lipoid type.
• 17-OHP is the most valuable test in 21-hydroxylase or 11-hydroxylase deficiency.
• Detectable amounts of pregnanetriol in urine or plasma after first week of life is usually diagnostic of CAH, but in some patients this may not appear until >1 month old.

Adrenocortical Insufficiency

See Table 13-22 and Figs. 13-12, 13-13.

Acute

• Primary (e.g., Waterhouse-Friderichsen syndrome [hemorrhagic necrosis] due to anticoagulant therapy, coagulopathy, antiphospholipid syndrome, sepsis [especially meningococcemia], postoperative state)
• Secondary to pituitary or hypothalamic disorders
• Following cessation of prolonged steroid therapy

♦ Blood cortisol is markedly decreased (<5 μg/dL).
Dehydration
Azotemia is due to dehydration and shock affecting renal function.

Table 13-22.   Laboratory Differentiation of Primary and Secondary Adrenal Insufficiency

Test	Primary Adrenal Insufficiency	Adrenal Insufficiency Secondary to Hypopituitarism
Blood ACTH level	Increased	Decreased
Urine 17-KS and 17-OHKS after ACTH stimulation	No responsive increase	Marked "staircase" response

Serum sodium and chloride are decreased and potassium is increased in some patients. Hypoglycemia occurs regularly.

Direct eosinophil count is >50/cu mm (<50/cu mm in other kinds of shock).

Chronic (Addison Disease)

Due to destruction of >90% of steroid-secreting cortex of both adrenal glands.

Due To
Chronic

- Primary adrenocortical insufficiency may be caused by CAH or associated with hypoaldosteronism.
- Primary

   Autoimmune adrenalitis: is most common cause; diagnosed by circulating adrenal antibodies in >70% of patients; typically associated with other autoimmune conditions (e.g., Hashimoto thyroiditis, pernicious anemia)

   Granulomas (e.g., TB [second most common cause], sarcoidosis)

   Metastatic carcinoma (lung, breast, kidney, GI tract, ovary), lymphoma

   Infiltrates (e.g., amyloidosis, hemochromatosis)

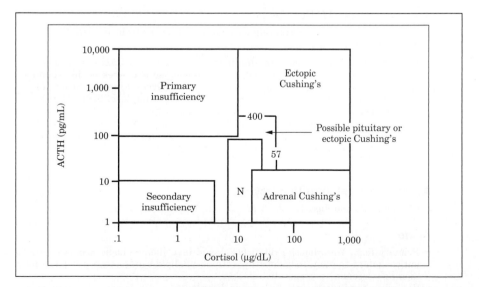

Fig. 13-12.   Adrenocorticotropic hormone (ACTH or corticotropin) and cortisol limits that are useful in diagnosis of Cushing syndrome. This figure shows the corticotropin versus cortisol area ambiguous for the differential diagnosis of pituitary-dependent and ectopic Cushing syndrome and the area diagnostic for ectopic Cushing syndrome. (NI, normal.) (From K Snow, et al. Biochemical evaluation of adrenal dysfunction. *Mayo Clinic Proc* 1992;67:1055, with permission.)

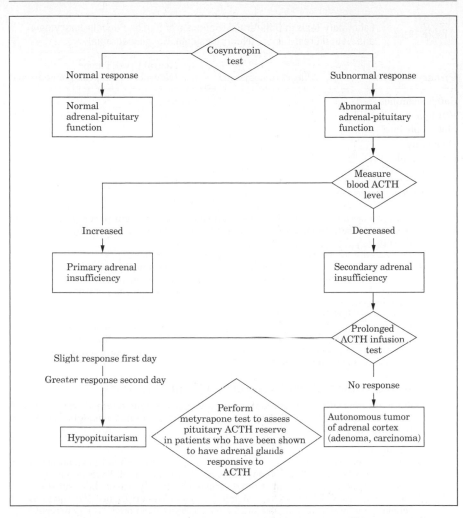

Fig. 13-13. Algorithm for diagnosis of adrenal insufficiency. (ACTH, adrenocorticotropic hormone.)

Systemic fungal infections (e.g., histoplasmosis, cryptococcosis, blastomycosis)
AIDS (e.g., opportunistic infections with CMV, bacteria, protozoa)
Adrenal hypoplasia (neonates)
Adrenoleukodystrophy
• Secondary to pituitary disease
Simmonds disease (idiopathic atrophy of pituitary)
Destruction of pituitary or hypothalamus by granulomas, tumor, etc.
May be associated with laboratory findings of hypothyroidism, hypogonadism, diabetes insipidus (DI), etc.

♦ Low supine levels at 8 AM are suggestive but not reliable. Random cortisol levels are only useful in excluding diagnosis of adrenal insufficiency if increased (>20 μg/dL).
♦ Low serum cortisol (<10 μg/dL) and marked increased ACTH is diagnostic of *primary* adrenal failure. In primary deficiency both cortisol and aldosterone are deficient with salt loss causing increased PRA; in secondary, aldosterone production is maintained but other secondary endocrine deficiencies may appear (e.g., hypothyroidism, hypogonadism).
♦ Increased blood ACTH (>150 pg/mL) with wide variation between morning and evening levels in primary adrenal hypofunction but decreased or absent ACTH in

Table 13-23.	Laboratory Tests in Differential Diagnosis of Benign Pheochromocytoma and Neural Crest Tumors (Neuroblastoma, Ganglioneuroma)	
Urinary Levels of	Pheochromocytoma	Neural Crest Tumor (Neuroblastoma, Ganglioneuroma)
Catecholamines	I	I
Vanillylmandelic acid	I	I
Metanephrines	I	I
Dopamine	N*	I
Homovanillic acid	N*	I

I = increased; N = normal.
*I in malignant pheochromocytoma.

pituitary (secondary) hypoadrenalism. Normal value rules out primary but not mild secondary insufficiency. Increased ACTH level is quickly suppressed by replacement therapy.
♦ Decreased ACTH with low cortisol indicates ACTH deficiency.
♦ Decreased blood cortisol (<5 μg/dL in 8 AM–10 AM specimen) is useful screening test. High or high-normal result excludes both primary and secondary adrenocortical insufficiency. Less than 3 μg/dL is said to indicate adrenal insufficiency and obviate need for further testing.
Borderline result is indication for ACTH stimulation test.
○ Hyponatremia (88% of cases), hyperkalemia (64% of cases), anemia (40% of cases) occur.
Monitor adequate steroid replacement therapy with serum sodium and AM plasma ACTH (for glucocorticoid replacement); monitor serum potassium and PRA (for mineral corticoid replacement).

Neuroblastoma, Ganglioneuroma, Ganglioblastoma

Malignant tumor arising in adrenal medulla or sympathetic chain. Seventy percent have metastases at time of diagnosis. Second most common malignant tumor in patients <3 yrs of age.

See Table 13-23.
♦ Urinary concentrations of catecholamines (norepinephrine, normetanephrine, dopamine, VMA, and HVA [homovanillic acid]) are increased. Excretion of epinephrine is not increased because of rapid catabolism. If only one of these substances is measured, only ~75% of cases are diagnosed. If VMA and HVA, or VMA and total catecholamines, are measured, 95% to 100% of cases are diagnosed. Ninety percent have increased HVA and ~75% have increased VMA at time of diagnosis.
Screening for catecholamines at age 6 months is said to detect neuroblastoma.
♦ These tests are also useful for differentiating Ewing tumor from metastatic neuroblastoma of bone and to show response to therapy (surgery, irradiation, or chemotherapy), which should return to normal in 1 to 4 months. Continued increase indicates need for further treatment.
♦ Increased plasma chromogranin A has S/S = 91%/100%. Correlated with tumor mass and response to treatment, survival.[13]
Cystathionine in urine suggests active disease but absence is not significant since it is not normally present.
Serum neuron–specific enolase may be increased in neuroblastoma; high level is associated with poor prognosis. Ratio of neuron-specific to non-neuronal enolase is reported to improve specificity to >85% for neuroblastoma.
Laboratory findings owning to metastases (e.g., anemia, tumor in biopsy of marrow, liver, etc.)

Pheochromocytoma

Tumor of chromaffin cells of sympathetic nervous system; may secrete catecholamines [epinephrine, norepinephrine, dopamine] and, uncommonly, ACTH

[13]Taupenot L, Harper KL, O'Connor DT. The Chromogranin-secretogranin Family. *N Engl J Med* 2003; 349:1134.

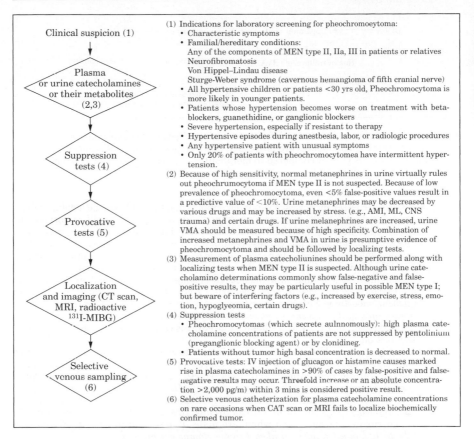

Fig. 13-14. Algorithm for diagnosis of pheochromocytoma. (MEA, multiple endocrine neoplasia; MI, myocardial infarction; MAO, monoamine oxidase; VMA, vanillylmandelic acid.)

and somatostatin. Occurs in 0.5% of hypertensive population of United States. Five percent of patients with pheochromocytoma have normal blood pressure most or all of the time. Sustained hypertension in 50% of cases.

See Figs. 13-14, 13-15, and Tables 13-23, 13-24.
♦ Diagnosis is best based on plasma free (unconjugated) metanephrines and normetanephrines by HPLC as the initial test. If both metabolites are normal (<61 ng/L; <0.31 nmol/L), tumor is highly unlikely. Metanephrine is the most sensitive of the metabolites for diagnosis because it is independent of episodic secretion, less likely to suffer from interferences, and close enough to 100% probability to not require confirmatory biochemical tests. Magnitude of increase above normal is related to tumor burden. Blood is drawn in the unstressed supine patient after an overnight fast, without interfering substances (e.g., caffeine, nicotine, acetaminophen, tricyclic antidepressants, alcohol). At 0.31 nmol/L, S/S = 99%/89%; at 1.20 nmol/L (adjusted for 100% specificity), sensitivity = 79%.[14-17] 4× URL of either metabolite is diagnostic. Most often test results are equivocal requiring a confirmatory test.

[14]Singh RJ. Advances in metanephrine testing for the diagnosis of pheochromocytoma. *Clin Lab Med* 2004;24:85. Includes S/S and reference ranges for metanephrines and catecholamines.
[15]Pacak K, et al. Recent advances in genetics, diagnosis, localization, and treatment of pheochromocytoma. *Ann Intern Med* 2001;134:315–329.
[16]Lenders JWM, Pacak K, Walther MM, et al. Biochemical diagnosis of pheochromocytoma. *JAMA* 2002;287:1427–1434.
[17]Eisenhofer GE, Sullivan P, Csako G. Pheochromocytoma. Improving diagnosis with plasma free metanephrines. *Clin Lab News* Feb 2001:6–8.

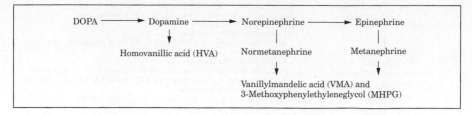

Fig. 13-15. Synthesis and breakdown of catecholamines. Because the hormones are broken down prior to release, metabolites are present in much larger amounts. When excretion of free catecholamines is greater compared to metabolites, it is said that tumor is likely to be very small and difficult to locate.

- ♦ If there are lesser increases, a clonidine suppression test will provide a definite diagnosis. A decrease >50% in plasma norepinephrine or to <2.96 nmol/L is normal, but increased concentrations before and after clonidine administration indicate a pheochromocytoma. Equivocal test results may occur with intermittently secreting tumors. False-positive results may occur due to diuretics or tricyclic antidepressants.
- ♦ A glucagon stimulation test may be used if plasma levels of normetanephrine or metanephrines are high and plasma catecholamine are normal or moderately increased. >3× increase in norepinephrine 2 minutes after IV glucagon indicates pheochromocytoma with high specificity but is not excluded by a negative test. *Take precautions against severe increase in blood pressure.*
- ♦ CT scan, MRI, or PET with radiopharmaceuticals can be used for confirmation and localization.
- ○ Usually sporadic. Familial inheritance in 10% to 20% of patients is associated with von Hippel-Lindau disease in ~20% of cases (see Chapter 9), von Recklinghausen disease, carotid body tumor, and MEN II. *All patients with pheochromocytoma should be screened for other components of MEN II present in ~4% of cases. Tumors associated with familial syndromes are more likely to be asymptomatic; 15% of pheochromocytomas are extra-adrenal; 10% are multiple. 70% are bilateral, 10% occur in children, 2/3 of whom are male. Two percent to 10% of adrenal and 20% to 40% of extra-adrenal pheochromocytomas are malignant.*
- ♦ Increased plasma chromogranin A has S/S = 83%/96%. (Chromogranin A is a protein stored and secreted with catecholamines by adrenal medulla and sympathetic chain.) Increased in 80% of pheochromocytomas but is not specific as secreted by other chromaffin tissues as is increased even with mild impairment of renal func-

Table 13-24.   Reference Range for Catecholamines and Metabolites

	Urine
Homovanillic acid	2–12 mg/24 hrs
Vanillylmandelic acid	2–7 mg/24 hrs
3-Methoxyphenylethyleneglycol	1.3–4.3 mg/24 hrs
Metanephrines	<1.6 mg/24 hrs
Dopamine	25–525 μg/24 hrs
Norepinephrine	10–64 μg/24 hrs
Epinephrine	0–36 μg/24 hrs
Norepinephrine + epinephrine	<100 μg/24 hrs
	Plasma
Dopamine	<100 pg/mL
Norepinephrine	65–400 pg/mL
Epinephrine	15–55 pg/mL

These data differ depending on source.
Source: Feldman JM. Diagnosis and management of pheochromocytoma. *Hosp Pract* 1989;(Jan 15): 175–198.

tion. Correlated with tumor mass. Not affected by drugs used in treatment.[18] Distinguishes malignant (10 × higher levels) from benign tumors. Useful for monitoring recurrence. Normal levels in factitious pheochromocytoma.

Diseases of Pituitary-Hypothalamus

Cushing Syndromes (Hypercortisolism)[19–21]

Hypercortisolism causes hypertension, truncal obesity, diabetes, hirsutism, acne, purple striae, psychiatric manifestations.

See Table 13-25, Figs. 13-12 and 13-16.
Due To (chronic glucocorticoid excess)
ACTH-dependent (plasma ACTH is increased): 80%
Pituitary (Cushing *disease*): 85%

- Pituitary tumor: 70% to 90% (may be part of MEN I)
- Hyperplasia of pituitary adrenocorticotropic cells: (rare)
- Ectopic CRH syndrome (nonhypothalamic secretion): <1%

Ectopic ACTH production: 15%

- Neoplasms (e.g., small-cell carcinoma of lung; carcinoids)
  Oat cell carcinoma: 50%
  Tumors of foregut origin: 35% (e.g., bronchial or thymic carcinoid, medullary thyroid carcinoma, islet cell tumors)
  Pheochromocytoma: 5%
  Others: 10%

ACTH-independent (plasma ACTH is suppressed): 20%
Adrenal (adrenal cause is predominant in children)

- Adenoma: >50%
- Carcinoma: <50%; 65% of patients aged <15 years
- Micronodular hyperplasia: ~1%
- Macronodular hyperplasia: <1%

Iatrogenic

- Iatrogenic (glucocorticoids or ACTH)
- Illicit use by athletes
- Factitious

Pseudo-Cushing syndrome

- Major depressive disorder: 1%
- Chronic alcoholism: <1%

◆ Definitive diagnosis or exclusion:
1. Establish autonomous hypercortisolism and loss of diurnal rhythm. May include increased plasma cortisol, salivary free cortisol, 24-hour urine free cortisol, overnight dexamethasone suppression test.
2. Determine etiology (see Fig. 13-16) by ACTH level, high-dose dexamethasone suppression test, metyrapone test.
3. Localize by imaging (adrenals, pituitary) and venous blood sampling (adrenal veins, jugular or petrosal sinuses with CRH stimulation).

---

[18]Taupenot L, Harper KL, O'Connor DT. The chromogranin-secretogranin family. *N Engl J Med* 2003; 349:1134.
[19]Orth DN. Cushing syndrome. *New Eng J Med* 1995;332:791.
[20]Freda PU. Differential diagnosis in Cushing syndrome. Use of CRH. *Medicine* 1995;74:74.
[21]Raff H, Findling JW. A physiologic approach to diagnosis of the Cushing syndrome. *Ann Intern Med* 2003;138:980.

ENDOCRINE

Table 13-25. Comparison of Different Causes of Cushing Syndrome

	Normal	Pituitary Cushing's	Adrenal			Ectopic ACTH Production	Other Illness
			Adenoma	Carcinoma	Hyperplasia		
Frequency		70%	9%	8%	Rare	15%	
Free cortisol							
Urine (μg/24 hr)	<100	>300 establishes diagnosis of Cushing's syndrome if increased					
Plasma (μg/dL)	7–25 at 8 a.m. 2–14 at 4 p.m.	>30 at 8 a.m. and >15 at 4 p.m.					False-positive may occur in alcoholism, depression, drug use, etc.
Low-dose dexamethasone suppression							
Urine free cortisol	Falls to <25 μg/24 hr	Does not fall to <25 μg/24 hr in Cushing's syndrome due to any cause		Not suppressed			
Plasma cortisol	Falls to <5 μg/dL			Not suppressed			
High-dose dexamethasone suppression	Suppressed in >90% of cases		Not suppressed but not reproducible			Not suppressed in 80% of cases	
Plasma ACTH (pg/mL)	60	I or high-normal range Not >200	Decreased or not detectable			>200 in ⅔ cases; 100–200 in ⅓ cases	
CRH stimulation	Rapid I in plasma ACTH and cortisol	ACTH increases		Flat plasma ACTH response to CRH			
ACTH ratio inferior petrosal sinus to peripheral blood		High; enhanced by CRH		Ratio = 1			

ACTH = adrenocoricotropic hormone; CRH = corticotropin-releasing hormone.

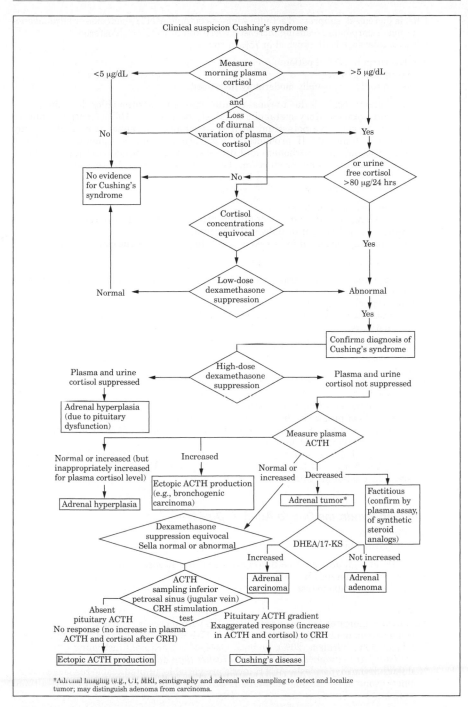

Fig. 13-16. Sequence of laboratory tests in diagnosis of Cushing syndrome (>90% of patients with Cushing syndrome are found to be categorizable using this scheme). (17-KS, 17 ketosteroids; CRH, corticotropin-releasing hormone; CT, computed tomography; DHEA, dehydroepiandrosterone; I, increased; MRI, magnetic resonance imaging; N, normal.) *Adrenal imaging (e.g., CT, MRI, scintigraphy and adrenal vein sampling to detect and localize tumor) may distinguish adenoma from carcinoma.

PRA is increased; suppressed activity suggests ectopic ACTH syndrome or adrenal adenoma or carcinoma (causing increased secretion of DOC or aldosterone).

Glucose tolerance is diminished in 75% of cases:

- Glycosuria in 50% of patients.
- DM in 20% of cases.
- Serum sodium is usually moderately increased.

○ Hypokalemic acidosis due to renal tubular loss of potassium chloride is characteristic but compensatory metabolic alkalosis occurs in ~10% of patients due to attempt to conserve potassium with H^+ exchange. Hypokalemic alkalosis may indicate ectopic ACTH production (e.g., bronchogenic carcinoma). Increased serum sodium and bicarbonate and decreased potassium and chloride are due to increased aldosterone production. Urine potassium is increased; sodium is decreased.

Hematologic changes:

- WBC is normal or increased.
- Relative lymphopenia is frequent (differential is usually <15% of cells).
- Eosinopenia is frequent (usually <100/cu mm).
- Hct is usually normal; if increased, it indicates an androgenic component.

Changes due to associated conditions

- Changes due to osteoporosis in long-standing cases. Serum and urine calcium may be increased.
- Kidney stones occur in 15% of cases.
- Polycystic ovary syndrome is common; Cushing syndrome should be ruled out in such patients.

Serum uric acid may be decreased due to uricosuric effect of adrenal steroids.

Urine creatine is increased due to muscle wasting, which may also cause increased BUN.

Serum gamma globulins may be decreased and alpha$_2$ globulin may be moderately increased.

80% of patients with Cushing disease have remission after removal of pituitary adenoma; tests of pituitary-adrenal axis may take weeks to months to become normal. Effectiveness of surgery is assessed by plasma cortisol and 24-hour urinary cortisol concentrations one week after surgery.

Pituitary imaging has false-negative scans because many functional tumors are so small (2–3 mms) and false-positive scans because 10% to 15% of normal persons have nonfunctioning tumors.

Cushing Syndrome Due To Adrenal Disease

See Fig. 13-16.

♦ Is suggested by:

- Failure of high-dose dexamethasone test to cause suppression
- Very low plasma ACTH
- Positive metyrapone test

Due To

Adenoma is indicated by low or normal 17-KS with increased cortisol.

Adrenal carcinoma is suggested by very high 17-KS. Carcinoma cases show hypercortisolism (50%), virilism (20%), or both (10%–15%); are nonfunctioning (10%–15%). *Virilism favors diagnosis of carcinoma rather than adenoma.*

Nodular adrenal hyperplasia: ACTH levels are variable, unpredictable response to dexamethasone suppression; therefore is difficult to distinguish from other adrenal causes.

- 50% of bilateral micronodular hyperplasia cases occur before age 30 years.
- 50% occur as autosomal dominant disorder associated with blue nevi, pigmented lentigines, myxomas (atrial, skin, mammary), pituitary somatotroph adenomas, testicular and other tumors.

Nonfunctioning adrenal adenoma may be found in 5% to 10% of normal persons.

Cushing Syndrome Owning To Ectopic ACTH Production

Due to ACTH-secreting neoplasm, e.g., small-cell carcinoma of lung (50% of cases), thymoma, islet cell tumor of pancreas (<5% of cases), medullary carcinoma of thyroid, bronchial carcinoid, pheochromocytoma, others. Occurs in 2% of patients with lung cancer. The primary tumor is often radiologically occult.

See Table 13-25 and Fig. 13-16.
♦ Plasma ACTH is markedly increased (500–1,000 pg/mL) compared (5×–10× higher) with pituitary Cushing disease (≤200 pg/mL) but overlap in 20% of ectopic ACTH cases. Morning basal level in normal persons is 20 to 100 pg/mL. Extreme increase suggests ectopic production rather than pituitary.
♦ Increased plasma and urine free cortisol, which may show marked spontaneous variation; lack of diurnal variation
♦ Increased ACTH in plasma from inferior petrosal sinus identifies ACTH-producing pituitary adenomas in ~88% of cases; combining with CRH stimulation improves the differentiation of pituitary from ectopic ACTH production.
♦ High-dose dexamethasone suppression does not occur in ectopic ACTH production but does occur in >90% of Cushing disease.
♦ Use of both dexamethasone suppression and CRH stimulation has diagnostic accuracy of 98% in distinguishing Cushing disease from ectopic ACTH production.
Metyrapone test may not be accurate in distinguishing this condition from Cushing disease.
○ Marked hypokalemic alkalosis (due to increased desoxycorticosterone and corticosterone occurs in ≤60% of such patients) rather than metabolic acidosis may suggest this diagnosis.

Cushing Syndrome Owning To Ectopic CRH Production

Usually due to bronchial carcinoids; may also be due to medullary thyroid cancer and metastatic prostate carcinoma. Clinically indistinguishable from ectopic ACTH production because most of these tumors also secrete ACTH.

♦ Plasma ACTH is increased. CRH is rarely measured.
CRH-stimulated secretion of ACTH is suppressed by high doses of dexamethasone; may not be present in many cases.

Cushing Syndrome, Factitious

♦ Increased plasma and urinary cortisol
♦ Plasma ACTH is low or undetectable.
♦ These findings may also occur in adrenal Cushing syndrome. Differentiate by history of ingestion or, in some cases, determination of synthetic steroid analogues by specific plasma assays.

Pseudo-Cushing Syndrome

Due To
Major depressive disorders: Cortisol secretion is abnormal in 80% of these patients but hypersecretion is usually minimal and transient; disappears with remission of depression.

• Evening nadir in plasma cortisol is preserved; <5 µg/dL rules out and >7.5 µg/dL indicates Cushing syndrome
• Plasma cortisol is low after administration of dexamethasone and remains low when CRH is given soon after, whereas in Cushing syndrome, plasma cortisol is not so low after dexamethasone and increases after CRH.
• Insulin-induced hypoglycemia causes increased plasma cortisol but not in chronic Cushing syndrome.
Chronic alcoholism—abnormal liver function tests; resolves during abstinence as liver function returns to normal.
Obesity

Tests for Cushing Syndromes

Interferences
More than one test may be needed because tests are misleading in *one third or more* of patients:

• Baseline measurements are increased by stress.

- Baseline measurements may vary daily and make dexamethasone suppression test difficult to interpret.
- Some drugs alter ACTH production or interfere with assays.
- Impaired renal function
- Cortisol production is somewhat proportional to obesity or large muscle mass.
- Cortisol production is pulsatile rather than uniform even in ectopic ACTH production or Cushing disease.
- Cortisol secretion may not be very increased on every determination.

◆ 24-Hour Urinary Free Cortisol

Use
Screening for

- Cushing syndrome (increased) and
- Adrenal insufficiency (decreased)

Interpretation
Increase is most useful screening test (best expressed as *per gram creatinine,* which should vary by <10% daily; if >10% variation, should collect two more 24-hour specimens). Should be measured in three consecutive 24-hour specimens to ensure proper collection and account for daily variability even in Cushing syndrome. Found in 95% of Cushing syndrome. <100 μg/24 hours excludes, and >300 μg/24 hours establishes, the diagnosis of Cushing syndrome. If values are intermediate, dexamethasone suppression test is indicated.

Interferences
False-positive or false-negative results were previously said to be rare, making 24-hour urine cortisol preferred test by some.

Increased values may occur in depression, chronic alcoholism, eating disorders, but do not exceed 300 μg/24 hours.

Various drugs (e.g., carbamazepine, phenytoin, phenobarbital, primidone)

Acute and chronic illnesses

Kidney function and fluid intake

Not affected by body weight

◆ Plasma Free Cortisol
Secreted by adrenal zona fasciculata

Use
Loss of normal diurnal variation for screening for Cushing syndrome; this diurnal variation disappears early and may be lost in almost all Cushing syndrome and 18% of patients without Cushing (due to depression, alcoholism, stress, etc.).

Interpretation
Blood levels vary with time of day, require standardized collection, are secreted in pulsatile fashion. False negatives are frequent if blood is drawn before 8 PM (PM blood is commonly drawn at 4 PM to coincide with hospital employee working hours.)

Because episodic rise and fall occurs in Cushing disease, ectopic ACTH production as well as in normal persons, should be measured on at least 2 separate days.

Samples every 30 minutes from 10 PM to midnight: ≤2 μg/dL exclude Cushing syndrome, ≤5.0 μg/dL are unlikely to represent Cushing syndrome, and >7.5 μg/dL strongly suggest Cushing syndrome.

Normal persons have highest concentration at 8 AM that declines by 50% to 80% between 10 PM and midnight.

Normal urine free cortisol and normal diurnal variation in plasma cortisol virtually exclude Cushing syndrome.

Midnight cortisol >7.5 μg/dL indicates Cushing syndrome, whereas <5 μg/dL virtually rules it out.

◆ Salivary Cortisol

5× a single day salivary cortisol is simple screen for hypercortisolism. >7 nmol/L at 11 PM is said to have S/S = >90% for Cushing syndrome; 3 to 7 nmol/L (requires additional confirmation).

◆ *Basal Plasma ACTH Concentration*

Interpretation

Cushing syndrome owning to autonomous cortisol production (e.g., adrenal tumor or exogenous steroids): Low or undetectable (<5 pg/mL)

Pituitary Cushing disease: High or high-normal range, but rarely >200 pg/mL. Hyper-response to chronic renal failure (CRF). Inferior petrosal sinus sampling (see next paragraph).

Ectopic ACTH syndrome (e.g., carcinoma of lung): Very high concentrations with no diurnal variation. Two thirds of patients have high concentrations (>200 pg/mL); the other one-third usually have moderately elevated values (100–200 pg/mL); no response to CRF. In these cases, difference in ACTH concentrations is measured in blood obtained simultaneously from both inferior petrosal sinuses and a peripheral vein before and after CRH stimulation. Ratio of inferior petrosal sinus:peripheral vein <2 indicates ectopic source of ACTH; has S/S = 95%/100%. Ratio ≥3.0 has S/S = 100%/100% for pituitary tumor.

Increased In

Primary adrenal insufficiency

Decreased In

Factitious Cushing syndrome

Secondary adrenal insufficiency

Interferences

ACTH has diurnal variation, episodic secretion, short plasma half-life.

Dexamethasone Suppression of Pituitary ACTH Secretion Test (DST)

Dexamethasone is a synthetic glucocorticoid not detected by cortisol assays. Dexamethasone should not fully suppress ACTH and therefore should not decrease adrenal secretion of cortisol.

Low-Dose Test

0.5 mg of dexamethasone is given orally every 6 hours for eight doses; specimen collection as for high-dose test below. A rapid overnight variation for screening uses a single 1-mg dose at 11 PM with plasma cortisol collection the following 8 AM. Followed in 2 hours by CRH stimulation improves diagnostic accuracy, S/S to ~100% in diagnosis of Cushing syndrome.

Use

Good screening test to rule out Cushing syndrome and to identify cases for further testing because there are few (1%–2%) false-negative results. Should be reserved primarily for cases with mildly increased urine cortisol or pseudo-Cushing syndrome.

Interference

False-positive results may occur in acute and chronic illness, alcoholism, depression, and due to certain drugs (e.g., phenytoin, phenobarbital, primidone); estrogens may cause a false-positive overnight dexamethasone test.

Noncompliance (check by measuring plasma dexamethasone)

Interpretation

Normal response is a fall in urine free cortisol to <25 μg/24 hours, plasma cortisol to <5 μg/dL. Fall in urine free cortisol >90% has reported specificity = 100%, i.e., normal result excludes hypercortisolism.

Patients with Cushing of any cause almost always have abnormal lack of suppressibility.

May require high-dose test because of interferences.

High-Dose Test

2 mg of dexamethasone is given orally every 6 hours for eight doses and plasma cortisol is measured 6 hours after last dose and urine free cortisol is measured on the second day; baseline specimens for 2 days before test.

Use

The high-dose test is the basic test to differentiate Cushing disease (in which there is only relative resistance to glucocorticoid-negative feedback) from adrenal tumors or ectopic ACTH production (usually complete resistance).

Interpretation

Cushing disease (pituitary tumor). S/S and accuracy = 80% with pretest probability of Cushing syndrome >90%.

- Suppression of plasma cortisol at 8 AM to <5 μg/dL excludes Cushing syndrome; 5.0 to 9.9 μg/dL is inconclusive; >10 μg/dL is abnormal.
- Suppression of urine free cortisol to <90% of baseline to is said to differentiate Cushing disease from ectopic ACTH production but not all pituitary tumor patients show such marked suppression. In obese children, must be based on weight or body surface area (e.g., normal maximum = 25–75 μg/M^2/24 hours).

Some patients with large ACTH-producing pituitary adenomas have marked resistance to high-dose dexamethasone suppression. In long-standing cases, nodular hyperplasia of adrenal may develop causing autonomous cortisol production and resistance to dexamethasone test.

Ectopic ACTH syndrome or nodular adrenal hyperplasia

- No suppression in 80% of cases

Adrenal adenoma or carcinoma or ectopic ACTH syndrome

- Urine and plasma cortisol are not decreased after high or low doses of dexamethasone.

Adrenal tumors do not reproducibly suppress.
Patients with psychiatric illness may be resistant.

Interferences

Atypical or false-positive responses may occur due to drugs (e.g., alcohol, estrogens, and birth-control pills, phenytoin, barbiturates, spironolactone), pregnancy, obesity, acute illness and stress, severe depression.

11-Deoxycortisol (Compound S), Serum

Present in blood as an intermediate in synthesis of cortisol from 17-hydroxyprogesterone; excretion in urine is included in 17-ketogenic steroid (17-KGS) and Porter-Silber 17-hydroxyketosteroid (17-OHKS) measurements. Originally used to provide some measure of cortisol production. 17-KS and 17-OHKS replaced by direct measurement of cortisol.

Use

In metyrapone test (see below)

Increased In

CAH (P450cII deficiency)
Following metyrapone administration in normal persons

Decreased In

Adrenal insufficiency

Metyrapone Test

Adrenal suppression of pituitary secretion of ACTH is inhibited by metyrapone, which blocks cortisol production thereby leading to increased ACTH secretion and therefore of 11-deoxycortisol.

750 mg of metyrapone is given every 4 to 6 hours beginning at midnight; baseline plasma levels are drawn at 8 AM and following 8 AM. Do not perform metyrapone test until ACTH test proves that adrenals are sensitive to ACTH.

Use/Interpretation

To distinguish Cushing disease from ectopic ACTH production.
To assess if adrenal insufficiency is secondary to pituitary disease. Some increase in 11-deoxycortisol indicates some pituitary reserve exists; in primary adrenal insufficiency, no rise occurs.
ACTH deficiency (secondary Addison disease)
Normal persons and pituitary Cushing disease: basal plasma 11-deoxycortisol increases ≥400× or >10 μg/dL if cortisol falls to <7 μg/dL and rise in plasma ACTH to >100 ng/L.
Blood level of 11-deoxycortisol

• Functioning pituitary-adrenal system shows increase from <200 ng/dL baseline to >7,000 ng/dL 8 hours after large dose of metyrapone, whereas in nonfunctioning system there is very little increase in blood level.

Adrenal tumor with excess cortisol production: no increase or fall in urinary 17-KS. Test is positive in 100% of adrenal hyperplasias without tumor, 50% of adrenal adenomas, and 25% of adrenal carcinomas.
Ectopic ACTH syndrome: May not be accurate in this condition.

Corticotropin-Releasing Hormone (CRH) Stimulation Test[22–24]

1 μg/kg of body weight of CRH is given IV; blood is then drawn at 2-, 5-, and 10-minute intervals for ACTH. ACTH concentrations are compared from both inferior petrosal sinuses and peripheral vein after CRH stimulation. Use of only peripheral plasma ACTH and cortisol has little value.

Use/Interpretation
Confirm diagnosis of Cushing disease when positive response to dexamethasone suppression, CRH administration or metyrapone stimulation.
Differentiates pituitary and nonpituitary causes of Cushing syndrome, especially ectopic ACTH production. Ratio of ACTH in jugular and peripheral veins >2 before, and >3 after, administration of IV CRH is diagnostic for Cushing disease. Bilateral petrosal and peripheral vein sampling has S/S and accuracy approaching 100%. Different values between right and left petrosal sinuses suggest on which side tumor is located. Especially useful when the high-dose dexamethasone suppression test is equivocal or when biochemical data indicate a pituitary source but radiographic examination is normal.
Cushing syndrome due to pituitary adenoma: Positive response is exaggerated increase above baseline of >50% in plasma ACTH and >20% in cortisol concentrations. After surgical removal of adenoma, basal concentrations of ACTH and cortisol are undetectable but response to CRH is normal.
Hypercortisolism of adrenal origin: Plasma ACTH is low (<30 pg/mL) or undetectable before and after CRH without any cortisol response.
Ectopic ACTH syndrome: No ACTH or cortisol response in ~92% of patients; positive response in ~8% of patients
Psychiatric states associated with hypercortisolism (e.g., depression, anorexia nervosa, bulimia): In uni- or bipolar depression, both peak and total ACTH response is decreased; only a normal small decrease in cortisol occurs; after recovery, response is not distinguishable from normal persons. Similar findings may occur in obsessive-compulsive disorders and alcoholism. Manic patients have response similar to controls.

♦ Urinary Steroid Findings in Different Etiologies of Cushing Syndrome
Isolated urine measurements of 17-KS are not recommended as screening tests for Cushing syndrome. In general, free cortisol is best for screening, free cortisol in dexamethasone suppression tests, 17-KS to screen for possible adrenal carcinoma or to help differentiate adrenal adenoma from pituitary or ectopic ACTH syndrome
Uses

Glucocorticoid Resistance Syndromes
Very rare autosomal recessive trait causing inability of target tissues to respond to glucocorticoids.

The resulting compensatory increase in pituitary corticotropin without any clinical stigmata of Cushing syndrome may cause any combination of excess secretion of:

• Adrenal androgens (may result in female masculinization with hirsutism, acne, oligomenorrhea, infertility; precocious puberty; abnormal spermatogenesis)

[22]Chrousos GP, et al. NIH conference. Clinical applications of corticotropin-releasing factor. *Ann Int Med* 1985;102:344.
[23]Kaye TB, Crapo L. The Cushing syndrome: an update on diagnostic tests. *Ann Int Med* 1990;112:434.
[24]Doppman JL, Oldfield EH, Nieman LK. Bilateral sampling of the internal jugular vein to distinguish between mechanisms of adrenocorticotropic hormone-dependent Cushing syndrome. *Ann Int Med* 1998;128:33.

- Mineral corticoid excess (may result in hypokalemic alkalosis, hypertension)
- Apparently normal glucocorticoid function (may be asymptomatic or have chronic fatigue)

♦ No evidence of Cushing syndrome but with elevated indices of plasma and urine cortisol normal with no loss of diurnal pattern
♦ Abnormal binding characteristics of glucocorticoid receptors in mononuclear leukocytes

Laboratory Tests for Diagnosis of Disorders of Pituitary and Hypothalamus

Growth Hormone, Human (GH)

Produced and secreted by pituitary somatotrope cells in response to hypothalamic secretion of growth hormone–releasing hormone (GHRH) and inhibited by somatostatin. Effects are mediated through insulin-like growth factors.

Use
Differential diagnosis of short stature, slow growth
Evaluation of pituitary function
Usually not clinically useful because of pulsatile secretion, variation in pulses, short half-life, age variation, overlapping values. Good sensitivity at 3 μg/L but only 60% specificity.

Increased In
Acromegaly and gigantism due to certain pituitary adenomas
Laron dwarfism (lack of GH receptors causes GH resistance; growth hormone–binding protein cannot be detected)
Renal failure
Uncontrolled DM
Drugs (e.g., estrogens, oral contraceptives, tranquilizers, antidepressants)
Starvation
2 hours after sleep

Decreased In
Hypothalamic defect causes most cases (e.g., tumors, infection, diseases such as hemochromatosis, perinatal insult such as birth trauma)
Hypopituitarism (e.g., familial isolated GH deficiency, tumors, infection, granulomas, trauma, irradiation)
Dwarfism
Corticosteroid therapy
Obesity
Low levels must be measured after stimulation (e.g., insulin, arginine).

Growth Hormone–Releasing Hormone (GHRH)

Hypothalamic secretion stimulates pituitary to release growth hormone.

Increased In
One percent of cases of acromegaly owning to GHRH by hypothalamus or ectopic secretion by neoplasms (e.g., pancreatic islet, carcinoid of thymus or bronchus, neuroendocrine tumors)

Normal In
Most cases of acromegaly owning to pituitary tumors

Somatomedin-C[25]

Also referred to as insulin growth factor-1 (IGF-1). Secreted by hypothalamus; release is mediated by GH in many tissues, especially hepatocytes. Values vary widely with age and gender.

See also Somatostatin.

---

[25]Pandian R, Nakamoto JM. Rational use of the laboratory for childhood and adult growth hormone deficiency. *Clin Lab Med* 2004;24:141.

Use

Diagnosis of acromegaly and pituitary deficiency; preferable to GH because it is constant after eating and during the day

Help determine optimum dosage of GH

Screening other growth disorders

Assessing nutritional status

Monitor effectiveness of nutritional repletion. Is more sensitive indicator than prealbumin, transferrin index, or retinol-binding protein.

Increased In

Acromegaly and gigantism

Pregnancy (2–3× nonpregnant values)

Decreased In

Pituitary deficiency

Laron dwarfism

Anorexia or malnutrition

Acute illness

Hepatic failure

Hypothyroidism

DM

Normal aging

Disorders of the Pituitary and Hypothalamus

The anterior pituitary contains cells that synthesize and secrete 5 different hormones, including growth hormone (GH), prolactin, thyroid-stimulating hormone (TSH), alpha- and beta-subunits of follicle-stimulating hormone (FSH), luteinizing hormone (LH), pro-opiomelanocortin, which is cleaved in the pituitary to form ACTH, and alpha-lipotropin. The hypothalamus secretes trophic hormones for each. The posterior pituitary does not synthesize hormones; hormones that it secretes are formed in the hypothalamus: antidiuretic hormone (ADH; arginine vasopressin); and oxytocin.

Pituitary Hormone Excess

Prolactinomas

Cushing syndrome

Acromegaly and gigantism

TSH-secreting adenomas

Pituitary Hormone Deficiency

Hypoadrenalism

Hypothyroidism

Hypogonadism

DI

Somatomedin deficiency

Effect of Sellar Mass

Hypopituitarism

Hypothalamic syndromes

Others (e.g., CSF rhinorrhea, hydrocephalus, neuropathies, visual field changes)

Acromegaly and Gigantism

Due To

Excess GH secretion

- Pituitary adenomas, hyperplasia, or carcinoma
- Ectopic pituitary tumor (sphenoid or parapharyngeal sinus)
- Ectopic hormone production (e.g., tumor of pancreas, lung, ovary, breast)

Excess GHRH secretion

- Hypothalamic tumor (e.g., hamartoma, ganglioneuroma)
- Ectopic hormone production (e.g., carcinoid of bronchus, GI tract, pancreas; pancreatic islet cell tumor, small-cell carcinoma of lung, adrenal adenoma, pheochromocytoma)

♦ Serum somatomedin C (insulin-like growth factor-I; IGF-I) is uniformly increased in untreated cases; is more precise and cost-effective screening test than serum GH since GH levels fluctuate and have short serum half-life (22 minutes).
♦ Autonomous serum GH is increased. (Avoid stress before and during venipuncture because stress stimulates secretion of GH; should perform several random measurements.) Annual random blood GH levels and ACTH are used for treatment follow up.

- Fasting levels >5 ng/mL in men or >10 ng/mL in women are suggestive but not diagnostic of acromegaly.

♦ Most patients show a fall of <50% or even an increase 60 to 90 minutes after glucose (50–100 g orally), whereas normal subjects show almost complete suppression of GH (or to <5 ng/mL) by induced hyperglycemia. This is the most reliable test. Failure to suppress GH to <2 ng/mL after oral glucose load is essential to diagnosis.
♦ If borderline response to hyperglycemia, perform TRH test. (500 μg TRH IV causes transient increase [>50% over basal levels] of GH in 15–30 mins in acromegaly patients but little effect in normal persons.)

- GHRH excess secretion (e.g., ectopic source such as pancreatic tumor or carcinoid causes <1% of acromegaly cases). Thus GHRH should be measured in all patients with acromegaly.

♦ All patients with acromegaly should have baseline serum prolactin measured since ≤40% of these adenomas may secrete both prolactin and GH.
IV ACTH administration may cause excessive increase in urine 17KS excretion.
Glucose tolerance is impaired in most patients. Mild insulin-resistant DM is found in <15% of patients.
Adrenal virilism and increased urine 17-KS are common in women.
Urine 17-KS, 17-KGS, and gonadotropins are usually normal or may be slightly changed but not diagnostically useful.
Hypogonadism develops in ≤50%.
Rare associated endocrinopathies are hyperthyroidism, hyperparathyroidism, pheochromocytoma, insulinoma.
In inactive cases, all secondary laboratory findings may be normal.
In late stage, panhypopituitarism may develop.
Serum phosphorus is increased for age of patient in 40% of cases.
Serum ALP may be increased.
Urine calcium is increased.
Urine hydroxyproline is increased.
Biopsy of costochondral junction evidences active bone growth.
CBC and ESR are normal.
♦ After successful surgery: basal plasma GH <5 ng/mL, should decrease to ≤2 ng/mL after glucose administration and insulin-like growth factor I should become normal.

Other Causes of Tall Stature in Children

Klinefelter syndrome
Marfan syndrome (inherited disorder with thin limbs, malformation of eyes and ears, medionecrosis of aorta, cardiac valve deformities, hypotonia, kyphoscoliosis)
Beckwith-Wiedemann syndrome (hypoglycemia, omphalocele, macrosomia, macroglossia)
Untreated CAH
Precocious secretion of androgens or estrogens
Obesity

Growth Hormone (GH) Deficiency[25]

Includes these analytes: GH (usually by stimulation testing), IGF-1, and IGF-binding protein-3.

---

[25]Pandian R, Nakamoto JM. Rational use of the laboratory for childhood and adult growth hormone deficiency. *Clin Lab Med* 2004;24:141.

There may be isolated deficiency with dwarfism or associated with TSH deficiency (should be ruled out first), with ACTH deficiency, or with TSH and ACTH deficiencies. GH deficiency is usually due to hypothalamic GHRH deficiency.

♦ Serum GH basal levels are decreased (<1.0 ng/mL). Use pooled or average of 3 samples. Less sensitive than stimulation tests. Increased basal or random serum level excludes this diagnosis but low levels do not distinguish normal persons from GH deficiency.

♦ Stimulation (functional) tests

• Draw serum at appropriate intervals for each test.
• Insulin-induced hypoglycemia (<40 mg/dL) (regular crystalline, IV, 0.05–0.3 unit/kg body weight) normally produces at least 2× increase in serum GH level and 3× increase in serum prolactin level at 60-minute peak. This is the most reliable challenge for GH secretion. Test of choice but beware of severe complications.
• Administration of arginine (0.5 g/kg body weight as 5% solution IV over 30 mins) should normally produce at least 3× increase in serum GH and at least 2× increase in serum prolactin level at 30- to 60-minute peak. May combine arginine with GHRH (cutoff value of 9 ug/L is most specific.)
• Administration of L-dopa (500 mg orally) should normally produce at least 2× increase in serum GH level at 60-minute peak.
• Also clonidine and glucagon stimulation tests
• Failure to produce these minimal responses indicates a lesion of pituitary or hypothalamus but does not differentiate between them.
• A normal response is at least 7 to 10 ng/ml peak value; 5 to 7 ng/mL is indeterminate; <5 ng/mL is subnormal. (A normal value rules out GH deficiency; in some labs the normal level is ≥7 ng/mL; some consider 3 ng/mL subnormal.)
• At least two of these tests should be used to confirm diagnosis of GH deficiency because approximately one fouth of patients with normal GH secretory capacity are unable to secrete GH in response to provocative tests indicated above, at any given time.
• Nonpituitary factors that impair GH response include obesity, primary hypothyroidism, thyrotoxicosis, primary hypogonadism, Kallmann syndrome, Cushing syndrome, use of various drugs (e.g., α-adrenergic antagonists, beta-adrenergic antagonists, serotonin antagonists, dopamine antagonists). Impaired GH response may even occur in presence of elevated GH basal level.
• *Normal response may also occur in patients with partial deficiency.*
• GH response is normal or exaggerated in growth failure due to lack of GH receptors (Laron dwarfism) or resistance to somatomedins (African pygmies).
• Exercise and sleep have been used for screening.

Decreased fasting blood sugar (<50 mg/dL) is frequent; responds to GH therapy.
Serum phosphorus and ALP are decreased in prepubertal child but normal in adult-onset cases.

♦ Serum prolactin baseline level is low and does not rise appropriately after TRH or other stimulation. In hypothalamic disease, basal prolactin level is increased and response may be normal or blunted.

Laboratory findings owning to involvement of other endocrines

• TSH deficiency (see Serum TSH; TRH Stimulation Test; Hypothyroidism; and Table 14-3)
• ACTH deficiency (see tests of adrenal function)
• Gonadotropins are decreased or absent from urine in postpubertal patients (but increased levels occur in primary hypogonadism).

For childhood growth hormone deficiency, IGF-1 and IGF-binding protein-3 are key tests.

Anorexia Nervosa

Eating and behavioral disorder meant to cause weight loss.

No diagnostic or typical laboratory profile; diagnosis is by exclusion. Findings may be compensatory changes secondary to nutritional deprivation (vomiting, purging, diuretic use) rather than primary hypothalamic dysfunction.

Vomiting may cause hypochloremic alkalosis (loss of H^+ and Cl^-; urine <10 mEq/day but higher in diuretic abuse).

Hypokalemia may be due to laxative and diuretic abuse as well as vomiting.

Laboratory findings of euthyroid sick syndrome

Anemia is unusual; leukopenia; thrombocytopenia. Vitamin deficiencies are rare.

Findings due to secondary hormonal changes may be present

- Persistent low gonadotropin levels (may be undetectable)
- Basal GH levels may be increased as in other forms of protein-calorie malnutrition; response to stimulation tests is usually normal.
- Increased plasma somatomedin C.
- Plasma prolactin level is normal.
- Plasma LH and FSH may be low with impaired response to LH-releasing hormone.
- Decreased serum estradiol; atrophic vaginal smear
- Decreased serum testosterone
- Adrenal function abnormalities may be found (e.g., normal or increased plasma corticoids, absence of diurnal variation of glucocorticoids, hyperresponsive ACTH test, incomplete suppression by dexamethasone, response to metyrapone may be intact or excessive, low 17-KS and 17-KGS in urine; no adrenal insufficiency)
- Secondary hyperaldosteronism
- TSH and T_4 are normal. Low T_3 and high rT_3.

Findings due to dehydration may be present

- ESR is low.
- Prerenal azotemia with increased BUN and serum creatinine may occur.
- Serum glucose, sodium, magnesium may be decreased.
- Renal calculi

Findings due to malnutrition may be present: with marked loss of body weight, serum protein, potassium, and phosphorus may be decreased.

Hypopituitarism

Due To
Pituitary disease

- Neoplasms (e.g., craniopharyngioma, chromophobe adenoma, eosinophilic adenoma, meningioma, metastatic tumor [especially breast, lung]); prolactin-secreting tumor is the most common pituitary neoplasm.
- Infiltrative diseases
  Granulomatous lesions (e.g., sarcoidosis, Hand-Schuller-Christian syndrome, histiocytosis X)
  Infection (e.g.—TB, mycoses)
  Hemochromatosis
  Autoimmune inflammation
- Hemorrhage
  Pituitary necrosis secondary to postpartum hemorrhage (Sheehan syndrome)
  Hemorrhage into pituitary tumor
- Infarction (e.g., sickle cell disease, cavernous sinus thrombosis)
- Miscellaneous
  Head trauma
  Internal carotid artery aneurysm
  Empty sella syndrome
- Idiopathic
  Isolated hormone deficiency (e.g., GH, ACTH, TSH, gonadotropin)
  Multiple hormone deficiency
- Iatrogenic (e.g., hypophysectomy, radiation, section of stalk)
- Familial pituitary deficiency (deficient hormone production or production of abnormal hormone)
- Partial GH deficiency (some forms of "constitutional short stature" with delayed onset of adolescence)

End-organ resistance to GH (normal or increased serum GH with low somatomedin level)

- Laron dwarfs (lack of GH receptors—somatomedin levels are often undetectable and fail to rise when GH is administered).

Hypothalamic dysfunction
Due To
- Neoplasms (primary or metastatic cancer, craniopharyngioma) (most frequent cause)
- Inflammation (e.g., TB, encephalitis)
- Head trauma (e.g., basal skull fractures, gunshot wounds)
- Granulomas (e.g., histiocytosis X, sarcoidosis)
- Releasing hormone deficiency, genetic or idiopathic
- Irradiation for childhood cancer

Manifestations of hypothalamic dysfunction
Sexual abnormalities are the most frequent manifestations of hypothalamic disease, e.g., precocious puberty, hypogonadism [frequently as part of Froehlich syndrome], diabetes insipidus is a frequent but not an early manifestation of hypothalamic disease.
Differentiate primary hypopituitarism from this secondary form due to hypothalamic disease by appropriate stimulation tests.
♦ *Serum somatomedin-C levels are 5% to15% of normal in most hypopituitary dwarfs and 4 to 12× normal in all active acromegaly patients.*
♦ Endocrinologic findings: Diagnosis is based on low serum level of target organ hormone and of the corresponding pituitary-stimulating hormone, e.g.,

- Hypogonadism:
  Men: Low sperm count, low serum testosterone, inappropriately low serum LH and FSH
  Women: Low serum estradiol, inappropriately low serum LH and FSH
- Hypothyroidism:
  Low serum T_4, inappropriately low serum thyrotropin
- Hypocortisolism:
  Low serum cortisol and ACTH.
  Low serum GH unresponsive to provocative tests
  Low serum prolactin unresponsive to provocative tests.
  Usually occurs late in course of hypopituitarism except in Sheehan syndrome, in which it may be the earliest manifestation. Rarely or never due to hypothalamic disease.

See sections on secondary insufficiency of gonads, thyroid, adrenals. Only one (usually gonadal first) or all of these may be involved.
♦ *Dynamic tests are usually needed to detect partial deficiencies.*
See Diabetes Insipidus (Central).

Pituitary Tumors

May be secretory or nonsecretory, microadenoma (<1 cm) or macroadenoma (>1 cm). Growth causes pressure on optic chiasma causing characteristic visual field defects or compression of cranial nerves or hydrocephalus; can compromise other pituitary-hormone production causing hormone deficiencies.

♦ Findings due to increased production of hormones or effect of growing mass. Most common tumors are:

- Prolactin-secreting tumors: 25% to 40% of pituitary tumors (see Prolactinomas, below)
- GH-secreting tumors: 10% to 15% of pituitary tumors (see Acromegaly and Gigantism)
- ACTH-secreting tumors: 10% to 15% of pituitary tumors (see Cushing syndrome)
- Nonfunctioning adenomas, which may produce findings of intracranial mass, especially with visual changes, hypopituitarism (sometimes with impaired hypothalamic function): 10% to 25% of pituitary tumors
- TSH-secreting tumors (<3% of pituitary tumors)

Microadenomas (<10 mm in size) may be present in 10% to 20% of the population by autopsy and x-ray studies ("incidentaloma"), but macroadenomas (>10 mm in size) are quite rare.

Prolactinomas

Most common functioning pituitary tumor. Circadian and pulsatile secretion with peak during sleep.

Serum Prolactin Reference Values

Normal <25 ng/mL in females; lower in males and children
Gradual increase from birth until adolescence
13 to 15 year old boys: 2.5× adult levels
13 to 15 year old girls: 3× adult levels
Serum samples should be collected under basal conditions with minimal stress and by pooling 3 blood samples collected at 20-minute intervals for one assay; all drugs should be discontinued for at least 2 weeks before testing.

Interpretation

40 to 85 ng/mL: Seen in craniopharyngioma, hypothyroidism, effect of drugs
50 ng/mL: 25% chance of a pituitary tumor
100 ng/mL: 50% chance of a pituitary tumor
>150 ng/mL: Usually indicates prolactinoma; degree of elevation correlates with tumor size <200 ng/mL with a macroadenoma, particularly with extrasellar extension, is most likely due to compression of pituitary stalk rather than prolactinoma.
200 to 300 ng/mL: Nearly 100% chance of a pituitary tumor; >200 ng/mL may indicate a macroadenoma rather than microadenoma and usually visible on CT or MRI but CT or MRI is normal in ≤20% of microadenomas
High levels may be seen with simultaneous multiple additive factors that usually cause lesser increases (e.g., chronic renal failure plus methyldopa)
♦ Immediate postoperative level <7.0 ng/mL indicates long-term cure but higher levels are associated with recurrence.
♦ Repeated serum levels in late morning or early afternoon increased 3 to 5× normal in men or nonlactating women are usually considered diagnostic of pituitary adenoma or rarely of hypothalamic disease of pituitary stalk section or hypothyroidism. One elevated level is not adequate for diagnosis. Normally increases sharply during sleep; higher in morning than in afternoon.

Increased Serum Prolactin In

Amenorrhea/galactorrhea

- 10% to 25% of women with galactorrhea and normal menses
- 10% to 15% of women with amenorrhea without galactorrhea
- 75% of women with both galactorrhea and amenorrhea/oligomenorrhea
- Causes 15% to 30% of cases of amenorrhea in young women

Pituitary lesions (e.g., prolactinoma, section of pituitary stalk, empty sella syndrome, 20%–40% of patients with acromegaly, ≤80% of patients with chromophobe adenomas). Concentrations are usually >200 ng/mL.
Hypothalamic lesions (e.g., sarcoidosis, eosinophilic granuloma, histiocytosis X, TB, glioma, craniopharyngioma). Concentrations are usually >200 ng/mL.
Other endocrine diseases

- ~20% of cases of hypothyroidism (second most common cause of hyperprolactinemia). *Therefore serum TSH and T-4 should always be measured.*
- Addison disease
- Polycystic ovaries
- Glucocorticoid excess—normal or moderately elevated prolactin

Ectopic production of prolactin (e.g., bronchogenic carcinoma, renal cell carcinoma, ovarian teratomas, acute myeloid leukemia)
Children with sexual precocity—may be increased into pubertal range
Neurogenic causes (e.g., nursing and breast stimulation, spinal cord lesions, chest wall lesions such as herpes zoster)
Stress (e.g., surgery, hypoglycemia, vigorous exercise, siezures)
Pregnancy (increases to 8–20× normal by delivery, returns to normal 2–4 weeks postpartum unless nursing occurs)
Lactation
Chronic renal failure (20%–40% of cases; becomes normal after successful renal transplant but not after hemodialysis)
Liver failure (due to decreased prolactin clearance)
Idiopathic causes (some probably represent early cases of microadenoma too small to be detected by CT scan)
Drugs—*most common cause*; usually subsides a few weeks after cessation of using drug; these concentrations are usually 20 to 100 ng/mL.

- Neuroleptics (e.g., phenothiazines, thioxanthenes, butyrophenones)
- Antipsychotic drugs (e.g., Compazine, Thorazine, Stelazine, Mellaril, Haldol)
- Dopamine antagonists (e.g., Metoclopramide, Sulpiride)
- Opiates (morphine, methadone)
- Reserpine
- Alpha-methyldopa (Aldomet)
- Estrogens and oral contraceptives
- Thyrotropin-releasing hormone
- Amphetamines
- Isoniazid

Serum Prolactin May Be Decreased In
Hypopituitarism

- Postpartum pituitary necrosis (Sheehan syndrome)
- Idiopathic hypogonadotropic hypogonadism

Drugs

- Dopamine agonists
- Ergot derivatives (bromocriptine mesylate, lisuride hydrogen maleate)
- Levodopa, apomorphine, clonidine

Interpretation
Normal value in child with growth retardation virtually rules out hypopituitarism but a low value is not diagnostic. Single blood value may be more reliable than multiple measurements of GH in diagnosis of active acromegaly.

TRH stimulation of patients with increased prolactin not due to pituitary tumors usually doubles serum prolactin level to peak >12 ng/mL in 15 to 30 minutes, but most patients with prolactinomas do not respond to TRH stimulation (< double baseline level). Enhanced responsiveness in hypothyroidism and blunted prolactin rise in chronic renal failure. Unresponsiveness to TRH (<2 × baseline level) also occurs in panhypopituitarism. Multiple basal prolactin levels have replaced stimulation tests for diagnosis of prolactinoma.

Microscopic examination of breast discharge shows numerous fat globules; if not seen, rule out intraductal breast carcinoma or infection.

Normal or decreased serum FSH, LH, and testosterone may occur in men.

Women may also present with hirsutism, infertility. Men may present with decreased libido, impotence, oligospermia, low serum testosterone levels, and sometimes galactorrhea.

Hypothyroidism

Acute fasting and chronic protein-calorie deprivation (when growth hormone often rises)

Thyroid-Stimulating Hormone (TSH)–Secreting Pituitary Adenomas
Rare type of pituitary adenoma that secretes TSH, causing hyperthyroidism.

- ◆ Laboratory findings of hyperthyroidism except serum TSH are increased and do not increase in response to TRH stimulation or do not decrease in response to suppressive doses of thyroid hormone.
- ◆ Increased molar ratio of alpha subunit of TSH to whole TSH.
- ○ Secretion of other hormones (e.g., prolactin, growth hormone) occurs in about 1/3 of these cases.

Disorders of Aldosterone, Plasma Renin Activity (PRA), and Angiotensin

---

Hypertension, Renovascular
See Fig. 14-5.

Sudden increase in serum creatinine and BUN, especially after onset of angiotensin-converting enzyme (ACE) inhibitor therapy. Less common with other antihypertensive therapy.

Hypokalemia (<3.4 mEq/L) in ~15% of patients

Proteinuria >500 mg/24 hours usually signifies complete occlusion of a renal artery in a patient with renovascular hypertension.

Captopril test causes

Stimulated peripheral PRA 12 μ/L(ng/mL)/hr and

Increases peripheral PRA ≥10 μg/L/hour and

Increases peripheral PRA ≥150%, or 400% if baseline value <3 μg/L/hour.

Does not differentiate unilateral and bilateral disease. Less reliable in azotemic patients.

Reported S/S >72%.

♦ Peripheral PRA (seated patient, drawn in AM, indexed against sodium excretion) has only S/S = 75%/66% but *a low PRA in untreated patients virtually rules out renovascular hypertension.*

♦ PRA is assayed in blood from each renal vein, inferior vena cava, and aorta or renal arteries.

The test is considered diagnostic when the concentration from the ischemic kidney is at least 1.5× greater than the concentration from the normal kidney (which is equal to or less than the concentration in the vena cava that serves as the standard) or as increment of PRA between each renal artery and vein. Reported S/S = 62% to 80%/80% to 100%; may be increased by repeating test after captopril administration. This is due to high PRA in the peripheral blood, increase in PRA in the renal vein compared to the renal artery of the affected kidney, and suppression of PRA in the other kidney. Maximum renin stimulation accentuates the difference between the two kidneys and should always be obtained by pretest conditions (avoid antihypertensive, diuretic, and oral contraceptive drugs for at least 1 month if possible; low-salt diet for 7 days; administer thiazide diuretic for 1–3 days; upright posture for at least 2 hours).

This is the most useful diagnostic test in renovascular hypertension as judged by surgical results but is not a sufficiently reliable guide to nephrectomy in patients with hypertension due to parenchymal renal disease. *In renovascular hypertension, if renal plasma flow is impaired in the "normal" kidney, surgery often fails to cure the hypertension.* With bilateral renal artery stenosis, most marked change on side with greatest degree of stenosis. Thus little value in patients with bilateral disease. Split renal function tests may show disparity between kidneys.

Aldosteronism

Primary[26,27]

Excessive mineralocorticoid hormone secretion causes renal tubules to retain sodium and excrete potassium.

See Figs. 13-17, 13-18, 13-19, Tables 13-26 and 13-27.

Due To

Solitary adrenal cortical adenoma (64% of patients)

Idiopathic bilateral adrenal hyperplasia (32% of patients)

Adrenal carcinoma (<5% of patients)

Ectopic production of aldosterone by adrenal embryologic rest within kidney or ovary (rare)

Ectopic production of ACTH or aldosterone by nonadrenal neoplasm (rare)

Glucocorticoid-suppressible hyperaldosteronism (<1% of patients)

♦ *Classic biochemical abnormalities are:*

• Decreased serum potassium (see Table 13-22)

• Increased aldosterone production that cannot be suppressed by volume expansion or increased sodium intake (sodium loading)

• Suppressed PRA

[26]Blumenfeld JD, Sealey JE, Schlussel Y, et al. Diagnosis and treatment of primary hyperaldosteronism. *Ann Int Med* 1994;121:877.

[27]Bornstein SR, et al. Adrenocortical tumors: recent advances in basic concepts and clinical management. *Ann Int Med* 1999;130:759.

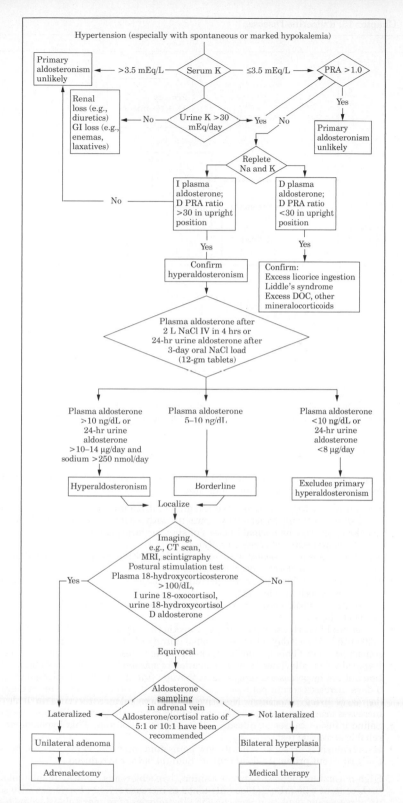

Fig. 13-17. Algorithm for diagnosis of aldosteronism. (D, decreased; DOC, deoxycorticosterone; I, increased; PRA, plasma renin activity.)

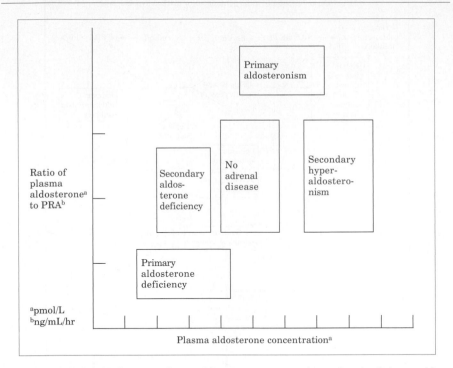

Fig. 13-18. Relationship between plasma aldosterone concentration and ratio of plasma aldosterone to plasma renin activity (PRA) in disorders of mineralocorticoid deficiency or excess.

♦ Hypokalemia (usually <3.0 mEq/L) not related to use of diuretics or laxatives in a hypertensive patient is a strong indicator.

• Present in 80% to 90% of cases; is often mild (3.0–3.5 mEq/L). Aldosteronism should be *suspected* in any hypertensive patient with spontaneous or easily provoked hypokalemia. May be normal in cases of shorter duration before classic clinical picture develops (~20% of cases initially).

• Hypokalemia is more severe with adenoma than with hyperplasia (normal in ~20% of latter) but considerable overlap occurs.

• Hypokalemia ≤2.7 mEq/L in a hypertensive patient is usually due to primary aldosteronism, especially adenoma.

• Intermittent hypokalemia or normokalemia may occur, especially in adrenal hyperplasia etiologies.

• In essential hypertensive patients on diuretic therapy, urine potassium decreases to <30 mEq/L 2 to +3 days after cessation of diuretics but continues in primary aldosteronism patients. (This should be checked several times after cessation of diuretics.)

• Hypokalemia is alleviated by administration of spironolactone and by sodium restriction but not by potassium replacement therapy. Administration of spironolactone for 3 days increases serum potassium >1.2 mEq/L. It also increases urine sodium and decreases urine potassium. Negative potassium balance reoccurs in 5 days. It increases urinary aldosterone (this is variable in hypertensive and normal people).

• Saline infusion causes significant fall in serum potassium. This hypokalemia is a reliable screening test.

• Hyperkaluria is present even with low potassium intake; <30 mEq/24 hours essentially rules out primary aldosteronism. Sodium output is reduced.

○ High-normal or increased serum sodium, hypochloremia, and metabolic alkalosis (CO_2 content >25 mEq/L; blood pH tends to increase >7.42); correlates with severity of potassium depletion. Are clues in all etiologies of primary aldosteronism.

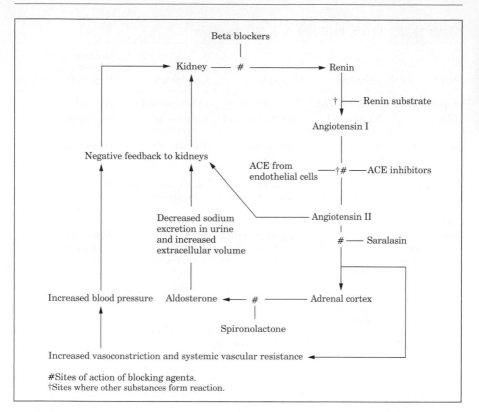

Fig. 13-19. Renin-angiotensin system and blocking sites. Angiotensin-converting enzyme (ACE) is produced primarily by endothelial and epithelial cells; may also be synthesized by activated macrophages in granulomas. Values vary between laboratories even with same method. See Sarcoidosis.

Table 13-26.	Differential Diagnosis of Causes of Hypertension and Hypokalemia		
Condition		PRA	Aldosterone
Primary hyperaldosteronism		D	I
Cushing's syndrome		D	D
Malignant hypertension		I	I
Renovascular hypertension		I	I
Licorice ingestion		D	D
Exogenous mineralocorticoids (e.g., in nasal spray or for orthostatic hypotension)		D	D
Liddle's syndrome		D	D
Congenital adrenal hyperplasia (11-beta- or 17-alpha-hydroxylase deficiency)		D	D

D = decreased; I = increased; PRA = plasma renin activity.

Table 13-27. Differential Diagnosis of Aldosteronism

Test	Adenoma	Idiopathic Hyperplasia	Adrenal Carcinoma	Glucocorticoid-Remediable Hyperaldosteronism
Hypokalemia	More marked	Less marked	Often profound	Normal
PRA	Suppressed; very low	Less suppressed	Suppressed; very low	Suppressed
Plasma or urine aldosterone	I	I is less marked	Usually very I	Often slightly I
Aldosterone response to postural test	D or not I in 70–80% of cases	I in almost all cases	Often unchanged or random I	D
Excess hormone production	I 18-oxocortisol and 18-hydroxy-cortisol in urine; occasionally cortisol	Only aldosterone and related corticosteroids	Androgen, estrogen, or cortisol often	Aldosterone, 18-oxocortisol, 18-hydroxy-cortisol

I = increased; D = decreased; PRA = plasma renin activity.

- ♦ *Proposed screening* tests are inappropriate kaliuresis, low PRA (<3.0 ng/mL/hour), high plasma aldosterone and aldosterone/PRA ratio (>30) (morning sample, upright posture).
- ♦ *Confirm diagnosis* by response of aldosterone and PRA excretion to sodium loading and depletion. Discontinue interfering drugs (for ≥2 weeks).
- Increased plasma and/or urinary aldosterone that is relatively nonsuppressible by salt loading or volume expansion. May be normal in 30% of cases (due to episodic secretion or chronic potassium deficiency, which can suppress aldosterone secretion; therefore must replete potassium before measurement if serum <3.0 mEq/L). Plasma aldosterone <8.5 ng/dL after morning saline infusion rules out primary aldosteronism. Reference values decline by 30% to 50% with increasing age. Plasma aldosterone is normal in recumbent hypertensive and nonhypertensive persons without aldosteronism and increases 2 to 4× after 4 hours of upright posture; increases ≥33% in aldosteronism due to adrenal hyperplasia, but no increase occurs if due to adrenal adenoma.
- Increased urinary aldosterone is best initial screening procedure (normal salt intake, no drugs; not detectable on all days). Cannot be reduced by high sodium intake or DOC administration. Therefore high NaCl intake (10–12 g/day) will cause 24-hr urine aldosterone >14 μg/24 hours and Na >250 mEq/24 hours; urine aldosterone <14 μg/24 hours rules out primary aldosteronism except for glucocorticoid-remedial type; S/S = 96%/93%.
- Volume expansion (by high salt intake, infusion of 2L of NaCl in 4 hours, or DOC) suppresses aldosterone level by >50% to 80% of baseline level in hypertensive patients without primary aldosteronism but not in patients with primary aldosteronism. (Plasma aldosterone level is first increased by having patient in upright position for 2 hours.) Since plasma aldosterone levels vary from moment to moment, a single specimen may not properly reflect adrenal secretion.
- PRA fails to rise to ≥4 ng/mL 90 minutes after stimulus of low-sodium diet, furosemide-induced volume contraction, and upright posture.
- Plasma aldosterone/PRA ratio ≥ 50 at 8 AM or in random blood sample after ambulating 2 hours in patient not on medication is said to indicate primary aldosteronism except in chronic renal insufficiency. Does not distinguish adenoma from hyperplasia.

♦ Captopril (ACE-inhibitor that blocks angiotensin II production) administered as 25 mg IV at 8 AM decreases aldosterone in plasma 2 hours later in normal persons and essential hypertension but remains elevated in primary aldosteronism (Fig. 13-19).

	Sensitivity (%)	Specificity (%)
Potassium <4.0 mEq/L	100	64
Stimulated renin <2.5 ng/mL/3 hours	100	88
Suppressed aldosterone >10 ng/dL	98	92
Sequential 1, 2, and 3	98	99

○ Basal plasma 18 hydroxycorticosterone >100 ng/dL at 8 AM supports diagnosis of aldosteronoma.

Urine is neutral or alkaline (pH >7.0) and is not normally responsive to ammonium chloride load. Its large volume and low specific gravity are not responsive to vasopressin or water restriction (decreased tubular function, especially reabsorption of water).

Plasma cortisol and ACTH are normal.

Serum magnesium falls.

♦ After diagnosis of aldosteronism is established, *cases due to adenoma (treated surgically) should be distinguished from idiopathic hyperplasia (treated medically)* (see Table 13-27, Fig. 13-16). Aldosterone concentration in adrenal vein plasma is higher on side of adenoma, preferably with corticotropin stimulation (90%–95% diagnostic accuracy). Cortisol should also be measured to evaluate accuracy of adrenal vein sampling. Adenomas can also be localized by CT, MRI, or scintigraphy with ^{131}I-labeled iodocholesterol after dexamethasone suppression (uptake increased in adenoma and absent in idiopathic and usually also in carcinoma). Rarely there is unilateral nodular adrenal hyperplasia similar in function to an adenoma. Patients with adenomas have higher plasma 18-oxocortisol (>15 µg/d) and 18-hydroxycorticosterone (>60 µg/d) concentrations which decrease on standing; plasma aldosterone also decreases or fails to increase >30% on standing. In patients with bilateral adrenal hyperplasia and normal persons, plasma aldosterone increases with upright position. A small subset of hyperplasia mimics adenoma because it is associated with angiotensin-independent aldosterone overproduction and is cured by unilateral adrenalectomy.

PRA

Use

Particularly useful to diagnose curable hypertension (e.g., primary aldosteronism, unilateral renal artery stenosis).

May help to differentiate patients with volume excess (e.g., primary aldosteronism) with low PRA from those with medium to high PRA; if latter group shows marked increase in PRA during captopril test, should be worked up for renovascular hypertension but patients with little or no increase are not likely to have curable renovascular hypertension.

• Captopril test criteria for renovascular hypertension: stimulated PRA ≥12 µg/L/hr, absolute increase PRA ≥10 µg/L/hr, increase PRA ≥150% (or ≥400% if baseline PRA <3 µg/L/hr)

In children with salt-losing form of congenital adrenal hyperplasia due to 21-hydroxylase deficiency, severity of disease is related to degree of increase. PRA level may serve as guide to adequate mineralocorticoid replacement therapy.

PRA Is Decreased (<1.5 ng/mL/3 hours) In

Ninety-eight percent of cases of primary aldosteronism. Usually absent or low and can be increased less or not at all by sodium depletion and ambulation in contrast to secondary aldosteronism. PRA may not always be suppressed in primary aldosteronism; repeated testing may be necessary to establish the diagnosis. Normal PRA does not preclude this diagnosis; not a reliable screening test.

Hypertension due to unilateral renal artery stenosis or unilateral renal parenchymal disease

Increased plasma volume due to high-sodium diet, administration of salt-retaining steroids

Eighteen percent to 25% of essential hypertensives (low-renin essential hypertension) and 6% of normal controls

Advancing age in both normal and hypertensive patients (decrease of 35% from the third to the eighth decade)

May also be decreased in CAH secondary to 11-hydroxylase or 17-hydroxylase deficiency with oversecretion of other mineralocorticoids.

Rarely in Liddle syndrome and excess licorice ingestion

Use of various drugs (propranolol, clonidine, reserpine; slightly with methyldopa)

Usually cannot be stimulated by salt restriction, diuretics, and upright posture that deplete plasma volume; therefore measure before and after furosemide and 3 to 4 hours of ambulation

Antihypertensive and hypotensive drugs should be discontinued for at least 2 weeks before measurement of PRA; spironolactone may cause an increase for up to 6 weeks; estrogens may cause an increase for up to 6 months. Blood should be drawn in an ice-cold tube and the plasma immediately separated in a refrigerated centrifuge. Renin level should be indexed against 24-hour level of sodium in urine.

PRA May Be Increased In

Secondary aldosteronism (usually very high levels), especially malignant or severe hypertension 50% to 80% of patients with renovascular hypertension. Normal or high PRA is of limited value to diagnose or rule out renal vascular hypertension. Very high PRA is highly predictive but has poor sensitivity. Low PRA using renin-sodium nomogram in untreated patient with normal serum creatinine is strongly against this diagnosis.[28]

Fifteen percent of patients with essential hypertension (high-renin hypertension)

Renin-producing tumors of the kidney (see Chapter 14)

Reduced plasma volume due to low-sodium diet, diuretics, hemorrhage, Addison disease

Some edematous normotensive states (e.g., cirrhosis, nephrosis, congestive heart failure)

Sodium or potassium loss due to GI disease or in 10% of patients with chronic renal failure

Normal pregnancy

Pheochromocytoma

Last half of menstrual cycle (twofold increase)

Erect posture for 4 hours (twofold increase)

Ambulatory patients compared to bed patients

Bartter syndrome

Various drugs (diuretics, ACE inhibitors, vasodilators; sometimes by calcium antagonists and alpha-blockers, e.g., diazoxide, estrogens, furosemide, guanethidine, hydralazine, minoxidil, spironolactone, thiazides)

	Primary Aldosteronism		Secondary Aldosteronism	
	Adenoma	Hyperplasia	Hypertension	Edema
Aldosterone	↑	↑	↑↑	↑
PRA	↓↓	N/↑	↑↑	↑
Serum sodium	N/↑	N	N/↓	N/↓
Serum potassium	↓	N/↓	↓	N/↓
Edema	0	0	0	Present
Hypertension	↑↑	↑	↑↑↑↑	N/↑

↑, increased; ↓, decreased; N, normal

Aldosteronism, Secondary

Due To

Decreased effective blood volume

- Congestive heart failure
- Cirrhosis with ascites (aldosteronism 2000–3000 mg/day)
- Nephrosis
- Sodium depletion

[28]Mann SJ, Pickering TG. Detection of renovascular hypertension. State of the art. *Ann Int Med* 1992;117:845.

Hyperactivity of renin-angiotensin system
- Renin-producing renal tumor (see Chapter 14)
- Bartter syndrome
- Toxemia of pregnancy
- Malignant hypertension
- Renovascular hypertension
- Oral contraceptive drugs

Secondary Normotensive Hyperaldosteronism (Bartter Syndrome)

Three inherited rare renal tubular disorders; associated with juxtaglomerular hyperplasia.

◆ Hypokalemia with renal potassium wasting is resistant to ADH. Maintaining normal plasma potassium levels is almost impossible despite therapy (supplement dietary potassium, limit sodium intake, drugs such as indomethacin or ibuprofen).
◆ Hyponatremia is not corrected by fluid restriction.
◆ Increased PRA is a characteristic feature.
◆ Increased plasma and urine aldosterone in the absence of edema, hypertension, or hypovolemia
○ Chloride-resistant metabolic alkalosis
Insensitive to pressor effects of angiotensin II (may occur in patients with prolonged hypokalemia due to any cause)
Hypercalciuria is common, often leading to nephrocalcinosis; decreased serum magnesium is uncommon in contrast to Gitelman syndrome (a variant of Bartter syndrome).
Excretion of large quantities of sodium and chloride in urine
Not due to laxatives, diuretics, or GI loss of potassium and chloride

Glucocorticoid Suppressible Hyperaldosteronism (Remediable)

Rare autosomal dominant defect of zona glomerulosa in which beta-methyloxidase produces aldosterone from precursor arising in zona fasciculate.

◆ Usual findings of primary aldosteronism with hypokalemia, increased aldosterone, and suppressed PRA.
◆ Reversal of clinical and laboratory findings (suppression of aldosterone secretion) by dexamethasone for 48 hours distinguishes this from primary hyperaldosteronism.
◆ Characteristic finding is large amounts of metabolites of 18-oxocortisol in urine.
Anomalous decrease in plasma aldosterone response to posture.
Normal CT and MRI of adrenals.

Pseudoaldosteronism (Liddle Syndrome)

Rare autosomal dominant collecting tubule disorder with clinical manifestations closely resembling those due to aldosterone-producing adrenal adenoma.

◆ Greatly reduced aldosterone secretion and excretion unresponsive to stimulation by ACTH, angiotensin II, or low-sodium diet causing:
Sodium retention
Low PRA
Hypokalemia due to renal potassium wasting, metabolic alkalosis, and hypertension
○ All are corrected by long-term administration of diuretics that act at distal tubule to cause natriuresis and renal potassium retention (e g , triamterene or amiloride) and by restriction of sodium.

Pseudoaldosteronism Due To Ingestion of Licorice (Ammonium Glycyrrhizate)

Excessive ingestion causes hypertension due to sodium retention.

◆ Urinary glycyrrhetinic acid can be measured by gas chromatography and mass spectrometry.

Unstimulated renin-aldosterone system may be suppressed for ≤4 months after cessation of chronic ingestion of licorice. Effect on electrolyte balance may persist for ≤1 week after cessation.
Decreased serum potassium
Decreased aldosterone excretion in urine
Decreased PRA

Hypoaldosteronism

Hypofunction of renin-angiotensin-aldosterone system.

Infrequent condition may be caused by

- Addison disease
- CAH
- Autosomal recessive deficiency of aldosterone synthase
- Prolonged administration of heparin (very rare)
- Removal of unilateral aldosterone-secreting tumor (usually transient)
- Autonomic nervous system dysfunction; aldosterone deficiency causes impaired renal sodium conservation but without hyperkalemia
- Idiopathic hyporeninism
- Associated with mild renal insufficiency (especially diabetic nephropathy, some interstitial nephropathies)

Hyperkalemia, hyponatremia, urinary sodium loss, hypovolemia corrected by administration of mineralocorticoids
Mild hyperchloremic metabolic acidosis
♦ Decreased aldosterone and PRA that are not increased by combined diuretic and posture establish the diagnosis.
Normal adrenal glucocorticoid response to ACTH stimulation test
Laboratory findings of associated diseases (e.g., DM, gout, pyelonephritis)

Pseudohypoaldosteronism

Autosomal recessive heterogeneous group of disorders due to resistance to aldosterone action with signs and symptoms of aldosterone deficiency, but aldosterone and PRA levels are markedly increased.

♦ Very high serum aldosterone, increased PRA associated with renal salt wasting; increases are resistant to mineralocorticoid therapy.
Hyponatremia, hyperkalemia
High sodium concentration in sweat, stool, saliva

Tests of Water and Electrolytes

Vasopressin (Antidiuretic Hormone [ADH])

Hormone secreted by posterior pituitary; regulates water permeability of renal collecting ducts and urine concentrating ability by increasing water reabsorption, which is mediated by transcellular water channels [aquaporins]. Reference range = 0.32–1.80 pmol/L (0.35–1.94 ng/L). Performed in reference labs. Should be correlated with plasma osmolality.

Use
Diagnosis and differential diagnosis of DI and psychogenic polyuria
Diagnosis of SIADH
Differential diagnosis of hyponatremias
Increased In Plasma
Nephrogenic DI (partial or complete): high ADH and low osmolality
Primary psychogenic polydipsia
SIADH inappropriately increased for degree of plasma osmolality, i.e., normal ADH relative to osmolality
Ectopic ADH syndrome
Certain drugs (e.g., chlorpropamide, phenothiazine, Tegretol)

Decreased In Plasma
Central DI (partial or complete): decreased for level of plasma osmolality

Osmolality, Plasma (see Chapter 3)
Osmolality, Urine (see Chapter 14)
Water Deprivation Test

Steps:

1. Restrict water intake after dinner (unless producing >10 L/day).
2. Spot urine until 3 successive urines are within 50–100 mmol/kg of each other.
3. Administer ADH.
4. Measure serum osmolality and plasma ADH.
5. Measure urine osmolality every 30 minutes for next 3 hours (to account for large-capacity bladder and/or time lag).

Normal: Water deprivation causes kidney to increase urine osmolality to 1,000 to 1,200 mmol/kg. ADH does not cause further increase in urine osmolality because endogenous ADH is already at maximum.

Complete DI: Water deprivation increases plasma osmolality but urine osmolality stays <290 mmol/kg and does not increase.

Partial DI: Water deprivation causes some increase in urine osmolality to 400 to 500 mmol/kg (less than normal).

Complete or partial nephrogenic DI or psychogenic polydipsia: Increased ADH levels. Giving ADH does not increase urine osmolality in complete nephrogenic DI.

Complete or partial central DI: Low ADH relative to plasma osmolality. Giving ADH increases urine osmolality ~200 mmol/kg but not in partial nephrogenic DI.

Does not distinguish partial nephrogenic DI from psychogenic polydipsia.

Disorders of Water and Electrolytes

Diabetes Insipidus (DI)

Characterized by excretion of abnormally large volumes [>30 mL/kg/day in adults] of dilute hypo-osmotic urine [<250 mmol/kg] in response to decreased production, secretion, or effect of ADH.

See Table 13-28.

Due To
Central (hypothalamic or pituitary): May be partial or complete. Usually acquired; less commonly is hereditary dominant appearing in childhood.

Nephrogenic: Renal insensitivity to antidiuretic effect of arginine vasopressin (ADH) due to renal disease, drugs, metabolic status, aging, etc.

Primary polydipsia: May be psychogenic or abnormal thirst mechanism

Gestational DI: Increased metabolism of ADH during pregnancy

High-set osmoreceptor

DI, Central

Due to failure of posterior pituitary to make or secrete vasopressin caused by lesions of hypothalamus/pituitary that impair osmotic regulation but maintain volume regulation of antidiuretic hormone secretion.

Due To
Primary

- Idiopathic (now causes <50% of cases)
- Hereditary (causes ~1% of cases)

Secondary

- Supra- and intrasellar tumors
    Neoplasms (suprasellar and intrasellar
    Primary (e.g., craniopharyngioma, cyst)
    Metastatic (e.g., carcinoma of breast, lung; leukemias)

Table 13-28.   Comparison of Different Types of Diabetes Insipidus

| | After Dehydration[a] | | | | |
	Urine Specific Gravity	Urine Osmolality (mOsm/kg)	Plasma Osmolality (mOsm/kg)	After Pitressin,[b] Urine Osmolality (% change)	Plasma Vasopressin (pg/mL)
Normal	≥1.015	700–1400	288–291	No change (<5%)	1.3–4.1
Central diabetes insipidus (complete)	<1.010	50–200	310–320	Doubles (>100%)[a]	<1.1
Central diabetes insipidus (partial)	1.010–1.015	250–500	296–305	Increases (9–67%)[c]	
Nephrogenic diabetes insipidus	<1.010	100–200	310–320	No change[d]	12–13 (>2.7 in high Ca/low K type)
High-set osmo-receptor diabetes insipidus	≥1.015	700–1400	300–305	No change	
Primary (psychogenic) polydipsia	Low	700–1200	Low	No change after medullary washout; normal increase after high-sodium diet	3.0–7.5

[a]Dehydration test: No fluid intake for 4–18 hrs, measure urine osmolality and/or specific gravity hourly, weigh patient (or urine) frequently to avoid loss of >3% of body weight (*if >3% of body weight, measure plasma and urine osmolality, and terminate test to avoid hypotension*). If three successive hourly urine osmolality determinations indicate no further change (i.e., a plateau has been reached), administer 5 U vasopressin (Pitressin) subcutaneously, and 60 mins later, measure urine osmolality.
[b]One hr after subcutaneous injection of 5 U of aqueous Pitressin.
[c]Useful to distinguish partial from complete central diabetes insipidus.
[d]Therefore differs from central diabetes insipidus.
Plasma, vasopressin levels must always be interpreted relative to plasma osmolality.

- Histiocytosis (eosinophilic granuloma is most common), Hand-Schuller-Christian disease
- Granulomatous lesions (e.g., sarcoidosis, TB, syphilis, Wegener granulomatosis)
- Trauma, with or without basal skull fracture; neurosurgical procedures
- Vascular lesions (e.g., aneurysms, thrombosis, sickle cell disease, Sheehan syndrome)
- Infections (e.g., meningitis, encephalitis, Guillain-Barré syndrome, CMV)
- Autoimmune
- Others (e.g., hypoxemic encephalopathy)

♦ Urine is inappropriately dilute (low specific gravity [usually <1.005] and osmolality [50–200 mOsm/kg]) in presence of increased serum osmolality (>295 mOsm/kg) and increased or normal serum sodium.
♦ Large urine volume (4–15/L/24 hours) is characteristic.
♦ Plasma ADH level is decreased relative to plasma osmolality. In contrast, complete or partial nephrogenic DI or primary psychogenic polydipsia have increased plasma ADH. Dehydration test fails to increase urine specific gravity or osmolality, and plasma osmolality remains elevated. After administration of vasopressin (ADH), urine osmolality will increase by 50%.
Partial central DI shows intermediate values between complete central and normal.
See Tables 13-28 and 13-29.

Table 13-29.   Comparison of Hyponatremia Due to Various Causes

Cause	Urine Sodium	Urine Osmolarity	BUN
Hypervolemic (e.g., congestive heart failure, cirrhosis, nephrotic syndrome)			
Early	D (usually <10–15 mEq/L)	I (usually >350–400 mOsm/L)	N
Late	D with isotonic urine is ominous finding	(>200 mmol/kg)	I disproportionate to creatinine
Hypovolemic			
Extrarenal Gastrointestinal Skin (burns, sweat) Third space	D (<10 mEq/L)	I (>400 mOsm/L)	N
Renal			
Diuretic (most common)	I (>20 mEq/L)	Isotonic to plasma	Usually I
Chronic renal disease (especially interstitial)		If severe volume contraction, 300–450 mOsm/kg	
Mineralocorticoid deficiency			
Normovolemic			
SIADH (almost always)	I (>20 mmol/L)	I (>200 mmol/kg)	Often D (<8–10 mg/dL)
Reset osmostat	V	V	N or D

D = decreased; I = increased; SIADH = syndrome of inappropriate antidiuretic hormone secretion; V = variable.

DI, Nephrogenic[29]

See Table 13-28.

Due To

Chronic renal failure (e.g., GN, pyelonephritis, gout, analgesic nephropathy, nephrosclerosis)

Other tubulointerstitial diseases (e.g., polycystic kidneys, medullary sponge disease, sickle cell disease or trait, amyloidosis)

Diuretic phase of acute tubular necrosis

Following renal transplant or relief of urinary tract obstruction

Hypergammaglobulinemia (e.g., multiple myeloma, amyloidosis, Sjögren syndrome)

Drugs (e.g., alcohol, some diuretics, lithium [55% of patients on long-term therapy], demeclocycline, amphotericin, propoxyphene, methoxyflurane, vincristine)

Prolonged potassium depletion and hypokalemia (condition is reversed by restoring potassium level to normal).

Prolonged hypercalciuria, usually with hypercalcemia (condition is reversed by restoring the calcium level to normal).

Hereditary renal tubular unresponsiveness to vasopressin due to X-linked genetic defect; severe form occurs in males; family history of this condition is frequent.

Primary hyperaldosteronism

Pregnancy

[29]Sands JM, Bichet DC. Nephrogenic diabetes insipidus. *Ann Intern Med* 2006;144:186.

Table 13-30. Comparison of Diabetes Insipidus (DI) and SIADH

	Normal	DI	SIADH
Serum sodium (mmol/L)	135–145	>145	<130
Plasma osmolality (mmol/L)	278–298	>295 (high-normal to slight increase)	<275
Urine osmolality (mmol/L)	50–1,200 Varies with fluid intake Usually >800	>300 300–800*	>1,200
Osmolality ratio U/P	1–3	<1	>3–4
Urine output	~2.5 L/day	>2.5 L/day	Decreased

*Partial central DI

♦ Laboratory findings are the same as in central DI except that nephrogenic type shows:

- Increased plasma vasopressin level
- Water deprivation test does not cause urine osmolality to increase above plasma osmolality.
- Administration of ADH causes urine osmolality to increase in central DI but not in nephrogenic DI.
- Dehydration test causes the plasma vasopressin level to increase.
- Urine osmolality does not increase with subsequent injection of vasopressin.

DI Due to High-Set Osmoreceptor

Rare entity in which the set point for stimulating release of ADH is ≥300 mOsm/kg instead of the normal 285 mOsm/kg level.

See Table 13-28.

As plasma osmolality increases, patient becomes thirsty and drinks fluids, thereby diluting the plasma before it reaches the higher set level to stimulate release of ADH, initiating cycle of polyuria and polydipsia. If thirst center is also impaired, patient develops essential hypernatremia.

♦ Plasma osmolality after dehydration is significantly higher than in normal state.

♦ Urine osmolality does not increase after administration of vasopressin.

Hypernatremia

Always denotes hypertonic hyperosmolality.

See Table 13-31.

Due To

Loss of water

   Renal (e.g., diuretics, renal disease)

   GI loss (e.g., vomiting, diarrhea, nasogastric drainage, bowel fistula, osmotic cathartics)

   Skin (excess sweating, burns)

   Lungs

   DI (see above)

Gain of sodium

   Hypertonic sodium infusion or ingestion

   Sea water ingestion

   Saline enemas or intrauterine injection

   Primary hyperaldosteronism

   Cushing syndrome

♦ Serum sodium and osmolality are increased.

Increased BUN, creatinine, BUN:creatinine ratio; usually albumin and Hct increased

Urine osmolality is increased to maximum, often >600 mOsmol/kg.

FeNa is usually <1%; may be normal in presence of metabolic alkalosis.

Metabolic alkalosis with low Cl⁻ and high bicarbonate is often present.

Table 13-31. Patterns in Hypernatremias

	Cause	Urine Tonicity	Urine Sodium (mmol/L)
Decreased total body water and sodium	Renal loss	N/D	>20
	Skin (e.g., Burns Sweating)	I	<10
	GI (e.g., diarrhea, fistulas)	I	<10
Normal total body water and sodium	Renal loss (e.g., DI) Hypodipsia	D/I/N	V
	Extrarenal loss (Skin, respiratory)	I	V
Increased total body water and sodium	1° hyperaldosteronism Cushing syndrome Hypertonic sodium infusion or ingestion (e.g., sea water; saline enemas or intrauterine injection)	I/N	>20

Total body water varies with size and fat: ~60% of body weight in younger men, ~50% of body weight in older men and younger women, ~40% of body weight in older women.
Extracellular fluid = 60% of body water. Intracellular fluid = 40% of body water.
N, normal; I, increased; D, decreased; V, variable.

Hyponatremia

See Table 13-29 and Fig. 13-20.

Due To

Isotonic (spurious or "pseudohyponatremia") when sodium is measured with flame photometer rather than ion-selective electrode. Plasma osmolality is normal. Abnormal retention of water responsible for low serum sodium.

- Hyperlipidemia "falsely" lowers serum sodium; measured plasma osmolality exceeds calculated plasma osmolality

  [Calculated plasma osmolality = $2 \times Na + (plasma\ glucose \div 18) + (BUN \div 2.8)$]

- Hyperproteinemia (e.g., myeloma, macroglobulinemia)

Table 13-32. Electrolyte Patterns in Hyponatremias

Condition	Preceding Condition	Urine Sodium	24-hr Urine Sodium	Urine Osmolality	Serum Potassium
Excess hydration	Excess intake of water	D	D	D BUN is D	N/D
Diuretic use/ abuse	Drug history	D	I	D	D
SIADH		I	I	I (>300 mOsm), but D serum osmolality	N/D
Adrenal insufficiency		Slightly I	I	N (>300 mOsm)	I
Bartter syndrome		D	I	D	D
Hyperosmolar diabetic coma	Blood glucose is very I	N	N	N.	I

N, normal; I, increased; D, decreased; V, variable.

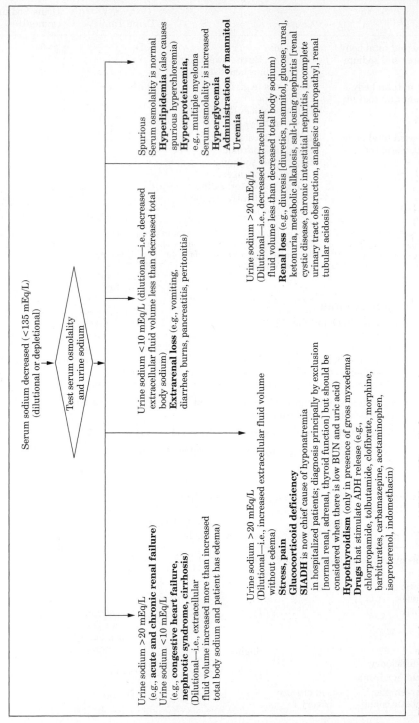

Fig. 13-20. Algorithm for hyponatremia. (ADH, antidiuretic hormone.)

- Hyperglycemia (each increase of blood sugar of 100 mg/dL decreases serum sodium by 1.7 mEq/L). Seen also with azotemia and after ethanol ingestion.
- Commonly caused by intravascular hemolysis with increased serum potassium resulting in reciprocal decreased in serum sodium. May occur with flame photometry or ion selective electrode.

Hypertonic

- Excess mannitol treatment

Hypotonic

- Hypervolemic usually with clinical edema.
  With low urine sodium (<10 mEq/L) may be due to congestive heart failure, cirrhosis with ascites, nephrotic syndrome With high urine sodium (>20 mEq/L) may be due to acute tubular necrosis or end-stage chronic renal failure where Na and H$_2$0 intake exceeds excretion. Serum uric acid and BUN tend to be increased.
- Hypovolemic
  Urine sodium <10 mEq/L. Due to extrarenal loss of sodium (e.g., GI tract, fistulas, pancreatitis, exercise, sweating, burns).
  Urine sodium >20mEq/L. Due to renal loss of sodium (e.g., diuretics such as furosemide or osmotic diuresis due to glucose or urea, diabetic ketoacidosis, renal tubular acidosis, salt-losing nephritis, adrenal insufficiency, hyporeninemia, hypoaldosteronism).
- Normovolemic—usually no edema is present.
  Large amounts of sodium appear in urine (>20 mEq/L). May be due to SIADH, hypothyroidism, hypopituitarism, low reset osmostat syndrome, physical or emotional stress, potassium depletion, renal failure, water poisoning, certain drugs (e.g., ADH analogues, amitriptyline, carbamazepine, chlorpropamide, cyclophosphamide, diuretics, haloperidol, thioridazine, vincristine).
Hyponatremic patients with BUN <10 mg/dL and uric acid <3.0 mg/dL should be considered to have SIADH or low reset osmostat until proved otherwise.
Correction of very low plasma sodium must be done cautiously to avoid central pontine myelinosis due to rapid correction of hyponatremia; not more than half of sodium deficit should be corrected at a time.

Dehydration, Hypertonic

Due To
Loss of water in excess of electrolyte loss (e.g., gastroenteritis with diarrhea, hyperventilation, high fever, DI)
Excessive intake of high-solute mixtures (e.g., accidental ingestion, iatrogenic infusion)
♦ Serum osmolality is increased
○ BUN is increased, often ≥60 mg/dL
○ Increased serum sodium to >150 mEq/L
○ Metabolic acidosis is almost always present.
Increased blood glucose is common, often >200 mg/dL.
Hypocalcemia is common and may persist if calcium is not administered.
Urine is concentrated with specific gravity usually >1.020.
Other laboratory findings of dehydration.
Rehydration with return of serum sodium to normal should not be completed in <48 hours because of risk of permanent CNS damage.

Dehydration, Hypotonic

Usually in children with vomiting and diarrhea treated with oral replacement of tap water.

○ Decreased serum sodium, usually <135 mEq/L
Other laboratory findings of dehydration
Urine pH is >7.0 (≤7.9) if potassium depletion is not severe and concomitant sodium deficiency (e.g., vomiting) is not present.
○ When urine chloride is low (<10–20 mEq/L) and the patient responds to NaCl treatment, the cause is more likely loss of gastric juice, diuretic therapy, or relief of chronic hypercapnia.

○ When the urine chloride is high (>10–20 mEq/L) and the patient does not respond to NaCl treatment, the cause is more likely hyperadrenalism or severe pulmonary deficiency.

Low Reset Osmostat

Due to production of ADH at lower plasma osmolality than normal.

Hyponatremia with mild volume expansion
Increased urine concentration and osmolality higher than plasma

Syndrome of Inappropriate Secretion of Antidiuretic Hormone (SIADH)

Syndrome of autonomous, sustained release of vasopressin in absence of stimuli (e.g., low plasma osmolality); kidney responds normally to ADH.

Due To

CNS disease of all types (e.g., neoplastic, degenerative, infective, trauma, vascular, psychogenic)

Advanced endocrinopathies (e.g., hypothyroidism, ACTH deficiency, adrenal insufficiency)

Neoplasms (most commonly small-cell carcinoma of lung; adenocarcinoma of lung, carcinomas of pancreas, duodenum, stomach, prostate, melanoma, lymphoma) some of which show ectopic production of ADH

Pulmonary diseases (e.g., cancer, pulmonary emboli, TB, pneumonia, chronic infections, lung abscess, aspergillosis)

Miscellaneous (e.g., acute intermittent porphyria, postoperative state)

Idiopathic

Various drugs:

- Oral hypoglycemic agents (chlorpropamide, tolbutamide, phenformin, metformin)
- Antineoplastic agents (vincristine, cyclophosphamide)
- Diuretics (chlorothiazide)
- Sedatives, analgesics (morphine, barbiturates, acetaminophen)
- Antidepressant drugs (amitriptyline, phenothiazines)
- Miscellaneous (clofibrate, isoproterenol, nicotine)

May be transient (acute) for 3 to 5 days postoperatively.

Etiology should be established since some causes are curable with resolution of SIADH. Cortisol deficiency and hypothyroidism should always be excluded.

♦ Characterized by high plasma ADH and low renin concentrations. High ADH causes increased tubular reabsorption of water resulting in the following:

♦ Dilutional hyponatremia (<130 mmol/L) with appropriately decreased osmolality (usually <270 mOsm/kg) when urine is not at maximum dilution; this is basis for diagnosis in patient with no evidence of cardiac, liver, kidney, adrenal, pituitary, or thyroid disease, or hypovolemia, and not on drug therapy (especially diuretics).

♦ Increased urine sodium (>20 mmol/L; >30 mmol/day) with inappropriately high urine osmolality (>500 mOsm/kg) is essential for diagnosis since it excludes hypovolemia as the cause of hyponatremia (in absence of abnormal renal function or causative drugs).

♦ Increased urine osmolality higher than plasma osmolality, usually by >100 mOsm/kg. Plasma osmolality is decreased to <279 mol/L.[2]

♦ Water load test—see Table 13-33. Plasma ADH.

Normal serum potassium, CO_2, BUN, and creatinine

Decreased serum chloride

Decreased anion gap

Decreased uric acid (due to dilution)

Increased plasma vasopressin that is inappropriately elevated for the degree of plasma osmolality is not helpful in diagnosis since most causes of true hyponatremia are associated with detectable or increased vasopressin (see Arginine Vasopressin [ADH]

Clinical and biochemical response to fluid restriction but not to administration of isotonic or hypertonic saline.

Table 13-33.	Water Load Test in SIADH*	
	Normal	SIADH
Water excretion in 4 hrs	90%	<90% In severe SIADH may be <40% in 5 hrs
Plasma osmolality	Baseline: 278–298 mmol/L Decreases ≥5 mmol/L	Decreases
Urine osmolality	Baseline: >800 mmol/L Decreases to ≤100 mmol/L	Remains >100 mmol/L
Ratio urine/plasma osmolality	>1	
Plasma ADH	Normal <2 pmol/L	Normal in most patients Only 2 hrs after water load, it is inappropriate in relation to low plasma osmolality thereby supporting the diagnosis of SIADH

*Water load test may be dangerous unless serum sodium >125 mmol/L. Patient drinks 20 mL/kg of water in 15–30 mins. Supine posture during test. Measure plasma and urine osmolality hourly for next 4–5 hrs and urine output. Measure urine creatinine to confirm complete collection.

Polydipsia, Psychogenic

Excessive intake of water owning to underlying psychoneurotic need causes loss of medullary sodium and urea to renal venous blood and abnormally reduced tonicity of renal medulla.

See Table 13-28.
○ Should be suspected when large volumes of very dilute urine occur with plasma osmolality that is only slightly decreased or low-normal.
Test dose of vasopressin often shows failure to concentrate urine, simulating nephrogenic DI. However, the test will be normal when performed after restoration of normal hypertonicity of renal medulla by a period of high-sodium and low-water intake.
Fluid deprivation test is least reliable in differentiating this from partial central DI; e.g., some increase in urine osmolality after dehydration with an inconclusive (~10%) further increase after vasopressin may be due to either condition.

Tests of Gonadal Function

Chromosome Analysis

Turner syndrome (gonadal dysgenesis)—usually negative for Barr bodies
Klinefelter syndrome—positive for Barr bodies
Pseudohermaphroditism—chromosomal sex corresponding to gonadal sex

Cytologic Examination of Vaginal Smear (Papanicolaou Smear) for Evaluation of Ovarian Function

Maturation index (MI) is the proportion of parabasal, intermediate, and superficial cells in each 100 cells counted.

• Lack of estrogen effect shows predominance of parabasal cells (e.g., MI = 100/0/0).
• Low estrogen effect shows predominance of intermediate cells (e.g., MI = 10/90/0).
• Increased estrogen effect shows predominance of superficial cells (e.g., MI = 0/0/100), as in hormone-producing tumors of ovary, persistent follicular cysts.

Some Patterns of Maturation Index in Different Conditions Index

	Index
Childhood	
Normal	80/20/0
Cortisone therapy	0/98/2
Childbearing years	
Preovulatory (late-follicular) phase	0/40/60
Premenstrual (late-luteal) phase	0/70/30
Pregnancy (second month)	0/90/10
Cortisone therapy	0/85/15
Amenorrhea after ovarian irradiation	0/30/70
Surgical oophorectomy	0/80/20–0/90/10
Bilateral oophorectomy and adrenalectomy	0/98/2
Postmenopausal years, early (age 60)	65/30/5
Postmenopausal years, late (age 75)	
Untreated	100/0/0
Moderate estrogen treatment	0/50/50
High-dose estrogen treatment	0/0/100
Years after bilateral oophorectomy	100/0/0
Postadrenalectomy, bilateral	6/94/0

Karyopyknotic index (KI) is the percentage of cells with pyknotic nuclei. Increased estrogen effect (e.g., KI ≥85%) is seen, as in cystic glandular hyperplasia of the endometrium.

Eosinophilic index is the percentage of cells showing eosinophilic cytoplasm; it may also be used as a measure of estrogen effect.

Combined progesterone/estrogen effect: No quantitative cytologic criteria are available. Endometrial biopsy should be used for this purpose.

The pattern may be obscured by cytolysis (e.g., infections, excess bacilli), increased red or white blood cells, excessively thin or thick smears, or drying of smears before fixation (artificial eosinophilic staining).

Estrogens (Total), Serum

Includes estradiol produced by ovaries, placenta, and smaller amounts by testes and adrenals; also includes estrone and estriol.

Use
Overall status of estrogens in females or males. Must be interpreted according to phase of menstrual cycle.

Increased In
Estrogen-producing tumors (e.g., granulosa cell tumor, theca-cell tumor, luteoma), secondary to stimulation by hCG-producing tumors (e.g., teratoma, teratocarcinoma)

Pregnancy

Gynecomastia

Decreased In
Ovarian failure

Primary hypofunction of ovary:

* Autoimmune oophoritis is the most common cause; usually associated with other autoimmune endocrinopathies (e.g., Hashimoto thyroiditis, Addison disease, IDDM). May cause premature menopause.
* Resistant ovary syndrome
* Toxic (e.g., irradiation, chemotherapy)
* Infection (e.g., mumps)
* Tumor (primary or secondary)
* Mechanical (e.g., trauma, torsion, surgical excision)
* Genetic (e.g., Turner syndrome)
* Menopause

Secondary hypofunction of ovary:

* Disorders of hypothalamic-pituitary axis

Follicular-Stimulating Hormone (FSH) and Luteinizing Hormone (LH), Serum

Glycoproteins produced by the anterior pituitary gland; regulated by hypothalamicGnRH (hypothalamic gonadotropin-releasing hormone that also initiates puberty and adrenal maturation) and feedback by gonadal steroid hormones. FSH stimulates follicular growth and stimulates seminiferous tubules and testicular growth. LH stimulates ovulation and production of estrogen and progesterone. LH controls production of testosterone by Leydig cells.

Use
Diagnosis of gonadal, pituitary, hypothalamic disorders
Diagnosis and management of infertility

Increased In
Primary hypogonadism (anorchia, testicular failure, menopause)
Gonadotropin-secreting pituitary tumors
Precocious puberty (secondary to a CNS lesion or idiopathic)
Complete testicular feminization syndrome
Luteal phase of menstrual cycle

Decreased In
Secondary hypogonadism

- Kallmann syndrome (inherited X-linked or autosomal isolated deficiency of GnRH; occurs in both sexes); Found in ~5% of patients with primary amenorrhea. Causes failure of both gametogenic function and sex steroid production (LH and FSH are "normal" or undetectable but rise in response to prolonged GnRH stimulation).
- Pituitary LH or FSH deficiency
- Gonadotropin deficiency

Inhibins A and B, Serum

Polypeptide hormones that belong to transforming growth factor family. Secreted by granulosa cells of ovary and Sertoli cells of testis. Inhibits pituitary production of FSH. Secreted by placenta during pregnancy.

Females

Inhibin A is mostly produced by corpus luteum.

- Undetectable before puberty
- Very low levels in postmenopausal state due to absent follicular secretions
- During pregnancy is secreted by placenta. Inhibin A peaks at 8 to 10 weeks, declines until 20 weeks, then increases gradually to term.

Inhibin B is produced by granulosa cells of small developing antral follicles.

- Rises to peak in early puberty; constant level thereafter.
- Gradually declines after age 40. In early menopause, follicular phase Inhibin B declines while Inhibin A and estradiol are still within normal range.
- May indicate low ovarian reserve in perimenopausal women and transition to menopause; useful for assisted reproduction. Measure on days 3 to 5 of menstrual cycle.

After menopause, Inhibin A and B fall to very low levels.
Also used as a serum marker for detecting Down syndrome pregnancies (see Chapter 12)
May be useful to screen for preeclampsia (see Chapter 14)

Males

Inhibin B is predominant in males and supports spermatogenesis by negative feedback of FSH.
Inhibin A is not significant in males(normal values <480 pg/mL); values remain fairly constant.
May be decreased in male infertility.

Müllerian Inhibiting Substance, Serum

Gonadal hormone produced by Sertoli cells that inhibits pituitary production of FSH. Detectable in normal boys from birth to puberty when concentration declines.

Use

Differentiate anorchia from nonpalpable undescended testes in boys with bilateral
  cryptorchidism

Presence indicates testicular integrity in children with intersexual anomalies

Supplement or replace response of serum testosterone to administration of hCG for
  gonadal evaluation in prepubertal children.

Decreased or Absent In

Anorchia

Negligible concentration in girls until puberty

Female pseudohermaphroditism

Interpretation

In prepubertal children, normal value in boys is sensitive and specific test predictive of
  testicular tissue (98%) and undetectable value predicts anorchia or ovaries (89%).

Values are better than serum testosterone alone; combined with serum testosterone,
  S/S = 62%/100% for absence of testes.[30]

Progesterone, Serum

**Hormone synthesized by ovary. Low in follicular phase but increases to 10 to 40
mg/day during luteal phase and ≤300 mg/day if pregnancy occurs.**

Increased In

Luteal phase of menstrual cycle

Luteal cysts of ovary

Ovarian tumors (e.g., arrhenoblastoma)

Adrenal tumors

Decreased In

Amenorrhea

Threatened abortion (some patients)

Fetal death

Toxemia of pregnancy

Gonadal agenesis

Testicle, Biopsy

Use

Infertility workup

Diagnosis of tumor

Interpretation

Normal spermatogenesis and normal endocrine findings in patient with aspermia and
  infertility suggest a mechanical obstruction to sperm transport that may be correctable.

Testosterone, Free, Serum

**Secreted by testes in male and by ovary and adrenal in females. Preferable to total
assay, which is bound to sex hormone–binding globulin [SHBG] and is not biologically functional and may result in underdiagnosis of hypogonadism.**

Use

Evaluation of gonadal hormonal function

Decreased In (Men)

Primary hypogonadism (e.g., orchiectomy)

Secondary hypogonadism (e.g., hypopituitarism)

Testicular feminization

Klinefelter syndrome levels lower than in normal male but higher than in normal
  female and orchiectomized male

Estrogen therapy

Total (but not free) testosterone decreased due to decreased SHBG (e.g., cirrhosis,
  chronic renal disease)

---

[30]Lee MM, et al. Measurements of serum Müllerian inhibiting substance in the evaluation of children with nonpalpable gonads. *NEJM* 1997;336:1480.

Increased In
Adrenal virilizing tumor causing premature puberty in boys or masculinization in women
Congenital adrenal hyperplasia
Idiopathic hirsutism—inconclusive
Stein-Leventhal syndrome—variable; increased when virilization is present
Ovarian stromal hyperthecosis
Use of certain drugs that alter thyroxine-binding globulins may also affect testosterone-binding globulins; however the free testosterone level will not be affected.

Gonadal Disorders

Ambiguous Genitalia

Sexual ambiguity occurs in 1 in 1,000 live-born infants.

Females [31]

Condition	Laboratory Finding
CAH with or without salt-losing	21-Hydroxylase deficiency, 11-Hydroxylase deficiency, 3-Beta-hydroxysteroid dehydrogenase mutations
Iatrogenic virilization	No diagnostic test; history of maternal ingestion of virilizing agents (i.e., progestins)
Maternal virilization	Increased androgens in maternal serum
Idiopathic virilization	Normal plasma and urine steroids; 46XX karyotype; gonadal biopsy may show Leydig tissue
Gonadal dysgenesis	No specific laboratory test. Laparotomy usually shows a streak gonad on one side and testicular tissue on other side. Karyotype may be nondiagnostic (46XX or 46XY), multiple mosaic (44XO/46XX/47XXY), or typical (45XO/46XY).
True hermaphrodite	No specific laboratory test. Biopsy of gonad shows ovarian follicles and testicular tubules. Karyotype may be 46XX, 46XY, or any mosaic included under gonadal dysgenesis. H-Y antigen is present.

Males [31]

Absent Müllerian inhibiting factor	46XY karyotype. Normal steroid levels. No specific laboratory tests. Testes and uterii inguinali present.
Undescended testes	Normal gonadotropin and hormone levels
Anorchia	May have low plasma testosterone and very high plasma FSH and LH. Later hCG stimulation is negative.
Leydig cell agenesis or hypoplasia	Plasma testosterone is very low and fails to rise following hCG stimulation. High LD. Normal FSH. Biopsy of testicle is diagnostic.
Unknown cause for unresponsiveness to androgens	Karyotype 46XY. Normal testosterone and dihydrotestosterone levels. No specific laboratory test.
Faulty androgen action	46XY karyotype. Normal testosterone level. *Sex-linked defect type* is diagnosed by in vitro binding study. LH may be high. Dihydrotestosterone level is normal. *Autosomal recessive type* has normal LH and FSH levels. Dihydrotestosterone level is low.

[31] MacLauglin DT, Donahoe PK. Sex determination and differentiation. *N Engl J Med* 2004;350:367.

Abnormal testosterone synthesis, no salt loss	Increased 17-KS in urine and low plasma testosterone in one type Decreased 17-KS in urine in other types
Abnormal testosterone synthesis, with salt loss	Decreased 17-KS in one type Increased plasma pregnenolone in other type
Hypopituitarism	Decreased growth hormone levels Other tropic hormones may be deficient. Neonatal hypoglycemia is usual.
Microphallus	No specific laboratory test.
Congenital malformations	No specific laboratory test.

Laboratory Differential Diagnosis

Gonads Palpable

Buccal smear chromatin positive and 17-KS normal

- True hermaphroditism
- Klinefelter syndrome variant

Buccal smear chromatin negative and 17-KS normal

- True hermaphroditism
- Anatomic defect
- Inherited enzyme deficiency syndrome affecting testosterone synthesis, metabolism, or action on target tissues

Buccal smear chromatin negative and 17-KS increased

- CAH (3-beta-hydroxysteroid dehydrogenase deficiency)

Gonads Not Palpable

Buccal smear chromatin positive and 17-KS normal

- True hermaphroditism
- Ovarian tumor (maternal 17-KS increased)
- Maternal exposure to androgens (history)

Buccal smear chromatin positive and 17-KS increased

- Congenital adrenal hyperplasia
  11-beta-hydroxylase deficiency
  21-hydroxylase deficiency
  3-beta-hydroxysteroid dehydrogenase deficiency

Buccal smear chromatin negative and 17-KS normal

- True hermaphroditism
- Gonadal dysgenesis (e.g., 45X/46XX, 45XY)

Precautions in Work-Up of Neonate with Ambiguous Genitalia

Buccal mucosal smear for nuclear sex chromatin determination may show false-negative patterns during first 2 days of life so all chromatin-negative smears should be repeated after the third day. Sex chromatin in >25% of cells from the buccal mucosa indicates presence of at least two X chromosomes. A leukocyte culture for karyotype preparation should begin immediately whenever possible to confirm the sex chromosome constitution. The Y chromosome fluorescence test may also be valuable.

A chromatin-positive newborn is almost always female.

External genitalia are normal in Klinefelter and most cases of Turner syndrome.

Amenorrhea/Delayed Menarche (Primary)

Absence of menstruation for ≥3 months in women with past menses or failure to menstruate by age 16.

See Fig. 13-21.

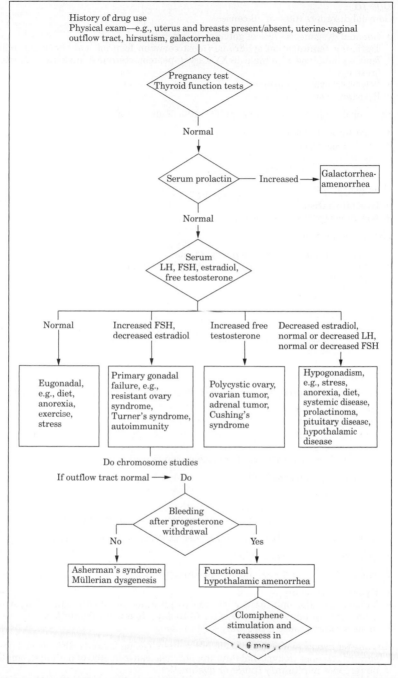

Fig. 13-21. Algorithm for workup of amenorrhea. Asherman syndrome is the obliteration of endometrial lining by adhesions due to pelvic inflammatory disease, tuberculosis, postabortal or puerperal endometritis, etc. Normal blood steroid levels that do not respond to progesterone administration by bleeding. Müllerian dysgenesis is a congenital deformity or absence of tubes, uterus, or vagina; normal karyotype and hormone levels. (LH, luteinizing hormone; FSH, follicle-stimulating hormone.)

Due To
Gonadal disorders (60% of all causes)

- Gonadal dysgenesis (75% of gonadal disorders)
  Testicular feminization syndrome (most common form of male hermaphroditism; female phenotype with male 46 XY karyotype, testosterone in male range; testes are present)
- Polycystic ovary syndrome
- Resistant ovary syndrome

Structural genital tract disorders (35%–40% of all causes)

- Imperforate hymen
- Uterine agenesis
- Vaginal agenesis
- Transverse vaginal septum

Pituitary disorders (rare)

- Hypopituitarism
- Adenomas (prolactin secreting)

Hypothalamic disorders (rare)

- Anatomic lesions (e.g., craniopharyngioma)
- Functional disturbance of hypothalamic-pituitary axis (e.g., anorexia nervosa, emotional stress)

Systemic disorders

- Hypothyroidism
- Congenital adrenal hyperplasia
- Debilitating chronic diseases (e.g., malnutrition, congenital heart disease, renal failure, collagen diseases)

Hormone Profiles
Normal LH, FSH, prolactin, estradiol, testosterone, T-4, and TSH (eugonadal)

- Drugs
- Diet, anorexia
- Exercise
- Stress, illness
- Structural genital tract disorders (see previous section)

Increased LH and normal FSH

- Early pregnancy
- Polycystic ovarian disease (Stein-Leventhal syndrome)
- Ectopic gonadotropin production by neoplasm (e.g., lung, GI tract)

Increased FSH (>30 mIU/mL) and LH, decreased estrogen (<50 pg/mL)

- Primary ovarian hypofunction

Normal or low LH and FSH, decreased estrogen

- Hyperprolactinemia
- Isolated gonadotropin deficiency due to pituitary or hypothalamic impairment. Administer clomiphene citrate is for 5–10 days; if gonadotrophin level increases or menses return, cause is probably hypothalamic.

Administer hypothalamic luteinizing hormone-releasing factor (LRF); normal or exaggerated response in hypothalamic amenorrhea (cause in 80% of patients); smaller or no response in pituitary tumor or dysfunction.

Increased androgen

- Polycystic ovarian disease (testosterone level usually <200 ng/dL)
- Tumor of adrenal or ovary (testosterone level may be >200 ng/dL)
- Testicular feminization
- Use of anabolic steroids (e.g., in athletes)

ENDOCRINE

Androgen Abuse

By athletes who use synthetic androgens to enhance performance or body building; effects depend on type and dose of drug used.

♦ When exogenous testosterone is used, urine testosterone:epitestosterone ratio >6:1 is often considered indicative of steroid abuse (normal ratio ~1:1 in men and women)
♦ Synthetic androgen or its metabolites are identified in urine.
Erythrocytosis may occur.
Serum testosterone may be low.
Decreased or normal LH and FSH.
Plasma HDL may be decreased and LDL may be increased.
Platelet counts and platelet aggregation may be increased.
Laboratory findings due to infertility and testicular atrophy.

Hypogonadism (Androgen Deficiency)[32]

See Fig. 13-22 and Tables 13-34, 13-35.
Due To
Secondary hypogonadism (hypogonadotropic)
Secondary to pituitary-hypothalamic disorders

* Hyperprolactinemia
* Panhypopituitarism (pituitary or hypothalamus)
  Tumor
  Granulomatous disease
  Hemochromatosis
  Trauma
  Infarction, vasculitis
* Isolated gonadotropin deficiency
  Isolated FSH or LH deficiency
  Idiopathic hypothalamic hypogonadism
  Kallmann syndrome
* Genetic disorders (e.g., Prader-Willi [deletion of paternal 15q11-q13 causing hypothalamic dysfunction; also mental retardation, hypotonia, obesity], Laurence-Moon-Biedl syndromes [with decreased GnRH secretion causing hypogonadism; other hypothalamic hormones usually intact])
* Systemic (e.g., chronic disease, nutritional deficiency, massive obesity)
* Drugs (e.g., glucocorticoids)

Constitutional (delayed puberty)
Usual in elderly men since testosterone levels decrease 1%/year beginning about age 40.
♦ Decreased serum testosterone (<300 ng/dL) with low or normal LH and FSH
♦ Decreased gonadotropin releasing hormone (GnRH)
♦ Administration of GnRH increases serum gonadotropin, testosterone, FSH and LH
Primary hypogonadism (hypergonadotropic)
Gonadal

* Genetic
  Klinefelter syndrome
  True hermaphroditism
  Defects in synthesis of androgens due to deficiency of various enzymes (e.g., 20-alpha-hydroxylase, 17,20-desmolase, etc.) Agenesis of testicles
  Miscellaneous (e.g., Noonan syndrome, streak gonads, myotonia dystrophica, cystic fibrosis)
* Acquired (e.g., chemotherapy, radiation, castration, drugs, alcohol, viral orchitis [especially mumps], cryptorchidism, chronic liver or kidney disease)

[32]Morgentaler A. A 66-year-old man with sexual dysfunction. *JAMA* 2004;291:2994.

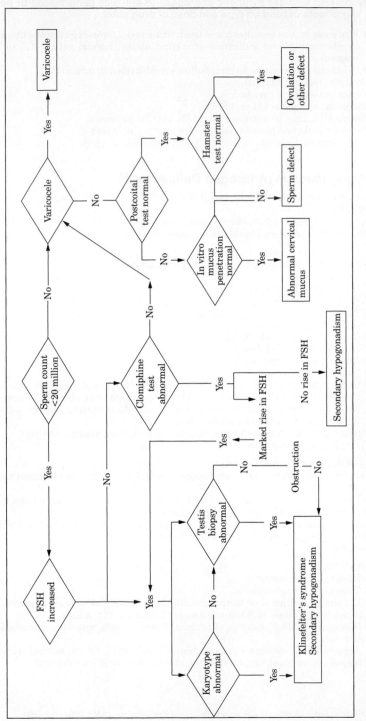

Fig. 13-22. Algorithm for evaluation of nonazoospermic infertility. (FSH, follicle-stimulating hormone.)

Table 13-34. Laboratory Differentiation of Primary and Secondary (to Pituitary Defect) Hypogonadism

Test	Primary Hypogonadism	Hypogonadism Secondary to Pituitary Defect
Level of FSH and gonadotropin in urine	High	Low
After administration of gonadotropins		
17-KS excretion	Does not increase	Increases

Clinical evidence of hypogonadism	Does not subside	Subsides with
		   Increased sperm count
		   Increased estrogenic
		     effect in Papanicolaou
		     smear

17-KS = 17-ketosteroid; FSH = follicle-stimulating hormone.

Hormonal

- Hormonal insensitivity (e.g., androgen or LH insensitivity)
- Defects in action of androgens (pseudohermaphroditism)

Complete (testicular feminization)
Incomplete
   Type I (defects in testosterone receptors)
   Type II (5-alpha-reductase deficiency)

Virilization in Females

Due To
CAH
Virilizing adrenal neoplasms
Virilizing ovarian neoplasms (e.g., arrhenoblastoma)

Feminization of Males

Due To
Adrenal or testicular neoplasms
Peutz-Jaeger syndrome
Increased extraglandular conversion of circulating steroids to estrogen (aromatase excess)
Adrenal feminization occurs in adult males with adrenal tumor [usually unilateral carcinoma, occasionally adenoma] that secretes estrogens.

Table 13-35. Serum Hormone Levels in Various Types of Androgen Deficiency

Disorder	FSH	LH	Testosterone
Primary testicular disease	I	I	D
Secondary to pituitary-hypothalamic disorders[a]	D	D	D
Testosterone resistance[b]	N to I	I to N	I to N
Isolated germinal cell disease	I to N	N	N

D = decreased; FSH = follicle-stimulating hormone; I = increased; LH = luteinizing hormone; N = normal.
[a]Decreased (less than twofold) or absent response of FSH and LH to administration of clomiphene (100 mg/day for 7–10 days) confirms pituitary-hypothalamic cause.
[b]Testosterone-receptor defects are the most common cause of testosterone resistance; characteristic pattern is increased serum testosterone and LH.

♦ • Urinary estrogens are markedly increased.
• May have evidence of hypercortisolism or hyperaldosteronism
• 17-KS is normal or moderately increased and cannot be suppressed by low doses of dexamethasone when due to adrenal tumor.

Biopsy of testicle shows atrophy of tubules.

Climacteric, Male

○ Decreased testosterone level in blood (<300 ng/mL) and urine (<100 μg/24 hrs)
Urinary gonadotropin level is elevated. (Gonadotropin is decreased when low testosterone level is due to pituitary tumor, gout, or diabetes.)

Corpus Luteum Deficiency

Corpus luteum produces insufficient progesterone for development of endometrium receptive for pregnancy.

Due To
Any condition that interferes with follicle growth and development, e.g.,

• Severe systemic illness including liver, kidney or heart dysfunction
• Hyperprolactinemia
• X-chromosome abnormalities
• Polycystic ovarian disease or other causes of inadequate FSH level early in cycle
• Deficient LH receptors on corpus luteum cells
• Inadequate LH level or deficient ovulatory surge

Endometrial biopsy on 26th day of cycle is less developed than menstrual day.
Serum progesterone measured on three different days during midluteal phase totals <15 ng/mL and random level is <5 ng/mL.

Germinal Aplasia

♦ Biopsy of testicle shows that Sertoli and Leydig cells are intact and germinal cells are absent.
○ Azoospermia
○ Buccal smears are normal (negative for Barr bodies).
○ Chromosomal pattern is normal.
Urinary gonadotropin is normal.
Urinary pituitary gonadotropin is increased.
17-KS is decreased.

Gynecomastia

See Fig. 13-23.
Due To
Neonatality
Puberty (25%)
Drugs (10%–20%)
    Hormones (e.g., estrogens)
    Altering androgen action or production (e.g., spironolactone, cimetidine)
    CNS-active (e.g., amphetamines, antihypertensive, antidepressant, sedative, tranquilizer)
Cirrhosis or malnutrition (8%)
Testicular tumors (3%) (e.g., Leydig cell, Sertoli cell, germ cell tumors containing trophoblastic tissue)
Ectopic production of hCG by tumors (e.g., lung, liver, kidney)
Primary gonadism (8%)
Secondary gonadism (2%)
Hyperthyroidism (1.5%)
Renal disease (1%)
Klinefelter syndrome
Feminizing adrenal cortical tumors
Idiopathic (25%)

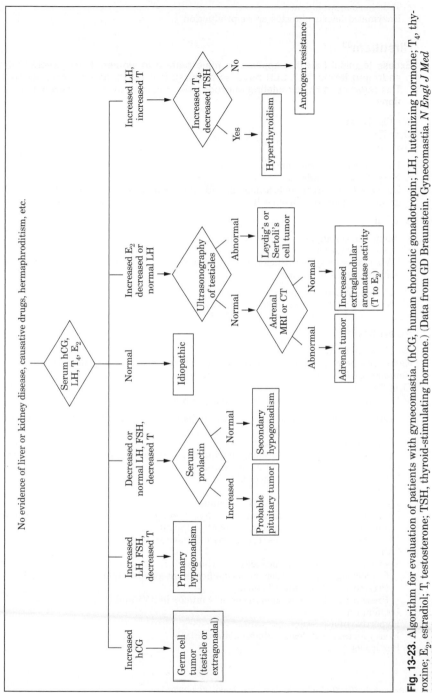

Fig. 13-23. Algorithm for evaluation of patients with gynecomastia. (hCG, human chorionic gonadotropin; LH, luteinizing hormone; T_4, thyroxine; E_2, estradiol; T, testosterone; TSH, thyroid-stimulating hormone.) (Data from GD Braunstein. Gynecomastia. *N Engl J Med* 1993;328:490.)

Conditions usually associated with ambiguous genitalia or deficient virilization

- Androgen-insensitivity syndromes
- True hermaphroditism
- Enzymatic defects of testosterone production

Hirsutism[33]

Excess terminal hair that appears in male pattern in women. Most patients with androgen levels >2× ULN have some hirsutism but does not correlate well. Testosterone is key circulating androgen derived from ovary and adrenal secretions.

See Fig. 13-24.
Due To
Ovarian

- Polycystic ovary syndrome
- Hyperthecosis syndrome
- Tumors (e.g., arrhenoblastoma, gonadoblastoma, dysgerminoma, Brenner cell, granulosa-theca cell, lipoid cell)

Adrenal

- Adenoma, carcinoma
- Cushing syndrome
- CAH (21-hydroxylase deficiency, 11-hydroxylase deficiency, 3-beta-hydroxysteroid dehydrogenase deficiency)

Drugs (e.g., anabolic steroids, androgens)
Idiopathic (e.g., increased 5 alpha-reductase activity)

Infertility[34–36]

See Figs. 13-22, 13-25, and 13-26.
Eighty-five percent of couples conceive after 12 months of unprotected intercourse. Remaining 15% warrant investigation for infertility.
Due To
Male factors (oligospermia in >16%; azoospermia in >7%)

- Testicular abnormalities (e.g., cryptorchidism, torsion, trauma, infection, varicocele)
- Coital factors (e.g., impotence)
- Drugs (e.g., anabolic steroids, marijuana, alcohol, medications [cyclosporine, spironolactone, cimetidine, nitrofurantoin])
- Infections (e.g., chlamydia, syphilis)
- Endocrine
  Hypothyroidism, various CAH syndromes
  Hypothalamic/pituitary disorders (e.g., hyperprolactinemia, Prader-Willi syndrome, Laurence-Moon-Biedl syndrome, panhypopituitarism)
- Chromosome abnormalities (e.g., Klinefelter syndrome, Down syndrome)
- Others:
  Sperm antibodies (numerous assay methods)
    Clinical significance of serum antibodies in men and women is controversial.
    Present in 10% of infertile men
    Present in infertile women in cervical mucus in 25% and in serum in 13%
  Irradiation
  Hyperthermia
  Heavy metals (e.g., lead, cadmium, manganese)
  Pesticides

[33]Rosenfield RN. Hirsutism. *N Engl J Med* 2006;353:2578.
[34]RESOLVE, The National Fertility Association [http://www.resolve.org].
[35]Smith S, et al. Diagnosis and management of female infertility. 2003;290:1767.
[36]Cook JD. Reproductive endocrinology in infertility. *Lab Med* 2004;35:558.

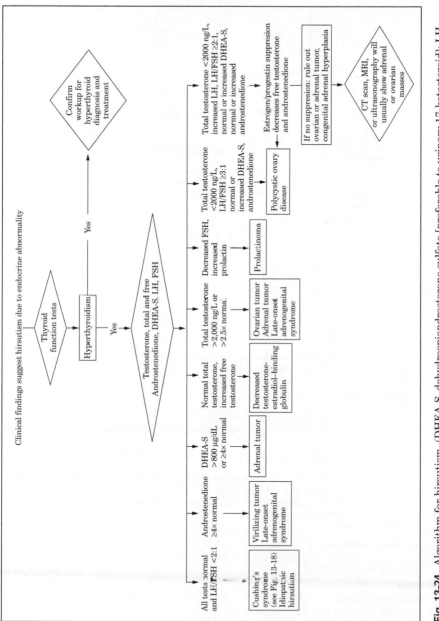

Fig. 13–24. Algorithm for hirsutism. (DHEA-S, dehydroepiandrosterone sulfate [preferable to urinary 17-ketosteroid]; LH, luteinizing hormone; FSH, follicle-stimulating hormone.)

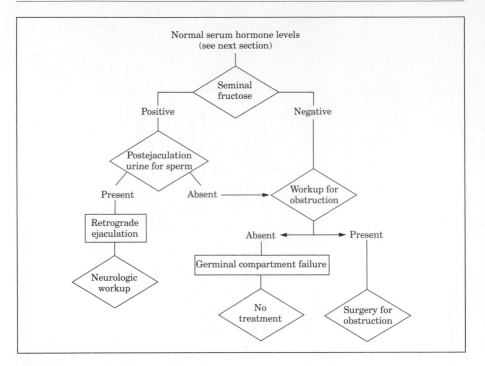

Fig. 13-25. Algorithm for evaluation of azoospermia.

Female factors (identified in ~40% of couples)

- Uterine factors
  Cervical (e.g., decreased cervical mucus quality or quantity, sperm antibodies)
  Uterine (e.g., endometriosis) in >6%
  Tube (e.g., salpingitis) in >23%
  Vaginal (e.g., aplasia, atresia, etc.)
- Endocrine
  Thyroid: e.g., hypothyroidism, hyperthyroidism
  Adrenal: e.g., CAH, virilizing adrenal tumors, Cushing syndrome, adrenal cortical
    insufficiency
  Pituitary: e.g., hypothalamic/pituitary disorders (e.g., hyperprolactinemia in >2%;
    hypopituitarism)
  Ovaries: e.g., disorders of ovulation in >15% (e.g., polycystic ovary syndrome),
    gonadal dysgenesis (e.g., XO, XX, XY)
  Other chromosome abnormalities: e.g., Turner syndrome
  Others, (e.g., irradiation)
- CNS disorders

Unidentified factors (in >25%)

Semen Analysis[37–39]

Use
Infertility studies
Absence of sperm to confirm vasectomy

[37]Adams JE. Infertility in men: diagnosis and treatment. ASCP Check Sample CC 87-9 (CC-187). 1987;27:1.
[38]Rothmann SA, Morgan BW. Laboratory diagnosis in andrology. *Cleve Clin J Med* Nov–Dec 1989;805.
[39]Ferrara F, Daverio R, Mazzini G, et al. Automation of human sperm cell analysis by flow cytometry. *Clin Chem* 1997;43:801.

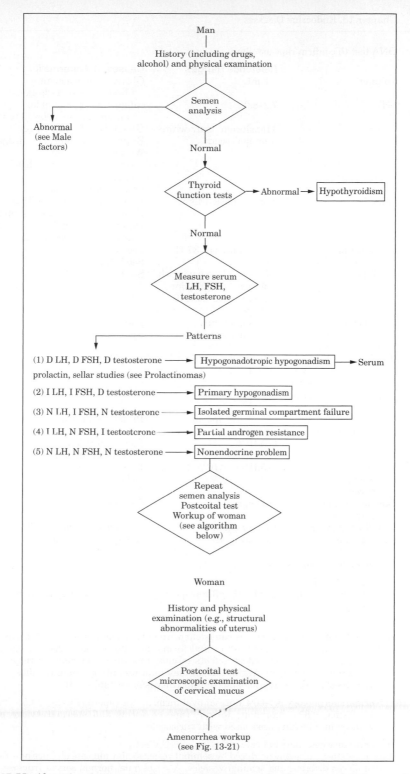

Fig. 13-26. Algorithm for investigation of the infertile couple. (D, decreased; I, increased; N, normal.) (Male portion of figure from RS Swerdloff. Infertility in the male. *Ann Intern Med* 1985;103:906.)

DNA test to confirm rape assailant

	Reference Ranges	Causes of Abnormality
Volume	>2 mL	Obstruction, congenital absence, retrograde ejaculation
pH	7.2–8.0	Inflammation, microbial contamination, delayed reading
Color	Translucent, gray-white, or opalescent.	Greenish: infection, drugs Bright yellow: bilirubin, drugs White-yellow: urine contamination, prolonged abstinence Other colors: drugs
Odor	None or bleach-like	Pungent: bacteria or WBCs Uriniferous: urine contamination Others: unacceptable container, drugs, prolonged abstinence
Liquefaction	<30 minutes at 37°C	See below
Viability	>65%	See below
Motility	>50% viable sperm with forward progression; progressive motility 3+ to 4+	See below
Sperm count	>20 million/mL	Possible testicular atrophy
Morphology of ≥200 sperm	>30% normal forms	e.g., abnormal head, neck, tail
Total motile functional sperm (= volume × % motility × sperm density × % normal morphology)	>40 million within 1 hr at 37°C.	See below
Vitality (Eosin Y stains only dead sperm)	≥75% live sperm	Prolonged abstinence. Dead sperm.
RBCs	0–5/HPF	Blood: infection, neoplasm of testes or prostate
WBCs	0–5/HPF (<10^6/mL)	Infection, inflammation
Clumping (aggregation)	None	Debris
Bovine cervical mucus penetration	>30 mm	See below
Test for organisms	No pathogens	E.g., bacteria, chlamydia
Aggregation	Negative	Antisperm antibodies

Sterile males usually show

- Volume <3 mL
- <20 million sperm/mL; only <5 million sperm/mL seems to reduce chance for pregnancy
- <25% motility

Abnormal motility or morphology can occur with normal sperm counts but are usually seen with decreased counts. Abnormal forms indicate impaired spermatogenesis. Decreased motility may reflect defects in cilia structure elsewhere (in respiratory and reproductive tracts). Agglutination may indicate anti-sperm antibodies (which can be measured, but relationship to infertility is not established).

- Normal morphology is >60% normal oval forms, <6% tapered forms, <0.5% immature forms, <8% amorphous forms. Tapered forms and spermatids are often increased in infertility associated with varicocele.

Inflammatory cells may indicate infection of GU tract.

Absent fructose (normally produced by seminal vesicles) may indicate absence or obstruction of vas deferens and seminal vesicles. Azoospermia, normal semen fructose, and normal serum FSH suggest obstruction proximal to entry of ejaculatory ducts.

Large numbers of sperm in postejaculation urine in these patients suggests retrograde ejaculation.

Repeated semen analysis (collected 7 days apart) are necessary to characterize average spermatogenesis.

Specimens should not be collected within 24 hours of, or >5 to 7 days later than previous ejaculation. Should be examined within 1 hour.

≤40% variability between different semen samples

Comparison of split ejaculate specimens is useful in patients with abnormal semen analysis associated with a high volume; specimens may show marked differences.

Antisperm antibodies (may test male serum or seminal fluid or female serum or cervical mucus; may occur in

- Testicular trauma (even minor)
- Almost all vasectomized patients
- Viral orchitis (permanent)
- Bacterial infections of GU tract (usually transient)

Cervical mucus penetration test measures greatest distance traveled by an individual sperm from a small aliquot of semen incubated 90 minutes in a capillary tube of bovine cervical mucus. 68% of infertile men had penetration scores <20 mm while 79% of fertile men has scores >30 mm.

Hamster egg penetration assay: hamster oocytes enzymatically treated to remove outer layers of egg (which prevent cross-species fertilization) are incubated with human sperm selected for their motile ability. Penetration rates <15% (number of eggs penetrated) indicate reduced fertility. May also be reported as number of sperm penetrations/egg (normal ≥5). Positive test indicates ability of sperm to propel itself to oocyte, bind to oocyte, and penetrate oocyte.

After vasectomy, spermatozoa are present for some time. To be certain, two centrifuged specimens properly collected 1 month apart should be sperm-free and fructose is absent.

Klinefelter Syndrome

Patients have two or more X chromosomes. Incidence = 1 in 500 males.

Azoospermia

Plasma LH and FSH are increased; high FSH is best demarcation between normal men and those with Klinefelter syndrome.

◆ Abnormal chromosomal pattern. XY males have an extra X; 47,XXY is the classic type; 10% of patients have the mosaic form (46,XY/47,XXY); may have additional X (e.g., XXXY, XXXXY).

◆ Urinary gonadotropin level is elevated; augmented response to FSH.

◆ Plasma testosterone levels are decreased to normal; no response to hCG.

Buccal smears are helpful if positive for Barr bodies but a negative does not rule out mosaicism. If negative, chromosome analysis should be performed, but in 70% of patients mosaic pattern may only occur in testes, requiring chromosomal analysis of testicular cells for definite diagnosis.

Biopsy of testicle shows atrophy, with hyalinized tubules lined only by Sertoli cells, clumped Leydig cells, and absent spermatogenesis.

Laboratory findings due to associated conditions, e.g., breast cancer, DM, thyroid dysfunction.

Menopause (Female Climacteric)

Triggered primarily by ovarian aging and depletion of ovarian follicles.

Serum estradiol <5 ng/dL and increased FSH >40 mIU/mL confirms primary ovarian failure; progesterone <0.5 ng/mL.

Urinary estrogens are decreased.

Dehydroepiandrosterone (DHEA) and dehydroepiandrosterone sulfate (DHEA-S) decrease with age along with adrenal corticotropin responsiveness.

Androstenedione and testosterone are decreased.

Plasma and urinary gonadotropin are increased.

Vaginal cytology shows menopausal pattern.

Laboratory changes due to osteoporosis, atherosclerotic cardiovascular disease, etc. may occur.

Ovarian Insufficiency, Secondary

Due To

Deficient estrogen production, e.g., diseases of the pituitary or hypothalamus (see separate sections)

Normal or increased estrogen production, e.g., ovarian tumors, functional cysts of ovary that suppress LH and FSH secretion

Disorders of adrenal (increased production of cortisol or androgens) or thyroid function.

Urinary gonadotropin is decreased or absent.

Plasma LH <0.5 mIU/mL.

Ovarian Tumors

Feminizing Ovarian Tumors

Granulosa cell tumor, thecoma, luteoma.

Pap smear of vagina and endometrial biopsy show high estrogen effect and no progestational activity; no signs of ovulation during reproductive phase.

Urinary FSH is decreased (inhibited by increased estrogen).

Pregnanediol is absent.

Masculinizing Ovarian Tumors

Arrhenoblastoma, hilar cell tumors, adrenal rest tumors.

♦ Androgen-secreting tumor of ovary or adrenal is highly likely if serum total testosterone >200 ng/dL or DHEA-S >800 μg/dL. Localization may require androgen measurement in blood from adrenal and ovarian veins.

Pap smear of vagina shows decreased estrogen effect.

Endometrial biopsy shows moderate atrophy of endometrium.

Urine FSH (gonadotropins) is low.

Urine 17-KS is normal or may be slightly increased in arrhenoblastoma. They may be markedly increased in adrenal tumors of ovary ("masculinovoblastoma"). The higher the urine 17-KS level, the greater the likelihood of adrenocortical carcinoma; >100 mg/24 hours is virtually diagnostic. It may be moderately increased in Leydig cell tumors, which may secrete androgens and estrogens and cause precocious puberty.

♦ In arrhenoblastoma there may be an increase of androsterone, testosterone, etc., excreted in urine even though the 17-KS is not much increased. Urine 17-KS normal or slightly increased associated with plasma testosterone in male range is almost certainly due to ovarian tumor.

♦ In adrenal cell tumors of ovary, laboratory findings may be the same as in hyperfunction of adrenal cortex with Cushing syndrome, etc.

In some cases there are no endocrine effects from these tumors. Some cases of arrhenoblastoma with masculinization also show evidence of increased estrogen formation.

Struma Ovarii

Approximately 5% to 10% of cases are hormone producing. Classic findings of hyperthyroidism may occur.

These tumors take up radioactive iodine. (Simple follicle cysts may also take up radioactive iodine.)

Primary Chorionepithelioma of Ovary

Urinary chorionic gonadotropins are markedly increased.

Estrogen and progesterone secretion may be much increased.

Nonfunctioning Ovarian Tumors

Only effect may be hypogonadism due to replacement of functioning ovarian parenchyma.

Granulosa Cell Tumors

May show increased total inhibin and may be useful to monitor for postoperative recurrence.[40,41]
See Chapters 12, 13.

Tumor Markers

CA-125, Serum

Monoclonal antibody against glycoprotein derived from coelomic epithelium. Increased in benign or malignant conditions that stimulate peritoneal synthesis.

Use/Interpretation

- Normal concentration does not exclude tumor.
- Not useful to distinguish benign from malignant pelvic masses even at high concentrations.
- Although may be increased ≤12 months before clinical evidence of disease, is not recommended for screening women for serous carcinoma of ovary since it is not increased in 20% of cases at time of diagnosis and <10% of Stage I and II cases (low sensitivity and specificity; high false-positive rate). Little benefit to early detection of late-stage cancers. Not helpful in early cases because related to tumor burden. May be used for screening with a hereditary cancer syndrome or a family history of first-degree relative with ovarian cancer.
- Postoperative monitoring for persistent or recurrent disease; poorer prognosis if elevated 3 to 6 weeks after surgery. Lower levels in patients with no residual tumor or <2 cms of residual tumor. Concentration >35 U/mL detects residual cancer in 95% of patients but a negative test does not exclude residual disease.
- Rising level during chemotherapy is associated with tumor progression and fall to normal is associated with response. Remains elevated in stable or progressive serous carcinoma of ovary.
- Rising concentrations may precede clinical recurrence by many months and may be indication for second-look operation, but lack of increased values does not indicate absence of persistent or recurrent tumor.
- Greater concentration is roughly related to poorer survival; >35 U/mL is highly predictive of tumor recurrence. With values >65 U/mL, 90% of women have cancer involving peritoneum. Higher levels are also seen in less-differentiated tumors (grade 2 and 3) and in serous cystadenocarcinoma. Not increased in mucinous adenocarcinoma.
- Sequential determinations are more useful than a single test since levels in benign disease do not show significant change but progressive rise occurs in malignant disease.
- CA-125 is positive in 80% of cases of common epithelial tumors, 50% of early stage disease, 0.6% of normal women over age 50 years.

Prognosis may be better if:

- 50% decline in concentration within 5 days after surgery.
- Ratio of 0.1 postoperative:preoperative concentrations within 4 weeks.
- Ratio of >0.1 to <0.5 may benefit from chemotherapy but recurrence rate is high.
- Ratio >0.8 should consider alternative therapy (e.g., radiation, different chemotherapy combinations).

Increased In
Upper limit of normal <35 U/mL.

Malignant disease

- Nonmucinous epithelial ovarian carcinoma (85%)
- Fallopian tube tumors (100%)

---

[40]Robertson DM, Cahir N, Burger HG, et al. Combined inhibin and CA125 assays in the detection of ovarian cancer. *Clin Chem* 1999;45:651–658.
[41]Robertson DM, Stephenson T, Pruysers E, et al. Characterization of inhibin forms and their measurement by an inhibin alpha-subunit ELISA in serum from postmenopausal women with ovarian cancer. *J Clin Endocrinol Metab* 2002;87:816–824.

ENDOCRINE

- Cervical adenocarcinoma (83%)
- Endometrial adenocarcinoma (50%)
- Trophoblastic tumors (45%)
- Non-Hodgkin lymphoma (40%) representing pleuropericardial or peritoneal involvement
- Squamous cell carcinomas of vulva or cervix (<15%)
- Cancers of pancreas, liver, lung

Conditions that affect the endometrium

- Pregnancy (27%)
- Menstruation
- Endometriosis

Pleural effusion or inflammation (see Chapter 6) (e.g., cancer, congestive heart failure)
Peritoneal effusion or inflammation (e.g., pelvic inflammatory disease). *Especially increased in bacterial peritonitis in which ascitic concentration is > serum concentration.*
Some nonmalignant conditions

- Cirrhosis, severe liver necrosis (66%)
- Other disease of liver, pancreas, GI tract (5%–8%), some disorders of GI tract
- Renal failure

Healthy persons (1%)
Not increased in mucinous adenocarcinoma.

Interferences
Human antimouse or heterophile antibodies.
Different assays do not produce equivalent values and should not be used interchangeably.

(2) Beta-hCG is positive in almost all cases of choriocarcinoma, 10%–30% of seminomas, and 5%–35% of cases of dysgerminoma. See Trophoblastic Neoplasms section.

(3) Alpha-fetoprotein is present in 80%–90% of cases of endodermal sinus tumors or immature teratomas.

(4) CEA is present in 50%–70% of cases of serous carcinoma. CA-125/CEA ratio is much higher in serous carcinoma (>10 and often >100) than in carcinomas of breast, lung, colon, or pancreas (usually <10), which may also cause increased levels of these markers.

(5) Osteopontin[42] (a glycophosphoprotein found in all body fluids) is a potential diagnostic marker.

RT-PCR for detection in tissue.
ELISA for detection in plasma. At cutoff value = 252 ng/mL, S/S = 80%/80% for Stage I/II cancer and S/S = 80%/85% for Stage III/IV cancer.

Germ Cell Tumors of the Ovary

Tumor	AFP*	hCG*
Seminoma	−	+
Seminoma with syncytiotrophoblastic giant cells (STGC)	−	+
Embryonal carcinoma	+	−
Embryonal carcinoma with STGC	+	+
Yolk sac tumor	+	−
Yolk sac tumor with STGC	+	+
Choriocarcinoma	−	+
Mature teratoma	−	−

*See Chapter 16.

When both markers are positive, both should be assayed after therapy as recurrence or metastases may be reflected by increase of only one marker.

[42]Kim J, et al. Osteopontin as a potential diagnostic biomarker for ovarian cancer. *JAMA* 2002;287;1671.

Polycystic Ovarian Disease (Stein-Leventhal Syndrome)[43]
Heterogeneous syndrome of multifactorial etiology characterized by androgen excess (hirsutism, acne), secondary amenorrhea, obesity, infertility.

♦ **Diagnostic Criteria** (2 of these 3 disorders confirmed):

- Oligo- or amenorrhea
- Hyperandrogenemia (increased free or total testosterone) with hirsutism, acne, male pattern baldness)
- Polycystic ovaries on ultrasound
- Exclusion of other etiologies (tumors of ovary and adrenals; pituitary disease, [e.g., Cushing syndrome, acromegaly hyperprolactinemia]; CAH [deficient 21-hydroxylase])

♦ Serum LH increased ~3× normal (>35 mIU/mL) in ~60% of patients in association with normal or slightly low FSH level. Abnormally high LH/FSH ratio (>2) is more consistently abnormal than is either measurement alone. Ratio ≥2 is considered highly suggestive; ratio ≥3 is considered diagnostic.

♦ Increased serum LH, LH/FSH .2, and mild increase of ovarian androgen level are sufficient for diagnosis in presence of the symptoms and clinical signs. *Because of erratic daily fluctuations of LH and androgens, daily plasma specimens for 3–5 days may be necessary.*

○ Serum free testosterone is increased ≤200 μg/dL in 40%–60% of cases; (>200 μg/dL; usually indicates an androgen-producing tumor); is not suppressed by dexamethasone. Sex hormone-binding globulin (SHBG) is decreased by ~50% due to 2× increased testosterone.

○ Plasma androstenedione (DHEA) is increased in ≤50% of cases.

○ Serum 3-alpha-androstanediol glucuronide (metabolite of dihydrotestosterone) is markedly increased in this and in idiopathic hirsutism.

Synthetic estrogens and progestins (as in oral contraceptives) for 21 days with before and after measurement of free testosterone and androstenedione:

- Free testosterone and androstenedione decrease by 50% or become normal in LH-dependent hyperandrogenism, e.g., polycystic ovaries.
- No suppression occurs in patients with ovarian tumors or adrenal disorders.
- Change in free testosterone accounts for estrogen-caused increase in sex hormone–binding globulin that could result in unchanged or increased total testosterone level.

○ Approximately 85% of these patients have one or more abnormalities of serum LH/FSH ratio, testosterone, or androstenedione. Hyperandrogenism does not differentiate condition from CAH but CAH is more likely if LH:FSH ratio is <2:1 and ovaries are normal in size.

Urinary 17-KS is somewhat increased (higher values occur in congenital virilizing adrenal hyperplasia and hyperadrenalism due to Cushing syndrome). (DHEA-S is preferable to evaluate adrenal disease.) Dexamethasone administration (0.5 mg q.i.d. for 5–7 days) causes partial suppression in cases of ovarian origin, but complete suppression suggests adrenal origin (e.g., late-onset CAH).

Administration of gonadotropin increases urinary 17-KS.

Biopsy of ovary is consistent with increased androgen effect but is not specific; biopsy is not part of routine diagnosis.

Plasma and urine cortisol and 17-KGS are normal.

Plasma prolactin is increased in ~30% of patients.

Hyperinsulinemia due to increased insulin resistance caused by increased androgens. ≤13% of these patients have partial 21-hydroxylase defects.

○ If testosterone is >2 ng/mL or DHEA >7,000 ng/mL, ovarian or adrenal tumor should be ruled out.

Laboratory tests may be helpful in following course of treatment, or ruling out adrenal or ovarian tumors.

[43]Ehrmann DA. Polycystic ovary syndrome. *N Engl J Med* 2005;352:1223.

Increased serum LH with normal or decreased FSH may also occur in simple obesity, hyperthyroidism, liver disease. Laboratory changes due to associated conditions:

- Insulin resistance, obesity (>50% of cases), impaired glucose tolerance (in one-third of obese patients), type 2 diabetes (in >10% of obese patients)
- Lipid abnormalities, especially low HDL-cholesterol, increased triglycerides
- Impaired fibrinolysis
- Infertility or complications of pregnancy
- Endometrial carcinoma
- Hirsutism is due to 5 α-reductase in skin.

Testicular Tumors

Tumor	Serum Tumor Marker
Seminoma	hCG increased in ~10%
	AFP not increased in pure seminoma without teratomatous component
Embryonal carcinoma	hCG or AFP or both increased in 90%
Yolk sac tumor	AFP increased in 100%
Choriocarcinoma (pure)	hCG increased in 100%
Teratoma	hCG or AFP or both increased in 50%
Mixed tumor	hCG and AFP increased in 90%

◆ Increased serum hCG (>1–2 ng/mL or >5–10 mIU/mL) is found in 40%–60% of patients with metastatic nonseminomatous tumors and in 15%–20% of patients with apparently pure metastatic seminoma. In the latter case, immunochemical staining of paraffin-embedded tumor should be performed, since isolated syncytiotrophoblastic cells may show the hormone but are not by themselves evidence of choriocarcinoma.

◆ Increased serum AFP (>20 ng/mL) is found in ≤70% of patients with metastatic nonseminomatous (embryonal carcinoma and yolk sac tumors) tumors.

◆ Both markers should always be measured simultaneously. 40% of patients with non-seminomatous tumors have increase of only one marker. 90% of patients with testicular tumors are positive for AFP or hCG or both; these are valuable for gauging efficacy of chemotherapy. 30% of patients receiving intensive chemotherapy apparently have a complete clinical remission; AFP levels may remain increased although lower than pretreatment levels.

Twenty percent to 30% of patients have false-negative results preoperatively despite tumor (usually microscopic) in the retroperitoneal lymph nodes. Therefore, lymphadenectomy should not be omitted simply because of normal marker levels.

Serum markers for AFP and beta-hCG may be increased in conditions other than testicular cancer. See Chapter 16. False-positive increase is rare.

◆ The most important use is for follow-up after surgery or chemotherapy. Failure of increased preoperative levels to fall after surgery suggests metastatic disease and the need for chemotherapy. Rise of levels that had previously declined to normal suggests recurrent tumor even with no other evidence of disease. Serum half-lives of α-fetoprotein = 5 to 7 days and of hCG = 30 hrs.

Negative markers are not useful for differential diagnosis of scrotal mass, but elevated levels indicate testicular cancer.

Serum LD is a third marker; not specific for testicular cancer; related to tumor burden and is an independent prognostic factor for advanced germ-cell tumors. Increased in ~60% of nonseminomatous germ-cell tumors and 80% of seminomatous germ-cell tumors.

Turner Syndrome (Ovarian Dysgenesis)[44]

Most common form of hypogonadism in females characterized by absence of all or part of normal second sex chromosome leading to a group of physical findings.

◆ Diagnosis is based on karyotype analysis. Chromosomal pattern includes wide spectrum of abnormalities, e.g., 45,X (50% of cases), duplication of long arm of one X (46,X,i(Xq)) (5%–10% of cases), mosaicism for 45,X (20%–35% of cases) with ≥1 additional cell lineages, and various deletions of part of an X chromosome. Female is phenotypic. Prenatal diagnosis by chorionic villus sampling or amniocentesis.

[44]Sybert VP, McCauley E. Turner's syndrome. *N Engl J Med* 2004;351:1227.

ENDOCRINE

♦ Prenatal screening combines maternal age >35 years with maternal serum analytes: β-hCG, AFP, unconjugated estriol levels, and fetal edema on ultrasound.
Barr bodies are absent (male pattern) in 80% of patients.
Because of the frequency with which 45,X cells are admixed with 46,XX cells, it is impossible to exclude the diagnosis (i.e., 45,X karyotype) by either buccal smear or chromosome analysis alone.
♦ Biopsy of ovary shows connective tissue stroma with rare follicular structure (gonadal dysgenesis).
Vaginal smear and endometrial biopsy are atrophic.
Increased FSH, LH, and gonadotropins because of gonadal failure.
ACTH and 17-KS are normal.
Glucose intolerance is common with mild insulin resistance.
Serum cholesterol is frequently increased.
Laboratory findings due to increased prevalence of associated conditions, e.g.,

* Autoimmunethyroiditis (10%–30%)
* Bicuspid aortic valves (≤50%), coarctation of aorta (≤20%), hypertension
* Horseshoe kidneys, duplication of collecting system (≤40%)
* Pyelonephritis due to anomalous obstruction of ureteropelvic junction
* Frequent otitis media

~60% of patients with primary amenorrhea have Turner syndrome or sometimes testicular feminization. 90% never menstruate. About 10% menstruate for a few years and then present as secondary amenorrhea.

Other Endocrine Conditions

Carcinoid Syndrome[45,46]

The syndrome in malignant carcinoids (argentaffinomas) includes flushing, diarrhea, bronchospasm, endocardial fibrosis, bronchospasm, arthropathy, glucose intolerance, hypotension produced by secretion of vasoactive peptides.

See Table 13-36.
Liver metastases are present in 95% of cases with syndrome except in lung and ovary primary sites but laboratory tests are not reliable indicators and serum ALP is frequently normal despite extensive metastases.
♦ Urinary level of 5-hydroxyindoleacetic acid (5-HIAA) (a metabolite of serotonin) is increased (>9 mg/24 hours in patients without malabsorption or >30 mg/24 hrs with malabsorption; normal <6 mg/24 hours) in 75% of cases, usually when tumor is far advanced (with large liver metastases, often 300–1000 mg/day), but may not be increased despite massive metastases. Sensitivity = 73%. Useful in diagnosis in only 5% to 7% of patients with a carcinoid tumor but in ~45% of those with liver metastases. Disease extent and prognosis correlates generally with urine 5-HIAA excretion; becomes normal after successful surgery. If urine HIAA is normal, check blood level of serotonin or a precursor, 5-hydroxytryptophan. Urine HIAA may be decreased in renal insufficiency.

Increased 5-HIAA In
Whipple disease
Nontropical sprue
Small increases may occur in pregnancy, ovulation, after surgical stress.
Various foods (e.g., pineapples, kiwi, bananas, eggplant, plums, tomatoes, avocados, plantains, walnuts, pecans, hickory nuts, coffee)
Drugs (e.g., acetanilid, acetaminophen, acetophenetidin, caffeine, glyceryl guaiacolate, heparin, L-dopa, mephenesin, methocarbamol, phenothiazine derivatives, Lugol's solution, reserpine, salicylates

Decreased 5-HIAA In
Use of certain drugs (e.g., chlorpromazine, promazine, imipramine, isoniazid, MAO inhibitors, methenamine, methyldopa, phenothiazines, promethazine)

[45]Kulke MH, Mayer RJ. Carcinoid tumors. *NEJM* 1999;340:858.
[46]Zuetenhorst JM, et al. Daily cyclic changes in the urinary excretion of 5-hydroxyindoleacetic acid in patients with carcinoid tumors. *Clin Chem* 2004;50:1634.

Table 13-36.	Carcinoid Tumors of GI Tract		
Tumor Site*	Frequency	Origin	Comment
Bronchus	32%	Foregut	Serotonin production low
Stomach[†]	3.8%		Mainly produces serotonin precursor
Duodenum	2.1%		(5-hydroxytryptophan)
Pancreas	<5%		Increased urine 5-HIAA
			May metastasize to bone
			Intense symptoms
Appendix	7.6%	Midgut	Mainly produce serotonin
Ileum	17%		Urine 5-HIAA normal/slightly increased
Jejunum	2.3%		Classical symptoms
Cecum	5%		Rarely metastasize to bone
Rectum	10.1%	Hindgut	Rarely produce serotonin or precursor
Transverse, descending, and sigmoid colon	6.3%		Rarely metastasize to bone
Other (e.g., thymus, ovary, kidney, breast)	12.5%		

*85% occur in GI tract, 10% in bronchi/lungs, 5% in thymus, ovary, kidney, breast, other. Cause 55% of GI tract endocrine tumors. ≤25% of cases have other malignancies.
[†]Type I constitutes ≤75% of gastric carcinoids, are associated with chronic atrophic gastritis type A, are often multiple and not associated with carcinoid syndrome. Type II constitutes 5%–10% of gastric carcinoids, are associated with Z-E syndrome and MEN-I, may be multiple, and are not associated with carcinoid syndrome. Type III constitutes 15%–25% of gastric carcinoids, are sporadic, frequently metastasize, and are associated with atypical carcinoid syndrome.

♦ Serum and urine serotonin may be increased (>0.4 μg/mL) in 20% of cases but without increased urine 5-HIAA.
♦ Platelet serotonin and urine serotonin are increased in 64% of cases.
♦ Plasma chromogranin A may be increased in many neuroendocrine tumors. Highest levels in metastatic carcinoid ≤1,000× upper range of normal.
Some tumors can produce various functionally active substances (e.g., histamine, ACTH, somatostatin, gastrin, catecholamines, prostaglandins, kinins), causing different paraneoplastic syndromes. Most are clinically silent because of small amounts secreted and rapid inactivation.
VMA and catecholamines levels in urine are normal.
Laboratory findings owning to other aspects of carcinoid syndrome (may include pulmonary valvular stenosis, tricuspid valvular insufficiency, heart failure, liver metastases, electrolyte disturbances).
Nonfunctioning tumors can only be diagnosed by histological examination.
Some patients may have decreased serum albumin and pellagra (due to diversion of tryptophan to synthesis of serotonin).

Table 13-37.	Characteristics of Markers for Carcinoid Tumors			
	Cutoff Value	S/S	PPV	NPV
Urine 5-HIAA	2.8	68–89	58	93
	6.7	52–98	87	90
Urine serotonin	55	64–68	70	62
	99	46–93	89	60
Platelet serotonin	5.4	74–91	63	95
	9.3	63–99	89	93

Data from Meijer WG , Kema IP, Volmer M, et al. Discriminating capacity of indole markers in the diagnosis of carcinoid tumors. *Clin Chem* 2000;46:1588–1596.

Chromogranin A, Plasma[47]

Widely distributed in endocrine, neuroendocrine, and central and peripheral nervous system. Increased in neuroendocrine tumors and hyperplasia but may not distinguish hyperplasia from tumor. EIA may have lower limit of detection than RIA.

Use
Aid in diagnosis of functioning neuroendocrine tumors; predicts response to treatment. Aid in diagnosis of nonfunctioning neuroendocrine tumors (e.g., thyroid carcinoma, small-cell lung cancer, anterior pituitary adenoma).

Increased In
Functioning neuroendocrine tumors

- Pheochromocytoma, aortic and carotid body tumors
- Neural tumors (e.g., neuroblastoma, ganglioneuroma, paraganglioma, medulloblastoma)
- Carcinoid tumors in various locations
- Gastroenteropancreatic tumors (e.g., gastinoma, insulinoma, VIPoma, etc.)
- Pararthyroid adneoma, carcinoma, hyperplasia
- Thyroid medullary carcinoma, hyperplasia
- Tumors with variable neuroendocrine differentiation (e.g., breast, prostate)—low sensitivity

Also increased in kidney, liver, or heart failure and correlates with severity of the CHF.

Not Increased In
Other tumors with possible neuroendocrine lineage (e.g., choriocarcinoma, thymoma, malignant melanoma, renal cell carcinoma).

Decreased In
CSF in Parkinson disease but does not increase after adrenal-to-caudate autografting and schizophrenia.

Nonendocrine Neoplasms Causing Endocrine Syndromes

Tumors secrete proteins, polypeptides, or glycoproteins that have hormonal activity.

♦ Diagnosed by arterio-venous gradient of hormone across tumor bed or between tumor and nontumor tissue; confirm by in vitro demonstration of hormone production by tumor cells and by resolution of endocrine syndrome after successful removal of tumor.

Cushing Syndrome

♦ Increased blood ACTH level (>200 pg/mL), inability to suppress with high dose dexamethasone test (except in bronchial carcinoids), loss of diurnal variation of cortisol levels (usually >40 μg/dL). Therefore cannot be distinguished from excessive pituitary secretion of ACTH by use of dexamethasone suppression test. Typically malignant disease causing ectopic ACTH production has acute effects on adrenals manifested predominantly by excess mineralocorticoid production with hypokalemia and hypertension. Patients with lung cancer may have elevated ACTH levels without Cushing syndrome.

- Bronchogenic oat cell carcinoma (causes ~50% of cases) and carcinoid
- Carcinoma of breast (occurs in 15% of patients with bone metastases)
- Also thymoma, hepatoma, carcinoma of ovary, kidney, medullary carcinoma of thyroid, islet-cell tumor of pancreas, squamous and large-cell carcinoma of respiratory tract, malignant lymphoma, myeloma, etc.

Hypercalcemia Simulating Hyperparathyroidism (See Humoral Hypercalcemia of Malignancy)

See Table 13-9.

[47]Taupenot L, Harper KL, O'Connor DT. The chromogranin-secretogranin family. *N Engl J Med* 2003;349:1134.

SIADH
Hypoglycemia

♦ Serum insulin is low in presence of fasting hypoglycemia. Not associated with decreased serum phosphorus as in insulin-induced hypoglycemia.

- Bronchogenic carcinoma (especially oat cell carcinoma)
- Carcinoma of adrenal cortex (6% of patients)
- Hepatoma (23% of patients)
- Retroperitoneal fibrosarcoma (most frequently)

Thyrotoxicosis—Signs and Symptoms Are Rare, but Laboratory Findings Are Present.

- Tumors of GI tract, hematopoietic, pulmonary, etc.
- Trophoblastic tumors in women
- Choriocarcinoma of testis

Precocious puberty in boys

- Hepatoma

Acromegaly

- Pancreatic tumors producing GH or growth hormone releasing factor (GHRF) in presence of normal sella; increased GH not suppressed by glucose
- Carcinoid

Erythrocytosis (Due to Erythropoietin Production) (see Chapter 11)

- Carcinoma of kidney, liver
- Fibromyoma of uterus
- Cerebellar hemangioblastoma

See also Carcinoid Syndrome, Precocious Puberty, SIADH.

Multiple Endocrine Neoplasia, (MEN Syndrome)[48]

MEN I (Wermer syndrome)

Inherited autosomal dominant triad of parathyroid, pancreatic islet cell, and anterior pituitary tumors.

○ Hyperparathyroidism (due to involvement of all 4 glands) in >88% of patients is usual presenting feature; associated renal and bone disease are infrequent. 15% of cases of hyperparathyroidism have MEN; frequently multicentric. 10% of parathyroid tumor patients have relatives with MEN.

○ Pancreatic endocrine tumors in ~60% of patients; most are functional; usually multiple.

- Gastrinomas with Zollinger-Ellison syndrome, occur in ~50% of cases and ~50% are malignant. 50% of cases of Z-E syndrome have MEN I.
- Insulinomas (beta cells) in ~25% of MEN I patients; usually benign; multiple foci are common
- Glucagonomas (alpha cells) syndrome of distinctive rash, DM, anemia, weight loss
- VIPomas occur less often.

○ Pituitary adenomas in 40%–50% of cases

- ~25% are prolactinomas.
- ~15% are eosinophilic adenomas causing acromegaly.
- ~5% are basophilic adenomas causing Cushing syndrome.
- ~10% are nonfunctional adenomas causing hypopituitarism due to space-occupying effect.

○ Tumors possible related to MEN 1

- Adrenal cortical adenomas or hyperplasia are incidental and nonfunctioning in ~10%, functioning in ~5% of cases. Adrenal medulla is not involved.
- Thyroid disease in ~20% of cases include benign and malignant tumors, colloid goiter, thyrotoxicosis, Hashimoto disease.

[48]NIH Conference. Multiple endocrine neoplasia type I: clinical and genetic topics. *Ann Int Med* 1998;129:484.

- Uncommon lesions include carcinoids [~16%], schwannomas, multiple lipomas, gastric polyps, testicular tumors.

Men II (or IIa) (Sipple Syndrome)

Autosomal dominant trait.

○ Medullary thyroid carcinoma in >90% of cases is usually multicentric bilateral, and preceded by C-cell hyperplasia (thereby differing from sporadic type). Produce calcitonin and sometimes ACTH or serotonin. Calcitonin response to IV pentagastrin stimulation has S/S >90%. 25% of these carcinomas occur as part of MEN II. May be asymptomatic but lethal.
○ Pheochromocytoma in ≤50% of cases; bilateral, often multiple and may be extra-adrenal. 10% of pheochromocytomas occur as part of MEN.
○ Hyperparathyroidism in ~30% of cases; due to hyperplasia in 84% and adenoma in 16%; occurs late in disease; may occur without medullary thyroid carcinoma. Often form kidney stones.
♦ DNA analysis detected carriers of the gene prior to biochemical manifestations (S/S = 100%).[49]

Men III (or IIb) (William Syndrome)

Features in common with MEN II but is a separate genetic syndrome. May be sporadic or familial.

○ Medullary thyroid carcinoma in 75% of cases; bilateral.
○ Pheochromocytoma in 33% to 50% of cases, bilateral; or diffuse or nodular hyperplasia. Hyperparathyroidism is rare (<5% of cases).
○ Other phenotypic lesions:

- Multiple mucosal gangliomas in >95% of cases appear early in life.
- Marfan syndrome habitus, hypertrophy of corneal nerves, ganglioneuromas of GI tract, characteristic retinal changes and facial appearance are frequent.

○ *All first-order relatives of MEN patients should have appropriate serial testing.*

Adipose Tissue Endocrine Secretion[50]

Newly recognized hormones that participate in regulation of energy metabolism; measured by RIA and ELISA.

Leptin (a proteohormone produced in adipose tissue)—satiety hormone regulates appetite and energy balance. Increased levels in obesity.
Adiponectin—produced in adipose tissue; may be an antiinflammatory hormone associated with increased insulin sensitivity and glucose tolerance. Decreased in type 2 DM, obesity, metabolic syndrome. Could suppress development of atherosclerosis and liver fibrosis. Plasma level increases 2× before a meal, decreases to trough within 1 hr after eating. Decreased levels in obesity.
Resistin—produced in stromovascular fraction of adipose tissue and in peripheral blood monocytes; may cause insulin resistance.
Ghrelin—peptide mainly produced in stomach; stimulates release of GH from anterior pituitary. Small amounts also produced in placenta, kidney, pituitary, hypothalamus.

Cardiac Endocrine Secretion

Natriuretic peptide produced by myocardial cells. See Chapter 5.

Polyglandular Syndromes (Polyendocrine), Autoimmune[51]

See Table 13-38.

[49]Lips CJM, et al. Clinical screening as compared with DNA analysis in families with multiple endocrine neoplasia type 2A. *New Eng J Med* 1994;331:828.
[50]Meier U, Gressner AM. Endocrine regulation of energy metabolism: review of pathobiochemical and clinical chemical aspects of leptin, ghrelin, adiponectin, and resistin. *Clin Chem* 2004;50:1511.
[51]Eisenbarth GS, Gottlieb PA. Autoimmune polyendocrine syndromes. *N Engl J Med* 2004;350:2068.

Table 13-38.	Comparison of Types of Polyglandular Syndromes		
	Prevalence (%)		
	Type 1 (rare)	Type 2 (common)	Type 3
Hypoparathyroidism	80–90	Rare	0
Adrenal insufficiency	60–70	100	0
Autoimmune thyroid disease	12*	70[†]	70
Insulin-dependent diabetes mellitus	≤4	50	Occasional
Ovarian failure	60	4	0
Testicular failure	14	2	0
Immunodeficiency (susceptibility to mucocutaneous candidiasis; asplenism)	≤100	0	0
Alopecia	20	Rare	Occasional
Pernicious anemia	16	1	Very common
Malabsorption	18	0	0
Vitiligo	10	5	>10
Chronic active hepatitis	11	0	0
Onset	Youth/infancy	Adult	
HLA associations	None	B8, DR3, DR4	?
Autosomal	Recessive	?	?
Family members affected	Only siblings	Multiple generations	

*Primary myxedema or Hashimoto thyroiditis.
[†]Hypo- and hyperthyroidism are equally prevalent.
Data from Q-G Ruan, J-X She. Autoimmune polyglandular syndrome type I and the autoimmune regulator. *Clin Lab Med* 2004;24:305; RJ Whitley. Polyglandular autoimmune syndromes: disorders affecting multiple endocrine glands. *Am Assoc Clin Chem Endocrinol* 1994;12:39; JR Baker. Autoimmune endocrine disease. *JAMA* 1997;278:1931.

Type I

♦ Requires ≥2 of the following: Hypoparathyroidism, Addison disease, chronic mucocutaneous candidiasis (all three are present in about one third of patients). Patient may also have associated immune disorders, e.g., autoimmune hypothyroidism, Type IA diabetes, pernicious anemia, gonadal failure, chronic hepatitis, etc.

Type II (Schmidt syndrome)

♦ Autoimmune thyroiditis or insulin-dependent diabetes (15% of all patients with IDDM have type II) with Addison disease. Interval between onset of endocrinopathies may be up to 20 yrs. Gonadal failure may sometimes occur independently.

Type III

♦ Autoimmune thyroid disease with two other autoimmune disorders, including PA, or a nonendocrine organ-specific autoimmune disorder (e.g., myasthenia gravis) but without Addison disease or type 1 diabetes.

Pineal Tumors

Germ cell [e.g., germinoma, embryonal cell], glial tumors, pineocytoma.

Effect is due to compression on hypothalamus, e.g., DI occurs occasionally, disorders of puberty.
Mass effect may compress/occlude cerebral aqueduct or germ cell tumors may secrete hCG.

14   Genitourinary Diseases

GU

GU

Renal Function Tests

See also Serum Urea Nitrogen, Serum Creatinine, BUN:Creatinine Ratio.

Renal Biopsy

Should be preceded by

- Confirmation that two kidneys are present
- No renal infection is present (urine Gram stain)
- There is no bleeding disorder (CBC, PT, aPTT, possibly a bleeding time)

Examination should include

- Histology—stained by H & E, trichrome, PAS, silver; other stains (e.g. for amyloid)
- Immunofluorescence—with antisera specific for IgG, IgA, IgM, C1q, C3, C4, fibrinogen, albumin, kappa and lambda light chains
- Electron microscopy—necessary for diagnosis of Alport syndrome, thin basement membrane nephropathy

Contraindicated In

Hemorrhagic diathesis is absolute contraindication until corrected.
Solitary kidney
Active kidney infections
Renal artery vasculitis with aneurysms
Hydronephrosis
Uncontrolled severe hypertension
Uncooperative patient

May Be Useful or Indicated In

Acute renal allograft dysfunction

- Primary nonfunction for >10 to 14 days
- Unexplained deterioration of graft function
- Unexplained proteinuria (usually months to years later; may indicate recurrent or new glomerular disease)
- Prior to beginning antilymphocyte therapy to prove diagnosis of rejection
- Cyclosporine nephrotoxicity

Persistent or recurrent hematuria with proteinuria
Nephritic syndrome to distinguish etiologies or to assess disease severity
Proteinuria >1 g/day or with abnormal urine sediment
Nephrotic syndrome. Biopsy if unresponsive to therapy or before therapy.
Nonnephrotic proteinuria with progressive disease
Evaluation or monitoring of collagen diseases, especially SLE
Others

Not Indicated In

Nonnephrotic proteinuria (<3.5 g/d) because of good prognosis and indications for therapy are rare.
Asymptomatic hematuria without proteinuria, decreased renal function, or hypertension (e.g., due to IgA nephropathy, hereditary nephritis, thin basement membrane nephropathy, isolated vascular C3 deposition) because no effective treatment.

Not Useful In
Polycystic kidney disease
Hepatorenal syndrome
Acute pyelonephritis
Malignant hypertension
End-stage renal disease with small kidneys

Concentration and Dilution

Concentration Test, Urine

Fluid deprivation may be contraindicated in heart disease or early renal failure.
May be used in the presence of edema or ascites. Contraindicated in coronary artery
   disease and pregnancy.

Interpretation
Normal: Urine specific gravity is ≥1.025.
With decreased renal function, specific gravity is <1.020.
As renal impairment becomes more severe, specific gravity approaches 1.010.
Fluid deprivation for 18 to 24 hours yields specific gravity ≥1.022 or osmolality ≥900
   mOsm/kg in 90% of normal persons.
Sensitive for early loss of renal function, but a normal finding does not necessarily rule
   out active kidney disease.
With specific gravity ≥1.022 or osmolality ≥900 mOsm/kg in absence of glucose, pro-
   tein, or radiopaque contrast material, concentration function is probably normal.
   Lower values suggest a defect.

Interferences
Unreliable in the presence of any severe water and electrolyte imbalance (e.g., adrenal
   cortical insufficiency, edema formation), low- protein or low-salt diet, chronic liver
   disease, pregnancy, lack of patient cooperation.

Concentration Test, Vasopressin (ADH; Pitressin)

May be used in the presence of edema or ascites. Contraindicated in coronary artery
   disease and pregnancy.

Use
Distinguish central from nephrogenic diabetes insipidus.
Tests renal concentration ability, not pituitary function.

Interpretation
Administration of 5 units of vasopressin causes osmolality to increase >10% above
   level caused by dehydration in complete or partial central diabetes insipidus with
   little or no response in nephrogenic diabetes insipidus. See Diabetes Insipidus.

Dilution Test, Urine

Water loading may be contraindicated in kidney and heart disease.
Interpretation (Normal)
Urine volume is >80% of ingested amount (1,200 mL).
Specific gravity is 1.003 in at least one specimen.
With decreased renal function, a smaller volume of urine is noted.
Specific gravity may not fall below 1.010.
Loss of dilution ability occurs later than loss of concentrating ability.

Cystatin C (CysC)[1]

**Low molecular weight cysteine protease inhibitor produced by nearly all nucleated
   cells and excreted into the blood. Filtered by glomerular filtration and metabolized by proximal tubules.**

Use
Newly approved marker to estimate glomerular filtration rate (GFR) independent of
   gender, age, and muscle mass, cirrhosis; does not need to be corrected for height or
   weight. Superior to serum creatinine.

[1]Laterza OF, et al. Cystatin C: an improved estimator of glomerular filtration rate? *Clin Chem*
2002;48:699.

Sensitive marker of allograft function. But may not be optimal marker in patients receiving glucocorticoids.

Risk factor associated with adverse cardiovascular events (CHF, ischemia, death) because kidney dysfunction is associated with such events.

Normal Range (varies slightly with assay method)

- Increases at birth then declines during next 4 months
- >1 yr old: 0.18–1.9 mg/L
- Healthy young persons: ≤0.95 mg/L
- Adult: 0.54–1.55 mg/L

Increased in

Glucocorticoid treatment

May also be affected by thyroid disorders

β-Trace Protein[2]

Also known as prostaglandin D synthase

Proposed as alternative marker for GFR in children, diabetics, various renal diseases

95% confidence interval = 0.40–0.74 mg/L

Increases when GFR <75 mL/min/1.73 m^2

Is also an accurate marker of CSF leakage

Glomerular Filtration Rate (GFR)

Creatinine is produced in muscle by conversion of creatine and phosphocreatine; ≤5 mg of creatine is derived from ingested meat. Produced at relatively constant rate, free filtered through glomerulus, not appreciably reabsorbed or secreted by tubules. Is sum of filtration rate of all functioning nephrons.

Use

The creatinine clearance test, particularly serial measurements, is the most reliable test of renal function; is independent of rate of urine flow. See cystatin (above). After baseline urine creatinine has been obtained, serum creatinine levels can be used to calculate clearance. Creatinine clearance overestimates GFR when GFR is <5% to 10% of normal; in these cases should average with urea clearance, which underestimates GFR. Is secreted by tubules as well as filtered by glomeruli and therefore may overestimate GFR; but is widely used and best measurement of GFR in most clinical instances. Low concentration of creatinine in serum makes test inaccurate for infants and young children.

Interpretation

Good estimate in patients with reduced GFR but underestimates GFR in persons with normal renal function.

Inaccurate if serum creatinine is not stable (e.g., onset or recovery from acute renal failure)

Unreliable in patients with extremes of age, body size, or composition (obesity, malnutrition)

- GFR decreases ~1% per year after age 40
- Diminished muscle mass (e.g., muscle wasting, amputation) may have a 30% decrease in GFR.
- Abnormal creatine intake (vegetarians)

Usually there is good correlation between urine concentrating function and GFR. A normal GFR in association with impaired concentrating ability may be found in sickle cell anemia, diabetes insipidus, nephronophthisis, and various acquired disorders (e.g., pyelonephritis, potassium deficiency, hypercalciuria).

Impairment may be more severe than indicated by laboratory studies if signs and symptoms are more disabling.

Increased GFR is a risk factor for progressive nephropathy in DM.

Creatinine clearance decreases ~8 mL/min/1.73 m^2/decade after age 30.

---

[2]Pöge U, et al. β-trace protein is an alternative marker for GFR in renal transplantation patients. *Clin Chem* 2005;51:1531.

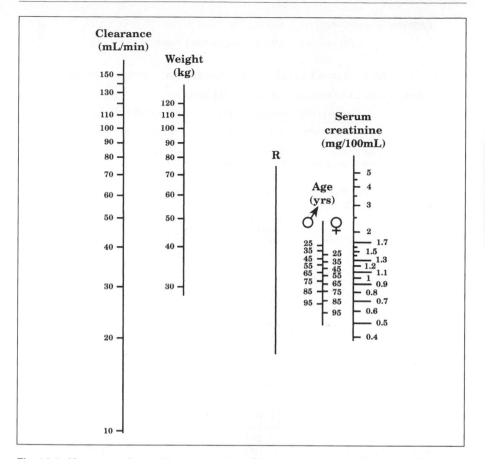

Fig. 14-1. Nomogram for rapid estimation of endogenous creatinine clearance. With a straight edge, join weight to age. Keep straight edge at crossing point of line marked "R." Then move the right-hand side of the straight edge to the appropriate serum creatinine value and read the patient's clearance from the left side of the nomogram. (From Appel GP et al. Antimicrobial agents in patients with renal disease. *Medical Times* 1977;105:116.)

Estimate of creatinine clearance from single serum creatinine clearance may be required for prompt therapy of nephrotoxic drug reaction or because of difficulty of accurate 24-hour urine collection. Can then estimate by following formulas or the nomogram (Fig. 14-1).

To *estimate* GFR from serum creatinine, these equations may be used but may only be accurate in patients with stable renal function who are not massively obese or edematous:

$$GFR = [(140 - \text{age in yrs}) \times (\text{weight in kg})] \div (72 \times \text{serum creatinine in mg/dL})$$

(Values for women are 85% of predicted. Multiply by 0.85.)

A more recent formula for calculating GFR from serum creatinine:

$$GFR = 186 \times (\text{serum creatinine})^{-1.154} \times (\text{age})^{-0.203} \times (0.742 \text{ if female}) \times (1.212 \text{ if African American})$$

$$\text{creatinine clearance (mL/min/1.73 m}^2) = [(9.8 - 0.8) \times (\text{age} - 20)] \div \text{serum creatinine in mg/dL}$$

(Values for women are 90% of predicted.)

Formulas for children:

$$GFR \text{ (mL/min)} = 0.55 \times \text{length (cm)} \div \text{serum creatinine}$$

or

$$GFR \text{ (mL/min/1.73 m}^2) = (0.43) \times \text{length (cm)} \div \text{serum creatinine}$$

calculation for 24-hr creatinine clearance (mL/min) =

$$\frac{(\text{urine creatinine concentration} \times \text{urine volume in mL})}{(\text{serum creatinine} \times \text{time period of collection}^\dagger)}$$

(†Calculation for 24-hour collection is 24 hours $\times$ 60 minutes = 1,440. Calculation for 6-hour collection is 6 hours $\times$ 60 minutes = 240 minutes.)

Normal Clearances (corrected to 1.73 m^2 body surface area)
Endogenous Creatinine

Age (yrs)	Mean Creatinine Clearance (mL/min/1.73 m^2 body surface area)	
0–1	72	
1	45	
2	55	
3	60	
4	71	
5	73	
6	64	
7	67	
8	72	
9	83	
10	89	
11	92	
12	109	
13–14	86	
	Males	**Females**
20–29	94–140	72–110
30–39	59–137	71–121
40–49	76–120	50–102
50–59	67–109	50–102
60–69	54–98	45–75
70–79	49–79	37–61
80–89	30–60	27–55
90–99	26–44	26–42
Inulin*	Males:	110–150 mL/minute
	Females:	105–132 mL/minute
Urea†	Maximum:	60–100 mL/minute
	Standard:	40–65 mL/minute

*Inulin is a fructose polymer. Is gold standard measure of GFR but requires continuous infusion to maintain adequate blood concentration during test. Normal inulin clearance = 25–30 mL/minute during first few days of life; ~50–60 mL/minute by end of first month. Adult values are reached by age 12–18 months. Considerable individual variation makes interpretation difficult unless clearly abnormal.
†Urea clearance: Marked variability in contributing factors (e.g., BUN, diet, urine flow) makes interpretation difficult and not useful in most clinical situations. Urea is mostly end product of dietary protein metabolism mainly synthesized in liver. Is normal until >50% of renal parenchyma is inactivated. With renal insufficiency, the clearance test parallels the parenchymal destruction.

Osmolality, Urine
Use
Measurement of urine osmolality during water restriction is an accurate, sensitive test of decreased renal function.
Interpretation
Normal: Concentration of >800 mOsm/kg

Table 14-1. Laboratory Guide to Evaluation of Renal Impairment

	Renal Function		
	GFR (mL/min/1.73 m²)*	Excretion of IV PSP in 15 Min (Renal Tubular Transport)	Condition
Stage 1	≥90. N or I	≥25%	Early kidney damage or I risk
Stage 2	60–89. Mild D	15%–25%	Kidney damage
Stage 3	30–59. Moderate D	10%–15%	Complications
Stage 4	15–29. Severe D	5%–10%	Refer to nephrologist Prepare for kidney replacement therapy
Stage 5	<15. Marked D	<5%	Renal failure

*For ≥3 months. N, normal; I, increase; D, decrease.

Minimal impairment of renal concentrating ability: 600–800 mOsm/kg
Moderate impairment: 400–600 mOsm/kg
Severe impairment: <400 mOsm/kg
Urine osmolality may be impaired when other tests are normal (concentration test, BUN, PSP excretion, creatinine clearance, IV pyelogram); may be especially useful in diabetes mellitus, essential hypertension, silent pyelonephritis.
It may be well to also measure serum osmolality and calculate urine:serum ratio (normal >3).
See Diabetes Insipidus.

Para-Aminohippurate (PAH) Clearance

Measures effective renal plasma flow (RPF) and, principally, tubular secretion. Is infrequently used because test requires continuous infusion of PAH to maintain steady-state plasma PAH level and timed urine and blood samples.

Males = 560–800 mL/minute
Females = 500–700 mL/minute
At age 20–29 yrs, 600 mL/minute; falls to 300 mL/minute by age 80–89 yrs

Phenosulfonpththalein (PSP) Excretion Test

Test is hazardous in severe renal insufficiency or heart failure because adequate prior hydration is required to obtain sufficient urine volume.

Use
Detect slight to moderate decrease in renal function; not useful in chronic azotemia with fixed specific gravity (serum creatinine and creatinine clearance are more useful in these cases).

Interferences
Use of small urine volumes magnifies errors.
Test is distorted by presence of residual bladder urine, abnormal drainage sites (e.g., fistulas), and interfering substances (e.g., hematuria).
Hepatic disease may lead to falsely elevated values (because 20% of the dye is normally removed by the liver).
False-positive results may also occur in multiple myeloma (because of excessive protein binding) and in hypoalbuminemia.
Certain drugs may interfere with PSP extraction (e.g., salicylates, penicillin, some diuretic and uricosuric drugs, and some radiographic contrast media).
False-positive results have been reported with kaolin, magnesium, methylene blue, nicotine acid, quinacrine (mepacrine), quinidine, quinine.

Interpretation
Normal: >25% in urine in 15 min: 55% to 75% in 2 hours

The 15-minute PSP excretion correlates with the GFR; a normal 15-min value indicates normal GFR. Progressive decrease of 15-minute value is proportional to decreased GFR (e.g., 15% PSP excretion in 15 minuntes approximates a 45% GFR). If the GFR is normal, the PSP test indicates renal blood flow or tubular function; better tests are available for measuring these two functions, and the PSP test is now rarely used.

Increased dye excretion in later time periods compared to the initial 15-minute period suggests increased residual urine due to obstructive uropathy or incomplete bladder emptying; the latter can be ruled out by placement of indwelling catheter during the test.

PSP that is normal with increased BUN and serum creatinine and decreased GFR suggest acute GN. PSP parallels these parameters in most chronic renal diseases.

Split Renal Function Tests

Interpretation
Affected kidney shows decreased urine volume and sodium excretion and decreased urine concentration of creatinine, inulin, or PAH.

Use
Aid in diagnosis of renal artery stenosis

Not useful in presence of GU tract obstruction (e.g., in men over age 50).

Other Renal Function Tests

Urinary acidification is impaired in chronic renal disease with azotemia. It is decreased without parallel impairment of GFR in renal tubular acidosis, some cases of Fanconi syndrome, and some cases of acquired nephrocalcinosis.

Proximal tubular malfunction is indicated by urinary excretion of substances normally reabsorbed by tubules: in renal glycosuria (blood glucose <180 mg/dL as in Fanconi syndrome, heavy metal poisoning), aminoaciduria, phosphaturia.

Kidney Diseases

Renal Failure, Acute

Defined as increased serum creatinine by ≥0.5 mg/dL or .50% over baseline value or 50% decrease in creatinine clearance or decreased renal function resulting in need for dialysis.

See Tables 14-3, 14-4, and 14-5, and Fig. 14-2.

Due To
Prerenal (causes 35%–40% of hospital-acquired and ~70% of community-acquired cases)

- Hypotension (e.g., shock, sepsis, drugs)
- Volume contraction (e.g., hemorrhage, dehydration, burns)
- Severe heart failure (e.g., myocardial infarction, cardiac tamponade, pulmonary emboli)
- Hepatorenal syndrome
- Drugs (e.g., cyclosporine, amphotericin B)
- Combinations of insults (e.g., NSAID treatment in presence of congestive heart failure, aminoglycoside exposure in patient with sepsis, radiocontrast agents in patients receiving ACE-inhibitors)
- Occlusion of renal artery or vein (e.g., due to thrombosis, embolism, severe arteriosclerotic stenosis, dissecting aneurysm)

Table 14-2.	Urine Sediment, Microscopic and Reagent Strips

	Normal No./HPF	Reagent Strip Detects	Some Causes
RBCs	≤5	Blood	Any source in GU tract Dysmorphic RBCs indicate glomerular source
Neutrophils	≤5	5–15/hpf in spun sediment ≥100 mg/dL of protein suggests renal disease; little/no protein suggests lower GU tract involvement	Infection, inflammation anywhere in GU tract
Eosinophils	<3	Not detected	Acute interstitial nephritis (due to drugs), atheromatous emboli, eosinophilic cystitis
Lymphocytes		Not detected	Early indicator of renal transplant rejection
Renal tubular epithelial cells	Few	Not detected	>15/10 HPF indicates active renal disease or tubular injury
Transitional cells	Few	Not detected	May be normal. Increased with inflammation, instrumentation. Rule out transitional carcinoma.
Squamous cells	0	Not detected	Contamination
Casts			Usually positive for protein
Hyaline	Few		Stress, exercise. May occur without proteinuria
RBC	0	Not detected	Indicates source of blood is within kidney
WBC	0	Not detected	Interstitial inflammation, e.g., acute pyelonephritis
Granular	0	Not detected	Strenuous exercise. Stasis in nephron; associated with tubulointerstitial disease
Completely degenerated granular cast	0	Not detected	Severe renal disease, e.g., chronic renal failure, malignant hypertension, diabetic nephropathy
Waxy ("renal failure casts")	0	Not detected	Chronic renal disease, amyloidosis
Fatty	0	Usually with proteinuria >300 mg/dL	Nephrotic syndrome, diabetic nephropathy, mercury or ethylene glycol toxicity
Epithelial	0	Usually + for protein	Serious disease such as acute tubular necrosis, virus (CMV) infection, toxicity (e.g., mercury, ethylene glycol, drug)

GU

(continued)

Table 14-2. *(continued)*

	Normal No./HPF	Reagent Strip Detects	Some Causes
Bacterial	0	May be + for WBC, bacteria	Infection within kidney
Crystal	0	Not detected	Crystals in tubules
Pigment	0	Positive for blood or bile	Hemoglobinuria, myoglobinuria, bilirubinuria, drugs
Bacteria	<20	May be + for protein, WBC, nitrite	
Glitter cells	0	May be + for protein, bacteria	Chronic pyelonephritis. Lower GU tract infection with dilute urine.
Clue cells	0	Not detected	*Gardnerella vaginalis* infection
Yeast	0	Not detected	Vaginal contamination; diabetes

Renal (causes ≤60% of inpatient and 11% of outpatient cases)

- Acute tubular necrosis
  Acute interstitial nephritis causes ~10% of cases
    Drugs (e.g., methicillin)
    Infection
    Cancer (e.g., lymphoma, leukemia)
    Other (e.g., sarcoidosis)
  Prolonged ischemia due to prerenal events causes ~50% of cases
  Toxic agents cause ~35% of cases
    Heavy metals (e.g., lead, mercury, cisplatin, arsenic, cadmium, bismuth)
    Organic solvents (e.g., carbon tetrachloride, ethylene glycol)
    Antibiotics (e.g., aminoglycosides [often nonoliguric], tetracyclines, penicillins, amphotericin)
    X-ray contrast media (especially in diabetic persons or preexisting renal insufficiency); tends to be oliguric

Table 14-3.   Some Renal Indices in Three Types of Postischemic Acute Renal Failure

	Type A[a]		Type B[b]		Type C[c]
Postischemic Time	1 hr	3 days	7 days	12 days	21 days
Urine flow rate (mL/min)	2.2–4.4	1.4–2.0	1.3–1.9	1.4–1.6	0.4–0.8
Inulin clear (mL/min/1.73 sq m)	18–28	27–33	10–14	26–32	3–7
U/P inulin	10–18	12–20	9–11	18–26	6–8
U/P osmolality	1.1–1.2	1.3–1.4	1.03–1.09	1.2–1.4	0.96–1.04
FE_{Na} (%)	8.8–17.2	0.6–1.0	4.6–5.6	0.8–2.0	4.6–11.6

U/P, urine/plasma ratio; FE_{Na}, fractional excretion of sodium.
[a]Isolated renal ischemic insult (e.g., suprarenal aortic clamping for 15–90 mins for repair of abdominal aneurysm) with preoperative (volume expansion and mannitol administration) and postoperative (furosemide and dopamine infusion) treatment. When >50 mins, acute renal failure is likely to occur.
[b]More severe and sustained partial renal ischemia (e.g., cardiopulmonary bypass for several days). When >160 mins, acute renal failure is likely to occur. Recovery after 2–3 wks. Values given are those that occur during nadir.
[c]Protracted acute renal failure (e.g., type B or C with additional or prolonged renal ischemia as in rupture of aortic aneurysm) is fatal in > 50% of patients.
Source: BD Myers, SM Moran. Hemodynamically mediated acute renal failure. *N Engl J Med* 1986;314:97.

Table 14-4. Urinary Diagnostic Indices in Acute Renal Failure

	Prerenal Azotemia	Postrenal (Acute Obstructive)	Acute GN and Vasculitis	Acute Interstitial Nephritis	Acute Tubular Necrosis		Renal Vascular Occlusion	
					Oliguric	Nonoliguric	Arterial	Venous
Urine volume (mL/24 hrs)	~500*	Usually <500; fluctuates from day to day	<500	V	<350	1,000–2,000	V; Anuria if bilateral/complete	V
Urine specific gravity	H (>1.015)				L; <1.010			
Urine osmolality (mOsm/kg H_2O)	>500	V; usually <500	<500	V	<350	350	V	V
Urine sodium (mEq/L)	L; <20	H; >40	L; usually <20	V	>40	V	V	V
U/P osmolality	>1.5	<1.2	<1.2		<1.2	<1.2		
U/P urea nitrogen	>8	Usually >8	>8		<3	<8		
U/P creatinine	>40	<20	>40		<20	<20		
Renal failure index	<1 (90% of cases)	>2 (95% of cases)	<1		>2 (95% of cases)	>3		
FENa	<1 (≤94% of cases)	>1	<1	V	>1	>1	V	V
BUN:creatinine ratio	>20:1	>20:1	>20:1	<20:1	<20:1	<20:1	<20:1	<20:1
Urine sediment	Hyaline casts	N; RBCs, WBCs, crystals may be present	RBCs, RBC casts	WBCs, WBC casts, eosinophils	Granular casts, renal tubular epithelial cells, cell debris, pigment, crystals		V	V
Comments	Decreased renal perfusion	Evidence of GU tract obstruction	Biopsy findings classify disease	Eosinophilia; thrombocytopenia	Renal hypoperfusion; nephrotoxin	Nephrotoxin	Aortic injury; atheromatous emboli	Renal vein occlusion with nephrotic syndrome

H, high; L, low; N, normal; U/P, urine/plasma ratio; V, variable.

*Polyuria may be present.

Sources: TE Andreoli, et al., eds. Cecil essentials of medicine, 2nd ed. Philadelphia: WB Saunders, 1990:212; DE Okun. On the differential diagnosis of acute renal failure. Am J Med 1981;71:916; RW Schrier. Acute renal failure: pathogenesis, diagnosis, and management. Hosp Pract 1981;(Mar):93; TR Miller, et al. Urinary diagnostic indices in acute renal failure: a prospective study. Ann Intern Med 1978;89:47.

GU

Table 14-5.   Comparison of Three Types of Renal Insufficiency

Laboratory Tests	Prerenal Azotemia	Hepatorenal Syndrome	Acute Renal Failure
Urine sodium (mEq/L)	<10	<10	>30 (may be less with sepsis)
Urine/plasma creatinine	>30:1	>30:1	<20:1
Urine osmolality	⊢————At least 100 mOsm > plasma————⊣ osmolality		Same as plasma osmolality
Urine sediment	Normal	Not remarkable	Cell debris, casts
Response to plasma expansion	Good	Absent	Variable

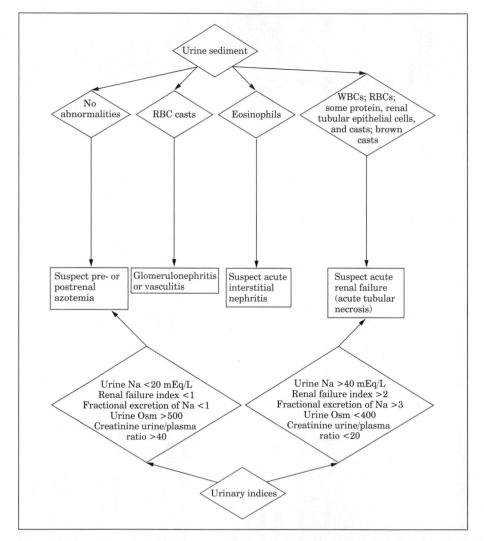

Fig. 14-2. Algorithm for differential diagnosis of acute renal failure. (Data from DW Schrier. Acute renal failure: pathogenesis, diagnosis, and management. *Hosp Pract*, March 1981, p. 93.)

Pesticides, fungicides
Others (e.g., phenylbutazone, phenytoin, calcium)
Pigment-induced (e.g., hemoglobin, myoglobin)
Intratubular obstruction (e.g., myeloma light chains; crystals such as uric acid, calcium oxalate, acyclovir, sulfonamide, methotrexate)
• Glomerulonephritis, causes ~5% of cases
Acute poststreptococcal
Rapidly progressive
SLE
Subacute bacterial endocarditis
Schönlein-Henoch purpura
Goodpasture syndrome
Malignant hypertension
Hemolytic-uremic syndrome
Thrombotic thrombocytopenic purpura
Drug-related vasculitis
• Large-vessel disease
Bilateral renal vein occlusion (thrombosis, tumor infiltration)
Renal artery occlusion (embolism, thrombosis, stenosis, aortic dissection, trauma to renal arteries)
• Small-vessel disease (e.g., malignant hypertension, vasculitis, sickle cell anemia, HUS, toxemia of pregnancy, scleroderma, atheroembolism, hypercalcemia, transplant rejection)
• Interstitial disease (e.g., acute interstitial nephritis, bilateral pyelonephritis, infiltration by leukemia, lymphoma or sarcoidosis, hypercalcemia)

Postrenal (causes 2%–5% of inpatient and 17% of outpatient cases)

• Bladder obstruction (e.g., BPH, carcinoma, urethral stricture)
• Bilateral obstruction of ureters or renal pelves (e.g., carcinoma, calculi, papillary necrosis, blood clots)

Sixty percent of acute renal failure cases occur during or immediately after surgery, most often with cardiac or aneurysm surgery.
Ten percent of cases are associated with obstetric problems.
Thirty percent of cases are associated with medical conditions, usually due to nephrotoxins or renal ischemic mechanisms.
Often, combined mechanisms (e.g., crushing injury with myoglobinemia plus shock, shock plus intravascular hemolysis from transfusion reaction or bacteremia)

Early Stage

♦ Urine is scant in volume (often <50 mL/day) for ≤2 weeks; anuria for >24 hours is unusual.
Usually bloody. Specific gravity may be high because RBCs and protein are present.
Urine sodium concentration is usually >50 mEq/L.
♦ BUN rises ≤20 mg/dL/day in transfusion reaction. It rises ≤50 mg/dL/day in overwhelming infection of severe crushing injuries.
♦ Serum creatinine is increased.
Serum uric acid is often increased; may be >20 mg/dL in some types (e.g., rhabdomyolysis)
Hypocalcemia may occur.
○ Disproportionately increased serum phosphorus and creatinine indicate tissue necrosis.
Serum amylase and lipase may be increased without evidence of pancreatitis.
Metabolic acidosis is present.
WBC is increased even without infection.

Second Week

♦ Urine becomes clear several days after onset of acute renal failure, and there is a small daily increase in volume. Daily volume of 400 mL indicates onset of tubular recovery. Daily volume of 1,000 mL occurs in several days or ≤2 weeks. RBCs and large hematin casts are present. Protein is slight or absent.

♦ Azotemia increases. BUN continues to rise for several days after onset of diuresis. Metabolic acidosis increases.

Serum potassium is increased (because of tissue injury, failure of urinary excretion, acidosis, dehydration, etc.). ECG changes are always found when serum potassium is >9 mEq/L but are rarely found when it is <7 mEq/L.

Serum sodium is often decreased, with increased extracellular fluid volume.

Anemia usually appears during second week.

Bleeding tendency is frequent, with decreased platelets, abnormal prothrombin consumption, etc.

Diuretic Stage

Large urinary potassium excretion may cause decreased serum potassium level.

Urine sodium concentration is 50 to 75 mEq/L.

Serum sodium and chloride may increase because of dehydration from large diuresis if replacement of water is inadequate.

Hypercalcemia may occur in some patients with muscle damage.

Azotemia disappears 1 to 3 weeks after onset of diuresis.

Later Findings

Anemia may persist for weeks or months.

Pyelonephritis may first occur during this stage.

Renal blood flow and glomerular filtration rate do not usually become completely normal.

Recovery from renal cortical necrosis complicating pregnancy may be followed by renal calcification, contracted kidneys, and death from malignant hypertension in 1 to 2 years.

Laboratory Findings Due to Complications

Infections develop in 30% to 70% of patients

GI bleeding occurs in 10% to 0% of patients

Anemia (Hct = 20%–30%)

Cardiovascular anomalies (e.g., pericarditis, heart failure, arrhythmias, hypertension)

Suspect urinary tract obstruction, bilateral renal vascular thrombi or emboli, cortical necrosis, or acute GN if there is complete anuria for >48 hours.

Suspect cortical necrosis if proteinuria is >3 to 4 g/L, BUN does not fall, and diuresis does not occur.

Suspect urinary tract obstruction if recurrent oliguria and increasing azotemia occur during period of diuresis.

Urinary Diagnostic Indices in Acute Renal Failure

See Table 14-4 and Fig 14-3.

Interpretation

Urinary sodium levels between 20 and 40 mEq/L may be found in all forms of acute renal failure.

$$\text{Fractional excretion of sodium } (FE_{Na}) = 100 \times (\text{urine sodium/plasma sodium}) \div (\text{urine creatinine/plasma creatinine})$$

Is an index of renal ability to conserve sodium and represents percent of filtered sodium to reach the urine. Is considered the most reliable test to distinguish prerenal azotemia from acute tubular necrosis with oliguria.

Some causes of $FE_{Na} < 1\%$

- Prerenal azotemia (e.g., blood volume loss, heart failure, dehydration)
- Renal vasoconstriction (e.g., NSAIDs, hepatorenal syndrome)
- Acute GN
- Early (few hours) acute urinary tract obstruction
- Sepsis
- Some cases of acute tubular necrosis due to x-ray contrast material or myoglobinuria due to rhabdomyolysis
- Early urinary tract obstruction
- 10% of cases of nonoliguric acute tubular necrosis

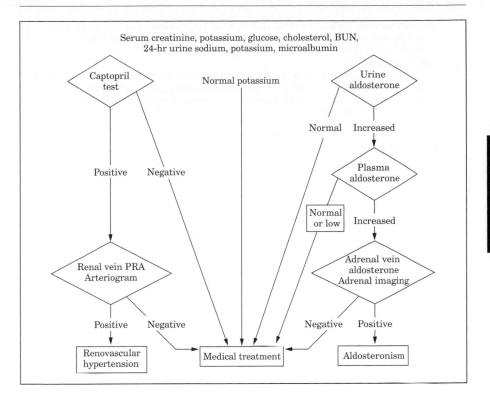

Serum creatinine, potassium, glucose, cholesterol, BUN,
24-hr urine sodium, potassium, microalbumin

Fig. 14-3. Algorithm for diagnosis of suspected renovascular hypertension. (PRA, plasma renin activity.)

Some causes of $FE_{Na} >1\%$ (injured tubules)

- 90% of cases of acute tubular necrosis
- Late urinary tract obstruction (days to months)
- Diuretic administration
- Mineralocorticoid deficiency
- Pre-existing chronic renal failure
- Diuresis due to mannitol, glycosuria bicarbonaturia, or radiocontrast agents

Renal failure index (RFI) = urine sodium/(urine creatinine/plasma creatinine); measures Na conservation and concentrating ability

Use

Indices (especially RFI and FE_{Na}) are chiefly of value in *oliguric* patients for the early differentiation of prerenal azotemia from acute tubular necrosis.

Indices are not useful for diagnosis of presence or absence of obstruction in cases of acute renal failure.

Interpretation

Values ≤ 1 for RFI and FE_{Na} strongly suggests prerenal azotemia and values ≥ 3 strongly suggest acute tubular necrosis with confidence level of 90%; values of 1 to 3 are less definitive but usually indicate tubular necrosis; nonoliguric acute renal failure patients frequently have intermediate values between prerenal azotemia and oliguric renal failure.

Values usually >1 in urinary obstruction or acute interstitial nephritis; values usually <1 in acute GN.

Diagnostic indices in patients with reversible acute obstructive uropathy often resemble indices in acute tubular necrosis or prerenal azotemia; indices in obstructive uropathy depend on duration of obstruction and severity of azotemia.

Differences between prerenal azotemia and acute tubular necrosis by these indices are particularly blurred in elderly patients as well as those with hypertensive or diabetic nephrosclerosis or other chronic parenchymal renal diseases.

These diagnostic indices are often intermediate, and considerable overlapping of values is frequent, especially at time of initial evaluation. Even the total profile may not be useful in the individual case.

Interferences

Specimens for urinary indices should be obtained before onset of treatment if possible; several therapies may make results uninterpretable, especially administration of dopamine, mannitol, or other diuretics. Glucose and radiographic contrast material in urine. It is not necessary to obtain a timed 12- or 24-hour urine specimen, since the patient with acute renal failure cannot vary urine sodium or osmolality significantly from hour to hour; a random specimen is sufficient.

Urine Sediment in Acute Renal Failure

Renal tubular cells (or cellular casts) and pigmented granular casts indicate acute tubular necrosis; present in ~80% of patients; urine Na >20 mEq/L.

Sediment may be normal in prerenal or postrenal causes with minimal or absent proteinuria.

Eosinophils may be found in acute interstitial nephritis; increased WBC and WBC casts; minimal proteinuria.

RBC casts indicate GN, vasculitis, or microembolic disease; increased RBCs and moderate proteinuria.

RBCs indicate blood from lower GU tract or from glomerulus.

Myoglobin casts indicate myoglobinuria.

WBCs in hyaline casts indicate renal parenchymal infection rather than lower GU tract infection.

In a patient with two functioning kidneys, obstruction of only one ureter should cause serum creatinine to rise ~50% to 2 mg/dL; acute renal failure that is postrenal with creatinine >2 mg/dL suggests that obstruction is bilateral or patient has only one functioning kidney.

Total anuria for more than two days is uncommon in acute tubular necrosis and should suggest other possibilities (e.g., ruptured bladder, GU tract obstruction, micro- or large-vessel disease, renal cortical necrosis, GN, allergic interstitial nephritis).

Renal Failure, Chronic

Chronic renal insufficiency defined as serum creatinine = 1.5 to 3.0 mg/dL. Chronic renal failure defined as serum creatinine >3.0 mg/dL.

♦ BUN and serum creatinine are increased and renal function tests are impaired. BUN:creatinine ratio usually = ~10

Creatinine clearance

>30 mL/min/1.73 m^2	usually asymptomatic
<30 mL/min/1.73 m^2	usually symptomatic
<15 mL/min/1.73 m^2	metabolic disturbances require intervention
<5 mL/min/1.73 m^2	end-stage renal disease requires dialysis and transplantation

♦ Loss of renal concentrating ability (nocturia, polyuria, polydipsia) is an early manifestation of progressive renal functional impairment. Specific gravity is usually same as that of glomerular filtrate.

♦ Abnormal urinalysis is usually the first finding. Variable abnormalities include proteinuria, hematuria, pyuria, granular and cellular casts and may be found in asymptomatic patients

♦ In nondiabetic renal diseases, protein/creatinine ratio[3]

• Glomerular disease (e.g., drug toxicity, autoimmune disorders, systemic infection, neoplasia): protein/creatinine ratio >1,000 mg/g

• Vascular disease (e.g. hypertensive nephrosclerosis, microangiopathy, large-vessel disease): protein/creatinine ratio <1,000 mg/g

• Tubulointerstitial diseases (e.g., GU tract infection, obstruction, stones, drug toxicity): protein/creatinine ratio <1,000 mg/g

• Cystic diseases: protein/creatinine ratio <1,000 mg/gm

---

[3]Levey AS. Nondiabetic kidney disease. *N Engl J Med* 2002;347:1505.

Hypotonic urine unresponsive to vasopressin may occur in

- Obstructive uropathy
- Chronic pyelonephritis
- Nephrocalcinosis
- Amyloidosis
- Familial nephrogenic diabetes insipidus

Serum sodium is decreased (because of tubular damage with loss in urine, vomiting, diarrhea, diet restriction, etc.). The decrease is indicated by increased urine sodium levels (>5–10 mEq sodium/L). It may occur in any renal disease, especially when polyuria is marked, but is more common with obstructive uropathy, chronic pyelonephritis, and interstitial nephritis than with chronic GN.

Serum potassium is increased (on account of dietary sodium restriction and increased potassium ingestion, acidosis, impaired potassium excretion, oliguria, tissue breakdown). Decreased serum potassium with increased loss in urine (>15–20 mEq/L) occurs in primary aldosteronism and may also occur in malignant hypertension, tubular acidosis, Fanconi syndrome, nephrocalcinosis, diuresis during recovery from tubular necrosis.

Acidosis is present (due to renal failure to secrete acid as NH_4^+ and to reabsorb filtered bicarbonate and to decreased tubular bicarbonate production).

Serum calcium is decreased (because of decreased calcium absorption in intestine, increased serum phosphorus, decreased serum albumin, etc.). Decreased renal production of calcitriol. Tetany is rare. Secondary parathyroid hyperplasia may occur, but hypercalcemia is not found.

Serum phosphorus increases when creatinine clearance falls to ~25 mL/min.

Serum ALP may be normal or may be increased with renal osteodystrophy.

Serum magnesium increases when glomerular filtration rate falls to <30 mL/min.

Increase in serum uric acid is usually <10 mg/dL. Secondary gout is rare. If clinical gout and family history of gout are present or if serum uric acid level is >10 mg/dL, rule out primary gout nephropathy.

Increased serum amylase occurs frequently; baseline level should be obtained in dialysis patients to evaluate episodes of abdominal pain, since these patients have an increased incidence of pancreatitis.

Serum CK and cTnT may be increased; a subset of uremic patients has a persistently increased CK-MB fraction without evidence of cardiac disease.

Increased serum triglycerides, cholesterol, and VLDL lipoprotein (prebeta) is common as renal failure progresses.

Serum homocysteine is often increased; correlated with cardiovascular complications,

Blood organic acids, phenols, indoles, certain amino acids, etc., are increased.

Normochromic normocytic anemia is usually proportionate to the degree of azotemia. Responds to erythropoietin. Burr cells or schistocytes are common.

Bleeding tendency is evident. There may be decreased platelets, increased capillary fragility, abnormal prothrombin consumption (possible platelet defect), normal bleeding and clotting time.

Gastrointestinal hemorrhage from ulcers anywhere in GI tract may be severe.

Laboratory findings due to uremic pericarditis, pleuritis, and pancreatitis are noted. (BUN is usually >100 mg/dL).

Laboratory findings due to uremic meningitis are noted (~50% of these patients have increased CSF protein or leukocytes; protein may be reduced by hemodialysis; pleocytosis is not related to degree of azotemia).

Serum albumin and total protein are decreased. When there is edema without hypoproteinemia or heart failure, rule out acute glomerulonephritis, toxemia of pregnancy, excess fluid intake in oliguria during acute tubular necrosis (ATN) or terminal renal failure.

Chronic Renal Failure with Normal Urine May Occur In

Nephrosclerosis (e.g., aging, hypertension)
Renal tubular acidosis
Interstitial nephritis
Hypercalcemia
Potassium deficiency
Uric acid nephropathy
Obstruction (including retroperitoneal fibrosis)

Table 14-6.	Chief Causes of Chronic Insufficiency in Patients Presenting for Dialysis
Glomerulonephritis	44%
Diabetic nephropathy	15%
Nephrosclerosis and renal vascular disease	12%
Congenital or hereditary disease (including polycystic kidney)	10%
Chronic pyelonephritis	6%
Others and unknown	15%

Dialysis for End-Stage Renal Disease (ESRD), Laboratory Tests for Management

See Table 14-6.

Conditions to Evaluate Routinely

Azotemia (creatinine and BUN; tests for residual renal functions including 24-hour urine volume)

Electrolyte and mineral balance (e.g., serum calcium, potassium, chloride, bicarbonate, phosphorus)

Liver function tests (serum total protein, albumin, LD, ALP, AST); HBsAg (if seronegative or if antibodies are present after HBV vaccination)

Renal osteodystrophy (osteomalacia) (serum calcium and phosphorus and quarterly serum PTH for secondary hyperparathyroidism)

Anemia (CBC)

Coagulation disorders (clotting time with each dialysis; weekly PT if on Coumadin)

Conditions to Evaluate Nonroutinely

See appropriate separate sections

* Tests for bleeding or clotting disorders
* Heart disease (e.g., uremic pericarditis, hypertension, hyperlipidemia)
* Bone disease (hyperparathyroid bone disease due to hyperphosphatemia and low $1,25(OH)_2$ vitamin D_3 levels)
* Hepatitis
* Symptomatic endocrine problems
* Uremic neuropathies
* Acute complications associated with dialysis (e.g., catheter infection, infective endocarditis, peritonitis if peritoneal dialysis)
* Tests for aluminum toxicity as cause of encephalopathy, Vitamin D-resistant osteodystrophy, and iron-resistant anemia. Histochemical staining of bone biopsy (if serum level >100 μg/L) or atomic absorption of serum (>200 μg/L = toxic; >100 μg/L "view with concern"; 60–100 μg/L appears to cause no problem). Serum assay every 6 to 12 months or every 3 months especially in pediatric patients; serum level may not reflect tissue content.
* Iron overload (due to frequent transfusions; now replaced by EPO therapy)
* Special tests for specific conditions (e.g., acquired renal cystic disease causing renal cell carcinoma, control of diabetes mellitus, etc.)

Interstitial Diseases

Interstitial Nephritis

Acute

Typical clinical triad of fever, rash, and eosinophilia in patients in acute renal failure.

Due To

Recent exposure to a causative drug ≤45% of cases
  Especially antibiotics, diuretics, NSAIDs, anticonvulsants, miscellaneous (e.g., allopurinol, street drugs)
Following infections

Especially Group A β-hemolytic streptococcal, diphtheria, brucellosis, leptospirosis, infectious mononucleosis, toxoplasmosis, Rocky Mountain spotted fever, measles
Metabolic (e.g., calcium, oxalate, uric acid)
Infiltrative (e.g., sarcoid, Sjögren syndrome, lymphoma, leukemia)
Idiopathic
Blood

- ◆ Eosinophilia (in 60%–100% of patients) with increased blood IgE
- Increased WBC, neutrophils, and bands
- Anemia with Hb as low as 6.5 g/dL; no evidence of hemolysis or iron deficiency; negative indirect Coombs' test; normal bone marrow. Anemia resolves when renal function becomes normal.
- Increased ESR
- Serum IgG is usually increased; serum complement is normal.
- Varying degrees of renal insufficiency with increased BUN and creatinine, hyponatremia, hyperchloremic metabolic acidosis, decreased serum albumin

Urine

- May be oliguric or nonoliguric
- Urinary indices similar to those seen in acute tubular necrosis
- ◆ Eosinophiluria reported in ≤100% of patients
- Microscopic hematuria
- Proteinuria is usually mild to moderate, <1.0 g/m²/24 hours, unless nephrotic syndrome is present.
- Sterile pyuria is minimal or absent.
- Casts are uncommon.
- Low osmolality and specific gravity
- Glycosuria without hyperglycemia and reduced TRP may occur.

Enlarged, poorly functioning kidneys may be demonstrated by IVP, ultrasound, or renal scan.
Nephrotic syndrome may occur.
◆ Biopsy of kidney establishes the diagnosis and is usually more severe than indicated by urinalysis and renal studies.

Chronic

Due infections

- Pyelonephritis

Not due to infections

- Analgesic abuse (see Phenacetin, Chronic Excessive Ingestion)
- Diabetes mellitus (see Kimmelstiel-Wilson disease)
- Drugs

    Allergic (e.g., antibiotics, diuretics, phenytoin, cimetidine, NSAIDs)
    Toxic (e.g., cyclosporine, lithium, cisplatin, amphotericin B)

- Toxic substances

    Exogenous (e.g., lead, mercury, cadmium)
    Endogenous, e.g.,
        Uric acid (see Kidney Disorders in Gout)
        Hypercalcemic nephropathy (see below)
    Oxalate

- Radiation nephritis
- Sarcoidosis
- Others

◆ Diagnosis is usually by exclusion. Renal biopsy may be helpful in undiagnosed cases.
May be associated with metabolic acidosis and hyperkalemia out of proportion to degree of renal insufficiency, decreased urine concentrating capacity, and renal salt-wasting.

Table 14-7.	Sensitivity, Specificity, and Predictive Values of Tests in Predicting Bacteriuria (10^5 colonies/mL)			
			Predictive Value (%) of	
Test	Sensitivity (%)	Specificity (%)	Positive Test	Negative Test
>5 WBC/HPF	80	83	46	96
>10 WBC/HPF	63	90	53	93
Nitrite	69	90	57	94
Leukocyte esterase	71	85	47	94
Nitrite + leukocyte esterase (either positive)	86	86	54	97

Pyelonephritis, Acute

Due To
Urinary outflow obstruction with ascending infection
Hematogenous (much less common)
Vesico-ureteric reflux
♦ **Tests for Bacteriuria and Pyuria**
In chronic pyelonephritis, bacteriuria and pyuria are usually absent.
See Table 14-7.

Use
Diagnosis of urinary tract infection (UTI) and determination of antibiotic sensitivity of
causative organism

Interferences
When urine is allowed to remain at room temperature, the number of bacteria doubles
every 30 to 45 minutes.
False-low colony counts may occur with a high rate of urinary flow, low urine specific
gravity, low urine pH, presence of antibacterial drugs, or inappropriate cultural
techniques (e.g., tubercle bacilli, *Mycoplasma*, *Chlamydia trachomatis*, anaerobes).
High doses of vitamin C may cause false-negative test for nitrite on dipstick.
Trichomonas may cause a positive leukocyte esterase reaction.

Interpretation
Dipstick test for pyuria for detection of WBC, sensitivity = 100% for >50 WBCs/HPF,
90% for 21 to 50 WBCs, 60% for 12 to 20 WBCs, 44% for 6 to 12 WBCs. For detection
of bacteria, sensitivity = 73% for "large" numbers, 46% for "moderate" numbers.

- Combined positive esterase and nitrate strips is sufficient indication for colony
count to identify bacteriuria.
- Dipstick of first-catch urine is a cost-effective way to detect asymptomatic
urethritis (*Chlamydia, Neisseria*) in males.
- Leukocyte esterase of neutrophil granules (intact or degenerated); does not detect
lymphocytes; has negative predictive value >90% and positive predictive value = 50%
for bacterial infection. False-negative reaction may be caused by glycosuria, large
doses of vitamin C, and some drugs. False-positive reaction may be caused by contaminated collection, indwelling catheters, foreign bodies, neoplasms, appendicitis, others.
- Dye tests (bacterial reduction of dietary nitrate to nitrite; tetrazolium reduction) do
not detect 10% to 50% of infections. False-negative reaction may be caused by some
important bacteria that do not reduce dye (Gram-positive) (e.g., coliforms are more
likely to be detected than enterococci; bacteria show great variability in rate of dye
reduction), urine has not incubated in patient's bladder for ≥4 hours, large doses of
vitamin C. False-positive reaction may be due to contaminated collection and artifacts (e.g., amorphous urates and phosphates).

Direct microscopic examination of uncentrifuged urine, either unstained or gram-
stained that shows 1 PMN or 1 organism/HPF has sensitivity of 85% and specificity
of 60% for bacteriuria. It may show >10% false-positive results.

- Uncentrifuged urine showing 1 organism/oil-immersion field (threshold of detection for microscopy) correlates with count ≥10,000 colonies/mL.
- Gram stain of cytospin specimen has >90% sensitivity and >80% specificity for ≥10^5/mL. With pyuria and bacteriuria, a Gram stain to differentiate Gram-positive cocci (e.g., *enterococci* or *staph.*) from Gram-negative bacilli will indicate appropriate immediate initial therapy.
- Fewer than 50% of patients with chronic UTI and asymptomatic bacteriuria may not show significant numbers of WBCs on urine microscopic examination; however, pyuria is associated with bacteriuria in ~90% of cases.
- Presence of both bacteria and WBCs has a higher predictive value than either alone.
- Large numbers of squamous epithelial cells may indicate a specimen that contains greater numbers of bacteria from the vagina or perineum rather than the urinary tract.
- High ratio of WBC to epithelial cells suggests infection.
- Bacteriuria and pyuria are often intermittent; in the chronic atrophic stage of pyelonephritis, they are often absent. In acute pyelonephritis, marked pyuria and bacteriuria are almost always present; hematuria and proteinuria may also be present during first few days.
- WBC casts are very suggestive of pyelonephritis. Glitter cells may be seen. A colony count should be performed under the following conditions: a midstream, clean-catch, first morning specimen is submitted in a sterilized container; the specimen is refrigerated until the colony count is performed; periurethral area has first been thoroughly cleaned with soap. Transport tubes have an inhibitory effect and should be used. Suprapubic sterile needle aspiration is the most reliable sampling technique, and the presence of any organisms on culture is virtually diagnostic of UTI (97% sensitivity); it is the only acceptable method in infants as urine collection bags have a very high false-positive rate; compared to urethral catheterization of adults, it is more accurate, simpler, and less traumatic.
- Count of >100,000 bacteria/mL indicates active infection (>85% sensitivity).
- Count of <10,000/mL in the absence of therapy largely rule out bacteriuria but pathogenic organisms may be clinically relevant.
- Count of 10,000 to 100,000/mL should be repeated and cultured.
- Count of <100,000/mL with clinical findings of acute pyelonephritis with no obvious explanation such as recent use of antibiotics, suggests urinary tract obstruction or perinephric abscess.

A culture should be performed for identification of the organism and determination of antibiotic sensitivity when these screening tests are positive. This antibiogram is useful to subsequently identify the same organism in relapsing infections.

- If culture shows a common Gram-positive saprophyte, it should be repeated because the second culture is often negative.
- Causative bacteria are usually Gram-negative rods (especially *E. coli*); 5% to 20% are Gram-positive cocci.
- Positive significant single culture or predominant organism should be considered positive in symptomatic patients (95% reliable) and repeat is unnecessary.
- Three or more species with none being predominant (i.e., >80% of the growth) almost always represents specimen contamination and culture should be repeated; but true mixed infections may occur after instrumentation or with chronic infection.
- Pseudomonas *or* Proteus *may indicate an anatomic abnormality in the patient. If organism other than* E. coli *is found, patient probably has chronic pyelonephritis even if this is the first clinical episode of infection.*
- In women, >80% of UTIs are caused by *E. coli;* smaller percent are caused by *Staphylococcus saprophyticus,* and less often to other aerobic Gram-negative bacilli. In men, Gram-negative bacilli cause ~75% of UTIs but *E. coli* causes only ~25% of infections in men and <50% of infections in boys.
- Other common Gram-negative bacilli are *Proteus* and *Providencia* species. Gram-positive organisms (especially enterococci and coagulase-negative staphylococci) cause about 20% of infections in men and boys but *S. saprophyticus* is rare. *Gardnerella vaginalis* is found in <3% of bacteriuric men.
- If *Candida* are isolated, should rule out contaminated specimen, diabetes mellitus, papillary necrosis, indwelling catheter, broad-spectrum antibiotic exposure, immunosuppressive chemotherapy, malignancy, malnutrition.

- "Sterile" (i.e., pyogenic infection is absent) pyuria ($\geq$10 WBCs/HPF in centrifuged urine) and absence of bacilli (<1 bacillus in multiple oil immersion fields or 20–40 bacteria/HPF in centrifuged sediments) should cast doubt on diagnosis of untreated bacterial UTI and may occur in renal TB, chemical inflammation, mechanical inflammation (e.g., calculi, instrumentation), early acute GN prior to appearance of hematuria or proteinuria, polycystic kidney disease, papillary necrosis, chronic prostatitis, interstitial cystitis, transplant rejection, sarcoidosis, GU tract neoplasm, uric acid and hypercalcemic nephropathy, lithium and heavy metal toxicity, extreme dehydration, hyperchloremic renal acidosis, genital herpes, nonbacterial gastroenteritis and respiratory tract infections, and after administration of oral polio vaccine; may persist for several months after transurethral prostatectomy.
- *When urine cultures are persistently negative in the presence of other evidence of pyelonephritis, specific search should be made for tubercle bacilli.*

○ With pyuria and bacteriuria, persistent alkaline pH may indicate infection with urea-splitting organism (e.g., *Proteus*; less often *Pseudomonas* or *Klebsiella*), suggesting a calculus.

Bacteria should be cleared from urine within 48 hours of antibiotic therapy; persistence indicates need to change antibiotic treatment or search for another explanation.

Asymptomatic bacteriuria occurs in $\leq$15% of pregnant women. Routine urinalysis is done on first prenatal visit because 20% to 40% of untreated patients with positive culture develop acute pyelonephritis during pregnancy (occurs in only 1% of women with negative cultures).

Persistent or recurrent infection may be caused by stones or obstruction. >10^5/mL colonies of a single organism found on culture of midstream specimen indicates significant bacteriuria.

Bacteriuria may be found in

- $\leq$15% of patients who are pregnant
- 15% of patients with diabetes mellitus
- 20% of patients with cystocele
- ~50% of patients with dysuria
- 70% of patients with prostatic obstruction
- $\leq$5% of patients during catheterization
- 95% of patients (untreated) with an indwelling catheter for >4 days
- Should be searched for in elderly patients with altered mental status and infants with failure to thrive, persistent fever, or lethargy
- Bacteriuria plus a positive dipstick test identified in specimens obtained by suprapubic aspiration, cystoscopy, nephrostomy, renal transplant, suggests infection but with a negative dipstick test suggests colonization.

♦ Acute pyelonephritis shows two consecutive colony counts $\geq$100,000 organisms/mL with or without upper GU tract symptoms (flank pain, fever, costovertebral angle tenderness, fever, chills, nausea, vomiting, leukocytosis).

♦ Acute urethral syndrome (AUS) and acute cystitis have colony count $\geq$100 organisms/mL and lower GU tract symptoms (dysuria, frequency, urgency, suprapubic pain). Urine dipstick for WBC (leukocyte esterase) detects 8 to 10 WBC/HPF. Pyuria is rarely present unless bacterial count >10,000/mL.

♦ Catheterization for <30 days or intermittent catheterization—criterion for bacteriuria is $\geq$100 organisms/mL; >95% of patients progress to >100,000 organisms/mL within days; multiple organisms are common

♦ Catheterization for >30 days—mixed infections >100,000 organisms/mL in >75% of cases; organisms constantly change with new ones appearing every ~2 weeks

Decreased glucose in urine (<2 mg/dL) in properly collected first-morning urine (no food or fluid intake after 10 PM, no urination during night) correlates well with colony count.

Positive test for antibody-coated bacteria (using fluorescein-conjugated antihuman globulin) is said to indicate bacteria of renal origin and be 81% predictive of upper GU tract infection but negative in bacteria from lower tract infection. False-positives may occur with heavy proteinuria, prostatitis, contamination with vaginal or rectal bacteria. False-negatives may occur in early infection. Test is less reliable in children and adults with neurogenic bladder. Test is not recommended for routine use.

Albuminuria is usually <2 g/24 hours ($\leq2+$ qualitative) and therefore helps to differentiate pyelonephritis from glomerular disease, in which albuminuria is usually >2 g/24
hours; may be undetectable in a very dilute urine associated with fixed specific gravity.
Beta$_2$ microglobulin is increased in 24-hour urine in pyelonephritis (due to tubular
damage) but not in cystitis.
LD-4 and LD-5 are increased in urine in renal medullary damage (pyelonephritis); less
useful than beta$_2$ microglobulin to distinguish upper from lower urinary tract damage.
Hyperchloremic acidosis (due to impaired renal acid excretion and bicarbonate reabsorption) occurs more often in chronic pyelonephritis than in GN.
Decreased concentrating ability occurs relatively early in chronic renal infection but
not bladder infections. Persistent dilute urine (low specific gravity or osmolarity)
suggests renal rather than bladder infection if patient is not forcing fluid. Not a
sensitive or specific test because of overlapping values even though is more
marked in bilateral than unilateral infection and concentrating ability increases
with cure.
Renal blood flow and glomerular filtration show parallel decrease proportional to
progress of renal disease. Comparison of function in right and left kidneys shows
more disparity in pyelonephritis than in diffuse renal disease (e.g., nephrosclerosis, GN).
Fluctuation in renal insufficiency (e.g., due to recurrent infection, dehydration) with
considerable recovery is more marked and frequent in pyelonephritis than in other
renal diseases.
There is a decrease in 24-hour creatinine clearance before a rise in BUN and blood creatinine takes place.
Laboratory findings of associated diseases, e.g., diabetes mellitus, urinary tract
obstruction (stone, tumor, etc.), neurogenic bladder dysfunction, are present. UTI in
infant <1 year old is associated with an underlying GU tract anomaly in 55% of
males and 35% of females.
Laboratory findings due to sequelae (e.g., papillary necrosis, bacteremia) are present.
*"Cured" patient should be followed with routine periodic urinalysis and colony count
for at least 2 years because asymptomatic recurrence of bacteriuria is common.*

Infections

Abscess

Perinephric

Laboratory findings due to underlying or primary diseases

- Hematogenous from distant foci usually due to staphylococci and occasionally strep-
tococci
- Direct extension from kidney infection (e.g., pyelonephritis, pyonephrosis) due to
Gram-negative rods and occasionally tubercle bacilli
- Infected perirenal hematoma (e.g., due to trauma, tumor, polyarteritis nodosa) due
to various organisms

Urine changes due to underlying disease

- Urine may be normal and sterile. *Do acid-fast smear and culture for tubercle bacilli.*

Increased WBC and ESR may be increased.
Blood culture may be positive.

Renal

Urine

- Trace of albumin
- Few RBCs (may have transient gross hematuria at onset)
- No WBCs

♦ • Very many organisms in stained sediment if connected to calyces
Increased WBC (may be $>30,000/\mu L$)
Laboratory findings due to underlying disease (e.g., obstruction, calculi, diabetes)

Tuberculosis (TB), Renal

○ Should be ruled out when there is unexplained albuminuria, pyuria, microhematuria with negative cultures for pyogenic bacteria, especially in presence of TB elsewhere.
♦ Urine culture for TB and molecular methods
See Tuberculosis, for general findings.

Metabolic Disorders

Renal Tubular Acidosis (RTA)

Nonuremic defects of urine acidification due to renal bicarbonate loss.

Proximal (Type 2)

Due to defective bicarbonate reabsorption in proximal tubule.

♦ Low plasma bicarbonate concentration with hyperchloremic acidosis
♦ Alkaline urine that becomes acid if extracellular bicarbonate level is decreased below the patient's maximum reabsorptive limit
Normal urine pH in the absence of bicarbonate in the urine
♦ IV $NaHCO_3$ ($\leq$1.0 mEq/kg/hr) causes rapid increase in urine pH even though plasma HCO_3^- has increased but is still less than normal (24–26 mEq/L).
Proximal RTA is diagnosed by fractional excretion of bicarbonate >15% when plasma bicarbonate >20 mEq/L.

Due To

Most commonly due to increased excretion of monoclonal Ig light chains in multiple myeloma or carbonic anhydrase inhibitor (e.g., acetazolamide for glaucoma) in adults and cystinosis or idiopathic cause in children.

Primary (defect in bicarbonate reabsorption)

• Usually occurs in males
• Only clinical manifestation is retarded growth; renal and metabolic complications are absent
• Good prognosis with clinical response to alkali therapy, which is usually not permanently required

Secondary

• Idiopathic or secondary Fanconi syndrome (cystinosis, Lowe syndrome [X-linked recessive disorder with congenital cataracts, neurological involvement], tyrosinemia, glycogen storage disease, Wilson disease, hereditary fructose intolerance, heavy-metal intoxication, toxic effect of drugs such as outdated tetracycline)
• Vitamin D–deficient rickets
• Medullary cystic disease
• Following renal transplantation
• Nephrotic syndrome, multiple myeloma, renal amyloidosis

Distal (Type 1)

Collecting ducts do not secrete sufficient H^+ to form ammonium or backleak of secreted H^+ out of collecting tubule lumen; occurs predominantly in females (70%).

♦ Hyperchloremic acidosis, low plasma bicarbonate concentration; should be suspected in any patient with metabolic acidosis with normal anion gap and inappropriately high urine pH (>5.3 in adults, >5.6 in children). Incomplete Type 1 RTA should be suspected with normal plasma bicarbonate concentration, urine pH persistently >5.3, and calcium stone disease, or positive family history.
♦ Alkaline urine (pH 6.5–7.0) that persists at any level of plasma bicarbonate
♦ Ammonium loading test (NH_4Cl 0.1 g/kg) shows inability to acidify urine below pH 6.5 and depressed rates of excretion of titratable acid and ammonium.
No other tubular defects
Often presents with complications (e.g., nephrocalcinosis, interstitial nephritis renal calculi, rickets, and osteomalacia) as well as growth retardation

Due To

Most commonly caused by autoimmune disorders (e.g., Sjögren syndrome) or hypercalciuria in adults and hereditary form in children

Hypokalemic or Normokalemic Type
Primary (inability of tubular cell to secrete enough H^+)
Secondary

- Increased serum globulins (especially gamma) (e.g., SLE, Sjögren syndrome, Hodgkin disease, sarcoidosis, chronic active hepatitis, cryoglobulinemia)
- Pyelonephritis
- Medullary sponge kidney
- Ureterosigmoidostomy
- Hereditary insensitivity to antidiuretic hormone (vasopressin)
- Various renal diseases (e.g., hypercalcemia, potassium-losing disorders, medullary cystic disease, polyarteritis nodosa, amyloidosis, Sjögren syndrome)
- Various genetically transmitted disorders (e.g., Ehlers-Danlos syndrome, Fabry disease, hereditary elliptocytosis)
- Starvation, malnutrition
- Hyperthyroidism
- Hyperparathyroidism
- Vitamin D intoxication

Hyperkalemic Type (Due to Impaired Na Reabsorption in Cortical Collecting Tubules)
- Hypoaldosteronism
- Obstructive nephropathy
- SLE
- Sickle cell nephropathy
- Cyclosporine toxicity

An incomplete or mixed tubular acidosis may be seen in obstructive uropathy and in hereditary fructose intolerance.

Aldosteronism (Type 4)
Consists of a variety of conditions characterized by:

- Mild to moderate renal impairment
- Hyperchloremic acidosis
- Hyperkalemia
- Acid urine pH
- Reduced ammonium secretion
- Frequently, tendency to lose sodium in urine
- Decreased mineralocorticoid secretion in some patients due to isolated hypoaldosteronism; others have decreased tubular response to aldosterone.

Hypercalciuria, Idiopathic
Generally defined as urine calcium >300 mg/24 hr in men and >250 mg/24 hr in women.

- ◆ Increased excretion of urinary calcium >350 mg/24 hr on diet containing 600 to 800 mg/day
  - >4 mg/kg (either sex)
  - >140 mg/gm of urinary creatinine is most useful in short or obese patients (either sex)

Normal blood calcium levels
Serum 1,25-dihydroxyvitamin D3 levels are usually high.
- ◆ Diagnosis requires exclusion of all other causes of hypercalciuria; may be familial. Occurs in ~40% of patients who form calcium renal stones. Occurs in 5% to 10% of general population.

Three types of hypercalciuria—2-hour urine collection after fasting

- **Renal**: Calcium/creatinine ratio >0.15. Hypercalciuria persists despite absent dietary calcium in intestine following fasting. One-tenth as common as absorptive type. Due to abnormality of renal tubular reabsorption.
- **Absorptive**: <20 mg calcium or calcium/creatinine ratio <0.15. Twenty-four-hour urine falls to <200 mg/24 hours following low-calcium diet (400 mg/day) for 3 to 4 days. Almost always due to primary increase in intestinal calcium absorption. Probably autosomal dominant. Is most common type.

- **Resorptive** (nonabsorptive): >30 mg calcium or calcium/creatinine ratio >0.15. Due to primary hyperparathyroidism.
- Indeterminate: Calcium 20 to 30 mg/2-hour urine

Hypercalcemic Nephropathy

Due to prolonged increase in serum and urine calcium (due to hyperparathyroidism, sarcoidosis, vitamin D intoxication, multiple myeloma, carcinomatosis, milk-alkali syndrome, etc.).

Early findings are decreased renal concentrating ability manifested by polyuria and polydipsia but no loss of ability to dilute urine. Decreased urine osmolality.

Urine is normal or contains RBCs, WBCs, WBC casts; proteinuria is usually slight or absent.

Later findings are decreased GFR, decreased renal blood flow, azotemia.

Renal insufficiency is insidious and slowly progressive; it may sometimes be reversed by correcting hypercalcemia.

Laboratory findings due to underlying disorders (e.g., hypercalciuria) and sequelae (e.g., stones)

Oxalosis

Secondary

Due To

Increased oxalate in diet (e.g., green leafy vegetables, chocolate, tea)

Ingestion of oxalate precursors (e.g., ascorbic acid, ethylene glycol)

Methoxyflurane anesthesia

Primary diseases of ileum with malabsorption (e.g., bypass surgery, Crohn disease, pancreatitis) causing increased absorption of dietary oxalate

Urinary oxalate is usually 50 to 100 mg/24 hours

Primary (Types 1 and 2)

Rare, autosomal recessive inherited disorders of glyoxylate metabolism causing recurrent calcium oxalate renal lithiasis, nephrocalcinosis, and uremia.

♦ Urinary oxalate is usually >100 mg/24 hours unless renal function is diminished.

Renal Transplant

Laboratory Criteria for Kidney Donation

Living Donor

- Three successive urinalyses and cultures must be negative.
- No evidence of HBV, HCV, HIV, CMV, malignancy, no history of renal disease or severe hypertension. Same for cadaveric donor.

Donor and recipient must show

- ABO and Rh blood group compatibility
- Leukoagglutinin, mixed lymphocyte culture compatibility
- Platelet agglutinin compatibility

Rejection

Total urine output is decreased.

Proteinuria is increased.

Cellular or granular casts appear.

Urine osmolality is decreased.

BUN and creatinine increase.

Hyperchloremic renal tubular acidosis may be an early sign of rejection or indicate smoldering rejection activity.

Renal clearance values decrease.

Sodium iodohippurate ^{131}I renogram is altered.
♦ Biopsy of kidney shows a characteristic microscopic appearance allowing definitive diagnosis.
♦ Sequential measuring of subsets of activated T cells by flow cytometry is useful for diagnosis of rejection and monitoring reversibility of rejection.
Messenger RNA recovered from cells in urine encoding cytotoxic proteins perforin and granzyme B are reported to be increased by PCR in acute rejection[4]

Recurrent Disease
Glomerulonephritis (GN), especially dense deposit disease, anti-glomerular basement membrane disease, focal glomerulosclerosis, membranous nephropathy
Diabetic intercapillary glomerulosclerosis (K-W syndrome)
Amyloidosis

Disorders of Immunity

Glomerulonephritis (GN), Classification

Defined as abrupt onset of hematuria, often with decreased GFR, proteinuria, edema, hypertension, and sometimes with oliguria.

See Tables 14-8, 14-9, and Fig. 14-4.

Antibody-mediated

* Anti-glomerular basement membrane (GBM) diseases
    Anti-GBM GN including Goodpasture syndrome
    Alport syndrome
    Following renal transplantation
* Immune complex–mediated diseases (typically show hypocomplementemia)
    IgA nephropathy
    Henoch-Schönlein purpura
    SLE
    Acute postinfectious GN
    Membranoproliferative (MPGN)
    Membranous GN
    Fibrillary GN

Cell-mediated

* Wegener granulomatosis
* Polyarteritis
* Churg-Strauss syndrome
* ANCA-positive GN
* Scleroderma

Also classified as:

Infectious

Acute poststreptococcal (group A beta-hemolytic GN)
Nonpoststreptococcal GN:

* Bacterial (e.g., infective endocarditis, bacteremias)
* Viral (e.g., HBV, HCV, CMV)
* Parasitic (e.g., trichinosis, toxoplasmosis, falciparum malaria)
* Fungal

Noninfectious

* Multisystem (e.g., SLE, Henoch-Schönlein purpura, Goodpasture syndrome, Alport syndrome)
* Primary glomerular disease (e.g., IgA nephropathy, MPGN, mesangial proliferative GN)

[4]Li B, Hartono C, Ding R. et al. Noninvasive diagnosis of renal-allograft rejection by measurement of messenger RNA for perforin and granzyme B in urine. *N Engl J Med* 2001;344:947.

GU

Table 14-8. Classification of Glomerulonephritis

Glomerular Disorder	Situations in Which May Be Found	Hematuria (% of cases)		Proteinuria (% of cases)		Renal Function Decreased	Comment
		Micro Present	RBC Casts Present	1–3 g Present	>3 g Present		
IgA nephropathy (Berger disease)	Focal proliferative GN	100	50	75	25	25% or NS; N in 75%	
IgM mesangial nephropathy		50	Rare	50	50	>75% or NS	
Acute GN secondary to infection (focal GN)	SBE, bacterial pneumonia, viral infections, infection of implanted devices	100	50	75	25	100%	
Crescentic (rapidly progressive) GN Anti-GBM	Goodpasture syndrome in 2/3 of patients	100	50	50	50	100%	90% have HLA-DR2 antigen
Immune complex	SLE, mixed cryoglobulinemia, Henoch-Schönlein purpura	100	50	50	50	100%	
Nonimmune complex	Wegener granulomatosis, polyarteritis						See Chapter 16.
GN and vasculitis	Wegener granulomatosis, Henoch-Schönlein purpura, mixed cryoglobulinemia; Goodpasture syndrome may occur	100	50	50	50	100%	

Disease	Etiology				Notes
SLE					
Mesangial		15	10	N	Most frequent type in SLE
Focal proliferative		50	25	N or D	
Membranous		50	85	N or D	
Diffuse proliferative (<25% of SLE patients)		75	75	Usually D; uremia develops in 50%–75%	
Minimal-change disease	Lipid nephrosis, nil disease	20	100	N	85% respond to steroid therapy. Most common cause of NS in children
Focal sclerosis		75	25	Usually D	Frequent cause of NS
Membranous nephropathy	Usually idiopathic; occasionally due to heavy-metal toxicity (e.g., gold, mercury), persistent hepatitis B infection, other viruses (e.g., measles, varicella, Coxsackie), other infections (e.g., malaria, syphilis, leprosy, schistosomiasis), neoplasias (e.g., colon carcinoma, lymphoma, leukemia), sarcoidosis, SLE, others	50	25	N early; D late	Frequent cause of NS. Strong association with HLA-DR3. Spontaneous remission in 25%–50%. Persistent proteinuria without progression in 25%. Progressive glomerular sclerosis causing renal failure in 50%. Common in adults; uncommon in children.

(continued)

Table 14-8. *(continued)*

Glomerular Disorder	Situations in Which May Be Found	Hematuria (% of cases)		Proteinuria (% of cases)		Renal Function Decreased	Comment
		Micro Present	RBC Casts Present	1–3 g Present	>3 g Present		
Membranoproliferative GN							
Type I (idiopathic)	SBE, essential cryo-globulinemia, Henoch-Schönlein purpura, SLE, sickle cell disease, hepatitis and cirrhosis, C2 deficiency, alpha$_1$-antitrypsin deficiency, infected shunts (*Staphylococcus*, *Corynebacterium*)	75	25	50	50	Usually D; NS at onset in 75%	Renal failure within 5 yrs common in adults but may be delayed 10–20 yrs. Persistent, marked protein-uria is poor prognostic sign. Renal vein thrombosis may occur.
Type II (idiopathic)	Infection with strepto-cocci, pneumococci, *Candida*, lipody-strophy						

D, decreased; GBM, glomerular basement membrane; N, normal; NS, nephrotic syndrome; SBE, subacute endocarditis.
Goodpasture syndrome occurs in <5% of cases of GN.
Source: WA Border, RJ Glassock. Progress in treating glomerulonephritis. *Drug Therapy* 1981;(Apr):97. TR Miller, et al. Urinary diagnostic indices in acute renal failure: a prospective study. *Ann Intern Med* 1978;89:47; DE Oken. On the differential diagnosis of acute renal failure. *Am J Med* 1981;71(Dec):916.

Table 14-9.	Serum Complement in Acute Nephritis

Disorder	Approximate Percentage of Cases
Depressed Serum C3 or Hemolytic Complement Levels	
Systemic disease	
SLE (focal)	75
SLE (diffuse)	90
Subacute bacterial endocarditis	90
"Shunt" nephritis	90
Cryoglobulinemia	85
Renal disease	
Acute poststreptococcal GN	90
Membranoproliferative GN	
Type I	50–80
Type II	80–90
Normal Serum Complement Level	
Systemic disease	
Polyarteritis nodosa	
Wegener granulomatosis	
Hypersensitivity vasculitis	
Henoch-Schönlein purpura	
Goodpasture syndrome	
Visceral abscess	
Renal disease	
IgG-IgA nephropathy	
Idiopathic rapidly progressive GN	
Anti–glomerular basement membrane disease	
Immune complex disease	
Negative immunofluorescence findings	

Also classified as:

Hypocomplementic

* Intrinsic renal diseases (especially postinfectious and MPGN)
* Systemic (e.g., SLE, bacterial endocarditis, cryoglobulinemia, serum sickness)

Normocomplementic (see Table 14-10)

IgA Nephropathy (Berger Disease)
An immunologically mediated, focal proliferative GN; is most common form of GN.

○ May present as

* Persistent or intermittent microscopic hematuria with and variable proteinuria
* Episodes of painless gross hematuria often associated with (rather than following) 4 to 10 days' infection of any type (usually upper respiratory).
* Nephrotic syndrome
* Henoch-Schönlein purpura

♦ Diagnosis is based on renal biopsy with immunofluorescence showing predominant mesangial IgA; IgG and C3 are variably present.
○ Plasma IgA increased in ≤50% of patients
Serum complement is normal.

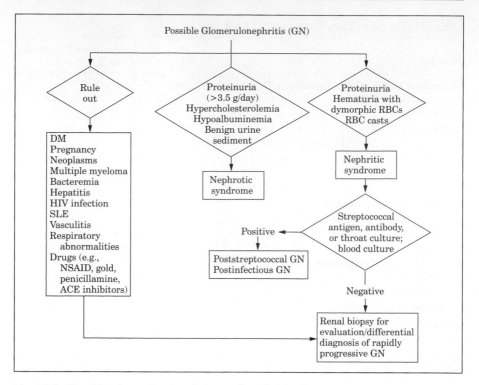

Fig. 14-4. Algorithm for evaluation of glomerulonephritis (GN).

Progressive decline in renal function in ≤40% of cases; half of these reach ESRD in 5 to 25 years. ≤30% have benign course with persistent microscopic hematuria, proteinuria <1 g/day, and normal serum creatinine.

IgA deposits may be associated with diseases of GI tract (e.g., celiac disease), skin (e.g., dermatitis herpetiformis), liver (e.g., cirrhosis); carcinomas (e.g., lung, pancreas), immunologic (SLE, RA), infections (e.g., HIV, leprosy).

Glomerulonephritis, Membranous

Antibody-mediated disease in which immune complexes localize between outer aspect of basement membrane and epithelial cells. These complexes are in situ or circulating and attach to intrinsic glomerular antigen or exogenous antigen on wall of capillary. Usually in adults, in whom it causes ≤50% of nephrotic syndrome.

Due To
Primary (≤75% of cases) or
Secondary

- Connective tissue diseases (e.g., SLE)
- Infections (e.g., HBV, syphilis, malaria, schistosomiasis, leprosy)
- Drugs (e.g., NSAIDs, penicillamine, gold)
- Neoplasms (non-Hodgkin lymphoma, leukemia, carcinomas, melanoma)

♦ Renal biopsy showing light microscopy, immunofluorescent antibody (IgG and C3) and EM diagnostic findings
○ Marked proteinuria with nephrotic type of syndrome is found in many patients; microscopic hematuria may be present.
≤25% of patients progress to ESRD in 20 to 30 years

Table 14-10.   Comparison of Primary Renal Diseases Presenting as Acute GN

	PSGN	IgA Nephropathy (Berger Disease)	MPGN	Idiopathic RPGN (Crescentic)
Acute nephritis	90%	50%	90%	90%
Hematuria	Gross or only microscopic	50%	Rare	Rare
Nephrotic syndrome	10%–20%	Rare	70% of patients	10%–20%
Acute renal failure	50% (usually transient)	Very rare	50%	60%
Laboratory findings	↑ASOT in 80% Positive streptozyme (95%) ↓C3-C9; normal C1, C4	↑IgA in serum in ≤50% Normal complement	↓C3; normal C4 Positive anti-GBM antibody ↑ASOT 20%	Positive ANCA Normal complement
Renal Pathology	Diffuse proliferation	Focal proliferation	Focal, diffuse proliferation	Crescentic GN
Immuno-fluorescence	Granular IgG, C3 deposits	Diffuse mesangial IgA, IgG, C3; IgA in dermal capillaries	Linear IgG, C3	
Electron microscopy	Subepithelial humps	Mesangial deposits	No deposits	No deposits
Course	95% resolve spontaneously; 5% get RPGN or slowly progress	Slow progression in ≤50% in 5–25 yrs	75% stabilize or improve with early treatment 50% of untreated have renal insufficiency in 10 yrs	75% stabilize or improve with early treatment
Hypertension	70%	30%–50%	Rare	25%

PSGN, poststreptococcal GN; MPGN, membranoproliferative GN; RPGN, rapidly progressive GN.
↓, decreased; ↑, increased.

Glomerulonephritis, Membranoproliferative (MPGN)

Types I, II, III are distinguished by morphology and immunofluorescence. Clinical course may be clinically active, or there may be periods of remission; 50% have chronic renal insufficiency in 10 years.

Marked proteinuria and nephrotic syndrome are found in 70% of patients.
○ Normal serum C4, but prolonged or permanent depression of C3 is found in 60% to 80% of patients; clinical course is not related to serum complement levels.
♦ Renal biopsy and immunofluorescent antibody findings
GFR <80 mL/min/1.73/m² in two thirds of patients
Associated with systemic diseases, neoplasms, infections (especially HCV with cryo-globulinemia)

Minimal Change Disease

Formerly called *lipoid nephrosis* or *nil lesion*.

May be associated with Hodgkin disease and non-Hodgkin lymphoma

♦ Shows fused epithelial podocytes by electron microscopy. No immune deposits by DFA. Light microscopy is normal.

Most common cause of nephrotic syndrome in children and ≤30% in adults

Microscopic hematuria in fewer than one third of patients

Glomerulonephritis, Postinfectious, Acute

Due to deposits of immune complexes in glomerulus basement membrane.

See Table 14-8.

♦ Evidence of infection, especially Group A β-hemolytic Streptococcus by

* Culture of throat
* Serologic findings indicative of recent infection (e.g., ASOT) Combined use of serologic tests will establish recent streptococcal infection in virtually all cases.

♦ Urine

* Hematuria—gross or only microscopic. Microscopic hematuria may occur during the initial febrile upper respiratory infection (URI) and then reappear with nephritis in 1 to 2 weeks. It lasts 2 to 12 months; usual duration is 2 months.
* RBC casts and dysmorphic RBCs show glomerular origin of hematuria.
* WBC casts and WBCs show inflammatory nature of lesion.
* Granular and epithelial cell casts are present.
* Fatty casts and lipid droplets occur several weeks later; not related to hyperlipemia.
* Proteinuria is usually <2 g/day (but may be ≤6–8 g/day). May disappear while RBC casts and RBCs still occur.
* Decreased urinary aldosterone occurs in the presence of edema.
* Oliguria is frequent.

GFR usually shows greater decrease than renal blood flow; therefore, filtration factor is decreased.

PSP excretion is normal in cases of mild to moderate severity; increases with progression of disease.

Blood

* Azotemia is found in ~50% of patients.
* Leukocytosis with increased PMNs; ESR is increased.
* There is mild anemia, especially when edema is present (may be caused hemodilution, bone marrow depression, or increased destruction of RBCs).
* Serum proteins are normal or there is nonspecific decrease of albumin and increase of alpha₂ and sometimes of beta and gamma globulins.
* Serum C3 and total hemolytic complement fall 24 hours before onset of hematuria and return to normal within ~8 wks when hematuria subsides. If C3 is low >8 wks, should consider lupus nephritis or MPGN.
* Antihuman kidney antibodies are present in serum in 50% of patients.
* Serum cholesterol may be increased.

♦ Renal biopsy shows characteristic findings with electron microscopy and immunofluorescence.

Chronic renal insufficiency reported in ≤20% of patients.

○ *Azotemia with high urine specific gravity and normal PSP excretion usually means acute GN.*

Glomerulonephritis, Rapidly Progressive (RPGN; Crescentic)

Syndrome (usually immunologically mediated) of rapid progression with severe oliguria and renal failure within weeks. Often preceded by multisystem diseases. Crescent formation is nonspecific response to severe inflammation. Takes ~30 days from initial injury to complete obliteration of glomerulus.

Due To

Infectious (bacterial [e.g., poststreptococcal GN, infective endocarditis], viral [e.g., HBV, HCV], fungal, parasitic)

Drugs (e.g., allopurinol, hydralazine, rifampin, D-penicillamine)

Multisystem diseases (e.g., SLE, Henoch-Schönlein purpura, Goodpasture syndrome, cancer of colon or lung, Wegener granulomatosis [see Chapter 5, cryoimmunoglobulinemia, others)

Primary diseases (e.g., anti-GBM GN, immune complex–mediated diseases, pauci-immune, mixed, idiopathic)

Superimposed on primary diseases (e.g., IgA nephropathy, MPGN)

○ Oliguria with urine volume often <400 mL/day

○ Hematuria is often gross; RBCs, WBCs, and casts are present; proteinuria is usually >3 g/day beginning about third day after injury.

○ Renal function may decline rapidly beginning ~1 to 2 weeks after injury. Azotemia is usually progressive, with BUN >80 mg/dL and serum creatinine >10 mg/dL (in poststreptococcal type, BUN is usually 30–100 mg/dL and serum creatinine 1.5–4.0 mg/dL).

○ Serum complement levels are normal.

♦ Renal biopsy and immunofluorescent antibody findings establish diagnosis and potential reversibility.

Laboratory tests to determine underlying cause

• Determine cause of infection
• ANCA (antineutrophil cytoplasmic antibody) positive and pauci-immune

ANCA-negative

• ANA

Prognosis and treatment of anti-GBM antibodies depend on renal function at presentation:

Renal Function	Treatment/Prognosis
Serum creatinine <2 mg/dL	Immunosuppressive Rx (glucocorticoids, cyclophosphamide)
Serum creatinine 2–6 mg/dL without oliguria	Immunosuppressive Rx plus plasma exchange
Serum creatinine >6 mg/dL especially with oliguria	Immunosuppressive Rx plus plasma exchange is unlikely to recover useful function.

Prognosis is poorer than in poststreptococcal GN.

Glomerulonephritis, Chronic

Syndrome characterized by proteinuria (may be <3.5 g/1.73 m²/day), variable abnormalities of urinary sediment, hypertension, decreased GFR, developing over years or decades, leading to irreversible EDRF.

Due To

Poststreptococcal GN	1%–2% progress to chronic GN
RPGN	90% progress to chronic GN
Membranous GN	50% progress to chronic GN
Focal glomerulosclerosis	50%–80% progress to chronic GN
MPGN	50% progress to chronic GN
IgA nephropathy	30%–50% progress to chronic GN

Various Clinical Courses

Early death after marked proteinuria, hematuria, oliguria, progressive increasing uremia, anemia

Intermittent or continuous or incidental proteinuria, hematuria with slight or absent azotemia, and normal renal function tests (may develop into late renal failure or may subside)

Exacerbation of chronic nephritis (with accentuation of proteinuria, hematuria, and decreased renal function) shortly following streptococcal upper respiratory infection

Nephrotic syndrome

○ *Compared to pyelonephritis, chronic GN shows lipid droplets and epithelial and RBC casts in urine, more marked proteinuria (>2–3 g/day), poorer prognosis for equivalent amount of azotemia.*

GU

Nephritic Syndrome

Immune disorder with acute onset of hematuria with dysmorphic RBCs, RBC casts, hypertension, oliguria, declining renal function (azotemia).

Due To

Renal, e.g., postinfectious (certain nephritogenic strains of streptococcal, staphylococcal, pneumococcal infections; mumps, measles, chickenpox, HBC, HBC) or MPGN, anti-glomerular membrane disease

Systemic (e.g., SLE, vasculitides, IgA nephropathy, Henoch-Schönlein purpura)

♦ Renal biopsy establishes the diagnosis.

♦ Decreased C3 complement

♦ Immunologic tests (e.g., antiglomerular basement, ASOT)

Some proteinuria but much less than in nephrotic syndrome

Congenital Disorders

Hematuria, Benign Familial or Recurrent

Common familial disorder. Some cases may be same as thin basement membrane disease.

♦ Asymptomatic isolated hematuria without proteinuria. Other laboratory and clinical findings are normal. Other family members may also have asymptomatic hematuria.

♦ Renal biopsy: EM with measurement of basement membranes shows thinning; is normal on light microscopy and immunofluorescence.

Should gradually clear spontaneously; annual screening for other abnormalities should be performed until condition clears.

Hereditary Nephritis

Classified into two types:

• Fabry disease
• Alport syndrome: Familial X-linked disease of type IV collagen associated with nerve deafness and lens defects is rare. Gene located at Xq13. Glomerular hematuria with normal complement. Nephrotic syndrome in 40% of cases. Renal disease is progressive to ESRD.

♦ Renal biopsy showing EM changes in glomerular basement membranes and IHC of skin biopsy.

♦ Prenatal and presymptomatic diagnosis by linkage analysis or by direct gene studies in previously tested families

Horseshoe Kidneys

Fusion of two kidneys across midline, usually at lower pole; usually associated with malrotation and other developmental abnormalties (e.g., Turner's syndrome).

Laboratory findings due to complications of ureteral obstruction (e.g., pyelonephritis, renal stones).

Polycystic Kidney Diseases (PKD)[5]

May be acquired or inherited.

Autosomal Dominant Form (ADPKD)

Usually slowly progressive and asymptomatic until >50 years old; accounts for ~10% of transplant or dialysis cases. Renal failure is inevitable.

---

[5]Wilson PD. Polycystic kidney disease. *N Engl J Med* 2004;350:151.

Type I comprises ≤90% of cases. Type II, ≤15% of cases has later onset symptoms, slower progression to renal failure, longer life expectancy. Autosomal recessive form is usually more severe and becomes manifest earlier with few survivors as adults.
Laboratory findings in ADPKD due to:

- Cysts that may occur in liver, ovary, pancreas, spleen, and CNS
- Associated intracranial aneurysms that cause cerebral hemorrhage and death in >10% of patients

Familial Nephronophthisis (Autosomal Recessive)

Cysts in medulla at border of cortex with bilateral shrunken kidneys

Medullary Cystic Kidney

Autosomal dominant traits with bilateral shrunken kidneys. First appear in adulthood and clinically milder than nephronophthisis. Renal failure is inevitable.

Medullary Sponge Kidney

- Findings due to complications (e.g., calculi in ≤50%; infection; hematuria)
- Disease is asymptomatic, not progressive. Renal failure is rare.

Other Inherited Conditions (Associated with Renal Cysts)

- Von Hippel-Lindau disease, tuberous sclerosis
- Acquired form: Simple cysts due to aging; multicystic may be seen due to drugs, hormones, chronic renal failure of any etiology, and ≤90% of dialysis (for >10 years) patients

May show polyuria, salt wasting, progressive renal insufficiency, hypertension, growth retardation. Anemia of renal failure is less severe than in other forms of kidney disease. Polycythemia may occur due to production of erythropoietin that may be increased.
Polyuria is common.
Hematuria may be gross and episodic or an incidental microscopical finding.
Proteinuria occurs in about one third of patients and is mild (<1 g/24 hours).
Renal calculi may be associated (≤30% of ADPKD patients).
Superimposed urinary tract infection is frequent (33% of patients).
Death occurs within 5 years after BUN rises to 50 mg/dL (33% of patients).
Death usually occurs in early infancy or in middle age when superimposed nephrosclerosis of aging or pyelonephritis has exhausted renal reserve.
Increased incidence of gout occurs in patients with polycystic kidneys.
- ◆ Prenatal diagnosis is possible using DNA obtained by amniocentesis or chorionic villus sampling.
- ◆ Diagnosis is usually made by ultrasound; MRI and CT are more sensitive.

Tumors of Kidney

Carcinoma of Renal Pelvis and Ureter, Leukoplakia

Hematuria is present.
Renal calculi are associated.
Urinary tract infection is associated.
- ◆ Cytologic examination of urinary sediment for malignant cells may be falsely negative in 20% of patients.

Leukoplakia of Renal Pelvis

- ◆ Cell block or Pap smear of urine may show keratin or keratinized squamous cells.
- ◆ High grade (aneuploid) tumors can be detected by flow cytometry of DNA on >90% of cases.

Metastases to kidneys occur in ~12% of cancer patients, most commonly with cancers of lung, breast, ovary, bowel, other solid cancers. >30% of patients with lymphomas have renal involvement.

Renal Cell Carcinoma

Originates from proximal tubule; ≤80% are clear cell type

○ Even in the absence of the classic loin pain, flank mass, and hematuria, renal cell carcinoma should be ruled out in the presence of these *unexplained* (paraneoplastic) laboratory findings, which are associated with a poorer prognosis.

* Abnormal liver function tests (in absence of metastases to liver) found in 40% of these patients, e.g., increased serum ALP or AST, prolonged PT, altered serum protein values
* Hypercalcemia
* Polycythemia in 5% to 10% of patients due to production of erythropoietin
* Thrombocytosis
* Leukemoid reaction
* Refractory anemia and increased ESR
* Amyloidosis
* Cushing syndrome
* Salt-losing syndrome
* Increased serum ferritin (due to hemorrhage within tumor)
* Von Hippel-Lindau disease
* ♦ Exfoliative cytology of urine for suspicious tumor cells
* Increased urine enzyme concentration
* Incidental finding of imaging of kidney

Needle biopsy is not recommended due to possible spread along needle tract as well as false-positive rate of 5% and false-negative rate of ≤25%.

Renin-Producing Renal Tumors

Extremely rare small hemangiopericytomas of juxtaglomerular apparatus are usually benign. Also Wilms' tumor; ectopic renin production by lung, pancreas, and ovary cancers.

♦ Plasma renin activity (PRA) is increased, with levels significantly higher in renal vein from affected side.
♦ PRA maintains circadian rhythm despite marked elevation; responds to changes in posture but not to changes in sodium intake.
♦ Secondary aldosteronism is evident, with hypokalemia, etc.
♦ Prorenin level may be >50× higher than active renin (normal = 3–5× higher), especially in ectopic renin production and Wilms' tumor.
Laboratory changes (and hypertension) are reversed by removal of tumor.

Wilms Tumor

Primary kidney tumor of children <5 years old associated with various groups of congenital malformations due to changes on chromosome 11p
Increased risk of Wilms' tumor in opposite kidney

Vascular Disorders

Nephrosclerosis

"Benign" nephrosclerosis ("essential hypertension")

* Urine contains little or no protein or microscopic abnormalities.
* 10% of patients develop marked renal insufficiency.

"Accelerated" nephrosclerosis ("malignant hypertension")

* Syndrome may occur in the course of "benign" nephrosclerosis, GN, unilateral renal artery occlusion, or any cause of hypertension.
* Increasing uremia is associated with minimal or marked proteinuria and hematuria.

Infarction of Kidney[6]

Due To

Renal artery embolism (e.g., atrial fibrillation, atheroemboli, after myocardial infarction, myxoma, paradoxical embolism)

Dissecting aneurysm of aorta or renal artery

Renal artery vasculitis (e.g., polyarteritis nodosa)

Renal artery thrombosis (e.g., atherosclerosis, hypercoagulability, angioplasty or catheterization, trauma)

O Microscopic or gross hematuria is usual.

Urine may show no protein or abnormal sediment unless emboli reach glomeruli. Proteinuria (≤4+) and pyuria may occur.

O Serum LD may be increased markedly (>400 U/dL); is the most sensitive laboratory abnormality; peaks on third day; returns to normal by tenth day. Urine LD may also be markedly increased.

Increases in serum transaminases, WBC, CRP, ESR are if area of infarction is large; similar in time changes to those in myocardial infarction.

Increased serum ALP (from vascular endothelium) occurs in about one third of cases and is the least discriminating enzyme abnormality.

BUN may increase but creatinine is normal unless other renal disease is present.

PRA may rise on second day, peak about 11th day, and remain elevated for more than a month.

Laboratory findings due to infarction of other organs (e.g., brain, heart, retina, mesentery)

♦ Atheromatous emboli cause eosinophilia (>350 eosinophils/μL) and eosinophiluria, which are characteristic, occurs in 70% to 80% of cases; increased ESR. Renal biopsy is specific for this diagnosis.

♦ Confirmed by renal angiography if surgery or fibrinolysis is planned, or CT scan.

Renal Artery Stenosis

See Fig. 14-3.

Mild proteinuria occurs often.

BUN and creatinine may show recent increase.

PRA in peripheral vein is increased and may cause hypokalemic metabolic alkalosis.

Urine sodium concentration may be low.

Asymmetrical renal function or size (e.g., scan, ultrasound, pyelogram)

IV pyelogram, arteriography, MRI, Doppler sonography of renal arteries may support diagnosis.

Late (> age 55) or early (< age 20) onset hypertension is often severe; stenosis is cause in >70%.

Ischemic nephropathy with irreversible parenchymal damage may occur.

Thrombosis, Renal Vein

Clinical syndrome depends on rate of occlusion and size of vessel.

Hematuria

Microscopic pyuria

Proteinuria and decreased creatinine clearance show marked variability from day to day.

Postprandial glycosuria

Nephrotic syndrome

Hyperchloremic acidosis (renal tubular acidosis)

Hyperosmolarity

Oliguria and uremic death if infarction is extensive

Anemia is common.

Platelet count may be decreased.

---

[6]Hazanov N, et al. Acute renal embolism: forty-four cases of renal infarction in patients with atrial fibrillation. *Medicine* 2004;83:292.

Increased fibrin degradation products in blood may be >3× normal limits (disseminated intravascular coagulation [DIC]).

Laboratory findings due to underlying causative conditions (e.g., nephrotic syndrome, hypernephroma, metastatic cancer, trauma, amyloidosis, diabetic glomerulosclerosis, hypertension, papillary necrosis, DIC, sickle cell disease, polycythemia, heart failure, other thrombophiliac causes)

Laboratory findings due to thromboembolic disease elsewhere (e.g., pulmonary)

Secondary Renal Diseases

Amyloidosis of Kidney, Primary or Secondary

Extracellular deposition of proteinaceous fibrillar material.

See Amyloidosis.

♦ Persistent proteinuria that varies from mild—with or without hematuria—to severe, with nephrotic syndrome

Approximately 25% of secondary amyloidosis cases present with proteinuria leading to nephrotic syndrome, azotemia, ESRD.

Vasopressin-resistant polyuria is present if the medulla alone is involved (rare).

Bacterial Endocarditis, Renal Changes

There are three types of pathologic changes: diffuse subacute GN, focal embolic GN, microscopic or gross infarcts of kidney.

Laboratory findings due to bacterial endocarditis are noted (see Chapter 5).

Albuminuria is almost invariably present, even when no renal lesions are found.

Hematuria (usually microscopic, sometimes gross) is usual at some stage of the disease, but repeated examinations may be required.

Renal insufficiency is frequent (15% of cases during active stage; 40% of fatal cases).

• BUN is increased (usually 25–75 mg/dL).
• Renal concentrating ability is decreased.

Calculi, Renal[7]

Collect two 24-hour urine specimens and routine blood chemistries to rule out underlying disorders. Helical CT is preferred imaging modality with S/S = 96%/100%; ultrasound S/S = 61%/96%.

Calcium oxalate alone (acid urine) or with phosphate is the constituent of kidney stones in 85% of male and 70% of female patients. Calcium phosphate stones form with hypercalciuria, hypocitraturia, and alkaline urine (see Fig. 14-5).

• Idiopathic hypercalciuria: ~50% of patients (see Table 14-11)
• Primary hyperparathyroidism in ~5% of patients with nephrolithiasis; 50%–75% of hyperparathyroidism patients have renal calculi.
• 20%–30% of patients have:
  Bone diseases—destructive (e.g., metastatic tumor) or osteoporosis (e.g., immobilization, Paget disease, Cushing syndrome)
  Milk-alkali (Burnett) syndrome
  Hypervitaminosis D
  Sarcoidosis
  Renal tubular acidosis—Type I (hypercalciuria, highly alkaline urine, serum calcium usually normal)
  Hyperthyroidism

Oxalate is present in 65% of stones but hyperoxaluria is a relatively rare cause of these calculi and may be primary or secondary hyperoxaluria.

Struvite stones (staghorn calculi): 10%–15% of stones. Only occur in UTI urea-splitting bacteria *Proteus* species (>50% of cases; but should rule out *Klebsiella, Pseudomonas, Serratia, Enterobacter*), and in patients with persistently alkaline urine. (Mg, NH_3, Ca, PO_4). Staghorn calculi should be cultured.

---

[7]Curhan GC. A 44-year-old woman with kidney stones. *JAMA* 2005;293:1107.

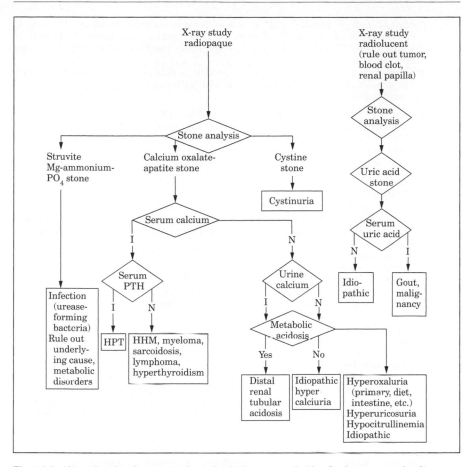

Fig. 14-5. Algorithm for diagnosis of renal calculi, as revealed by flank pain, renal colic, hematuria, fever, and urinalysis findings. (I, increased; N, normal; PTH, parathyroid hormone; HPT, hyperparathyroidism; HHM, humeral hypercalcemia of malignancy.)

Table 14-11.   Comparison of Types of Idiopathic Hypercalciuria

	Resorptive	Absorptive	Renal
Due to	Primary hyper-parathyroidism	Primary increase in intestinal absorption; autosomal dominant	Abnormal renal tubular reabsorption
Frequency	Least common	Most common	1/10 as common as absorptive type
2-hr urine after fasting			
Calcium	30 mg	<20 mg	Increased
Calcium/creatinine ratio	>0.15	<0.15	>0.15

Cystine stones (present in 1%–2% of stones) form when urine contains >300 mg/day of cystine in congenital familial cystinuria. Cystine-only stones form only in homozygotes. Tend to have bilateral obstructive staghorn calculi with associated renal failure.
♦ Urine showing characteristic cystine crystals is diagnostic. Cyanide-nitroprusside test is positive (false-positive may occur with sulfur-containing drugs).
Uric acid is present in 5% of stones.

• Gout: 25% of patients with primary gout and 40% of patients with marrow-proliferative disorders have calculi. Stones precede joint symptoms in 40% of cases.
• Urine is more acid than normal, often <5.5 (e.g., patients with chronic diarrhea, ileostomy); only form in persistently acid urine.
• >50% of patients with urinary calculi have normal serum and urine uric acid levels.

Hereditary glycinuria is a rare familial disorder associated with renal calculi.

In Children
Infections account for 13% to 40% of stones.
Hypercalciuria is most common noninfectious cause (especially idiopathic but also caused by distal renal tubular acidosis and therapy with furosemide, prednisone, or ACTH).
Oxaluria accounts for 3% to 13% of stones.
Uric acid stones account for 4% of stones.
Cystinuria is found in 5% to 7% of children with stones.
Hypocitraturia is found in 10% of children with stones.
Xanthine is present in children with inborn error of metabolism.
Deficiency of adenine phosphoribosyltransferase

In All Patients
Anatomic abnormalities
Microscopic hematuria is found in 80% of patients.
In renal colic, hematuria and proteinuria are present, and there is an increased WBC due to associated infection.
Crystalluria is diagnostically useful when there are cystine crystals (occurs only in homozygous or heterozygous cystinuria) or struvite crystals. Calcium oxalate, phosphate, and uric acid should arouse suspicion about possible cause of stones but they may occur in normal urines.
WBC may be increased if there is infection or stress.

Diabetic Nephropathy (Intercapillary Glomerulosclerosis; Kimmelstiel-Wilson [K-W] Syndrome)

Recognized after diabetes mellitus has been present for years. Occasionally is associated only with prediabetes. Incidence of end-stage renal disease is nearly 30% in insulin-dependent diabetes mellitus (IDDM) and 4% to 20% in non–insulin-dependent diabetes mellitus (NIDDM).

See Table 14-12.
♦ Defined as persistent proteinuria (present in at least two of three urine collections over a 3- to 6-month period) in absence of other renal disease. Proteinuria may be earliest clinical clue and may be marked (often >5 g/day). Nephrotic syndrome may be associated. Periodic protein testing of urine should be part of routine treatment of all diabetics; dipstick assay detects >200 to 300 mg/dL. Present in ~25% of Type I and 36% of Type II diabetes mellitus patients with negative dipstick test. In IDDM, microalbuminuria has S/S = 82%/96% specific and PPV = 75% for subsequent overt nephropathy; lower values in NIDDM.
Microalbuminuria (see Chapter 4) is associated with longer duration of diabetes, poorer glycemic control, higher blood pressure, development of more advanced retinopathy and neuropathy, and overt nephropathy and subsequent renal failure, increased vascular damage, and risk for cardiovascular disease.
Urine shows many hyaline and granular casts and double refractile fat bodies. RBC casts are inconsistent with this diagnosis; if present, should rule out HIV, hepatitis, other disorders with, serum and urine protein electrophoresis, ANA antibodies. Hematuria is rare.
Serum protein is decreased.
Azotemia develops gradually after several years of proteinuria.

Table 14-12.   Evolution of Renal Disease in Insulin-Dependent Diabetes Mellitus (IDDM)

Stage	Time of Onset	Laboratory Findings*	Morphologic Findings	% of Cases that Progress
Early	At time of diagnosis	I GFR	Kidney size I	100
Renal lesions; no clinical signs	2–3 yrs after diagnosis	I GFR; albuminuria cannot be detected	I thickness of glomerular and tubular capillary basement membrane; glomerulosclerosis	35–40
Incipient nephropathy	7–15 yrs after diagnosis	Albuminuria 0.03–0.3 g/day. N or sl I GFR; beginning to decline	Glomerulosclerosis progressing	80–100
Clinical diabetic nephropathy	10–30 yrs after diagnosis	Albuminuria >0.3 g/day. N or sl I D GFR; steady fall	Glomerulosclerosis widespread	>75
End-stage renal disease	20–40 yrs after diagnosis	GFR <10 mL/min; serum creatinine ≥10 mg/dL		

D, decreased; GFR, glomerular filtration rate; I, increased; N, normal; sl, slightly.

*When albuminuria s 0.075–0.1 g/day in IDDM, significant renal disease is present and albuminuria will progress to clinical nephropathy. GFR declines −10 mL/min/yr after nephropathy is established.

Source: JV Selby, et al. The natural history and epidemiology of diabetic nephropathy. *JAMA* 1990;263:1954.

GU

♦ Biopsy of kidney is diagnostic.

Diabetic nephropathy includes K-W lesions, urinary tract infection (including papillary necrosis), renal vascular lesions (principally arteriolosclerosis).

Course

Type I

Onset	Hyperfiltration with increased GFR
2–5 yrs	Changes in basement membrane and mesangium
5–10 yrs	Microalbuminuria, often with hypertension
>20 yrs	Overt proteinuria; GFR declines
Then	Increasing creatinine
Next 10 yrs	50% of patients need dialysis or renal transplant

Type II

At time of diagnosis	Microalbuminuria in ≤20%, overt proteinuria in ≤5% GFR can decline when microalbuminuria is present
5 years earlier than Type I	Overt nephropathy 10% to 35% with overt proteinuria develop end-stage renal disease

Stage I: Asymptomatic. Hyperfiltration with increased GFR. Reversible microalbuminuria.

Stage II: Sustained microalbuminuria that is risk factor for progressive nephropathy and cardiovascular complications.

Stage III: GFR approaching normal. Overt proteinuria. Hypertension.

Stage IV: Declining GFR. Increasing proteinuria. Decreasing renal function.

Stage V: Progressive decline in renal function with increasing proteinuria. Edema. Difficult-to-control hypertension. Metabolic disturbances of chronic renal failure (e.g., secondary hyperparathyroidism, metabolic acidosis, anemia). Dialysis or renal transplant.

Gout, Kidney Disorders In

See Chapter 10.

Due To

Kidney stones occur in 25% of patients with gout; may occur in absence of arthritis (see Chapter 13).

Predisposes to GU tract infection

Tubular obstruction

Interstitial crystal deposition with tophi formation

Arteriolar nephrosclerosis and pyelonephritis are usually associated.

Early renal damage is indicated by decreased renal-concentrating ability, mild proteinuria, and decreased PSP excretion.

Later renal damage is shown by slowly progressive azotemia with slight albuminuria and slight or no abnormalities of urine sediment.

Renal disease causes death in ≤50% of patients with gout.

It has been suggested that acute uric acid nephropathy may be differentiated from other forms of acute renal failure if ratio of urine urate:urine creatinine >1.0 in an adult (many children under age 10 years have ratio >1.0).

Hemolytic-Uremic Syndrome (HUS)

See Thrombotic Thrombocytopenic Purpura.

Hepatorenal Syndrome

Usually appears in patients with laboratory findings of decompensated cirrhosis with moderate to marked ascites, especially following fluid loss (e.g., GI hemorrhage, diarrhea, forced diuresis).

See Table 14-5.

Oliguria is marked (urine volume <500 mL/day).

Progressive azotemia (serum creatinine >2.5 mg/dL)

Urine sodium is decreased to almost absent (<10 mEq/L; often 1–2 mEq/L).

Concentrated urine with high specific gravity and urine:plasma osmolality ratio >1.0

Urine is acid; small amount of protein (<500 mg/day)

O Bland urine sediment with few hyaline and granular casts, few RBCs (<50/HPF)

O Urine indices resemble those of prerenal azotemia and contrast with acute tubular necrosis in which urine has low fixed specific gravity and high sodium content and a characteristic sediment may be found.

Hyponatremia, hyperkalemia, hepatic encephalopathy, coma may be present.

Must be differentiated from renal failure caused by toxins, drugs (e.g., NSAIDs, acetaminophen, CCl_4), infection, acute tubular necrosis, obstructive nephropathy

Henoch-Schönlein Purpura[8]

Hypersensitivity systemic vasculitis of small vessels with IgA deposition. Called *Henoch purpura* when abdominal symptoms are predominant and *Schönlein purpura* when joint symptoms are predominant. Renal picture varies from minimal urinary abnormalities for years; ESRD within months in <2%.

See Vasculitis, Chapter 5.

Diagnosis is clinical; there are no pathognomonic laboratory findings.

♦ Renal biopsy supports the diagnosis; shows focal segmental necrotizing GN that becomes more diffuse and crescentic with IgA and C3 deposition.

Urine contains RBCs, casts and slight protein in 25% to 50% of patients. Gross hematuria and proteinuria are uncommon.

	Hematuria	**Proteinuria**	**Renal function**
Minor urinary abnormality	Microscopic, intermittently gross	<1 g/24 h	Normal
Active renal disease		>1 g/24 h	Normal
Renal insufficiency			GFR <60 mL/min/1.73 m^2

Nonthrombocytopenic purpura. Hematologic tests are normal. Serum complement is usually normal.

BUN and creatinine may be increased.

Myeloma Kidney

♦ See Multiple Myeloma.

Renal function is impaired in ≤50% of patients: usually there is loss of renal-concentrating ability and azotemia.

Proteinuria is very frequent due to albumin and globulins in urine; Bence Jones (BJ) proteinuria may be intermittent. BJ protein occurs in <50% of myeloma patients but in almost all patients with renal failure due to myeloma kidney.

Severe anemia out of proportion to azotemia.

Occasional changes due to altered renal tubular function are present.

• Renal glycosuria, aminoaciduria, decreased serum uric acid, renal potassium wasting

• Renal loss of phosphate with decreased serum phosphorus and increased ALP

• Nephrogenic diabetes insipidus

• Oliguria or anuria with acute renal failure precipitated by dehydration

O *Hyperchloremia or hyperbicarbonatemia with normal or low serum sodium values reduces anion gap and should suggest myeloma in an appropriate clinical setting.*

O Changes due to associated amyloidosis or hypercalcemia.

Nephrotic Syndrome

Defined as proteinuria >3.5 g/1.73 m^2/24 hr, hypoalbuminemia, hyperlipidemia, lipiduria, edema.

Due To

Renal (causes 95% of cases in children, 60% in adults)

[8]Calviño MC, et al. Henoch-Schönlein purpura in children from northwestern Spain. *Medicine* 2001;80:279.

Primary glomerular disease (>50% of patients):

- Membranous GN: ~65% have spontaneous complete or partial remission of proteinuria and ~15% develop end-stage renal disease
- Membranoproliferative GN
- Other proliferative GN (e.g., focal, IgA nephropathy, pure mesangial): 10% in children, 23% in adults
- Rapidly progressive GN
- Minimal change disease (formerly called *lipoid nephrosis* or *nil lesion*)
- Focal segmental glomerulosclerosis

Relative Frequency (%) of Primary Glomerular Diseases Underlying Nephrotic Syndrome in Children and Adults[9]

Primary Glomerular Disease	Children	Adults <60 yrs	Adults >60 yrs
Minimal change disease	76	20	20
Membranous GN	7	40	39
Membranoproliferative GN	4	7	0
Focal segmental glomerulosclerosis	8	15	2
Other diseases	5	18	39

Systemic (most common)

- Diabetic glomerulosclerosis (15% of adult patients): most common cause of nephrotic proteinuria
- SLE (20% of adult patients)
- Amyloidosis (primary and secondary)

Systemic (less common)

- Henoch-Schönlein purpura
- Multiple myeloma
- Goodpasture syndrome (rare)
- Berger disease
- Polyarteritis (rare)
- Takayasu syndrome
- Sarcoidosis
- Sjögren syndrome
- Wegener granulomatosis (rare)
- Dermatitis herpetiformis
- Cryoglobulinemia
- Myxedema

Venous obstruction

- Obstruction of inferior vena cava (thrombosis, tumor)
- Constrictive pericarditis
- Tricuspid stenosis
- Congestive heart failure

Infections

- Bacterial (poststreptococcal GN, bacterial endocarditis, syphilis, leprosy, etc.)
- Viral (HBV, HCV; also HIV, CMV, infectious mononucleosis, varicella)
- Protozoal (quartan malaria)
- Parasitic (schistosomiasis, filariasis, toxoplasmosis)

Allergic (e.g., pollens, poison ivy and oak, bee sting, vaccines, antitoxins)

Neoplasm-associated in 10% of adults and 15% >age 60 yrs (e.g., Hodgkin disease; carcinomas of colon, lung, stomach and others; lymphomas and leukemia); paraproteinemia (multiple myeloma, light chain nephropathy). *In adult with minimal-change nephrotic syndrome without evident cause, first rule out Hodgkin disease. With membranous lesion, carcinoma may be more likely.*

Drugs, toxins (e.g., heavy metals, heroin, captopril, probenecid, NSAIDs, penicillamine, mephenytoin, ampicillin, anticonvulsants, chlorpropamide, lithium, rifampin,

[9]Orth SR, Ritz E. The nephrotic syndrome. *NEJM* 1998;338:1202.

interferon alfa). Heroin may cause focal segmental glomerulosclerosis and progressive renal insufficiency.

Hereditary/familial (e.g., Alport syndrome, Fabry disease, sickle cell disease). In atypical familial nephrotic syndrome, course is benign; more than one sibling is involved.

Miscellaneous

- Toxemia of pregnancy
- Chronic allograft rejection
- Renal artery stenosis
- Malignant nephrosclerosis
- Ulcerative colitis

Others

Urine immunoelectrophoresis should always be performed to rule out myeloma and renal primary (AL) amyloidosis.

Characterized By

♦ Marked proteinuria: >3.5 g/1.73 square meter body surface/day—usually >4.5 g/day
♦ Hyperlipidemia: Increased serum cholesterol (free and esters)—usually >350 mg/dL (low or normal serum cholesterol occurs with poor nutrition and suggests poor prognosis); increased serum triglycerides, phospholipids, neutral fats, low-density beta-lipoproteins, and total lipids
♦ Decreased serum albumin (usually <2.5 gm/dL) and total protein
♦ Serum α_2 and β-globulins are markedly increased, γ-globulin is decreased, α_1 is normal or decreased. If γ-globulin is increased, rule out systemic disease (e.g., SLE).
♦ Urine containing doubly refractive fat bodies seen by polarizing microscopy; many granular and epithelial cell casts

Hematuria: Present in 50% of patients but is usually minimal and not part of syndrome

Azotemia: May be present but not part of syndrome

Changes secondary to proteinuria and hypoalbuminemia (e.g., decreased serum calcium, decreased serum ceruloplasmin, increased fibrinogen)

Increased ESR due to increased fibrinogen

Serum C3 complement is normal in idiopathic lipoid nephrosis but decreased when there is underlying GN.

Laboratory findings due to:

- Primary disease
- Increased susceptibility to infection (especially pneumococcal peritonitis) during periods of edema
- Hypercoagulability with thromboembolism; abnormalities in coagulation factors, clotting inhibitors, fibrinolytic system, platelet function have been described. Associated renal vein thrombosis has been reported in ~35% of patients (≤40% of these will have pulmonary emboli), especially when due to membranous nephropathy, MPGN, rapidly progressive GN.

♦ Renal biopsy establishes the diagnosis.

Acute Tubular Necrosis (ATN)[10,11]

Sudden 50% decline in GFR, azotemia, inability of kidney to regulate balance of Na, electrolytes, water, and acid.

See Table 14-4.

Due To

Sepsis, ischemic, or toxic insults. Usually multiple causes (e.g., hypotension, volume depletion, nephrotoxic drugs, x-ray contrast material).

Nonoliguric form (one third to two thirds of all cases of ATN) is usually due to nephrotoxic agents. Mortality ~25%.

Oliguric form is usually due to ischemic events (e.g., renovascular occlusion, bilateral cortical necrosis), rapidly progressive GN, obstructive uropathy. Mortality ~50%.

Sudden progressive increase in BUN and serum creatinine with ratio <20:1.

[10]Esson ML, Schier RW. Diagnosis and treatment of acute tubular necrosis. *Ann Int Med* 2002;137:744.
[11]Herget-Rosenthal S, et al. Prognostic value of tubular proteinuria and enzymuria in nonoliguric acute tubular necrosis. *Clin Chem* 2004;50:552.

Table 14-13. Comparison of Diagnostic Indices in Acute Renal Failure

	Prerenal	Renal
Serum		
BUN, creatinine, BUN/creatinine, ratio	Creatinine rarely >4 mg/dL even when BUN >100 mg/dL in pure prerenal azotemia with ratio >20:1	Sudden progressive increase in BUN and serum creatinine with ratio ~10:1
Urine		
Sediment	May contain granular or hyaline casts, but cellular or pigmented casts are conspicuously absent	Many renal tubular cells and casts and many narrow (often pigmented) casts
Specific gravity	>1.020	~1.010
Urine$_{osm}$ (mOsm/kg H$_2$O)	>500	~300
Urine$_{Na}$ (mEq/L)	<20	Usually high (40–80 mEq/L)
FE Na (%)	<1	>2
FE Uric acid (%)	<7	>15
FE Lithium (%)	<7	>20
Brush border enzymes (e.g., alanine aminopeptidase, ALP)	Low	High
Low molecular weight proteins (e.g., lyzozyme, retinol binding protein, alpha-1 microglobulin)	Low	High
Proteinuria	Excretion is frequently increased but rarely >2 g/24 h	Often >2 g/24 h

In oliguric type without recent diuretic therapy, urine <400 mOsm/kg H$_2$O, spot Na >20 mEq/L

Urine sodium usually >40 mEq/L but may be <20 mEq/L in nonoliguric patients. FE$_{Na}$ is usually >2% in both oliguric and nonoliguric patients.

Increased excretion of cystatin and microglobulinuria may predict unfavorable prognosis in nonoliguric form of ATN.

Polyarteritis Nodosa

Necrotizing vasculitis of medium-sized or small arteries without GN or vasculitis in arterioles, capillaries, or venules causes renal involvement in 75% of patients.

See Chapter 5.

Azotemia is often absent or only mild and slowly progressive.

Albuminuria is always present.

Hematuria (gross or microscopic) is very common. Fat bodies are frequently present in urine sediment.

There may be findings of acute GN with remission or early death from renal failure.

Always rule out polyarteritis in any case of GN, renal failure, or hypertension that shows unexplained eosinophilia, increased WBC, or laboratory evidence of involvement of other organ systems.

Prerenal Azotemia

Occurs commonly in CHF. May occur in other functional forms of decreased renal perfusion (e.g., hepatorenal syndrome).

Serum creatinine rarely >4 mg/dL, even when BUN >100 mg/dL in pure prerenal azotemia. BUN/creatinine ratio >20.

Urine is hypertonic (increased osmolality) with low sodium concentration (<10 mEq/L).
Protein excretion is frequently increased but rarely >2 g/24 hours.
Urine sediment may contain granular or hyaline casts, but cellular or pigmented casts
are conspicuously absent.
In contrast, in *acute tubular necrosis,* which may complicate cardiac failure or be due
to cardiogenic shock, excessive use of diuretics or vasodilators

* Urine osmolality approaches that of plasma.
* Urine sodium is usually high (40–80 mEq/L).
* Urine sediment contains many renal tubular cells and casts and many narrow (often
  pigmented) casts.

Radiation Nephritis

**Exposure (one or both kidneys) to >2,000 rads for 2 to 5 weeks. Injury related to
total dose and duration.**

Latent period is >6 to 12 months.

Acute:

Abrupt onset hematuria, proteinuria, severe hypertension, severe normochromic, normocytic anemia (may be disproportionate); after >10 years, most progress to
chronic nephritis with diminishing renal function and severe hypertension

Chronic:

Stable isolated proteinuria, mild-to-moderate hypertension, slow progression to renal
failure
Laboratory findings due to other complications of radiation (e.g., retroperitoneal fibrosis obstructing ureters, radiation neuropathy causing neurogenic bladder)

Scleroderma (Progressive Systemic Sclerosis [PSS]), Renal Disease

Renal involvement occurs in two thirds of patients; one-third die of renal failure.

See Chapter 16.
Clinical cause of slowly progressive renal insufficiency with moderate proteinuria often
<2 g/day and hypertension, or less commonly, acute renal failure, which may be
associated with malignant hypertension, CHF, microangiographic hemolytic anemia, and marked increase in PRA

Sickle Cell Nephropathy

Renal functional abnormalities are very common.

Albuminuria (macro- and micro-) in $\leq68\%$ of patients; usually 1 to 2 g/day
Gross hematuria is relatively common.
Early decrease of renal concentrating ability is evident in heterozygotes as well as
homozygotes; more pronounced in HbSS and HbSC. Progressively decreases with
age. The decrease is temporarily reversed in children by transfusion but not in
adults.
Even with normal BUN, GFR, and renal plasma flow; it occurs in sickle cell trait as
well as anemia but
Chronic renal failure occurs only with SS (4.2%) or SC (2.4%).
Papillary necrosis occurs in 39% of patients.
Renal tubular acidosis may produce severe hypokalemia.

Systemic Lupus Erythematosus (SLE), Nephritis

See Table 14-14.
Renal involvement occurs in two thirds of patients with SLE.
Nephritis of SLE may occur as acute, latent, or chronic GN, nephrosis, or asympto-
matic albuminuria or hematuria.

Table 14-14.	Comparison of Clinical and Morphologic Types of Systemic Lupus Erythematosus Nephritis			
	Mesangial Changes (% of patients)	Focal Proliferative GN (% of patients)	Diffuse Proliferative GN (% of patients)	Membranous GN (% of patients)
% of total patients	39	27	16	18
Hematuria, pyuria	13	53	78	50
Proteinuria	36	67	89	100
Nephrotic syndrome	0	27	56	90
Azotemia	13	20	22	10
Decreased complement	54	77	100	75
Increased anti-DNA	45	75	80	33
Decreased complement and increased anti-DNA	36	63	80	33
Hypertension	22	40	56	50
Prognosis	Better	Worse	Worse	Better

Source: GB Appel. The course of management of lupus nephritis. *Intern Med* 1981;2:82.

Urine findings are as in chronic active GN. Azotemia or marked proteinuria usually indicates death in 1 to 3 years.

Laboratory findings of SLE may disappear during active nephritis, nephrosis, or uremia.

♦ Examination of needle biopsy should always include immunofluorescent and EM as well as light microscopy. May show normal or minimal disease, mesangial lesions, focal or diffuse proliferative GN, or membranous GN.

Laboratory findings due to drug therapy:

• Prednisone
• Cytotoxic drugs (e.g., azathioprine, cyclophosphamide)

    Leukopenia—nadir WBC kept at 1,500 to 4,000/μL
    Infection (e.g., herpes zoster, opportunistic organisms)
    Gonadal toxicity
    Hemorrhagic cystitis
    Neoplasia

Nonrenal Genitourinary Diseases

Bladder

Bladder Carcinoma

Hematuria may be gross or only microscopic.

♦ Biopsy of tumor confirms the diagnosis.

♦ Cytologic examination of urine for tumor cells is useful for Grades II, III, and IV carcinoma but not for Grade I, which has a high false-positive rate. Positive cytology with negative cystoscopy correlates with eventual development of transitional cancer. It may be of value in screening dye workers in chemical industry.

	Cytology Sensitivity*	
	First Urine Specimen	**Cumulative Third Urine Specimen**
Grade I	None	20% (many false positives)
Grade II	30%	80%
Grade III	65%	85%
Grade IV	92%	98%

*False positives may occur due to atypia in chronic cystitis, calculi, irradiation, chemotherapy (e.g., myleran).

Table 14-15.   Comparison of Sensitivity and Specificity of Four Bladder Tumor Markers*

	New Tumors				Recurrent Tumors			
	NMP22	BTA Stat	UBC	Cytology	NMP22	BTA Stat	UBC	Cytology
Sensitivity	65%	75%	60%	41%	45%	55%	40%	NA
Specificity	74%	75%	75%	94%	64%	54%	40%	NA

*Data from: Boman H, Hedelin H, Holmang S. Four bladder tumor markers have a disappointingly low sensitivity for small size and low grade recurrence. *J Urol* 2002;167:80–83.

GU

♦ Flow cytometry of urine quantitatively measures DNA content or ploidy; cells with normal DNA content are diploid and cells with abnormal DNA content are aneuploid, which is found only in neoplastic cells although diploidy is found in both normal and neoplastic cells. Aneuploidy is early indicator of neoplasia and may be present before microscopic evidence of tumor. Seventy-eight percent sensitivity for bladder cancer; specificity for nonneoplastic disease = 2%.
○ Tumor markers in urine:[12,13]

• Bladder tumor antigen (BTA Stat) in urine is a qualitative latex agglutination test and a quantitative test (BTA TRAK) with S/S = ~25%/90%. Positive BTA may occur within 14 days of prostate biopsy or resection, with renal or bladder calculi, symptomatic sexually transmitted disease, other GU tract cancers (e.g., penis, ovary, endometrium, cervix).

BTA is approved by FDA *only* to detect recurrence of bladder cancer, in conjunction with cystoscopy.

• NMP22 (*n*uclear *m*itotic apparatus *p*roteins): A component of the nuclear matrix is measured in urine. Immunoassay value >10 U/mL has reported S/S = 55%/85%. 86% had no bladder cancer with <10 U/mL. NMP22 is approved by FDA for initial detection of bladder cancer.
• Fibrin degradation product (FDP) dipstick identifies fibrinogen and fibrin degradation products in urine. Sensitivity = 70%; sensitivity = 100 % with muscle invasion. May not be available in the United States.
• Antigen detection in urine using fluorescence microscopy (commercial name is ImmunoCyt).
• Surviving (member of family of apoptosis inhibitors) gene detected in urine can be confirmed by RT-PCR and WB.
• Hepatoma unregulated protein (HURP) (a cancer-related gene) found in RNA to transitional cell carcinomas detected in urine has reported S/S = 88%/100%.
• UBC and ELISA-CYFRA 21-1 assays measure soluble cytokeratins in urine by immunoradiometric assay.
• Telomerase assay had reported S/S = 70%/99%.
• Hyaluronic acid and hyaluronidase combined have reported high S/S; also found in other cancers (e.g., breast, colon).
• Le^x blood group–related antigens have reported S/S = 80%/86%.
• Many others (e.g., oncogenes, growth factors, CD44. BLCA-4, etc). S/S will vary according to grade of tumor. Newest tests may not be available or approved yet in the United States.

The large number of tumor marker tests indicate that this is a field still developing.
Urinary LD level may be useful in screening studies to discover asymptomatic patients with neoplasm of GU tract (e.g., occupational exposure).
Laboratory findings due to complications will stem from infection or from obstruction of ureter.

[12]Getzenberg RH. Urine-based assays for bladder cancer. *LabMed* Aug 2003;34:613.
[13]Grossman HB, et al. Detection of bladder cancer using a point-of-care proteomic assay. *JAMA* 2005;293:810.

Laboratory findings due to pre-existing conditions (e.g., schistosomiasis, stone, or infection)

Epididymitis

Due To
Acute

- STD: Chlamydiae (DFA and ELISA have S/S = 70%/>80%) or gonococci
- GU tract infection due to Gram-negative pathogens found in urine, urethra or prostate

Chronic

- Chlamydiae
- *Mycobacterium tuberculosis* (only 35% have history of previous TB)
- *Coccidioides immitis*
- *Blastomyces*
- *Idiopathic*

Pyuria
Evidence of urethritis (see Fig. 14-6) or aspirate or biopsy material for appropriate organisms
Laboratory findings due to complications (e.g., abscess formation, infarction of testicle)
Should test for other sexually transmitted diseases

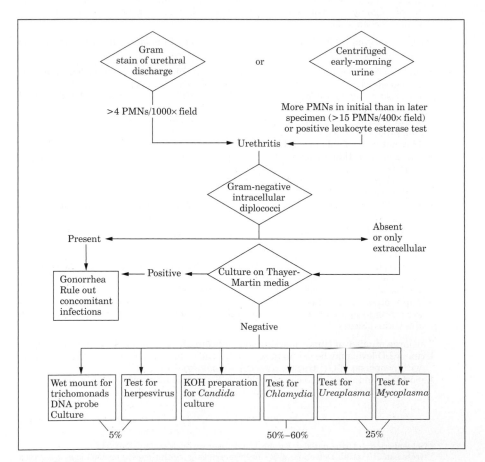

Fig. 14-6. Algorithm for diagnosis of urethritis in males.

Fibrosis, Retroperitoneal

Due To
Primary (70% of cases)

- Angiomatous lymphoid hamartoma

Secondary (30% of cases)

- Infection
- Trauma
- Connective tissue disease
- Aortic aneurysm
- Irradiation
- Drugs (e.g., methysergide; also methyldopa, ergotamine, phenacetin, hydralazine, propranolol)

ESR is increased.
Anemia, leukocytosis, and increased ESR may be present.
Occasionally eosinophilia occurs.
Serum protein and A/G ratio are normal; if the person is chronically ill, total protein may be decreased and γ-globulins may be increased.
○ Laboratory findings due to ureteral obstruction

Postvasectomy Status

Sperm Count
May fall to low levels after three or four ejaculations and then rise abruptly before falling again.
Fifteen to 20 ejaculations may be required before sperm count reaches 0.
—Twenty-five to 50 HPFs are examined microscopically (e.g., phase contrast) for motile and nonmotile sperm.
If none seen, examine sediment after centrifugation.
♦ Two consecutive azoospermic specimens 6 to 10 weeks after surgery, 1 month apart are recommended before dispensing with contraception.
Recanalization of the vas deferens may occur.

Priapism

Persistent erection for >4 hours with pain and tenderness but without sexual desire

Due To
Thromboembolic disease (e.g., sickle cell disease or trait, polycythemia, pelvic thrombophlebitis)
Infiltrative diseases (e.g., leukemia, bladder or prostate carcinoma)
Penile trauma
CNS infection (e.g., syphilis, TB) or spinal cord injury or anesthesia
Drugs (e.g., antihypertensives, hydralazine, testosterone, phenothiazine, heparin, ethanol, marijuana) or treatment of impotence by penile drug injection (e.g., papaverine, prostaglandin, phentolamine)
Others (e.g., prostatitis, retroperitoneal bleeding)
♦ Intracorporeal pO_2 determination differentiates dangerous low-flow priapism from high-flow priapism, which is less of a medical emergency.

Prostate

Benign Prostatic Hypertrophy (BPH)
Laboratory findings are those due to urinary tract obstruction and secondary infection.
Serum PSA may be increased 4 to 10 ng/mL in 20% of patients and >10 ng/mL in occasional patient, confusing its use for screening for prostate cancer. Is more common cause of increased PSA than prostate carcinoma. Returns to reference range after resection.
Finasteride treatment causes a median decrease of ~50% in PSA.

GU

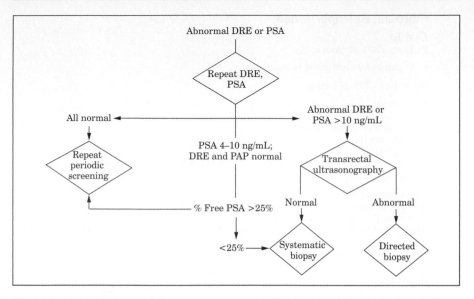

Fig. 14-7. Algorithm for prostate cancer screening. (DRE, direct rectal examination; PSA, prostate-specific antigen; PAP, prostatic acid phosphatase.)

Prostate Carcinoma[14]

Prevalence of ~25% in third decade increases to 65% in seventh decade

♦ Needle biopsy or incidental finding in prostate resection for BPH. Gleason histologic grade of adenocarcinoma is considered most powerful predictor of biologic behavior; often has important role in patient treatment.

♦ *Serum Prostate Specific Antigen (PSA)*

Also known as *human kallikrein* 3. Serine protease produced by prostate acinar cells; also by periurethral glands and breast in women; pancreas and salivary gland in both sexes. Reference range ≤4 ng/mL, increases with age; ≤6.5 ng/mL over age 70; higher in black men than in white men.

See Fig. 14-7.

Use

Monitor response to total prostatectomy for cancer (failure to decline at least to normal range indicates residual prostatic tissue or metastases; increasing levels indicate recurrent disease) or radiation therapy. Third generation tests measure concentration down to 0.2 to 0.4 ng/mL but resulting in diagnosis of earlier recurrence by months to years but prognostic and therapeutic implications are unclear.[15]

Now approved for screening by FDA but is problematical because:

• PSA detects only ~2% of cancers in screening healthy asymptomatic men. Cases detected by PSA and digital rectal exam (DRE) may not be the same ones. Not recommended without DRE.
• 4 to 10 ng/mL in 20% of patients with BPH
• DRE alone detects ~50% of organ-confined cancer; increased by combining with PSA.
• PSA is not sufficiently specific or sensitive to be used alone for screening.
• ~45% of confined cancers and 25% of unconfined cancers have PSA <4.0 ng/mL.
• <4 ng/mL occurs in 20% of men with localized cancer.
• >10 ng/mL occurs in 2% of cases of BPH and 44% of cases of cancer.
• PPV in otherwise asymptomatic men = ~65%.

[14]Kantoff PW, Carroll PR, D'Amico AV, eds. Cancer: principles and practice. Philadelphia: Lippincott Williams & Wilkins, 2002.
[15]Bock JL, Klee GC. How sensitive is a prostate-specific antigen measurement? *Arch Pathol Lab Med* 2004;128:341.

- Cost benefit of early diagnosis and treatment of prostate carcinoma is questionable since not likely to cause symptoms or affect survival in 30% of men > age 50 because prostate cancer is an incidental finding in >50% of these men.[16]
- Lifetime risk of diagnosis of cancer is ~16% but risk of death from cancer is ~3.4%. Doubling time of prostate cancer is >3 years.
- Not recommended in asymptomatic men > age 75.

Staging of patients with prostate carcinoma

- <4 ng/mL, have organ-confined disease
- <10 ng/mL, bone metastases are rare
- >10 ng/mL, >50% have extracapsular disease
- >50 ng/mL, most have positive lymph nodes
- >100 ng/mL predicts bone metastases with >90% accuracy, S/S = >66%/96%, PPV = 73%.

Superior to and replaces PAP for routine monitoring at each stage of disease. PSA is more sensitive but less specific than PAP. Useful in advanced cancer when PSA is increased, whereas PAP is normal in >20% of cases.

Interpretation
Monitoring
Successful radiation or antiandrogen therapy reduces PSA in patients with residual disease.

Failure of radiation to decrease PSA to <1 ng/mL means substantial likelihood of recurrence; some reports suggest <0.5 ng/mL to predict long-term disease-free status.

With successful radiation, PSA may not return to normal or baseline for 2–6 mos.

After removal of all tumor, PSA may not return to normal or baseline for >2 wks. PSA ≥0.2 ng/mL indicates recurrence.

Doubling time

- Occurs 4 to >33 months in ~67% of patients before treatment
- Correlates with recurrence of disease after radiation therapy
- After radical prostatectomy, doubling time reflects aggressiveness of original cancer.

Diagnosis
In cancers diagnosed by careful pathologic examination, 80% had a normal PSA; if tumor volume = 0.5–1.9 cc, 50% had a normal PSA.

Percent of Patients with Prostate Cancer

	Total PSA (ng/mL)			
	0–2	**2–4**	**4–10**	**>10**
DRE negative	1%	15%	25%	>50%
DRE positive	5%	20%	45%	>75%

PSA 4 to 10 ng/mL is gray zone when fPSA may be most useful (see below).

Ambulatory values are higher than sedentary values that may decrease ≤50% (mean = 18%).

Different assays yield different values.

◆ Increased In
Transient increases return to normal in 2 to 6 weeks.

Prostate diseases
- Cancer
- Prostatitis   5–7×
- BPH
- Prostatic ischemia
- Acute urinary retention   5–7×

Manipulations
- Prostatic massage   ≤2×
- Cystoscopy   4×
- Needle biopsy   >50× for ≤1 month
- Transurethral resection   >50×

[16]See also *Am J Med* 2002;113:663 and *Brit Med J* 325, online at bmj.com.

- DRE increases PSA significantly if initial value is >20 ng/mL and is not a confusing factor in falsely elevating PSA
- Radiation therapy
- Indwelling catheter
- Vigorous bicycle exercise ≤2–3× several days
  Treadmill stress test no change
  Drugs (e.g., testosterone)
Physiologic fluctuations ≤30%
- PSA has no circadian rhythm but 6%–7% variation can occur between specimens collected on same day.
- Ambulatory values are higher than sedentary values which may decrease ≤50% (mean = 18%).
- Ejaculation causes transient increase <1.0 ng/mL for 48 hours.

Analytic factors

- Different assays yield different values
- Antibody cross-reactivity
- High titer heterophile antibodies

Other diseases/organs

- Also found in small amounts in other cancers (sweat and salivary glands, breast, colon, lung, ovary) and in Skene's glands of female urethra and in term placenta
- Acute renal failure
- Acute MI

Decreased In
Ejaculation within 24 to 48 hours.
Castration
Antiandrogen drugs (e.g., finasteride)
Radiation therapy
Prostatectomy
PSA falls 17% in 3 days after lying in hospital
Artifactual (e.g., improper specimen collection; very high PSA levels)
Finasteride (5-α-reductase inhibitor) reduces PSA by 50% after 6 months in men without cancer.
♦ *Free:Total PSA (fPSA:tPSA) Ratio (%)* is lower in cancer than in BPH patients and lower % may suggest more aggressive cancer.
Chief utility is when tPSA = 4 to 10 ng/mL.

- In most healthy men, 10% to 40% is free.
- Repeat of negative biopsy is indicated in high-risk populations if fPSA suggests high probability because ~20% of cancers are missed on first biopsy.

PSA Velocity (rate of change): more rapid rate of increase (>0.75 ng/mL/year or >20%/year) in early cancer may distinguish carcinoma from BPH (reported S/S = 90%/100%). Requires ≤3 measurements over 18-month period. Is not useful for staging. Additional data are needed.
PSA Density (quotient of serum PSA to prostate gland volume measured by transrectal ultrasound) may help to distinguish BPH and cancer, especially when PSA is 4.0 to 10.0 ng/mL; low PSA density is unlikely to be cancer but increased density (>0.15) is more likely to be cancer. Additional data are needed.
The following are among markers being actively evaluated for their utility:

- BPSA is a degraded form of free PSA that appears to be specific for BPH may assist monitoring medical or surgical treatment of BPH.
- Truncated PSA. Intact PSA.
- Human glandular kallikrein (hK2)

♦ Increased Serum Acid Phosphatase (PAP) Activity
Use
Identify local extension or distant metastases from prostate carcinoma. It is increased in 60% to 75% of patients with bone metastases, 20% of patients with extension into periprostatic soft tissue but without bone involvement, 5% of patients with carcinoma confined to gland. Occasionally it remains low despite active metastases.

Monitor response to treatment. Increased PAP shows pronounced fall in activity within 3 to 4 days after castration or within 2 weeks after estrogen therapy is begun; may return to normal or remain slightly elevated; failure to fall corresponds to failure of clinical response that occurs in 10% of patients. Increased PAP should return to normal 1 week following surgery or radiotherapy for carcinoma palpable on rectal examination; failure to do so suggests the presence of metastatic lesions.

Interpretation

Most patients with invasive carcinoma show a significant increase in PAP after massage or palpation; this rarely occurs in patients with normal prostate, BPH or in situ carcinoma, or in patients with prostate carcinoma who are receiving hormone treatment.

PAP by immunoassay is nearly always increased with a palpable prostatic carcinoma. Specificity >94% but may be normal in poorly differentiated or androgen-insensitive prostate carcinomas. More frequently increased with advancing stage and grade of cancer and in presence of lymph node or bone metastases. If PAP assay is elevated in presence of a negative biopsy, the biopsy should be repeated. If PAP is elevated with a normal PSA, the diagnosis lies elsewhere; rule out disseminated malignancy, myeloproliferative or chronic infectious disease. Not increased in nonprostate diseases listed below.

May be increased in ≤8% of prostate carcinoma patients with normal PSA.

♦ Increased In

Prostate carcinoma

Infarction of the prostate (sometimes to high levels)

Operative trauma, instrumentation of the prostate, or prostatic massage may cause transient increase

Gaucher disease (only when certain substrates are used in the analysis)

Excessive destruction of platelets, as in idiopathic thrombocytopenic purpura with megakaryocytes in bone marrow

Thromboembolism, hemolytic crises (e.g., sickle cell disease) due to hemolysis (only when certain substrates are used in the laboratory determination); is said to occur often

Leukemic reticuloendotheliosis ("hairy") cells using a specific assay

In the absence of prostatic disease, occurs occasionally in

- Partial translocation trisomy 21
- Diseases of bone
- Advanced Paget disease
- Metastatic carcinoma of bone
- Multiple myeloma (some patients)
- Hyperparathyroidism
- Various liver diseases (slight) (e.g., hepatitis, obstructive jaundice, Laennec cirrhosis)
- Acute renal impairment (not related to degree of azotemia)
- Other diseases of the reticuloendothelial system with liver or bone involvement (e.g., Niemann-Pick disease)
- In-vitro hemolysis

Decreased In

Not clinically significant

Serum ALP is increased in 90% of patients with bone metastases. Increases with favorable response to estrogen therapy or castration and reaches peak in 3 months, then declines. Recurrence of bone metastases causes new increase in ALP.

♦ Needle biopsy of prostate confirms diagnosis.

♦ Carcinoma cells may appear in bone marrow aspirates.

♦ Molecular detection (PCR based on tissue specific RNA) can detect 1 cell in >10^6 peripheral nucleated blood cells. Research technique at present.

Anemia may be present.

Fibrinolysins are found in 12% of patients with metastatic prostatic cancer; occur only with extensive metastases and are usually associated with hemorrhagic manifestations; they show fibrinogen deficiency and prolonged prothrombin time.

Urinary tract infection and hematuria occur late.

Cytologic examination of prostatic fluid is not generally useful.

Prostatitis

Bacterial form is most frequently due to

- *Escherichia coli*
- *Proteus mirabilis*

* *Pseudomonas*
* *Klebsiella*
* *Streptococcus faecalis*
* *Staphylococcus aureus*

Acute

♦ WBCs in centrifuged sediment of last portion of voided urine specimen
♦ Urine usually shows positive colony count and culture.
Blood cultures should be done.
Semen may also show organisms.

Chronic Bacterial

♦ To differentiate from urethritis, compare specimens from initial urine, mid-stream urine, prostatic secretions (by prostatic massage), and first urine after prostatic massage. All show a greater (usually 10×) colony count compared to the first urine specimen, but finding is reverse in urethritis. Shows >10 WBC/HPF.
Laboratory findings due to associated or complicating conditions (e.g., epididymitis) may be present.

Chronic Nonbacterial

Much more common than chronic bacterial prostatitis.

♦ Prostatic fluid usually shows >10 WBC/HPF with negative cultures of urine, semen, and prostatic fluid; do not respond to antibiotic therapy. Many lipid-laden macrophages are suggestive.
May be caused by organisms that are difficult to culture (e.g., *Ureaplasma, Chlamydiae*, trichomonads, CMV, or herpes virus) or to treatment.
Serum PSA may be increased, causing confusion in the screening for prostate cancer.

Sexually Transmitted Diseases (STDs) (Including Urethritis)

See Fig. 14-6.
Due To
Bacteria

* *Neisseria gonorrhoeae*
* *Treponema pallidum*
* *Mycoplasma hominis*
* *Calymmatobacterium granulomatis*
* *Campylobacter fetus*
* Others

* *Chlamydia trachomatis*
* *Haemophilus ducreyi*
* *Shigella* sp.
* *Gardnerella vaginalis* (?)
* *Streptococcus* Group B (?)

Viruses

* HIV
* Hepatitis A and B
* Papilloma virus (genital wart)

* Herpes simplex
* Cytomegalovirus
* Molluscum contagiosum

Protozoa

* *Trichomonas vaginalis*
* *Giardia lamblia*

* *Entamoeba histolytica*

Ectoparasites

* Crab louse

* Scabies mite

♦ Both *Chlamydia* and *Neisseria gonorrhoeae* can be identified in same urine or genital swab specimen by amplification techniques with S/S ≥90%. Some kits may be inhibited by Hb, nitrates, others, crystals.
♦ Urethritis is diagnosed if smear of urethral discharge shows >4 PMNs/1000× field.
♦ In absence of urethral discharge,
  • First-void urine specimen showing >10 WBC/HPF or positive leukocyte esterase test
  • Early-morning urine specimen is collected in 3 sequential containers. The initial 10-mL specimen container is centrifuged and compared to the rest of the sample. If the first specimen shows more PMNs (>15 PMNs/400× field) than the later sample, urethritis is diagnosed. If equal numbers of PMNs are present in both specimens, the inflammation is higher up in the GU tract. If no PMNs are present,

urethritis is unlikely. Sediment of the first specimen should also be examined for *Trichomonas vaginalis*.

♦ Gram stains will show Gram-negative intracellular diplococci in >95% of cases of gonorrhea. When only some extracellular diplococci are seen, subsequent cultures are positive for *Neisseria gonorrhoeae* in <15% of patients.

♦ In males, a positive Gram-stained smear establishes the diagnosis of gonorrhea and a culture is not necessary, but in females, a positive smear should be confirmed by culture on appropriate media (i.e., Gram stains are highly sensitive and specific in males but not in females).

Chlamydia cannot be identified on Gram stains; cultures must be done at specialized laboratories.

When Gram stains and cultures for gonorrhea are negative, the presumptive diagnosis is nongonococcal urethritis, and *Chlamydia trachomatis* causes about 50% of such cases. This is the most frequent venereal disease and is estimated to be >2× more frequent than gonorrhea.

In venereal disease (VD) clinics, up to 50% of males with gonococcal urethritis have concomitant *C. trachomatis* present. *Chlamydiae* are responsible for 70% of post-gonococcal urethritis. In VD clinics, *C. trachomatis* can be cultured from 25% to 50% of females.

In sexually active men with no symptoms or laboratory findings of urethritis, chlamydial infection is found in <3%.

In sexually active young men, acute epididymitis is almost always caused by STD; 10% are caused by to gonorrhea; 50% to 80% are caused by to *C. trachomatis* in heterosexuals but *E. coli* is more common in homosexual men and men >35 years old. Laboratory findings of urethritis will usually be found even if patient is asymptomatic.

Women infected with *C. trachomatis* show infection of urethra (50% of cases), rectum (25% of cases), and cervix (75% of cases). Present in <50% of women with cervical gonococcal infection.

Sexually active women with symptoms of lower urinary tract infection, pyuria (>15 WBCs/HPF), but sterile urine cultures probably have chlamydial infection. If coliforms or staphylococci are found, bacterial cystitis is likely even if <100,000/mL.

Ureaplasma urealyticum is no longer considered a cause of urethritis in males or PID.

Mycoplasma hominis may cause pyelonephritis (5% of cases), pelvic inflammatory disease (10% of cases), and postpartum febrile complications (10% of cases). *M. hominis* is usually diagnosed by culture; DNA probes are less sensitive. Serological methods are not widely used for various reasons (lack of specificity, complexity, etc.); diagnosis requires 4× rise in IgG titer; increased IgM titer may be reliable in urethritis or salpingitis.

Candida albicans, T. vaginalis, herpes simplex, and CMV probably cause 10% to 15% of cases of nongonococcal urethritis.

Laboratory findings of complications

- Prostatitis (20% of patients)
- Epididymitis (<3% of patients)
- Urethral stricture (<5% of patients)
- Reiter syndrome (2% of patients)
- Cervicitis, cervical erosion, cytologic atypia on Pap smear, salpingitis
- Sterility
- Acute proctitis

Gynecological Disorders

Menstruation, Altered Laboratory Tests

Platelet count is decreased by 50% to 70%; returns to normal by fourth day.
Hemoglobin is unchanged.
Fibrinogen is increased.
Serum cholesterol may increase just before menstruation.
Urine volume, sodium, and chloride decrease premenstrually and increase postmenstrually (diuresis).
Urine protein may increase during premenstrual phase.
Urine porphyrins increase.
Urine estrogens decrease to lowest level 2 to 3 days after onset.

Uterine Cancer

Cancer of Cervix

See Human papillomavirus infection.

♦ Pap Smear

Use

Routine screening of asymptomatic women to detect carcinoma of cervix or various atypias. Combined with human papillomavirus (HPV), DNA testing is being evaluated as primary screening test for uterine cervical abnormalities.

Also used to monitor response to therapy for carcinoma, infections, etc.

Occasionally detects carcinoma from other sites (e.g., endometrium, ovary, tube)

Often detects presence of various previously undiagnosed infectious agents (e.g., *Trichomonas vaginalis*, HSV, Candida)

Occasionally useful in chromosome studies

May be used to estimate ovarian functional hormonal status

Interferences

False-negative results in ~5% to 10% of cases

Sparse cells—100 abnormal cells is threshold for reliable screening; usual Pap smear contains 50,000 to 300,000 cells.

Sampling problems (poor fixation or staining), mislabeling, floating cells, obscured cells due to exudate, blood, degeneration, drying, etc. Malignant cells may not be present if smear is repeated too soon after previous abnormal smear.

Certain tumor types are less readily diagnosed (e.g., adenocarcinoma, lymphoma, sarcoma, verrucous carcinoma).

Human error in interpreting difficult cells; <3% of preventable cervical cancer are due to misread smears.

Interpretation

Routine screening in the general population may be positive for ~6 of every 1,000 women (prevalence); only 7% of these lesions are invasive. The prevalence rate is greatest in certain groups:

* Women ages 21 to 35 years, with peak in 31st to 35th year
* Black and Puerto Rican women
* Women who use birth control pills rather than diaphragm for contraception
* Women with early onset or long duration of sexual activity
* *Vaginal pool Pap smear has an accuracy rate of ~80% in detecting carcinoma of the cervix. Smears from a combination of vaginal pool, exocervical, and endocervical scrapings have an accuracy rate of 95%.*
* *After an initial abnormal smear, the follow-up smear taken in the next few weeks or months may not always be abnormal; there is no clear explanation for this finding.*

♦ *Biopsy shows important lesions of the cervix in some of these patients. Therefore an abnormal initial smear requires further investigation of the cervix regardless of subsequent cytologic reports.*

For high-grade lesions of cervix S/S = 55% to 80%/>90%.

HPV-DNA

S/S = 84%–100%/64%–95%.

Laboratory findings due to

* Obstruction of ureters with pyelonephritis, azotemia, etc.
* General effects of cancer

Cancer of Uterine Body

Pap smear of vagina/cervix is positive in ≤70% of patients with endometrial adenocarcinoma; a false-negative result occurs in 30% of patients. Therefore, a negative Pap smear does not rule out carcinoma.

Pap smear from aspiration of endometrial cavity is positive in 95% of patients.

Endometrial biopsy may be helpful, but a negative result does not rule out carcinoma. Diagnostic curettage is the only way to rule out carcinoma of the endometrium.

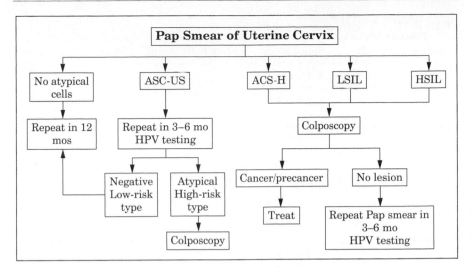

Fig. 14-8. Routine screening for cancer of cervix. (ASC-US, atypical squamous cells unknown significance; ASC-H, atypical squamous cells; cannot exclude squamous intraepithelial lesion; LSIL, low-grade squamous intraepithelial lesion; HSIL, high-grade squamous intraepithelial lesion.)

Trophoblastic Neoplasms

Hydatidiform mole—10% become invasive moles; 2.5% progress to choriocarcinoma

- Complete mole—normal amount of DNA that is all of paternal origin (due to fertilization of an anucleate ovum). Seventy-five percent to 85% are homozygous 46 XX; rest are heterozygous, mostly 46 XY with few 46 XX.
- Partial mole—paternal and maternal DNA present but overabundance of paternal DNA. Fertilization of oocyte by 2 haploid sperm causes triploid 69 XYY, 68 XXY, 69 XXY karyotypes in two thirds of cases; rest have diploid karyotype (46 XX or 46 XY). β-hCG is not usually very increased and spontaneously regresses in >95% of cases requiring chemotherapy.
- hCG (secreted by placenta synctiotrophoblasts) is important to identify 15% to 20% of hydatidiform moles that persist after curettage.
- Increased incidence of preeclampsia

Choriocarcinoma—50% are preceded by molar pregnancy, 25% by term pregnancy, 25% by abortion or ectopic pregnancy. β-hCG corresponds to tumor burden.

◆ hCG is used for diagnosis and management of both benign and malignant types.

- Persistently elevated or slowly declining level by end of first trimester indicates persistent trophoblastic disease and the need for systemic therapy for invasive mole or choriocarcinoma. >500,000 mIU/L is virtually diagnostic.
- After evacuation of the uterus, hCG is negative by 40 days in 75% of cases. If test is positive at 50 days, 50% have trophoblastic disease.
- Repeat test every 1 to 2 weeks with clinical examination for 6 mos. Disease remits in 80% without further treatment.
- Plateau or rise of titer indicates persistent disease. Chemotherapy is indicated if disease persists or metastasizes.
- Repeat negative titer should be rechecked every 3 months for 1 to 2 yrs. High-risk patients are indicated by initial serum titer >40,000 mIU/L.
- Frequent follow-up titers are indicated after radiation therapy with lifelong titers every 6 months.

◆ Measurement of hCG in CSF (ratio of serum:CSF <60:1) is used in diagnosis of brain metastases.

Table 14-16.	Comparison of Various Causes of Vaginitis				
Condition	pH	Saline Mount	10% KOH Mount	Culture	Amine Test
Normal	4.0–4.5	PMN/EC <1; rods dominant; 3+ squames	—		—
Bacterial vaginosis	>4.5	Clue cells; PMN/ED <1; D rods; I coccobacilli	—	No value	>70%+
Vulvovaginal candidiasis	4.0–4.5	PMN/EC <1; hyphae in ~40%; rods dominant; 3+ squames	Hyphae in 70%	If wet mount is –.	—
Trichomoniasis	5.0–6.0	Motile trichomonads in ~60%; 4+ PMNs: mixed flora	—	Use if wet mount is –.	Often +
Atrophic vaginitis	>6.0	1–2+ PMNs; I cocci and coliforms; D rods; parabasal cells	—		—

+, positive; −, negative; D, decreased; I, increased; PMN/EC, ratio of PMNs to epithelial cells.

Laboratory findings due to treatment (e.g., hemorrhage, infection, perforation of uterus, radiation, chemotherapy)

♦ Diagnosis by histologic examination of tissue removed by curettage

RhD-negative patients should receive RhIg at the time of evacuation.

Clinical and biochemical evidence of hyperthyroxemia may occur because alpha subunits of TSH and hCG are identical.

Beware of false lows due to artifactual "hook effect" of immunoassays due to large antigen excess ($>1 \times 10^6$ mIU/L); eliminated by 2-stage immunoassay.

Vulvovaginitis

Laboratory confirmation is necessary for reliable diagnosis.

See Table 14-16.

Due To

♦ Fungi, especially Candida albicans (causes 20%–25% of cases)

• Normal vaginal pH (4.0–4.5)
• Wet mount in KOH or Gram stain of vaginal fluid may not detect 15% of cases
• May be seen on Pap smears
• Culture on Nickerson's or Sabouraud's medium is most sensitive; is needed for definitive identification.
• Sexual transmission plays a very minor role.
• Underlying conditions may be present, especially uncontrolled diabetes mellitus, use of antibiotics, vaginal sponges intrauterine devices

♦ Trichomonas vaginalis

• Wet-mount preparation of freshly examined vaginal fluid. Sensitivity = 50% to 70% compared with culture; requires 10^4 organisms/mL; specificity is almost 100%. DFA is more sensitive but more complex to perform.
• Frequently an incidental finding in routine urinalysis.
• Frequently found in routine Pap smears. S/S = ~70%/~95%, PPV = 75%, NPV = 38%. The organism is often not identified but may be associated with characteristic concomitant cytologic changes. Not recommended for screening.

- Qualitative immunochromatographic kit has reported S/S = 99%/98%.
- Culture is the gold standard; results in 3 to 7 days.
- Urine PCR has high sensitivity may be useful for screening males.
- DNA probe test kit allows prompt results; excellent method.

Douching within 24 hours decreases sensitivity of tests. Do not test during first few days of menstrual cycle.

- Occasionally detected in material from male urethra in cases of nonspecific urethritis. Found in 40% of male sexual partners of infected women. Prostatic fluid usually contains few organisms.
- Increased PMNs are present.
- pH is increased.

Serologic tests are not useful.

◆ Bacterial Vaginosis

Due to complex polymicrobial interaction between anaerobic and aerobic organisms, including *G. vaginalis* and/or *Mobiluncus curtisii*, and concomitant decrease in lactobacilli

Diagnosis is based on ≥3 of the following:

- Vaginal pH >4.5 (using pH indicator paper) in >80% of these cases (found in one third of normal women)
- Wet mount of vaginal discharge shows curved rods and "clue cells" (>20% of vaginal squamous cells coated with small coccobacilli) found in 90% of these cases
- Positive culture on HB or chocolate agar for *G. vaginalis* in 95% of clinical cases but not recommended for diagnosis or test of cure because may also be found in 40% to 50% of asymptomatic women with no signs of infection.
- DNA probe kit allows prompt results
- Gram stain and Pap smear may also suggest this diagnosis: Gram-negative curved rods and decreased-to-absent Gram-positive rods resembling lactobacilli
- Homogeneous adherent discharge: When mixed with 10% potassium hydroxide on slide produces a fishy amine odor; this has a PPV = 70%.

Local cause is most common (e.g., endocrine, poor hygiene, pinworms, scabies, foreign body, irritants [e.g., soaps, perfumes, spermicides], hypersensitivity reaction [e.g., antimycotic creams, latex condoms]).

Atrophic Vaginitis

Increased pH (5.0–7.0)
Wet smear shows increased PMNs and parabasal epithelial cells
Mixed nonspecific Gram-negative rods with decreased lactobacilli
Vaginal cytology shows atrophic pattern

Desquamative Inflammatory Vaginitis

Purulent discharge
Increased pH
Gram stain shows absent Gram-positive bacilli replaced by Gram-positive cocci
Massive vaginal cell exfoliation with increased number of parabasal cells

Other Organisms

Neisseria gonorrhea
Chlamydia
Streptococcal group A vaginitis
Staphylococcus aureus with toxic shock syndrome
Idiopathic associated with HIV infection

Other Causes

Collagen vascular disease, Behçet's syndrome, pemphigus, lichen planus
Multiple causes may be present and should be sought in each case.

Tests During Pregnancy

Altered Laboratory Tests in Pregnancy

By term unless otherwise specified.

RBC mass increases 20%, but plasma volume increases ~40% causing RBC, Hb, and Hct to decrease ~15%.

WBC increases 66%.

Platelet count decreased by average 20%.

ESR increases markedly during pregnancy, making this a useless diagnostic test during pregnancy.

Respiratory alkalosis with renal compensation. Normal pCO_2 = ~30mEq/L, normal HCO_3^- = 19 to 20 mEq/L.

Serum osmolality decreases 10 mOsm/kg during first trimester.

Increased GFR 30% to 50% early until ~20 weeks postpartum

Renal plasma flow increases 25% to 50% by mid-pregnancy.

Creatinine clearance

BUN and creatinine decrease 25%, especially during first half of pregnancy. *BUN of 18 mg/dL and creatinine of 1.2 mg/dL are definitely increased (abnormal) in pregnancy, although normal in nonpregnant women. Beware of BUN of >13 mg/dL and creatinine of >0.8 mg/dL.*

Serum uric acid decreases 35% in first trimester (normal = 2.8–3.0 mg/dL); returns to normal by term.

No changes are found in serum levels of sodium (normal = ~135 mEq/L), potassium, chloride, phosphorus, amylase, AST, ALT, LD, ICD, acid phosphatase, α-hydroxybutyrate dehydrogenase.

Urine volume is not increased.

Fasting blood glucose decreases 5 to 10 mg/dL by end of first trimester. Glycosuria occurs in >50% of patients due to impaired tubular resorption. Lactosuria should not be confused with glucose in urine.

Proteinuria (200–300 mg/24 hr) is common (~20% of patients); worsens with underlying glomerular disease.

Serum aldosterone, angiotensins I and II, renin are increased although normal women are resistant

Pressor effects (see toxemia)

Occasionally cold agglutinins may be positive and osmotic fragility increased.

Serum iron decreases 40% in patients not on iron therapy.

Serum transferrin increases 40% and percent saturation decreases ≤70%.

Serum total protein decreases 1 g/dL during first trimester; remains at that level.

Serum albumin decreases 0.5 g/dL during first trimester; decreases 0.75 g/dL by term.

Serum α-1 globulin increases 0.1 g/dL.

Serum α-2 globulin increases 0.1 g/dL.

Serum β-globulin increases 0.3 g/dL.

Serum ceruloplasmin increases 70%.

Serum cholesterol increases 30% to 50%.

Serum triglycerides increase 100% to 200%.

Serum phospholipid increases 40% to 60%.

Serum CK decreases 15% by 20 weeks; increases at beginning of labor to peak 24 hours postpartum, then gradually returns to normal. CK-MB is detected at onset of labor in ~75% of patients with peak 24 hours postpartum, then returns to normal. Serum LD and AST remain low.

Serum ALP increases (200%–300%) progressively during the last trimester of normal pregnancy caused by an increase of heat-stable isoenzyme from the placenta.

Serum leucine aminopeptidase (LAP) may be moderately increased throughout pregnancy.

Serum lipase decreases 50%.

Serum pseudocholinesterase decreases 30%.

Serum calcium decreases 10%.

Serum magnesium decreases 10%.

Serum vitamin B_{12} level decreases 20%.

Serum folate decreases 50% or more. Overlap of decreased and normal range of values often makes this test useless in diagnosis of megaloblastic anemia of pregnancy.

Serum T_3 uptake is decreased and T_4 is increased. T_7 ($T_3 \times T_4$) is normal. TBG is increased. (See Endocrine-Maternal Thyroid Disease)
Serum progesterone is increased.
Urine porphyrins may be increased.
Urinary gonadotropins (hCG) are increased (see Pregnancy Test).
Urine estrogens increase from 6 months to term (≤ 100 μg/24 hours)
Urine 17-ketosteroids rise to upper limit of normal at term.

Amniotic Fluid (AF) Embolism

Laboratory findings due to pulmonary embolism (see Chapter 6)
○ Identification in maternal lung tissue at postmortem

- Morphologic identification of fetal products (e.g., fat from vernix caseosa, mucin derived from meconium)
- Immunohistochemical identification of fetal isoantigen A[30] and mucin-type glycoprotein derived from meconium and AF

○ Consumptive coagulopathy

Fibronectin, Fetal

Is secreted by chorionic trophoblast throughout pregnancy.

Use
Indicates risk of preterm labor/birth (>50 ng/mL), e.g., marker for decidual disruption.
Interpretation
Normally absent from cervicovaginal fluid after 20 weeks. Normally present in early pregnancy and within 1 to 2 weeks of onset at labor on term.
For high-risk patients, sensitivity = 70%, specificity = 75%

Hormones

Maternal Serum Unconjugated Estriol
See Chapter 12.

Maternal Urine Unconjugated Estriol

Use
Reflects both placental and fetal adrenal cortical function and fetal liver function. Monitoring is usually begun at 34 weeks, but may begin at 28 weeks in high-risk pregnancy (e.g., severe maternal hypertension, intrauterine growth retardation).
Interpretation
Reliable evaluation requires *serial* (rather than *isolated*) determinations (at least 2×/wk) to detect an abrupt fall. A fall less than 50% is generally considered significant but may be affected by variable maternal renal function.
Twenty-four-hour urine level of estriol normally shows a progressive increase during gestation. *May show a 25% variation from day to day in an individual patient. Therefore need two values in same direction.*
>12 mg/24 hours at term indicates a healthy neonate
4 to 12 mg/24 hours or decrease >50% indicates infant in jeopardy
<4 mg/24 hours indicate fetal death or severe jeopardy
Decrease Due To
Fetus
  Intrauterine death
  Fetal abnormalities (e.g., anencephaly, adrenal hypoplasia)
Placenta
  Sulfatase deficiency
  Infarcts
  Placental dysfunction
  Hydatidiform mole
Mother
  Oral antibiotics (values may be two thirds of normal)
  Renal disease
  Liver disease

Corticosteroid administration (values may be 50% of normal)
Incomplete urine collection
Laboratory
Mandelamine in urine (prevents bacterial splitting or reabsorption of estriol)

Plasma Progesterone and Urinary Pregnanediol (Its Chief Metabolite)

Increases progressively during pregnancy.
Reflects only adequate placental function but not fetal status.

Human Chorionic Gonadotropin (hCG)

Glycoprotein secreted first by trophoblastic cells of conceptus and later by placenta. Prevents degeneration of corpus luteum. Amount of hCG produced correlates with amount of trophoblastic tissue.

* **Blood:** Sensitivity <10 mIU/mL; positive in ~95% of patients. Normal value for nonpregnant woman <3 mIU/mL; ≤50 mIU/mL during first week after conception. In normal pregnancy, detectable 6 to 18 days after ovulation; doubles every 2 days in first few weeks of first trimester to peak at tenth week (~100,000 mIU/mL). Then declines slowly to constant level (10,000 mIU/mL) at 17 weeks until delivery.
* Slower rate of rise (<2 day doubling of titer or increase <66%) suggests ectopic pregnancy or spontaneous abortion.
* Much higher values may indicate multiple pregnancy, hydatidiform mole, or hCG-secreting tumors.

Urine: Becomes positive as early as 4 days after expected date of menstruation (~9 days after implantation); by day 10 to 14 is >95% reliable. hCG increases to peak at day 60 to 70, then decreases progressively.

* Urine qualitative test to determine presence of pregnancy; test can confirm pregnancy in 30 minutes. By 24 to 26 days after last menses, urine hCG is usually >200 mIU/mL and urine tests will be positive (sensitivity = 20–25 mIU/mL).
* Urine quantitative test to detect hydatidiform mole or hCG-secreting tumor; test negative ≥1 or more times in >60% and negative at all times in >20% of these patients, for whom more sensitive methods should be used. Quantitative titers should be performed for diagnosis and for following the clinical course of patients with these conditions. Serum is preferred test.

Urine hCG concentration is approximately half of serum level.

Urine False Positive Due To
Drugs (e.g., chlorpromazine, phenothiazines, promethazine, methadone)
Bacterial contamination
Protein or blood in urine

Urine False Negative Due To
Drugs (e.g., promethazine [DAP test])
Dilute urine
Missed abortion
Dead fetus syndrome
Home pregnancy and POC tests that do not measure H-hCG (hyperglycosylated hCG).

Urine Interferences
False-negative results may occur with dilute urine or in cases of missed abortion, dead fetus syndrome, ectopic pregnancy.
False-positive results may occur in:

* Heterophile antibodies ~1 in 3,300 women can have positive hCG ≤900 mIU/mL.
* Bacterial contamination or protein or blood in urine or in patients on methadone therapy.
* Marijuana smokers
* Postorchiectomy patients (secondary to decreased testosterone)

Leukocyte alkaline phosphatase scoring has also been used as a pregnancy test.

Prenatal Screening

At first prenatal visit, all pregnant women should have:
CBC, blood type, Rh type, antibody screen, rubella screen

Tests for sexually transmitted diseases

- RPR test for syphilis
- HBsAg for HBV infection
- Pap smear if not done in preceding year
- HIV test should be offered
- High-risk women—test for *Neisseria gonorrhoeae, Chlamydia trachomatis*, HBsAg; repeat at 28 weeks

At 15 to 22 weeks: Triple or quadruple screen and sonogram for Genetic Disorders (see Chapter 12).

Optional screen for Group B streptococcus at 36 weeks.

Obstetric Disorders

Abortion

Threatened

In threatened abortion during the first 20 weeks of pregnancy, progressive increase in serum diamine oxidase is usually associated with continuation of pregnancy.

Septic

Due To

Mixed aerobic and anaerobic Gram-negative and Gram-positive bacteria

E. coli

Bacteroides fragilis

Enterococcus

Beta-hemolytic streptococcus

Clostridium perfringens and *C. tetani*

Laboratory findings due to sequelae (e.g., endometritis, parametritis, salpingo-oophoritis, uterine perforation, peritonitis, septic thrombophlebitis, septicemia)

Laboratory findings due to complications or sequelae

- Renal failure
- DIC
- Septic shock

Amniotic Infection

Due To

Bacteria (in congenital pneumonia and chorioamnionitis, two thirds are Gram negative) Most common organisms are *Gardnerella vaginalis, Candida albicans,* Group B streptococcus, diphtheroids, genital mycoplasmas, anaerobic bacteria.. Most dangerous are *E. coli* and Group B streptococcus. Twenty percent of intraamniotic infections cause two thirds of maternal or neonatal bacteremia.

Virus (e.g., rubella, CMV, HSV, simplex)

Bacterial Infection

AF glucose level ≤5 mg/dL has PPV = 90% but 10 mg/dL has PPV = 52%; >20 mg/dL is 98% predictive of negative culture. Six to 20 mg/dL is not helpful in ruling out infection.

Gram stain is highly specific; sensitivity of only 50% to 79%.

WBC may be increased; >50 WBC/μL predicts clinical infection.

AF culture may demonstrate causative bacteria.

Maternal PMNs and shift to left may be seen.

Increased maternal serum CRP may precede clinical findings by 12 hours.

Presence in AF of acetic, propionic, butyric, and succinic acids (by gas-liquid chromatography) produced by bacteria is said to be >94% sensitive and specific for infection.

Serological tests for viruses.

Histologic examination of fetal membranes establishes diagnosis.

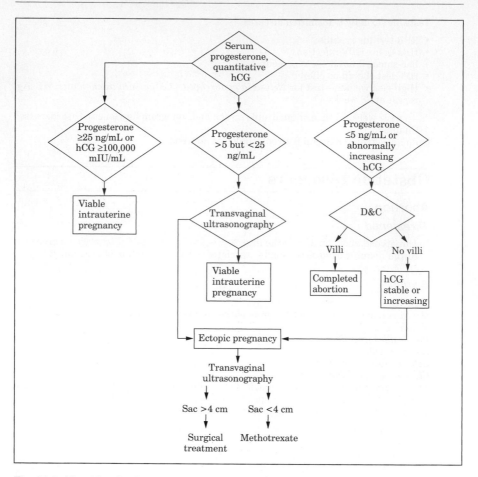

Fig. 14-9. Algorithm for diagnosis of unruptured ectopic pregnancy. (From Carson SA and Buster JE. *N Engl J Med* 1993;329:1174, with permission.)

Ectopic (TUBAL) Pregnancy

Implantation of blastocyst elsewhere than endometrium.

See Fig. 14-9.

♦ Tests for hCG should recognize three important forms: Intact hCG, H-hCG (hyperglycosylated hCG produced by invasive cytotrophoblasts; is key component in early pregnancy), and free β-hCG that many kits and POC tests do not recognize.

• hCG titer doubles about every 2 to 3.5 days during first 40 days of normal pregnancy (at least two measurements 48 to 72 hours apart are needed to calculate this); an abnormally slow increase in hCG (<66% in 48 hours during first 40 days of pregnancy) indicates ectopic pregnancy (S/S = 80%/91%) or abnormal intrauterine pregnancy in ~75% of cases.

• >6,500 mIU/mL (equivalent to ~6 weeks gestation) without an intrauterine gestational sac by transabdominal sonography favors ectopic pregnancy since at this titer an intrauterine pregnancy should be visualized. May also occur with spontaneous abortion.

• Intrauterine gestational sac by sonography may not be identified conclusively until 28 days after conception.

• <6,000 mIU/mL without a sac = unknown diagnosis; absent gestational sac at this hCG concentration is associated with ectopic pregnancy in >85% of cases.

- <6,000 mIU with a sac suggests either ectopic or an early normal/abnormal pregnancy.
- ~2,000 mIU/mL, transvaginal sonography should identify viable intrauterine pregnancy.
- Decrease of hCG of ≥15% 12 hours after curettage is diagnostic of completed abortion but hCG that rises or remains the same indicates ectopic pregnancy.
- hCG level >50,000 mIU/mL in ectopic pregnancy is rare. Normally rise to 100,000 mIU/mL, then plateaus.

Serum hCG is used to monitor methotrexate treatment of ectopic pregnancy (performed weekly until undetectable).

Urine pregnancy test is more variable.

♦ Serum progesterone should be used to screen all patients at risk for ectopic pregnancy at time of first positive pregnancy test. ≥25 ng/mL is said to indicate normal intrauterine pregnancy (sensitivity = 98%) and ≤5 ng/mL confirms nonviable fetus (100% sensitivity) permitting diagnostic uterine curettage to distinguish ectopic pregnancy from spontaneous intrauterine abortion.

WBC may be increased; usually returns to normal in 24 hours. Persistent increase may indicate recurrent bleeding. 50% of patients have normal WBC; 75% of the patients have WBC <15,000/μL. Persistent WBC >20,000/μL may indicate pelvic inflammatory disease (PID).

Anemia depends on degree of blood loss; often precedes the tubal pregnancy in impoverished populations. Progressive anemia may indicate continuing bleeding into hematoma. Absorption of blood from hematoma may cause increased serum bilirubin.

Culdocentesis fluid with Hct >15% indicates significant intraperitoneal hemorrhage.

D & C shows decidua without chorionic villi.

Multiple Pregnancy

May be caused by fertility drug therapy (e.g., clomiphene, gonadotropins). One-third are monozygotic.

Increased maternal serum AFP
Laboratory findings due to associated conditions (e.g., polyhydramnios)
hCG may be increased.

Sequelae

- Preeclampsia
- Twin-to-twin transfusion
- Others, e.g., intrauterine growth retardation

Pelvic Inflammatory Disease (PID)

Infection of upper genital tract; may include endometrium, myometrium, parametrium, uterine tubes, ovaries, peritoneum. Common and most important complication of STD (85%); 15% arise postoperatively.

See Sexually Transmitted Diseases (STDs).

Includes

Urethritis
Cervicitis
    Cervical Gram stain >10 PMNs/HPF (1,000×) in nonmenstruating women
    Tests for appropriate organism
        Culture may not correlate with intraabdominal culture.
        Direct antigen test (e.g., *Chlamydia*)
Vulvovaginitis (see above)
Pelvic abscess—usually polymicrobic (≥3 organisms), aerobic (e.g., *Streptococcus*, *E. coli*) and anaerobic (e.g., *Peptococcus*, *Bacteroides*). *Chlamydia* and *N. gonorrhoeae* recovered from cervix in approximately one third of cases.
Perihepatitis (Fitz-Hugh-Curtis syndrome), see *C. trachomatis*
Laboratory findings due to complications (e.g., infertility, ectopic pregnancy, premature birth, neonatal conjunctivitis, infant pneumonia, septicemia, septic shock, peritonitis, pelvic thrombophlebitis)

GU

Due To

Chlamydia trachomatis (see Chapter 15). *PID due to C. trachomatis causes less severe symptoms than that due to N. gonorrhoeae.*

Neisseria gonorrhoeae infection is found in 8% of acute cases (see Chapter 15).

Mycoplasma hominis (see Chapter 15)

Anaerobic bacteria (e.g., *Clostridium* sp., *Actinomyces* sp.)

Coliform bacilli

Many cases are polymicrobial.

See causes of vulvovaginitis (above).

Placentae Abruptio and Previa

Placenta Abruptio

Premature separation of normally implanted placenta after 20th week of gestation; causes hemorrhage and 15% of third-trimester stillbirths.

No diagnostic laboratory findings

Laboratory findings due to hypovolemic shock, acute renal failure, DIC (is most common cause of DIC in pregnancy)

Placenta Previa

Abnormal implantation of placenta into lower uterine segment; covers part (partial) or all (complete) of the internal os. May cause painless vaginal bleeding.

Laboratory findings due to blood loss. Maternal Hct should be maintained ≥35%.

Beware of DIC that occurs in >15% of cases.

Determine lung maturity by amniocentesis for preterm delivery.

May be complicated by placenta accrete (placenta attached to myometrium).

Preterm Delivery

Gestational age <37 weeks or 259 days; premature infant weighs <2,500 g. *Term infant is* defined as born between 38 and 42 weeks after onset of mother's last period.

Fibronectin

Fetal fibronectin in cervical secretions >50 ng/mL (immunoassay) or rapid test identifies women who deliver before term with S/S = 60% to 93%/52%–85%, PPV = 25%. With high-risk patients, S/S = 70%/75%.

♦ NPV = 96% rules out labor within 7 days[17]

Normally present in early pregnancy and within 1 to 2 weeks of onset of labor at term but normally absent from cervicovaginal fluid after 20 weeks. If present between 24 and 36 weeks, precedes preterm labor/birth by ≥3 weeks.

Laboratory findings due to associated conditions (e.g., hyaline membrane disease, intraventricular hemorrhage)

See section on amniotic fluid—fetal lung maturity.

Prolonged Pregnancy

Pregnancy lasting >294 days or 42 weeks' gestation.

AF L/S ratio <2 in 6% of cases. High ratio (~4) can occur before 42 weeks' gestation. Thus, L/S ratio not useful for this diagnosis.

Progressively falling rather than a rising estriol (E3) is usually found.

Squalene (derived from fetal sebaceous glands) is markedly increased in AF after 39 weeks.

Squalene/cholesterol ratio in AF

- <0.40 before 40 weeks
- >0.40 after 40 weeks
- >1.0 after 42 weeks

---

[17]Foxman EF, Jarolim P. Use of the fetal fibronectin test in decisions to admit to hospital for preterm labor. *Clin Chem* 2003;50:663.

Ruptured Membranes, Detection

♦ Direct observation of fluid leaking from cervical os is best proof.
○ Laboratory diagnosis of fluid from posterior fornix as AF rather than urine

* Detection of fetal isoform of fibronectin (immunoassay) in vaginal secretions indicates presence of AF; sensitivity >98% but low specificity. Is 5 to 10× greater in AF than in maternal plasma; not present in normal vaginal secretions or urine.
* Other laboratory methods for detecting AF in the vagina

    "Fern" test is most reliable test (>96% accuracy) (AF air-dried on a glass slide shows a characteristic fernlike pattern microscopically). False positive in presence of cervical mucus or semen and false negative in presence of blood, dry swab, or insufficient drying time; not affected by meconium or pH.

    Nitrazine paper changes from blue to yellow if pH >6.5. Accuracy ~93%. False positive due to blood, semen, alkaline urine, trichomoniasis, bacterial vaginosis. Normal vaginal pH in pregnancy = 4.5–4.7; AF pH = 7.1–7.3.

Reagent strip test pH ≥7 and protein ≥100 mg/dL indicate AF.

	Sensitivity	Specificity
pH alone	85%	83%
Protein alone	90%	87%
Either or both	95%	91%

Blood, meconium, renal disease, infection interfere with accuracy
Microscopic detection of fat-laden fetal squamous epithelial cells (Nile blue sulfate stain)

To detect premature rupture of membranes in any trimester, saline washings of vaginal fornix reportedly show hCG >50 mIU/mL with high S/S and PPV.[18]

Measurement of α-fetoprotein in vaginal secretions is unreliable. Same concentration in AF and maternal plasma in third trimester.

Toxemia of Pregnancy

Preeclampsia

Hypertension and proteinuria, edema (of face, hands, legs) after 20th week of pregnancy on ≥2 occasions 6 hours but <1 week apart. Etiology is unknown; many theories. One theory: Renin (produced in kidney) acts on angiotensins I and II. Normal pregnant women are resistant to vasoconstriction and increase in BP but in toxemia this is not the case.

Mild Preeclampsia

♦ **Diagnostic criteria**
Hypertension >140/90 but diastolic <110 mm Hg *and*
Proteinuria (collected by catheter if membranes have ruptured or in presence of vaginitis)

* >300 mg/24 hours or >1+ on dipstick on 2 occasions >6 hours but <1 week apart *or*
* 2 specimens ≥1+ by dipstick 6 hours but <1 week apart *or*
* Single specimen ≤2+ by dipstick *or*
* Single specimen with protein/creatinine ratio ≤0.35

Proteinuria is variable and usually late sign (1+ dipstick correlates with 30 mg/dL).
Increased serum Inhibin A (at 15–20 weeks) and Activin A (at ~30 weeks) may indicate preeclampsia and preterm labor.[19]

[18]Anai T, et al. Vaginal fluid hCG levels for detecting premature rupture of membranes. *Obstet Gynecol* 1997;89:261.
[19]Cukle H, et al. Maternal serum Inhibin A can predict preeclampsia. *Br J Obstet Gynaecol* 1998;105:1101.

Severe Preeclampsia

♦ **Diagnostic criteria**

Hypertension >160/110 mm Hg or diastolic ≥110 mm Hg on 2 occasions >6 hours apart on bed rest

Proteinuria (collected by catheter if membranes have ruptured or in presence of vaginitis) *or*

- >500 mg/24 hours or >3+ on dipstick on two occasions >6 hours apart *or*

Significant new onset proteinuria

- ≥3.0 to 5.0 g/24 hours *or* >3+ by dipstick on two occasions

Oliguria—urine output ≤500 mL/24 hours

Platelet count <100,000/μL

Abnormal liver function tests with persistent RUQ or epigastric pain

Persistent severe visual or cerebral disturbances

Pulmonary edema

Biopsy of kidney is pathognomic (swelling of glomerular and mesangial endothelial cells) and also rules out primary renal disease or hypertensive vascular disease.

Includes eclampsia

♦ Serum uric acid is increased in virtually all cases of preeclampsia; correlates with disease severity.

Creatinine clearance is decreased causing increased BUN and creatinine.

○ HELLP syndrome occurs in 4% to 12% of cases. May increase cellfree fetal and maternal DNA in maternal blood.

○ Serum creatinine >1.2 mg/dL. BUN may be normal unless the disease is severe or there is a prior renal lesion. *(BUN usually decreases during normal pregnancy because of increase in glomerular filtration rate.)*

RBCs and RBC casts are not abundant; hyaline and granular casts are present.

Eclampsia

▶ **Diagnostic criteria**

Is indicated by new onset of grand mal seizures without other identifiable cause occurring in woman who meets criteria for preeclampsia.

Approximately 20% of women who develop eclampsia have only mild hypertension and often without proteinuria or edema.

Laboratory findings due to complications (e.g., cerebral hemorrhage, pulmonary edema, renal cortical necrosis)

$MgSO_4$ treatment requires urine output ≥100 mL/4 hours.

Beware of associated or underlying conditions (e.g., hydatidiform mole, twin pregnancy, prior renal disease, diabetes mellitus, nonimmune hydrops fetalis).

Obstetric Monitoring of the Fetus and Placenta

Amniotic Fluid (AF)

Use

Determination of increased bilirubin level in severe Rh disease (see Hemolytic Disease of the Newborn)

Determination of L:S ratio to estimate fetal lung maturity (see below)

Gram stain for organisms and WBC for diagnosis of amnionitis

Diagnosis of congenital anomalies (e.g., Down syndrome, neural tube defect)

Prenatal diagnosis of genetic disorders, e.g.,

   Wilms' tumor may be associated with deletion of chromosome 11, aniridia, and other malformations (e.g., overgrowth of one side or parts of one side of body); may be indicated when other children in family have Wilms' tumor. Chromosome studies and renal investigation are also indicated in presence of aniridia in newborn since Wilms' tumor is often curable.

   See Chorionic Villus Sampling (Chapter 12).

Assess intrauterine growth retardation

Assess postdate pregnancies (>40 weeks)
Others (e.g., fetal death)
May contain abnormal metabolites (e.g., excess methylcitrate in propionic acidemia) or enzyme activity (e.g., N-acetyl-D-hexosaminidase A activity in Tay-Sachs disease) but usually tissue culture of AF cells is used with analysis for specific deficient enzyme.

Volume

At 16 weeks = ~250 mL
At 32 to 35 weeks = ~800 mL
After 35 weeks = ~500 mL

Decreased (Oligohydramnios)

Less than fifth percentile for gestational age

Due To

Fetal anomalies
Renal agenesis
Fetal obstructive uropathies
Postmaturity syndrome
Placental insufficiency (e.g., preeclampsia)
Donor-twin transfusion syndrome

Increased (Hydramnios)

◆ **(More than 1,000 mL at any gestational age)**

Due To

Idiopathic (35%)
Maternal diabetes[1] (25%)
Erythroblastosis fetalis (10%)
Multiple gestation[1] (10%)
Congenital malformations (20%)
- CNS malformation with exposed meninges, anencephaly, hydrocephaly, microcephaly[1,2]
- Chromosomal anomalies e.g., trisomies 13, 18, 21[2]
- Volvulus with atresia or congenital bands of upper jejunum or with common mesentery and herniation of liver, esophageal atresia, pyloric stenosis, duodenal atresia, imperforate anus, cleft palate[2]
- Congenital heart disease[1]
- Disease of genitourinary tract[1]
- Others (e.g. CMV, toxoplasmosis, syphilis; twin-to-twin transfusion)

[1]Increased production
[2]Decreased AF absorption (e.g., impaired swallowing, impaired absorption at amnion-uterine interface).

Color

May be milky or turbid (due to vernix caseosa and squamous debris) until centrifuged, which should give a clear colorless-to-light straw color supernatant.
Yellow

- Usually due to bilirubin (normal maximum occurs at 20–28 weeks); may be increased with fetal RBC hemolysis (e.g., erythroblastosis fetalis); increase correlates with fetal condition and prognosis.
- May also occur from fetal ascitic fluid, amniotic cysts, maternal urine (accidental puncture of mother's bladder).
- Yellow-brown color may be caused by traces of meconium. Meconium staining occurs in ≤20 of deliveries and may indicate fetal distress.

Green (may be with brown or black hue) is due to biliverdin from meconium that may indicate fetal distress.
Red to brown—usually caused by RBCs or Hb. Special stain (Kleihauer-Betke) or electrophoresis distinguishes fetal Hb from maternal blood due to trauma.
Bright red indicates recent intrauterine hemorrhage or hemolysis; may be port wine color in placenta abruptio.
Brown may be caused by oxidized Hb from degenerated RBCs.
Brown-black may be caused by fetal maceration.

Amniotic Fluid, Maternal and Fetal Serum: Normal Values[20]

	AF*	Maternal Serum*	Fetal Serum*
Glucose (mg/dL)	10.7 (5.2)	66.6 (8.7)	48.7 (10.4)
Creatinine (mg/dL)	2.4 (0.3)	1.1 (0.2)	1.1 (0.3)
Urea (mg/dL)	33.9 (11.7)	17.1 (8.7)	16.5 (8.14)
Uric acid (mg/dL)	7.5 (0.3)	3.1 (0.8)	2.6 (0.9)
Total protein (gm/dL)	0.28 (0.3)	6.5 (0.6)	5.8 (0.7)
Albumin (%)	65.2 (4.8)	46.4 (3.1)	60.8 (4.8)
A/G ratio	1.9 (0.7)	0.8 (0.1)	1.5 (0.3)
Total cholesterol (mg/dL)	42.8 (3.2)	258.6 (47.2)	83.5 (39.7)
Triglycerides (mg/dL)	19.3 (9.4)	153.7 (51.4)	16.1 (10.7)
LD (U/mL)	112.3 (64.8)	199.5 (46.4)	328.2 (114.0)
Aldolase (U/mL)	10.1 (7.5)	9.5 (7.0)	23.2 (9.4)

*Values are mean values. Numbers in ( ) represent one standard deviation.

Amniotic Fluid and Urine Differences

	AF	Urine
Specific gravity	1.025	1.005–1.030
pH	Neutral or alkaline	Usually acidic
Protein	Significant quantity	Absent
Urea	Similar to plasma	High
Bilirubin	May be present	Absent
Chloride	Moderate to high	Low to high
Creatinine	Similar to plasma	High
Uric acid	Similar to plasma	High
ALP	High	Low
Ascorbic acid	Low	Low to high

Amniotic Fluid, Normal Chemical Components

	Second Trimester	At Term
Uric acid	3.7 mg/dL	9.9 mg/dL (due to increased muscle mass and increased urinary output of fetus)
Creatinine	0.9 mg/dL	2.0 mg/dL (due to increased muscle mass of fetus)
Total protein	0.6 g/dL	0.3 g/dL
Albumin	0.4 g/dL	0.95 g/dL
AST	17 IU	40 IU
ALP	25 IU	80 IU (≤350 IU in some cases)

Levels of glucose, bilirubin, urea nitrogen, calcium, phosphorus, cholesterol, LD do not change significantly during gestation.

Amniotic Fluid to Monitor Fetal Lung Maturity[21, 22]

Use
Determination of fetal maturity to predict likelihood of respiratory distress syndrome (RDS) and determine when it is safe to interrupt gestation because of threat to fetus (e.g., erythroblastosis fetalis) or mother (e.g., toxemia, hypertension).

Incidence of RDS by 37 weeks gestation is <1%. Thus, no fetal lung maturity testing is done after 37 weeks gestation except with poorly controlled maternal diabetes.

At 34 weeks gestation, risk of RDS = 20%, increasing to 60% at 29 weeks. Thus, most difficult decision time is at 34 to 37 weeks gestation.

[20]Castelazo-Ayala L, Karchmer S, Shor-Pinsker V. The biochemistry of amniotic fluid during normal pregnancy. Correlation with maternal and fetal blood. In Hodari AA, Mariona F, eds. *Physiological biochemistry of the fetus. Proceedings of the international symposium.* Springfield IL: Charles C. Thomas, 1972:32–53.

[21]Dubin SB. Assessment of fetal lung maturity. Practice parameter. *Am J Clin Path* 1998;110:723.

[22]Natelson S, Scommegna A, Epstein MB, eds. *Amniotic fluid. Physiology, biochemistry, and clinical chemistry.* New York: John Wiley & Sons, 1974.

◆ *Lecithin:Sphingomyelin (L:S) Ratio (determined by thin-layer chromatography [TLC])*

Is the single most accurate test of fetal maturity.

L:S ratio	(Some laboratories use these values)	Lung Maturity
<1	<2.0	Very immature lungs (up to 30th wk of gestation); severe RDS is expected; lung maturity may require many wks; do not resample before 2 wks.
1.0–1.49		Immature lungs; moderate to severe RDS is expected; lung maturity may occur in 2 wks; resample in 1 wk.
1.5–1.9	2.0–3.0	Lungs on threshold of maturity (within 14 days); mild to moderate RDS may occur. Test should be repeated in 1 wk.
≥2	>3.0	Mature lungs (35th wk of gestation); low incidence of RDS even if PG is absent. S/S = 80%–85%.
Abundant lecithin with trace or no sphingomyelin		Postmature lungs

Definite exceptions to prediction of pulmonary maturity with L:S ratio >2.0

• Infant of diabetic mother (L:S ratio >2.0 has been frequently seen in cases in which RDS developed)
• Erythroblastosis fetalis

Possible exceptions

• Intrauterine growth retardation
• Toxemia of pregnancy
• Hydrops fetalis
• Placental disease
• Abruptio placentae

◆ *Foam (Shake) Test*

Reliable simple bedside qualitative expression of L:S ratio that gives prompt results. Commercial kit said to have S/S = 87%/97%.

Interferences (L:S ratio and Foam Tests)

Contamination of AF with meconium, blood, vernix, or vaginal mucus makes L:S determinations unreliable (should be leukocyte esterase–negative using urine dipstick). Whole blood L:S ratio ~1.5.
Collection in siliconized tubes
Dilution due to oligo- or polyhydramnios may make foam test unreliable.

Interpretation

Although an L/S ratio >2 and a positive foam test indicate pulmonary maturity and absence of RDS in >95% of cases, a ratio <2 and a negative foam test have a high false-negative rate in predicting RDS and therefore are unreliable.
If AF is not available, L:S ratio or foam test can be done on gastric aspirate of infant during first 6 hours of life if no milk has been given and the trachea is not occluded by intubation. Can also use tracheal fluid or hypopharyngeal secretion.

Other Tests

◆ Phosphatidylglycerol (PG) >2% (0.5 μg/mL by new immunoagglutination kit) and phosphatidylinositol >15% in AF indicate fetal lung maturity and are not affected by contamination of AF or by diabetes mellitus or erythroblastosis fetalis and are thus more sensitive than L:S although more laborious to perform (commercial rapid slide agglutination test is now available). Absence of both indicates high risk of RDS for at least 3 to 4 weeks. PG does not appear in AF until after 36 weeks gestation; therefore absence has poor predictive value for RDS. If these and L:S ratio

GU

are available, little is added by other measurements. However, the total profile of
tests provides the most reliable results.

○ Optical absorbance at 650 nm to measure AF turbidity; maturity criterion ≥0.1.
Interference by blood, meconium, dilution due to oligo- or polyhydramnios.
Corresponds to the gross pearly opalescence of mature AF and to a count of lamellar
bodies (derived from fetal lung) using automated platelet counter.

○ Nile-blue stain of AF differentiates fetal squamous cells from anucleated fat cells;
>50% fat cells indicates mature fetus (40 weeks) and also correlates with occurrence
of RDS. Low counts should be interpreted with caution and correlated with other
findings. *Maternal diabetes may cause spurious elevation of fat cell count.*

♦ Creatinine ≥2 mg/dL (represents muscle mass of fetus and the presence of 1 million
functioning glomeruli) and corresponds to pregnancy ≥37 weeks in >90% of cases.
Values 1.6 to 2.0 mg/dL are considered equivocal, and <1.6 mg/dL indicates fetal
weight <2,500 g and <37 wks' gestation. May be decreased in mature but low-birth
weight infants. May be spuriously increased by hypertensive disorders of pregnancy
(e.g., preeclampsia) and maternal renal disease; therefore maternal serum creatinine should also be determined. Ratio of maternal serum to AF creatinine ≥3 suggests gestational age of about 36 weeks in 97% of cases. Urea and uric acid levels
show more fluctuation and therefore are less useful than creatinine.

○ Bilirubin virtually disappears by 36 weeks' gestation. May be increased due to
maternal hyperbilirubinemia (e.g., hepatitis, hemolytic anemia, cholestasis) or to
administration of drugs (e.g., phenothiazides) that make the test useless. Meconium
results in positive interference. Oligohydramnios may have false-positive results
and polyhydramnios may have false-negative results.

♦ Osmolarity <250 mOsm/L indicates term pregnancy.

♦ Lamellar bodies (lamellated phospholipids that carry surfactant; are secreted into
AF by fetal pneumocytes) in AF can be counted as platelets in electronic cell
counter. <30,000/μL S/S = 100%/64%, NPV = 100%. At 10,000/μL, S/S = 75%/95%,
NPV = 96%.[23]

These tests are valid indicators of fetal maturity (low false-positive rates) but less reliable indicators of immaturity (appreciable false-negative rates). In general, multiple
tests give more reliable results than any single test.

GGT:ALP ratio >2.0 in AF has been reported to indicate pulmonary maturity.

Fetal Death in Utero

Due To

Antepartum (86% of deaths)

• Chronic hypoxia of different etiologies (30%)
• Congenital malformations/chromosomal anomalies (20%)
• Complications of pregnancy e.g., abruptio placentae, Rh immunization (25%)
• Fetal infections (5%)
• Idiopathic (25%)

Intrapartum deaths
♦ AF may be brown with markedly increased CK level.
Intrauterine fetal death has been said to be reliably indicated by increased CK.
DIC may occur especially if >16 weeks' gestation and retained dead fetus ≥4 weeks.

Neonatal Monitoring

Neonatal Screening

See Chapter 12.

Infection in Neonates and Young Infants

○ Gram stain of gastric aspirate within 6 hours of birth should be done on any infant
at risk of infection. Presence of PMNs and bacteria is suspicious for infection. AF
gram stain, culture, tests for lung maturity in prenatal period may also indicate risk
of infection.

[23]Dalence CR, et al. Amniotic fluid lamellar body count: a rapid and reliable fetal lung maturity
test. *Obstet Gynecol* 1995;86:235.

ESR (normal <15 mm/hr on first day) increase is suspicious for infection but beware of false-positive results (e.g., DIC, Coombs'-positive hemolytic disease and Rh disease, clot in tube). CRP has also been used.

Total WBC <5,000/μL, total neutrophil count <1,000/μL or >20% bands are consistent with infection. Decreased WBC may also occur with toxemia and increased WBC may also be associated with maternal glucocorticoids.

♦ Detection of bacterial antigen (CIE) are most sensitive and specific; urine, CSF, AF, and (least desirable) blood can be used.

♦ Cultures of blood, CSF, and urine (do all 3) and tracheal aspirate. Do not use heel stick for blood culture. Urine should be obtained by bladder tap or catheter.

♦ Abnormal urinalysis or CSF examination; but these are often normal in presence of infection.

♦ Gram stain of buffy coat of spun Hct may show bacteria.

Platelet count <100,000/μL.

Laboratory findings due to site of infection:

- Pneumonia
- Umbilical cord—staphylococci, Gram-negative organisms
- UTI—often same organism as in mother. Gram stain of unspun urine may identify organism. Colony count >10,000/μL of one organism is diagnostic in bladder tap urine.
- Skin—staphylococci
- Bone—staphylococci, group B streptococci, Gram-negative organisms, gonococci, *Candida*
- Joint—gonococci, Gram-negative organisms, staphylococci, *H. influenzae*
- GI tract—enteropathogenic *E. coli, Salmonella, Pseudomonas, Klebsiella, Enterobacter, Proteus, S. aureus, Campylobacter* fetus, viruses; *Shigella* is rare
- Otitis media—*Staph. aureus*, Gram-negative enteric bacteria
- Indwelling catheter sites—*Candida,* staphylococci
- Sepsis may be present with, or without, any of these—group B streptococci, *E. coli, L. monocytogenes, Staph. epidermidis, anaerobes* (including *clostridia* and *Bacteroides fragilis*)
- Viral (e.g., CMV, varicella zoster, parvovirus B19, rubella, HAV, HBV, HCV, rubeola) and parasitic (e.g., *Toxoplasma*) infections—see Chapter 15

Newborn, Well-Baby, Recommended Routine Laboratory Tests

Hct/Hb, WBC and differential
Urinalysis
Standard bacteriologic tests
Cord blood should be saved for 2 weeks

- Blood type and hold and Coombs' tests if mother is Rh-negative or if jaundice develops by 24 hours
- Serologic test for syphilis and for HBV if mother not tested antepartum
- Possible screening for toxoplasma or viral infection if requested

Blood chemistries: Direct and total bilirubin, glucose, sodium, potassium, chloride, calcium at appropriate intervals

Newborn screening on day of discharge or follow-up at age 4 days as mandated by state law, e.g., PKU, thyroid function tests, others

Infants at Increased Risk, Laboratory Tests

Due To

During pregnancy: Infants born before 38th wk of gestation. Low birth weight = <2,500 g; very low birth weight = <1,500 g; extremely low birth weight = <1,000 g. Gestational age may not parallel birth weight although most low–birth weight infants are preterm. Other infants at increased risk include high–birth weight infants (>4,000 g) postmaturity infants, infants of high-risk mothers (toxemia, diabetes, drug addiction, cardiac or pulmonary disease), polyhydramnios, oligohydramnios, cesarean section delivery, infection, other major illnesses such as hepatitis, thyrotoxicosis.

During labor and delivery: Fetal pH <7.2, pulmonary immaturity, amnionitis, meconium staining of AF, others

Table 14-17.   Base Deficit and Blood pH Measurements

	Maternal pH (mean)	Fetal pH (mean)	Base Deficit (mEq/L)
Normal mother and fetus	7.42	7.25	7.0
Normal mother and acidotic fetus	7.42	7.25	2.6
Acidotic mother and vigorous fetus	7.36	7.15	4.8

Neonatal:
Tests for RDS, chronic lung disease, e.g., blood gases (pO_2, pCO_2, and pH) indicated by baby's color, condition, and respiratory symptoms
   Pneumothorax/pneumomediastinum occurs in ≤3% in full-term newborns.
Metabolic function
   Hypoglycemia and hypocalcemia
Anemia of prematurity due to
   Insufficient Ep production (most)
   Shorter RBC life span = ~35 to 50 days (term infant = 60–70 days)
   Physiologic anemia at 10 to 12 weeks occurs earlier; more marked than in term newborns
      Phlebotomy
         >10 nucleated RBCs is highly suggestive of fetal ischemic encephalopathy[24]
   Rh/ABO immunization
Nonimmune hydrops fetalis due to various causes (e.g., cardiovascular, respiratory, hematologic, GI, GU, others)
Infections are more common than in term newborns, e.g., late-onset nosocomial infection by coagulase-negative staphylococci and fungi with central venous catheters; sepsis or pneumonia due to amnionitis
Gastrointestinal, e.g., necrotizing enterocolitis, cholestasis with prolonged parenteral feeding
Neonatal hyperbilirubinemia (see Chapter 8)

Chromosome Analysis (Karyotyping), Indications
See Chapter 12.

pH, Fetal Blood
Fetal scalp blood is rarely used in current practice.[25]
When fetal scalp blood is acidotic, maternal acidosis should be differentiated from fetal acidosis, since maternal acidosis does not have the same serious implications. Base deficit and blood pH measurements are shown in Table 14-17. Fetal pH is usually ~0.04 units below maternal pH. pH >7.25 is normal during labor; pH = 7.20 to 7.25 is worrisome and another should be done promptly; pH ≤7.20 suggests significant fetal hypoxia and prompt delivery.
After age of 3 hours, capillary blood from infant's warmed heel correlates well with arterial blood samples for measurements of acid-base status.
Umbilical cord arterial blood pH in uncomplicated pregnancy has normal lower limit of 7.10.[26] *Blood pH is the only objective measure of asphyxia available at delivery by which this diagnosis can be made.*
In general, mean blood pH of 7.27 in the newborn is associated with an Apgar score ≥7. Mean blood pH of 7.22 is associated with an Apgar ≤6. Fetal acid-base status is valuable index of fetal asphyxia or oxygenation; should be evaluated with other evidence of fetal distress. Fetal blood pH provides best correlation with fetal outcome. In almost 20% of infants, the fetal acid-base status may be misleading (e.g., due to fetal edema, contamination with AF).

[24]Phelan JP. Nucleated red blood cells: a marker for fetal asphyxia? *Am J Obstet Gynec* 1995;173:1380.
[25]Henderson Z, Ecker JL. Fetal blood sampling: limited role in contemporary obstetric practice. *Lab Med* 2003;34:548–553.
[26]Orth SR, Ritz E. The nephrotic syndrome. *N Engl J Med* 1998;338:1202.

False Normal

Normal blood pH but depressed infant function.

Due To

Medications administered
Obstetrical manipulation (e.g., difficult forceps delivery)
Precipitous delivery
Prematurity (especially <1,000 g with noncompliant lungs)
Congenital anomalies preventing normal onset of good lung function at birth (e.g., laryngeal web, choanal atresia, hypoplastic lungs associated with diaphragmatic hernia, edematous cyst of lung)
Aspiration syndromes
Previous episodes of asphyxia with resuscitation
Intrauterine infection

False Abnormal

Maternal acidosis is usual cause.

GU

15 | Infectious Diseases

INFECTIOUS

INFECTIOUS

INFECTIOUS

INFECTIOUS

Laboratory Tests for Infectious Diseases

Cytology Detection Tests

Aspergillus species
Blastomyces dermatitis
Candida species
Coccidioides immitis
Cryptococcus species
Histoplasma capsulatum
Pneumocystis jiroveci (formerly *carinii*)
Zygomycetes

Smears

- More than 1 organism on drop of unspun body fluid (e.g., urine) is equivalent to $>10^5$/mL on culture.
- Presence of PMNs is likely to indicate purulent specimen rather than colonization.
- Abundant epithelial cells (>10/low power field) with relatively few PMNs suggests poor sputum sample.

Gram stain separates bacteria into two groups: Gram-positive (retain crystal violet) or Gram-negative (do not retain crystal violet) offers an initial clue to identity of organism.

Giemsa/Wright

- Stains for malaria and babesiosis.
- Tzanck preparations for herpes simplex and varicella-zoster

Acid-fast

Stains for mycobacteria (poor sensitivity—requires 5×10^3 bacilli/mL) and *Nocardia* species.

Special Stains

- Silver stains (e.g., *Treponema pallidum, Bartonella henselae, Pneumocystis carinii*)
- PAS stains for fungi
- Fluorescent antibody and immunocytochemical stains

Wet Mounts

- Saline for trichomonads
- KOH for fungi
- India ink for *Cryptococcus neoformans*
- Darkfield microscopy for syphilis

Diseases That May Be Detected By Finding Organisms On Peripheral Blood Smear

Malaria (*Plasmodium*)
Plague *(Yersinia)*
Relapsing fever (*Borrelia*)
Ehrlichiosis
Babesiosis
Meningococcemia
Disseminated histoplasmosis
Lymphatic filariases
Acute stage of trypanosomiasis.

Blood Cultures

See Table 15-1
Perform as soon as possible after onset of chills or fever.
Before antimicrobial therapy is started.
Use resin-assisted blood cultures if patient is already on antimicrobial therapy.
Take 2 to 3 cultures at least 30–60 minutes apart if possible; shorter time interval if urgent need to begin therapy.
Take 2 to 3 cultures per septic episode or per 24 hour period.
Draw 20 to 30 mL of blood per culture. Some organisms may require a larger volume.
Use aerobic and anaerobic techniques.

Do not draw blood from IV catheter unless no vein sites are available or from umbilical artery catheter in infants.

Special methods should be used if suspected organisms are fungi or mycobacteria; routine methods are negative in 66% of cases of disseminated mycotic disease.

Use strict aseptic technique; contamination rate should be <3% per month.

Suspect contamination if:

- Only one of several cultures is positive (90% of cases)
- Type of organism
    - True infection is almost always present if organism is streptococci (non-viridans group), aerobic and facultative Gram-negative rods, anaerobic cocci and Gram-negative rods, yeasts (possible exception is *Candida tropicalis*).
    - Common contaminants are *Staphylococcus epidermidis*, *Bacillus* spp., *P. acnes*, *Corynebacterium* sp., *Clostridium perfringens*, viridans streptococci, *Candida tropicalis*.

When automated blood cultures are positive, FISH targeting ribosomal RNA allows rapid identification of most common pathogens (*Staphylococcus* sp., *Streptococcus* sp., *Enterococcus* sp., Enterobacteriaceae, *Pseudomonas aeruginosa, Candida* sp.).

Antibody Detection Tests

Presence of IgM antibodies or > fourfold rise in IgG titer between acute and convalescent phase sera drawn within 30 days of each other indicates recent infection. Generally, presence of IgG indicates past exposure and possible immunity. Congenital infections require serial sera from both mother and infant. Passively acquired antibodies in infant will decay in 2 to 3 months (see AIDS). Antibody levels that are unchanged or increased in 2 to 3 months indicate active infection. Absence of antibody in mother rules out congenital infection in infant.

Requires a 4× increase in titer using paired acute and convalescent stage sera tested at the same time or an increased IgM in acute illness (usually >1:8 but may vary with organism). In some instances, a very high IgG titer may be diagnostic.

Cross reaction and nonspecific precipitation may occur with some antisera and among various organisms.

Bacteria

Bartonella henselae
Bordetella pertussis
Borrelia spp. (relapsing fever)
Borrelia burgdorferi (Lyme disease)
Brucella spp.
Clostridium botulinum toxin
Clostridium tetani toxin
Corynebacterium diphtheriae toxin
Anaplasma phagocytophilum [formerly *Ehrlichia*] (human monocytic ehrlichiosis)
    Ehrlichia chaffeensis (human monocytic ehrlichiosis)
E. coli O157 toxin
Francisella tularensis
Haemophilus influenzae type b
Helicobacter pylori
Legionella pneumophila
Leptospira spp.
Salmonella typhi
Treponema pallidum
Yersinia pestis

Chlamydia/Mycoplasma

Chlamydia spp.
Mycoplasma pneumonia
Rickettsia
Coxiella burnetii (Q fever)
Rickettsia typhi (Murine typhus)
Rickettsia rickettsii (Rocky Mountain spotted fever)
Rickettsia tsutsugamushi (Scrub typhus)

Fungi
Aspergillus spp.
Blastomyces dermatidis
Candida spp.
Coccidioides immitis
Cryptococcus neoformans
Histoplasma capsulatum
Penicillium marneffei
Sporothrix schenckii
Zygomycetes
Parasites
Babesia microti
Echinococcus spp.
Entaboeba histolytica
Fasciola hepatica
Filariasis
Giardia lamblia
Leishmania spp.
Paragonimus westermani
Plasmodium spp.
Schistosoma spp.
Strongyloides stercoralis
Taenia solium
Toxocara canis
Toxoplasma gondii
Trichinella spiralis
Trypanosoma cruzi

Antigen Detection Tests

Provide rapid, specific, reliable detection of certain antigens. In bacterial meningitis, CSF is best specimen; urine is occasionally useful in establishing diagnosis; serum is usually not helpful. Sensitivity may be improved by testing serum, urine, and CSF.

For bacteria, is most useful for identification of *Haemophilus influenzae* type B, *Streptococcus pneumoniae*, *Neisseria meningitidis* (groups A and C), group B streptococcus. A negative test does not, however, unequivocally exclude infection caused by that organism.

- CIE (countercurrent immunoelectrophoresis) and latex agglutination are being replaced by more sensitive and specific molecular biology tests that can be used to detect certain bacterial antigens in virtually any body fluid (CSF, serum, urine, joint).
- ELISA have largely replaced radioimmunoassays (RIA). Simple ELISA kits for group A β-hemolytic streptococci. Less S/S than culture.
- Compared to ELISA, immuno-PCR enhances detection sensitivity 100-fold to 10^5-fold for *Staphylococcus aureus*,[1] *Escherichia coli*, group A *Streptococcus*.

For viruses, see later discussion.

Use

Increased S/S of identification. Better sensitivity than culture for viruses.

Early diagnosis prior to appearance of antibodies in serological tests

Faster report turn-around-time

Confirmation of culture

Fastidious transport may not be required

Identification of organisms that are nonviable or cannot be cultured (e.g., HBV, HCV, HPV, *Anaplasma phagocytophilum* [formerly *Ehrlichia*], *Tropheryma whippelii*, parvoviruses, astroviruses, caliciviruses)

Is especially valuable when patient has received antibiotics before cultures and gram stains are taken and whenever smear and culture are negative.

---

[1]Huang SH, Chang TC. Detection of *Staphylococcus aureus* by a Sensitive Immuno-PCR Assay. *Clin Chem* 2004;50:1673.

Identification of fastidious, slow-growing organisms (e.g., *Mycobacterium tuberculosis*, *Mycoplasma pneumoniae*, *Legionella pneumophiliae*, some pathogenic fungi)

Identification of organisms that are dangerous to culture (e.g., *Francisella tularensis*, HIV, *Brucella* spp., hemorrhagic fever viruses, *Coccidioides immitis*, *Coxiella burnetii*)

Identification of previously unknown infectious agents

Identification of organisms present in small numbers (e.g., CMV in transplanted organs, HSV in CSF in encephalitis, HIV in antibody-negative patients) or in small-volume specimens (e.g., intraocular fluid for HSV, CMV, EBV, herpes virus, VZV; or forensic samples)

Density of amplifiable DNA correlates with microbial density (e.g., *Plasmodium vivax*, *Borrelia burgdorferi*, *Chlamydia trachomatis*, HSV)

Monitor disease progression or initiate or monitor therapy (e.g., HIV viral load)

Larger amounts of antigen correlate with more complications and poorer prognosis.

Drug susceptibility testing (e.g., detect antimicrobial resistance genes or mutations as in methicillin-resistant *Staphylococcus*)

Differentiate antigenically similar organisms (e.g., HPV types 16 and 18 compared to types 6 and 11 associated with cervical cancer)

Molecular epidemiology and infection control (identify source of disease outbreak in hospital or community)

Disease diagnosis by characterization of genetic materials without direct identification of infectious agent (e.g., toxins of *Clostridium difficile*, *E. coli* O157:H7, staphylococcal toxic shock syndrome, staphylococcal enterotoxins, streptococcal pyogenic exotoxins)

Relationship of organisms to neoplasms (e.g., HHV-8 to Kaposi sarcoma)

Bacteria

Bacillus anthracis
Bartonella henselae
Bordetella pertussis
Borrelia spp. (relapsing fever)
Borrelia burgdorferi (Lyme disease)
Brucella spp.
Chlamydia trachomatis
Clostridium difficile toxins A and B
Francisella tularensis
Klebsiella pneumoniae
Legionella spp.
Listeria monocytogenes in CSF
Mycobacterium tuberculosis
Neisseria gonorrhoeae
Pseudomonas aeruginosa
Staphylococcus aureus in pleural fluid
Tropheryma whippelii (Whipple disease, see Chapter 7)
Yersinia pestis

Viruses

Adenovirus
Colorado tick fever virus
Coronavirus
EBV
HBV, HCV
HSV
HPV
HIV-1
HTLV-1 and -2
Influenza A virus
Jacob-Creutzfeldt syndrome
Parainfluenza virus
Parvovirus B19
RSV
Rotavirus
VZV

Fungi

Candida sp.
Cryptococcus neoformans meningitis in CSF, urine, or serum
Pneumocystis jiroveci (formerly *carinii*) pneumonitis

Parasites

Cryptosporidium parvum
Entamoeba histolytica, especially in liver abscess material
Giardia lamblia
Taenia solium (cysticercosis)
Toxoplasma gondii
Trichinella spiralis

Molecular Biology

Techniques include nucleic acid testing (e.g., HSV types 1 and 2, HPV, *N. gonorrhoeae*, *Chlamydia trachomatis*) and genotype-based methods for resistance studies (e.g., *mec A* gene for methicillin resistant Staphylococcus and strain typing).
MEC A Gene predicts methicillin susceptibility in *Staphylococcus aureus*.

Drug Resistance/Susceptibility Testing

May increasingly be performed using molecular biology methods.

Bactericidal Titer, Serum

That dilution of serum able to kill >99.9% of the original bacterial inoculum in 18 to 24 hours when patient is on antibiotic therapy (usually for bacterial endocarditis; has also been recommended for osteomyelitis, septic arthritis, empyema, patient receiving multiple antimicrobials, immunosuppressed patients with sepsis). Using CSF or urine instead of serum has been adapted for bacterial meningitis and GU tract infections. Generally correlates with in vitro broth concentration that kills microorganism. Can also determine serum inhibitory activity. Assays effect of antimicrobial level. Method is not standardized. Requires three days. Many doubt clinical value of test.

Beta-Lactamase Testing

Iodometric, acidometric, chromogenic cephalosporin methodologies.

Positive test

- Predicts resistance to penicillin, ampicillin and amoxicillin among *Haemophilus* spp., *N. gonorrhoeae* and *M. catarrhalis*.
- Predicts resistance to penicillin, acylamino-, carboxy-, and ureidopenicillins among staphylococci and enterococci.

Table 15-1.	Etiology of Bacteremia	
Organism	% of Cases	Predisposing Factors
Staphylococcus epidermidis	34	Contaminated IV catheters, heart valve prostheses, shunts
Escherichia coli	22	GU indwelling catheters and instruments, perforated bowel, septic abortion
Staphylococcus aureus	15	Abscess, decubitus ulcer, osteomyelitis, staphylococcal pneumonia
Pseudomonas species	6	Burns, immunosuppressive chemotherapy
Alpha *Streptococcus*	6	Dental procedures, gum disease
Streptococcus pneumoniae	6	Alcoholism, chronic obstructive pulmonary disease, pneumococcal pneumonia
Bacteroides species	3.5	Trauma, GI or GU tract disease
Haemophilus influenzae	3	*H. influenzae* nasopharyngitis
Candida species	1.5	Burns, immunosuppressive chemotherapy, parenteral alimentation
Streptococcus pyogenes	1.4	Streptococcal pharyngitis/tonsillitis
Clostridium species	1.4	Septic abortion, biliary tract disease/surgery
Salmonella species	0.8	Contaminated food/water

One-third of staphylococcal bacteremias are primary; predisposing factors are decreased immune defenses (e.g., diabetes mellitus, neoplasms, steroid therapy, hemodialysis).

Drug Monitoring, Therapeutic

See Table 19-1

Use

Where margin between therapeutic and toxic concentrations is narrow (e.g., aminoglycosides, vancomycin).

Patients with renal failure.

Endotoxin Detection

Present in all species of Gram-negative organisms. New test detects enhanced chemiluminescent response of neutrophils to complexed antibody.

Infectious Disease Indicators, Nonspecific

Acute phase reactants (see Chapter 3)

Limulus lysate assay detects trace amounts of endotoxin from all Gram-negative bacteria (including *E. coli*, *Neisseria meningitidis*, *H. influenzae*) in body fluids (e.g.,. blood, urine, BAL). Presence in CSF is sensitive indicator of Gram-negative bacterial meningitis but rapid clearance from blood may make serum test less reliable. (See Chapter 9).

Infectious Diseases

Anaerobic Bacterial Infections

The most common anaerobic organisms cultured are *Bacteroides* and *Clostridia* species and streptococci. Frequently, several anaerobic organisms are present simultaneously and are often associated with aerobic bacteria as well. If cultures from suspicious sites are reported as negative, the culturing for anaerobic organisms has not been performed properly. The most commonly associated aerobic bacteria are the gram-negative enteric bacteria [*Escherichia coli*, *Klebsiella*, *Proteus*, *Pseudomonas*, enterococci]. *Mixed aerobic-anaerobic infections are often successfully treated by suppressing only the anaerobes*.

○ Clues to anaerobic infection include gram stain showing polymicrobial flora, putrid odor, gas formation, tissue necrosis or abscess formation (e.g., lung, brain, dental, skin), culture failure (due to failure to culture anaerobically), toxin production, or clinical features.

○ Anaerobic organisms should be sought particularly in cultures from intra-abdominal infections (e.g., bowel perforations, acute appendicitis, biliary tract disease), obstetric and gynecologic infections (e.g., pelvic abscess, Bartholin gland abscess, postpartum, postabortion, posthysterectomy infections), chest infections (e.g., bronchiectasis, lung abscess, necrotizing pneumonia), urinary tract, soft tissue infections, <5% of endocarditis cases (especially streptococci), 10% of cases of bacteremia.

○ *Bacteremia due to anaerobic organisms is characterized by high incidence of jaundice, septic thrombophlebitis, and metastatic abscesses; the GI tract and the female pelvis are the usual portals of entry (in aerobic bacteremia, the GU tract is the most common portal of entry).*

Bacteroides infection is usually a component of mixed infection with coliform bacteria, aerobic and anaerobic streptococci or staphylococci.

Local suppuration or systemic infection is secondary to disease of the female genital tract, intestinal tract, or tonsillar region.

Laboratory findings due to complications (e.g., thrombophlebitis, endocarditis, metastatic abscesses of lung, liver, brain, joint) are present.

Laboratory findings due to underlying conditions (e.g., recent surgery, cancer, arteriosclerosis, diabetes mellitus, alcoholism, prior antibiotic treatment, and steroid, immunosuppressive, or cytotoxic therapy) are present.

Cellulitis[2]

Cellulitis is acute spreading pyogenic inflammation of dermis and subcutaneous tissue, usually a complication of ulcer, wound, dermatosis. Erysipelas is

[2]Swartz MN. Cellulitis. *N Engl J Med* 2004;350:904.

Table 15-2.   Some Organisms Commonly Present in Various Sites

Site	Normal Flora	Pathogen	Disease
External ear	Aerobic corynebacteria, α-hemolytic streptococci, *Bacillus* spp., *Staphylococcus epidermidis Candida* spp.	α-hemolytic streptococci	Otitis media
		<u>Fungi</u> *Candida* spp., *Aspergillus* spp., <u>Viruses</u> e.g.,	
		HSV	Herpes
		Molluscum contagiosum virus	Molluscum contagiosum
		Papovavirus	Warts
		Varicella zoster virus	Varicella
Middle ear	Sterile	*H. influenzae, Strept. pneumoniae, Moraxella catarrhalis,* β-hemolytic strept. <u>Viruses</u> e.g., RSV, influenza virus, enterovirus, adenovirus	Acute otitis media
		Staphylococcus aureus *Proteus* spp., *Pseudomonas* spp., other Gram-negative bacilli α-hemolytic streptococci <u>Viruses</u> e.g., RSV, influenza virus	Chronic otitis media
Nasal passages	*Staphylococcus epidermidis, Staphylococcus aureus,* diphtheroids, *Strept. pneumoniae,* α-hemolytic streptococci, nonpathogenic *Neisseria* spp., aerobic corynebacteria	*Staphylococcus aureus, Strept. pneumoniae, Klebsiella-Enterobacter* spp., α-hemolytic streptococci, β-hemolytic streptococci, *Moraxella catarrhalis*	Acute sinusitis
		Staphylococcus aureus α-hemolytic streptococci β-hemolytic streptococci *Strept. pneumoniae* <u>Fungi</u>: *Mucor* and *Aspergillus* spp. (especially in diabetics)	Chronic sinusitis

Table 15-2.	*(continued)*		
Site	Normal Flora	Pathogen	Disease
Pharynx and tonsils	α-hemolytic streptococci, *Neisseria* spp., *Staphylococcus epidermidis*, *Staphylococcus aureus* (small numbers), *Strept. pneumoniae*, nonhemolytic (gamma) streptococci, diphtheroids, coliforms, β-hemolytic streptococci (not Group A), *Actinomyces israellii*, *Haemophilus* spp.	Group A β-hemolytic streptococci. *Bordetella pertussis*, *Bordetella parapertussis*, *Chlamydia pneumoniae*, *Neisseria meningitides*, *H. influenzae*, *Staphylococcus aureus*, *Mycoplasma pneumoniae*, *Neisseria gonorrhoeae*	Upper respiratory infection (pharyngitis, tonsillitis). *Marked predominance of one organism may be clinically significant even if it is a normal inhabitant.*
		Strept. pyogenes *Corynebacterium diphtheriae* <u>Viruses</u>: Respiratory viruses <u>Fungi</u> *Candida albicans*	Scarlet fever Diphtheria
Epiglottis Larynx		*H. influenzae* Viruses: EBV, Respiratory viruses <u>Fungi</u> *Candida albicans,* *Corynebacterium diphtheriae* *Mycobacterium tuberculosis*	Croup Laryngitis Diphtheria TB of larynx
Bronchi		*Mycoplasma pneumoniae,* *Corynebacterium diphtheriae* *Strept. pneumoniae*	Bronchitis, acute; chronic
Bronchioli Lungs		<u>Viruses</u> e.g., RSV *Bordetella pertussis* *Mycoplasma pneumoniae*[†] *Legionella pneumophila*[†] *Chlamydia* spp.,[†] *E. coli, Francisella tularensis, H. influenzae,*[†] *Klebsiella*[†]- *Enterobacter-Serratia,** Nocardia asteroides, Proteus mirabilis,*	Bronchiolitis Whooping cough Primary atypical pneumonia Legionnaire's disease Pneumonia

(continued)

INFECTIOUS

Table 15-2.   Some Organisms Commonly Present in Various Sites

Site	Normal Flora	Pathogen	Disease
		*Pseudomonas pneumoniae,** *Staphylococcus aureus,** *Streptococcus pneumoniae,*[†] *Yersinia pestis*	
		Mycobacterium tuberculosis[†]	TB
		Parasites *Paragonimus westermani*	Paragonimiasis
		Rickettsiae (e.g., *Coxiella brunetti, R. typhi, R. prowazeki)*	Q fever, typhus
		Protozoans (e.g., *Toxoplasma gondi)*	Toxoplasmosis
		Fungi[†] (e.g., *Aspergillus* spp., *Blastomyces, Coccidioides, Histoplasma, Pneumocystis jiroveci* [formerly *carinii*])	Granulomas, pneumonia
		Viruses[†] (e.g., SARS, adenoviruses, CMV, coxsackievirus, echovirus, hantavirus, HSV, influenza, parainfluenza, reovirus, RSV, viruses of exanthems)	Pneumonia, bronchiolitis, bronchitis
Pleura	Sterile	*Mycobacterium tuberculosis*	TB granuloma, effusion
		Anaerobic streptococci	Exudative effusion, empyema
		E. coli	
		H. influenzae	
		Staphylococcus aureus	
		Staphylococcus epidermidis	
		Klebsiella pneumoniae	
		Streptococcus pneumoniae	
		Streptococcus pyogenes	
		Actinomyces spp, *Nocardia asteroides*	Exudative effusion
GI tract			
Mouth	α-hemolytic streptococci, *Bacteroides* spp.,	*Candida albicans* ??	Thrush Trench mouth

Table 15-2. *(continued)*

Site	Normal Flora	Pathogen	Disease
Teeth	diphtheroids, enterococci, fusobacteria, lactobacilli, *Neisseria* spp., staphylococci	*Strept. mucans*	Tooth decay (caries)
Parotid glands		Mumps virus	Mumps
Esophagus		Viruses (e.g., CMV, HSV)	
		Candida albicans	Thrush
Stomach	Sterile	*H. pylori*	Gastritis, peptic ulcer
Small intestine	Sterile in one third. Scant bacteria in two thirds (e.g., α-hemolytic streptococci, diphtheroids, enterococci, *E. coli*, *Klebsiella-Enterobacter*, *Staphylococcus . epidermidis*)	*H. pylori*	Peptic ulcer
		E. coli (EHEC, ETEC), *Yersinia*, *Campylobacter*	Diarrhea
		Salmonella spp.	Typhoid
		Vibrio spp.	Cholera
		Brucella spp.	Brucellosis
		Clostridium perfringens, *Bacillus cereus*, *Staph. aureus*	Diarrhea
		Protozoans e.g., *Giardia lamblia*, *Cryptosporidium*, *Microsporidium*, *Isospora belli*, *Cyclospora*	Diarrhea
		Viruses e.g., Norwalk agent, rotavirus, CMV	
Colon	Abundant bacteria (e.g., *Bacteroides* spp., enterococci, *E. coli*, *Klebsiella-Enterobacter*, *Proteus* spp.). Yeasts	*Campylobacter jejuni*, *Chlamydia* spp., *Clostridium difficile*, (antibiotic-associated), *Cl. perfringens* (food poisoning), enteropathogenic *E. coli*, *Salmonella* spp., *Shigella* spp., *Staphylococcus. aureus*, *Vibrio* spp., MAI, *Yersinia enterocolitica*	Colitis, dysentery
		Fungi: *Candida albicans*	
		Protozoans e.g.,	
		Balantidium coli	Balantidiasis
		Cryptosporidium parvum, *Cyclospora cayetanensis*, *Isospora belli*	Coccidiosis
		Cryptosporidia spp.	Cryptosporidiosis
		Entamoeba histolytica	Amebiasis
		Giardia lamblia	Giardiasis

(continued)

INFECTIOUS

Table 15-2.   Some Organisms Commonly Present in Various Sites

Site	Normal Flora	Pathogen	Disease
		Helminths: Nematodes, trematodes, cestodes, etc.	Infections
		Viruses (e.g., astroviruses, adenoviruses, caliciviruses, rotavirus, Norwalk virus)	Gastroenteritis
Rectum/Anus	Same as colon	*Neisseria gonorrhoeae*	Proctitis
		Chlamydia trachomatis	Lymphogranuloma venereum
		Haemophilus ducreyi bacillus	Chancroid
		Trepenoma pallidum	Chancre
		Enterobius vermicularis	Pinworm
		Papillomavirus	Warts
Peritoneum	Sterile	May be polymicrobial. Anaerobic bacteria *Clostridium* spp. *E. coli* *Pseudomonas* spp., *Staphylococcus aureus* Streptococci spp., *Streptococcus pneumoniae*, etc.	Peritonitis
Liver		Bacteria *Brucella* spp.	Brucellosis
		Protozoans e.g., *Entamoeba histolytica*	Amebic abscess
		Helminths (e.g., *Taenea* spp., *Schistosoma* spp., *Clonarchis sinensis)*	Infestations
		Viruses (e.g., HAV, HBV, HCV, HDV, HEV)	Hepatitis. Hepatocellular carcinoma
		Yellow fever virus	Yellow fever
		Epstein Barr virus	Infectious mononucleosis
		CMV	CMV inclusion disease
Gall bladder	Sterile	Bacteria (e.g., *E. coli, Enterococci, Klebsiella- Enterobacter- Serratia)* Occasionally: Coliforms *Proteus* spp. *Pseudomonas* spp. *Salmonella*	Cholecystitis

Table 15-2.	(continued)		
Site	Normal Flora	Pathogen	Disease
CNS (see Chapter 9)	Sterile CSF	<u>Bacteria</u> e.g., *Neisseria meningitides* *Haemophilus influenzae* *Listeria monocytogenes* *Streptococcus pneumoniae* *Mycobacterium tuberculosis*, etc.	Meningitis
		Trepenoma pallidum	Tertiary syphilis
		Clostridium tetani	Tetanus
		Clostridium botulinum	Botulism
		Mycoplasma pneumoniae	Encephalitis
		<u>Viruses</u> e.g.,	
		HIV	AIDS
		Rabies virus	Rabies
		Arbovirus e.g., West Nile, St. Louis, Japanese viruses	Encephalitis
		Herpes simplex (HSV)	Encephalitis
		Enterovirus (Coxsackie, echo viruses)	Most common cause of aseptic meningitis
		Coxsackie	Poliomyelitis
		Echo	Subacute sclerosing panencephalitis
		Polio	Encephalitis
		Varicella-zoster	Shingles
		Measles, mumps, Epstein Barr virus	
		<u>Prions</u> e.g.,	
		Variant Creutzfeldt-Jakob (vJC) Disease	CJ disease (dementia)
		Kuru	Kuru
		<u>Fungi</u>, e.g.,	
		Cryptococcus neoformans, Coccidiodes immitis	Meningitis
		<u>Protozoal</u> e.g., *Naegleria, Acanthamoeba*	"Aseptic" meningitis
		Trypanosoma spp.	Sleeping sickness (trypanosomiasis)
		Toxoplasma gondii	Toxoplasmosis
		<u>Helminths</u> (e.g., *Schistosoma*)	Space-occupying mass

INFECTIOUS

(continued)

Table 15-2.	Some Organisms Commonly Present in Various Sites		
Site	Normal Flora	Pathogen	Disease
Blood	Sterile	<u>Bacteria</u> *Haemophilus influenzae,* *Leptospira* spp., *Listeria monocytogenes,* *Neisseria meningitides,* *Salmonella* spp., *Streptococcus pneumoniae*	Bacteremia, endocarditis, etc.
		<u>Protozoons</u> e.g., *Babesia microti* *Plasmodium* spp. *Trypanosoma cruzi* *Leishmania tropica,* *L. braziliensis*	Babesiosis Malaria Chagas' disease Leishmaniasis
		<u>Opportunistic fungi</u> e.g., *Blastomyces dermatidis, Candida* spp., *Histoplasma capsulatum)*	
IV Catheter	Sterile	Coagulase-negative staphylococci, *Staphylococcus aureus,* Gram-negative bacilli, *Candida* spp.	
Cardiovascular	Sterile	Also see Blood. <u>Bacteria</u> (e.g., *α-hemolytic streptococci)*	Subacute bacterial endocarditis
		Staphylococcus aureus, Gram-negative bacteria	Acute bacterial endocarditis
		Treponema pallidum	Aortitis, gummas, aortic insufficiency
		<u>Viruses</u> e.g., Coxsackieviruses Yellow fever virus Dengue virus	Myocarditis Yellow fever Dengue fever
		<u>Rickettsia</u> e.g., *Rickettsii prowazeki,* *Rickettsii typhi*	Typhus
		Rickettsii rickettsii	Rocky Mountain Spotted Fever
		Rickettsii tsutsugamushi	Scrub typhus
Pericardium	Sterile	*Haemophilus influenzae* *Neisseria meningitides* *Streptococcus pneumoniae* *Pseudomonas* spp. *Streptococcus* spp.	

Table 15-2.	*(continued)*		
Site	Normal Flora	Pathogen	Disease
Eye	Usually sterile. Occasionally small numbers of diphtheroids and coagulase-negative staphylococci.	<u>Bacteria</u> *Neisseria gonorrhoeae*	Ophthalmia neonatorum
		Chlamydia trachomatis	Trachoma
		Haemophilus spp.	Pink eye (conjunctivitis)
		Staphylococcus aureus, Staphylococcus epidermidis, Streptococcus spp.	Ophthalmitis
		Bacillus cereus	Endophthalmitis
		<u>Viruses</u> HSV type 1	Herpetic kerato-conjunctivitis
		Adenoviruses	Epidemic kerato-conjunctivitis
		Echoviruses and coxsackieviruses	Acute hemorrhagic conjunctivitis
		Acanthamoeba	Keratitis
		<u>Fungi</u>: *Candida* spp.	Endophthalmitis
		<u>Helminths</u> *Loa loa*	Loiasis (eyeworm)
		Onchocerca volvulus	Onchocerciasis (river blindness)
		Toxocara canis	Larva migrans
Skin	*Staphylococcus aureus, Staphylococcus epidermidis*	<u>Bacteria</u> e.g., *Staphylococcus aureus*	Impetigo, folliculitis, furunculosis. Scalded skin syndrome.
		Group A streptococcus	Erysipelas, impetigo
		Bacillus anthracis	Anthrax
		Francisella tularensis	Tularemia
		Treponium pallidum	Chancre, secondary syphilis
		Mycobacterium leprae	Leprosy
		Mycobacterium tuberculosis	TB
		Mycobacterium marinum	Swimming pool granuloma
		<u>Viruses</u> e.g., *Papillomavirus*	Warts
		Poxviruses	Smallpox. Variola. Vaccinia. Cowpox. Molluscum contagiosum
		Varicella-zoster virus	Varicella (chickenpox), herpes zoster (shingles)
		Rubella virus	German measles
		HSV, type 1	Cold sores
		<u>Fungi</u> e.g., *Candida albicans*	Candidiasis

(continued)

INFECTIOUS

Table 15-2.	Some Organisms Commonly Present in Various Sites		
Site	Normal Flora	Pathogen	Disease
		Trichophyton, Microsporum, Epidermophyton spp.	Superficial mycoses
		Malassezia furfur, Exophiala werneckii, Trichosporon beigelii, Piedraia hortae	Cutaneous mycoses
		Sporothrix schenckii, Rhinosporidium seeberi, etc.	Subcutaneous mycoses (e.g., sporotrichosis, rhinosporidiosis, mycetoma, chromoblastomycosis)
		<u>Protozoans</u> e.g., *Leishmania tropica, L. braziliensis*	Leishmaniasis
G-U tract			
Urethra, male	*Staphylococus aureus, Staphylococus epidermidis*	*Chlamydia trachomatis* *Neisseria gonorrhoeae* *Gardnerella vaginalis* *E. coli* *Klebsiella-Enterobacter* *Haemophilus ducreyi* *Staphylococcus aureus* *Bacteroides* spp. Enterococci Anaerobic and microaerophilic streptococci	Sexually transmitted diseases. Urethritis.
Urethra, female and vagina	Lactobacillus (large numbers) Coli-aerogenes, Staphylococci. Anaerobic and aerobic streptococci *Ureaplasma urealyticum* *Bacteroides* spp. *Candida albicans*	*Chlamydia trachomatis* *Neisseria gonorrhoeae* *Gardnerella vaginalis* Group B streptococci *Trichomonas vaginalis* *Listeria monocytogenes* <u>Fungi</u>: Yeasts and *Candida albicans.* (See also Urethra, male.)	Sexually transmitted diseases. Urethritis. Vaginitis.
Prostate	Sterile	*Strept. faecalis* *Staphylococcus epidermidis* *Pseudomonas* spp. Anaerobic and micro-anaerophilic streptococci (alpha, beta, gamma types) *Bacteroides* spp. *Enterococci*	Prostatitis

Table 15-2.	(continued)		
Site	Normal Flora	Pathogen	Disease
		Beta-hemolytic streptococci (usually group B), Staphylococci *Clostridium perfringens* E. coli, *Klebsiella-Enterobacter-Serratia* *Proteus* spp. *Listeria monocytogenes*	
Urine	α- and β-hemolytic streptococci Coagulase-negative staphylococci diphtheroids Enterococci, Lactobacilli *Proteus* spp.	Coagulase-negative and positive staphylococci *E. coli* *Klebsiella-Enterobacter-Serratia* *Proteus* spp. *Providencia* spp. *Pseudomonas* spp. *Salmonella* and *Shigella* spp. *Mycobacterium tuberculosis* *Trichomonas vaginalis*	G-U tract infection TB Vaginitis
Wound	–	Coliform bacilli and other Gram-negative rods *Clostridium* spp. *Pseudomonas* spp. *Serratia* spp. *Staphylococcus aureus* *Staphylococcus epidermidis* *Strept. pyogenes*	
Bones	Sterile	Acute Hematogenous *Staphylococcus aureus* *H. influenzae* Gram-negative bacilli (e.g., *Pseudomonas aeeruginosa, Serratia marcescens, E. coli*) *Mycobacterium tuberculosis* *Neisseria gonorrhoeae* Streptococci (groups A and B) *Salmonella* spp. especially in sickle cell disease	Acute osteomyelitis

(continued)

Table 15-2.	Some Organisms Commonly Present in Various Sites

Site	Normal Flora	Pathogen	Disease
		Contiguous Anaerobic bacteria (e.g., *bacteroides,* cocci, fusobacteria)	Chronic osteomyelitis
Joints	Sterile	β-hemolytic streptococci *H. influenzae* *Klebsiella pneumoniae* *Neisseria gonorrhoeae* *Staphylococcus aureus* *Staphylococcus epidermidis* *Streptococcus pneumoniae*	Suppurative arthritis
		Gram-negative pathogens	In newborns
		Mycobacterium tuberculosis	E.g., Pott's disease
		Salmonella spp.	Especially in sickle cell disease
Skin	*Staphylococcus aureus* *Staphylococcus epidermidis* *Peptostreptococcus* and spp. Varies with area (e.g., perineum contains colon flora), *Propionibacterium* in hair follicles and sebaceous glands.	Viruses (e.g., HBV, mumps, parvovirus B, varicella-zoster) Fungi (e.g., *Blastomyces dermatitidis, Candida, Coccidioides immitis, Sporothrix schencki*)	

†Community-acquired pneumonia. *Hospital-acquired pneumonia.

superficial cellulitis with prominent lymphatic involvement. Pathogen is isolated in <30% of needle aspirates; Gram-positive in 70% of cases.

Type of Cellulitis	Usual location	Commonly Caused By
Bites, dog/cat	Limbs	Pasteurella sp., *Staphylococcus aureus* and other *Staphylococcus* species, anaerobes, others
Bites, human	Various	Oral anaerobes, *Staphylococcus aureus, Streptococcus viridans*, others
Body piercing	Ear, nose, umbilicus	*Staphylococcus aureus,* group A streptococcus
Buccal	Cheek	*Haemophilus influenzae*
Crepitant	Trunk, limbs	Clostridia or nonspore forming anaerobes alone or mixed with facultative organisms (e.g., *E. coli*)
Diabetic ulcers	Feet	Aerobic Gram-negative bacilli (Enterobacteriaceae, *Pseudomonas aeruginosa,* Acinetobacter), anaerobes (bacteroides, Peptococcus)

Erythema migrans	Trunk, limbs	*Borrelia burgdorferi*
Immunocompromised	Cutaneous	Gram-negative (e.g., *E. coli*)
Immunocompromised	Bacteremic, AIDS	Proteus and pseudomonas sp., *Cryptococcus neoformans,* others
Liposuction	Abdominal wall, thigh	Group A streptococcus, Peptostreptococcus
Lumpectomy	Breast	Non-group A streptococcus
Occupational (butcher, fish handler, veterinarian)	Hands	*Erysipelothrix rhusiopathiae*
Perianal	Perineum	Group A streptococcus
Periorbital	Periorbital	*Staphylococcus aureus,* pneumococcus, group A streptococcus
Radical mastectomy	Arm	Non-group A streptococcus
Saphenous vein harvest for coronary artery bypass	Leg	Group A or non-group A streptococcus
"Skin popping" (illicit drugs)	Limbs, neck	*Staphylococcus aureus,* various streptococci, others
Very early post-operative wound	Abdomen, chest, hip	Group A streptococcus
Water exposure, salt	Abrasion, laceration	*Vibrio vulnificus*
Water exposure, fresh	Abrasion, laceration	Aeromonas sp.

Fever of Unknown Origin

Temperature ≥101°F (38.3°C) for ≥3 weeks that is undiagnosed after 1 week in hospital.

Due To
> age 65, in order of decreasing frequency: collagen vascular diseases (≤20%), infections, neoplasms, especially lymphomas (30%), undiagnosed (10%)
In younger patients: undiagnosed (≤10%), miscellaneous (26%), infection (21%), collagen vascular diseases
Liver biopsy yields diagnosis in ~15% of cases.
Infections: TB, GU tract, endocarditis, abscesses (e.g., subdiaphragmatic, pelvic). Less common are *Salmonella,* brucellosis, HIV, osteomyelitis, sinusitis, dental, cat-scratch disease, malaria, and the like; ≤50% of cases in all age groups
Neoplasms (e.g., lymphoma, leukemia, renal cell carcinoma, liver or brain metastases). Less common are hepatoma or cancer of pancreas or colon. Rarely—atrial myxoma.
Collagen vascular diseases (e.g., temporal arteritis, Still's disease, polyarteritis nodosa, RA, SLE, vasculitis). Less common are granulomas (e.g., sarcoidosis).
Miscellaneous, especially due to drugs; also hepatitis, Crohn disease, factitious, etc.

Sepsis[3,4]

Systemic response to presence of microorganisms or their toxins.

Due To
Pathogenic Gram-negative and Gram-positive bacteria, fungi, yeast
Culture from blood, urine, CSF, bronchial materials may be negative.
Application of biomarkers (e.g., CRP, TNFα, IL-6, IL-8, others) and gene polymorphisms are not yet useful for routine clinical application.

[3]Schrier RW, Wang W. Acute Renal Failure and Sepsis. *N Engl J Med* 2004;351:159.
[4]Carrigan SD, et al. Toward Resolving the Challenges of Sepsis Diagnosis. *Clin Chem* 2004;50:1301.

Table 15-3.

Bacteria	Sample	Diagnotic Assay		
B. anthracis	Blood. CSF. Sputum. Pleural fluid. Skin lesions.	Gram stain. ELISA-Ag. ELISA serology.		
Brucella spp.	Blood. Bone marrow. Paired sera.	Culture. Serology: agglutination.		
Yersinia pestis	Blood. Sputum. LN aspirate.	Gram Wright stain. ELISA-AG. Culture. Serology: ELISA, IFA.		
Francisella tularensis	Blood. Sputum. Serum.	Culture is difficult. Serology: agglutination.		
Campylobacter jejuni				
E. coli				
Mycobacterium avium intracellulare				
Salmonella				
Salmonella				
Shigella				
Vibrio cholerae				
Yersinia enterocolitica				
Clostridium difficile, Cl. perfringens				

Ag, antigen; LN, lymph node.

May be associated with acute renal failure, acute respiratory distress syndrome, etc. (see Chapter 16).

Mortality rate is higher when a positive culture is associated with acute renal failure.

	Laboratory Findings	Clinical Findings	% Association with Acute Renal Failure
Moderate sepsis	Arterial CO_2 <32 mm Hg or respirations >20/min.	Evidence of infection. T° >38°C or <36°C. Pulse rate >90/min.	19%
Severe sepsis	WBC >12,000 or <4,000/μL or >10% bands.		23%

	Sepsis-associated lactic acidosis, oliguria, or →→→→→→→→	Altered mental status	
Septic shock	Includes sepsis findings.	Sepsis-induced hypotension	51%

Solid Organ Transplant Infections

Significant cause of morbidity and mortality in recipients.

Nosocomial bacterial infections.
Latent infection in transplanted tissue or host. May be activated by immunosuppressive therapy and therefore similar to those superimposed in AIDS.

* Cytomegalovirus
* EBV
* Toxoplasma gondii (especially in heart transplants)
* BK virus (especially in renal transplants)
* *Pneumocystis jiroveci* (formerly *Pneumocystis carinii)* reported incidence ≤10%
* *Strongyloides stercoralis*

Bacterial Diseases

Classification of Bacterial Diseases

* Gram-positive cocci
    * Staphylococci (coagulase-positive and coagulase-negative)
    * Streptococci
        * • *Group A β-hemolytic (S. pyogenes)*
        * • *Group B β-hemolytic*
        * • *Group C β-hemolytic*
        * • *Group F β-hemolytic*
        * • *Streptococcus pneumoniae*
        * • *Streptococcus viridans*
        * • *Enterococcus*
* Gram-negative cocci
    * *Neisseria meningitides; Neisseria gonorrhoeae* (meningitis; gonorrhea)
* Gram-positive bacilli (aerobic and facultative anaerobic)
    * *Listeria monocytogenes* (listeriosis)
    * *Bacillus anthracis* (anthrax)
    * *Corynebacterium diphtheriae* (diphtheria)
    * *Gardnerella vaginalis* (bacterial vaginosis)
    * *Lactobacillus* (various infections e.g., endocarditis, abscess)
    * *Nocardia asteroides* (nocardiosis)
    * *Tropheryma whipplei* (Whipple disease)
* Gram-negative bacilli
    * *Pseudomonas aeruginosa, Burkholderia, Pseudomallei* (melioidosis)
    * *Bordetella* (whooping cough)
    * *Moraxella* (respiratory infections)
    * *Campylobacter* (e.g., gastroenteritis)
    * *Helicobacter pylori* (gastritis, ulcer)
    * *Vibrio* (cholera, wound infections)
    * *Haemophilus influenzae* (respiratory infections)
    * *Pasteurella* (infected animal bites, CNS)
    * *Brucella* (brucellosis)
    * *Francisella* (tularemia)
    * *Bartonella* (angiomatosis, cat-scratch disease, Oroya fever)
    * *Legionella* (Legionnaire disease)
    * *Yersinia pestis* (plague)
    * *Yersinia enterocolitica* (enterocolitis)
    * *Borrelia, Bacteroides, Campylobacter, Fusobacterium, Treponema* (anaerobes)
    * *Lactobacillus* (non-spore forming anaerobes)

INFECTIOUS

- Mycobacteria
  - *Mycobacterium tuberculosis hominis, M. tuberculosis bovis; M. avium; M. intracellulare* (TB)
  - *Mycobacterium leprae* (leprosy)
- Mycoplasma and Ureaplasma
  - *Mycoplasma pneumoniae* (pneumonia)
  - *Mycoplasma hominis; Ureaplasma urealyticum* (e.g., GU, GYN infection)
- Spirochetal Infections
  - *Treponema* (syphilis [*T. pallidum*], yaws [*T. pertenue*], pinta [*T. carateum*], bejel [*T. endemicum*])
  - *Borrelia recurrentis* (relapsing fever), *B. burgdorferi* (Lyme disease)
  - *Leptospira* (Leptospirosis [*Leptospira interrogans*])
  - *Spirillum Minor* (Rat-bite fever)

Gram-Positive Organisms

Staphylococcal Infections

Gram-positive cocci in grapelike clusters. Causes of human diseases are classified as coagulase positive (*S. aureus*) or coagulase negative (*S. epidermidis, S. saprophyticus, S. hemolyticus*).

Pneumonia

Often secondary to measles, influenza, mucoviscidosis, debilitating diseases, such as leukemia and collagen diseases, or to prolonged treatment with broad-spectrum antibiotics.

- WBC is increased (usually >15,000/μL).
- ◆ Sputum contains very many PMNs with intracellular Gram-positive cocci.
- ◆ Bacteremia occurs in <20% of patients.

Acute Osteomyelitis, Septic Arthritis, Pyomyositis

Due to hematogenous dissemination

- ◆ Bacteremia occurs in >50% of early cases.
- WBC is increased.
- Anemia develops rapidly.
- ○ Secondary amyloidosis occurs in long-standing chronic osteomyelitis.

Endocarditis

Occurs in valves without preceding rheumatic disease and showing little or no previous damage; causes rapid severe damage to valve, producing acute clinical course of mechanical heart failure (rupture of chordae tendineae, perforation of valve, valvular insufficiency) plus results of acute severe infection

- Metastatic abscesses occur in various organs.
- Anemia develops rapidly.
- WBC is increased (12,000–20,000/μL); occasionally is normal or decreased.
- *From 1% to 13% of cases of bacterial endocarditis are caused by coagulase-negative* Staphylococcus albus; *bacterial endocarditis due to* S. albus *is found following cardiac surgery in one third and without preceding surgery in two thirds of patients.*
- Bacteremia is common.
- Teichoic acid antibodies are found in titer ≥1:4 in about two thirds of patients with S. aureus endocarditis or bacteremia with metastatic infection, about one half of patients with nonbacteremic staphylococcal infections. May be found in ~10% of other infections or in normal persons. Titer ≥1:4 is said to suggest current or recent serious staphylococcal infection; positive result without suppuration at primary site of infection suggests endocarditis or metastatic infection. May also be useful when cultures are negative because of prior antibiotic therapy or when deep-tissue infection is inaccessible to culturing (e.g., osteomyelitis, abscesses of brain, liver, etc.). Major value is to determine length of treatment of bacteremia, since lack of rise of

titer during 14 days of therapy makes it unlikely that undetected metastatic seeding has occurred.

Food Poisoning

Due to enterotoxin.

♦ Culture of staphylococci from suspected food, especially custard and milk products and meat.

Necrotizing Enterocolitis of Infancy as seen in Hirschsprung disease

Impetigo especially in infants between ages 3 weeks and 6 months

Meningitis (see Chapter 9)

Toxic Shock Syndromes

Due to toxin-producing strains of *Staphylococcus aureus* or Group A streptococci. Fever, hypotension, rash, with no evidence of drug reaction, or autoimmune disorder.

Disease diagnosis by characterization of genetic materials without direct identification of infectious agent (e.g., toxins of staphylococcal toxic shock syndrome, staphylococcal enterotoxins, streptococcal pyogenic exotoxins)

Anemia is normocytic, normochromic, nonhemolytic, moderate, progressive and may persist for ≤1 month after onset of illness; resolves without treatment; occurs in ~50% of cases.

ESR may be normal or very high.

Table 15-4. Toxic Shock Syndrome Due To Streptococcal and Staphylococcal Toxins

	Streptococcal	Staphylococcal
Usually associated with:	Invasive tissue infection	Use of tampons in healthy menstruating women
	Bacteremia (60%)	No
	Pneumonia, peritonitis, osteomyelitis, myometritis	Rarely
	Local soft tissue necrosis (e.g., cellulitis, fasciitis)	Not usually
Culture	*S. pyogens* (usually)	*Staphylococcus aureus*
Serological tests	Positive for ASOT, DNAse B, other streptococcal toxins	
Diagnostic Criteria	Isolation of β-hemolytic streptococcus from a sterile site, hypotension and ≥2 of these: • Renal impairment, coagulopathy, abnormal liver chemistries (see *Staphylococcus,* toxic shock syndrome) • Acute respiratory distress syndrome • Soft-tissue necrosis	• Negative serologies for measles, leptospirosis, Rocky Mountain spotted fever, and negative blood or CSF cultures for other organisms • Laboratory findings involving ≥3 organ systems. Increased serum bilirubin, AST, LD, CK, BUN or creatinine >2× ULN or pyuria without GU tract infection are found in ~60% of cases about the seventh day of illness, at which time clinical improvement begins to occur and these changes rapidly become normal. Platelets <100,000/μL in ~25% of cases.

INFECTIOUS

Moderate leukocytosis with predominance of immature granulocytes in 70% of cases and toxic granulation. Usually increases for several days and then rapidly returns to normal.

Decreased serum albumin,* total and ionized calcium,* phosphorus.

Hypokalemia, hyponatremia, and metabolic acidosis frequently accompany vomiting and diarrhea.*

Proteinuria, and RBCs resolve within 2 weeks.

Increased PT and PTT in two thirds of patients.

DIC causing hemorrhage is not a significant clinical problem.

*Abnormalities usually become normal by fifth day of illness.

Streptococcal Infections

Uncommon in children younger than age 2 years.)

Classification of Streptococci

Lancefield Group	Name	
None	*S. pneumoniae*	See previous section
None	Viridans streptococci	Show α-hemolysis. Causes SBE (see Chapter 5).
A	*S. pyogenes*	β-hemolytic (Lancefield group A.) Cause scarlet fever, URI. Are the most frequent type of streptococci causing otitis media, mastoiditis, sinusitis, meningitis, cerebral sinus thrombosis, pneumonia, empyema, pericarditis, bacteremia, suppurative arthritis, puerperal sepsis, lymphangitis, lymphadenitis, erysipelas, cellulitis, impetigo (in older children, is often mixed infection with staphylococci that overgrow the culture plate).
B	*S. agalactiae*	Colonizes ≤30% of vagina and rectum in pregnancy causing septic abortion, premature rupture of membranes, chorioamnionitis, postpartum endometritis. Especially infects neonates during delivery (sepsis, pneumonia, meningitis), and elderly. Most are nosocomial. Involves devitalized soft tissues, decubiti, pneumonia, GU tract. Should screen women after 35th week of pregnancy. RT-PCR has PPV and PNV >98% in 2 hours. Culture is gold standard. Rapid latex screen for antigen (replaces CIE) sensitivity >70% for neonatal meningitis.
C	*S. equisimilis* and *S. zooepidemicus*	Colonizes <3% of normal persons. Causes pharyngitis (which may be followed by GN); occasional cases of bacteremia, endocarditis, meningitis, puerperal sepsis, pneumonia
D	*E. faecalis* and *S. bovis*	Both are important causes of endocarditis. *(Half of adults with S. bovis endocarditis have anatomic lesion of colon, e.g., carcinoma, polyp, adenoma). S. bovis rarely causes other infection. E. faecalis* causes infections of GU tract, peritoneal cavity, pneumonia in elderly persons, infection of damaged tissues (e.g., decubiti, burns, diabetic tissues), polymicrobial bacteremia
F	*S. milleri*, others	
G	No name	Comprise 5%–10% of streptococci in blood cultures. Cause polymicrobial bacteremia, bacteremia with no known primary focus,

<table>
<tr><td>Anaerobic
streptococci</td><td>major underlying diseases, serious infection of compromised skin and soft tissue (e.g., radiation, edema). Clinically indistinguishable from *S. pyogenes* infection. Can increase ASOT and cause GN.
Associated with coliform bacilli, clostridia, bacteroides in compound fractures and soft-tissue wounds, puerperal and postabortion sepsis, visceral abscesses (e.g., lung, liver, brain). Associated with *Staphylococcus aureus* in gangrenous postoperative abdominal incision.
Without associated bacteria in burrowing skin and subcutaneous infection.</td></tr>
</table>

♦ Throat swab for rapid direct antigen for group A streptococci have S/S >75%/>95% depending on criteria; allows identification within minutes. (Take two swabs: if first is positive, treat as streptococcal pharyngitis; if first is negative, use second swab for routine culture method.) Positive means patient has streptococcus pharyngitis or is a carrier.

♦ Streptococci appear in smears and cultures from appropriate sites.

♦ Blood culture may be positive.

WBC is usually increased (14,000/μL) early in scarlet fever and URI. It becomes normal by end of first week. (If still increased, look for complication, e.g., otitis.) Is often more markedly increased ($\leq$20,000–30,000/μL) with other sites.

Increased eosinophils appear during convalescence, especially with scarlet fever.

Urine may show transient slight albumin, RBCs, casts, without sequelae.

♦ Serological tests (e.g., ASO titer [see also Chapters 3, 5, and 14]) are gold standard for diagnosis of antecedent infection.

Acute GN follows streptococcal infection after latent period of 1 to 2 weeks; preceding infection of pharynx. Latent period prior to onset of acute rheumatic fever is 2 to 4 weeks; preceding infection is pharyngeal but rarely of the skin.

Recently approved rapid test for Group B streptococci detects DNA in swabs from vagina or rectum.

See Rheumatic Fever, Chapter 5, and Acute GN, Chapter 14.

Streptococcus Pneumoniae (Pneumococcal) Infections

Gram-positive lancet-shaped α-hemolytic diplococci.

Pneumonia

♦ Gram stain of sputum—many PMNs, many Gram-positive cocci in pairs and singly; direct pneumococcus typing using capsular swelling (quellung reaction) method.

♦ Sputum culture sensitivity = 45%.

♦ Blood culture positive for pneumococci in 25% of untreated patients during first 3 to 4 days

♦ Pleural effusion contain organisms in ~15% of patients

♦ Rapid urine kit that tests for *S. pneumoniae* antigen has S/S = >60%/$\leq$100%.

Laboratory findings due to complications (pleural effusion [$\geq$60% endocarditis], empyema [~15%] meningitis, peritonitis, arthritis, etc.)

○ Increased WBC of 20,000/μL correlates with good prognosis; normal or low WBC correlates with poor prognosis (e.g., overwhelming infection, in aged patients, or with other causative organisms (e.g., Friedländer's bacillus)

Endocarditis

See Chapter 5

Meningitis

Is the most common cause of meningitis in adults and children >4 years old. See Table 9-3. Laboratory findings due to associated or underlying conditions (pneumococcal pneumonia, endocarditis, otitis, sinusitis, multiple myeloma)

♦ Kit that tests for *S. pneumoniae* antigen in CSF is said to have 97% accuracy.

Peritonitis

Positive blood culture
Increased WBC
♦ Ascitic fluid—identification of organisms by gram stain and culture (see Chapter 7).
○ *Increased susceptibility to pneumococcus infection in hyposplenism (e.g., post-splenectomy, sickle cell disease, congenital abnormalities of spleen, children with nephrotic syndrome)*

Diphtheria

Upper respiratory infection due to *Corynebacterium diphtheriae,* a pleomorphic Gram-positive rod that produces an exotoxin.

♦ Smear from involved area stained with methylene blue is positive in >75% of patients.
♦ Culture from involved area is positive within 12 hours on Loffler's medium (more slowly on blood agar) (toxin-producing strain). Nose cultures should always be obtained. *If there has been prior antibiotic therapy, culture may be negative or take several days to grow.* Penicillin G eliminates *C. diphtheriae* within 12 hours; without therapy, organisms usually disappear after 2 to 4 weeks. PCR allows rapid diagnosis of suspicious isolates.
♦ Fluorescent antibody staining of material from involved area provides more rapid diagnosis, with a higher percentage of positive results.
WBC is increased (≤15,000/μL). If >25,000/μL are found, there is probably a concomitant infection (e.g., hemolytic streptococcal).
Albumin and casts are frequently present in urine; blood is rarely found.
Moderate anemia is common.
Decreased serum glucose occurs frequently.
Laboratory findings of peripheral neuritis are present in 10% of patients, usually during second to sixth week. Increased CSF protein may be of prolonged duration.
Laboratory findings of myocarditis (which occurs in up to two thirds of patients) are present.
Serologic tests (EIA) are used for epidemiological studies or to assess immune function by comparing pre- and postimmunization sera. Toxoid antibody by EIA ≥0.1 AU/mL indicates immunity and eliminates need for antitoxin; titers decrease with age. Cannot be used for diagnosis.

Ehrlichiosis

Due to obligate intracellular rickettsialike coccobacilli with clinical picture similar to Rocky Mountain spotted fever or Lyme disease.

♦ Ehrlichia inclusion bodies (morulae) may be seen within monocytes (~3% of cases) or buffy coat leukocytes or, rarely, CSF mononuclear cells with Wright stain.
♦ *Ehrlichia* may be isolated in culture but test is not widely available.
♦ PCR positive for *Ehrlichia* DNA in serum or CSF in acute stage (sensitivity = 60%–85%).
♦ IFA ≥256 or that shows ≥4× change in specific IgG titer 3 to 6 weeks apart or negative to positive titer ≥1:64 suggests recent infection; is often only useful in retrospect.
Antibodies may persist >1 year in ≤50% of patients. More than 60% are seronegative in acute phase. There may be some cross-reactivity. Clinician must indicate to the lab which organism is being sought. No specific serology for *Ehrlichia ewingi.*
CSF may show increased lymphocytes and protein.
Varying combinations of anemia, thrombocytopenia and leukopenia in 50% to 75% of cases.
Laboratory findings due to specific organ involvement (e.g., liver, CNS, marrow).

Listeriosis

Due to *Listeria monocytogenes*, Gram-positive, nonspore-forming, short bacillus. May occur during pregnancy especially in third trimester, and may cause amnionitis, septic abortion, bacteremic flulike syndrome, and the like. Usually

Table 15-5.   Comparison of Ehrlichioses

Disease	Human Monocytic Ehrlichiosis	Human Granulocytic Anaplasmosis	"Ehrlichiosis Ewingi" Ehrlichiosis	Sennetsu Fever
Organism	*Ehrlichia chaffeensis*	*Anaplasma phagocytophilum*	*Ehrlichia ewingi*	*Ehrlichia sennetsu*
Vector	Lone Star tick (*Amblyomma americanum*), *Ixodes scapularis*, *Dermacentor variabilis*	*Ixodes scapularis*	Lone Star tick (*Amblyomma americanum*)	Not known
Animal Host	White-tailed deer, dogs, foxes, wolves, coyotes	White-footed mouse, other mammals	White-tailed deer, dogs, foxes, wolves, coyotes	Not known
Infected Cell	Monocytes	Neutrophils	Neutrophils	
Region	SW, south-central, mid-Atlantic US	NE, upper-midwest US, California, Europe	SW, south-central, mid-Atlantic US	Japan, Malaysia

Adapted from JH Stone, et al. Human monocytic ehrlichiosis. *JAMA* 2004;292:2263.

asymptomatic or mild during pregnancy. Infection of adult nonpregnant patients is associated with being debilitated or immunocompromised. No screening test available.

♦ Neonatal infection from maternal infection
• Meningitis
  Purulent CSF with 100 to 10,000 WBC/μL; 70% show preponderance of PMNs; protein is usually increased; glucose is normal in 60% of cases. Gram stain is positive in <20% but cultures are usually positive. Negative gram stain and monocytic response may lead to misdiagnosis as viral, syphilis, Lyme disease, TB, etc. Positive blood cultures in 60% to 75% of cases. CNS involvement without meningitis is based on blood cultures as <50% of CSF cultures are positive.
• Granulomatosis infantiseptica: Abscesses or granulomas of viscera may occur (e.g., endophthalmitis, septic arthritis, osteomyelitis, liver abscess, pleuro-pulmonary infection).
• Increased WBC and other evidence of infection.
• Gram stain of meconium may show Gram-positive bacilli. *This should be done whenever mother is febrile, before or at onset of labor.*

♦ Diagnosis requires isolation of organism from a normally sterile site (e.g., blood, CSF).
♦ Isolation of pure culture from food may require days to weeks. Monoclonal antibodies or nucleic acid hybridizations do not require pure culture; they identify the genus but are not specific for *L. monocytogenes*.
♦ Serological tests

• CF showing ≥4× rise in titer after absorption of reactive sera with *S. aureus* to remove cross-reacting agglutinins. Titer 1:8 has high predictive value.
• EIA for specific antibodies, antigen detection in CSF are in development.

Laboratory findings due to bacteremia, endocarditis (in presence of underlying cardiac lesion), skin infection, or the like, are present.
Epidemic cases are usually food-borne. Food role in sporadic cases is unknown. Food borne organism present in feces of some healthy persons.

INFECTIOUS

Nocardiosis[5]

Due to *Nocardia* now reclassified as a higher bacterium rather than a fungus. Soil-dwelling, Gram-positive, facultative, intracellular, aerobic, opportunistic organisms.

Clinical types: Acute, subacute, or chronic suppurative disease usually begins in respiratory tract.

* Pulmonary disease (pneumonitis, abscess) is most common; metastatic brain abscesses in one third of cases.
* *Nocardia asteroides* species in human infections; occurs predominantly in immunosuppressed patients.
* *Nocardia brasiliensis* is predominantly a skin disease in immunocompetent persons.

♦ Recognition of organism in sputum or pus

* Sputum positive in only 30% of cases; bronchial washings, tracheal aspirate or tissue biopsy are preferred. Blood culture is rarely positive.
* Direct smear—Gram-positive or Gram-variable and weakly acid-fast stain. Not significant in gastric washings as may be present in foods. *May be saprophytic in sputum.*
* Positive culture on Sabouraud's medium and blood agar. (*Beware of inactivation by concentration technique for tubercle bacillus.*)
* Species differentiated by HPLC, gene analysis.

♦ Serologic tests

* EIA is sensitive (titer >1:256) and specific.
* CF (titer = 1:16–1:32 3–4 weeks after infection; sensitivity = 80%) and immunodiffusion (positive 2 weeks after infection; sensitivity = 50%–70%) are sometimes useful in systemic nocardiosis.

Laboratory findings due to predisposing immunocompromised conditions (e.g., AIDS, alcoholism, diabetes mellitus, lymphoma, organ transplant, long-term corticosteroid therapy) or underlying pulmonary disease (e.g., COPD).

Whipple Disease (Intestinal Lipodystrophy)

Chronic relapsing multiorgan disease due to facultative, intracellular Gram-positive Actinomycete named *Tropheryma whippelii*.

♦ Biopsy of proximal intestine (especially duodenum) and mesenteric lymph nodes establishes the diagnosis by light (using special stains) and characteristic electron microscopy showing bacilli. Has also been observed in other tissues (e.g., liver, lymph nodes, heart, CNS, eye, kidney, synovium, lung). Immunohistochemistry identifies *T. whippelii* antigens in duodenal biopsy.
♦ Organism has recently been cultured.
♦ PCR detects bacterial 16S ribosomal RNA in infected tissues, mononuclear cells of peripheral blood, many body fluids; is highly sensitive; rare in patients without characteristic histologic features.

IgM antibodies are more specific than IgG.

Laboratory findings due to involvement of various organs

* Malabsorption syndrome with steatorrhea occurs in most patients
* Anemia of chronic disease in 90% of cases; occasionally due to iron deficiency; rarely due to folate or B_{12} deficiency.
* Hypogammaglobulinemia is usual.
* Wasting syndrome
* Seronegative arthritis
* Sarcoidlike illness
* Culture negative bacterial endocarditis

Many patients are anergic with impaired immune function.

---

[5]Lederman ER, Crum NF. A Case Series and Focused Review of Nocardiosis. *Medicine.* 2004;83:300.

Gram-Negative Organisms

Bartonellosis

Zoonotic infections mainly transmitted by vectors due to tiny fastidious Gram-negative bacilli of genus *Bartonella*.

Cat-Scratch Disease

Due to *Bartonella* [formerly *Rochalimaea*] *henselae* in ~85% of cases and *Afipia felis* in ~15% of cases.

◆ PCR is sensitive and specific for detection organisms in blood, CSF, and tissue.
◆ Organisms can be isolated using special culture techniques. Has low sensitivity; usually is impractical because bacilli are slow-growing, fastidious, poorly staining.
◆ Serologic tests—varying reports of S/S.

• EIA for detection of IgG antibodies to *B. henselae*; sensitivity; may be higher if test for IgM or use paired sera. More sensitive than IFA.
• IFA for *B. henselae* (≥1:64)
• Antibodies react in serologic tests for *Chlamydia* and *Coxiella burnetii*.

◆ Histologic appearance of excised lymph node, skin lesions, etc. may be characteristic but are nonspecific. Demonstration of organisms in tissue by special stains is most efficient and rapid.
○ EM has low sensitivity.
○ Blood cultures from infected cats may be positive for prolonged periods. Widely distributed among pet cats; transmitted by cat flea.
ESR is usually increased. WBC is usually normal but occasionally is increased ≤13,000/μL; eosinophils may be increased.
Laboratory findings due to organ involvement:

• Liver (e.g., increased serum GGT and ALP), peliosis in 25% of patients
• Endocarditis
• CNS (brain abscess, aseptic meningitis)

Trench Fever; Endocarditis; Bacillary Angiomatosis; Peliosis

Trench fever is caused by body louse-borne *Bartonella* (formerly *Rochalimaea*) *quintana*. Endocarditis is caused by *B. elizabethae* transmitted by sandfly.

◆ Blood culture may be positive in cases with bacteremia which may be prolonged. Should be suspected in endocarditis when blood culture is negative. Reported to cause ~3% of cases of endocarditis. Both *B. quintana* and *B. henselae* have been found in patients with bacillary angiomatosis and endocarditis.
◆ Species identification by direct immunofluorescence of isolate and DNA hybridization studies and analysis of restriction-fragment-length polymorphisms.
◆ Demonstration of *B. quintana* in heart valves or lymph nodes by gram stain and identification by immunofluorescence and immunohistochemistry.
◆ PCR of blood and tissue in culture negative endocarditis.
◆ Histology, Warthin-Starry stain, and culture of tissue biopsy in bacillary angiomatosis.
◆ Increased serologic IgG titer against *B. quintana*. Frequently cross-reacts with *Chlamydia* species. Bacillary angiomatosis occurs primarily in immunocompromised patients.

Oroya Fever

Endemic South American infection due to *B. bacilliformis*; sandfly is vector.

◆ Blood smears may show bacilli in ≤90% of RBCs (Giemsa stain); they are also present in monocytes. Bacteria are also present in phagocytes of RE system.
◆ Blood culture is positive.
○ Sudden very marked intravascular hemolytic anemia occurs; negative Coombs test.
Susceptible to superimposed Salmonella infection.

INFECTIOUS

Veruga Peruana

Is chronic bartonellosis. Vascular proliferative phase of Oroya fever.

♦ Blood culture may be positive in apparently healthy persons.
♦ Culture of skin lesions and bone marrow may be positive.
Is histologically similar to bacillary angiomatosis.
Moderate anemia is found.

Brucellosis (Undulant Fever)[6,7]

Zoonotic chronic granulomatous intracellular infections due to small, Gram-negative aerobic coccobacilli *Brucella melitensis* (primarily goats and sheep), *B. suis* (primarily swine) *B. abortus* (primarily cattle) and *B. canis* (primarily dogs). Transmitted by contact with infected animals or eating contaminated animal products. Malodorous perspiration is almost pathognomonic.

♦ Serologic tests are most common diagnostic modality

• Agglutination reaction becomes positive during second to third week of illness; 90% of patients have titers of ≥1:160. Rising titer is of diagnostic significance. False-negative results are rare. False-positive test results may occur with tularemia or cholera or with cholera vaccination or after brucellin skin test. In chronic localized brucellosis, titers may be negative or ≤1:200. They may remain positive long after infection has been cured. Antibodies due to *B. canis* are not detected with the usual antigens; *B. canis* antigen must be used.

• EIA is method of choice to detect specific IgM and IgG antibodies. Opsonophagocytic test and CF test are not generally useful.

• Failure of titers to decline may indicate incomplete cure as may nucleic acid amplification methods.

♦ Multiple blood cultures are more likely to be positive with high agglutination titer. *Brucella abortus* requires 10% CO_2 for culture. Must be incubated for at least 4 weeks. About 70% are positive.
♦ Bone marrow culture is occasionally positive when blood culture and serologies are negative.
It may show microscopic granulomas.
♦ Biopsy of tissue may show nonspecific granulomas suggesting a diagnosis of brucellosis. Tissue may be used for culture.
Laboratory abnormalities tend to be more severe in *Brucella melitensis* infections.
Laboratory findings due to involvement of various organ systems

• Liver (>50% have increased serum LD, AST, ALT).
• CNS in ≤7% of cases
• Endocarditis usually involving aortic valve; principal cause of death.
• Hematologic
    • Decreased WBC occurs with a relative lymphocytosis.
    • ESR is increased in <25% of patients and usually in nonlocalized type of brucellosis.
    • Thrombocytopenia in ≤20% of patients.
    • Anemia appears in <75% of patients often with localized type of disease.

Burkholderia Infection

Due to Gram-negative aerobic nonspore forming bacilli with preference for watery environment.

Glanders

Very rare infection principally of equines due to *Burkholderia* (formerly *Pseudomonas*) *mallei*. Clinical types include acute or chronic suppurative soft tissue, pulmonary, and septicemic forms.

---

[6]Troy SB, et al. Brucellosis in San Diego. Epidemiology and species-related differences in acute clinical presentations. *Medicine* 2005;84:174.
[7]Pappas G, et al. Brucellosis. *N Engl J Med* 2005;352:2325.

Table 15-6. Comparison of Syndromes Due To *Bartonellae*

Syndromes	*Bartonellae*	Special Stains	Serology	Detection*	Comment
Cat scratch disease	*B. henselae*	Direct smear and fluorescent antibody detection. Infrequent	Acute infection: one titer = ≥512, or 4× increase in titer or seroconversion.	Blood culture is rarely positive; requires special techniques. PCR to confirm serology and clinical diagnosis. IgM/IgG EIA has S/S >85%.	EIA may cross react with *Chlamydia* and *Coxiella burnetii*.
Conjunctivitis	*B. henselae*				
Afebrile, "culture-negative" endocarditis	Disseminated *B. henselae, B. quintana,* others			Blood culture positive in 50% of cases.	
Bacillary angiomatosis	Disseminated *B. henselae, B. quintana*	Warthin-Starry stain and culture of tissue biopsy		Blood culture positive in 10%–50% of cases.	Immuno-compromised
Peliosis	Disseminated *B. henselae, B. quintana*				Immuno-compromised
Trench fever (chronic bacteremia)	*B. quintana*		IgM occurs within 1–2 weeks of symptoms; peak by 4 weeks; not detectable >2 weeks. IgG detected >2 weeks, peak by 8 weeks, then persist or decline. Blood culture may require prolonged incubation.	IFA, EIA, immunoblot	
Oroya fever (fulminant bacteremia with hemolysis)	*B. bacilliformis*	Organisms within RBCs seen with Warthin-Starry stain.	Acute infection: one titer = ≥256, or 4× increase in titer.		

*Culture of blood and tissue may require prolonged incubation ≤45 days and special media and techniques.

INFECTIOUS

♦ Culture or animal inoculation of infected material from appropriate sites is performed.
○ Agglutination (titer >1:640 by second week) and CF tests are positive in chronic disease.
WBC is variable.

Melioidosis

Due to *Burkholderia pseudomallei*. Clinical infectious forms include acute suppurative soft tissue, pulmonary, and septicemic.

♦ Culture or animal inoculation of infected material from appropriate sites is performed (e.g., pus, urine, blood, sputum).
♦ Serologic tests

• EIA for IgG antibodies is >90% sensitive and specific; EIA for IgM is 92% sensitive for active disease and can be used to monitor therapy.
• Agglutination test is positive in chronic disease; infection can be inactive for many years. May be negative in fulminant septicemic form.

WBC is normal or increased.
Infection is occasionally transmitted among narcotic addicts using needles in common.

Pseudomonas Infections

Due to *Pseudomonas aeruginosa*, a motile Gram-negative bacillus that prefers moist environments.

Occur in many sites.
Associated With
Replacement of normal bacterial flora or initial pathogen because of antibiotic therapy (e.g., urinary tract, ear, lung)
Burns
Debilitated condition of patient (e.g., premature infants, the aged, patients with leukemia)
♦ Bacteremia is most common in patients with acute leukemia; usually acquired in hospital. Overall mortality ~40%.

• Positive blood culture in 80% of cases.
• Laboratory findings due to associated factors (e.g., shock and pneumonia each occur in one third of patients).
• Shock, pneumonia, persistent neutropenia are each associated with poorer prognosis.

Decreased WBC during bacteremia in patients with leukemia or burns is more frequently caused by Pseudomonas *than to other Gram-negative rods.*

Campylobacteriosis

Usually due to Gram-negative bacteria, *Campylobacter jejuni*; few cases due to *C. coli* and *C. fetus*.

Clinical Types
Disseminated Form Without Diarrhea
Meningitis—occurs in infants less than 2 months old, usually premature or with congenital CNS defects; 50% mortality.
Pediatric bacteremia—rare disorder, usually secondary to malnutrition or diarrhea; usually recover.
Disseminated adult infection—commonly have predisposing conditions (e.g., immunosuppression, malignancy, cardiovascular, endocrine disease, etc.).
♦ • 90% of cases have positive blood culture.
♦ • IHA shows antibody titers of 1:1,600 to 1:6,400 in acute phase and 1:40 to 1:320 six months after cure.
Gastroenteritis
Most common bacterial cause in developed countries.
♦ Stool culture using microaerophilic incubation and selective media
♦ Microscopic examination of stool shows "seagull" organisms. Few to moderate number of WBC

Stools become negative in 3 to 6 weeks even without therapy, but 5% to 10% of patients have organisms in stool for a year or longer.
Blood culture positive in <1% of cases
PCR of stool may become useful.
CF and EIA have good S/S are used epidemiologically. High EIA titer may indicate recent or ongoing infection.

Chancroid

Sexually transmitted disease due to small, Gram-negative, bipolar staining *Haemophilus ducreyi.*

♦ Gram stain of smear from genital ulcer shows bacteria.
♦ Gram stain and cultures of lymph node aspirate are usually negative; only after rupture is culture likely to be positive. Culture requires special media not widely available; sensitivity ≤80%; limited practical value.
○ Biopsy of genital ulcer or regional lymph node may be helpful.
Serologic tests and PCR are not presently available.
Syphilis, AIDS, herpes simplex and granuloma inguinale should be ruled out in ulcerative genital lesions (see separate sections).

Chlamydial Infections

Gram-negative obligate intracellular organisms that require cell culture but classified as bacteria because contain both DNA and RNA.

♦ Serologic tests

• Not useful for superficial infections; 4× rise in antibody titer between acute and convalescent sera or random titer >1:32 may be useful in diagnosis of invasive and systemic infections (e.g., infantile pneumonia, pelvic inflammatory disease, lymphogranuloma venereum).
• Microimmunofluorescence (MIF) to detect specific antibodies; CF is used as an alternative. Primarily used for lymphogranuloma venereum and psittacosis. Not useful for definitive diagnosis in most oculogenital infections.
• In neonates, antibody may be derived from mother rather than caused by neonatal infection. The only syndrome in which serologic tests are method of choice is neonatal pneumonia in which high IgM levels should be diagnostic.

Genital Tract Infection

Sexually transmitted disease due to *Chlamydia trachomatis*; at least 10 major immunotypes. Incidence of chlamydial cervicitis and urethritis is 10× greater than *N. gonorrhoeae* infection. Fifty percent of the latter have concomitant chlamydia infection. Most *C. trachomatis* genital infections are asymptomatic.

See Nonspecific Urethritis, Chapter 14.
♦ DNA probe tests are highly sensitive and specific with rapid turnaround time. Also tests for *N. gonorrhoeae* in same specimen of urine or genital swab. Coexistent *Chlamydiae trachomatis* infection is present in 20% to 60% of cases.
♦ Isolation in cell culture (obligate intracellular pathogen) is the most sensitive (≤90%) and specific (~100%) test but is technically difficult and may not be easily available. Culture requires sample of infected epithelial cells rather than discharges, urine or semen. Longest turnaround time (2–3 days). Is only acceptable method in cases of suspected sexual assault or abuse or when diagnosis is in dispute.
♦ Serologic tests

• Antigen detection provides high S/S by EIA of secretions (>79%/>95%) or staining of smears by direct IF (>90%/>95%) in symptomatic or high prevalence groups; PPV and MPV are >80%, >90% and >87%, >98% respectively.

♦ Giemsa or immunofluorescent staining of scrapings from genital lesions to detect elementary bodies within epithelial cells has low sensitivity but high specificity. Has been replaced by immunologic procedures.

Table 15-7. Comparison of Diagnostic Methods for Chlamydial Species

	Chlamydia trachomatis Trachoma biovar	*Chlamydia trachomatis* LGV biovar	*Chlamydia pneumoniae*	*Chlamydia psittaci*
Disease in Humans	Trachoma, conjunctivitis, ophthalmia neonatorum, infant pneumonia, lymphogranuloma venereum	Lymphogranuloma venereum	Respiratory illness	Psittacosis
Culture in cells show intra-cytoplasmic inclusions	48–72 hrs		5–10 days	Difficult to grow
Microscopic exam of stained smear	Used in conjunctivitis, ophthalmia neonatorum; sensitivity >90%.			Not useful
DIF	Rapid test. Useful for cervical, urethral specimens. Titer usually >1:512.			Not specific
EIA	Lesser S/S than DIF.		Cross reacts with normal respiratory flora.	
CF	Patients usually have titer of ≥1:64 but titer ≤1:16 tends to exclude LGV. Not useful.		4× rise in antibody titer between acute and convalescent sera or random titer >1:32 may be useful in diagnosis of invasive and systemic infections.	
PCR	Can be done on urine (in males) and swabs.		NA.	Respiratory specimens (also for *Mycoplasma pneumoniae*).

DIF, direct immunofluorescence; EIA, enzyme-linked immunoassay; CF, complement fixation; NA, not available.

Diagnosis should be sought and tests performed for:

- All symptomatic patients (e.g., acute urethritis, mucopurulent cervicitis, endometritis, PID, acute proctitis, etc.)
- Asymptomatic women
    Those in various high risk groups
    Those with abnormal vaginal Pap smear
    IV drug abuse
    Pregnant women, specifically screening in cases of premature labor
    Those with high-risk sexual partners
- Tests should be performed on men in appropriate groups if resources permit; otherwise treat empirically.

Reiter syndrome—*Chlamydia trichomatosis* has been isolated from the urethra in ≤60% of men with Reiter syndrome, but tetracycline does not change the clinical course, and etiologic role is speculative. See Chapter 10.

Acute proctitis—see Chapter 7.

Mucopurulent cervicitis—cervical material shows >10 PMNs/HPF (1,000×) in non-menstruating women, positive culture or direct antigen test.

Acute urethral syndrome in women show pyuria with bacteriuria, positive culture or direct antigen test from cervix or urethra.

PID—findings of mucopurulent cervicitis, acute urethral syndrome; endometrium may show positive culture or direct antigen test and endometritis on biopsy.

Perihepatitis may show findings of PID and high titer of IgM (44% of cases) or IgG antibody to *C. trachomatis*.

Increased WBC and ESR in <20% of patients.

Frei test is no longer recommended.

Adult form of inclusion conjunctivitis is associated with genital tract infections.
- ◆ • Typical intracytoplasmic inclusions in epithelial cells on Giemsa-stained smears from conjunctival scrapings are found in 50% of cases. Immunofluorescent staining of inclusions has S/S = 70% to 95%/98% in conjunctival lesions (sensitivity <50% in genital lesions). Inflammatory response shows both neutrophils and mononuclear cells compared to viral conjunctivitis, which shows predominantly lymphocytes and allergic conjunctivitis that shows predominantly eosinophils. Immunofluorescent stains are commercially available and significantly increase sensitivity.
- ◆ • Tissue culture of *Chlamydia* is the most sensitive and specific test and positive cultures are usually detectable within 48 hours. May not be available locally.
- ◆ • Detection of antigen in secretions by EIA or direct immunofluorescent staining of smears.

Distinctive Pneumonia Syndrome of Infants

Afebrile, chronic diffuse lung involvement, slight eosinophilia, and distinctive cough.

The major cause of pneumonia before age 6 months with incidence of 8/1,000 live births.
- ◆ Presence of IgM in infants with pneumonia is diagnostic of *Chlamydia* pneumonia.

Ophthalmia Neonatorum

Occurs in 18% to 50% of infants of mothers with genital infection; fathers often have urethritis.

Trachoma

- ◆ Detection of *Chlamydia* antigen (EIA, DFA) or DNA (PCR) is becoming increasingly useful.
- ◆ Typical cytoplasmic inclusion bodies are in epithelial cells scraped from conjunctiva of upper eyelid (Giemsa stain).
- ◆ Presence of serum IgM or rise in IgG (EIA) replaces CF.

Psittacosis

- ◆ With compatible clinical illness, diagnosis is *confirmed* by

- Culture from respiratory secretions or
- Antibody increase ≥4× (to ≥1:32) by CF or MIF in paired specimens 2 weeks apart or
- IgM detected by MIF titer ≥1:16

◆ With compatible clinical illness, diagnosis is *probable* by

• Single antibody titer by CF or MIF ≥1:32

Positive CF test in early stage is presumptive; is usually also positive with other *Chlamydia* species and sometimes other infections (e.g., brucellosis, Q fever). Rising titer (≥4×) between acute and convalescent sera is diagnostic but not species-specific. MIF is species-specific.

◆ Detection of IgM or rising IgG titer (EIA, IFA) indicates recent infection; IgM can last for 4 weeks after infection. May cross react with *C. trachomatis* and LGV.

Tetracycline treatment can delay or diminish antibody response.

◆ Culture of sputum, pleural fluid or clotted blood may be positive during acute illness before antimicrobial treatment; performed by few laboratories.

Cold agglutination is negative.

Albuminuria is common.

Sputum smear show normal flora.

WBC may be normal or decreased in acute phase and increases during convalescence.

ESR is increased or frequently is normal.

Respiratory Illness

Causes pharyngitis, tonsillitis, sinusitis, pneumonia similar to clinically to infection

Lymphogranuloma Venereum

Sexually transmitted disease.

◆ Nucleic acid amplification tests (e.g., PCR) can use urine specimens; have high S/S useful for screening program.

◆ High (≥1:32) or increasing (4×) CF titers or conversion of negative to positive may indicate recent infection; also present in psittacosis.

◆ Detection of antibody by microimmunofluorescence.

○ Biopsy of regional lymph node shows stellate abscesses.

○ Serum globulin is increased with reversed A/G ratio during period of activity.

Biologically false-positive reaction for syphilis that becomes negative in a few weeks appears in 20% of patients. If titer increases, beware of concomitant syphilitic infection.

WBC is normal or increased <20,000/μL. There may be relative lymphocytosis or monocytosis.

ESR is increased.

Cholera

Water-borne infection due to motile Gram-negative enterotoxigenic strain of *Vibrio comma.*

◆ Motile vibrios identified in "rice water" stool by immunofluorescence, darkfield and phase-contrast microscopy immobilized by specific antisera allows rapid specific diagnosis. Absent WBCs and RBCs.

◆ Stool culture is positive.

◆ Serologic tests

• EIA for antitoxin antibodies shows ≥4× increase in titer in paired sera. Increases by 12 days; may persist for months. Does not occur because of vaccination. May cross-react with some *E. coli* enterotoxins. Not positive with nontoxigenic strains of *V. cholerae.*

• Direct agglutination and vibriocidal antibody tests show ≥4× rise in titer in >90% of patients; vaccination also elicits vibriocidal antibodies. Agglutination detects non-toxigenic strains.

Laboratory findings due to marked loss of fluid and electrolytes

• Loss of sodium, chloride, and potassium
• Hypovolemic shock
• Metabolic acidosis
• Uremia

Table 15-8. Laboratory Methods for Diagnosis of Chlamydial Infection

Method	Application	Sensitivity/Specificity
Tissue culture. Requires special transport media. Results in 2–3 days.	All chlamydia infections. Is only acceptable method for medicolegal cases (e.g., suspected sexual assault or abuse).	Gold standard; most valuable to screen low risk patients. ≤80% sensitivity.
Cytology	Inclusion conjunctivitis, trachoma.	~95% sensitivity.
Serology In neonates, antibody may be derived from mother rather than caused by neonatal infection.	The only syndrome in which serologic tests are method of choice is neonatal pneumonia in which high IgM levels should be diagnostic. Primarily used for lymphogranuloma venereum and psittacosis (4× rise in antibody titer between acute and convalescent sera may be useful). Not for genital or superficial eye infections.	
Complement fixation	*Chlamydia psittaci* infection; not for infantile pneumonia.	
Microimmunofluorescence. Results in 4–6 weeks.	Not widely available; CF is used as alternative. IgM ≥1:16 or single IgG ≥1:512. Pneumonia: 4× increase in acute and convalescent titers.	Sensitivity—50%–90%. Specificity is unknown.
Antigen detection		
Direct fluorescent antibody	Specimens from GU tract, conjunctiva, nasopharynx, rectum.	S/S = 60%–100%/>95%.
Enzyme immunoassay Rapid turn around.	Specimens from GU tract, conjunctiva. Needs confirmation with a blocking antibody to rule out false-positive.	S/S = 48%–98%/>90% from endocervix.
Nucleic acid DNA probes	Method of choice for genital specimens. Not good for urine specimens. Same specimen can be used to test for *N. gonorrhoeae*.	Sensitivity ~85%. Specificity same as direct fluorescent antibody and culture.
Amplification (PCR or ligase chain reaction)	Specimens from GU tract. Method of choice for urine specimens.	S/S = 85%/>95%.

Positive nonculture results should be verified by culture or another nonculture technology.
Data from: Traditional and New Molecular Methods in the Diagnosis of Chlamydia Trachomatis. ASCP Check Sample MPAT 95-3.

Infections Due To Other *Vibrio* Species

Short, curved, aerobic Gram-negative bacilli; at least 10 species are pathogenic for humans; often difficult to classify; most are found in marine or estuarine water.

♦ Diagnosis by culture of appropriate site.
Causes three types of infection:

Gastroenteritis Infection

From eating uncooked seafood, especially oysters or clams. Some (e.g., *V. vulnificus*) may rapidly progress to bacteremia with 50% fatality rate. Due to *V. comma*, others (e.g., *V. vulnificus, V. alginolyticus, V. fluvialis, V. parahaemolyticus*)

Wound Infection and Sepsis

Usually associated with seawater (e.g., while fishing or swimming). Twenty percent mortality rate. Often rapidly progresses to bacteremia. Superficial localized type of wound infection of eyes, ears, skin due to *V. alginolyticus*.

Occurs in presence of pre-existing disease (e.g., *V. vulnificus*)

V. vulnificus septicemia occurs most often (75% of cases) in immunocompromised patients especially with iron overload (e.g., hemochromatosis, thalassemia major, cirrhosis).

Skin

Coliform Bacteria Infections

Escherichia coli is principal species of *Escherichia* genus; Gram-negative, facultatively anaerobic, rod-shaped bacilli. *Klebsiella pneumoniae* are Gram-negative, aerobic bacilli belonging to *Enterobacteriaceae* family. *Enterobacter* species (e.g., *E. cloacae*) of *Enterobacter* genus are Gram-negative, aerobic bacilli.

Bacteremia

Secondary to infection elsewhere; occasionally caused by transfusion of contaminated blood

Secondary to debilitated condition in 20% of patients (e.g., malignant lymphoma, irradiation or anticancer drugs, steroid therapy, cirrhosis, diabetes mellitus)

Early diagnosis and treatment reduces mortality

Polymicrobial in 6% to 21% of cases. Higher mortality than when caused by one organism. Most common sources are GI tract and intravascular. Most often mixed Gram-negative; occasionally Gram-negative and positive; mixed Gram-positive are infrequent.

Gram-negative shock occurs in 20% to 40% of patients.

*   Increased serum potassium
*   Decreased serum sodium
*   Metabolic acidosis
*   Increased serum amylase (decreased renal perfusion)
*   Renal findings due to shock (e.g., oliguria, proteinuria, azotemia, acute tubular necrosis). Renal insufficiency in sepsis without shock may be caused by GN, interstitial nephritis, bacterial endocarditis, etc. (see appropriate separate chapters)
*   Hematologic findings: leukocytosis with shift to left, Döhle bodies, toxic granules, eosinopenia. DIC in 10% of cases, usually associated with shock.
*   Adult respiratory distress syndrome with hypoxemia; tachypnea (an early sign) is usually associated with respiratory alkalosis; metabolic acidosis is much less common and occurrence is usually late.
*   GI manifestations—stress ulcers of stomach with or without bleeding; mild cholestatic jaundice with increased bilirubin (up to 10 mg/dL), mildly increased alkaline phosphatase and increased AST may occur several days before positive blood cultures or clinical recognition of infection.
*   Hypoglycemia is relatively uncommon; hyperglycemia in diabetics may be early clue to infection.
*   Infection is most frequently from GU tract, GI tract, uterus, lung (in that order).
*   *E. coli* is the most frequent organism; it causes the lowest mortality (45%) and the lowest incidence of shock. *Pseudomonas aeruginosa* has the highest mortality (85%). *Klebsiella-Enterobacter*, paracolon bacilli, and *Proteus mirabilis* are intermediate, with 70% mortality.

GU Tract Infection

Seventy-five percent of cases due to *E. coli*.

See Chapter 14.

Wound Infections, Abscesses, etc.

Sepsis Neonatorum

Bacterial infection during the first 30 days of life with primary involvement of blood and, frequently, meninges.

◆ Positive blood culture—*E. coli* and *Klebsiella-Enterobacter* cause ~75% of cases. Group B and Group D streptococci and *Listeria monocytogenes* cause most of the other cases. May also be caused by a large variety of other bacteria. *Incidence of contaminated blood cultures is high in newborns. Negative blood culture does not rule out this condition; should take cultures from umbilical stump, skin lesions, mucous membranes, urine.*
◆ Positive culture of CSF occurs frequently. *There may be no WBC increase early in the course of the disease.*
WBC is variable; leukopenia is often associated with a high mortality.
Anemia and decreased platelets may occur.
Laboratory findings due to involvement of other organs (e.g., kidney, with albumin, cells, or casts increased in urine; liver, with increased direct or indirect bilirubin).

Gastrointestinal and Biliary Tree Infections

Verotoxin-producing *E. coli* (VTEC)—associated with two separate diseases:

• Hemolytic uremic syndrome (HUS) and hemorrhagic colitis.
• O157:H7 (primarily from undercooked beef; also raw milk, apple cider; especially in elderly and children. Most common cause of renal failure in children.

◆ Specific enteropathogenic strains identified by genetic probes (especially O157:H7 serotype). Is an important cause of HUS in children and thrombotic thrombocytopenic purpura in adults. (See Chapter 11) Requires special media. EIA to identify toxin. Latex agglutination to determine O157 antigen.
Enterotoxigenic *E. coli* (ETEC)—toxins cause cholera-like secretory diarrhea in third world countries.
Enteroinvasive *E. coli* (EIEC)—cause inflammation of colon; resembles bacillary dysentery.
Enteropathogenic *E. coli* (EPEC)—diarrhea in infants and children
Appendicitis, cholecystitis, etc.

Pneumonia

One percent of primary bacterial pneumonias due to *Klebsiella* [Friedländer's bacilli], especially in alcoholics.

WBC is often normal or decreased.
◆ Sputum is very tenacious, brown or red ("currant jelly"). Smear shows encapsulated Gram-negative bacilli. (*Gram stain of sputum in lobar pneumonia allows prompt diagnosis of this organism and appropriate therapy.*) Bacterial culture confirms diagnosis.
Bacteremia in 25% of cases of Klebsiella pneumonia.
Laboratory findings due to complications (lung abscess, empyema) or underlying diseases are present.
Rarely chronic lung infection due to Klebsiella simulates TB.

Dysentery, Bacillary

Enteric infection due to Gram-negative nonmotile rods of *Shigella* species; four groups and ~40 serotypes.

• Stool culture is positive in >75% of patients. Rectal swab can also be used.

Microscopy of stool shows mucus, RBCs, and WBCs.
Serologic tests are not useful. EIA and PCR techniques are not in clinical use.
WBC is normal.
Blood cultures are negative.
Laboratory findings due to complications

• Marked loss of fluid and electrolytes (hyponatremia, hypokalemia, hypoproteinemia, hypoglycemia)
• Intestinal bleeding
• Relapse in 10% of untreated patients
• Carrier state
• Acute arthritis—especially untreated disease due to *Shigella shigae* (culture of joint fluid is negative)
• Hemolytic-uremic syndrome may occur in severe infections

INFECTIOUS

Enterococci

There are many different species. Due, principally, to aerobic Gram-negative *Enterococcus faecalis*. Normal inhabitant of bowel.

Endocarditis—causes 5% to 15% of cases of bacterial endocarditis.
Bacteremia
GU tract infection
Intraabdominal and pelvic infections
Others (e.g., neonatal, CNS)
♦ Culture organism from appropriate site.

Gonococcal Infections

Due to Gram-negative cocci *Neisseria gonorrhoeae*.

Genital Infection

See also Sexually Transmitted Diseases, Chapter 14
♦ Gram stain of smear from involved site, especially urethra, prostatic secretions, cervix, pelvic inflammatory disease. Consider smear positive only if intracellular, Gram-negative diploici are found; extracellular, Gram-negative diplococci are considered equivocal, correlate poorly with culture results, and should always be confirmed with culture. Smear is positive in only 50% of asymptomatic patients; asymptomatic patients should always be cultured. *Smear may become negative within hours of antibiotic therapy.* In women, Gram stain has sensitivity of 45% to 65% from endocervical canal and 16% from urethra with >90% specificity; smears from vagina, anal canal and pharynx are not recommended. Gram stain from urethra has S/S >95% in symptomatic men, S/S = 69%/86% in asymptomatic men; from anal canal S/S = 57%/>87%.
♦ Bacterial culture (*use special media such as Thayer-Martin*) is the gold standard; should always be taken at the same time as smear (before beginning antibiotic therapy). In ~2% of male patients, Gram stain of urethral exudate is negative when a simultaneous culture of the same material is positive.
♦ Fluorescent antibody test on smear of suspected material.
♦ Detection of antigen (EIA) in centrifuged sediment of urine has S/S >80%/>97%. Antigen detection is sensitive and specific for urethral infection in men but less sensitive than culture in women. Present methods are useful for screening high-risk patients when distant from the lab and should be considered presumptive. Confirm with culture if medicolegal implications.
♦ DNA probe tests are highly sensitive and specific with rapid turnaround time. Tests for *Chlamydia trachomatis* in some commercial kits. Coexistent *Chlamydia trachomatis* infection is present in 20% to 60% of cases.
♦ DNA amplification (e.g., PCR) are most S/S tests and have rapid turnaround time. Can be used with urine as well as swab specimens.

Proctitis

Is symptomatic in ~5% of cases. See also Chapter 7.
Gram-stained smears are not sufficiently reliable because of presence of nonpathogenic *Neisseria* species; not recommended unless there is mucopurulent exudate.
♦ Bacterial culture on special media (e.g., Thayer-Martin) is required for confirmation; avoid fecal contamination.
Rectal biopsy shows mild and nonspecific inflammation. In a few cases, gram stain of tissue section may reveal small numbers of Gram-negative intracellular diplococci after prolonged examination.
♦ *Rectal gonorrhea accompanies genital gonorrhea in 20% to 50% of women and is found without genital gonorrhea in 6% to 10% of infected women. Therefore, rectal cultures for gonococcus should be taken in all suspected cases of gonorrhea.*

Oropharyngeal Infection

Is present in 10% of women and 20% of homosexual men.

♦ Bacterial cultures are required for diagnosis as gram-stained smears are not sufficiently reliable because of presence of nonpathogenic *Neisseria* species.

Arthritis

Synovial fluid (see Table 10-4)

♦ • Gonococci identified in about one third of patients

• Variable; may contain few WBCs or be purulent

Gonococcal CF test for differential diagnosis of other types of arthritis is not a reliable test in urethritis but may rarely be helpful in arthritis, prostatitis, and epididymitis. Test results become positive at least 2 to 6 weeks after onset of infection and remain positive for 3 months after cure. If test is negative, it should be repeated; two negative tests help to rule out gonococcus infection. False-positive test may occur after gonococcus vaccine has been used. Test is of limited value and is seldom used.
Associated nonbacterial ophthalmitis in ≤20% of patients

Ophthalmitis of Newborn

Acute Bacterial Endocarditis

Bacteremia

Resembles meningococcemia; occurs in 1% to 3% of patients. CNS and cardiac infection occur in 1% of these cases.
Only 40% of blood cultures are positive.
Gram stain of skin lesions may be useful.

Peritonitis and Perihepatitis Following Spread from PID

♦ Cultures should always be done on contacts of known cases of gonorrhea, for suspected extragenital gonorrhea, and to evaluate test of cure. Culture for test of cure should be from all sites cultured before therapy and from both endocervix and anal canal in women 3 to 4 days after treatment; if pharynx culture was positive, at least two posttherapy cultures should be taken from this site because of the difficulty in eradicating from here.

Granuloma Inguinale

Sexually transmitted disease due to Gram-negative intracellular coccobacilli *Calymmatobacterium granulomatis.*

♦ Wright- or Giemsa-stained smears of lesions show intracytoplasmic Donovan bodies in large mononuclear cells in acute stage; they may be present in chronic stages.
♦ Biopsy of lesion shows suggestive histologic pattern and is usually positive for Donovan bodies in acute stage, which may also be seen on crush preparation.
Cultures are not useful for routine diagnosis as cannot be cultured on standard media.
No serologic tests are available.
Serologic tests and dark-field examination for syphilis are negative unless concomitant infection is present.

Haemophilus Influenzae

Due to small, pleomorphic, aerobic nonmotile, fastidious, and Gram-negative coccobacilli; humans are only known hosts.

Strains	Type of Infection
Encapsulated forms (Types a–f particularly Type B) have increased virulence. Types a, c, d, e, and f are similar to nonencapsulated forms Less common.	Associated with invasive disease. Meningitis and pneumonia occur primarily in infants <2 years old. Epiglottitis occurs mainly in children 2–7 years old. Bacteremia, otitis, cellulitis
Nonencapsulated forms (nontypeable)	Bronchitis, sinusitis, otitis media. Bacteremia and meningitis are rare. Occurs in children and adults.

♦ Culture and gram stain from appropriate sites
♦ Positive blood culture in ~50% of patients with meningitis

♦ Latex agglutination can detect Type B bacterial capsular antigen in CSF and urine. Has replaced CIE. (See Chapter 9).

Increased WBC (15,000–30,000/μL) and PMNs.

Presence of nontypeable strain (especially unencapsulated) in CSF may indicate immunodeficiency or defect in meninges.

In community-acquired pneumonia, rule out COPD and AIDS.

Infants >1 year in age commonly have empyema, bacteremia, and meningitis concomitantly; therefore CSF should always be examined in infants with empyema.

Helicobacter Pylori Infections

Due to spiral urease-producing, microaerophilic, Gram-negative rod formerly classified as *Campylobacter pylori*. *H. pylori* is found in ≤95% of persons with duodenal ulcer (except Zollinger-Ellison syndrome), 80% of non-NSAID-induced gastric ulcer, 60% of persons with gastric cancer. Found in >50% of persons over age 50. Independent risk factor for gastric carcinoma and lymphoma.

♦ These tests have >90% sensitivity and good specificity. Except for serology, tests may be false-negative if patients have taken antibiotics, bismuth, or proton-pump inhibitors recently.

Test	Comment
Endoscopic biopsy	Invasive. Expensive. ≥2 specimens are needed for best sensitivity.
Histology, touch Cytology	Histologic demonstration of the organism. Superficial chronic active gastritis is almost characteristic infection even if organism is not identified and absence excludes infection. Exclude or detect cancer. Immunocytochemistry.
Culture	Not routinely for initial diagnosis but after failure of therapy. Use to determine antibiotic resistance. Least sensitive but most specific.
Rapid urease test kit	S/S = 90%/>90%
PCR	Most sensitive. May have false-positive due to poor cleaning of endoscopes. Can also use on gastric juice.
Nonendoscopic tests	Noninvasive
Serology	S/S = >90%. Indicates infection unless antibiotic therapy has been given. Does not distinguish current and past infection. Available in rapid kit form. Titer slowly decreases; can be used after 6–12 months to determine cure limiting its use. Not reliable in children <5 years old.
Urea breath test uses oral ^{14}C- or ^{13}C-labeled urea; radiolabeled CO_2 measured in breath before and after ingestion is produced in presence of *H. pylori* urease.	Useful to indicate successful therapy. Represents global sample of gastric mucosa. Can determine if infection is active. Test of choice to determine cure within 4–6 weeks. Can use in children.
Antigen in stool	Rapid EIA test detects active infection. Use to indicate successful therapy after 1 week. Useful in children.

Some tests presently used in research settings: detection of IgG in saliva, measurement of serum ^{13}C-bicarbonate after ingestion of ^{13}C-labeled urea, stool culture, DNA in saliva or stool.

Routine monitoring for eradication after therapy is not presently recommended unless symptoms recur or ulcer is complicated.

Legionnaire Disease

Due to *Legionella pneumophila*, a faintly staining Gram-negative bacillus that is a facultative aerobic, intracellular, opportunistic pathogen widely disseminated in environment; at least 12 serogroups are known.

♦ Optimal diagnosis combines culture, detection of antigen, and DFA or PCR of sputum, BAL, or pleural fluid.
♦ Urinary antigen assay is S/S = 90%/100% in severe disease but only ~50% sensitive in mild disease; can be detected for weeks following acute illness. Detects only serogroup 1 which accounts for large majority of cases; can provide results in 15 minutes.
♦ Organism may be cultured in 3 to 7 days on special media from pleural fluid, lung biopsy, transtracheal or bronchial aspirate, blood; isolate can then only be identified by special tests (e.g., DFA).
♦ PCR can detect *Legionella* in urine, serum, BAL fluid. Used on clinical specimens or culture material; reported S/S =74%/100%. Detects all species; rapid. Negative result does not exclude diagnosis.
♦ DFA may demonstrate the organism in sputum, pleural fluid, lung, or other tissue within 2 to 3 days of onset of clinical disease; is extremely useful for rapid specific diagnosis (S/S = ≤70%/88%). May be negative with few organisms present in early or mild cases or after antibiotic treatment. Hence negative test is of little value and does not substitute for culture.
♦ IFA (allows detection of IgM versus IgG antibody)
♦ ELISA titers <1:64 are considered negative. Single titers of 1:64-1:256 suggests prior infection at undetermined time. Single IFA titer of >1:256 is strong presumptive evidence. Antibody titers (by IFA, ELISA or agglutination) show 4× increase to 1:128 in two thirds of patients in 3 weeks and all patients in 6 weeks and is evidence of recent infection. Paired acute and convalescent sera is most useful for retrospective diagnosis or epidemiological study but too late for clinical use.
○ Pleural effusion in ≤50% of patients may be bilateral; are usually small exudates; culture and test for antigen (as in urine) should be performed.
Gram stain of sputum is of little use; shows few to moderate number of PMNs; bacteria are not seen because *Legionella* stains poorly in clinical specimens.
Increased WBC (10–20,000/μL) in 75% of cases; leukopenia is a bad prognostic sign.
○ Diagnosis should be suspected in pneumonia patients with decreased serum phosphorus, abnormal liver function tests and bradycardia. Mild to moderate increase of serum AST, ALP, LD, or bilirubin is found in ~50% of patients. Decreased serum phosphorus and sodium occurs in ~50% of patients.
Hypoalbuminemia <2.5 g/dL.
Proteinuria occurs in ~50% of patients; microscopic hematuria.
Renal failure and DIC are unusual complications.
CSF is normal.

Meningococcal Infections
Due to Gram-negative cocci *Neisseria meningitides.*

Clinical syndromes

* In cases of blood stream invasion, ~55% have only meningitis, ~30% have meningitis with meningococcemia, and ~15% have only fulminant meningococcemia without meningitis.
* Meningitis (see Chapter 8)—CSF must be examined in all suspected cases of meningococcal disease; >90% of adults with meningococcal infections have meningitis.
* Waterhouse-Friderichsen syndrome occurs in 3% to 4% of cases (see Chapter 13)

♦ Gram-stained smears of body fluids (e.g., CSF, buffy coat of blood, nasopharynx, skin lesions
♦ Culture (use chocolate agar incubated in 10% CO_2)—blood, CSF, skin lesions, nasopharynx, other sites of infection may take ≤1 week to grow.
♦ Latex agglutination
♦ PCR assay of blood or CSF is most sensitive method and may allow serogroup typing during outbreaks.
CSF (see Table 9-2)

* Markedly increased WBC (2,500–10,000/μL), almost all PMNs
* Increased protein (50–1,500 mg/dL)
* Decreased glucose (0–45 mg/dL)
♦ • Positive smear and culture. Gram stain is diagnostic in 50% to 70% of patients with positive cultures. Pyogenic meningitis in which bacteria cannot be found in smear is more likely to be caused by meningococcus than to other bacteria.

INFECTIOUS

♦ • Detection of antigen by EIA has S/S >80%/>95%; is especially useful if antibiotic therapy has begun before CSF is obtained or if gram stain is negative; detects 10^5 organisms/mL. CIE detects 50 ng/mL of purified polysaccharide of certain serogroups. LA can detect certain serogroups.

Increased WBC (12,000–40,000/μL)
Urine may show albumin, RBCs; occasional glycosuria
Laboratory findings due to complications (e.g., DIC, myocarditis) and sequelae (e.g., subdural effusion)
Laboratory findings of predisposing conditions such as asplenic (e.g., sickle cell anemia) or IgM immunodeficient.

Moraxella (Branhamella) Catarrhalis Infections

Aerobic, gram-negative coccobacilli, formerly *Micrococcus catarrhalis* and *Neisseria catarrhalis.*

Acute Purulent Tracheobronchitis and Pneumonia

♦ Diagnosis is by culture from appropriate site.
♦ Sputum shows many WBCs and intra- and extracellular Gram-negative diplococci.
Increased WBC (~15,000/μL)
May also cause bacteremia (usually with pneumonia), otitis media, or sinusitis.

Pasteurella Multocida Infections

Gram-negative minute coccobacilli; colonize upper respiratory tract and mucous membranes of animals. Human infection usually from dog or cat bites or scratches.

♦ Gram stain and culture of bacteria from appropriate sites (e.g., blood, skin, CSF). WBC is increased.

Pertussis (Whooping Cough)[8]

Most cases are due to Gram-negative *Bordetella pertussis;* ≤30% are caused by *Bordetella parapertussis.*

♦ PCR for detection of *Bordetella pertussis* target (e.g., toxin, Rec A). Much more sensitive than culture; is test of choice. Reported to detect ten organisms, which do not need to be viable. May be positive in asymptomatic persons, especially children. Can distinguish between species.
♦ Detection of antigen on nasopharyngeal smears or serum by DFA allows a presumptive diagnosis; should be confirmed by culture, serology or DNA detection.
♦ Positive cultures from nasopharynx or cough plate in 20% of patients; differentiates organisms; may be positive only during catarrhal and early paroxysmal stage. Nasopharyngeal swab cultures are negative in >50%. Negative blood cultures.
♦ Serologic tests have poor sensitivity; not standardized.

• Serum IgM and IgG (EIA) establishes diagnosis from first sample in 75% of cases; paired sera are needed before 6 months of age. IgM may persist for months after infection or vaccination.
• Direct agglutination (correlates with IgG) usually requires paired acute and convalescent phase sera 2 to 4 weeks apart; persists after illness; insensitive in infants <6 months old.

♦ CDC recommends using culture and PCR at least 3 weeks after onset of cough or 4 weeks after any symptoms appear. After 4 weeks of cough, serologic tests alone are most useful.
○ Marked increase in WBC (≤100,000/μL; usually 12,000–25,000/μL) and ≤90% mature lymphocytes.

[8]Hewlett EL, Edwards KM. Pertussis—not just for kids. *N Engl J Med* 2005;352:1215.

Proteus Infections

Due to aerobic Gram-negative bacilli (e.g., *Proteus vulgaris, P. mirabilis*).

♦ Culture of bacteria from appropriate sites (e.g., blood, skin).
Proteus infections usually follow other bacterial infections.

* Indolent skin ulcers (decubital, varicose ulcers)
* Burns
* Otitis media, mastoiditis
* Urinary tract infection especially with nephrolithiasis
* Bacteremia

Characteristic spreading growth on culture plate may obscure associated bacteria since Proteus infection frequently is part of mixed infection; antibiotic sensitivity testing may not be possible.

Salmonella Infections

Facultative anaerobic Gram-negative rods in Enterobacteriaceae family. Transmitted by food contaminated with animal feces.)

Typhoid Fever

Due to *Salmonella typhi* and *S. paratyphi*. Other nontyphoidal salmonella serotypes usually cause gastroenteritis. *S. typhi* is only present in humans; no animal reservoir.

♦ Diagnosis is based on culture.

* Blood (best if >15 mL) cultures are positive during first 10 days of fever in 90% of patients and during relapse; <30% are positive after third week.
* Bone marrow is more sensitive; positive in 80% to 95% of patients regardless of duration of illness and even if antibiotic treatment for several days.
* Stool cultures are positive after tenth day, with increasing frequency up to fourth or fifth week, in <50% of cases. Positive stool culture after 4 months indicates a carrier; occurs in ~3% of cases.
* Urine culture is positive during second to third week in 25% of patients, even if blood culture is negative.

Serological criteria for diagnosis of ≥4× increase in O titer in unvaccinated patients in nonendemic areas is rarely useful. Serologic diagnosis is unreliable and Widal reaction has been largely abandoned for these reasons:

* Positive Widal test may occur because of typhoid vaccination or previous typhoid infection; nonspecific febrile disease may cause this titer to increase (anamnestic reaction). False-positive results may occur in autoimmune diseases.
* Early treatment with chloramphenicol or ampicillin may cause titer to remain negative or low.
* Increase in O titer may reflect infection with any organism in the Group D salmonellae (e.g., *S. enteritidis, S. panama*) and not just *S. typhosa*.
* Because of differences in commercially manufactured antigens, there may be a 2× to 4× difference in O titers on the same sample of serum tested with antigens of different manufacturers.
* H titer is very variable and may show nonspecific response to other infections; it is, therefore, of little value in diagnosis of typhoid fever.
* >10% of cases in endemic areas are seronegative.
* EIA and DNA probes continue to be developed.

WBC is decreased—4,000 to 6,000/μL during first 2 weeks, 9,000 to 5,000/μL during next 2 weeks; ≥10,000/μL suggests perforation or suppuration.
Decreased ESR is found.
Normocytic anemia is frequent; with bleeding, anemia becomes hypochromic and microcytic.
Laboratory findings due to complications

* Increased serum LD, ALP, and AST are frequent; increased CK occurs in some patients

- Intestinal hemorrhage is occult in 20% of patients, gross in 10%; it occurs usually during second or third week. It is less frequent in treated patients.
- Intestinal perforation occurs in 3% of untreated patients.
- Relapse occurs in ≤20% of patients, usually 1 to 2 weeks after defervescence.

  > Blood culture becomes positive again.
  > Widal titers are unchanged.

- Secondary suppurative lesions (e.g., pneumonia, parotitis, furunculosis) are found.
- Abnormal liver function tests (e.g., serum bilirubin, AST) occur in ~25% of patients as an incidental finding. Hepatitis is the chief clinical feature in ~5% of patients.

Enteritis

♦ Stool culture remains positive for 1 to 4 weeks; occasionally longer.
WBC is normal.

Paratyphoid Fever

Usually due to *Salmonella paratyphi* A or B or to *Salmonella choleraesuis.*

♦ Cultures of blood and stool and decreased WBC show same values as indicated in preceding section.

Bacteremia

Especially due to *Salmonella choleraesuis.*

♦ Blood cultures are intermittently positive.
Stool cultures are negative.
WBC is normal. It increases (≤25,000/μL) with development of focal lesions (e.g., pneumonia, meningitis, pyelonephritis, osteomyelitis).

Local Infections

Meningitis, especially in infants.
Local abscesses with or without preceding bacteremia or enteritis.
One third of patients are predisposed by underlying disease (e.g., malignant lymphoma, SLE). Nontyphoid strains are recognized with increasing frequency as an opportunistic infection in AIDS. Patients with GI salmonellosis at risk for AIDS should be treated with antibiotics even in absence of bacteremia.
Bacteremia and osteomyelitis are more common in patients with sickle hemoglobinopathy. Bacteremia is more common in patients with acute hemolytic Bartonella infection.
Agglutination tests on sera from acute and convalescent cases are often not useful unless present in high titer (>1:560) or rising titer is shown.

Tularemia

Due to *Francisella tularensis,* small, Gram-negative coccobacilli which is primarily an animal pathogen.

Clinical types (frequency)

- Ulceroglandular (75%)
- Typhoidal (25%)
- Overlapping syndromes: Glandular, oropharyngeal, oculoglandular, pneumonic, gastrointestinal, endocardial, meningeal, osteomyelitic, etc.

♦ Detection of tularemia antigens by DFA or IHC staining of appropriate specimens (e.g., lymph node, mucocutaneous lesions, sputum, gastric washings) in reference laboratories permits rapid diagnosis.
♦ ELISA and PCR antigen detection are replacing agglutination tests and allow rapid diagnosis; performed in reference laboratories.
♦ Biopsy of involved tissues shows granulomas (may be caseous); organisms may be seen with silver impregnation bacterial stains or IFA.
♦ Silver impregnation bacterial stains and cultures of suspected material from appropriate sites require special techniques. Cultures should be held at least 10 days.

♦ A single microagglutination titer ≥1:128 or a tube agglutination titer ≥1:160 indicates recent or past infection. A 4× increase in paired titers taken 7 to 10 days apart is diagnostic. Antibodies are demonstrable beginning at 10 days, peak at 4 weeks; both IgG and IgM may persist for years.

WBC is usually normal.

ESR may be increased in severe typhoidal forms; it is normal in other types.

Serum AST is commonly elevated.

Yersinia Infections

Enterocolitis[9]

Enteric infection due to high- or low-virulent strains *Yersinia enterocolitica*, which are facultative anaerobic Gram-negative coccoid bacillus; transmitted primarily by ingestion of contaminated food, milk, and water.

Stool may contain WBCs and RBCs; gross blood in ≤25% of cases.

♦ PCR targeting *ail* gene present only in pathogenic strains.

♦ Stool culture requires special techniques; should be interpreted cautiously because of low-virulence environmental strains not related to human disease; serotyping may be useful to distinguish these.

♦ Serologic tests

• Tube agglutination, ELISA, RIA increase 1 week after onset of symptoms and peak in second week. Titer ≥1:200 present in most cases but 4× increases are rare. Titer ≥1:128 at time of complications is presumptive evidence of yersiniosis. May be useful for retrospective diagnosis in patients with reactive arthritis.

• Limitations
Antibodies may be detected for years after infection.
Cross reactions may occur with *Brucella abortus, Rickettsia* spp., *Salmonella* spp., *Morganella morganii,* and enterohemorrhagic *E. coli.*

Titers ≥1:32 present in ≥1.5% of healthy persons with no previous history of infection.

Laboratory findings due to focal infection in many extraintestinal sites without detectable bacteremia (e.g., pharyngitis, lymphadenitis, liver and spleen abscesses, endocarditis).

Laboratory findings due to reactive disease (e.g., arthropathy, erythema nodosum, Reiter syndrome, myocarditis, glomerulonephritis).

Plague

Due to *Yersinia pestis*, small Gram-negative coccobacilli transmitted from rodents by fleas.

♦ Identify bacteria in stained blood smear (e.g., Wright, Giemsa).

♦ Identify bacteria in gram-stained smear (characteristic "safety-pin"), culture or rapid assay (ELISA, PCR, DFA) of suspected material from appropriate site (e.g., lymph node aspirate, blood, sputum) in government reference laboratories.

♦ Serum may be positive for WB, hemagglutination antibodies, protein microarray analysis. A ≥4× increase in titer or a single titer ≥1:16 is presumptive evidence of infection.

WBC is increased (20,000–40,000/mm^3), with increased PMNs showing toxic granulations.

Laboratory findings due to involvement of organ systems (e.g., lung, liver, septicemia, meninges, DIC).

Variable Gram Stain Reaction

Clostridial Infections

Anaerobic spore-forming, toxin-producing bacilli; gram stain reaction is variable.

[9]Lamps LW, et al. Molecular biogrouping of pathogenic *Yersinia enterocolitica*. Development of a diagnostic PCR assay with histologic correlation. *Am J Clin Path* 2006;1255:658.

INFECTIOUS

Botulism[10]

Due to *Clostridium botulinum* toxins. Clinical types are food, wound, infant, biological warfare.

Usual laboratory tests are not abnormal or useful. CSF is normal.
♦ Diagnosis is made by injecting suspected food, serum, gastric contents, and stool intraperitoneally into mice, which will die in 24 hours unless protected with specific antitoxin.
♦ In addition to serum toxin assay, anaerobic culture of wound exudate or tissue sample or stool should be performed.
♦ Antigen detection is reported to have a high negative predictive value.

Clostridial Gas Gangrene, Cellulitis, and Puerperal Sepsis

Due to *Clostridium perfringens, C. septicum, C. novyi*, and the like that live in soil and animals. Clinical types: Soft tissue and intraabdominal wounds, intestinal food poisoning, pseudomembranous colitis, bacteremia.

♦ Smears of material from appropriate sites show Gram-positive rods, but spores are not usually seen and other bacteria are often also present.
♦ Anaerobic culture of material from appropriate site is positive. *Clostridia are frequent contaminants of wounds caused by other agents. Other bacteria may cause gas formation within tissues.*
WBC is increased (15,000–>40,000/μL).
Platelets are decreased in 50% of patients.
In postabortion sepsis, sudden severe hemolytic anemia is common with hypoglobulinemia, hemoglobinuria, increased serum bilirubin, spherocytosis, increased osmotic and mechanical fragility, etc.
Protein and casts are often present in urine.
Renal insufficiency may progress to uremia.
Laboratory findings due to underlying diseases (diabetes mellitus) or complications (hemolysis).

Tetanus

Due to *Clostridium tetani* toxin.

Diagnosis is clinical.
WBC, urine, CSF, imaging studies are normal.
Identification of organism in local wound is difficult and not usually helpful.
Serologic tests (EIA) are used to assess immunity and to assay immune function by assay of pre- and postimmunization sera. Antibody level $\geq$0.1 IU/mL is protective. Cannot be used for diagnosis.

Pseudomembranous Colitis

Antibiotic/antineoplastic drug-associated diarrhea and colitis due to *C. difficile* toxins A and B.

♦ Toxin detected in stool in >95% of patients with pseudomembranous colitis but may also be found in some asymptomatic patients or those with uncomplicated diarrhea.
• EIA for toxins A and B and cytotoxin B tissue culture assay. S/S= >65%/>75%.

Asymptomatic carrier rates:

• Cystic fibrosis patients = $\leq$50%
• Children 2 years old = 7% to 60%
• Children >2 years old and healthy adults = <4%
• Healthy adults given antibiotics or hospitalized >4 weeks = $\leq$50%
• Elderly persons in acute or chronic care facilities = 14% to 21%.

---

[10]Clostridium botulinum and the Clinical Laboratorian. *Arch Pathol Lab Med* 2004;128:653.

Fecal leukocytes in stool (see Chapter 7)

Recent drug exposure (especially cephalosporin) followed within 8 weeks by onset of diarrhea.

Only test liquid stools should be tested.

Acid-Fast Stain Positive

Leprosy (Hansen Disease)

Chronic infection due to *Mycobacterium leprae* that is of low infectivity; incubation period >3 years. Bacteria accumulate mostly in skin and peripheral nerves.

♦ Ziehl-Neelsen stained bacilli are found in smear or tissue biopsy from nasal scrapings or lepromatous lesions. Acid-fast diphtheroids are not infrequently found in nasal septum smears or scrapings in normal persons, and *M. leprae* is not found here in two thirds of early lepromatous cases. Therefore, nasal smear may have very limited diagnostic value. Bacilli may show a typical granulation and fragmentation that precede the clinical improvement due to sulfone therapy. Larger, more nodular lesions are more likely to be positive. In lepromatous lesions (patients with poor immune response), enormous numbers of bacilli may be present in skin lesions and may be found in peripheral blood smears. Bacilli are usually very difficult to find in skin lesions of tuberculoid leprosy (patients with good immune response).

○ Histologic pattern of the lesions is used for classification of type of leprosy.

○ Number of bacilli (graded 0–6+) in six skin sites is used to measure response to therapy as well as classification.

♦ ELISA is positive in lepromatous but not tuberculoid disease; declines after chemotherapy is initiated.

Laboratory findings due to complications are noted.

○ • Amyloidosis occurs in 40% of patients in the United States.

• Other diseases (e.g., TB, malaria, parasitic infestation) may be present.

• Sterility caused by orchitis is very frequent.

○ False-positive serologic test for syphilis occurs in >10% of patients.

Mild anemia—Sulfone therapy frequently causes anemia, which indicates dosage change is needed.

CRP, ESR and other acute phase reactants are increased.

Serum albumin is decreased, and serum globulin is increased. Thirty percent have cryoglobulinemia.

Serum cholesterol is slightly decreased.

Serum calcium is slightly decreased.

Tuberculosis

Communicable disease caused by *Mycobacterium tuberculosis hominis* or *Mycobacterium tuberculosis bovus;* may be caused by *M. avium* and *M. intracellulare* (MAI) in immunosuppressed persons.

♦ Acid-fast stained smears and cultures of concentrates of suspected material from clinical sites (e.g., sputum, effusions, urine, CSF, pus) should be performed on multiple specimens. Reported sensitivity of smears compared to culture are 22% to 78%; multiple sputum smears more than doubles sensitivity. Acid-fast smears are highly specific but do not differentiate from other mycobacteria species. 10^4 acid-fast bacilli/mL of sputum are required for detection on smear. When sputum is not available or smears are negative, can use gastric aspirates (especially in children), bronchoscopy (especially useful for endobronchial lesions) with bronchial washings, lavage, brushings or transbronchial biopsy, pleural fluid or biopsy. Fluorochrome stain is faster and more sensitive for screening than Ziehl-Neelsen stain.

♦ Culture on conventional solid media (e.g., Lowenstein-Jensen) is required for conventional biochemical tests and nucleic acid probes. Therefore, it should be inoculated along with BACTEC radiometric method within 2 weeks; conventional culture requires ≤10 weeks. Eighty percent to 85% sensitivity in detecting all cases. Culture

INFECTIOUS

is essential for drug susceptibility testing, detection of nontuberculosis mycobacteria, epidemiologic studies, specimen cross-contamination.

♦ Molecular techniques show S/S ~88%/~95%.

• Direct detection of specific mycobacterial DNA by PCR has greater sensitivity (can detect ~10 bacilli/specimen) than Ziehl-Neelsen stain. May also detect mutations that confer rifampin resistance.
• Same-day detection is possible.
• Identify multidrug resistant strains.
• May identify some newly infected persons before tuberculin conversion.
• Nucleic acid probes in cultures are S/S ≤100% except for *M. kansasii*, with identification in 8 days.
• Mycobacterial genus and species identified by DNA probes permits epidemiological surveillance and transmission studies.

♦ Gas-liquid or high-performance liquid chromatography of isolate measures characteristic fatty acids; identifies 90% of mycobacteria rapidly.
♦ Characteristic histologic pattern appears in random biopsy of lymph node, liver, bone marrow (especially in miliary dissemination), or other involved sites (e.g., bronchus, pleura).
♦ Increased adenosine deaminase (>30 U/L) in various body fluids may aid in early diagnosis. >40 U/L has S/S = >91% for TB pericarditis.
♦ Urine—rule out renal TB in presence of hematuria (gross or microscopic) or pyuria with negative cultures for pyogenic bacteria. Routine urine cultures are positive in ~7% of TB patients with normal urinalysis and no GU symptoms.

Laboratory findings due to extrapulmonary TB

• Tuberculous meningitis
   CSF shows
      ♦ Acid-fast smear (positive in 20% of cases) and culture (positive in <75% of cases) from pellicle; detection by PCR is more sensitive 100 to 1,000 WBC/μL (mostly lymphocytes)
   Increased protein (slight in early stages but continues to increase); >300 mg/dL associated with advanced disease; much higher levels when block of CSF occurs.
   Decreased glucose (<50% of blood glucose)
   Decreased chloride is not useful in diagnosis
   Increased tryptophan
   Serum sodium may be decreased (110–125 mEq/L) especially in aged; may also occur in overwhelming TB infection.
   Detection of anti-BCG-IgG by ELISA or of antibody-secreting cells by solid immunospot assay has been reported recently.
      ♦ Detection of mycobacterial antigen and antibody by ELISA provides rapid identification.
   ≤33% of cases have miliary TB
• Miliary TB
      ♦ Sputum smears and cultures positive in 30% to 60% of patients
      ♦ Culture from liver, marrow, urine may be positive
      ♦ Bone marrow is positive in 30% to 70% of cases with miliary TB.
      ♦ Liver biopsy shows granulomas in 50% to 90% of cases with ~10% positive for AFB.
• Tuberculoma
• Tuberculous pleural or pericardial effusions (see Chapter 6)
   Pleural effusions occur in ≤5% of all TB patients, >15% of patients with extrapulmonary TB, and in >20% of TB patients with negative sputum smears.
   Fluid is an exudate with increased protein (>3 gm/dL) and increased lymphocytes.
      ♦ Acid-fast stained smears are rarely positive.
      ♦ Pleural fluid culture is positive in 25% of patients.
      ♦ Tissue biopsy for histology and culture is usually needed for diagnosis.
      ♦ Sputum is positive on culture in ~25% of patients.
• Lymph nodes
      ♦ Culture is important to rule out infection caused by other mycobacteria atypical or anonymous (e.g., *M. intracellulare-avium* in AIDS).

♦ • Positive smear of tissue for AFB by direct microscopy requires ~1,000 to 10,000 mycobacteria/g of tissue.

WBC is usually normal. Granulocytic leukemoid reaction may occur in miliary disease. Active disseminated disease is suggested by more monocytes (10%–20%) than lymphocytes (5%–10%) in peripheral smear.

ESR is normal in localized disease; increased in disseminated or advanced disease. It is not used as index of activity.

Moderate anemia may be present in advanced disease.

Laboratory findings due to complications (see appropriate separate sections):

O • Amyloidosis
O • Addison disease

Laboratory findings due to underlying diseases (e.g., diabetes mellitus, sickle cell anemia, AIDS)

In AIDS, *M. avium* and *M. intracellulare* (MAI) are the major problem (present in 20%–60% of AIDS autopsies) but *M. tuberculosis* is also increased. Fifty percent of active TB in late AIDS cases are extrapulmonary.

♦ Persistent prolonged bacteremia is characteristic; blood culture is sensitive means of diagnosis.

♦ Direct exam of Kinyoun-stain of buffy coat smear may be helpful; marrow cultures are frequently positive. Blood culture is positive in <20% of AIDS patients with CD4 count >100/μL but in ≤50% of cases with CD4 <100/μL. May involve lymph nodes, spleen, liver, GI tract, lung, and brain. *All patients with TB should be tested for HIV coinfection.*

Environmental Mycobacteria

Soil and water are reservoir for these organisms in contrast to *M. tuberculosis* which is an obligate human pathogen.

	Diagnosis	Comment
	Takes acid fast, weak Gram-positive, fluorescence stains. Culture at lower incubation temperature; single positive unconfirmed culture is not sufficient to diagnose disease. Should be heavy smear-positive or heavy culture-positive of sputum or BAL or three positive cultures over 1 year regardless of smear positivity. PCR is not yet commercially available. HPLC identifies mycolic acid patterns from uncultured specimens.	
Pulmonary disease Common	Histology	
M. kansasii M. avium intracellulare (MAI)	Positive culture, absence of other etiologic agents, compatible clinical picture. DNA probe to detect RNA.	Rarely a contaminant.
M. chelonae Rare M. xenopi M. szulgai M. fortuitum M. simiae	Lung biopsy may be needed.	
AIDS-associated MAI	May be found in many sites (e.g., lymph nodes, blood, marrow, liver, spleen, GI tract). Histology	Disseminated infection in ~50% of AIDS cases relatively late; CD4 count usually <100/μL. Most common bacterial infection in AIDS.
Lymphadenitis Common	Histology	
MAI M. scrofulaceum		95% involve unilateral cervical nodes; most common in 2–5-year-old children.

INFECTIOUS

Rare
  M. kansasii
  M. fortuitum
  M. chelonae

Cutaneous	Culture of skin biopsy. Histology	
Common		
M. marinum	Incubate culture at low temperature (28°C–30°C).	Swimming pool granuloma
M. fortuitum	Culture skin biopsy	Postsurgical or environmental wound contamination
M. chelonae		

Rare
  M. avium complex
  M. kansasii
  M. smegmatis
  M. haemophilum

Bacteria That Lack a Cell Wall

Mycoplasma Pneumoniae Pneumonia

Small aerobic coccoid bacteria lacking a rigid cell wall. Epidemics every 4–6 years; also endemic and sporadic.

♦ Serologic tests are preferred tests. Many kits are available.

- IgM increases in first week, peaks in third to fifth week, begins to decrease in 4 to 6 months, and may persist ≤1 year. S/S = 75% to 80%/80% to 90%; may also be associated with other infections, neoplastic and connective tissue diseases.
- IgG peaks in ~5 weeks; not found in first week; increases for 3 to 4 years; indicates previous exposure.
- Presence of IgM (>1:64) or 4× rise in IgG indicates recent infection.
- CF measures mostly IgM; begins to rise in 7 to 10 days, peaks in 4 to 6 weeks. A 4× increase in CF titer occurs in ~50% of patients; if only a convalescent serum is available, a single titer ≥1:32 has sensitivity = 89%. False-positive results may occur in acute inflammatory diseases (e.g., bacterial meningitis), autoimmune disorders, other mycoplasma infections.
- IFA has S/S = 78%/92%, PPV = 57%.
- EIA depending on kit may measure IgM or IgM and IgG. Should be performed in acute and convalescent (1–3 weeks) sera.
- Antigen detection by immunoblotting, RNA by hybridization, and PCR may not be routinely available. Detection by PCR may not indicate current disease; serologic tests should be used to distinguish acute from persistent infections.
- Increased cold hemagglutination (IgM autoantibody that agglutinates I antigen on RBCs at 4°C) occurs late in course in ≤75% of patients; becomes positive at about seventh day, rises to peak at 4 weeks, then disappears by 5 months. Poor S/S (<50%). Not helpful diagnostically. Also occurs in infectious mononucleosis.
- Increased streptococcal MG agglutination occurs in 25% of patients; higher titer in more severe illness.

♦ Culture of organism from sputum, nasopharynx, etc. by special techniques may require 7 to 10 days. S/S = >90%/50% to 90%. Isolates need DNA probe for speciation. Difficult to interpret as it may persist in throat following infection. Limited availability.

WBC is slightly increased (in 25% of patients) or is normal.

ESR is increased in 65% of patients.

Mycoplasma pneumoniae may cause encephalitis; implicated in immune-mediated diseases (e.g., Guillain-Barré syndrome, transverse myelitis).

Mycoplasma hominis may cause pyelonephritis, PID, and postpartum febrile complications (see Chapter 14). *Mycoplasma* infection should also be considered in the differential diagnosis of acute arthritis, hemolytic anemia, various dermatologic disorders, myocardial or cerebral disease, as well as severe bilateral pneumonia.

Ureaplasma Urealyticum

Small aerobic coccoid bacteria lacking a rigid cell wall associated with PID, amnionitis and perinatal morbidity, and mortality and GU tract in males.

♦ Culture of organism by special techniques may require 7 to 10 days.

Spirochetal Infections

Syphilis

Chronic disease due to spirochete *Treponema pallidum;* usually sexually transmitted or congenital.

See Figures 15-1 through 15-3.

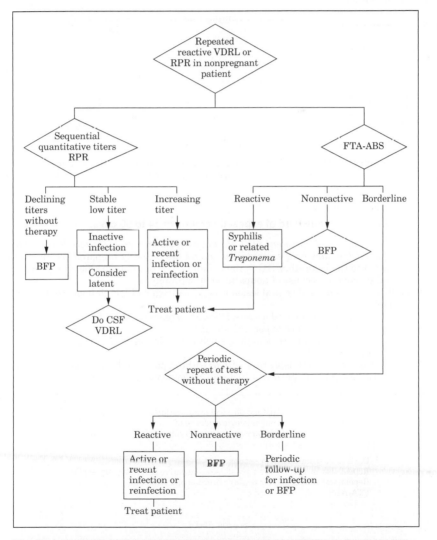

Fig. 15-1. Algorithm for positive serologic test for syphilis. Rule out underlying causes of biologic false-positive (BFP). RPR, rapid plasma reagin test.

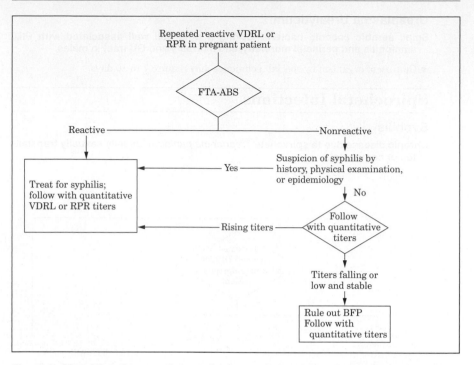

Fig. 15-2. Algorithm for reactive serologic test for syphilis in the pregnant patient. BFP, biologic false-positive; FTA-ABS, fluorescent treponemal antibody absorption test; RPR, rapid plasma reagin test.)

Primary Syphilis

Occurs in about one third of exposed persons in 14 to 90 days.

- ♦ *Direct immunofluorescent (IF) staining of smears from lesion has essentially replaced the dark-field examination* and allows properly prepared specimens to be mailed to the laboratory. S/S = 100%. Can use IF, but not dark-field examination on oral specimens because of nonpathogenic saprophytes.
- ♦ If IF examination of genital lesion is negative, regional lymph node aspirate may be used.

Is particularly useful on oral lesions. *IF will be negative if there has been recent therapy with penicillin or other treponemicidal drugs.*

- ♦ PCR on genital ulcers can simultaneously detect *Haemophilus ducreyi* and HSV (not in United States.)
- ♦ Serologic test shows rising titer with or without positive IF examination. VDRL does not become positive until 7 to 10 days after appearance of chancre.

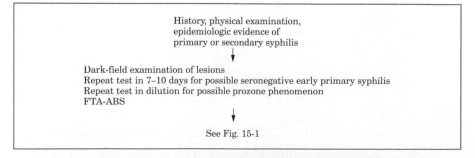

Fig. 15-3. Algorithm for nonreactive serologic test for syphilis in the nonpregnant patient. FTA-ABS, fluorescent treponemal antibody absorption test.

Table 15-9. Comparison of Different Stages of Syphilis

Stage	Symptom	Time after Exposure	VDRL, RPR	FTA-ABS*	MHA-TP*	EIA for IgM	WB for IgM	WB for IgG
Primary	Darkfield on chancre. Lymph node.	11–90 days (Av = 3 w) Av = 4 w	Poor sensitivity. Rising titers.	Sensitivity >80%. To confirm or instead of VDRL or RPR.		Confirmatory test especially in untreated primary syphilis.		
Secondary	Darkfield on skin, mucous membranes lesions.	6–20 wks	Peak titers. For screening. False + = <1%. Must use confirmatory tests.	To confirm positive VDRL or RPR.		Not useful since IgM declines in a few wks.		Confirmatory test; S/S ≤100%.
Latent	NA	Early: 3–12 mos. Late: >12 mos.	Screening test.	Confirmatory test; sensitivity ≤100%. Decreased in late latent.	Confirmatory test; sensitivity ≤100%.	Confirmatory test; sensitivity ≤100%.		Confirmatory test.
Late	NA	Usually >4 y.	Screening blood test. CSF VDRL diagnoses CNS neurosyphilis but negative does not rule it out.	FTA may still be useful to rule out neurosyphilis.		Not useful as IgM levels are low.		Can use to confirm positive RPR or VDRL. Sensitivity ≤100%.
Congenital	NA	Immediately	Test useless as maternal IgG crosses placenta.	Use modified FTA-ABS that measures IgM.	Test useless as maternal IgG crosses placenta.	Diagnostic as IgM does not cross placenta.		Test useless as maternal IgG crosses placenta.

Treponema pallidum particle agglutination (TPPA) test has replaced the microhemagglutination test (MHA-TP) and is the only confirmatory test for a positive VDRL or RPR.
If TPPA is negative and RPR is positive, is a false-positive RPR.
FTA-ABS, fluorescent treponemal antibody absorption test (does not distinguish syphilis from yaws or pinta);
MHA-TP, microhemagglutination assay for *Treponema pallidum* (does not distinguish syphilis from yaws or pinta);
EIA, enzyme immune-assay; WB, western blot; NA, not applicable.

INFECTIOUS

♦ Biopsy of suspected lesion for histologic examination using silver stain or DFA-Tp may be useful in certain seronegative cases (e.g., HIV infections).

Secondary Syphilis

Dissemination occurs.

♦ Dark-field or IF examination of mucocutaneous lesions is positive.
♦ Serologic tests are almost always positive in high titer (>1:32).
Prozone reaction may cause false-negative test.

Latent Syphilis

No symptoms or signs of syphilis within 12 months.

♦ A positive serologic test is the only diagnostic method.

Congenital Syphilis

Nearly all infants born of mothers with primary and secondary syphilis will have congenital infection; 50% will be clinically symptomatic.

♦ IF examination of mucocutaneous lesions or scraping from moist umbilical cord is positive.
♦ Nontreponemal *test may be positive because of maternal antibodies but without congenital syphilitic infection.* Titer ≥4× maternal titer or rising (4×) titer or a stable titer at age 3 months establishes diagnosis of congenital syphilis If mother has been adequately treated during pregnancy, infant's titer falls steadily to nonreactive level in 3 months because passively transferred antibodies should not be detected after 3 months. If mother acquires syphilis late in pregnancy, infant may be seronegative and clinically normal at birth and then manifest syphilis 1 to 2 months later.
Because infection may occur as early as ninth week of gestation, high risk women should be tested during first and third trimesters. In early congenital syphilis, treatment causes VDRL to become nonreactive. After age 2 years, titer decreases slowly but may never become nonreactive.
Only the quantitative VDRL is recommended for the diagnosis of congenital syphilis (performed serially to detect rise or fall in titers).
At delivery, use maternal blood rather than cord blood for screening because of false-positive (due to Wharton jelly) and false-negative (due to infection acquired late in pregnancy) reactions.
♦ IgM immunoblotting and PCR can detect syphilis in newborns (*New Eng J Med* 2002;346:1792).

Tertiary Syphilis

Usually becomes evident 10 to 25 years after primary infection.

CNS (see Table 9-1)

♦ • VDRL on CSF is highly specific but lacks sensitivity (40%–60%); therefore, it should be used to rule in not rule out neurosyphilis. VDRL cannot be used to follow response to therapy. VDRL is the only accepted serologic test for CSF specimens.
Meningitis

• ≤2,000 lymphocytes/µL

♦ • Positive serologic test in blood and CSF

Meningovascular disease

• Increased cell count (≤100 mononuclear cells/µL) in 60% of cases
• Increased protein (up to 260 mg/dL) in 66% of cases; increased γ-globulin in 75% of cases
♦ • Positive serologic test in blood and CSF
• Laboratory findings due to cerebrovascular thrombosis

Tabes dorsalis

• Early—increased cell count and protein
• Positive serologic test in blood and CSF (titer may be low).

- Increased γ-globulin is less marked than in general paresis.
- Late— ~25% of patients may have normal CSF and negative serologic tests in blood and CSF

General paresis (CSF always abnormal in untreated patients)

- Increased cell count ≤175 mononuclear cells/μL
- Increased protein ≤100 mg/dL with marked increase in γ-globulin
- ◆ • Positive serologic test (titer usually high)
- CSF cell count should return to normal within 3 months after therapy; otherwise retreatment is indicated.

◆ Asymptomatic CNS lues

- May have negative blood and positive CSF serologic test
- Increased cell count and protein are index of activity.

◆ Cardiovascular syphilis-VDRL is usually reactive but titer is often low
◆ Gummatous lesions-VDRL is almost always reactive, usually in high titer
    Involvement of other organs (e.g., liver, skin, bone)
◆ Biopsy of skin, lymph node, larynx, testes, etc.
Adequately treated primary and secondary syphilis usually show decreasing titer and become serologically nonreactive in about 9 and 12 months, respectively; 2% of patients remain positive for several years. Therapy causes a negative reagin test in 75% of patients with early latent syphilis in 5 years, but <25% of patients with late syphilis become nonreactive although titers may fall steadily over a long period.
◆ PCR has been used to detect treponemal DNA in CSF and amniotic fluid.

Serologic Tests for Syphilis

Nontreponemal Tests (e.g., VDRL, RPR, ART) detect IgG and IgM antibodies to a cardiolipin-lecithin-cholesterol antigen.

Use and Interpretation
Routine screening of asymptomatic persons. Simple, convenient; frequent local requirement for premarital and prenatal serology. False-positive rate of 1% to 2% in pregnant women.
Diagnosis of symptomatic infection. Does not become positive until 7 to 10 days after appearance of chancre.

- High titer (>1:16) usually indicates active disease.
- Low titer (≤1:8) indicates biologic false-positive (BFP) test in 90% of cases or occasionally due to late or late latent syphilis.

Following titers to determine effect of therapy. Quantitation of VDRL should always be performed before onset of treatment.

- A 4× decrease in titer indicates response to therapy. Treatment of primary syphilis usually causes progressive decline (2-tube at 6 months, 3-tube at 12 months, 4-tube at 24 months) to negative VDRL within 2 years. Treatment of secondary syphilis usually causes 3-tube decline at 6 months and 4-tube decline at 12 months. In early latent syphilis, may not show 2-tube decline until 12 months. In secondary, late, or latent syphilis, low titers persist in ~50% of cases after 2 years despite fall in titer; this does not indicate treatment failure or reinfection and these patients are likely to remain positive even if retreated. Titer response is unpredictable in late and latent syphilis. First infections are more likely to serorevert than repeat infections. Falling titer indicates response to treatment. Adequate treatment of primary and secondary syphilis should cause a 4× decline in titer by fourth month, and a 8× decline by eighth month. Treatment of early syphilis usually results in little or no reaction after 1 year.
- Rising titer (4×) indicates relapse, reinfection or treatment failure and need for retreatment.

Differentiation of congenital syphilis from passive transfer of maternal antibodies.
Interferences
May be nonreactive in early primary, late latent, and late syphilis (~25% of cases)
VDRL may be nonreactive in undiluted serum in presence of an actual high titer ("prozone" phenomenon) in 1% of patients with secondary syphilis.

INFECTIOUS

Reactive and weakly reactive tests should always be confirmed with FTA-ABS. One third of patients with only weakly reactive VDRL are reactive with more sensitive test.

Twenty percent or fewer of reactive screening tests may be BFP. Two thirds of these are low titer (<1:8) and revert to normal within 6 months.

Acute (<6 months duration) false-positive tests may occur in the following cases:

* Various acute viral illnesses (e.g., infectious mononucleosis, hepatitis, measles)
* *Mycoplasma pneumoniae*
* Chlamydia
* Malaria
* Some immunizations
* Pregnancy (rare)

Chronic (>6 months duration) false-positive tests may occur in:

* 50% are shown to have syphilis or other treponemal infections.
* 25% have serious underlying disease (e.g., collagen vascular diseases, leprosy, malignancy).
* BFP occurs in 20% to 25% of IV drug users.
* >20% of patients with BFP also show positive tests for RA, antinuclear antibodies, antithyroid antibodies, cryoglobulins, elevated serum gamma globulins; they may show ITP, autoimmune hemolytic anemia, antiphospholipid syndrome, Sjögren syndrome, AIDS, thyroiditis.
* ≤10% of patients over age 70 may show BFP.
* Some antihypertension drugs

Treponemal Tests

Uses treponemal antigen.

Use and Interpretation

To confirm nontreponemal tests that conflict with clinical findings (i.e., to distinguish true from false-positive nontreponemal tests).

Diagnosis of late syphilis when nontreponemal tests may be negative.

Not to be used for screening.

Are qualitative tests that cannot be used to monitor efficacy of treatment. Are less likely to become negative because of treatment than nontreponemal tests.

Nonreactive test generally indicates no past or present infection unless treated in early primary stage when 10% to 25% will be nonreactive 2 to 3 years later. One percent are false-positive (same percent as nontreponemal).

Passively transferred antibodies disappear from noninfected infant in 6 to 8 months but persist in congenital syphilis.

Interferences

Positive in presence of antibodies of related treponematoses (e.g., yaws, pinta, bejel). Once antibodies develop, they may remain positive despite therapy. (This is the mechanism for one type of BFP.)

If therapy is given before antibodies develop, these tests may never be positive.

TPI (Treponemal pallidum immobilization) has been replaced by these tests:

* **MHA-TP** (microhemagglutination), **TP-PA** (particle agglutination), and **HATTS** (hemagglutination treponemal test)

Compares well with FTA-ABS in S/S as a confirmatory test with fewer false-positive reactions but is less sensitive in early primary syphilis. Sensitized or unsensitized cells may occasionally be reactive with sera from patients with SLE, autoimmune diseases, viral infections, leprosy, drug addicts.

* **FTA-ABS-IgG (Fluorescent treponemal antibody absorption)**

Use

Test of choice to confirm VDRL or confirmation of diagnosis (e.g., BFP).

Most sensitive and specific test.

More sensitive than MHA-TP in primary syphilis; parallels findings in other stages.

If late syphilis of any type is suspected, always do FTA-ABS, even if VDRL is nonreactive.

Table 15-10.   Sensitivity/Specificity for Serologic Tests for Syphilis

	Sensitivity (%)			
	Primary	Secondary	Latent	Specificity (%)
VDRL slide	78 (74–87)	100	98 (85–100)	98 (96–99)
RPR card	86 (77–99)	100	96 (88–100)	98 (93–99)
FTA-ABS	84 (70–100)	100	100	87 (84–100)
TP-PA	90–100			50–100

From CS Hall, JD Kllausner. Diagnostic Tests for Common STDs and HSV-2. *MLO*. Feb 2004;pg. 10.

Titers are not correlated with clinical activity.

Remains positive indefinitely in ~95% of patients reflecting previous infection any time in past, except for early primary syphilis.

Not used to document adequacy of treatment, as remains positive for 2 years after adequate therapy in 80% of cases of seropositive early syphilis; thus, a positive test does not separate active from inactive disease.

Not done on CSF.

Beaded pattern is common in collagen diseases (e.g., SLE) but is considered negative for syphilis.

No longer recommended for early detection of congenital syphilis in infants because of passive transfer of IgG across placenta; for these cases, FTA-ABS-IgM is used, which has 35% false-negative and 10% false-positive rate.

Nonsyphilitic Spirochetal Diseases

Chronic skin diseases transmitted by human skin contact. Yaws is caused by *T. pallidum pertenue*, pinta is caused by *T. carateum*.

♦ Dark-field microscopy of early skin lesions.
♦ Serologic tests (e.g., VDRL) are positive after 2 weeks (see Syphilis).

Leptospirosis

Zoonosis most frequently due to spirochetes *Leptospira icterohaemorrhagiae*, *L. canicola*, *L. Pomona*, *etc.* after exposure to mammal-contaminated body fluids (especially urine), water, or soil.

♦ PCR can quickly establish diagnosis; most sensitive and specific test especially in early stage. Also useful for epidemiologic studies.
♦ Blood and CSF cultures may be positive during first 10 days of disease in ≤90% of patients. Urine cultures may be positive after first week and only intermittently; are difficult because of contamination and low pH; rarely positive after the fourth week. Special culture techniques are needed.
♦ Serologic tests

• ELISA to detect IgM may be positive in 4 to 5 days. An increasing titer (≥4× in 2 weeks) is diagnostic.
• Microscopic agglutination test shows 4× increase between acute and convalescent sera. Probable positive is titer ≥200:1. Is standard for serologic diagnosis but difficult to perform and not widely available (refer to CDC via State Health Departments).
• CF has been used for screening; may become positive in 10 to 21 days; positives should be confirmed by agglutination because of cross-reaction with HAV, CMV, scrub typhus and mycoplasma antibodies.

○ Characteristic morphology and motility by dark field or phase-contrast must be confirmed by serology, culture, or immunofluorescence.

Normochromic anemia is present.

WBC may be normal or ≤40,000/μL.

ESR is increased.

INFECTIOUS

Urine is abnormal in 75% of patients: proteinuria, WBCs, RBCs, casts.
Liver function tests are abnormal in 50% of patients.

* Increased serum bilirubin, ALP, reversed A/G ratio
* Increased AST and ALT, but average levels are not as high as in viral hepatitis

○ *Increased CK-MM in one third of patients during first week may help to differentiate condition from hepatitis.*
○ CSF is abnormal in cases with meningeal involvement (up to two thirds of patients)

* Increased cells (≤500/μL), chiefly mononuclear type
* Increased protein (≤80 mg/dL)
* Glucose and chloride normal
* Organisms are not found in CSF.

Dark-field examination of body fluids is not helpful.
Laboratory findings due to complications (e.g., renal failure, hemorrhage).

Lyme Disease

Due to spirochete *Borrelia burgdorferi*; primary tick vector is *Ixodes scapularis* in the northeast United States and *I. pacificus* in the western United States.

Stage 1: About 1 week (varies 3–33 days) after tick bite; nonspecific febrile "viral syndrome;" ≤85% have characteristic erythema migrans ("target") rash. Serologic test is not helpful or necessary at this stage since only 40% to 60% sensitive at this stage and diagnosis is not ruled out by a negative test. Early antibiotic therapy often prevents antibody response. Antibiotic therapy is critical to prevent long-term involvement of various organs.

Stage 2: About 4 weeks after tick bite, ~5% develop cardiac involvement (causes most deaths); 15% have neurologic findings (triad of aseptic fluctuating meningoencephalitis, Bell palsy, and peripheral neuropathy is very suggestive).

Stage 3: Six weeks to several years after tick bite; occurs in 60% of untreated cases, principally as arthritis frequently mistaken as juvenile RA.

Reinfection causing recurrence of clinical disease is recognized.

♦ **Diagnostic Criteria**

Isolation of organism from clinical specimen *or*
Diagnostic titers of IgG and IgM in serum or CSF *or*
Significant change in serum titers of IgG or IgM in paired acute- and convalescent-phase.

♦ **Serologic tests**

Should be ordered *only* to support clinical diagnosis; not for screening persons with nonspecific symptoms. Serological tests have poor S/S. Are generally not clinically useful if pretest probability is <0.20 or >0.80; if <0.20, positive ELISA is more likely to be false than true-positive; if >0.80, positive ELISA rules in diagnosis of Lyme disease.

Recommended protocol is ELISA (S/S = 89%/72%) or IFA that should be followed by WB. Assay for IgM, IgG or both.

A positive serology does not necessarily indicate current infection or establish the diagnosis and a negative serology, especially within 2 weeks of onset of symptoms, should not be only basis for excluding diagnosis.

Vaccination produces seropositivity.

Specific IgM antibodies usually appear 2 to 4 weeks after erythema migrans, peak after 3 to 6 weeks of illness, decline to normal after 4 to 6 months; only positive in 40% to 60% of stage 1 cases. In some patients, IgM remains elevated for many months or reappears late in illness which predicts continued infection. IgM titer ≥1:200 is considered positive, IgM titer = 1:100 is considered indeterminate. IgM <1:100 is considered negative. A negative test within 2 weeks of onset of symptoms does not rule out infection.

IgG titers rise more slowly (appear ~4–8 weeks after rash), peak after 4 to 6 months, may remain high for months or years, even with successful antibiotic therapy.

Almost all patients with complications of stage 2 and 3 have positive IgG on first specimen. A single increased IgG titer only indicates previous exposure but not timing of infection or cause of current symptoms. IgG titer ≥1:800 is considered positive, 1:200 to 1:400 is indeterminate, and 1:100 is considered negative.

Paired acute and convalescent sera at 4 to 6 week intervals showing conversion or significant rise in titer indicates infection and is principally useful for ill patients without a known tick bite or rash who have been in endemic area.

Interferences (ELISA)

Rheumatoid factor may cause false-positive result for IgM.

False-positive IgG in high titers may be caused by antibodies from spirochetal diseases (syphilis, relapsing fever, yaws, pinta); low titers may be found in infectious mononucleosis, hepatitis B, autoimmune diseases (e.g., SLE, RA), periodontal disease, ehrlichia, rickettsia, other bacteria (e.g., *Helicobacter pylori*), and 5% to 15% of normal persons in endemic areas.

Low concordance between test kits.

Western Blot (WB) is more sensitive and specific than ELISA and is used to distinguish true- and false-positive ELISA, to confirm an indeterminate ELISA, or for an undiagnosed antibiotic-treated patient and is the present gold standard; positive WB indicates past or current infection. However, WB may not become positive until after many months of illness; negative WB should be repeated in 2 to 4 weeks if Lyme disease is strongly suspected. Test is expensive, has limited availability, technically difficult, not standardized, and has many cross-reacting antibodies.

True seronegativity is uncommon with disseminated or chronic Lyme disease. Serologic tests cannot judge therapy efficacy or test of cure (unlike VDRL in syphilis). Absence of titer does not rule out Lyme disease.

♦ PCR to identify specific DNA in blood, CSF, skin biopsy, urine is usually not helpful except in joint fluid and synovial tissue.

♦ Culture is usually not useful clinically as it may take several weeks; organism is infrequently found even using special stains in known positive tissues. Low yield except in biopsy of erythema migrans lesions (60%–80% sensitivity) which is rarely necessary.

T-cell proliferative assay needs further evaluation.

Organism is not detected in peripheral smears.

Laboratory findings due to organ involvement

- Neurologic: 80% with meningitis may show increased lymphocytes (≤450/μL), increased protein and IgG, oligoclonal bands, normal glucose. May have encephalitis (tends to involve white matter), myelitis, radiculitis, cranial or peripheral neuritis in various combinations.
    - ♦ Intrathecal antibody may be demonstrated by higher titer in CSF than serum. IgG and IgM may be present in CSF but not in serum. Almost all of these patients will have positive serum serologic tests.
- Arthritis: Joint fluid may show increased WBC (up to 34,000/μL), PMNs (≤96%), and protein (up to 6.6 gm/dL). Most with Lyme arthritis are seropositive.
    - ♦ Lyme antibodies in fluid differentiates this from other arthritides. PCR on synovial fluid has sensitivity = 23% to 45% (median = 65%). Culture is insensitive.
- Anicteric hepatitis
- Diffuse fasciitis with eosinophilia

Nonspecific findings of mild increase of ESR, lymphopenia, cryoglobulinemia, mild increase of
AST, increased serum IgM, etc.

FTA-ABS may be positive, but nontreponemal tests (VDRL, RPR) should be nonreactive.

Morphologic changes in tissues are not specific.

Coinfection with babesiosis may occur.[11]

Relapsing Fever

Spirochetal infections that are endemic due to *Borrelia hermsii* transmitted by Ornithodoros tick or epidemic due to *Borrelia recurrentis* transmitted by human body louse.

[11]Tugwell P, Dennis DT, Weinstein A, et al. Laboratory evaluation in the diagnosis of lyme disease. *Ann Int Med* 1997;127:1109.

INFECTIOUS

♦ Identification of organism by
>   Wright stain of peripheral blood smear or buffy coat or dark-field or phase-contrast
>   microscopy of plasma wet mounts (platelet fraction) during febrile episode.
>   Intraperitoneal injection of guinea pigs or mice
>   Culture on special medium is most specific but is not widely performed

Serologic tests are not routinely available

- A 4× rise in titer between acute and convalescent sera.
- IFA using monoclonal antibody has been reported.
- Biologic false-positive serologic test for syphilis in ≤25% of patients

Increased WBC (10,000–15,000/μL); moderately increased ESR; thrombocytopenia
Protein and mononuclear cells sometimes increased in CSF
Laboratory findings due to complications (e.g., DIC, rupture of spleen, secondary infection)

Laboratory Tests for Rickettsial Infections

Gram-negative obligate intracellular bacteria transmitted by arthropod vectors.

♦ Indirect immunofluorescence (IFA) or ELISA detection of rickettsial-specific IgG
and IgM. ELISA is more sensitive and specific for IgM and is now the test of choice;
specimens taken at 3- to 4-day intervals will show seroconversion.

♦ CF or agglutination tests are positive in most cases when group-specific and type-
specific rickettsial antigens are used. These tests permit differentiation of various
rickettsial diseases. No test is available for trench fever. Rising titer during convalescence is the most important criterion. Early antibiotic therapy may delay appearance of antibodies for an additional 1 to 4 weeks, and titers may not be as high as
when treatment is begun later. Low titers of CF antibodies may persist for years. CF
is less sensitive than IFA.

Weil-Felix reaction to *Proteus vulgaris* strains OX-2 and OX-19 has poor S/S; replaced
by ELISA.

Guinea pig inoculation—scrotal reaction following intraperitoneal injection of blood
into male guinea pig. Test is not often used at present.

- Marked in Rocky Mountain spotted fever and endemic typhus
- Moderate in boutonneuse fever
- Slight in epidemic typhus and Brill-Zinsser disease
- Negative in scrub typhus, Q fever, trench fever, and rickettsialpox

♦ Microscopic examination of organisms following animal inoculation; test is not often
used.

In less severe cases, blood findings are not distinctive.
In severe cases, the following changes are found:

- Early in disease WBC is decreased and lymphocytes are increased (usually
  4,000–6,000/μL; as low as 1,200/μL in early scrub typhus). Later WBC increases to
  10,000 to15,000/μL with shift to the left and toxic granulation. If count is higher,
  rule out secondary bacterial infection or hemorrhage.
- Mild normochromic normocytic anemia (as low as Hb = 9 gm/dL) appears around
  tenth day.
- Decreased platelets (<150,000/μL) is frequent.
- ESR is increased.
- Total protein and serum albumin are decreased.
- Serum sodium is frequently decreased.
- BUN may be increased (prerenal). Urine may show slight increase in albumin,
  hematuria, granular casts.
- CSF is normal despite symptoms of meningitis.
- Blood cultures for bacteria are negative (to rule out other tickborne diseases, e.g.,
  tularemia).

Laboratory findings due to specific organ involvement (e.g., pneumonitis, hepatitis) or
due to complications (e.g., secondary bacterial infection, hemorrhage) are present.
Acute GN occurs in 78% of patients with epidemic typhus, 50% of patients with Rocky
Mountain spotted fever, and 30% of patients with scrub typhus.

Rickettsial Infections

- *Rickettsia prowazekii* (epidemic typhus)
- *Rickettsia typhi* (murine typhus)
- *Coxiella burnetii* (Q fever)
- *Rickettsia rickettsii* (Rocky Mountain spotted fever)
- *Rickettsia conorii* (Boutonneuse Fever)
- *Rickettsia akari* (Rickettsialpox)
- *Orientia* (formerly *Rickettsia) tsutsugamushi* (scrub typhus)

Epidemic Typhus (Brill-Zinsser Disease; Recrudescent Typhus)

Due to *Rickettsia prowazekii* transmitted by body louse from humans.

♦ Assay of paired sera for specific IgM and ≥4× rise in IgA (IFA, EIA) are best methods and indicate recent infection. Single IFA titer of ≥1:128 is strongly suggestive. Specificity of these tests is close to 100%.
CF has insufficient S/S.
Presence of IgG generally indicates previous exposure and present immunity.

Murine Typhus

Due to *R. typhi* transmitted by rat flea from rats.

♦ Paired sera for specific IgM and ≥4× rise in IgG (IFA, EIA) are best methods and indicate recent infection. Single IFA titer ≥1:128 is strongly suggestive. Specificity of these is close to 100%.
♦ In house species-specific PCR under development.
CF has insufficient S/S.
Presence of IgG generally indicates previous exposure and present immunity.

Q Fever

Due to *Coxiella burnetii* that is classified as *Rickettsia* but phylogenetically closest to *Legionella*. Gram-negative intracellular bacterium. Transmitted by aerosol or ingestion of contaminated unpasteurized milk.

♦ Single phase IgG titer ≥1:800 by microimmunofluorescence or any IgM titer is diagnostically significant. Phase 1 IgG titer ≥1:800 strongly suggests *Coxiella burnetii* endocarditis.
♦ ELISA is sensitive (>84%) in early convalescence; is replacing CF, IFA, and agglutination.
♦ Detection of *Coxiella burnetii* by PCR, EM, or immunohistologic staining are research tests.
♦ Elevated IFA antibody response to *Coxiella burnetii* phase 1 or 2 antigens.
○ High specific-IgM titer suggests hepatitis; high specific IgA titer is common in chronic Q fever and suggests culture-negative endocarditis.
Serology determines duration of antibiotic treatment for chronic disease; >10% of US population is seropositive.
Cannot be cultured by routine methods. Laboratory findings due to various organ involvement

- Hepatitis: Serum transaminases usually 100 to 200 U/L in <75% of patients and alkaline phosphatase and bilirubin increased in ≤15% of patients.
- "Doughnut" granuloma in liver biopsy or bone marrow in osteomyelitis is highly indicative but not pathognomonic.
- CNS, joints, pulmonary, etc.
- Endocarditis, infected vascular prosthesis or aneurysm

Rocky Mountain Spotted Fever

Infectious vasculitis due to *Rickettsia rickettsii* transmitted by infected ticks.

♦ DFA of skin biopsy for antigen has S/S = ~70%/100%; is only specific test in early stages of disease. Available from CDC.
♦ Culture requires special conditions and is rarely performed.

♦ PCR has been used to detect *R. rickettsii* DNA in blood and tissues.
♦ Paired sera show ≥4× increase in IgG or total antibody by IFA or specific-IgM is evidence of recent infection. IgM appears by day 3 to 8, peaks at 1 month, may last 3 to 4 months.
IgG appears within 3 weeks, peaks at 1 to 3 months, and may last for 12 months or more. Demonstrable IgG usually indicates previous exposure and immunity. Paired sera for both IgG and IgM should always be done early and 10 to 14 days later.
CF is too insensitive to be used alone and appears too late (8–12 days) for early diagnosis and treatment. CF and IgG titers may be decreased by early treatment.
Infection may be life-threatening in patients with G6PD deficiency.
Laboratory findings due to involvement of various organs (e.g., encephalitis, myocarditis, kidneys, liver, etc.)

Boutonneuse Fever

Due to *Rickettsia conorii* transmitted by ticks.

♦ Immunocytologic demonstration of organism in circulating endothelial cells by monoclonal antibodies to surface antigen of circulating endothelial cells.
♦ Biopsy at site of rash for immunohistologic diagnosis.

Rickettsialpox

Due to *Rickettsia akari* transmitted by mites from house mice.

♦ Paired early and later (2–3 weeks) sera (showing 4× increase in titer) for CF and for IgM and total Ig (IFA) should be used. Should be absorbed with *R. rickettsii* and *R. akari* antigens to prove specificity of reaction.
♦ Direct immunofluorescence antibody reaction can be used on fixed tissue from presumed site of inoculation.

Scrub Typhus

Due to *Orientia* (formerly *Rickettsia*) *tsutsugamushi* transmitted by chiggers.

♦ Presence of specific IgG and IgM (ELISA, IFA) 4× increase in titer to 1:200 strongly favors diagnosis.
Diagnostic Weil-Felix agglutination shows ≥4× rise in titer to *Proteus* OX-K and no reaction to *Proteus* OX-2 or OX-19 (in 50%–70% of patients); a single titer ≥1:160 is also diagnostic; normal is ≤1:40. Better S/S than CF.

Viral Diseases

Laboratory Tests for Viral Infections

***Direct Methods*:** Viral culture, *p24* antigen assay, PCR.
Indirect Methods: Enzyme immunoassay (EIA), enzyme-linked immunosorbent assay (ELISA), Western blotting (WB; immunoblotting), indirect immunofluorescence assay (IFA), radioimmunoprecipitation assay (RIPA)
♦ *Viral cultures*

• Inoculation of animals and eggs have been supplanted by cell culture.
• Standard viral "tube" culture showing typical cytopathologic changes is the gold standard for proving etiology but may require 10 days to weeks and limited range of viruses that can be detected. Uses animal (e.g., monkey or rabbit kidney) or human (e.g., fibroblast, HeLa, blood cells) cells. Cultures can be confirmed with hemadsorption (e.g., influenza, parainfluenza, mumps) or with FA antibodies. Shell viral cultures can be confirmed with specific FA antibody to detect specific antigen (e.g., CMV, HSV, VZV, respiratory and enteroviruses) can provide results in 1 to 2 days.
• Some viruses cannot be cultured and require other methods or special techniques (e.g., arenaviruses, astrovirus, calicivirus, coronaviruses, Coxsackievirus Type A, flaviviruses, filovirus, hepatitis A-E, Lassa, Molluscum contagiosum, noravirus, papillomaviruses, parvoviruses, polyomavirus, rabies, rotaviruses).

- Finding enterovirus in stool supports diagnosis but does not prove it is the cause of present illness (e.g., aseptic meningitis, myopericarditis).
- Some viruses can be shed for months in asymptomatic persons (e.g., adenoviruses, HSV, CMV) and their presence may not indicate disease but this is unusual for other viruses whose presence does indicate disease (e.g., measles, mumps, influenza, parainfluenza, RSV).
- Wood and cotton are toxic to viruses and should not be used for culture specimens.

Clinical Specimen	Virus Commonly Isolated
Blood	CMV, HSV, VZV, enteroviruses*
CSF, brain, spinal cord	CMV, HSV, enteroviruses*, mumps
Skin	HSV, VZV, enteroviruses*, adenovirus
Mucosa	
Oral	HSV, VZV
Genital	HSV, CMV, *Chlamydia*
Rectal	HSV, VZV, enteroviruses*
Eye	HSV, VZV, CMV, *Chlamydia,* adenovirus, enteroviruses*
Respiratory (Sputum is not acceptable)	
Upper	Adenovirus, HSV, enteroviruses*, influenza, parainfluenza, RSV, rhinovirus, reovirus
Lower	Adenovirus, influenza, parainfluenza, RSV, CMV
Urine	CMV, enteroviruses*, adenovirus, mumps
Stool	Enteroviruses*, adenovirus, Norwalk, astrovirus, rotavirus
Tissue	CMV, HSV, enteroviruses*

*Enteroviruses include Coxsackievirus, poliovirus, echovirus, and enterovirus.

◆ Antigen Detection Tests
Provide diagnosis within a few hours. Do not require viable virus.
Direct detection of viral antigens by DFA, IFA, EIA (commercial kits for RSV, rotavirus, adenovirus, influenza A, HSV), and agglutination kits (for rotavirus)

- Respiratory tract (nasopharyngeal, tracheal, BAL) (e.g., adenovirus, respiratory syncytial virus, influenza A and B, parainfluenza virus, measles, rhinovirus varicella-zoster virus, HSV, enterovirus)
- Conjunctiva/cornea (e.g., adenovirus, HSV)
- Stool (e.g., adenovirus [enteric serotypes], rotavirus)
- Urine—CMV, mumps, adenovirus. Increased sensitivity by using several specimens.

Useful in mumps encephalitis when other sites are negative.

- Blood (hepatitis B virus, HIV [*p24*], arborvirus, enterovirus)
- Peripheral blood leucocytes (e.g., CMV pp65)
- Tissue—lung (CMV, influenza, adenovirus) and brain (HSV) are the most productive.
- CSF—Nucleic acid amplification tests are most reliable for detection of herpesviruses.
- Skin (e.g., HSV, VZV)

◆ Nucleic acid detection
of amplified specific sequences of DNA. Used for RNA viruses (e.g., HIV, HCV, RSV, enterovirus influenza and parainfluenza viruses, rotavirus, etc). PCR is particularly useful for viruses that grow slowly, are not viable, or only a small sample is available.

- Serum (e.g., HBV, parvovirus B19)
- Plasma (e.g., HIV RNA, HCV [qualitative and quantitative], CMV)
- Leukocytes (e.g., CMV, EBV; HIV DNA in infant of infected mother)
- Amniotic fluid (e.g., parvovirus B19)
- CSF (e.g., HSV, CMV, enteroviruses, VZV, EBV, JC virus)
- Ocular fluid (e.g., HSV, VZV, CMV)
- Genital secretions (e.g., papillomavirus virus)
- Saliva (e.g., HIV)

◆ Electron microscopic (EM)
identification of viral antigen in patient tissues (e.g., brain biopsy for HSV particles in encephalitis, Jakob-Creutzfeldt virus) or specimens (e.g., urine for CMV in congenital infection of infants; feces for rotaviruses, Norwalk

viruses, adenoviruses, coronaviruses, caliciviruses; vesicle fluid for HSV and poxviruses). Is often enhanced by other techniques (e.g., antibody binding).

♦ *Light microscopy* identifies inclusions in nucleus (e.g., HSV, VZV, CMV, adenovirus, measles) and cytoplasm (e.g., CMV, measles, rabies).

Cytology

- HPV: Koilocytes, other changes in uterine cervical Pap smears, respiratory, and urine specimens.
- HSV, VZV: Tzanck smears
- CMV: "Owl eye" nucleus in gynecologic, respiratory, and urine specimens.
- HPV: Cytologic changes in gynecologic, respiratory, and urine specimens.
- Polyoma viruses: Urine sediment showing intranuclear inclusion.
- *Molluscum contagiosum*: Gynecologic and skin scrapings.

Other inclusion bodies (e.g., measles; "smudge" cells for adenovirus, RSV); virus identification can be confirmed by FA and immunoenzyme specific antibody staining.

Histology

- Inclusions in biopsy or autopsy is gold standard for diagnosis of significant CMV infection. Enhanced by immunohistochemistry; in situ hybridization to detect specific nucleic acids; in situ PCR.

♦ *Serologic*

(1) Evidence of recent infection may be based on the following:

- Seroconversion from negative to positive test or $\geq 4\times$ rise in antibody titer in paired serum samples collected 2 to 4 weeks apart is usually diagnostic of recent infection but is usually too late to be useful for a particular episode. *Paired sera should always be submitted for diagnosis of viral disease; acute phase serum should be obtained as early as possible in clinical course.* Some exceptions are anamnestic reactions, cross-reactions to related antigens; some specific exceptions (e.g., high CMV antibody titers in influenza A or *Mycoplasma pneumoniae* infections).
- Single serum specimens that show specific IgM antibody early in the infection (e.g., EBV, CMV, VZV, rubella, mumps, measles, coxsackieviruses, rabies, dengue, HIV, HTLV I and II, hepatitis viruses A through E.
- Various IgM exceptions must be remembered:
  IgM responses may be transient, weak or absent limiting their use in some illnesses (e.g., measles, mumps, *Mycoplasma pneumoniae*).
  Some may recur with reactivation or reinfection (e.g., HSV, CMV, EBV, VZV).
  Some antibodies may persist for ≥ 6 months (e.g., CMV, rubella).
  Heterotypic response of one virus antibody to another infection (e.g., CMV, EBV)
- False-positive titers are frequent in sera that contain rheumatoid factor. *Spurious results may also occur in other conditions (e.g., SBE, chronic liver disease, TB and other chronic infections, sarcoidosis, some healthy persons).*
- False-negative titers may occur in immunocompromised patients, neonates, infants.

(2) Determine immune status (e.g., EBV, HSV, rubella, measles, HVA, anti-HBs, parvovirus B19).

(3) For diagnosis of congenital infection, serial sera from mother and infant should be submitted.

- Infants' passive antibody acquired transplacentally decreases markedly in 2 to 3 months; unchanged or increasing titer indicates active infection although maternal HIV antibodies may persist for ≤ 18 months in infant.
- Specific IgM in neonatal blood or cord blood can diagnose congenital infection since mothers' IgM does not cross placenta.
- Single maternal serum negative for IgG may be useful to exclude that particular congenital infection in neonate (e.g., rubella, CMV).
- Positive IgG titer that does not rise indicates previous exposure and often immunity.

Tests to determine immune status may be used for viruses of rubella (in women of childbearing age), CMV (in women of childbearing age working in high-risk environments [e.g., hemodialysis, transplant, pediatric and nursery units]), measles, mumps, chickenpox (VZV), HAV (IgG), HBV (anti-HBs), EBV, HSV, parvovirus B19.

- Preferred to culture where virus does not grow well in cell culture (e.g., rubella, EBV) or are hazardous.

Rapid assays for HIV have S/S >99%.
Assays:

- Genotypic assay for drug resistance (e.g., HIV; CMV resistance to ganciclovir)
- WB (e.g., to confirm positive HIV EIA; determine type specificity of HSV antibodies).
- RIBA to confirm positive HCV EIA.
- Rapid latex agglutination for varicella immune status in exposed healthcare workers.
- Hemagglutination-inhibition, CF, neutralizing antibodies are rarely used now.

Diagnosis by
PCR detection of virus in blood mononuclear cells, CSF, autopsy tissues (vitreous humor, spleen, liver, lymph nodes).
Virus isolation after animal inoculation (mice, mosquitoes, tissue culture).
Antigen detection in tissue or culture by IF, hemagglutination-inhibition, neutralization or CF.
Virus-specific ELISA IgM antibody in serum or CSF after 5 to 14 days or increasing IgM antibody titer.

Routine Laboratory Tests

Generally, leukopenia, particularly lymphopenia, is present in contrast to bacterial infections where there is often leukocytosis unless bacterial infection is superimposed.

Viral Infections

Acquired Immune Deficiency Syndrome (AIDS)[12]

Due to human immunodeficiency virus, [HIV-1], RNA retrovirus subfamily of lentiviruses. Formerly called Human T-cell lymphotropic virus III (HTLV III). HIV predominantly infects CD4 T-lymphocytes where it is uncoated and forms multiple copies of enzymes (e.g., reverse transcriptase, protease) that make a DNA copy of viral RNA and ultimately viral messenger RNA.

HIV-2 is a recently described virus that causes a disease not distinguishable from AIDS in Africans and small numbers of Europeans and South Americans. Current screening tests for HIV-1 do not consistently and reliably detect antibody due to HIV-2 infection. All blood donations must be tested for HIV-2 as well as HIV-1.
See Tables 15-13, 15-14 and Figures 15-4, 15-5, 15-6 and 15-7 and appropriate separate section for each disease or test referred to below.
♦ **Laboratory evidence of HIV infection (any of the following)**
Repeated reactive screening test for HIV antibody (e.g., ELISA) confirmed by WB, IFA, culture, or molecular testing for HIV DNA or RNA. Diagnosis should always be based on presence of antibodies.
Positive test for HIV serum antigen but levels may fluctuate.
Positive HIV culture confirmed by both PCR and a specific HIV antigen test or in situ hybridization using a nucleic acid probe.
Positive result with any other highly specific test for HIV (e.g., nucleic acid probe of peripheral blood lymphocytes)
Child <15 months old whose mother had HIV infection during perinatal period with repeated reactive screening test, plus increased serum Ig levels, and at least one of the following abnormal immunologic tests: Reduced absolute lymphocyte count, depressed CD4+ count, if subsequent confirmatory antibody tests are positive.
Neonatal infection (see below).

Antibody to Human Immunodeficiency Virus Type I (HIV-I)

- HIV antibody develops in all patients infected with this virus and is taken as evidence of past or present infection other than perinatal and neonatal periods. Presence of antibody does not cause immunity. ELISA is usual initial screening test for HIV-1 and HIV-2; antibodies appear in circulating mononuclear cells 1 to several

[12]Some data from *Clin Lab Med* 2002;22

Table 15-11.   Summary of Clinically Most Significant Human Viral Infections

Virus Family DNA/RNA*	Virus/Disease	Diagnosis	Chapter Number
Arenaviridae Single-stranded Enveloped RNA	*Arenavirus* Lymphocytic choriomeningitis. Aseptic meningitis	IFA for IgM (within first week) and IgG appear very early making increased titer hard to detect. Culture is difficult; not routinely done. CSF changes.	9
	Arenavirus Lassa virus. Lassa fever (meningoencephalitis)	ELISA Ag + in 3–5 days. IgM + in 5–7 days; peaks by ~12 day. Lasts for weeks. Not found with antigen. IgG is + in ~3 weeks and past infection. + in acute illness rules out this diagnosis. PCR has been used. Blood culture is + with acute fever.	
	Argentine, Bolivian, and Venezuelan hemorrhagic fever viruses. South American hemorrhagic fevers	ELISA Ag + with symptoms. IgM + when Ag disappears; may last for months. IgG + in ~3 weeks and in past infection; + in acute illness rules out this diagnosis. PCR has been used. Cell culture of blood + with acute fever.	
Retroviridae HIV single-stranded RNA is reverse transcribed to DNA in host cell.	*Lentivirus* HIV. AIDS	EIA Ab confirmed by WB. *p24* Ag in blood, other body fluids.	15
	Oncovirus Human T-cell leukemia viruses (HTLV) 1 and 2). HTLV-1 causes adult T-cell leukemia. HTLV-2—not known if causes human disease.	ELISA Ab (S/S >97%) confirmed by WB and RIP. Identify DNA by Southern blot.	15
Bunyaviridae Single-stranded RNA.	*Phlebovirus* Rift Valley fever *Hantavirus* Hantavirus pulmonary syndrome (HPS) occurs within America. Hemorrhagic fever with renal syndrome (HFRS) occurs outside of Americas. *Bunyavirus* La Crosse	ELISA for antigen and specific IgM have S/S >90%; ELISA IgG peaks during first week and remains detectable. Serology is less useful in parts of South America where there is high seroprevalence of antibodies. IFA replaced by ELISA. WB and neutralization to confirm diagnosis if necessary. Blood culture is difficult. IHC on autopsy tisssues. PCR for RNA and	15

Table 15-11.	*(continued)*		
Virus Family **DNA/RNA***	**Virus/Disease**	**Diagnosis**	**Chapter** **Number**
		immunohistochemical staining for antigen in tissue. Tests in reference laboratories.	
Picornaviruses Single-stranded RNA.		Stool, throat, CSF viral culture confirmed by type-specific antisera neutralization. ELISA for specific IgM. PCR direct detection (e.g., CSF) is rapid; replaces nucleic acid probes. Paired serum titers.	10
Enterovirus	Polio, coxsackie, echo viruses. CNS	IgM and total anti-HAV in acute infection, transaminases. Total anti-HAV for immune status or risk assessment in travelers.	9
Hepatovirus	HAV. Hepatitis	RT-PCR. ELISA can detect IgG and IgA in serum and IgA in secretions. NP secretions for viral isolation. Serology (e.g., neutralization, IHA, CF).	
Rhinovirus	Human rhinovirus; many serotypes. "Common cold"		
Calciviridea Single-stranded RNA.	Hepatitis E. Hepatitis E. Norovirus ("Norwalk-like"). Gastroenteritis. "Sapporo-like". Gastroenteritis	Serology RT-PCR of stool, vomitus, food, water, fomites. ELISA to detect viral antigen in clinical specimens. Older methods: Immune EM of stool, 4× rise in IgG antibodies.	9 8
Astroviridae Single-stranded RNA.	Human astroviruses. Gastroenteritis, especially in children.	EM of stool detects ~10^6 virons/gm stool. EIA for viral antigen and antibody. S/S >90%.	
Togaviridae Single-stranded RNA.	*Rubivirus* Rubella. Exanthem ("German measles")	Amniotic fluid: Culture is gold standard. IgM for acute disease. Viral isolation is rarely needed. Serum: IgM: recent exposure. IgG 4× increase in titer in paired serum. IgG >1:10: confirms immunity in pregnancy. In infant at birth: IgM indicates congenital	15

(continued)

INFECTIOUS

Table 15-11.   Summary of Clinically Most Significant Human Viral Infections

Virus Family DNA/RNA*	Virus/Disease	Diagnosis	Chapter Number
		infection; absent IgG excludes congenital infection.	
	Alphaviruses. Eastern, Western, Venezuelan Equine encephalitis	Specific IgM in serum or CSF, isolate virus in cell culture, RT-PCR of serum or CSF.	15
Flaviviridae Single-stranded RNA.	*Hepacivirus* HCV Hepatitis	EIA antibody confirmed by RIBA.	8
	HGV Hepatitis	HCV RNA by PCR. Serum ALT is *not* increased.	8
	Flavivirus West Nile encephalitis. Meningoencephalitis.	ELISA for IgM should be + by 8th day 90% of cases. Increasing acute and convalescent IgG titers is confirmatory. RT-PCR of blood, CSF, tissue detects RNA. Plaque reduction neutralization test by CDC for confirmation.	15
	Flavivirus St. Louis, Japanese Virus. Encephalitis	ELISA IgM is + in 3-5 days. HI serology for whole group; single CF is presumptive evidence.	
	Flavivirus Dengue virus. Hemorrhagic fever (fever, rash, arthritis)	ELISA IgM is + within 5 days; may last for months; is test of choice. ELISA IgG appears soon after IgM; lasts for life.	15
	Flavivirus Yellow fever virus. Yellow fever (hepatitis, fever, rash, arthritis)	Commercial ELISA Ig kit for dengue. ELISA Ag: sensitivity varies. Culture blood is + within 5 days.	15
	Tick-borne encephalitis, Omsk hemorrhagic fever, Kyasanur Forest disease	Post-mortem liver culture is +.	
Coronaviri- dae Positive- stranded RNA	Mild upper respiratory infections	IEM. Increase in antibody titer by CF or NA. RT-PCR. In-situ hybridization.	
	SARS virus. *Severe Acute Respiratory Syndrome*	Culture of virus in NP, BAL, blood. RT-PCR. Detection of antibody by IFA after 10 days. EM.	15
Rhabdo- viridae Negative- stranded RNA.	*Lyssavirus* Rabies virus Rabies	Virus in saliva injected into mice. FA of cornea. CSF antibodies if no prior vaccination. PCR in saliva, tissues for RNA.	15

Virus Family DNA/RNA*	Virus/Disease	Diagnosis	Chapter Number
		Skin biopsy of face /neck for antigen. VNA in serum late in course if no prior vaccination. Autopsy CNS tissue for FA or avidin-biotin IHC test.	
Filoviridae Single-stranded RNA.	*Filovirus* Ebola, Marburg hemorrhagic fevers	ELISA Ag + in blood within hours. Viral antigen and RNA by PCR. Blood culture +. IHC for antigen in frozen tissue. EM of cultures or tissues.	
Paramyxoviridae Enveloped Single-stranded RNA.	*Rubulavirus* Mumps virus. Parotitis Parainfluenza types 2, 4	ELISA specific IgM and IgG.	15
RNA.	*Morbillivirus* Measles virus. Exathem	Cytology for giant cells and inclusions in NP, saliva, urine. EIA for IgM and IgG in serum and saliva. Culture of saliva (first 4–5 days), urine (≤2 weeks) is difficult, rarely used. CSF in 50% of cases (first 8–9 days of CNS symptoms).	15
	Paramyxovirus Parainfluenza virus types 1,3. Respiratory infections (e.g., pneumonia, croup, bronchiolitis, tracheobronchitis)	Viral culture, RNA or antigens in respiratory secretions. Serology: 4× increase in titers of acute and convalescent sera.	15
	Pneumovirus Respiratory syncytial virus (RSV). Acute lower and upper respiratory infections Human metapneumovirus. Acute lower respiratory infections in infants and elderly.	DFA rapid screen; S/S >90%. Culture. RT-PCR of nasal secretions. Culture.	15
Orthomyxoviridae Single-stranded RNA.	*Influenzavirus* Influenza A, B. Respiratory infections	Rapid diagnostic tests for influenza A and B by antigen, enzyme, or nucleic acid in doctor's offices. Culture and IFA. RT-PCR, RNA isolation.	15
Hepadnaviridae Double-stranded DNA.	*Orthohepadnavirus* HBV. Hepatitis B	Serology	9

(continued)

Table 15-11. Summary of Clinically Most Significant Human Viral Infections

Virus Family DNA/RNA*	Virus/Disease	Diagnosis	Chapter Number
Herpesviridae Enveloped Double-stranded DNA.	*Simplexvirus* Herpes simplex virus (HSV-1 and HSV-2.) Neonatal infection. Recurrent cold sores, genital lesions.	Tzanck smear: EM, indirect IFA, immunoperoxidase approach sensitivity of culture. Antigen detection (EIA or direct fluorescence) is rapid (<4 hours) and as sensitive as culture. PCR for antigen, shell viral culture from nasopharynx, skin, eyes, tissue. DFA in skin lesions. ELISA, IFA, EIA, WB, CF to detect gG or gC epitopes.	15
	Aseptic meningitis. Encephalitis.	PCR of CSF to detect DNA in CNS and disseminated. Has S/S >98%/>94%; has supplanted brain biopsy. Culture may be + in meningitis but rarely + in encephalitis.	
	Varicellovirus Varicella-zoster virus (HSV-3). Varicella (chickenpox). Herpes zoster (shingles).	Antigen detection by FA or shell virus culture of skin lesions. ELISA, FAMA to determine immunity.	15
	Lymphocryptovirus Epstein-Barr virus (EBV) (HSV-4). Infectious mononucleosis.	Monospot. ELISA EA-IgM, EA-IgG; EBNA-IgG (to determine immunity) in serum.	15
	Burkitt lymphoma Nasopharyngeal carcinoma T-cell lymphoma Hodgkin disease Gastric carcinoma, other neoplasms	Histology. Virus identified in tissue. Patients have + serological tests.	
Enveloped Double-stranded DNA.	*Cytomegalovirus* CMV (HSV-5). Infectious mononucleosislike illness. Congenital infection. Infection in immuno-compromised hosts (e.g., bone marrow and organ transplant patients). May cause marrow suppression (varies from transient to fatal aplastic anemia),	Rapid shell vial assay is gold standard; only reliable method to diagnose active infection; can detect infection within 72 hours with S/S = 86%/100% in marrow and liver transplant patients. Tissue-cell cultures show specific cytopathic effects (requires 5–21 days).	15

Table 15-11.	(continued)		
Virus Family DNA/RNA*	<u>Virus</u>/Disease	Diagnosis	Chapter Number
	encephalitis, interstitial pneumonitis, susceptibility to other viral infections (e.g., EBV, CMV, RSV, adenovirus).	Serum IgM antibody titer rises 3 weeks after onset of exanthema subitum limiting its usefulness. Useful to detect latent infection or sero-prevalence but not reliable indicator of reactivation. PCR to detect HHV-6 DNA in blood cells has limited value in diagnosing active infections. PCR on cell-free sample of CSF is gold standard; has low sensitivity. IHC stains can detect HHV-6 in tissues or cytology (e.g., BAL) has moderate sensitivity.	
	Roseolovirus <u>HSV-6A, HSV-6B, HSV-7</u> Roseola, febrile illness	Culture is gold standard for active infection. Serology: ELISA IFA, etc. IgG: not useful to detect active infection. IgM: active infection recently; does not indicate current infection. PCR for DNA or mRNA. CSF: Positive culture indicates active infection but has low sensitivity. PCR of is gold standard; indicates active infection.	15
	<u>HSV-8</u> Kaposi's sarcoma (classic, endemic, AIDS-associated, posttransplant forms). Primary effusion lymphomas. Multicentric Castleman disease (a reactive lymph-adenopathy).	Microscopic examination of tissue and IHC. PCR can detect virus DNA in various tissues, body fluids, serum, blood mononuclear cells; does not distinguish active from latent infection. Serology e.g., IFA to detect antigens. Gene detection by IFA, ELISA.	15
Parvoviridae Single-stranded DNA	*Parvovirus B19* <u>Parvovirus B19.</u> > 100 genotypes. Fifth disease. Pure RBC aplasia. Transient RBC crisis. Transient arthopathy.	Antigen, ELISA, FA, culture of nasopharynx, trachea, eye.	15

(continued)

Table 15-11.   Summary of Clinically Most Significant Human Viral Infections

Virus Family DNA/RNA*	Virus/Disease	Diagnosis	Chapter Number
Adenoviridae Nonenveloped Double-stranded DNA	*Mastadenovirus* At least 51 serotypes. Respiratory, eye, GI tract especially in children; infrequently in other organs.		
Rotaviridae Double-stranded DNA.	Numerous strains. Gastroenteritis	Direct EM of stool. Virus or viral antigen in stool or serological response. LA is less sensitive than EIA.	15
Polyomaviridae Double-stranded DNA	*Human papillomavirus (HPV)* Genital and anal warts. Dysplasia and carcinoma of uterine cervix (high-risk types are 16, 18, 45, 58; intermediate-risk types are 31, 33, 35, 39, 51, 52, 69). Nongenital warts. *JC virus.* Progressive multifocal leukoencephalopathy in immuno-compromised hosts (e.g., AIDS). *BK virus* Hemorrhagic cystitis especially in marrow and renal allograft transplant recipients.	Koilocytes. PCR and nucleic acid hybridization for HPV DNA. PCR to detect DNA in CSF or brain tissue. PCR to detect DNA in urine, blood, renal tissue. Viral inclusions in uroepithelial cells in urine. Renal biopsy to evaluate nephropathy.	14
Reoviridae Double-stranded RNA	*Coltivirus* Colorado tick fever *Rotavirus* Group A and B rotaviruses *Orthoviruses* Reoviruses	ELISA to detect antibodies. IFA detects antigen. PCR detects RNA. Culture of body fluids.	15
Poxiviridae Double-stranded DNA	*Orthopoxvirus* Smallpox (Variola). Vaccinia. Monkeypox in humans. Cowpox. *Molluscipoxvirus* Molluscum contagiosum.	PCR, EM, culture, IHC of skin lesions.	15

*Bold, Family; *Italics*, Genus; Underlined, name of virus; Normal print, Disease.
IHC, immunohistochemical; ELISA, enzyme-linked immunoabsorbent assay; FA, fluorescent antibodies; WB, western blot; PCR, polymerase chain reaction; RT-PCR, reverse transcription PCR; HAI, hemagglutination; CF, complement fixation; RIBA, recombinant immunoblot assay; EM, electron microscopy; RIP, radioimmune precipitation; RIA, radioimmunoassay; S/S, sensitivity and specificity; Ag, antigen; Ab, antibody; +, positive.
Paired, acute and convalescent sera; = 4× increase in titer of acute and convalescent samples.
NP, nasopharynx; HTLV, human T-cell leukemia viruses; RSV, respiratory syncytial virus.
Hemorrhagic fevers show varying degrees of thrombocytopenia (except Lassa fever), leukopenia (except Lassa and Hantaan fevers), increased clotting time, DIC, azotemia, increased transaminases. Rapid EIA and cultures are available only at CDC.

Table 15-12. Diagnosis of Congenital Viral Infections

Virus	Diagnosis In-utero	Diagnosis in Newborn
CMV	Culture or PCR on AF	Culture urine during first week
VZV	PCR on AF	Culture or FA stain of lesion
HSV	—	Culture lesion; culture body fluids, nasopharynx, mouth. PCR on blood in disseminated infection.
Parvovirus B19	PCR on AF	PCR on serum. Specific IgM
HBV	NA	HBsAg
HIV	Contraindicated	HIV DNA PCR
Rubella	Culture or PCR on AF. Specific IgM.	Specific IgM, persistent specific IgG. Culture body fluids.
Enteroviruses	NA	Culture stool, NP, blood, urine
HCV	No information	PCR
Lymphocytic choriomeningitis virus	No information	Specific IgG and IgM

AF, amniotic fluid; NP, nasopharynx; NA, not applicable.

weeks after infection and usually appear in plasma 6 to 8 weeks and, rarely >6 months; found in >95% of patients within 3 months. Third-generation assays include subtype O antigens, detects IgM and IgA as well as IgG. S/S >99%.
* *Positive ELISA tests means that each positive test has been repeatedly positive in duplicate on the same serum specimens. Degree of test reactivity is important.*

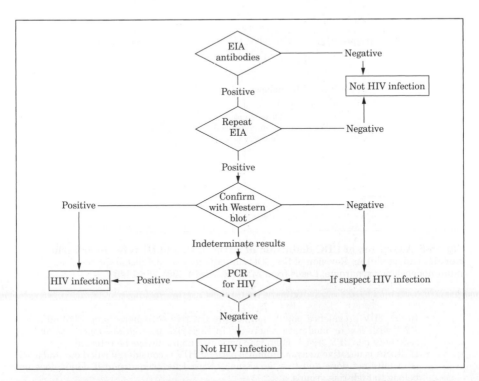

Fig. 15-4. Algorithm for serologic testing for AIDS. PCR, polymerase chain reaction.

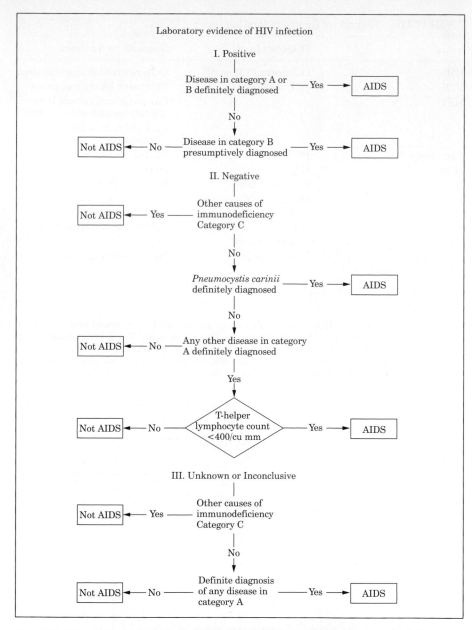

Fig. 15-5. Algorithm of CDC definition of AIDS. I, II, and III refer to criteria herein. (Adapted from Revision of the CDC surveillance case definition for acquired immunodeficiency syndrome: Leads from MMWR. *JAMA* 1987;258:1143.)

- In low HIV prevalence population, highly reactive specimens have PPV 86%, but <2% with low or moderate reactivity. In high-risk population, moderate or high reactivity has PPV >95%. High-risk patients should always be retested.
- If ELISA is negative in asymptomatic patient, HIV is considered ruled out and a WB is usually not done and this blood may be used for transfusion if donor does not belong to high-risk groups.

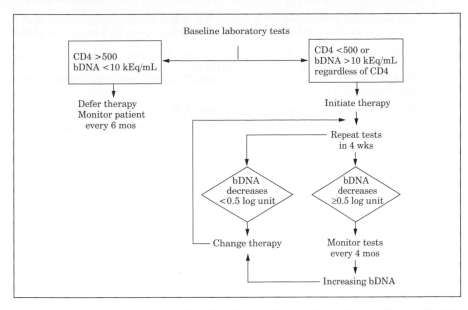

Fig. 15-6. Laboratory tests to assist therapy decisions. (From *Signals*. Emeryville, CA: Chiron reference Testing Laboratory, 1966 March.)

- Rare patient with AIDS/ARC defining illness and a negative antibody test should have RNA quantitative testing and/or p24 antigen testing.
- Incidence of HIV antibody in donated blood in the United States is <0.22%.
- If ELISA is positive it must be confirmed by WB or IFA; if WB or IFA are positive, the individual has been infected with HIV. ≤10% to 20% of repeat reactive ELISA HIV-1 have indeterminate WB or IFA that may be caused by false-positive results or

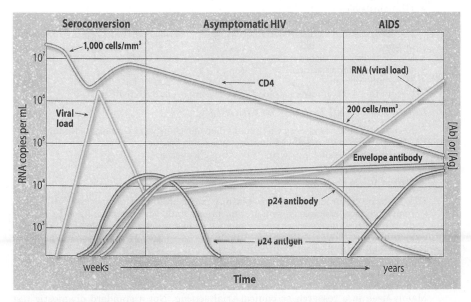

Fig. 15-7. Kinetic characteristics of HIV infection. (From NT Constantine. Quantifying viremia. *Clinical Laboratory News*, 1997, with permission.)

not completed seroconversion; if repeat WB is still indeterminate during next 6 months, patients are usually not infected. This person should not be used as a blood donor.
- If ELISA is positive and WB is negative the patient's blood should not be used for transfusion although the diagnosis of AIDS is not confirmed.
- PCR for HIV is used to confirm indeterminate WB results or negative results in persons suspected of infection.

False-Positive ELISA Results May Be Caused By

- Many of these have been eliminated since use of synthetic or recombinant HIV peptides.
- Patients in HIV vaccine trials.
- Administration of influenza vaccine up to 3 months prior to test.
- Administration of immune globulin (e.g., for HBV) manufactured before 1985 within 6 weeks of testing from products (antibody is present but cannot transmit HIV).
- Presence of HLA-DR antibodies in multigravida women.
- Presence of RF
- Autoimmune disorders
- Hemodialysis
- Hypergammaglobulinemia (e.g., multiple myeloma)
- Positive RPR test
- Alcoholic hepatitis
- Unknown causes
- Subclinical infections that are asymptomatic.

False-Negative ELISA or WB Results May Be Caused By

- Advanced AIDS disease (but there is usually other evidence of AIDS)
- Early infection before antibodies are detectable. *This donated blood may transmit HIV.*
- Immunosuppression due to malignancy or chemotherapy.
- Agammaglobulinemia
- Infection with HIV-1 subtype strains with little genetic homology with HIV-1 subtype M.

False-Positive WB Test May Be Caused By

- HLA antibodies
- Presence of antibody to another human retrovirus (e.g., HIV-2).
- Poorly understood cross-reaction with other nonvirus-derived proteins in healthy persons.
- Connective tissue disorders
- Polyclonal gammopathies
- Hyperbilirubinemia
- Occurs in ≤4.8% of low-risk blood donors compared to RNA-PCR.

Indeterminate WB Test May Be Caused By

- Recent HIV infections; test will usually become positive in 6 weeks to 6 months.
- AIDS patients with advanced immunodeficiency because of loss of antibodies.
- Simian immunodeficiency virus (SIV) in ≤2% of cases.

◆ *HIV-1 Virus Culture*

HIV-1 can be cultured from serum, plasma, peripheral blood monocytes, CSF, saliva, semen, cervical specimens, semen, and breast milk. Viremia begins ~4 to 11 days after exposure, peaks by 3 weeks, then declines rapidly to stabile set point by 3 months.

Use

Confirm diagnosis of AIDS when serological tests are inconclusive (e.g., infant of HIV infected mother).

Only a positive result is conclusive. False-negative results may occur.

Mainly used in a research or clinical trial setting. Not a standard diagnostic test because expensive, time-consuming, and potentially dangerous; may be useful in unusual cases.

Table 15-13.	Correlation of CD4 Count and Disease in HIV Infection

CD4 Count (per cu mm)	Disease
500–800	Aggressive bacterial, respiratory, skin, enteric infections
>500	Kaposi's sarcoma
200–500	Weight loss, fever, sweats
	Hairy leukoplakia
	Candida (oral, esophageal)
	TB reactivation
<200	Pneumocystosis
	Mycobacterium avium-intracellulare
	Cryptococcosis
	Dementia
<50	Toxoplasmosis
	CMV
	Death

Source: Shelhamer JH, et al. Respiratory disease in the immunosuppressed patient: NIH Conference. *Ann Intern Med* 1992;117:415.

New divergent strain of HIV-1 group O identified in Africa is rare in United States and may be difficult to detect; presently only two kits are FDA-approved.

◆ *Quantitative HIV-1 RNA Assay*
Measures viral load by RT-PCR, bDNA, nucleic acid sequence based amplification or transcription-mediated amplification with different detection ranges of 40–10,000,000 copies/mL.

Use (Should be combined with CD4+ count. Should perform each of these tests, 1–2 weeks apart.)
Superior to CD4+ count. Correlates with CD4+ count, response to therapy, clinical stage, disease progression, and death.
Guideline for treatment

• Should establish baseline for individual patient.
• Is best measure of effective therapy. Gauge response to therapy and long-term outcome during antiviral therapy or during latent periods.
• Should decline 1 to 2 log within 4 to 8 weeks of effective therapy. Failure to achieve <50 copies/mL (level of detection) within 16 to 24 weeks or rebound after suppression should raise concern about drug resistance, poor drug absorption, or noncompliance. Goal is sustained decrease below level of detection.
• Begin therapy in HIV-infected patients depending on HIV, RNA, and CD4+.

Table 15-14.	1993 Revised Classification System for HIV Infection and Expanded AIDS Surveillance Case Definition for Adolescents and Adults (≥13 Yrs)

CD4+ T-Cell Categories		Clinical Categories		
Number	%	A	B	C
(1) ≥500/cu mm	≥29	A1	B1	C1
(2) 200–499/cu mm	14–28	A2	B2	C2
(3) <200/cu mm	<14	A3	B3	C3

Notes: Groups A3, B3, C3 with CD4+ T-cell counts <200/cu mm are reported as AIDS. Groups C1, C2, C3 with AIDS-indicator conditions are reported as AIDS. T-cell count <200/cu mm is an AIDS indicator. The lowest accurate CD4+ T-cell count is used for classification; need not be the most recent count.

INFECTIOUS

- Before initiating or changing therapy (on two occasions) and at intervals thereafter (e.g., 4 weeks, 3–4 months)
- Do not use during or within 4 weeks after successful treatment of intercurrent infection, resolution of symptomatic illness, or immunization.
- Change in clinical status or decline in CD4+ cell count
- Predictive value improves when combined with CD4+ cell counts at same time.
- Patients with higher viral loads are likely to benefit from antiretroviral treatment.
- Surrogate marker for drug resistance.
♦ • CD4+ T-cell count is the most valuable test for evaluation of immune status; is essential for care of HIV infections; is usually combined with HIV-1 RNA assay.
- Should be obtained immediately after positive virologic test and then every 3 months in children; every 3 to 6 months in adults.
- Vaccination or mild intercurrent illness can cause transient decrease of CD4+ cell number and percent.
- Antiretroviral therapy is recommended if CD4+ count <500/μL.
- Lymphopenia is largely caused by progressive decrease in CD4+ and increased CD8+ (by flow cytometry).

Lymphopenia is found in 50% of patients with Kaposi sarcoma and almost all patients with opportunistic infections.
Total B-cell and natural killer cell counts are usually normal.

- Infected infants with CD4+ count <1,900/μL have more rapid disease progression.
- CD4+ counts may change ≤30% without change in clinical status due to biological and methodologic variation. Therefore, monitor trends over time rather than change results on one specific test.
- CD4+ counts decline ~50 to 100 cells/μL annually without treatment of HIV.
- CD4+ counts rapidly increase during first 4 to 12 weeks of HAART (highly active antiretroviral therapy).

Prognosis and monitor effectiveness of therapy

- Initial peak during primary infection, then rapid decline (≤3 log copies) of titer to steady-state within 6 to 12 months after seroconversion, lasting months or years indicates effectiveness.
- Viral load after 6 to 12 months predicts long-term progression to AIDS. Viral load >50,000 copies/mL are at greatest risk and shortest time to clinical progression and death; <500 copies/mL has little risk.
- Any child with >100,000 copies/mL is at high risk for mortality.

Interpretation

- Only changes >3× (or 0.5 $\log_{(10)}$) in adults and >5× (or 0.7 $\log_{(10)}$) at age <2 years are significant because of biologic variation within same person.
- Values are not interchangeable between assays; may be a ≥2× difference; same assay should be used for same patient or new baseline should be established if change from one assay to another.
- HIV-infected persons with viral load below detectable limits should be considered infectious.
- HIV replication may be continuing in various tissues.

Table 15-15.   Risk of Developing AIDS or Dying in Next 10 Years

Plasma HIV-1 RNA copies/mL	Risk of Developing AIDS or Dying in Next 10 Years
≤500	5%
500–3,000	17%
3,000–10,000	33%
10,000–30,000	55%
>30,000	80%

Table 15-16.   Laboratory Indications for Treatment in Chronic HIV-1 Infection

Clinical	CD4+ T cell count/μL	Plasma HIV-1 RNA copies/mL	Treatment
Symptomatic	Any	Any	Treat
Asymptomatic	<200	Any	Treat
Asymptomatic	200–350	Any	Treat but different opinion about treatment if viral load <10,000 copies/mL.
Asymptomatic	>350	>55,000	Treat because 3-year risk of AIDS without treatment is >30%.
Asymptomatic	>350	>55,000	Defer treatment and monitor because 3-year risk of AIDS without treatment is <15%.

From: Guidelines for the use of antiretroviral agents in HIV-infected adults and adolescents. 2002. http://www.hivatis.org.

Interferences

May not include other subtypes than B, which is most common in North America.
Prone to contamination causing false-positive reactions
Improper specimen collection, handling (e.g., separation of plasma within 4 hours and prompt freezing) may cause acute degradation of HIV-1 RNA. Heparin anticoagulant rather than EDTA causes lower quantities. Lower values in serum than in plasma.
Intercurrent infection or illness (e.g., TB, pneumonia, HSV, *Candida*, *Pneumocystis jiroveci* [formerly *carinii*]), or vaccination (e.g., tetanus, influenza, pneumococcus) cause transient increase; therapeutic decisions should be based on long term trends.
Not affected by antiretroviral drugs, triglycerides, Hb, etc.
Diagnosis

- Make presumptive diagnosis of HIV infection and initial evaluation of newly diagnosed HIV infection. Is earliest marker of HIV infection; may be detected 2 weeks after infection is established before antibody production begins but not intended as a primary diagnostic test for HIV infection.
- Patients with syndrome consistent with acute HIV infection
- Confirmation of indeterminate WB results
- Differentiate between HIV-1 and HIV-2
- During latent periods
- In high-risk seronegative patients
- Neonates born to HIV-seropositive mothers

♦ HIV-1 DNA Assay

Reported S/S >95% but less reliable for nonsubtype B HIV.

♦ Antigen Assay (for p24 Antigen in Blood)[13]

Is very specific, but low sensitivity in asymptomatic seropositive persons. Antigens decline and disappear as antibodies arise. Can be detected in serum, plasma, CSF. Is the first clinically detectable antigen to appear. Increasingly supplanted by HIV-1 RNA assay.
50 RNA copies of HIV-1 = 25 virions. ~3,000 molecules of p24 antigen per HIV-1 virion. Therefore, 75,000 p24 molecules for detection at 50 viral RNA copies.

[13]Barletta JM, et al. Lowering the detection limits of HIV-1 viral load using real-time immuno-PCR for HIV-1 *p*24 antigen. *Am J Clin Pathol* 2004;122:20.

INFECTIOUS

Use

Developed as interim test to screen blood donors but not used for HIV diagnosis.

Detection of early HIV infection before seroconversion, especially in high-risk persons.

Diagnosis of HIV infection in infants born of seropositive mothers or in persons with indeterminate confirmatory antibody results.

Monitoring antiviral drug therapy in AIDS and AIDS-related complex; less reliable than HIV-RNA and not clinically useful.

Differentiation of AIDS from primary immunodeficiency syndrome in HIV-1-negative children.

Single Use Diagnostic System

Subjective qualitative test using serum or plasma.

Rapid test results within 30 minutes.

Reported S/S comparable to blood ELISA.

◆ Other HIV-1 Antibody Tests

Useful for prompt use in ER, clinic, or cases of occupational exposure. High S/S, PPV, and NPV.

Home Sample Collection—Patient can mail test card to lab containing three drops of blood from finger prick. Reported S/S comparable to blood ELISA. Results in 3 to 7 days. Allows for anonymity. Reactive result must be confirmed by WB.

◆ Saliva and Urine Test for HIV-1 Antibodies

Uses rapid test kits on random sample of urine, oral fluids; also vaginal secretions or seminal fluid (e.g., in case of rape). S/S >99%. Must be confirmed by WB.

Assay for only the gp160 band in contrast to blood, which requires two out of three protein bands associated with HIV to be considered positive.

Fewer indeterminate results than serum WB.

May be positive when serum is HIV negative.

Laboratory Evidence Against HIV Infection

Nonreactive screening test for serum HIV antibody without any other positive laboratory test for HIV infection (e.g., antibody, antigen, culture).

Inconclusive Laboratory Evidence (either item below)

Repeatedly reactive screening test for serum HIV antibody (e.g., EIA) followed by a negative or inconclusive test (e.g., WB, IFA) without a positive serum antigen or culture.

Child <15 months old whose mother had HIV infection during perinatal period with repeatedly reactive HIV antibody screening test, even if positive by supplemental test but without additional evidence of immunodeficiency and without a positive serum antigen or culture.

◆ Drug resistance

• Tests (>17 antiretroviral drugs are now available; no established therapeutic ranges)

• Genotyping: Patient's blood sample is examined for genetic mutations indicating resistance and checked by computer program to a list of >70 mutations linked to resistance to specific drugs.

• Phenotyping: Culture of patient's virus in presence of individual drugs and the inhibitory zone is measured analogous to traditional bacterial resistance testing. Aims to identify drugs still active against the virus of that patient. Performed in specialized labs.

• Recommendations for testing:
  • Acute-symptomatic HIV infection or evidence of recent infection.
  • Before starting treatment of established infection.
  • To guide therapy after failure of various drug regimens.
  • Pregnant HIV-positive women especially with previous drug regimens to optimize therapy of mother and infant.

Acute infection:
>In first 2 weeks, lymphopenia involving CD4+ and CD8+ cells.
>In 3 to 4 weeks, lymphocytosis with CD8+ >CD4+ cells and mild thrombocytopenia.

Chronic infection:

Leukopenia, anemia, idiopathic thrombocytopenia are common; thrombocytosis also occurs.

Hypoalbuminemia. Increased serum γ-globulins early in course of HIV infection, especially IgG and also IgA; slight IgM increase may occur associated with opportunistic infection.

Increased serum transaminase.

Complement C3 and C4 levels are usually normal

Decreased T-cell function evidenced

- In vivo by
    Decreased delayed-type hypersensitivity (skin test reactivity)
    Opportunistic infections
    Neoplasms
- In vitro by various tests that are not routinely available

Other serologic findings (not used in clinical diagnosis): increased levels of

- Acid-labile α-interferon (previously known in patients with autoimmune disease; found in 63% of homosexual AIDS patients and 29% without AIDS) (more studies are needed to determine value as screening test)
- $α_1$ thymosin (found in <1% of normal persons, 70%–80% of AIDS patients, and 60%–70% of patients with chronic reactive lymphadenopathy syndrome)
- β-2-microglobulins appear to correlate with clinical course of HIV infection (also increased in patients with hepatitis, kidney diseases, B-cell malignancies such as multiple myeloma)
- Circulating immune complexes

Laboratory findings due to coexisting infection. Should monitor serological tests especially for HBV, HCV, syphilis, CMV, *T. gondii*.

- HBcAg is positive in >90% of AIDS patients and 80% of patients with lymphadenopathy syndrome. Hepatitis B rate is 10× to 30× that of general population in United States
- Epstein Barr virus (EBV) and human T-cell leukemia virus

CD4+ Count and Opportunistic Infections

- CD4+ count decreased (>500/μL): Bacterial infections, oral candidiasis, TB, VZV
- CD4+ count = 250 to 500/μL: All of above plus esophageal candidiasis, Kaposi sarcoma
- CD4+ count = 50 to 250/μL: All of above plus *Pneumocystis jiroveci* [formerly *carinii*]) pneumonia, toxoplasmosis, extra-CNS lymphoma, HIV encephalopathy, progressive multifocal leukoencephalopathy, refractory candidiasis
- CD4+ count = <50/μL: All of above plus CMV retinitis, disseminated *MAI*, protozoon enteritides, cryptococcal meningitis, disseminated VZV, CNS lymphoma invasive aspergillosis

Laboratory findings due to involvement of organ systems

- Pneumonia
    Parasites (*Pneumocystic jiroveci* [formerly *carinii*]), *Toxoplasma gondii*) Viruses (CMV, herpes simplex)
    Fungi (*Cryptococcus neoformans, Histoplasma capsulatum, Coccidioides immitis, Candida* spp.)
    Bacteria (*Mycobacterium tuberculosis* and *M. avium-intracellulare* [may have positive culture and antigen detection of blood and marrow]),
    Streptococcus pneumoniae, Haemophilus influenzae, Staphylococcus aureus, Legionella species, *Nocardia asteroides*)
    Others (lymphoma, Kaposi sarcoma, lymphocytic interstitial pneumonitis)
- Nervous system (see Chapter 9).
    Dementia occurs in >50% of cases. Correlates CSF viral load. No correlation between CSF and plasma viral load.
    Aseptic meningitis
    Meningitis due to various organisms (*Cryptococcus neoformans, T. gondii*)
    Myelopathy

INFECTIOUS

      Peripheral neuropathy

      CNS lymphoma

      CSF should be examined for syphilis routinely in all patients with AIDS. AIDS causes treatment failures, relapses after treatment and increased incidence of early neurosyphilis. AIDS also alters serologic response to spirochete.

- Gastrointestinal

      Oropharyngeal candidiasis

      Cryptosporidiosis

      M. avium intracellulare causing diarrhea, or malabsorption or hepatitis

      CMV esophagitis or colitis or hepatitis

      Isosporosis causing diarrhea

      Coccidia—may cause acute, self-limited diarrhea in immunocompetent hosts; HIV hosts with CD4+ cell counts >180/μL had self-limited disease, but <180/μL did not clear the parasite. In HIV infection, reported prevalence rates of >20%. Is one of the "indicator" diseases for AIDS and can be a major factor leading to death; may involve stomach, pancreas, biliary tract, lungs.)

- Nephropathy—resembles nephrotic syndrome with very poor prognosis and rapid progression to end-stage renal disease; death usually within 6 months even with dialysis. Acute renal failure may be caused by drugs, sepsis, and the like. May also occur in asymptomatic carriers or ARC. Patients may have acute tubular necrosis, chronic tubulointerstitial nephritis, nephrocalcinosis, or heroin nephropathy.

- Neoplasms

      Kaposi sarcoma— ≥50% probability of occurrence within 10 years in men infected with both HIV and human herpesvirus 8 (HHV-8)

      Non-Hodgkin B-cell lymphoma—rapid course, poor prognosis, frequent extranodal and CNS involvement.

      Hodgkin Disease, Stage III/IV—mixed cellularity, nodular sclerosis

      Possible HIV association (T-cell non-Hodgkin lymphomas, cervical dysplasia/neoplasia, pediatric smooth muscle tumors)

- Lymph node aspirate

      Mycobacterial infection in 17%

      Lymphoid hyperplasia in 50%

      Non-Hodgkin lymphoma in 20%

      Kaposi sarcoma in 10%

      Occasional cases of Hodgkin disease, squamous cell and other carcinomas

- Other: Infectious mononucleosislike syndrome (rash, pharyngitis, enlarged spleen, etc.) may occur during initial viremia period with hematological picture of infectious mononucleosis but serological tests for EBV and CMV are negative; meningeal signs with CSF pleocytosis may occur. Most patients are asymptomatic during initial HIV viremia.

- Because of diminished immune function, AIDS patients

      With syphilis with positive VDRL may have negative FTA-ABS and have accelerated course and be refractory to standard therapy.

      Have high rates of salmonella infection.

      Have lower seroconversion rates and shorter duration of protection after HBV vaccination.

Laboratory findings due to treatment

- Anemia, leukopenia, thrombocytopenia
- Altered liver and renal function tests
- Increase in MCV often occurs with zidovudine and is useful to confirm patient compliance.
- Severe hemolysis may occur in G-6-PD deficiency after exposure to TMP-SMZ

Laboratory findings that should heighten suspicion in patients at risk:

- Lymphopenia
- Positive serologic test for syphilis
- Increased ESR
- Increased serum LD
- Low serum cholesterol
- Indicator diseases
- HCV coinfection in HIV patients averages 35%.
- HIV coinfection in HCV patients estimated at 5% to 10%.

In the absence of laboratory evidence of HIV infection, any of these known causes of immunodeficiency disqualify the indicator diseases:

- High-dose or long-term corticosteroid or other immunosuppressive/ cytotoxic therapy within 3 months of onset of indicator disease
- Genetic (congenital) immunodeficiency syndrome or an acquired syndrome atypical of HIV infection (e.g., with hypogammaglobulinemia)
- Any of the following diseases diagnosed <3 months after diagnosis of indicator disease: Hodgkin disease, non-Hodgkin lymphoma (other than primary brain lymphoma), lymphocytic leukemia, multiple myeloma, any other cancer of lymphoreticular or histiocytic tissue, angioimmunoblastic lymphadenopathy.

Indicator diseases that are considered evidence of AIDS when laboratory evidence of AIDS is present in a child age <13 years: Multiple or recurrent bacterial infections, septicemia, pneumonia, meningitis, bone or joint infection, abscess of internal organ or body cavity, due to *Haemophilus*, *Streptococcus* (including *pneumococcus*) or other pyogenic bacteria.

Clinical Category A

- Asymptomatic patients with none of the disorders of category B or C
- Documented HIV infection and ≥1 of the following:
    Asymptomatic HIV infection
    Persistent generalized lymphadenopathy
    Acute HIV infection

Clinical Category B

- Symptomatic patients with none of the disorders of Category (A) or (C) with conditions due to HIV infection or defect in cell-mediated immunity or where clinical course or management is complicated by HIV infection.
- Examples of conditions include (but are not limited to): Bacillary angiomatosis; Candidiasis, oropharyngeal (thrush); Candidiasis, vulvovaginal; frequent, persistent, or poorly responsive to therapy. Cervical dysplasia, moderate or severe or carcinoma in situ. Constitutional symptoms (e.g., fever or diarrhea) for >1 month. Hairy leukoplasia, oral. Herpes zoster of >1 dermatome or a least two episodes. Idiopathic thrombocytopenic purpura. Listeriosis, PID, especially if with tubo-ovarian abscess. Peripheral neuropathy.

Clinical Category C—AIDS-indicator conditions

Candidiasis or trachea, bronchi, lungs, or esophagus. Cervical cancer, invasive*. Coccidioidomycosis, extrapulmonary or disseminated. Cryptococcosis, extrapulmonary. Cryptosporidiosis, intestinal for >1 month. CMV other than liver, spleen, or lymph nodes. CMV retinitis with loss of vision. Encephalopathy, HIV-related. Herpes simplex ulcer for >1 month or bronchitis, pneumonitis, esophagitis. Histoplasmosis, disseminated or extrapulmonary. Isosporiasis, intestinal for >1 month. Kaposi sarcoma. Lymphoma, Burkitt or immunoblastic or primary of brain. *Mycobacterium* tuberculosis, any site*. *Mycobacterium*, any species, disseminated or extrapulmonary. *Pneumocystis carinii* pneumonia. Pneumonia, recurrent (more than 1 episode in a year).* Progressive multifocal leukoencephalopathy. Salmonella septicemia, recurrent. Toxoplasmosis of brain. Wasting syndrome due to HIV.

*= Added to list since 1991.

Recommended for HIV blood testing are persons who:

- Have a history of identifiable risks (e.g., IV drug use, prostitution, homosexual or bisexual men, infected sex partners) or have sexual partners with such risks
- Inmates of correctional institutions
- May have a sexually transmitted disease, TB, hepatitis B or C
- Received transfusions of blood or blood products (e.g., Factor VIII) between 1978 and 1985, but transfusion did not include immune serum globulin or albumin.
- Are planning marriage
- Women of childbearing age
- Patients admitted to hospitals
- Consider themselves at risk
- Donors of blood, organs, sperm

A repeat positive test requires the blood donor facility to inform the donor.

INFECTIOUS

About 22% to 50% of HIV antibody-positive persons develop AIDS at 5 years and 50% to 70% at 10 years.

Prediction of which seropositive persons will develop AIDS or show clinical symptoms is not possible. Antibody-positive persons are potentially infectious.

It may become possible to distinguish new infection from longer term infection by using highly diluted serum in immunoassay or by measuring different appearance times of antibodies to various HIV proteins and epitopes (e.g., early infection anti-*gag* (p24) and anti-*env* (gp41/gp120) antibodies appear but later in infection anti-*pol* develops; anti-p24 declines with development of clinical AIIDS).

Neonatal infection

IgG antibodies can cross placenta during third trimester; all infants born to HIV-1-infected women will be HIV-1 seropositive for ≤18 months.

Diagnostic testing should be done by age 48 hours.

Pregnant women with HIV-1 RNA <1,000 copies/mL have 0% transmission rate but with HIV-1 RNA >100,000 copies/mL have >40% transmission rate.

Increased risk of vertical HIV-1 transmission if maternal CD4+ cell count is low, HIV-1 RNA is high and prolonged rupture of membranes. PPV = 55% in neonates and 83% in infants >30 days old but the probability of HIV infection <3% if PCR is negative; thus, positive DNA PCR must be interpreted cautiously in neonates but negative tests are informative. HIV-1 DNA PCR is preferred method during infancy. HIV-1 infection is excluded if DNA PCR is negative after 6 months.

Diagnosis of vertical HIV-1 infection is indicated if one blood specimen is culture positive and a separate blood specimen is positive by DNA PCR or culture or (if infant >28 days) plasma *p24* antigen. Do not use umbilical cord blood to avoid contamination with maternal blood.

Most infected neonates have related symptoms within 1 year and ~50% have AIDS by 5 years; therefore, early diagnosis and therapy is essential.

Less than or equal to 40% of infants born to HIV infected women acquire HIV infection.

Less than or equal to 30% of infected infants are DNA PCR-positive at birth indicating in-utero infection while ≤70% are DNA PCR-negative at birth but positive after 7 days. More thand 90% of infected infants are DNA PCR-positive at 14 days.

HIV-1 DNA may still be detected in peripheral blood mononuclear cells in treated children with undetectable HIV-1 RNA, normal humoral and cellular immune function.

HIV RNA may be more sensitive than DNA PCR for early diagnosis of infants.

p24 antigen tests have high specificity but less sensitivity than other tests. Not recommended as sole test in infants <1 month caused by false-positive results.

HIV infection is diagnosed if two positive virologic tests on separate blood samples.

HIV is excluded if results are negative ≥2 virologic tests at >1 month and >4 months or ≥2 IgG antibody tests 1 month apart are negative after age 6 months if no clinical evidence of HIV infection or hypogammaglobulinemia.

Infants infected in utero have higher viral load than infants infected in peripartum period.

Infants' viral load increases rapidly during first 1 to 2 months and slowly declines for next 2 years. Maintains >100,000 copies/mL during first year.

High viral load at 1 month that remains high at 6 months predicts disease progression in next years without therapy.

Viral loads >10^5 copies/mL correlate with growth retardation, encephalopathy, opportunistic infection, death.

Children who are treated have same viral load response as adults. HAART treatment results in 2 to 3 $\log_{10}$/mL reduction to <500 copies/mL in 4 to 8 weeks and <50 copies/mL within 6 months.

Retroviral Syndrome, Acute

Syndrome of fever, malaise, lymphadenopathy, skin rash occurring in first few weeks after HIV infection in 20%; 80% are asymptomatic. HIV DNA has been detected in cryopreserved lymphocytes ≤3 years before seroconversion. Mean time from infection to symptoms is >8 years.

Antibody test is not yet positive.

Viral load assay should not be sole test as false positives may occur.

♦ *p24* ELISA.

AIDS-Related Complex (ARC, Chronic Lymphadenopathy Syndrome)

♦ Defined as lymphadenopathy for >3 months involving >2 extra inguinal sites in homosexual men without other illness or drug use known to cause lymphadenopathy. Lymph node biopsy shows reactive hyperplasia.

CD4+ T-Lymphocytopenia, Idiopathic

♦ Low CD4+ T-cell count (usually <300/μL) and <20% on ≥1 occasion; counts are stable rather than progressive depletion.
♦ HIV-1, HIV-2, HTLV-I, HTLV-II are not identified by serologic, immunologic, or virologic studies; no other obvious causes (e.g., SLE, sarcoidosis) can be identified.
Immunoglobulins are normal or slightly decreased in contrast to AIDS.
Opportunistic infections may be present
Syndrome not present in sex partners, household contacts, or blood donors and other epidemiologic and clinical differences from AIDS.

Antibody to Human T-Lymphotropic Virus Type I (HTLV-I)

HTLV-I is a retrovirus but not closely related to HIV. HTLV-I does not cause depletion of T-helper lymphocytes and is not generally associated with immunosuppression. HTLV-I does not cause AIDS and presence of antibody does not imply HIV infection or risk of AIDS. HTLV-I and HIV antigens do not cross react. HTLV infection and positive serology are lifelong.
Positive screening test (by ELISA) is recommended for screening for whole blood and cellular components and should be confirmed by more specific tests (Western blot; if indeterminate, then radioimmune precipitation). S/S of ELISA >97%. Source plasma need not be screened for HTLV-I. Repeatedly positive donors should be permanently deferred and counseled against blood donation, sharing needles, breast feeding, etc. Neither the screening nor more specific tests distinguish between antibodies to HTLV-I and HTLV-II (a closely related human retrovirus). HTLV-II has been isolated from patients with hairy-cell leukemia but has not been proved to cause any disease. Seroconversion occurs in 63% of blood transfusion recipients containing cells but not plasma fractions, 25% of breastfed infants of seropositive mothers and fewer nonbreastfed infants. Smaller percent in sexual partners.
Viral culture and PCR for research use only.
May Be Positive In
Adult T-cell leukemia/lymphoma (see Chapter 11). Risk of disease estimated at 2% to 4% after infected 20 years
Degenerative neurological disease called tropical spastic paraparesis in Caribbean and HTLV-I-associated myelopathy in Japan. Latent period of clinical disease occurs about 4 years after blood transfusion.
In United States, female prostitutes, and recipients of multiple blood transfusions, incidence occurs in up to 49% of IV drug users. Rare in homosexual men and patients in sexually transmitted disease clinics; nonexistent in hemophiliacs. A 0.025% incidence in random blood donors.
In Caribbean islands, occurs in 5% of general population and 15% of older persons.
In Japan, ≤15% of general population and ≤30% of older persons.

Choriomeningitis, Lymphocytic

Due to zoonotic arenavirus acquired from mice or hamsters; causes <10% of "aseptic meningitis".

○ CSF

• Cell count is increased (100–3,000 lymphocytes/μL, occasionally ≤30,000).
• Protein is normal or increased to 50 to 150 mg/dL.
• Glucose is decreased in 25% of patients.

♦ Serologic tests

- IgM (IFA) may be detected in serum and CSF within first week of illness.
- Increasing CF antibody titer between acute and convalescent sera (2–3 weeks). Disappears in a few months.
- IgG (IFA) may appear very early (therefore, sera should be drawn early) making 4× increase in titer difficult to detect; slowly declines over months.
- Neutralizing antibodies appear in 1 to 2 months, last for many years; therefore useful to document past infection.

Viral isolation by animal inoculation is not routinely performed.
WBC is slightly decreased at first; normal with onset of meningitis.
ESR is usually normal.
Thrombocytopenia develops during first week.

Colorado Tick Fever

Due to a coltivirus in the *Reoviridae* family transmitted by tick *Dermacentor andersoni*.

♦ Serologic tests show an increase in antibodies (EIA, IFA, CF and neutralizing) in acute and convalescent phase sera. EIA and IFA titers are larger and appear earlier, often within 10 days and persist for life. IFA for IgG is 90% sensitive and for IgM is 66% sensitive. CF antibodies last only a few months so presence of CF suggests recent infection.
♦ DFA method can demonstrate antigen in peripheral RBCs in 40% of cases 8 weeks after onset and sometimes up to 6 months. During first week, 50% of cases show false–negative results.
♦ Virus isolation is the most reliable test. Blood may be inoculated into suckling mice.
WBC is decreased (2,000–4,000/μL); decreased PMNs but with shift to the left.

Coxsackievirus and Echovirus

An enterovirus that may cause epidemic pleurodynia, "grippe," meningitis, myocarditis, herpangina.

Laboratory findings are not specific.
CSF

- Cell count ≤500/μL, occasionally ≤2,000/μL; predominantly PMNs at first, then predominantly lymphocytes.
- Protein may increase ≤100 mg/dL.
- Glucose is normal.

WBC varies but is usually normal.
Serologic tests may show increasing titer of neutralizing or CF antibodies between acute and convalescent phase sera. Are generally not clinically helpful because of many serotypes and extensive cross-reaction with other enteroviruses. With Coxsackie A or B infection, CF antibodies are often increased in acute phase making a 4× rise in titer difficult to demonstrate.
♦ Culture is required for certain syndromes (e.g., chronic meningoencephalitis with agammaglobulinemia may show echovirus 11 in CSF).

Encephalitis

See Tables 9-1 and 15-2.
Due To
Virus:

- Flaviviridae (e.g., West Nile, Japanese, St. Louis)
- Togaviridae (e.g., Eastern and Western and Venezuelan equine)
- Bunyaviridae (e.g., Rift Valley fever)
- Herpesviridae (e.g., HSV, CMV, VZV)
- Others (e.g., HIV, adenovirus, influenza, rabies, mumps, influenza, adenovirus enterovirus [e.g., coxsackievirus, echovirus, poliovirus])

Bacteria
Fungi
Amoebae (e.g., *Naegleria*)
♦ CSF findings. See Chapter 9.
♦ Appropriate culture and serologic tests for specific organism identification and additional laboratory tests (see separate sections for each agent).

Erythema Infectiosum (Fifth Disease)[14]

Due to parvovirus B19, a single-stranded DNA virus.

♦ Diagnosis by

* IgM antibodies appear 10 to 12 days after infection; indicates recent current infection.
  Peaks in ~1 month, undetectable after 2 to 3 months but may last for 6 months.
* IgG appears in ~2 weeks; high concentrations of IgG persist for >1 year. Present in 10% of children <5 years and >50% of adults. Indicates previous infection and immunity.

IgG	IgM	Interpretation
–	–	No exposure/immunity
+	–	Past infection and immunity
–	+	Recent infection
+	+	Recent infection

* Giant pronormoblasts in marrow biopsy have prominent intranuclear inclusions confirmed by IHC staining with antibody to virus.
* In situ DNA hybridization or PCR applied to maternal or fetal blood or amniotic fluid.

Also causes

* Pure erythrocyte aplasia and persistent infection in patients with underlying hemolytic anemias (sickle cell disease, hereditary spherocytosis, pyruvate kinase deficiency, β-thalassemia) and immunosuppressed hosts. Usually transient but may be chronic.
* Arthropathy in adults; "slapped cheek" rash in children with fifth disease.
* Chronic infection may cause severe anemia in immunocompromised persons.
* ≤20% of cases of nonimmune hydrops fetalis; congenital anemia. Specific IgM present in cord blood.

Gastroenteritis

See Chapter 7.

Hemorrhagic Epidemic Fevers

Due to hantavirus, a genus in single-stranded RNA family *Bunyaviridae*.

Hemorrhagic Fever with Renal Syndrome (HFRS)

Occurs in South America.

Laboratory findings due to renal damage (e.g., proteinuria, oliguria with azotemia and hemoconcentration and abnormal electrolyte concentrations. *Return of normal tubular function may take 4 to 6 weeks.*
WBC is increased, with shift to the left.
Coagulopathy

* Platelet count is decreased (<100,000/μL) in 50% of patients.
* Increased PT and aPTT may be present.
* DIC may occur.
* Increased serum LD and decreased albumin and total protein.

[14] Young NS, Brown KE. Parvovirus B19. *N Engl J Med* 2004;350:586.

INFECTIOUS

Hantavirus Pulmonary Syndrome (HPS)

Recently described in southwest United States; causes rapidly progressive non-cardiac pulmonary edema. Primarily carried by deer mice. Mortality >55%.

In both syndromes:
♦ Immunohistochemical staining for hantaviral antigens or RT-PCR for DNA can be identified in formalin fixed (e.g., autopsy) tissues.
♦ Serology is less useful in parts of South America where there is high seroprevalence of antibodies in persons with no history of exposure.

• Rapid test using recombinant antigens detects IgG and IgM antibodies. Positive tests are confirmed at CDC which is distributing ELISA assays to state laboratories to detect IgG and IgM.
• ELISA for antigen and specific IgM have S/S >90%; ELISA IgG peaks during first week and remains detectable. IFA replaced by ELISA. PCR should not be used alone. WB and neutralization to confirm diagnosis if necessary.

Blood culture is difficult and hazardous.
CBC shows thrombocytopenia, hemoconcentration, presence of immunoblasts.
Other viral hemorrhagic fevers (e.g., Philippine, Thailand, Singapore, Argentinian, Bolivian, Crimean, Omsk, Kyasanur Forest) show much less severe renal damage, and WBC is normal (Philippine, Thailand) or decreased.

Hepatitis
See Chapter 8.

Human Herpesviruses (HSV)[15]
Due to double-stranded DNA herpesvirus. See Chapter 8.

Virus	Genus	Disease
HSV 1	*Simplexvirus*	Herpes labialis (predominantly)
HSV 2		Herpes genitalis (predominantly)
Varicella-zoster	*Varicellovirus*	Chickenpox, herpes zoster (shingles)
Epstein-Barr	*Lymphocryptovirus*	Infectious mononucleosis
Cytomegalovirus	*Cytomegalovirus*	Infectious mononucleosis-like
HSV 6	*Roseolovirus*	Roseola, febrile illness
HSV 7		
HSV 8		Kaposi sarcoma

(1,2) Herpes Simplex
Due to HSV-1 and HSV-2 found in ≤90% and 10% to 30% of population respectively. Each may be associated with encephalitis.

♦ Direct cytologic examination of scrapings of lesions (Wright-Giemsa stain) show multinucleated giant cells with intranuclear inclusions (Tzanck smear). Skin vesicles produce a positive smear in 66% and positive viral culture in 100% of cases; pustules produce a positive smear in 50% and a positive viral culture in 70% of cases; crusted ulcers produce a positive smear in 15% and a positive viral culture in 34% of cases. Permits rapid diagnosis. Does not differentiate HSV-1, HSV-2, and zoster-varicella. May also be identified in routine Pap smear of cervix by multinucleated cells showing typical intranuclear inclusions and halo. Direct EM can also be used. Other microscopy-based tests include indirect IFA and immunoperoxidase that approach sensitivity of culture. Negative test does not rule out this diagnosis.
♦ Culture of vesicles or ulcers is reference method and confirmation by staining with specific monoclonal antibodies establishes the diagnosis. Culture from recurrent late disease is much less sensitive.

[15]Zerr DM, et al. Primary human herpesvirus 6 infection. *N Engl J Med* 2005;352:768.

♦ Antigen detection (EIA or direct fluorescence) in clinical specimen (e.g., vesicles, ulcers) distinguishes HSV-1 and HSV-2, is more rapid (1–4 hours) and as sensitive (70%–94%) in asymptomatic persons as culture and is significantly more sensitive and specific (>92%) than Tzanck test or direct EM.

♦ PCR detection of DNA identifies HSV in tissue, CSF, or cell samples, is sensitive, specific, rapid but may not be commercially available.

ELISA IgM and IgG.

○ Serologic tests: ELISA, WB, or immunoblot for glycoprotein G can distinguish HSV-1 (gG1) and HSV-2 (gG2). Positive result indicates prior exposure; negative result indicates no prior exposure. WB is gold standard for antibody detection. Immunoblot IgG has S/S = >80%/96%. Primary infections show seroconversion or a ≥4× increased titer in paired serum.

♦ In encephalitis, PCR of CSF (S/S = 98%/>94%) has supplanted brain biopsy.

♦ For neonatal infection, antigen detection or virus culture of buffy coat of blood establish the diagnosis. Seroconversion or increasing IgG/IgM titers are less useful. Specific IgM antibodies can be detected within 2 weeks of onset of infection.

(3) Chickenpox (Varicella-Zoster; VZV) and Herpes Zoster (Shingles)

Primary infection due to human DNA herpesviruses. Shingles is reactivation of latent varicella virus in dorsal root ganglia.

Lab tests are usually not needed except to possibly differentiate it from smallpox.

♦ Demonstration of DNA sequences by PCR is 88% sensitive in stained smears and 97% sensitive in unstained smears.

♦ Light microscopic demonstration of Wright-stained epithelial giant cells with intranuclear inclusion in fluid or base of vesicle (Tzanck smear) has 75% sensitivity. Also positive in herpes simplex. EM shows similar particles in vesicle fluid.

♦ Demonstration of VZV antigen by immunofluorescent staining in material from a lesion is diagnostic of acute infection; is more sensitive than culture (in contrast to HSV and CMV), especially in crusted lesions. Allows prompt diagnosis.

♦ Isolation of VZV by cell culture of vesicle fluid or scrapings of lesion; usually positive in 3 to 5 days.

♦ Immunohistochemical staining visualizes infected cells in 4 to 10 hours.

♦ Serologic tests (e.g., CF) are mostly supplanted by the above tests. Presence in CSF is diagnostic of aseptic meningitis caused by VZV even without skin lesions. LA is sensitive, commercially available, rapid, and simple to perform. Acute and convalescent serum showing a 4× increase in titer can confirm the diagnosis.

♦ In situ hybridization can demonstrate VZV virus in peripheral blood mononuclear cells in primary infection in 24 hours. Forty percent of zoster patients show increased cells (<300 mononuclear/µL) in CSF. Culture is rarely positive in HSV encephalitis; PCR-based detection is useful. Forty percent of bone marrow transplant recipients develop infection or reactivation.

WBC is decreased with absolute and relative lymphocytosis after 72 hours.

Liver function tests may be slightly abnormal.

(4) (6,7) Roseola Infantum (Exanthema Subitum; Sixth Disease) See Chapter 8

Due to human herpesvirus-6 [HHV-6] and HHV-7. >90% of infants are infected by second year of life.

HHV-6 infection occurs in 30% to 60% of bone marrow and organ transplant patients. May cause marrow suppression (varies from transient to fatal aplastic anemia), encephalitis, interstitial pneumonitis, susceptibility to other viral infections (e.g., EBV, CMV, RSV, adenovirus).

♦ Rapid shell vial assay of blood can detect infection within 72 hours. Reported S/S = 86%/100% in marrow and liver transplant patients. Is only reliable method to diagnose active infection. CSF and tissue cultures have low sensitivity.

♦ Tissue-cell cultures show specific cytopathic effects (requires 5–21 days).

♦ PCR to detect HHV-6 DNA in blood cells has limited value in diagnosing active infections. PCR on cell-free sample has low sensitivity. PCR on CSF is gold standard and shows active infection. Can be detected in saliva for >12 months after initial infection.

♦ IgM antibody titer to HHV-6 rises in 3 weeks after onset of exanthema subitum limiting its usefulness. Useful to detect latent infection or seroprevalence but may not be reliable indicator of reactivation. IgG can also be detected.

♦ Immunohistochemical stains that detects HHV-6 in tissues or cytology (e.g., BAL) shows active infection with moderate sensitivity.

WBC is increased during fever, then decreased during rash, with relative lymphocytosis.

Epstein-Barr Virus (EBV) Infections

Due to human herpesvirus 4 [HHV-4] of DNA viruses; infects B lymphocytes and epithelial cells; long lasting, usually latent, frequent reactivation is common.

Infectious Mononucleosis (IM)

♦ **Diagnostic criteria:**

• Compatible clinical syndrome
• Hematologic findings of absolute (>4,500/μL) and relative lymphocytosis ($\geq$50%) in >70% of cases and $\geq$10% (often $\leq$70%) characteristically atypical lymphocytes.
• Serologic findings. See Heterophil Agglutination (Paul-Bunnell test).

♦ EBV can be confirmed in liver biopsy by in situ hybridization or PCR.

♦ PCR can be used to detect EBV nucleic acid in tissue from undifferentiated nasopharyngeal carcinoma and for early diagnosis of lymphoproliferative disease.

○ Evidence of mild hepatitis (e.g., increased serum transaminases, increased urine urobilinogen) is very frequent at some stage but may be transient. Increased serum bilirubin in $\leq$30% of adults and <9% of children. Bilirubin/enzyme dissociation (serum bilirubin normal or <2 mg/dL with moderate increase of ALP, GGT, AST, ALT) occurs in 75% of cases. If no liver function abnormalities can be found, another diagnosis should be sought.

Leukopenia and granulocytopenia are evident during first week. Later, WBC is increased (usually 10,000–20,000/μL) because of increased lymphocytes; peak changes occur in 7 to 10 days; may persist for 1 to 2 months. Increased number of bands and >5% eosinophilia are frequent.

Serologic tests for syphilis RA, and ANA may show transient false-positive results.

Mild thrombocytopenia is seen in about 50% of early cases, and platelet dysfunction is frequent.

Hemolytic anemia is rare.

Heterophile-negative mononucleosis syndrome may be found in other infections diseases, especially CMV, toxoplasmosis, and HSV. Atypical lymphocytes may be seen in other acute illnesses (e.g., rubella, roseola, mumps, acute viral hepatitis, acute HIV, drug reactions).

Heterophile Agglutination (Paul-Bunnell Test)

Agglutination of sheep RBCs by serum of patients with infectious mononucleosis due to EBV.

Commercial slide agglutination ("spot") tests are now performed as the usual initial test and tube dilution tests are only done if necessary for confirmation; spot test S/S $\leq$92%/>96%, except in children <4 years old when slide test is less sensitive. False-positive slide tests may occur in leukemia, malignant lymphoma, malaria, rubella, hepatitis, pancreatic carcinoma and may be present for years in some persons with no known explanation. False-positive results in ~2% and false-negative results in ~5% to 7% of adults.

Titers $\leq$1:56 may occur in normal persons and in patients with other illnesses.

A titer of $\geq$1:224 is presumptive evidence of IM but may also be caused by recent injection of horse serum or horse immune serum. Therefore, a differential absorption test should be performed using guinea pig kidney and beef cell antigens. See Table 15-17.

Guinea pig absorption will not reduce the titer in IM to <25% of the original value; most commonly the titer is not reduced by more than 1 or 2 tube dilutions. If >90% of the agglutination is removed by guinea pig adsorption, the test is considered negative.

Beef red cell absorption takes most (90%) or all of the sheep agglutinations and does reduce the titer in IM; failure to reduce the titer is evidence against a diagnosis of IM.

Heterophil agglutination is positive in 60% of young adults by 2 weeks and 90% by 4 weeks after onset of clinical IM; thus may be negative when positive hematologic and clinical findings are present and a second heterophil agglutination 1 to 2 weeks later may be positive. The heterophil agglutination may have become negative even though some residual hematologic findings are still present. Low titers may persist for a year.

When horse RBCs are used for the test, results may still be positive up to 12 months after the acute illness in up to 75% of cases.

Heterophil antibodies are found in only 30% of children <2 years old, 75% of children 2 to 4 years old and >90% of older children with IM.

False-positive tests are very rare and occur in relatively low titers. A resurgence of heterophil antibody titer may occur in response to other infections (e.g., viral upper respiratory infection). Occasionally positive in other diseases (e.g., lymphoma, hepatitis, autoimmune disease [rheumatoid arthritis], rubella).

Is not specific for EBV. Titer does not crossreact with or correlate with antibodies for EBV; neither correlates with severity of illness. Not useful for evaluating chronic disease.

Heterophile agglutination is almost never positive in Japanese patients with IM for unknown reasons.

Heterophile-negative IM-like may occur in 10% of patients (mostly young children), toxoplasmosis, viral infections (e.g., CMV, hepatitis, rubella, acute HIV). Negative heterophile must be confirmed by EBV-specific antibodies.

Chronic Mononucleosis Syndrome

Three types are described; many question the existence of this syndrome.

* Rare distinct entity marked by acute mononucleosis >6 months duration, abnormal EBV antibody titers, histologic evidence of organ disease (e.g., pneumonitis, hepatitis) containing EBV DNA or antigens.
* True chronic mononucleosis is caused by EBV in >90% of cases, typical clinical picture with positive heterophile and serologic evidence of primary EBV infection but caused by CMV in 5% to 7% of cases, and *Toxoplasma gondii* in <1% of cases. Less common causes include AIDS, HSV II, varicella, viral hepatitis, adenovirus, rubella, and certain drugs (e.g., PAS, phenytoin, sulfasalazine, dapsone).

Table 15-17.   Sample Titers in Heterophil Agglutination

Presumptive Test	After Guinea Pig Kidney Absorption	After Beef RBC Absorption	Interpretation of Diagnosis of Infectious Mononucleosis
1:224	1:112	0	+
1:224	1:56	0	+
1:224	1:28	0	+
1:224	1:14 or less	0	−
1:224	1:56	1:56	−
1:224	0	1:112	−
1:56	1:56-1:7	0	+
1:56	1:56	1:28	−
1:28	1:28-1:7	0	+

INFECTIOUS

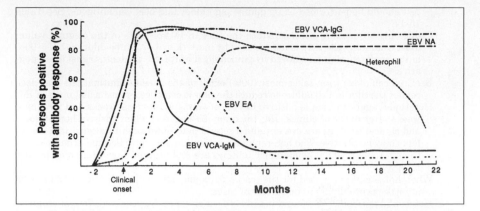

Fig. 15-8. Percentage of persons with positive antibody response at specified time intervals. (EBV, Epstein-Barr virus; VCA, viral capsid antigen; EA, early antigen; NA, nuclear antigen.) [Ortho Diagnostic Systems, Raritan, NJ.]

- Severe, chronic, active EBV infection (very rare) with very high EBV antibody titers and persistent serious disease (e.g., pancytopenia, agranulocytosis, chronic hepatitis, pneumonia); may coexist with true chronic mononucleosis. Heterophile is positive in ~10% of cases. No definitive diagnostic.

Posttransplantation Lymphoproliferative Disease

Spectrum of EBV-related disorders that range from IM to lymphoma due to immunosuppressive drugs.

◆ Biopsy of involved lymph nodes is diagnostic.
◆ Measure EBV viral load by PCR in peripheral blood or tissue. Fewer than 4,000 copies/mL of blood is very high and consistent with diagnosis. Serial measurements to follow the course; <200 copies/mL suggests resolution of posttransplantation lymphoproliferative disease and return of host immunity. Serology is not useful.

◆ Serologic Tests for Epstein-Barr Virus (EBV)

EBV antibody tests are rarely required, because 90% of cases are heterophile-positive and false-positive results are rare, and because illness is usually self-limited and relatively mild. Test may be useful in atypical or very severe cases with negative heterophile tests, especially in young children or immunocompromised patients. (See Table 15-18 and see Fig. 15-8.)

IgG-VCA (viral capsid antigen): Indicates past infection and immunity. May be present early in illness, usually before clinical symptoms are present, detected at onset in 100% of cases; only 20% show a 4× increase in titer after visiting a doctor. Decreases during convalescence but detectable for many years after illness; therefore, not helpful in establishing diagnosis of IM.

IgM-VCA: detected at onset in 100% of cases, high titers present in serum 1 to 6 weeks after onset of illness, starts to fall by third week and usually disappear in 1 to 6 months; sera are often taken too late to be detected. Is almost always present in active EBV infection and, thus, most sensitive and specific to confirm acute IM. May be positive in other herpesvirus infections (especially CMV); therefore confirmation with IgG and EBNA assays is recommended.

Early antigen (EA) anti-D titers rise later (3–4 weeks after onset; is transient) in course of IM than AB-VCA and disappear with recovery; combined with IgG-VCA suggests recent EBV infection; only found in 70% of patients with IM due to EBV. High titers are found in nasopharyngeal carcinoma due to EBV.

IgA antibodies against EBV capsid antigen and neutralizing antibodies against EBV DNAse together are reported to predict nasopharyngeal carcinoma.[16]

[16]NEJM 12/27/2001.

Early antigen (EA) anti-R antibodies rarely occurs in primary EBV infection, 2 weeks to months after onset, may persist for a year; more often in atypical or protracted cases. No clinical significance; high titers are found in chronic active EBV infection or Burkitt lymphoma.

Epstein-Barr nuclear antigen (EBNA) are the last antibodies to appear and is rare in acute phase; develops 4 to 6 weeks after onset of clinical illness and rises during convalescence (3–12 months); and persist for many years after illness. Absence when IgM-VCA and anti-D are present implies recent infection. Appearance early in illness excludes primary EBV infection. Appearance after previous negative test evidences recent EBV infection. ELISA kits detect EBNA IgG and IgM simultaneously; IgM > IgG indicates acute infection but IgG > IgM indicates previous exposure to EBV. Absent EBNA and presence of VCA indicates acute infection.

Acute primary EBV infection is indicated by ≥1 of these serologic findings:

• IgM-VCA that is found early and later declines
• High titer (≥1:320) or ≥4× rise in IgG-VCA titer during the illness
• Transient rise in anti-D titer (≥1:10)
• Early IgG-VCA without EBNA and later appearance of EBNA

Acute or primary EBV infection is excluded when IgG-VCA and EBNA titers are unchanged in acute and convalescent serum samples.

Current or recent infection is indicated by IgM anti-VCA or IgM/IgG early antigen with low or absent EBNA antibodies.

Persistence of early antigen and IgG-VCA in high titer indicate chronic EBV infection.

• *>90% by age 20, >95% by mid-20s. EBNA is often absent in immunosuppressed patients. EA-D and EA-R may be increased with no change in VCA. EBV is associated with Burkitt's lymphoma, nasopharyngeal carcinoma, 40% to 60% of cases of Hodgkin disease, hairy leukoplakia of tongue; in immunosuppressed patients (e.g., AIDS, organ transplant) is associated with B-cell lymphoma and leiomyosarcoma.*
• Severe, often fatal, mononucleosis occurs in patients with X-linked lymphoproliferative syndrome; predisposes to subsequent lymphoma.
• *Anti-VCA titers increased 8× to 10×.*
• *Anti-EA-R is high and correlated with tumor burden in Burkitt lymphoma.*
• *Anti-EA-D is high and correlated with tumor burden nasopharyngeal carcinoma.*

(5) Cytomegalic Virus (CMV) Inclusion Disease

DNA virus; member of herpesvirus family.

♦ Less than 40% of population has lifelong latent infection that is only significant in immunocompromised persons. Quantitative determination of CMV DNA may determine presence of active infection. Detection of CMV messenger RNA may indicate active rather than latent infection.

♦ • BAL fluid for diagnosis of interstitial pneumonitis in immunocompromised patients for shell culture and monoclonal antibody testing is more sensitive than

Table 15-18. Serologic Antibody Patterns in EBV Infection

	Susceptible/ No Infection	Primary Acute Infection	Established Infection	Convalescence	Past (remote) Infection
Heterophile Ab	−	+	+	Decreasing	−
VCA-IgM	0 or <1:10	+ >1:10	+ or >1:10	Decreasing	0 or ≤1:10
VCA-IgG	0 or <1:10	−; + early	+ or >1:10	Increasing	+ or ≥1:10
EA-IgM	−	+	+	Decreasing	−
EA-IgG	−	−; + early	+	Decreasing	+
EBNA-IgG	0 or <1:5	0 or <1:5	0 or <1:5	Increasing	+ or ≥1:5

routine cytology and can be combined with nucleic acid hybridization assay or routine cell culture.

♦ • GI tract disease is confirmed by biopsy showing presence of typical inclusions, immunological stain for CMV antigen, or in situ DNA probe for CMV DNA.

♦ Pregnancy and congenital infection

• Intrauterine CMV infection caused by infection of mother during pregnancy causes obvious CMV inclusion disease in 10% to 15% of infants at birth; many affected infants die soon after birth and others may require lifelong institutionalization. Fetal infection in ~20% of these (≤2/1,000 births). In 5 years, 25% have sequelae (e.g., CNS, chorioretinitis).

• Special culture techniques using urine specimens gives earlier results in congenital CMV infection than in other populations; within first 2 weeks, is most sensitive and specific means for diagnosis of congenital CMV infection.

• PCR to detect CMV is rapid, sensitive, specific.

• CMV-IgM (>1:32) antibodies are found in about two thirds of infants infected in utero; presence in single infant serum specimen is diagnostic.

• Intranuclear inclusions in epithelial cells in urine sediment and liver biopsy is diagnostic; more useful in infants than adults.

• Negative CMV-IgG in mother and child excludes CMV infection.

• In newborns, viral isolation is more accurate than IgM. Isolation in standard cell culture (shows cytopathic effects in 3–7 days) of urine, saliva or tissue within first 21 days of life is gold standard for intrauterine infection. After 21 days, perinatal infection cannot be ruled out.

• Amniotic fluid viral culture is sensitive and specific indicator of intrauterine CMV infection.

• Shell-vial culture (see below). Maximum sensitivity uses both culture systems.

• CMV-IgM by EIA (S/S = 69%/94%) or RIA (S/S = 89%/100%) in first 2 to 3 weeks of infection. Should be confirmed by culture.

• EM of urine has ~66% sensitivity. Cannot distinguish CMV from other herpesviruses.

• Microscopic examination of tissue showing intranuclear inclusions and giant cell formation in stillborn infants.

• PCR assay for CMV DNA in urine, CSF, serum has excellent S/S.

• 50% of infants have hemolytic anemia with icterus and 75% have thrombocytopenia.

• CSF normal except for protein >120 mg/dL in 50% of cases.

○ Screening and diagnosis of recipient and donor of blood products and organ transplants

• CMV infection occurs in >50% of bone marrow transplant patients, usually in 1 to 3 months; CMV pneumonia causes significant mortality. Seronegative patients should be given CMV seronegative blood products. Filtration to reduce leukocytes to <10^6/unit and platelets prevents transmission by transfusion of unscreened blood.

♦ Syndrome of heterophil-negative infectious mononucleosis in immunologically competent adults (due to CMV in 50% of cases) is characterized by:

• Hematologic and hepatic test findings identical with those in heterophil-positive infectious mononucleosis due to Epstein Barr virus.

• Immunologic findings
    Increased cold agglutinin titer (same as in heterophil-positive patients)
    Cryoglobulinemia is common (mixed IgG-IgM).
    Increased RF (cold-reactive more common than warm-reactive)
    Positive direct Coombs test is common.
    Polyclonal hypergammaglobulinemia is common.
    False positive serologic test for syphilis in <3% of cases
    ANA (speckled pattern) commonly present transiently

♦ Serological tests are not useful in immunocompromised patients.

• Latex agglutination to detect CMV antibody is rapid assay with sensitivity of 98%; useful for blood and organ donor screening; negative tests are confirmed by EIA. About 50% of adults in North America are seropositive for CMV antibodies; in urban areas may be >80%.

- Presence of CMV-IgM 10 to 14 days after primary infection using a single test during acute illness (>1:32); titer <1:16 may persist for 12 months in 24% of patients.
- 4× increase in serial CMV-IgG antibody titer in 2 to 4 weeks in primary but only occasionally in reactivation or reinfection limits value in adults.

♦ Confirmatory tests for CMV

- Isolation of virus in standard cell culture may take weeks. CMV may be shed in absence of disease for up to 2 years after primary infection, tests must be interpreted carefully.
- Active CMV infection is most accurately diagnosed by rapid tissue culture (shell vial) with DFA staining; permits detection in urine, blood, secretions, tissues in <48 hours.
- CMV pp65 antigenemia can be detected within hours; antigenemia test kit is said to have S/S = 83%/89%; peripheral blood WBCs are frequently positive in immunocompromised patients and those with CMV mononucleosis and indicates viremia.
- Identification of CMV inclusion bodies or CMV antigen in infected tissue (e.g., BAL) by IFA is more rapid but less sensitive than culture.
- DNA and RNA hybridization techniques have high S/S.
- PCR detects DNA/RNA within a few hours from blood, plasma, CSF, BAL.

Laboratory changes due to involvement of liver, kidney, brain.

- Encephalitis found in 16% of HIV-infected patients; 85% of cases are infected with HIV.
    PCR S/S = 79%/95%.
    Viral cultures of CSF are usually negative.
    Other techniques include detection of pp65 antigen in CSF WBCs, CMV DNA in CSF, in situ hybridization of CSF WBCs, increased CMV antibody CSF/serum ratio.
- Disseminated CMV disease occurs in immunosuppressed patients (e.g., retinitis-induced blindness occurs in 10%–45% of AIDS patients).

Laboratory findings due to predisposing or underlying conditions (e.g., immunocompromised state or after receiving transfusions of fresh blood); may be associated with other opportunistic pathogens. Confirmation of opportunistic infection is important in immunocompromised patients. Most severe disease occurs in patients with AIDS and bone marrow transplants. Acquired active CMV infection is found in >60% of solid organ transplant recipients and >35% of stem cell transplant recipients. Important to monitor for CMV in recipients to distinguish from transplant rejection.

(6, 7) Roseola Infantum (Exanthema Subitum; Sixth Disease)

Due to human herpesvirus-6 [HHV-6] and HHV-7. >90% of infants are infected by second year of life. HHV-6 infection occurs in 30% to 60% of bone marrow and organ transplant patients. May cause marrow suppression (varies from transient to fatal aplastic anemia), encephalitis, interstitial pneumonitis, susceptibility to other viral infections (e.g., EBV, CMV, RSV, adenovirus).

♦ Rapid shell vial assay of blood can detect infection within 72 hours. Reported S/S = 86%/100% in marrow and liver transplant patients. Is only reliable method to diagnose active infection. CSF and tissue cultures have low sensitivity.
♦ Tissue-cell cultures show specific cytopathic effects (requires 5–21 days).
♦ PCR to detect HHV-6 DNA in blood cells has limited value in diagnosing active infections. PCR on cellfree sample has low sensitivity. PCR on CSF is gold standard and shows active infection. Can be detected in saliva for >12 months after initial infection.
♦ IgM antibody titer to HHV-6 rises in 3 weeks after onset of exanthema subitum limiting its usefulness. Useful to detect latent infection or seroprevalence but may not be reliable indicator of reactivation. IgG can also be detected.
♦ Immunohistochemical stains that detects HHV-6 in tissues or cytology (e.g., BAL) shows active infection with moderate sensitivity.
WBC is increased during fever, then decreased during rash, with relative lymphocytosis.

INFECTIOUS

Human Papillomavirus (HPV)[17]

Due to subgroup of papovaviruses; >200 distinct types of double stranded DNA viruses. Infects squamous epithelium causing spectrum of diseases of skin, respiratory and genital tracts from warts, to dysplasia to carcinoma.

♦ Molecular methods can detect HPV DNA or RNA by in situ hybridization or PCR.
♦ Routine histology or immunohistochemistry are less sensitive indicators.
HPV antibodies are not sensitive enough for diagnostic purposes.

Lesion	HPV Type
Common warts	1, 2
Plantar warts	1
Flat warts	3
Butcher warts	3, 7
Epidermodysplasia	3, 5, 8, 9, 10, 12, 14,15, 17, 19, 20, 21, 22, 23, 24, 25
Verruciformis	28, 29
Respiratory	6, 11, 30, others
Genital, low risk	6, 11, 42, 43, 44
Genital, high risk	16, 18, 31, 33, 35, 39, 45, 51, 52, 56, 58, 59, 68

See Pelvic Inflammatory Disease, Chapter 14, pp. 760, 765.

Measles (Rubeola)

Exanthem due to virus family Paramyxoviridae, genus *Morbillivirus*.

Diagnosis is usually made clinically.
♦ Wright stain of sputum or nasal scrapings show measles multinucleated giant cells, especially during prodrome and early rash.
♦ Papanicolaou stain of urine sediment after appearance of rash shows intracellular inclusion bodies; more specific is FA demonstration of measles antigen in urine sediment cells.
♦ Viral serologic tests

• Serum IgM (EIA) is detectable with onset of rash and usually persists for 4 weeks; 50% become negative by 2 to 4 months. Presence of IgM or ≥4× rise in IgG indicates recent infection. Presence of IgG generally indicates present immunity.
• Within 6 days after onset of rash, antibodies are found in >80% of cases (HAI, EIA, IFA, CF; HAI is most sensitive). Maximum titers are reached in 2 to 3 weeks. Paired sera show significant increases in titer.

RT-PCR for detection of RNA has been used.
Virus recovery from respiratory secretions, conjunctiva, urine, or blood mononuclear cells is difficult and rarely used.
CNS

• Measles encephalitis: There is a marked increase in WBCs. CSF may show slightly increased protein and ≤500 mononuclear cells/μL. Fewer than or about ≤10% of all measles patients have a significant increase in cells in CSF.
• Postmeasles encephalitis is an autoimmune disorder; virus is not detected in brain.
• Persistent CNS infection causes subacute sclerosing panencephalitis (progressive fatal illness in children 5–14 years old). Diagnosed by presence of IgM or ≥4× rise in IgG titers in CSF.

WBC shows slight increase at onset, then falls to ~5,000/μL with increased lymphocyte count. Increased WBC with shift to the left suggests bacterial complication (e.g., otitis media, pneumonia, appendicitis).
Mild thrombocytopenia in early stage.
Measles may cause remission in children with nephrosis.

[17]Anderson SM. Human papillomavirus and cervical cancer: an update. *Advance/Laboratory* 2005:92.

Mumps

Salivary adenitis due to enveloped single-stranded RNA virus of family Paramyxoviridae, genus *Rubulavirus*.

Uncomplicated salivary adenitis

* WBC and ESR are normal; WBC may be decreased, with relative lymphocytosis.
* Serum and urine amylase are increased during first week of parotitis; therefore, increase does not always indicate pancreatitis.
* Serum lipase is normal.

◆ Serologic tests
   IgM (EIA) is present by day 2 in 70% of patients and by day 5 in 100% of patients; may last >5 months in 50% of patients. Presence of IgG indicates immunity due to past infection or vaccination. Serum IgG and IgM should be taken as early as possible and again in 10 to 14 days (EIA, IFA). ≥4× rise in IgG (88% sensitivity) or presence of IgM indicates recent infection. Serum neutralization, CF, and HAI tests that become positive later and are much less sensitive have been largely replaced.
◆ Virus culture from urine, saliva or CSF or direct fluorescent antibody on urine or saliva.

Laboratory findings due to complications of mumps

* Meningitis or meningoencephalitis (see Chapter 9)—aseptic meningitis occurs in 4% to 6% of clinical cases of mumps; causes >10% of cases of aseptic meningitis. Clinical mumps may be absent in 20% to 60% of patients. The disease may be clinically identical with mild paralytic poliomyelitis. WBC is usually normal. CSF contains 0 to 2,000 mononuclear cells/μL (average = 250); protein ≤100 mg/dL but rarely >700 mg/dL; decreased glucose in ≤29% of cases.

◆ Simultaneous serum and CSF specimens show increased mumps IgG antibody index (in 83% of patients) and mumps IgM antibody index (in ~67% of patients with IgM in CSF). Oligoclonal Ig in CSF in 90% of cases. Virus can be isolated from CSF. PCR has been reported to provide rapid diagnosis.

* Orchitis (in 20% of postpubertal males but rare in children)—WBC is increased, with shift to the left. ESR is increased. Sperm are decreased or absent after bilateral atrophy.
* Pancreatitis (see Chapter 8) is much less frequent in children. Serum amylase and lipase are increased even if no abdominal symptoms are present. Patient may have hyperglycemia and glycosuria.
* Ovaries are involved in 5% of adult females. Thyroiditis, myocarditis, arthritis, etc.

Phlebotomus Fever (Sandfly Fever)

Due to single stranded RNA virus of Bunyaviridae family transmitted by *Phlebotomus* flies.

WBC <5,000/μL in 90% of patients by third day. Lymphopenia early followed by relative lymphocytosis.
Liver function tests and urine are normal.
Aseptic meningitis in ~10% of patients

Poliomyelitis

Due to single stranded RNA enterovirus.

CSF

* Cell count is usually 25 to 500/μL; rarely is normal or <2,000/μL. At first, most are PMNs; after several days, most are lymphocytes.
* Protein may be normal at first; increased by second week (usually 50–200 mg/dL); normal by sixth week.
* Glucose is usually normal.
* AST is always increased but does not correlate with serum AST; reaches peak in 1 week and returns to normal by 4 weeks; level of AST does not correlate with severity of paralysis.

INFECTIOUS

- *CSF findings are not diagnostic but may occur in many CNS diseases due to viruses (e.g., Coxsackie, mumps, herpes), bacteria (e.g., pertussis, scarlet fever), other infections (e.g., leptospirosis, trichinosis, syphilis), CNS tumors, multiple sclerosis, etc.*

Blood shows early moderate increase in WBC ($\leq$15,000/μL) and PMNs; normal within 1 week.

Laboratory findings of associated lesions (e.g., myocarditis) or complications (e.g., secondary bacterial infection, stone formation in GU tract, alterations in water and electrolyte balance caused by continuous artificial respiration) are present.

Increased AST in 50% of patients is caused by the associated hepatitis.

Serologic tests may show $\geq$4$\times$ increase in CF antibody types 1, 2, 3 titer between acute and convalescent sera (after 3 weeks), but titer may have already reached peak at time of hospitalization. Not useful to determine immune status for which neutralization test is used. EIA, IF, and neutralization tests have also been used.

♦ Virus may be cultured from stool up to early convalescence

Rabies (Hydrophobia)

Due to a Lyssavirus causing lethal neurotropic infection in mammals. Encephalitis due to bite of rabid animal; in United States, skunks (62%), bats (12%), raccoons (7%), cattle (6%), cats (4%), dogs (3%); in Africa and Asia, dog rabies is endemic.

♦ Earliest tests are virus culture (using saliva, CSF, brain) and antigen detection using FA or nucleic acid amplification and can sometimes be reported in 48 hours. Detection of rabies antigen in corneal impressions, cutaneous nerve fibers in biopsy of hair-bearing skin.

♦ PCR may be positive on nuchal skin biopsy, saliva, tears, CSF. Viral RNA can indicate variant associated with various animal sources.

♦ FA antibody staining for antigen in skin and buccal mucosa biopsies, and brain biopsy material can also be used for diagnosis during clinical phase.

♦ Antibody in CSF is conclusive evidence of infection. Serum IgG antibodies usually require rising titer for accurate diagnosis; does not appear until >8 days after onset of clinical symptoms which may be months after exposure; almost all patients have antibodies by 15 days; are diagnostic if patient has not received immunization.

Intradermal prophylactic immunization may not be adequate and should be checked with serologic tests.

♦ Microscopic examination of brain tissue sections or imprint smears of rabid animal shows Negri bodies (intracytoplasmic inclusions) in ~80% of cases which has largely been supplanted.

Rabid animal dies within 7 to 10 days.

♦ Brain tissue of suspected animal is inoculated into brain of white mice, which is later examined by FA. S/S >96%.

CSF is usually normal or has a slight increase in protein and an increased number of mononuclear cells (usually <100/μL).

WBC is increased (20,000–30,000/μL), with increased PMNs and large mononuclear cells.

Urine shows hyaline casts; reaction for albumin, sugar, and acetone may be positive.

Rotavirus Infection

Due to double-stranded DNA virus; many strains. Causes gastroenteritis.

Direct EM examination of stool for virus is >80% sensitive; IEM is not needed. Can be confirmed by ELISA that is highly sensitive.

Serological tests: EIA for IgG, IgM and IgA; IFA.

Commercial kits are available for EIA, latex agglutination, hemagglutination, immunoblot, dot hybridization. Latex agglutination screening must be confirmed by other tests (e.g., EIA).

PCR is most sensitive methodology and permits genotyping.

Rubella (German Measles)

Due to single-stranded RNA *Rubivirus*. Identifying exposure to rubella infection and verifying immunity in pregnant women is important because infection in the

first trimester of pregnancy is associated with congenital abnormalities, abortion, or stillbirth in ~30% of patients; during first month ≤80% of patients show this association. Twenty-five percent to 50% of cases are subclinical.

♦ ELISA tests for IgG and IgM are >97% sensitive and specific. For antenatal patients, IgG titer >1:10 confirms immunity; is present in >90% of population in USA; lower titer is considered nonimmune. After vaccination high levels last for 8 to 12 weeks.

♦ IgM is detected 11 to 25 days after onset of rash in all patients and may persist for ≤1 year. Detected 15 to 25 days after vaccination in ≤80% of cases. In congenital infection IgM can be detected at birth and persists for ≤6 months in >90% of infants. During first 6 months of life, IgM is the best test for congenital or recent infection. After age 7 months, assess persistence of IgG. IgG appears 15 to 25 days after infection and >25 to 50 days after vaccination; less than one third of persons may show no detectable IgG after 10 years. Absence of IgG in infant excludes congenital infection.

Low levels of IgM may occur in infectious mononucleosis; cross reaction may occur with parvovirus IgM. Some pregnant women with IgM antibodies to rubella may also have IgM to CMV, varicella-zoster, and measles virus.

♦ With rubella rash, diagnosis is established if acute sample titer is >1:10 or if convalescent-phase serum taken 7 days after rash shows increase in titer.

♦ Even if no rash develops in a patient exposed to rubella, a convalescent-phase serum taken 14 to 28 days after exposure that shows ≥4× increase in titer indicates rubella exposure but not necessarily recent infection.

♦ Reinfection (occurs occasionally but usually asymptomatic) can be suspected if sera drawn ≥2 weeks apart show ≥4× increase in IgG titer and IgM does not develop.

♦ Rubella virus isolated from amniotic fluid indicates congenital infection.

Smallpox (Variola)

Due to double-stranded DNA virus of Poxviridae family.

Testing is only available at CDC.
Skin vesicles or fluid, scabs, pharyngeal swab:
♦ Microscopic findings of cytoplasmic elementary bodies (Guarnieri bodies) in scrapings from base of skin lesions; does not discriminate from vaccinia.
♦ Electron microscopy showing virions from skin lesions; does not discriminate from vaccinia.
♦ Viral antigen identified by immunohistochemistry from skin lesions.
♦ PCR and fluorescent antibody staining of virus from skin lesion.
♦ Viral serologic tests

• Increasing titer of neutralizing antibody in acute and convalescent-phase (2–3 weeks later) sera to distinguish recent infection from prior vaccination.
• Rapid technique using vesicular fluid in hemagglutination, precipitation, or CF tests
• Newer methods to detect IgM may enhance S/S

♦ Characteristic pocks on chorioallantois culture is antiquated.
WBC decreased during prodrome, increased during pustular rash.

Respiratory Viral Infections

♦ New rapid kits (EIA) for influenza and RSV have S/S = 50–90%/80–90%.
♦ Commercial kits are available for qualitative detection of 7 respiratory viruses by FA in direct patient specimens or after growth in cell culture. Includes RSV, influenza A and B, adenovirus, parainfluenza 1, 2, and 3.

Due to Respiratory Syncytial Virus (RSV)
Major cause of bronchiolitis and pneumonia in infants and young children.

♦ RT-PCR is commercially available with better sensitivity than culture or antigen detection.
♦ Direct detection of antigen in clinical specimens by EIA or FA have high sensitivity and specificity and is test of choice.
♦ Presence of serum IgM or ≥4× increase in IgG (EIA) indicates recent infection.
♦ Viral culture of NP is gold standard; requires 4 to 6 days.

ESR and WBC may be increased in children.

Pharyngeal smears may reveal many epithelial cells that contain cytoplasmic inclusion bodies.

Due to Adenovirus

May cause at least six clinical syndromes: Respiratory infection, conjunctivitis, gastroenteritis in children, acute hemorrhage cystitis, genital ulcers and urethritis, and CNS disease.

♦ PCR assay in various body fluids and tissue detects adenovirus antigens or nucleic acid.

♦ Cell culture can take 10 to 20 days. Rapid centrifugation culture can take 2 to 5 days.

♦ Latex agglutination tests of stool is less sensitive than culture.

♦ Direct EM has been useful for diagnosis of gastroenteritis in children.

Direct examination of defoliated cells by cytopathology affords rapid diagnosis but not generally successful.

Serology (e.g., CF, ELISA, IF) to identify culture isolates. A 4× titer increase in paired specimens.

Due to Rhinoviruses

♦ EIA provides simple rapid diagnosis.

WBC may be slightly increased.

ESR is increased in ~5% of patients.

Due to Parainfluenza Virus

♦ Type-specific diagnosis requires recovery of virus in tissue-culture.

EIA is more sensitive but less specific than CF. Not useful for routine clinical studies.

WBC is variable at first; later becomes normal or decreased.

Due to Influenza A, B

♦ Serologic tests

• Rapid diagnostic tests for influenza A and B by antigen, enzyme, or nucleic acid in doctor's offices. Has replaced following tests.

• Presence of IgM or ≥4× increase in IgG (EIA, IFA) indicates recent infection. IgM peaks at 2 weeks and IgG at 4 to 7 weeks. IgG indicates past exposure and immunity.

• CF and HAI may show 4× increase in sera taken during acute phase and 3 weeks later.

♦ IFA stain of cells in nasopharyngeal swab.

♦ RT-PCR has better sensitivity than culture.

♦ Culture may take 3 days but rapid method followed by ELISA gives results in <24 hours or IFA.

WBC normal (5,000–10,000/μL) with relative lymphocytosis. Leukopenia occurs in 50% of patients. WBC >15,000/μL suggests secondary bacterial infection.

Avian influenza (H5N1) is subtype of *Influenza A*. FDA has recently cleared a RT-PCR assay.

Severe Acute Respiratory Syndrome (SARS)[18,19]

Pandemic due to a novel coronavirus that causes acute diffuse alveolar damage.

♦ RT-PCR for detection of viral RNA.

♦ Virus can be cultured or seen on EM; corroborated by IFA and RT-PCR.

Maximum recovery (>90%) during second to fourth weeks in feces and respiratory material and in urine ≤45%. Viremia level reaches maximum 4 to 5 days after onset of fever. Found in plasma or serum in ≤78% of cases within 3 days; 25% by day 14. May be detectable for >30 days in all specimens.

♦ Serology detects specific IgG antibody after ~21 days (e.g., IFA and ELISA); shows 4× increase. Not useful for early diagnosis.

Serologic tests and urinary antigens for other respiratory organisms (e.g., *Chlamydia pneumonia* and *psittaci*, *Mycoplasma pneumoniae*, *Streptococcus pneumoniae, and L. pneumophila*) are negative.

---

[18]Chan PKS, et al. Laboratory diagnosis of SARS. *Emerg Infect Dis* 2004;10:825.
[19]Chan KH. Detection of SARS coronavirus in patients with suspected SARS. *Emerg Infect Dis* 2004;10:294.

Lymphopenia with normal neutrophil and monocyte count in ~70% of cases, thrombocytopenia in ~45% of cases, increased aPTT in ~45% of cases, increased D-dimer in 45% of cases.

Increased serum AST (in ~78% of cases), ALT (in 56% of cases), LD (in ~80% of cases), CK (in ~56% of cases) and decreased O_2 saturation.

Vaccinia

Vaccine virus skin infection during vaccination against smallpox.

♦ Guarnieri bodies (cytoplasmic inclusions) in skin lesions
   Laboratory findings due to complications

- Progressive vaccinia. Rule out malignant lymphoma, chronic lymphatic leukemia, neoplasms, hypogammaglobulinemia, and dysgammaglobulinemia
- Superimposed infection (e.g., tetanus)
- Postvaccinal encephalitis

West Nile Virus Encephalitis[20]

Due to member of *Flavivirus* genus; transmitted by mosquitoes from birds; also by blood products/organ transplants, laboratory exposure, and intrauterine transmission. Two thirds have encephalitis and one third have meningitis.

♦ Most useful and usual test is ELISA for IgM in CSF occurs earlier than serum; usually (90%) detectable by third to fifth day when patient is symptomatic but RNA may have disappeared from blood. Should repeat test if initially negative. Can remain positive for ≤1 year. Is more specific than IgG which may represent prior infection. IgG appears ~5 days after IgM; conversion to positive or increase between acute and convalescent phases confirms diagnosis. May cross react with other flaviviruses (e.g., St. Louis encephalitis, dengue) or yellow fever vaccination necessitates confirmation with viral neutralization. ELISA has better S/S than IFA. Neutralization antibody tests are more specific but require specialized laboratory.

♦ PCR of CSF identifies virus in ≤60% of cases. Is most useful when IgM is negative. CSF shows elevated protein, lymphocytic pleocytosis and normal glucose; positive culture is rare. May be positive for IgG (rare) and IgM.

♦ Detection of viral RNA (by RT-PCR) is used for diagnosis and screening blood donors. More useful in seronegative immunocompromised patients. Detection of viral RNA in urine may also establish the diagnosis.

♦ Plaque reduction neutralization test (PRNT) is used for confirmation by CDC and public health laboratories.

♦ Culture is used for screening mosquitoes and birds; human viremia level is low and brief.

Inoculation of heart blood in neonatal mice can also be used.

♦ Brain tissue from autopsy is positive by PCR in >80% of cases; also specific IHC staining.

One in 5 infected persons develops mild flu-like illness; 1 in 150 develops meningoencephalitis.

Should first rule out treatable causes of meningitis/encephalitis that can be rapidly diagnosed (e.g., bacteria, herpes virus, enteroviruses).

Donated blood should also be screened (e.g., nucleic acid amplification tests).

Dengue[21]

Endemic tropical disease due to single-stranded RNA member of *Flavivirus* genus transmitted by (e.g., *Aedes aegypti*) mosquitoes. Four distinct serotypes: DEN-1, 2, 3, 4 distinguishable by CF and neutralization tests; immunity is specific to each serotype.

[20]Solomon T. Flavivirus encephalitis. *N Engl J Med* 2004;351:37.
[21]Wilder-Smith A, Schwartz E. Dengue in Travelers. *N Engl J Med* 2005;353:924.

> **Probable diagnosis**
> ♦ Serologic tests ELISA for IgM (appears within 5 days, persists for months); is test of choice and ELISA IgG appears soon after IgM; persists for life single titer ≥1,280.
> **Confirmed diagnosis**
> ♦ Culture is positive within first 5 days (sensitivity <50%); can also culture from liver at autopsy.
> ♦ Detection of virus in tissue, serum, or CSF by IHC, IFA, or ELISA. ELISA for specific viral antigen have supplanted IFA.
> ♦ Increase specific IgG or IgM ≥4× by HAI. Cross-reacts with other flaviviruses and previous vaccinations.
> ♦ Detection of genomic sequence of virus by RT-PCR (sensitivity >90% early; <10% in 7 d.) still a research tool.
> ♦ WB and neutralization tests can be used to confirm acute infection if necessary.

WBC decreased (2,000–5,000/μL) with toxic granulation of leukocytes and neutropenia; may have marked atypical lymphocytes.
Complications
    Dengue hemorrhagic fever

- Decreased platelets (<100,000/μL) with impaired aggregation, prolonged PT and aPTT. DIC may occur.
- Increased transaminases (500–1,000 U/L) and bilirubin.

    Dengue shock syndrome

Yellow Fever

Due to member of *Flavivirus* genus; transmitted by Aedes aegypti mosquito.

♦ Serologic tests

- ELISA for IgM (appears within 5 days, persists for months); is test of choice and ELISA for specific viral antigen have supplanted IFA.
- WB and neutralization tests can be used to confirm acute infection if necessary.
- IHC can make post-mortem diagnosis.
- ELISA IgG appears soon after IgM; persists for life.
- RT-PCR is still a research tool.

♦ Culture is positive with first 4 days; can also culture from liver at autopsy.
○ Increased transaminases and bilirubin.
○ Biopsy of liver for histologic examination.
Decreased WBC (2,000–5,000/μL) is most marked by sixth day, associated with decrease in both leukocytes and lymphocytes.
Decreased platelets with impaired aggregation, prolonged PT and aPTT. DIC may occur.
Proteinuria and azotemia occur in severe cases.
Laboratory findings are those due to GI hemorrhage, which is frequent; there may be associated oliguria and anuria.

Fungus/Yeast Infections

See Table 15-19
Most disseminated or CNS fungal infections occur primarily in immunosuppressed patients.
Fungus/Yeast Infections

- *Aspergillus fumigatus* and other species (aspergillosis)
- *Blastomyces dermatides* (blastomycosis)
- *Candida albicans* (candidiasis)
- *Coccidioides immitis* (coccidiomycosis)
- *Cryptococcus neoformans* (cryptococcosis)
- *Geotrichosis candidum*

Table 15-19. Summary of Laboratory Findings in Fungus Infections

Disease	Causative Organism	Blood	CSF	Stool	Urine	Nasopharynx, throat	Sputum, lung	Gastric washings	Vagina, cervix	Exudates, lesions, sinus tracts, etc.	Skin, nails, hair	Bone marrow	Lymph node	Fresh unstained material	Stained material	Culture	Animal inoculation	Serologic tests	Histologic examination
		Source of Material												Microscopic examination		Diagnostic Methods			
Cryptococcosis	*Cryptococcus neoformans*	+	+	+	+		+				+	+	+		+	+	+	+	+
Coccidioidomycosis	*Coccidioides immitis*	+	+	+			+	+			+	+	+	+		+	+	+	+
Histoplasmosis	*Histoplasma capsulatum*	+					+	+			+	+			+	+	+	+	+
Actinomycosis	*Actinomyces israelii*						+			+					+	+			+
Nocardiosis	*Nocardia asteroides*										+			+	+	+	+		+
North American blastomycosis	*Blastomyces dermatitidis*						+				+				+	+		+	+
South American blastomycosis	*Paracoccidioides brasiliensis*					+					+		+	+					+
Moniliasis	*Candida albicans*	+				+			+		+				+	+		+	+
Aspergillosis	*Aspergillus fumigatus,* others						+							+		+		+	+
Geotrichosis	*Geotrichum candidum*						+								+	+			+
Chromoblastomycosis	*Fonsecaea pedrosoi, Phialophora verrucosa, compactum,* etc.										+			+		+			+
Sporotrichosis	*Sporotrichum schenckii*										+					+	+	+	+
Rhinosporidiosis	*Rhinosporidium seeberi*					+													+

- *Histoplasma capsulatum* (histoplasmosis)
- *Pneumocystis jiroveci (formerly carinii)*
- *Rhinosporidiosis seeberi*
- *Sporothrix schenckii* (sporotrichosis)

Aspergillosis

Due to ubiquitous fungus *Aspergillus fumigatus* and other species.

Clinical Types of Lung Disease

- Invasive aspergillosis in immunocompromised individuals with invasion of bronchial wall. Serologic tests may be negative.
- Allergic bronchopulmonary aspergillosis occurs in 1% to 2% of patients with chronic asthma. EIA has S/S ~90%. Should be confirmed by immunoblotting. Can be monitored by changes in increased serum IgE.
- Fungus ball (pulmonary aspergilloma)—saprophytic aspergilloma superimposed on an preexisting cavity or bronchiectasis. Serum IgG may be increased but IgE is not.
- Is one cause of hypersensitivity pneumonitis (farmer's lung)
  Eosinophilia (>1,000/μL; often >3,000/μL)
  Serum IgE antibody for *A. fumigatus* is markedly increased but not specific; significantly higher than in uncomplicated bronchial asthma.
  Expectorated mucus plug contains eosinophils, mycelial elements, and Charcot-Leyden crystals.

- ◆ Recognition of organism in material (especially sputum) from sites of involvement (especially lung; also brain, sinuses, orbit, ear). *Organisms occur as saprophytes in sputum and mouth. Confirm by staining organisms in biopsy specimens.*
- ◆ Positive culture on most media at room temperature or 35°C. Blood cultures are usually negative.
- ◆ PCR assay of blood and/or BAL for *Aspergillus* DNA is being evaluated. Also positive in some other invasive mold infections. PCR for detection of galactomannan antigen.
- ◆ Serologic tests

- EIA for galactomannan antigen (polysaccharide in wall of *Aspergillus* species) in blood has S/S >90%.
- CF for detecting recent or active disease; has good specificity but less sensitive than immunodiffusion.
- Immunodiffusion has high specificity but is often negative in invasive disease in immunocompromised patients for whom EIA for IgG is best choice.
- Antigen detection has good specificity but variable sensitivity.
- Specific ELISA IgG levels useful for early diagnosis and monitoring treatment. Precedes x-ray appearance of lung lesions and cytologic or microbiological identification by weeks.

Laboratory findings due to underlying or primary disease

- Aspergilloma—Superimposed on lung cavities caused by TB, bronchiectasis, carcinoma
- Invasive aspergillosis—Immunocompromised patients (e.g., AIDS, malignant lymphoma, acute leukemia, cystic fibrosis)

Blastomycosis

Due to dimorphic fungi; North American blastomycosis due to *Blastomyces dermatitidis*; South American blastomycosis due to *Paracoccidioides brasiliensis*.

Clinical types

- North American—involvement of skin and lungs
- South American—involvement of nasopharynx, lymph nodes, cecum, CNS
- Later, visceral involvement may occur in both types.

- ◆ Recognition of organism in material (e.g., pus, sputum, biopsied tissue) with special and immunohistochemical stains, DNA hybridization

- Positive culture on Sabouraud's medium at room temperature and blood agar at 37°C; slow growth of *P. brasiliensis* on blood agar ≤1 month; is the only certain diagnostic method. Seeing typical yeasts in tissue sections is less satisfactory.
- Wet smear preparation in 20% KOH
- Negative animal inoculation

◆ Serologic tests for *B. dermatitidis*

- Antibodies are usually detectable within 25 days of onset of illness; rise to peak at 51 to 75 days and then decrease. In chronic pulmonary disease, may peak within 25 days and then decrease.
- EIA is most sensitive and specific, especially in early disease; is initial test of choice. Initial titers are often negative; therefore serial titers should be performed. Titer ≥1:32 supports diagnosis and falling titers indicate improvement. Positive test should be confirmed with immunodiffusion.
- RIA may be slightly less sensitive and specific.
- Immunodiffusion assay for precipitin antibodies against antigen A is 17% to 65% sensitive and 95% specific; may be negative in early disease.
- CF test is positive in high titer with systemic infection and high titer is correlated with poor prognosis but test is not useful for diagnosis; sensitivity <25%. CF show 17% cross-reaction with histoplasmosis.

◆ ELISA detection of antibodies in CSF in cases with CNS involvement.
WBC and ESR are increased. Mild normochromic anemia is present.
Serum globulin is slightly increased.
Serum ALP may be increased with bone lesions.
Skin tests are positive in 40% of patients; false-positive results may occur in other fungal diseases (e.g., histoplasmosis) caused by cross-reactivity.

Coccidioidomycosis

Due to soil-dwelling dimorphic fungus (saprophytic yeast and parasitic mold)
***Coccidioides immitis* endemic to hot desert of southwest United States. Is acquired by inhalation of spores.**

◆ Positive culture (e.g., sputum, bronchoalveolar lavage) is diagnostic.
◆ Serologic tests are especially useful in this disease for both diagnosis and prognosis. Positive results are highly specific but false-negatives may occur, especially early in illness. Repeat testing during first 2 months may be needed.

- ELISA can detect antigen before appearance of antibodies.
- Determination of IgG and IgM by ELISA has S/S >92% in serum and CSF and is method of choice. Minimal cross-reaction with other diseases and are rare. IgM occurs temporarily in 75% of cases of primary infection. IgG appears later and usually disappears in several months if infection resolves. Increased IgG titer indicates disseminated extrapulmonary disease but may not be found in meningitis.
- Tube precipitin and immunodiffusion are used to detect IgM antibodies of early acute infection. Appear early, decrease after the third week, are uncommon after the fifth month. They occur at some stage of the disease in 75% of patients and usually indicate early infection. In primary infection, they are the only demonstrable antibodies in 40% of patients. If tests are negative, repeat three times at intervals of 1 to 2 weeks. *Beware of occasional cross-reaction with primary histoplasmosis and cutaneous blastomycosis.*
- CF is used to detect IgG antibodies that persist throughout disease course. Appear later (positive in 10% of patients in first week), and the titer rises with increasing severity.
    Less than one third of cases are positive in the first month; most positive reactions occur between the fourth and fifth weeks. Antibodies decrease after 4 to 8 months but may remain positive in low titer for years. The titer parallels severity of infection and is useful for following the course. Low titers may be found early in disease and are significant; low titers may be seen in pulmonary, limited extrapulmonary or inactive disease. Titers of 1:16 to 1:32 are highly suggestive of disease. Titers >1:32 indicate active disease and suggest extensive, disseminated disease. Fall in titer suggests effective therapy but rising titer is diagnostic and denotes disease progression. High titer not always present in disseminated disease. May

be found in other body fluids, usually 1 to 2 dilutions less than serum. In CSF, is diagnostic of meningitis (occurs in 75% of these cases). May cross-react with other mycoses, notably histoplasmosis.

♦ Wet preparation in 20% KOH and culture on mycologic media of sputum, gastric contents, CSF, urine, blood, marrow biopsy, liver biopsy, exudate, skin scrapings, etc., or intraperitoneal injection of mice.
♦ Biopsy of skin lesions, affected lymph nodes, lung, etc showing mature spherule with endospores is pathognomonic.
♦ DNA probe now commercially available allows confirmatory testing in hours.
CSF in meningitis shows 100 to 200 WBCs/μL (mostly mononuclear), increased protein, frequently decreased glucose.
♦ Positive IgG-specific antibody is diagnostic of meningitis in undiluted CSF; any titer is significant; is also used to indicate response to amphotericin B as well as relapse for 1 to 2 years after end of therapy. Serum titers are often negative or borderline in meningitis. CF antibodies are present in 75% of meningitis patients; latex agglutination parallels CF.
○ Eosinophilia in ≤35%; >10% in 25% of patients.
WBC (with shift to the left) and ESR are increased.
Laboratory findings due to underlying immunosuppression (e.g., AIDS patients who may have concurrent disseminated and aggressive pulmonary disease; Hodgkin disease, immunosuppressive drugs); also late stages of pregnancy and diabetes.
♦ Skin test conversion strongly indicates recent infection; skin testing does not cause serologic response.

Cryptococcosis

Systemic infection due to encapsulated yeast-like fungus *Cryptococcus neoformans*. Usual manifestation is CNS although lung is usual portal of entry.

♦ Serologic tests

• Antigen detection test is test of choice. Latex slide agglutination on serum and CSF detects specific cryptococcal *antigen* (specificity = 100%). Measurement of cryptococcal capsule antigen in serum and CSF is the most valuable test in meningitis. Use for screening of suspected cryptococcosis, because it is more sensitive (>90%) than India ink smears of CSF, it may be positive in 30% of cases without meningitis. Serum or CSF is positive in most cases; when negative, agglutination test may be positive. Antigen titers reflect extent of disease; is rarely positive with local involvement other than CNS (e.g., lung, skin); increasing titer suggests progressive disease and failure to decrease with treatment suggests insufficient therapy. EIA antigen detection has higher S/S.
• Antibody detection (IFA, direct agglutination) is most useful in early disease when antigen production is small. Beware of false positives caused by RF, other fungi, neurosyphilis, bacterial meningitis and false-negative results due to immune complexes, prozones, nonencapsulated variants, very early disease.
• Antibody testing in serum and CSF is positive only in early CNS or no CNS involvement; may become positive only after institution of therapy. May be found in healthy persons. Rising titer may be a favorable prognostic sign.

♦ Cultures should always be done because false-positive antigen tests may occur because of other fungi (e.g., *Trichosporon beigelii*). Culture of CSF for *C. neoformans* on Sabouraud's medium becomes positive in 1 to 2 weeks (positive in 97% of cases) followed by mouse inoculation; 20% of cases require multiple cultures. Culture is commonly positive even without chemical changes in CSF. Repeated fungal cultures are often necessary; cisternal fluid is sometimes superior to lumbar CSF. One may also get positive cultures from blood (25%), urine (37%), stool (20%), sputum (19%), and bone marrow (13%). Sputum cultures are most often positive when there is no x-ray evidence of pulmonary disease. Urine cultures are commonly positive with little kidney involvement. Positive blood culture indicates extensive disease and an extremely poor prognosis.
○ CSF

• Cell count is almost always increased ≤800 cells (more lymphocytes than leukocytes).

- Protein is increased in 90% (<500 mg/dL).
- Glucose is moderately decreased in ~55% of patients.
- Relapse is less frequent when increase in protein and cells is marked rather than moderate. Poor prognosis is suggested if initial CSF examination shows positive India ink preparation, low glucose (<20 mg/dL), low WBC count (<20/μL).
- Positive culture is related to CSF volume; should be ≥10 mL.
- Positive antigen serologic test without other CSF changes should be viewed with suspicion except in immunosuppression (e.g., AIDS). Should always confirm low titer serology with culture. Repeat CSF exam to evaluate therapy.

◆ India ink slide

- CSF is positive in ~80% of AIDS patients ~50% of non-AIDS patients with meningitis (usually more acute onset); thus, half of cases will be missed if India ink preparations are used as the sole criterion; rarely seen in other fungal types. Lower limit of detection is 1,000 organisms/cu mL.
- India ink preparations are also used on sputum, pus, skin scrapings.

◆ In biopsy material, mucicarmine, Alcian blue, silver, Giemsa, and the like, stains are positive; also positive on intraperitoneal injection of white mice.
CBC and ESR usually remain normal.
Increased risk of failure of amphotericin B treatment if positive culture from sites other than CSF (e.g., blood, sputum, urine), anticryptococcal antibodies are absent, CSF or serum cryptococcal antigen titer initially is >1:32 or posttreatment is ≥1:8, immunosuppressed states.
There is evidence of coexisting disease affecting T-lymphocytes in ~50% of patients (e.g., AIDS, diabetes mellitus, steroid therapy, Hodgkin disease, lymphosarcoma, leukemia). Occurs in ≤9% of patients with AIDS. In AIDS, cryptococcal disease most commonly appears as meningitis but typical signs in only ~50% of cases; dissemination to lungs, marrow, skin is common. In AIDS patients are more likely to find organisms in blood cultures and blood smears; CSF changes may be very slight and organisms may have smaller capsules making recognition with India ink more difficult; while CSF antigen titer declines with treatment, serum antigen level often remains constant or increases.
Laboratory findings due to involvement of other organs (e.g., heart, adrenals).

Geotrichosis

Rare infection due to a filamentous fungus [mold], *Geotrichum candidum*; disseminated in patients with neutropenia.

◆ Recognition of organisms from material from sites of involvement (respiratory tract; possibly colon)
◆ Positive culture on Sabouraud's medium (room temperature). *Organisms occur as saprophytes in pharynx and colon.*
◆ Microscopic visualization of organisms in biopsy material.

Histoplasmosis[22]

Due to *Histoplasma capsulatum*, a dimorphic fungus whose spores are inhaled from soil contaminated by bat or bird droppings. Primarily affects lungs.

◆ Biopsy (specially stained) of skin and mucosal lesions, bone marrow, and RE system provides initial diagnosis in ~45% of cases.
◆ Demonstration of *H. capsulatum* in specially stained smears of peripheral blood, buffy coat, bone marrow (25%–60% positive), respiratory secretions is often the most rapid method of diagnosis but are insensitive and should be performed with cultures.
◆ Culture of lung, skin and mucosal lesions, sputum, broncho-alveolar washings, gastric washings, blood or bone marrow may be difficult (Sabouraud's medium at room temperature; blood agar at 37°C not specific). Blood and bone marrow cultures are

[22]Goulet CJ, et al. The Unturned Stone. *N Engl J Med* 2005;352:489.

positive in 50% to 70% of patients. Culture is positive in <10% of asymptomatic self-limiting cases, 65% of cavitary pulmonary cases, and 75% of disseminated cases. Large volumes of CSF (30–40 mL) may be needed. Culture may require 2 to 6 weeks. Mouse inoculation, especially from sputum, may give a positive subculture from spleen on Sabouraud's medium in 1 month.
♦ Serologic tests

• Antigen detection
    In urine in 90% of disseminated cases, ~20% of acute self-limited disease, <10% of chronic pulmonary cavitary disease. Especially useful in disseminated disease in which patients may not show significant antibody response. Absent or low levels after amphotericin B therapy. Increase in serum or blood heralds relapse.
    In serum is less sensitive; found in 70% of disseminated cases.
    In CSF in <50% of meningitis cases; may cross-react with coccidioidal meningitis (CSF antibodies may also cross-react).
    In bronchoalveolar lavage, sensitivity = 70%.
• CF titers
    A single serum titer ≥1:32 or 4× increase in titer is highly suggestive of active histoplasmosis; <1:8 is considered negative. Rising CF titers occur in >95% of symptomatic primary infections. Increased titer is less common in disseminated primary infection. CSF titer ≥1:8 is evidence for meningeal histoplasmosis. They appear during the third to sixth week. Higher titers tend to be found in chronic pulmonary cavitary disease and lower titers in disseminated disease. Positive titers persist for months or years if disease remains active. Prognosis is not indicated by level or changes in titers.
• IgG and IgM detection by is not clinically useful because high (25%–50%) false-positive rates in other infections and false-negative rates in immunocompromised patients.
• Skin testing can cause conversion of antibody titers within 1 week. Skin tests are negative in 50% of disseminated cases. Frequent cross-reactivity with blastomycosis and coccidioidomycosis. Not helpful in clinical diagnosis but useful in epidemiologic studies.

Anemia, leukopenia, and thrombocytopenia are more common (60%–80% of cases) in acute than in subacute or chronic disseminated types.
Laboratory findings due to involvement of various organ systems (e.g. meningitis, endocarditis [particularly aortic valve], adrenal insufficiency, which are occasionally seen in subacute and less often in chronic disseminated histoplasmosis).
Since coinfection is common, specimens should be examined for other opportunists, especially mycobacteria. Underlying AIDS should be ruled out.
Very increased serum LD may be clue to disseminated form in AIDS patients.

Moniliasis

Due to fungus (yeast) *Candida albicans*.

♦ Definitive diagnosis by histopathology showing organisms invading tissue.
♦ Positive culture on Sabouraud's medium and on direct microscopic examination of suspected material.
♦ PCR detection of *Candida* DNA may replace culture.
♦ Serum antibody tests showing seroconversion, sharply rising titers, production of multiple precipitins usually indicate deep-seated infection in patients who are not immunosuppressed but may not distinguish transient candidemia. Precipitin titer = 1:8 or 4× increase in titer indicates invasive candidiasis rather than *Candida* colonization.
○ *In vaginitis, rule out underlying diabetes mellitus*; also antimicrobial drugs, pregnancy, oral contraceptives, corticosteroids, exogenous hormones, AIDS, local allergy caused by perfumes, nylon underwear. Gram stain or 10% KOH preparation confirms diagnosis but negative finding does not rule it out.
○ *In skin and nail involvement in children, rule out congenital hypoparathyroidism and Addison disease.*
○ *In septicemia with endocarditis, rule out IV drug abuse, prosthetic heart valve. Persistent positive blood culture after removal of a central venous catheter indicates endocarditis rather than catheter contamination.*

○ *In myocarditis, rule out corticosteroid or intensive antibiotic therapy, or abdominal surgery.*
○ *In GI tract overgrowth, rule out AIDS or chemotherapy suppression of normal bacterial flora.*
○ *In positive blood culture, which is rare, rule out serious underlying disease (e.g., malignant lymphoma), multiple therapeutic antibiotics, and plastic IV catheters.*
♦ Ratio of serum D-arabinitol (in μmol/L) to creatinine in mg/dL of ≥4.0 in fungemia and deeply invasive tissue or mucosal candidiasis (S/S = 74%/>40%); highest values in persistent fungemia. Therapy that reduces tissue burden of *Candida* causes decline in DA/Cr ratio.

Mucormycosis

Due to ubiquitous opportunistic fungus of Mucorales family.

♦ Histopathological detection is the gold standard.
♦ Mycologic cultures from brain and CSF are rarely positive; may be positive from infected nasal sinuses or turbinate.
No reliable serologic tests at present.
Clinical types

• Cranial (acute diffuse cerebrovascular disease and ophthalmoplegia in uncontrolled diabetes mellitus with acidosis)
• Pulmonary (findings due to pulmonary infarction) occurs in neutropenic patients (e.g., lymphoma, leukemia)
• In abdominal blood vessels (findings due to hemorrhagic infarction of ileum or colon)
• Disseminated form (dialysis patients on deferoxamine therapy are predisposed)
• Cutaneous

Laboratory findings of underlying disease or complications are present (e.g., neoplasms, IV drug users, malnutrition).

Pneumocystis Jiroveci (formerly Carinii)[23,24]

Usually an opportunist infection. Recently classified as fungus closely related to yeasts.

♦ Diagnosis requires demonstration of organism.

• Induced sputum (nebulization with saline) is very effective for diagnosis, inexpensive and can be done as outpatient. Use of routine and special stains and IFA stain allows diagnosis in ~95% of cases.
• Bronchoalveolar lavage is equally successful in diagnosis (sensitivity 60%–95%); rarely needed.
• The organism is rarely found in routine sputum, bronchial washings or brushings.
• Transbronchial lung biopsy is very effective way to make a definite diagnosis. Also allows diagnosis of other infections (e.g., fungi) or diseases (e.g., lymphoma), use of various stains, touch preparations. Open lung biopsy is rarely needed.
• Organisms can be found in postmortem histologic material.
• Immunologic stain with monoclonal antibodies is useful to diagnose extrapulmonary lesions.

♦ PCR has greater S/S than conventional staining.
♦ The morphology of the lung lesions suggests the diagnosis.
Organism does not stain with routine H & E stains; requires immunofluorescence or special stains (e.g., Giemsa, Schiff).
Seropositivity is almost universal by age 2 years.
No culture techniques are available.
○ Laboratory findings of associated diseases; found in >55% of sputum specimens from patients with various types of immunosuppression.

[23]Thomas CF, Jr., Limper AH. Pneumocystis Pneumonia. *N Engl J Med* 2004;350:2487.
[24]Wazir JF, Ansari NA. Pneumocystis carinii Infection. *Arch Pathol Lab Med* 2004;128:1023.

INFECTIOUS

- Is the primary presenting opportunistic infection in 55% to 65% of AIDS cases; is twice as common in IV drug users as in homosexuals.
- Administration of cytotoxic drugs and corticosteroids.
- Premature or debilitated infants.
- Underlying diseases (e.g., immunoglobulin defects; malignant lymphoma and leukemia patients more susceptible than other tumors)
- Other infections (especially CMV, systemic bacterial infections [especially *Pseudomonas* or *Staphylococcus*], TB, cryptococcosis).
- 25% of patients who die after renal transplant.

Laboratory findings due to organ system involvement (e.g., Pulmonary disease)

- Hypoxemia and hypercapnia
- Increased serum LD
- Pleural effusion may occur but should consider a second condition (e.g., Kaposi sarcoma, mycobacterial disease)

May affect other organs (e.g., liver spleen, marrow, eye, skin).
Leukopenia indicates a poor prognosis. Lymphopenia and anemia are common.

Rhinosporidiosis
Rare fungus infection due to *Rhinosporidium seeberi*.

♦ Recognition of organism (sporangia containing sporangiospores) in biopsy material from polypoid lesions of nasopharynx or eye (cannot be cultured)

Sporotrichosis
Endemic fungus infection due to *Sporotrichum schenckii*. Clinical forms: lympho-cutaneous, fixed cutaneous, disseminated cutaneous, systemic.

♦ Recognition of organism in skin, pus, or biopsy material

- Positive culture on Sabouraud's medium from unbroken pustule.
    Intraperitoneal mouse inoculation of these colonies or of fresh pus produces organism-containing lesions.
- Direct microscopic examination is usually negative.

♦ Serologic tests

- EIA is 100% sensitive at titer ≥1:128. Titer much higher in extracutaneous disease compared to cutaneous disease.
- Tube and latex slide agglutination shows 94% sensitivity; persistent elevation or rising titer is common in pulmonary disease. Low titer (e.g., <1:16) in non-fungal disease (e.g., leishmaniasis). CSF titer of 1:32 in meningeal infection. CF is less sensitive; (titer of ≥1:16) antibodies can be demonstrated in extracutaneous disease (e.g., pulmonary, disseminated). Cross-react with other mycotic and bacterial infections.
- Sera and CSF antibodies are present in meningeal disease (EIA ≥1:8 is positive); titers decrease after onset of therapy. CSF may show oligoclonal IgG bands and elevated IgG index in meningeal infection.

Laboratory Tests for Parasitic Diseases

See Tables 15-20 and 15-21
♦ Diagnosis usually depends on demonstrating the causative organism in appropriate specimens concentrated and stained appropriately (e.g., sedimentation or flotation of stools; stained thick and thin smears of peripheral blood can detect parasites of malaria, babesiosis, lymphatic filariases, acute stage of trypanosomiasis).

Stool Examination
Interferences
Foreign materials in stools (e.g., barium, bismuth, mineral oil, nonabsorbable antidiarrheal agents).

Use of antimicrobial agents that may modify intestinal flora (e.g., tetracycline) for one week before examination.

Serologic Tests include IHA, CIE, EIA, ELISA, CF.

Use
Epidemiologic studies.
Complementary when primary diagnostic method is negative.
Less expensive than direct microscopy.
Negative test is useful to rule out certain diseases (e.g., invasive amebiasis).
Positive test in a traveler who has not previously been in an endemic area can be helpful.

Disadvantages
May not distinguish between present and past infection.
Do not identify the causative species which may be important for therapy (e.g., malaria).
Do not identify drug-resistant strains (e.g., malaria).
Not widely available in kit form or performed only in research or reference laboratories.
May require special equipment (e.g., flow cytometry).
Newer technology (e.g., DNA probes, monoclonal antibodies for detection of antigen in stool) improves diagnostic utility when available but genetic and molecular diversity of population of organisms (e.g., trypanosomes) makes it difficult to construct reliable serologic tests.
○ Eosinophilia may be a clue to parasitic infection.
○ Increased IgE in helminth infections.
○ Increased globulin (IgG) with reversed A/G ratio may be a clue to parasitic infection.

Parasitic Infections

Helminth Infections

* Nematodes
    * *Ascaris lumbricoides* (ascariasis) round worms
    * *Enterobius vermicularis* (pinworm) round worms
    * *Trichuris trichiura* (trichuriasis; whipworm)
    * *Strongyloides stercoralis* (strongyloidiasis; hookworm)
    * *Onchocerca volvulus* (onchocerciasis)
    * *Dracunculus medinensis* (dranculiasis)
    * *Dirofilaria immitis* (dirofilariasis; dog heartworm)
    * *Toxocara canis* or *T. cati* (larval migrans)
    * *Trichinella spiralis* (trichinosis)
* Cestodes
    * *Taenia solium* (pork tapeworm; cysticercosis of brain), *T. saginata* (beef tapeworm)
    * *Diphyllobothrium latum* (giant fish tapeworm)
    * *Hymenolepis nana* (dwarf tapeworm)
    * *Echinococcus* (hydatid disease)
* Trematodes
    * *Schistosome mansoni, S. haematobium, S. japonicum)* (schistosomiasis)
    * *Fasciola hepatica, Clonorchis sinensis* (liver flukes)
    * *Fasciolopsis buski* (giant intestinal fluke)
    * *Paragonimus westermani* (lung fluke)

Ascariasis

Common nematode infection due to roundworm *Ascaris lumbricoides*.

♦ Stools contain ova. Occasionally, adult worms are spontaneously passed in stool.
○ Eosinophils are increased during symptomatic phase.
Serologic tests are not useful.
Laboratory findings due to malabsorption, intestinal obstruction, biliary or pancreatic disease.

Table 15-20. Helminths and Protozoa

Helminths	Organism	Bld	CSF	Stool	Urine	Urethra	Vag	BM	Other
Cestodes (Tapeworms)	*Diphyllobothrium latum*								
	Hymenolepis nana								
	Echinococcus granulosus								
	Echinococcus multilocularis								
	Taenia saginata								
	Taenia solium								
Nematodes									
Roundworms	*Ascaris lumbricoides*			+					
	Enterobius vermicularis			+					
Filariae	*Wuchereria bancrofti*	+							
	Onchocerca volvulus								**Conjunctiva**
	Loa Loa	+							
Hook-worms	*Ancylostoma duodenale*			+					
	Necator americanus								
	Strongyloides stercoralis			+					
Whipworm	*Trichinella spiralis*								
	Trichuris trichu'ra			+					
Trematodes									
Intestinal fluke	*Fasciolopsis buski*								
Liver flukes	*Fasciola hepatica*								
	Clonorchis sinensis								
Lung fluke	*Paragonimus westermani*			Occ.					
Blood flukes	*Schistosoma haematobium*				+				
	Schistosoma japonica			+					
	Schistosoma mansoni			+					

Protozoa

Microsporidia	e.g., *Encephalitozoon, Enterocytozoon*
Amoebae	*Entamoeba histolytica* *Naegleria fowleri* *Acanthamoeba*
Ciliate	*Balantidium coli* *Giardia lamblia*
Coccidia	*Cryptosporidium parvum* *Cyclospora cayetanensis* *Isospora belli*

Bld, blood; CSF, cerebrospinal fluid; Vag, vagina; BM, bone marrow; SPL, spleen; LN, lymph node; Oth, other sites.

Table 15-21. Serologic Tests to Diagnose Protozoa and Helminth Infections?

	Serology (Antibody)	DNA (Antigen)	Stool	Other Body Sites	Chapter Number	Other Features
Protozoans						
Amoebae						
Entamoeba histolytica	DD, EIA, IHA	EIA	+	Endoscopic biopsy	15	Liver abscess
Naegleria fowleri						
Acanthamoeba						
Babesiosis (*Babesia microti*)	IFA	DNA in blood.		Blood smear: DFA or Giemsa	15	Hemolytic anemia
Chagas disease (*Trypanosoma brucei cruzi*)	EIA, IFA, CF, IHA				15	
Coccidia: *Cryptosporidium Cparvum, Isospora belli, Cyclospora cayetanensis*	EIA (Ag in stool)	EIA, DFA, IFA	Acid fast stain		15	
Ciliate						
Giardiasis *Giardia lamblia*	EIA, CF	EIA, DFA, IFA	Cysts		15	Malabsorption
Balantidium coli						
Microsporidia e.g., *Encephalitozoon, Enterocytozoon*						
Leishmaniasis (*Leishmania donovani, L brasiliensis, L tropica* and others)	IFA, CF, IHA, CIE			Smear, cultures from blood, tissues	15	↑↑↑↑ IgG
Malaria (*Plasmodium vivax, P malariae, P. falciparum, P. ovale*)	IFA	IC		Blood smear	15	Blackwater fever
Toxoplasmosis (*Toxoplasma gondii*)	EIA, IFA, EIA-IgM	DFA, IP			15	Sabin-Feldman dye test
Trichomoniasis (*Trichomonas vaginalis*)		Ag, DFA, EIA		Wet mount from vagina. Pap smear	14	

Helminths
Nematodes

Ancylostoma duodenale, Necator americanus (hookworms)	Not useful		O		15
Ascaris lumbricoides	Not useful		O, A	Rare L in sputum early	15
Dracunculus medinensis			None		15
Filariasis	EIA, IHA	Ag in urine		Blood smear	15
Loa Loa (filaria)			None	MF in blood smear, tissue	15
Onchocerca volvulus (filaria)	EIA, IHA		None	MF in skin	15
Strongyloides stercoralis (Strongyloidiasis)	EIA, IHA		O		15
Trichuris trichura	Not useful				15
Trichinella spiralis (Trichinosis)	BF, EIA, IHA	None		L in muscle	15
Ancylostoma or Toxocara canis (Toxocariasis; larva migrans)	EIA		O		15
Cestodes					
Echinococcus multilocularis (canine tapeworm)	IB, IHA, IEP, DD	Ag in cyst fluid	Not found	Biopsy	15
Diphyllobothrium latum (fish tapeworm)			O	Megablastic anemia	15
Hymenolepis nana (dwarf tapeworm)			O		15
Taenia saginata (beef tapeworm)			G, O, S	O in perianal cellophane tape	15
Taenia solium (pork tapeworm) (Cysticercosis)	EIA, IHA, IB		G, O, S; after treatment	Biopsy of lesion	15

Table 15-21. (Continued)

	Serology (Antibody)	DNA (Antigen)	Stool	Other Body Sites	Chapter Number	Other Features
Trematodes						
Liver flukes						
Clonorchis sinensis		EIA	O	O in duodenal contents	15	Cholangitis, cirrhosis, cholangio-carcinoma
Fasciola hepatica	EIA, CIE IFA	Ag in serum	O		15	
Opistorchis felineus			O	O in duodenal contents	15	
Intestinal flukes						
Fasaciolopsis buski			O, occasionally A		15	Diarrhea, ascites, intestinal ulcers
Tissue flukes						
Paragonimus	EIA, IB		O	O in sputum	15	Lung abscess, GI ulceration, seizures
Blood flukes						
Schistosoma mansoni	EIA, IB, IFA		O	O in biopsied granulomas	15	Liver fibrosis, portal hypertension, splenomegaly
S. japonicum			O		15	
S. haematobium				O in urine	15	Hematuria, proteinuria. Pyelonephritis, hydronephrosis, carcinoma

A, adult; G, gravid segments; L, larvae; O, ova; S, scolex; Neg, negative; Ag, antigen; BF, bentonite floculation; CF, complement fixation; DD, double diffusion; EIA, enzyme immunoassay; IM, immunoblot; IF, indirect immunofluorescence; IHA, indirect hemagglutination; IP, immunoperoxidase; IEP, immunoelectrophoresis; MF, microfilariae.

Enterobiasis (Pinworm Infection)
Due to intestinal nematode *Enterobius vermicularis*.

♦ Ova and occasionally adults are found on cellophane tape swab of perianal region which *should be taken on first arising early in morning*. Three tests will find 90% and five tests will find 95% of cases.

Stool is usually negative for ova and adults.

Eosinophil count is usually normal or may be slightly increased.

Serologic tests are not useful.

Trichinosis
Nematode infection due to *Trichinella spiralis* from eating meat containing larvae.

○ Eosinophilia appears with values of ≤85% on differential count and 15,000/μL on absolute count. It occurs about 1 week after the eating of infected meat and reaches maximum after third week. It usually subsides in 4 to 6 weeks but may last up to 6 months and occasionally for years. Occasionally it is absent; it is usually absent in fatal infections.

♦ Stools do not contain adults or larvae.

♦ Identification of larvae is made in suspected meat by acid-pepsin digestion followed by microscopic examination.

♦ Muscle biopsy may show the encysted larvae beginning 10 days after ingestion. Direct microscopic examination of compressed specimen is superior to routine histologic preparation.

♦ Serologic tests become positive 1 week after onset of symptoms in only 20% to 30% of patients and reach a peak in 80% to 90% of patients by fourth to fifth week. Rise in titer in acute and convalescent phase sera is diagnostic. Titers may remain negative in overwhelming infection. False-positive results may occur in polyarteritis nodosa, serum sickness, penicillin sensitivity, infectious mononucleosis, malignant lymphomas, and leukemia.

• EIA is method of choice; peaks in 3 months; may still be detected at 1 year. Specificity >95%. IHA is also used. Previously used tests include CF, bentonite flocculation, precipitin and latex fixation.

• Antigen detection is said to have S/S = <50%/100%.

Decrease in serum total protein and albumin occurs in severe cases between 2 and 4 weeks and may last for years.

Increased (relative and absolute) gamma globulins parallel titer of serologic tests. The increase occurs between 5 and 8 weeks and may last 6 months or more.

ESR is normal or only slightly increased.

Decreased serum cholinesterase often lasts 6 months.

Serum muscle enzymes may be increased (e.g., creatine kinase).

Urine may show albuminuria with hyaline and granular casts in severe cases.

With meningoencephalitis, CSF may be normal or ≤300 lymphocytes/μL with increased protein with higher antibody level in CSF than serum.

Trichostrongylosis
Usually asymptomatic enteric infection due to nematode *Trichostrongylus* species.

♦ Stools contain ova. Usually a concentration technique is required; *ova may be mistaken for hookworm ova*.

○ Increased in WBC and eosinophils (≤75%) when patient is symptomatic.

Trichuriasis
Usually asymptomatic infection of colon due to nematode (whipworm) *Trichuris trichiura*.

▲ Stools contain ova.

○ Increased eosinophils (≤25%), leukocytosis, and microcytic hypochromic anemia may be present.

Serologic tests are not useful.

Larva Migrans

Cutaneous

Due to nematode hookworms *Ancylostoma caninum* and *A. braziliense* from dogs, cats, or other carnivores.

Serological tests and biopsy are not useful.

Visceral

Due to nematode roundworms *Toxocara canis* or *T. cati*; past exposure in humans is ~10%.

♦ Tissue biopsy showing larvae is only definite way to make diagnosis; usually from liver which shows granulomas.
♦ ELISA is 78% sensitive and poor specificity since it may also detect infection with other nematodes and flukes; negative predictive value >95%. May be less sensitive in ocular than in visceral disease. IHA and bentonite flocculation tests are insensitive and nonspecific.
○ WBC is increased; increased eosinophils (usually >30%) may be vacuolated and contain fewer than normal granules; persists for several months.
Serum γ-globulin is often increased, especially IgE.
Increased anti-A and anti-B antibodies in most cases caused by stimulation of isohemagglutinins.
Laboratory findings due to organ system involvement (e.g., liver in 85% of cases and lung in 50% of cases—may cause Löffler syndrome).

Hookworm Disease[25]

Due to intestinal nematode *Necator americanus* or *Ancylostoma duodenale* transmitted by contact with contaminated soil.

♦ Stools (even unconcentrated) contain hookworm ova after ~5 weeks. Ova of *A. duodenale* and *N. americanus* cannot be distinguished except by PCR. Quantitation for epidemiologic studies.
WBC is normal or slightly increased, with 15% to 30% eosinophilia begins at 4 weeks; peaks at 5 to 9 weeks (coincides with appearance of adults in intestine) when ≤75% eosinophils are present.
Iron deficiency anemia caused by blood loss. *A. duodenale* causes greater blood loss than *N. americanus*. When anemia is more severe, eosinophilia is less prominent. Generally burden of 40 to 160 worms is associated with Hb <11 g/dL. Hb decreases in proportion to infection.
Hypoalbuminemia may occur with heavy infection.
Stools are usually positive for occult blood. Charcot-Leyden crystals are present in >50% of patients.
Serologic tests are not useful for diagnosis or monitoring infection.
Laboratory findings are those due to frequently associated diseases (e.g., malaria, beriberi).

Strongyloidiasis

Due to intestinal nematode *Strongyloides stercoralis*; found in ~4% of rural Kentucky children.

♦ Stools contain hookworm ova after ~5 weeks.
♦ Stools contain larvae (sensitivity = 30%–60% for direct examination, 70%–80% after Baermann concentration). Larvae may also be found in duodenal washings (sensitivity = 60%–70%); string test (Entero-Test) sensitivity is 60% to 80%. Filariform larvae may suggest hyperinfection.
♦ Larvae appear in sputum, BAL with pulmonary involvement; eosinophils may also be present; indicates hyperinfection.
♦ Serological tests (ELISA) for antibodies show S/S, NPV >95%. Thus, a positive test indicates need for examination of stool and duodenal contents, especially if a patient

[25]Hotez PJ, et al. Hookworm infection. *N Engl J Med* 2004;351:799.

is to be treated with cytotoxic or immunosuppressive therapy but may cross-react with *Ascaris lumbricoides, Loa loa* or hookworm. A negative test without symptoms or other laboratory findings suggests no infection.

♦ Stool on agar plate for 3 days shows tracks, moving larvae or adults; confirm microscopically.

○ Increase in eosinophils is almost always present, but the number usually decreases with chronicity; is most marked in patients with prominent skin manifestations; may be absent with immunosuppression.

○ Leukocytosis is common. Leukopenia and absence of eosinophilia are poor prognostic signs. *Condition may be encountered in orphanages and mental institutions.*

Filariasis
Due to tissue-dwelling nematodes transmitted by insect bites.

Lymphatic Filariasis
Due to *Wuchereria bancrofti* or *Brugia malayi* primarily transmitted by mosquitoes.

♦ Microfilariae are found in thick blood smear (Wright or Giemsa stain) or wet preparation; can be concentrated (e.g., centrifugation, membrane filtration). Collect blood after 8 PM. *Persons with microfilariae in blood may be asymptomatic; circulating microfilariae may be absent in patients with this disease.*

♦ Eosinophils are increased.

♦ Biopsy of lymph node may contain adult worms.

♦ Serologic tests

• Antigen detected in serum (50% of cases) and urine (100% of cases) in *W. bancrofti* infection. Can monitor treatment and relapse by level in urine but not by serum antibody levels.

• Antibody detection lacks S/S

Chyluria may occur.

Nonlymphatic Filariasis

Loaiasis
Due to *Loa loa* transmitted by *Chrysops* spp. deer flies.

♦ Marked increase of eosinophils (50%–80%) may occur.

♦ Identify microfilariae in thick blood smears or concentrated filtrate of hemolyzed blood stained with Giemsa; collect blood between 10 AM and 2 PM.

♦ Identification of excised migrating subconjunctival adults.

♦ Identification of microfilariae in CSF in cases of meningoencephalitis.

♦ Serologic tests (see Lymphatic Filariasis).

Onchocerciasis (River Blindness)
Due to *Onchocerca volvulus* transmitted by *Simulium* spp. blackflies.

♦ Identify microfilaria in skin

Tropical Pulmonary Eosinophilia
Due to *Wucheria bancrofti* filarial transmitted by mosquitoes.

♦ Eosinophilia is extreme (usually >3,000/μL) and persists for weeks.

♦ Serum IgE levels are markedly elevated (usually >1,000 U/mL).

No microfilaria can be found in blood but may be found in enlarged lymph nodes when adenopathy is present.

Other laboratory abnormalities (e.g., increased ESR) are not diagnostically useful.

Dirofilariasis (Pulmonary)
Due to dog heartworm *Dirofilaria immitis*; (insect transmission, usually mosquito; rarely some fleas or ticks). Is rare in humans.

INFECTIOUS

Filariform larvae transmitted by bite of intermediate host, migrate to heart and die resulting in pulmonary emboli and infarcts.
♦ Diagnosis is made by open lung biopsy.
Eosinophilia is not significant.
Cross-reactions make EIA serologic tests difficult to interpret.

Clonorchiasis
Due to trematode liver fluke *Clonorchis sinensis* endemic in Asia.

♦ Ova appear in stool or duodenal contents.
♦ EIA for antigen detection in stool has sensitivity, specificity, and PPV >90% when prevalence = 50%. Cross-reactions may occur.
Clonorchiasis may cause laboratory findings due to cholangitis, cholecystitis, pancreatitis, etc.

Fascioliasis
Rare infection due to trematode liver fluke *Fasciola hepatica* in livestock. Humans are accidental hosts.

♦ Ova may appear in stool or duodenal contents.
♦ Serologic tests

• Antibodies appear within 2 to 4 weeks after infection (5–7 weeks before eggs appear in stool).
• Antibodies by EIA and CIE have high sensitivity but may show cross-reaction with schistosomiasis and trichinosis. CIE becomes negative with cure and is useful for therapeutic monitoring.
• EIA can detect antigen in serum. More antigen identification and serologic tests are becoming available.
• IFA is positive in ~80% of cases; frequent cross-reaction with infections caused by other helminths, *Clonorchis sinensis* and *Opisthorchis* species.
• CF is positive in only 14% of cases.

○ Eosinophils may be marked.
○ Liver function tests may be abnormal.

Fasciolopsiasis
Due to trematode intestinal fluke *Fasciolopsis buski* endemic to southeast Asia.

♦ Ova appear in stool.

Fasciolopsiasis
Due to trematode intestinal fluke *Fasciolopsis buski* endemic to southeast Asia.

♦ Ova appear in stool.

Opisthorchiasis
Due to human infection with trematode cat and dog liver fluke *Opisthorchis felineus* and *O. viverrini*, chiefly in Asia.

♦ Ova appear in stool or duodenal contents.
♦ EIA for IgG and IgE antibodies are useful.
♦ Antigen detection assay and DNA-based diagnosis should be useful.
May cause obstructive jaundice, cholangitis, and ultimately cholangiocarcinoma.

Paragonimiasis
Due to trematode lung fluke *Paragonimus westermani* and others. Transmitted to humans by eating infected crustaceans.

○ Eosinophilia is usual.
♦ Ova appear in stool or sputum, which may contain blood.
♦ Serologic tests

• ELISA is method of choice; antibody levels decrease after treatment. Cross-reactions may occur.
• Antigen detection methods are under development.

Schistosomiasis

Due to trematode blood flukes *Schistosoma mansoni, S. japonicum, S. haematobium* that parasitize human venous channels; transmitted by fresh water snails.

Acute

○• Eosinophilia occurs in 20% to 60% of cases.
• ESR is increased.
• Hematuria is first sign of *S. haematobium* infection; also occurs in chronic infection.
• Serum globulin is increased.

♦ Chronic

• Diagnosis depends on detection of ova in stools or urine; only viable eggs indicate active infection. Quantification by egg count per gram of feces or per 10 mL of urine gives some indication of severity of infection. Species identification depends on egg morphology and is needed to select drug dosage or choice of drugs.
• Ova appear in urine sediment and in biopsy of vesical mucosa in infection with *S. haematobium*. *S. haematobium* ova are sometimes found in stool and *S. mansoni* eggs are sometimes found in urine, especially in heavy infection.
• Unstained rectal or bladder mucosa examined microscopically showing living or dead ova when stools are negative is most sensitive test; granulomatous lesions may be present.

Changes secondary to clay pipestem fibrosis of liver with portal hypertension, esophageal varices, splenomegaly, etc. Liver function changes are quite minimal; increased serum bilirubin is rare, even with advanced cirrhosis. Increased serum globulin is frequent.
Serum ALP is elevated in 50% of adult patients but is not useful in children.
♦ Ova may be found within granulomas.
Pulmonary involvement

♦ • Ova in sputum is very rare.
♦ • Lung biopsy may be positive in advanced cases.
• Changes secondary to pulmonary hypertension

Multiple granulomatous lesions may appear in uterine cervix.
♦ Serologic tests are particularly useful for chronic infections when stools contain no ova; they are not useful to assess chemotherapeutic cure. Does not determine activity or intensity of current infection and may not distinguish new and old infections. Positive serology is most useful to support the diagnosis of acute schistosomiasis. Not useful for diagnosis in adults from endemic areas because specificity for active infection is too low. Cross-reaction with other helminths may occur.

• IFA test is useful when IHA titer 1:64 +IHA >1:256 in >90% of acute *S. mansoni* cases; cross-react with other Schistosoma, filariasis, trichinosis.
• Screen sera with ELISA and confirm and speciate with EITB (Western blot) are most sensitive and specific methods.
• Antigen detection of adult worms and ova is promising method. Immunoblot assay to detect worm antigen is reported to have S/S =95%/100%.

Anemia, eosinophilia, increased serum globulin and decreased albumin, hematuria, proteinuria, hydronephrosis, azotemia, squamous cell carcinoma of bladder may occur.

Tapeworm

Due to infection with cestode larval cysts.

Beef Tapeworm

Due to *Taenia saginata* which lives in jejunum of humans.

♦ In stool, ova cannot be distinguished from those of *Taenia solium*.

• Proglottids establish species diagnosis. Stool examination is positive in 50% to 75% of patients.

♦ Cellophane tape swab of perianal region is positive in ≤95% of patients. Eosinophils may be slightly increased.

Pork Tapeworm

Due to *Taenia solium* found in human small bowel. Pig is intermediate host.

♦ Biopsy of solitary lesions may establish the diagnosis when serologic tests are negative.

♦ Stool (single specimen detects 50% to 75% of carriers) and cellophane tape swab of perianal region (may detect >75% of infections) are both used. 3 to 6 specimens are examined over 1 to 2 weeks.

○ Eosinophils may be increased (up to 10%–15%). Marked increase in ESR is unusual and suggests another diagnosis.

♦ With CNS involvement (cysticercosis), CSF may show increased eosinophils (in 10% to 77% of cases) increased mononuclear cells (≤300/μL), slightly increased protein, normal or mildly decreased glucose; parasites are not found. Serologic tests are used in conjunction with CT scan or MRI. Older tests (e.g., IHA, IFA, CIE, immunoelectrophoresis) have sensitivity ~80%. ELISA detects antibody in serum or CSF in 75% to 80% with few or calcified cysts and 93% with severe CNS disease. Enzyme-linked immunoelectro-transfer blot (EITB) on serum or CSF has S/S >94% with multiple CNS lesions and ~72% with single lesions. Change in titers is not reliable to judge cure. *Solitary CNS lesions may not produce antibodies consistently.* Status of antigen assays, ELISA, PCR, DNA probes, monoclonal antibodies awaits future studies.

Dwarf Tapeworm

Due to *Hymenolepis nana* transmitted from feces of rats and mice contaminating food and water and hands.

♦ Stool shows ova, occasionally adults.

Fish Tapeworm

Due to *Diphyllobothrium latum*.

♦ Stool shows ova.

○ Macrocytic anemia (see Chapter 11) may occur when worm is in proximal small intestine.

○ Increased eosinophils and leukocytes are found.

Canine Tapeworm

Zoonotic infection due to *Echinococcus granulosus*, *Echinococcus multilocularis* causes cystic hydatid disease in humans.

♦ Identification of scolices and hooklets in cyst fluid and on histologic examination.

♦ Serologic tests indicate current or previous infection.

• High titers (>1:256) IHA has S/S = 90%/≤100% in cases with hydatid cysts of liver or peritoneum; 60% sensitivity in cases of lung and bone; 10% sensitivity in cases of calcified cysts. ≤10% false positives (in cysticercosis, schistosomiasis, collagen disease, neoplasia); titers can persist for years after surgical removal.

• Precipitation assays (e.g., immunoelectrophoresis, immunoblotting, double diffusion are more specific.

• EIA is method of choice. EIA, but not IHA, can differentiate *E. granulosus* from *E. multilocularis* in test for antigen on cyst fluid.

○ Laboratory findings due to cystic lesion of liver in 65% of cases (see Space-Occupying Lesions of Liver, Chapter 8); cysts are widely scattered in 10%; multiple in 20% to 40% of cases.
○ Eosinophils are increased in 33% of cases; rises dramatically if cyst leaks.
Stool examination is not helpful.

Protozoan Disease

* Intestinal Protozoa
  * *Entameba histolytica* (amebiasis)
  * *Balantidium coli*
  * *Cryptosporidium parvum, Isospora belli, Cyclospora cayetanensis* (cryptospidiosis)
  * *Giardia lamblia*
  * *Encephalitozoon intestin alis* (microsporidiasis)
* Tissue and Blood Protozoa
  * *Plasmodium falciparum, P. vivax, P. malariae, P. ovale* (malaria)
  * *Babesia microti* (babesiosis)
  * *Leishmania donovani* (kala-azar), *L. tropica* (cutaneous leishmaniasis), *L. braziliensis* (mucosal leishmaniasis)
  * *Trypanosoma gambiense* (African trypanosomiasis; sleeping sickness), *T. cruzi* (Chagas disease; South American trypanosomiasis)
  * *Toxoplasma gondi* (toxoplasmosis)

See Table 15-22

Intestinal Protozoa

Amebiasis[26]

Due to protozoal GI tract infection caused by *Entamoeba histolytica* and sometimes by *E. dispar*. Asymptomatic self-limiting in 90%, invasive in 10%, extraintestinal in <1% of cases.

♦ Microscopic examination of stool for *E. histolytica;* ingested RBCs are pathognomonic. Six daily consecutive stools concentrated and stained will identify 20% to 60% of positive cases. Must be examined fresh or fixed immediately and stained. (*Beware of interfering substances in feces, e.g., bismuth, kaolin, barium sulfate, soap or hypertonic-salt enema solutions, antacids and laxatives, sulfonamides; antibiotic, antiprotozoal, and antihelmintic agents.*) *Abundant RBCs but minimal WBCs on microscopic examination of stool helps to differentiate condition from bacillary dysentery.*
♦ PCR for detection of *E. histolytica* antigen or DNA in stool in 90% of colitis cases and in serum in 65% of early colitis cases. Can detect 1 trophozoite per sample. Can distinguish pathogenic and non-pathogenic species. Can simultaneously detect *E. histolytica, G. lamblia* and *Cryptosporidium* with 100% sensitivity.
♦ Endoscopic biopsy or smear of exudate of intestinal ulcers may show *E. histolytica* in 50% of cases.
♦ Culture is gold standard of research.
♦ Antigen detection kit have S/S = 95%/93% compared to culture.
♦ Serologic antibody tests are primarily used for amebic liver abscess or symptomatic patients or acute infections; absent during first week of infection.

* EIA/ELISA are most sensitive and specific and are method of choice. IgG is present in all patients with invasive amebiasis and indicates current or previous infection; less sensitive in noninvasive disease. IgM is found in >90% of cases of liver abscess; usually disappear within 6 weeks of successful treatment.
* Indirect hemagglutination test (>1.128) is sensitive and specific (>95% each) in patients with liver abscess or invasive intestinal disease but cannot distinguish these from noninvasive intestinal infection and can persist for years after infection.

---

[26]DiMiceli L. Distinguishing Between Pathogenic and Non-Pathogenic Species of Entamoeba. *Lab Medicine* 2004;35:613.

Table 15-22. Summary of Laboratory Findings in Protozoan Diseases

Disease	Causative Organism	Blood	CSF	Stool	Urine	Vagina	Urethra	Exudates, ulcers, skin lesions	Bone marrow	Spleen	Lymph node aspirate	Fresh unstained material	Stained material	Culture	Animal inoculation	Xenodiagnosis	Histologic examination	Anemia	WBC decreased	Monocytosis	Serum globulin increased	CSF abnormalities	Renal function abnormalities	Liver function abnormalities	Skeletal muscle abnormalities	Cardiac abnormalities	Other
		Source of Material										**Microscopic examination**		**Diagnostic Methods**				**Other Significant Laboratory Abnormalities**									
Malaria	*Plasmodium* species	+							+				+					+	+		+	+	+	+			
Babesiosis	*Babesia microti*	+											+		+		+	+			+		+	+			
Trypanosomiasis Acute sleeping sickness	*Trypanosoma rhodesiense*	+	+						+		+		+	rare	+		+	+			+			+			
Chronic sleeping sickness	*T. gambiense*	+	+						+		+	+	+	rare	+		+	+			+						
Chagas' disease	*T. cruzi*	+							+	+	+		+	+	+	+	+[a]				+	+	+	+	+	+	
Leishmaniasis Kala-azar	*Leishmania donovani*	+									+		+	+	+		+	+	+		+		+				
American mucocutaneous	*L. brasiliensis*							+					+	+	+		+	+									
Oriental sore	*L. tropica*							+					+	+	+		+[c]										
Toxoplasmosis	*Toxoplasma gondii*		+										+		+		+				+						+[b]

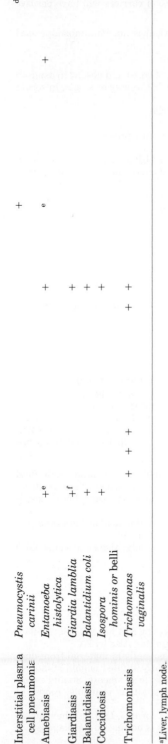

Disease				
Interstitial plasma cell pneumonia (*Pneumocystis carinii*)[d]			+	
Amebiasis (*Entamoeba histolytica*)	+[e]	+	+	[e]
Giardiasis (*Giardia lamblia*)	+[f]	+		
Balantidiasis (*Balantidium coli*)	+	+		
Coccidiosis (*Isospora hominis or belli*)	+	+		
Trichomoniasis (*Trichomonas vaginalis*)	+ + +	+		

[a] Liver, lymph node.
[b] Hemagglutination Sabin-Feldman dye test.
[c] Lymph node, muscle.
[d] Special stains
[e] Intestine.
[f] Also duodenal washings.

Notes: Serologic tests can be performed at the Centers for Disease Control and Prevention (Atlanta, GA) on specimens submitted through state health department laboratories that do not perform such tests.

- When severe diarrhea is caused by *E. histolytica*, serologic tests will be positive in >90%; when diarrhea has never been present, <50% of carriers will have positive serologic tests.

Negative tests are unlikely with invasive disease if patient is not immunosuppressed and, thus, useful for ruling out invasive amebiasis.
Liver abscess

◆ • Needle biopsy of abscess shows organism in <20% of cases and absent in aspirate *but should not be done.* Antigen detection in ~40% of abscesses or stools; in serum in 100% of untreated cases.
- Stool is also usually negative; bacterial culture is sterile.
- Normochromic, normocytic anemia
- Leukocytosis (5,000–33,000/μL); eosinophilia is not usually present.
- ESR is markedly increased.
- Increased serum AST, ALT (2–6× normal) and normal ALP in acute liver abscess; in chronic liver abscess ALP (usually 2–3× normal) tends to be increased with normal ALT.
- Serum albumin may be decreased and globulin increased.
- Total bilirubin may be increased if complications occur.
- Liver scanning
- Serologic tests (see previous paragraph).

Balantidiasis
Due to intestinal protozoa *Balantidium coli*.

◆ Recognition of organisms in stool. *Intermittent appearance requires repeated examinations.*
No serologic tests are available.

Cryptosporidiosis
Due to obligate coccidian intracellular protozoons including *Cryptosporidium parvum, Isospora belli, Cyclospora cayetanensis* that infect microvillus epithelial cells of GI tract. Usually transmitted by contaminated water supply causing watery diarrhea. Most US surface water is contaminated. In immunocompetent persons, reported prevalence rates of 1% to 2% in Europe, ≤4.3% in North America, 3% to 20% in Asia, Africa, Latin America. Seroprevalence rates are higher.

◆ Diagnosis by identification of organism in concentrated stool or other body fluid sample that has been acid-fast stained or unstained is insensitive. Phase contrast requires 10,000 to 100,000 organisms for positive response. Routine O & P examination is inadequate. WBCs are absent.
◆ IFA microscopy is method of stool has S/S >98% compared to acid fast staining.
◆ PCR for identification of *Cyclospora cayetanensis* DNA in stool.
Immunofluorescent antibody assay is used to test water supply; algae may cause false positive.

Giardiasis
Due to *Giardia lamblia*, motile flagellated protozoan.

◆ Detection of *Giardia* antigen in stool (method of choice) by EIA has S/S >80%/>98% compared to microscopy. Should examine ≥2 stool samples. Also by FA.
◆ Recognition of cysts or trophozoites in stools, or occasionally in material from duodenum, which have been concentrated and permanently stained is gold standard. Sensitivity ~50% for microscopic recognition of cysts in fecal smears. Should examine ≥2 stool samples. IFA detection using commercial kits is available. Biopsy of small intestine may occasionally show trophozoites.
◆ Serologic tests by CF and ELISA are available. ELISA for IgG, IgM, IgA have negative predictive value >98% but presence of antibodies is not useful for diagnosis of recent infection.

Chronic infection may cause malabsorption syndrome.
♦ Identification of *Giardia* DNA in stool by PCR.

Babesiosis

Due to intracellular protozoan *Babesia microti* transmitted by bite of nymphal *Ixodes* tick, which can also transmit Lyme disease and granulocytic ehrlichiosis; has been transmitted by blood transfusion.

♦ Diagnosis is established by

- Identification of parasite within or outside of RBCs on Wright- or Giemsa-stained thick and thin peripheral blood smears or by DFA staining is the gold standard.
- Serologic studies become positive in 2 to 4 weeks (from CDC). IFA IgM indicates acute infection. IgG ≥1:64 is considered positive for current or past infection but ≥1:1024 in most patients with acute illness; or 4× increase in serum titer between acute and convalescent phase. Increased titer may persist months after resolution of symptoms. May cross-react with Colorado tick fever, *Plasmodium* sp. Increased titer may occur in *R. rickettsii* infection. False-positive results may occur with autoimmune and connective tissue diseases.
- PCR based identification of *B. microti* DNA in blood is more sensitive than microscopy; is rapidly cleared from blood after successful therapy and presence indicates active parasitemia. May be indicated to monitor course of infection; may persist for ≥6 months along with symptoms. Best done in reference laboratory.
- Blood smears in intraperitoneally inoculated hamsters are positive for ≤2 months.
- Immunohistochemical assay on formalin-fixed, paraffin-embedded tissues and blood smears identifies organism.[27]

Hemolytic anemia may last days to months; most patients have thrombocytopenia. Laboratory changes caused by complications

- Renal failure
- Liver dysfunction (e.g., increased serum AST, LD). ~20% of patients have clinical and serologic evidence of concurrent Lyme disease. Ehrlichiosis may also be found.

Microsporidia

Encephalitozoon intestinalis causes 10% to 20% of cases of intestinal microsporidiosis but should be distinguished from more common *E. bieneusi* because of propensity to cause disease in other organs and responsiveness to treatment. These are common opportunistic eukaryotic intracellular protozoal parasites of intestinal epithelium that may cause acute or chronic, life-threatening diarrhea in immunocompromised hosts (e.g., AIDS patients); may also cause keratoconjunctivitis (gram stain of sputum for spores), hepatitis, sclerosing cholangitis, peritonitis, respiratory tract infection, sinusitis, myositis, kidney disease.

♦ Identified by cytology, biopsy and touch preparations of intestinal mucosa. EM is still the best diagnostic method.
♦ Microscopy of stool wet-mounts, UV fluorescence, or acid-fast or other special stains
♦ Molecular methods (e.g., PCR), cell culture, serology testing are in development in research settings.

Tissue and Blood Protozoa

Malaria

Protozoan infection of RBCs due to *Plasmodium vivax, P. malariae, P. falciparum,* or *P. ovale.*

♦ Organism is identified in thin or thick smears of peripheral blood or bone marrow. Thick smear sensitive to 2 parasites/1,000,000 uninfected RBCs. Smears should be

[27]Torres-Velez FJ, et al. *Am J ClinPathol* 2003;120:833.

made every 6 to 12 hours for 3 consecutive days. Fluorescent stains have also been used. Cytocentrifugation improves yield. Determines parasite density, confirms species identification, and negative test results.

♦ Serologic tests—useful when there are few parasites in blood or when smears are obtained after therapy or to screen blood donors; not useful to determine species. Not useful in acute malaria because requires ≤3 weeks to produce increase in titer.

• Indirect fluorescent antibody test (for IgG) shows high S/S ≤99% and is useful for diagnostic purposes. Titer >1:256 suggests recent infection (>1:64 in nonendemic areas). Titers rise ~1 to 2 weeks after fever onset and remain increased for duration of infection. Titers fall ~6 months after cure except in endemic areas where 1:64 may be present with subclinical infection.
• Monoclonal antibodies to detect IgM and detection of antigen in serum have S/S ≤100% but do not distinguish past and present infection.
• Indirect hemagglutination can detect antibody many years after infection and is useful for prevalence studies.
• Nucleic acid probes using DNA can identify *P. falciparum* (50 parasites/L of blood) and identify drug-resistant strains.

♦ PCR-based assay is >90% sensitive and specific; allows species confirmation.
♦ Rapid immunochromatographic antigen capture tests can detect >100 parasites/μL (.002% parasitemia) within 20 minutes for various antigens. Not licensed in USA.[28]
♦ Methods presently not generally available include:

• Flow cytometry to detect infected RBCs
• Rapid dipstick tests for various antigens are not yet approved by FDA. Hemolytic anemia (average 2.5 million RBCs/μL in chronic cases) is usually hypochromic; may be macrocytic in severe chronic disease. There is increased serum indirect bilirubin and other evidence of hemolysis. Reticulocyte count is increased.

○ Thrombocytopenia and relative monocytosis is a common pattern.

WBC is decreased. There may be pigment in large mononuclear cells occasionally.

Bone marrow shows erythroid hyperplasia, RBCs containing organisms, and pigment in RE cells. Marrow hyperplasia may fail in chronic phase.

• Agranulocytosis and purpura may occur late.

Serum globulin is increased (especially euglobulin fraction); albumin is decreased.

ESR is increased.

Biologic false positive test for syphilis is frequent.

Osmotic fragility of RBCs is normal.

P. malariae may cause acute hemorrhagic nephritis (albuminuria, hematuria); causes chronic renal disease in West Africa.

Blackwater fever (massive intravascular hemolysis) due to *P. falciparum*

• Severe acute hemolytic anemia (1–2 million RBCs/μL) with increased bilirubin, hemoglobinuria, etc.
• May be associated with acute tubular necrosis with hemoglobin casts, azotemia, oliguria to anuria, etc.
• Parasites absent from blood

Laboratory findings due to involvement of organs

• Liver—vary from congestion to fatty changes to malarial hepatitis or central necrosis; malarial pigment in Kupfer cells; moderate increase in AST, ALT, and ALP
• Pigment stones in gallbladder
• Cerebral malaria

Persistence of parasite for years may contaminate donor blood.

Toxoplasmosis

Latent infection due to intracellular protozoan *Toxoplasma gondii*. Common in cats who are infected by eating other animals or insufficiently cooked meat; oocysts excreted in stool.

[28]Marx A, et al. Meta-analysis: accuracy of rapid tests for malaria in travelers returning from endemic areas. *Ann Intern Med* 2005;142:836.

♦ Serologic tests are diagnostic methods of choice.

Presence of antibody is primary method of diagnosis since <10% of normal adults in USA has evidence of past infection. Causes 15% of unexplained lymphadenopathy. Thirty percent to 80% of domestic cats have evidence of past infection.

- IgM and IgG by ELISA have fewer false positives or negatives (major test presently in use). Detectable within 1 to 2 weeks; IgM lasts 3 to 5 months; IgG remains at low level for life.
- FDA recommends confirmation of positive Ig M test. May include toxoplasma serological profile (IgG, IgM, IgA, IgE) to distinguish remote and recent infection and recently developed high-IgG avidity EIA test: high avidity excludes infection during past 3 to 4 months.
- IgG (IFA, DT, IHA, or CF) test that shows a 2× rise in titer at 3 week interval indicates acute infection. IgG peak occurs within 1 to 2 months, so initial specimen must be drawn early to demonstrate the rise in titer. Titers eventually reach 1:1,000; IgG or dye test is rarely <1:1,000 in acute toxoplasmosis. IgG antibodies at low level may persist for many years.
- IgM (IFA) appears in first week of infection, peaks within 1 month, disappears in 3 to 5 months (as early as 1 month). Occurs in 75% of congenitally infected infants and 97% of acute adult infections. A negative test rules out infection of <3 weeks duration but does not exclude infection of longer duration. A single titer (≥1:80) or serial rise in titer (>4×) indicates recent, new, or reactivated infection. (High titer ≥1:16, low titer <1:16, negative titer <1:8; levels; titers vary with laboratory). Antinuclear antibodies and RF may cause false-positive IgM-IFA test. Not test of choice.
- CF detects IgG later than IFA test, returns to normal earlier, is less sensitive than other tests and is not widely used now.
- Indirect hemagglutination (IHA) titer detects IgG antibodies; follows the same course as DT but lags by a few days. Is useful for screening and population studies but not helpful in diagnosis of acute infection. Is less sensitive than IFA or CF tests.
- Direct agglutination and latex agglutination tests are not available in United States.
- Tests for specific antigen in serum, CSF, and urine are not commercially available. In immunocompromised patients, IgM is usually absent and IgG only confirms chronic infection.
- Sabin-Feldman dye test (DT) detects primarily IgG antibodies; is benchmark for evaluating new tests but is superseded by other tests due to complexity and need for live organisms. Dye test detects antibodies 1 to 2 weeks after onset of infection, and peak to ≥1:1,000 in the 6 to 8 weeks, then declines during months or years to low level (1:4–1:64) for life of patient; false-positive or false-negative tests are rare.

Serologic tests are often not helpful since IgM is usually negative and IgG is often moderately elevated and 4× rise is uncommon. Titer = 1:1,024 strongly supports the diagnosis but is not usually found. Disease activity does not correlate with antibody titer or with changes in titer. Will occur in 5% to 10% of AIDS patients; absence of IgG in serum occurs in 3% of AIDS patients with toxoplasmic encephalitis. All AIDS patients with CNS symptoms should be tested for *T. gondii* antibodies.

♦ Determination of immune status

Acute infection is indicated seroconversion or ≥4× increase in titer or DT or IFA titer ≥1:1,024 or rising IgG in presence of compatible clinical illness.

Flat IgG titers in absence of IgM titers suggests infection more than 6 months ago.

High IgM and high IgG together indicate infection within past 3 months.

Low-to-medium IgM and high IgG may indicate infection 3 to 6 months ago.

In organ transplantation, serology profile of both patient and donor are important; seronegative recipient should be monitored for disseminated toxoplasmosis if donor is seropositive.

♦ Mouse inoculation or tissue culture (e.g., from tissue, blood or CSF) are most reliable methods.

♦ Only rarely is diagnosis made by recognition of trophozoite in appropriate material (CSF, lymph node, muscle) with Wright or Giemsa stain. Confirmation by IFA antibody technique is often needed. May be aided by immunoperoxidase technique. Demonstration of organism in Giemsa-stained BAL or CSF may be significant.

♦ Cysts may be incidental finding of chronic asymptomatic infection.

♦ PCR amplification of gene fragments is most sensitive for detection in both paraffin-embedded tissue and aqueous humor.

INFECTIOUS

♦ Detection of DNA in amniotic fluid, CSF, or brain tissue. Demonstration of antigen in blood, urine or CSF is helpful in immunocompromised patients with low/absent antibody titers.

Adult Patients

○ Heterophil agglutination is negative, but hematologic picture may exactly mimic infectious mononucleosis; eosinophilia in 10% to 20% of patients.
WBC varies from leukopenia to leukemoid reaction; atypical lymphocytes may be found.
Anemia is present.
Serum gamma globulins are increased.
Laboratory findings are those due to involvement of various organ systems:

♦ • Lymph node shows distinctive marked hyperplasia; organism may be identified in histologic section.
♦ • CNS shows CSF changes (typically mild increase in number of mononuclear cells, normal glucose, moderate increase in protein, and organism can be identified in smear of sediment). Occasionally biopsy of brain may be needed. Immunoperoxidase stain may be very valuable when histopathology is not definitive.
• Coomb negative hemolytic anemia.
• Disseminated form (e.g., hepatitis, myositis, meningoencephalitis) is an important complication of the immunologically compromised patient but positive or changing titers may not be present.
• If ocular findings are the only clinical disease, many patients show only very low titers that are not useful.

♦ Antibody titer may be greater in aqueous humor from anterior chamber tap than in serum.

Congenital Infection

Maternal infection in 1 to 5/1,000 pregnancies. Occurs in 1:1,000 live births in United States. Infection rate = 11% in first trimester, 90% in late third trimester. With primary infection, risk varies from 25% in first trimester to 65% in third trimester. Severe disease is more likely with infection in first trimester. High mortality; 90% have CNS sequelae. In mild infections, 80% have sequelae (e.g., chorioretinitis, CNS).

♦ Diagnosis by demonstrating toxoplasma-IgM in fetal serum but may be found in ~20% of cases or isolating parasite from fetal WBCs or clotted blood inoculation into mice or tissue culture.
Nonspecific changes may include increased WBC, eosinophil and platelet counts, increased serum total IgM, GGTP and LD.
♦ Prenatal diagnosis

• Tissue culture of chorionic villi (in first trimester)
• Fetal cord blood, amniotic fluid at 2 to 22 weeks gestation
• PCR of amniotic fluid (sensitivity >97%, NPV >99%).

Neonatal Infection

♦ Organism isolated in placenta from 95% of untreated mothers and 81% of treated mothers.
♦ Screening has been performed by detection of specific IgM (ELISA) antibody or antigen in neonatal blood on same filter paper used for detection of metabolic disorders.
♦ Diagnosis can also be made by isolating *T. gondii* in blood, CSF or histological examination of tissue.
♦ Persistent or increasing serum IgG titer in infant compared to mother; untreated newborn produces IgG by 3 months; treatment delays production until 9 months and sometimes prevents production.
♦ Demonstration of IgM antibody or of local production of IgG in CSF or eye fluid (body fluid titer/serum titer) × (serum γ-globulin/body fluid γ-globulin).
♦ Demonstration of toxoplasma antigen in blood, urine, or CSF.
♦ Persistence of IgG in infant's serum after 1 year indicates congenital infection.

Specific IgM is detected in <60% of cases. IgA may be detected more frequently.

Posttransplant Infection

Latent infection of solid organs, especially myocardium (heart transplants).

♦ Diagnosis by biopsy demonstrating tachyzoites in tissue.
♦ Serology can be useful.

Leishmaniasis

Endemic infection of tropics and subtropics transmitted by bite of sandflies.

Visceral Leishmaniasis (Kala-Azar)

Systemic parasitism of RE system by _Leishmania donovani_ and others.

♦ Diagnosis is mainly morphological. Organism identified in Giemsa-stained smears of aspirate or biopsy from bone marrow (safest; diagnostic in 90% of cases), peripheral blood, spleen, lymph node, or liver.
♦ PCR of tissue or WBC buffy coat has also been used (at NIH).
♦ Culture to CDC (incubate at 26°C) from same sources may take up to 4 weeks
♦ Serologic tests (ELISA, IFA, CIE, direct agglutination, IHA) do not distinguish recent from remote infection. May be done in immunosuppressed patients from endemic areas with appropriate clinical findings. Primarily for epidemiological surveys. Tests are not generally available. May cross-react in trypanosomiasis, malaria, leprosy.
○ Markedly increased serum globulin (IgG) with decreased albumin and reversed A/G ratio
Increased ESR caused by increased serum globulin
Anemia, leukopenia, thrombocytopenia due to hypersplenism and decreased marrow production
Frequent urine changes (proteinuria, hematuria)
Laboratory findings due to amyloidosis in chronic cases

Mucosal Leishmaniasis

Due to _Leishmania brasiliensis_ and others.

♦ Organism identified by histologic examination in scrapings or biopsy from lesions by direct microscopy (in 30% of patients), culture (with special techniques in 50% of cases).
♦ Positive immunofluorescent antibody test.
♦ PCR gene amplification for _Leishmania_ DNA or culture.
Prior cutaneous leishmaniasis.

Cutaneous Leishmaniasis (Oriental Sore)

Due to _Leishmania tropica_ and others.

♦ Organisms identification by direct microscopy and culture in scrapings from lesion

Trypanosomiasis

Due to flagellate protozoan _Trypanosoma_.

Sleeping Sickness

Acute Rhodesian due to protozoan _T. brucei rhodesiense_; chronic Gambian due to _T. brucei gambiense_ transmitted by tsetse flies.

♦ Identification of organism in appropriate material (blood, bone marrow, lymph node aspirate, CSF, chancre) by thick or thin smears or concentrations, wet mounts, animal inoculation, rarely culture. In Gambian, lymph node aspirate is more likely to reveal organism than blood.

INFECTIOUS

♦ Serologic tests are useful to establish suspicion of disease but histologic confirmation of diagnosis is required because present drug therapy is not innocuous. IFA test or card agglutination test are particularly useful for early diagnosis of chronic infection. Other methods (e.g., ELISA, IHA, CIE) are not available commercially.
○ Increased serum globulin producing increased ESR, rouleaux formation, etc.
Mass spectrometry is said to produce a "proteomic signature" with S/S = >98%.[29]
Increased monocytes in peripheral blood
Thrombocytopenia is usual. DIC, hemolytic anemia are uncommon.
CSF

♦ • Organisms may be identified by microscopic examination of CSF sediment. If organisms are not found, increased WBC and protein or increased IgM or presence of morula (Mott) cells is strongly suggestive.
• Increased number of cells (mononuclear type): ≤30/μL during second month; later 100 to 400/μL.
• Increased protein (use as index to severity of disease and to therapeutic response)— 60 to 100 mg/dL with considerable increase in γ-globulin.
• Latex agglutination or immunofluorescence tests of CSF give best results.

Chagas Disease (American trypanosomiasis)

Due to *Trypanosoma brucei cruzi* causes disease in ≤30% of those infected. Transmitted by feces of kissing bug, blood transfusions, and in-utero to man and animals.

♦ Identification of organism

• Definitive diagnosis is based on demonstration of parasite in blood, CSF or lymph fluid but is difficult to demonstrate in latent or chronic stages.
• Buffy coat or anticoagulated blood for motile forms or Giemsa-stained thin and thick smears will usually demonstrate parasites.
• Biopsy of lymph node or liver (shows leishmanial forms)
• Culture on blood broth at 28°C from lymph node aspirate
• Intraperitoneal injection of mouse that is killed after 1 to 2 weeks
• Xenodiagnosis (laboratory-bred reduvid bug fed on patient develops trypanosomes in gut in 4 weeks that are identified in feces) is only useful method during chronic stage; highly specific but sensitivity = 50%

♦ Serologic tests—specific IgG increases soon after infection and usually remains increased for life.

• IHA and direct agglutination tests at titers >1:64 have good S/S. IFA has poor specificity. Frequently cross-react in leishmaniasis, infection with other parasites, fungi, bacteria. Therefore, it is often recommended that serum test be positive by two different assays. In United States, tests accepted by FDA for clinical testing but not for blood bank screening include EIA, ELISA. CF test is less reliable.
• Gel tests (e.g., CIE) are most reliable, but no commercial reagents are available.
• Newer methods (e.g., DNA probes) are being developed and may be available through CDC or state laboratories or for research.
• Antigenuria can be detected in ~85% of chronic cases.

Laboratory findings due to organ involvement (e.g., heart, CNS, GI tract, skeletal muscle).

Prion Infections[30]

Due to proteinaceous infectious particles that do not utilize nucleic acids to mediate transmission. Protease-resistant infectious proteins devoid of nucleic acids that cause fatal untreatable disease. Is conformationally altered form of a normal

[29]*Lancet* 2004;363:1358.
[30]Source: Johnson RT, et al. Case 27-2005. *N Engl J Med* 2005;353:1042. *Clin Lab Med* 2003;23:43.

plasma membrane protein called PrPc. Abnormal form (PrPsc) is very resistant to proteases and can form rod-shaped multimers that precipitate as amyloid. Different pathogenic conformations are associated with different disease phenotypes. Neurodegenerative changes [characteristic spongioform changes in gray matter] are caused by accumulation of prion protein. Incubation period of months to years [formerly called slow viruses]. Causes chronic, progressive, and fatal neurodegenerative disease.

Human prion diseases include kuru, iatrogenic, vCJD, sporadic (six types), fatal insomnia (familial and sporadic), and Gerstmann-Sträussler-Scheinker syndrome (a familial prion disease).

Animal prion diseases include bovine spongioform encephalopathy ("mad cow disease"), scrapie (sheep), chronic wasting disease (deer, elk in United States), feline spongioform encephalopathy (cats), transmissible encephalopathy (mink).

Variant Creutzfeld-Jakob Disease (vCJD; Transmissible Spongioform Encephalopathy)

Fatal disease caused by eating the meat of cows with bovine spongioform encephalopathy ("mad cow disease"), blood transfusions, tissue grafts (cornea, dura mata), contaminated neurosurgical instruments or in response to biological products (human growth hormone, chorionic gonadotropin).

♦ Diagnosis based on biopsy showing pathologic changes and demonstration of prions or a known prion gene mutation. Histologic changes in brain tissue (spongioform vacuolar degeneration of gray matter with accumulation of protease-resistant protein and little or no amyloid accumulation). Is confirmed by immunohistochemical and WB analysis and DNA extracted from various tissues. Also found in appendix, lymph nodes, spleen, tonsils of patients with vCJD but not in classic CJD patients. For premortem diagnosis, tonsil may be preferred biopsy site.

♦ Highly suggestive of CJD are:
CSF protein is normal.
Presence of 14-3-3 protein in CSF which is marker for some prion diseases.
MRI changes with hyperintense signals in basal ganglia.

Congenital and Neonatal Infections

Antenatal/Neonatal/Perinatal Infections[31]

Other Significant Infections

- Toxoplasmosis (chorioretinitis, CNS, others)
- Congenital syphilis
- *Neisseria gonorrhoeae* (e.g., ophthalmia, septicemia)
- *Chlamydia trachomatis* (e.g., ophthalmia, pneumonia)
- Group B streptococcus
- Mycoplasma (e.g., *Ureaplasma urealyticum, Mycoplasma hominis* [GU, GYN, other infections)
- Others (e.g., listeriosis)

Tick-borne Infections

Ixodes (deer tick)
    Lyme disease
    Babesiosis
    Human granulocytic ehrlichiosis
Dermacentor
    Tularemia

[31]Gilbert GL. Diagnosis, prevention and management of infectious diseases in the fetus and neonate. In: Trent RJ (ed). *Handbook of Prenatal Diagnosis*. Cambridge: Cambridge University Press, 1995.

Table 15-23. Congenital Viral Infections

Virus	Diagnosis In-utero	Diagnosis in Newborn
CMV (multiorgan involvement)	Culture or PCR on AF	Culture urine during first week
Varicella-zoster (chickenpox)	PCR on AF	Culture or FA stain of lesion
Herpes simplex virus (skin, eye, CNS, multiorgan)	–	Culture lesion; culture body fluids, nasopharynx, mouth. PCR on blood in disseminated infection.
Parvovirus B19	PCR on AF	PCR on serum. Specific IgM
Hepatitis B Virus	NA	HBsAg
Hepatitis C Virus	No information	PCR
HIV	Contraindicated	HIV DNA PCR
Rubella (e.g., CNS, congenital heart, eye, pneumonitis, etc.)	Culture or PCR on AF. Specific IgM.	Specific IgM, persistent specific IgG. Culture body fluids.
Enteroviruses	NA	Culture stool, NP, blood, urine
Lymphocytic choriomeningitis virus	No information	Specific IgG and IgM

AF, amniotic fluid; NP, nasopharynx; NA, not applicable.

Table 15-24. Commonly Associated Pathogens in Patients with Immunosuppression (e.g., Organ Transplantation, Treatment of Malignancies, AIDS)

Immune Response Depressed	Underlying Condition	Commonly Associated Pathogens
Humoral	Lymphatic leukemia	Pneumococci
	Lymphosarcoma	*Haemophilus influenzae*
	Multiple myeloma	Streptococci
	Congenital hypogammaglobulinemias	*Pseudomonas aeruginosa*
	Nephrotic syndrome	*Pneumocystis carinii*
	Treatment with cytotoxic or antimetabolite drugs	*Pneumocystis carinii*
Cellular	Terminal cancers	Tubercle bacillus
	Hodgkin's disease	*Listeria*
	Sarcoidosis	*Candida* species
	Uremia	*Toxoplasma*
	Treatment with cytotoxicor antimetabolite drugs or corticosteroids	*Pneumocystis carinii*
Leukocyte bactericidal	Myelogenous leukemia	Staphylococci
	Chronic granulomatous disease	*Serratia*
	Acidosis	*Pseudomonas* species
	Burns	*Candida* species
	Treatment with corticosteroids	*Aspergillus*
	Granulocytopenia due to drugs	*Nocardia*

Table 15-25. Commonly Associated Pathogens in Patients with Neoplasms

Neoplasm	Infection	Commonly Associated Pathogens
Acute nonlymphocytic leukemia	Sepsis with no apparent focus, pneumonia, skin, mouth, GU tract, hepatitis	Enterobacteriaceae, *Pseudomonas*, staphylococci, *Corynebacterium*, *Candida, Aspergillus, Mucor*, non-A, non-B hepatitis virus
Acute lymphocytic leukemia	Disseminated disease, pneumonia, pharyngitis, skin	Streptococci, *Pneumocystis carinii*, HSV, CMV, varicella-zoster virus
Lymphoma	Disseminated disease, sepsis, GU tract, pneumonia, skin	*Cryptococcus neoformans*, mucocutaneous *Candida*, HSV, herpes zoster virus, CMV, *Pneumocystis carinii, Toxoplasma gondii*, mycobacteria, *Nocardia, Strongyloides stercoralis, Listeria monocytogenes, Brucella, Salmonella*, staphylococci, Enterobacteriaceae, *Pseudomonas*
Multiple myeloma	Sepsis, pneumonia, skin	*Haemophilus influenzae, Streptococcus pneumoniae, Neisseria* meningitis, *Pseudomonas*, Enterobacteriaceae, herpes zoster virus, *Candida, Aspergillus*

Table 15-26. Pulmonary Infections

<30 days	30–120 days	>120 days
Following organ transplantation (continuing immunosuppressive therapy)		
Usually nosocomial gram-negative bacteria (e.g., *Pseudomonas aeruginosa, Klebsiella, Escherichia coli, Serratia*) Anaerobes Opportunistic organisms are uncommon	Opportunistic organisms (e.g., CMV, *Pneumocystis Aspergillus, carinii*, *Nocardia*, mycobacteria, HSV, varicella-zoster virus)	Routine bacterial and viral pathogens *P. carinii* *Cryptococcus neoformans* Nocardia Legionella
Following bone marrow transplantation (initial immunosuppressive therapy)		
(Prolonged neutropenia, progressive decrease in humoral and cell-mediated immunity)		(Delayed maturation of donor immune system leads to defective humoral immunity. Also graft-versus-host disease and use of chemotherapeutic drugs)
Gram-negative bacilli (*P. aeruginosa, Klebsiella, E. coli, Serratia*) Anaerobes *Candida Aspergillus* HSV	CMV, HSV, *P. carinii*, adenovirus	Encapsulated bacteria (*Streptococcus pneumoniae, Haemophilus influenzae, Staphylococcus aureus*) Varicella-zoster virus

INFECTIOUS

Rocky Mountain spotted fever
Colorado tick fever
Human monocytic ehrlichiosis (lone star tick [*Amblyomma americanum*]).
Soft tick
Tick-borne relapsing fever

Opportunistic Infections

See Tables 15-24, 15-25, 15-26.
Laboratory findings due to acquired underlying diseases (e.g., AIDS, malignant lymphoma and leukemia, diabetes mellitus, immunoglobulin defects, following renal transplant, uremia, hyposplenism, hypoparathyroidism, hypoadrenalism) or inherited (e.g., sickle cell disease, various primary immune deficiency diseases [see Chapter 11]).
Laboratory findings due to administration of drugs (antibiotics, corticosteroids, cytotoxic and immunosuppressive drugs)

Table 15-27. Pathogens and Infectious Diseases Recognized in Past 25 Yrs

Viruses

Parvovirus B19 (aplastic crisis in chronic hemolytic anemia)
Rotavirus (infant diarrhea)
Hepatitis C, E
Human T-lymphotrophic virus 1 (T-cell lymphoma–leukemia)
Human T-lymphotrophic virus 2 (hairy cell leukemia)
Human immunodeficiency virus (acquired immunodeficiency syndrome [AIDS])
Herpesvirus 6 (roseola subitum)
Hemorrhagic fever viruses
  Ebola (Ebola hemorrhagic fever)
  Hantaan (hemorrhagic fever with renal syndrome)
  Guaranito (Venezuelan hemorrhagic fever)
  Sabia (Brazilian hemorrhagic fever)
Sin Nombre virus (adult respiratory syndrome)
Human herpesvirus 8 (associated with Kaposi's sarcoma in AIDS patients)

Bacteria

Campylobacter jejuni (enteric pathogen)
Toxin-producing strains of *Staphylococcus aureus* (toxic shock syndrome)
Legionella pneumophila (legionnaire's disease)
Escherichia coli O157:H7 (hemolytic-uremic syndrome; hemorrhagic colitis)
Borrelia burgdorferi (Lyme disease)
Helicobacter pylori (peptic ulcer)
Ehrlichia chaffeensis (ehrlichiosis)
Vibrio cholerae O139 (new strain; epidemic cholera)
Bartonella henselae (cat-scratch disease; bacillary angiomatosis)

Parasites

Cryptosporidium parvum (diarrhea)
Enterocytozoon bieneusi (persistent diarrhea)
Cyclospora cayatanensis (persistent diarrhea)
Encephalitozoon hellum (conjunctivitis; disseminated disease)
Encephalitozoon cuniculi (disseminated disease)
Babesia—new species (atypical babesiosis)

Table 15-28. Some Human Diseases that May Be Transmitted by or from Animals

Disease	Pathogen	Arthropod Vector[a]	Animal Reservoir[b]								
			D	C	B	F	P	R	M	X	H
Bacterial											
Campylobacter jejuni infections	*C. jejuni*		+	+	+	+	+	+	+		
Salmonella infections	*Salmonella* spp.	F, roaches	+	+	+	+	+	+	+		
Bacillary dysentery	*Shigella* spp.	F, roaches							+		
Yersinia infections	*Y. enterocolitica*		+	+		+	+	+			
Anthrax	Anthrax bacillus		+			+	+				
Brucellosis	*Brucella* spp.		+	+		+	+	+			
Tularemia	*Francisella tularensis*	T, biting flies	+	+		+		+			
Leptospirosis	*Leptospira* spp.		+	+		+		+			
Tuberculosis	*Mycoplasma tuberculosis*		+	+	+						
Lyme disease	*Borrelia burgdorferi*	T						+		+	
Relapsing fever	*Borrelia hermsii, B. parkeri, B. turicatae, B. recurrentis*	T / L						+			+
Ehrlichiosis	*Ehrlichia chaffeensis*	T						+			
Plague	*Yersinia pestis*	Fl						+			
Viral											
Rabies	Lyssavirus		+	+		+					
Cat-scratch disease	*Bartonella* spp.			+							
Psittacosis	*Chlamydia psittaci*				+			+			
Lymphocytic choriomeningitis			+								
St. Louis encephalitis	Flavivirus	M			+						
Western equine encephalitis	Alphavirus	M			+						
Eastern equine encephalitis	Alphavirus	M			+						
Venezuelan equine encephalitis	Alphavirus	M				+		+			
La Crosse encephalitis	Bunyavirus	M						+		3	
Dengue	Flavivirus	M									
Yellow fever	Flavivirus	M							+		
Colorado tick fever	Orbivirus	T						+			+
Hemorrhagic fever with renal and pulmonary syndrome	Hantavirus							+			+
California encephalitis	Arbovirus	M						+			

(continued)

INFECTIOUS

Table 15-28. (continued)

Disease	Pathogen	Arthropod Vector[a]	Animal Reservoir[b]								
			D	C	B	F	P	R	M	X	H
Rickettsial											
Q fever	*Coxiella burnetii*	T								1	
Rocky Mountain spotted fever	*Rickettsia rickettsii*	T								2	
Rickettsialpox	*R. akari*	T						+			
Murine typhus	*R. typhi*	Fl						+			
Epidemic typhus	*R. prowazekii*	L								4	+
Fungal											
Ringworm	*Microsporum, Tricophyton, Epidermophyton* spp.			+			+	+			
Histoplasmosis	*Histoplasma capsulatum*				+					+	
Parasitic											
Leishmaniasis	*Leishmania mexicana*	F						+		6	
Roundworm infestation	*Toxocara* sp.			+	+						
Tapeworm infestation	*Taenia* spp.			+	+						
Echinococcus				+	+						
Visceral larva migrans	*Toxocara canis, T. cati*		+	+							
Cutaneous larva migrans	*Ancylostoma caninum, A. braziliense*		+	+							
Dirofilariasis	*Dirofilaria immitis*	M	+	+							
Scabies	*Sarcoptes scabiei*		+	+							
Chagas' disease	*Trypanosoma cruzi*	O, kissing bugs (reduviids)						+		5	
Toxoplasmosis	*Toxoplasmosis gondii*	M	+	+							
Malaria	*Plasmodium* spp.	M									+
Babesiosis	*Babesia microti*	T						+			

Anisakiasis (nematode) from eating raw fish (e.g., sashimi).

Trichinosis from eating poorly prepared pork or exotic meats (e.g., bear, walrus, wild boar).

Capnocytophaga canimorsus (gram-negative bacteria) transmitted by dog bite or saliva causing acute overwhelming cellulitis, septicemia, meningitis, endocarditis; diagnosis by culture of blood, CSF, or tissue.

[a]Arthropod vector: F = fly; Fl = flea; L = louse; M = mosquito; O = other; T = tick or mite.

[b]Animal reservoir: B = birds; C = cat; D = dog; F = farm animals; H = human; M = monkeys; R = rodents; X = other; 1 = domestic livestock ticks; 2 = *Dermacentor* sp.; 3 = *Aedes triseriatus* mosquito; 4 = flying squirrels; 5 = opossums, raccoons, armadillos; 6 = opossums, cotton rats, armadillos.

Table 15-29.	Weapons of Biological Warfare and Terrorist Agents*	
Category A	Category B	Category C
Highest priority	**Second highest priority**	**Third highest priority**
Easily transmitted or disseminated. High mortality.	Moderately easy to disseminate. Moderate morbidity; low mortality.	Emerging pathogens. Could be engineered for mass dissemination.
Smallpox	Q fever *(Coxiella burnetti)*	Hantaviruses
Anthrax	Brucellosis (Brucella species)	Nipah virus
Plague *(Yersinia pestis)*	Glanders *(Burkholderia mallei)*	Yellow fever
Clostridium botulinum toxin	Alpha viruses	Multidrug-resistant TB
Tularemia *(Francisella tularensis)*	Venezuelan encephalomyelitis	Tickborne encephalitis viruses
Filoviruses (e.g., Ebola and Marburg hemorrhagic fevers)	Eastern and Western equine encephalomyelitis	Tickborne hemorrhagic fever viruses
Arenaviruses (e.g., Lassa fever)	Ricin toxin from castor beans *(Ricinus communis)*[†]	
	Clostridium perfringens epsilon toxin	
	Staphylococcal enterotoxin	
	Food or water borne agents	
	Salmonella species	
	Shigella dysenteriae	
	E. coli O157:H7	
	Vibrio cholerae	
	Cryptosporidium parvum	

*Adapted from Biological and chemical terrorism: strategic plan for preparedness and response. MMWR. April 21,2000[RR4]:1-14.
†www.bt.cdc.gov/agent/ricin/index.asp

Associated with other factors (e.g., plastic intravenous catheters, narcotic addiction)
Laboratory findings due to particular organism (see appropriate separate sections)

- *Cryptococcus neoformans*
- *Candida albicans*
- *Aspergillus*
- *Mucorales* fungi
- *Staphylococcus aureus*
- *Staphylococcus albus, Bacillus subtilis, Bacillus cereus*, and other saprophytes
- Enteric bacteria (*Pseudomonas aeruginosa, Escherichia coli, Klebsiella-Enterobacter, Proteus*)

See Table 15-27 for infectious diseases and pathogens that have been recognized in the past 25 years.
See Table 15-28 for a guide to human diseases that may be transmitted by or from animals.

Diseases Which Must Be Reported

Diseases which must be reported (confirmed or suspected cases) to most health departments
Anthrax, Botulism, Brucellosis, Diphtheria, *Haemophilus influenza*, Hepatitis A in institutions, Measles, Meningococcal invasive disease, Outbreaks (foodborne,

Table 15-30. Some Biological Warfare and Terrorist Agents*

Agent	Common Specimen Sources	Stains	Cultures	ELISA	PCR	Others	See Page
Bacteria							
Bacillus anthracis[1] (anthrax: cutaneous; inhalational; GI)	Blood, skin lesions, pleural fluid	X	X	X	X		736
Brucella species[2] (brucellosis)	Blood, bone marrow, liver, spleen		X	X	X	IFA	733–734
E. coli O157:H7[2]	Stool		X	X	X		
Yersinia pestis[1] (plague: pneumonic; septicemic; bubonic)	Blood, BAL, sputum, lymph node aspirate	X	X	X	X	IFA	734
Coxiella burnetti[2] (Q fever)	Blood		X	X	X	IFA	752
Salmonella species[2] (salmonellosis)	Stool		X	X	X		
Shigella species[2]	Stool		X	X	X		
Vibrio cholerae (cholera)	Stool		X	X	X		
Francisella tularensis[1] (tularemia: septicemic; lymphocutaneous)	Blood, tissue		X	X	X		734

Agent	Specimen			Detection methods	Page
Burkholderia species[2] (glanders; mellioidosis)	Blood, urine, sputum, skin, tissue depending on clinical presentation	X	X X	Microscopy	803
Parasites					
Plasmodium species	Blood	X	X X	Microscopy	875
Cryptosporidium parvum[2]	Stool	X	X X	Microscopy	874
Toxins					
C. botulinum[1] (botulinism) Clinical, epidemiological.	Nasal swab, induced respiratory secretions for first 3 days, serum, stool, food. Postmortem liver, spleen.	X	X	Bioassay	736
Staphylococcal enterotoxins.[2] Clinical (food poisoning or respiratory syndrome), epidemiological	Stool (first 24 hours), nasal swab.	X	X	Paired acute and convalescent sera. PCR for toxin genes in respiratory secretions. ELISA antigen capture in lung, kidney at autopsy.	160–162
Shigatoxin[2]	Stool		X	Bioassay	
Aflatoxins			X	HPLC. Mass spectrometry.	

(*continued*)

Table 15-30. (continued)

Agent	Common Specimen Sources	Stains	Cultures	ELISA	PCR	Others	See Page
Mycotoxins of filamentous fungi (e.g., *Fusarium*, *Myrotecium*, *Trichoderma*, *Stachybotrys* genera)	Autopsy tissues					HPLC. Mass spectrometry.	
Ricin toxin[2] (from castor beans). Clinical, epidemiological.				X		Swabs, sera for ELISA antigen capture, IgG, PCR. >6 days, urine for toxic metabolites.	
Bioregulators (e.g., cytokines, hormones, neuro-transmitters)	Various	Various					

[1]Highest priority. Easily transmitted or disseminated. High mortality.
[2]Second highest priority. Moderately easy to disseminate. Moderate morbidity; low mortality.
[3]Third highest priority. Emerging pathogens. Could be engineered for mass dissemination.
*Sources include: DR Franz, et al. Clinical recognition and management of patients exposed to biological warfare agents. *JAMA* 1997;278:399.
Marty AM. Laboratory aspects of biowarfare. *Clin Lab Med* 2001.
Peruski LF, Peruski AH. Rapid diagnostic assays in the genomic biology era; detection and identification of infectious disease and biological weapon agents. *Bio Tech* 2003;35:840.
Biological and chemical terrorism: strategic plan for preparedness and response. *MMWR* 2000(RR4):1–14.

waterborne, SARS, acts of bioterrorism), Pertussis, Plague, Poliomyelitis, Rabies, Rubella, Smallpox, Tularemia, Viral hemorrhagic fevers.

Biological Warfare and Terrorist Weapons

Chemical Warfare Agents[32]

Nerve agents (e.g., sarin, soman, tabun, VX) are indicated by decreased cholinesterase activity in serum in acute exposure and decreased in RBCs in chronic exposure. Also by gas chromatography-mass spectrometry.

Vesicants (blistering agents) (e.g., Lewisite, nitrogen mustard, sulfur mustard) can be measured by gas chromatography.

Pulmonary agents (e.g., chlorine, phosgene) can be measured by automated portable sensors. Also hydrogen chloride, nitrogen oxides.

Cyanides (e.g., arsine, hydrogen cyanide) can be measured by gas chromatography and other techniques. Usual levels in plasma and whole blood in nonsmokers are 0.004 mg/L and 0.016 mg/L; in smokers usual levels in plasma and whole blood are 0.006 mg/L and 0.041 mg/L, respectively.

INFECTIOUS

[32]Jortani SA, et al. The role of the clinical laboratory in managing chemical or biological terrorism. *Clin Chem* 2000;46:1883–1893.

16 Autoimmune and Miscellaneous Diseases

MISC

Laboratory Tests for Autoimmune Diseases

Antinuclear Antibodies (ANAs)

Use
Mainly to exclude SLE (see Tables 16-1 and 16-2)

Interpretation
ANA is the most sensitive laboratory test for detecting SLE (detects ≤95% of cases); specificity is as low as 50% in rheumatic disease in general. May be present in healthy persons, aged, other rheumatic diseases, infectious mononucleosis, unrecognized chronic infections, use of certain drugs (e.g., hydralazine, isoniazid, chlorpromazine), or family of SLE patients. Negative ANA in patient with active multisystem disease is strong (but not absolute) evidence against SLE; positive ANA without other manifestations is not diagnostic. High titers are most often associated with SLE; <1:160 often have minimal clinical significance and may not be related to patient's symptoms. ANA may become negative during remission. Titers correlate poorly with remission/relapse; usually not useful to follow course or response to therapy. Titer of <1:40 is considered negative, titer of 1:40 to 1:80 is considered low positive, and titer of ≥1:160 is considered positive. Persistently negative ANA tests occur in about 5% of SLE patients because of congenital deficiency of early complement component (usually C4 or C2); detected by absent total hemolytic complement (CH50). These patients tend to have prominent skin disease and low incidence of serious renal and CNS disease.

Pattern of ANA immunofluorescence (IFA) is of limited value in discriminating SLE from other collagen vascular diseases but may suggest subsequent tests.

• Homogeneous (diffuse or solid) pattern is associated with antibodies to DNA-histone (deoxyribonucleoprotein); high titers are more strongly associated with SLE than with other diseases and correlate with activity of SLE; also found in drug-induced SLE, and many connective tissue diseases.
• Rim (peripheral) pattern is associated with anti-dsDNA and has the highest specificity for SLE.
• Speckled pattern detects numerous antigens (e.g., ENA, Sm, nRNP, SS-A, SS-B); antibodies to these antigens should be ordered when a speckled pattern is found.
• Nucleolar pattern is associated with anti-RNP; characteristic of scleroderma; rarely in other immune disorders.

Anti-extractable nuclear antigen (ENA) (by EIA or gel diffusion) detects only two ENAs: ribonucleoprotein (RNP) and Sm.

• Anti-RNP is found in 25% to 30% of SLE, 10% of RA, 22% of scleroderma, 100% of mixed connective tissue disease (MCTD) patients.
• Anti-Sm (speckled IFA pattern) is found in 25% to 30% of SLE patients and *is the most specific diagnostic test for SLE*; occurs almost exclusively in SLE. Serum levels remain fairly constant and not related to disease activity.

Anti- native double-stranded DNA (dsDNA) is found in 40% to 80% of SLE patients and rarely in other diseases; *high specificity* is almost same as anti-Sm (rim or peripheral nodular IFA pattern). Absence of anti-dsDNA throughout clinical course is associated with improved prognosis and severe clinical disease frequently correlates with a high initial titer which declines with clinical improvement; however, it may be present for prolonged periods without clinical activity. *High titers are characteristic of SLE and rarely in other conditions*; low titers (e.g., 1:10–1:20) are found in other rheumatic diseases.

Anti-single-stranded DNA (ssDNA) are found in all other rheumatic diseases and many chronic inflammatory conditions, is not specific for SLE but presence in almost all SLE patients makes it a sensitive indicator.

Autoimmune Diseases

Lupus, Systemic Erythematosus (SLE)[1]

Multisystem autoimmune disease with broad spectrum of polyclonal autoantibodies (average ≥3).

[1]Wallace DJ, Hahn BH (eds). *Dubois' Lupus Erythematosus*, 6th Ed. Philadelphia: Lippincott Williams & Wilkins; 2002.

Table 16-1. Antinuclear Antibody Disease Profiles*

ANAs	SLE	Drug-Induced Lupus Erythematosus	Mixed Connective Tissue Disease	Scleroderma Syndrome	CREST Syndrome	Sjögren's Syndrome	Dermatomyositis and Polymyositis	RA
ANA screen	>95	>95	>95	70–90	70–90	75–90	40–60	R
Native DNA	**60**	R	R	R	R	R	R	40
Histones	30	**>95**	R	R	R	R	R	20
Sm	**30**	R	R	R	R	R	R	R
Nuclear RNP	40–50	R	**>95**	15	10	R	15	10
Scl-70	R	R	R	**30–70**	R	R	R	R
SS-A (Ro)	40–60	R	R	R	R	**≤90**	10	R
SS-B (La)	15	R	R	R	R	**≤60**	R	R
Centromere	R	R	R	30	**70–85**	R	R	R
Nucleolar	25	R	R	**40–70**	R	R	R	R
PM-Scl (PM-1) and Jo-1	R	R	R	~20	R	R	**10–50**	R

CREST = calcinosis, *Raynaud's syndrome, esophageal dysmotility, sclerodactyly, telangiectasia*; DNA = deoxyribonucleic acid; PM-Scl = polymyositis-scleroderma; R = rare; RNP = ribonucleoprotein; Scl = scleroderma; Sm = Smith; SS = Sjögren's syndrome.
*Reported frequency of ANAs in various diseases is given as a percentage. Boldface indicates significant correlation.
Source: Tan EM, Robinson CA, Nakamura RM. ANAs in systemic rheumatic disease: diagnostic significance. *Postgrad Med* 1985;78:141.

MISC

Table 16-2.	Comparison of Idiopathic and Drug-Induced Lupus	
	Idiopathic SLE	Drug–Induced Lupus
Renal, CNS involvement	Common	Rare
ANA pattern	Rim	Homogeneous
Immune complexes	Present	Rare
Low complement level	50–70%	5%
Antihistone antibodies	≤70% of patients	>95% of patients; if negative, drug–induced lupus is unlikely
Other antibodies (e.g., anti–dsDNA and anti–Sm)	Frequently present	Usually absent

dsDNA = double-stranded deoxyribonucleic acid.
Drug-induced ANA is histone dependent, but in idiopathic SLE, histone dependence is found in only 30% of patients and histone–dependent ANAs are never the only ones.

Criteria for Classification of SLE[2]

♦ Presence of ≥4 criteria at same or different times allows the diagnosis of SLE and excludes other disorders.

	Sensitivity (%)	Specificity (%)
Malar rash	57	96
Discoid lupus	18	99
Oral/nasopharyngeal ulcers	27	96
Photosensitivity	43	96
Arthritis, nonerosive, involving ≥2 peripheral joints	86	37
Proteinuria (>0.5 g/day or 3+ qualitative) or cellular casts	51	94
Seizures or psychosis not due to other causes	20	98
Pleuritis or pericarditis	56	86
Cytopenia (any of these 4 findings)	59	89
Autoimmune hemolytic anemia	15	
Neutropenia (<4,000/cu mm on ≥2 occasions)		
Lymphopenia (<1,500/cu mm on ≥2 occasions)		
Thrombocytopenia (<100,000/cu mm in absence of causative drugs)		
Immunologic findings (any of these 4 findings)	85	93
1. Anti-dsDNA antibodies		
2. Anti-Sm antibodies		
3. Positive test for antiphospholipid antibodies based on:		
(a) Abnormal serum IgM or IgG anticardiolipin antibodies		
(b) Lupus anticoagulant		
(c) False positive serological test for syphilis ≥6 months duration confirmed by FTA-ABS or TPI		
4. Abnormal ANA titer in the absence of known causative drugs	99	49
Overall =	96	96

Hochberg MC. Updating the American College of Rheumatology revised criteria for the classification of systemic lupus erythematosus. *Arthritis Rheum* 1997;40:1725.

♦ ANA profile in SLE

• *ANA is the most sensitive laboratory test for SLE* (detects ≤95% of cases). Best single test to rule out SLE.

    Most patients with SLE will have multiple (≥3 antibodies) present; this is *characteristic of SLE*. Drug-induced lupus and other connective tissue diseases are

[2]Hochberg MC. Updating the American College of Rheumatology revised criteria for the classification of systemic lupus erythematosus. *Arthritis Rheum* 1997;40:1725.

likely to have fewer ANA present. *Combination of positive ANA test, positive dsDNA antibodies, and hypocomplementemia has diagnostic specificity of virtually 100%. Negative IFA ANA rules out SLE in 99% of cases.* Positive ANA present in 20% to 40% of healthy persons.

- *High titers of anti-dsDNA are characteristic of SLE;* very specific for SLE; occur in 50% to 60% of patients; may be present in chronic active hepatitis. Low titers should be viewed with suspicion. Not found in drug-induced lupus. Indicates degree of lupus nephritis. Can be used to predict or monitor disease flares. Less than 50% of SLE patients may be negative; ~58% of these have antibody to Ro/SS-A.
- *High titers of anti-Sm are very specific for SLE but not sensitive.* (Present in 30% of patients; 50%–60% by ELISA). Virtually absent in normal persons. May be found in absence of anti-dsDNA. Titers remain constant. Does not correlate with disease activity.
- ssDNA has low specificity; poor correlation with disease activity.
- DNP in ≤70% of patients
- Histones in ≤60% of patients
- SS-A in 25% of patients
- SS-B in 15% of patients
- RNP in ≤34% of patients, usually associated with anti-Sm.

Recommended sequence of tests: Screen for SLE with ANA; if positive, follow with anti-dsDNA, confirm with anti-Sm.

♦ Current indicators of disease activity

- No single test predicts exacerbation; most useful are anti-dsDNA and serum complement.
- Decrease in early complement components (C3, C4; C4 is most sensitive) and total hemolytic complement (THC) occur in ~70% of patients with active; is not specific for diagnosis but is helpful in managing patients who are at risk for renal and CNS involvement; C3 and/or C4 may be helpful in following response to therapy. THC should be part of initial evaluation of SLE patients.

♦ Reduced C3, C4 are rarely seen without immune complex diseases; therefore their reduction strongly supports diagnosis of SLE in patient with suggestive history and physical exam. Complement activation products (e.g., C3a, C4a, C3d, C4d) may be superior to C3 and C4.

- Increasing titers of anti-DNA; serial monitoring is probably not of value.
- Presence of circulating immune complexes.
- Presence of cryoglobulins (see Chapter 11) correlates well with disease activity.
- High anti-dsDNA and low serum complement values predict lupus nephritis.
- Monoclonal RF assay.
- C1q binding.
- Raji cell assay is not recommended as indicator of SLE disease activity.
- Traditional parameters of disease activity (Hb, WBC, ESR, CRP, urinalysis, serum creatinine) do not distinguish activity from superimposed infection or drug toxicity and may not be sensitive enough to detect early exacerbation.

These indicators do not predict which manifestations are likely to become active or the time interval (may be weeks to months), and some patients with these laboratory abnormalities never manifest active disease. The strongest correlation is with active nephritis, but these tests may be normal in 10% to 25% of cases and in any case do not substitute for renal biopsy.

SLE may present as "idiopathic" thrombocytopenic purpura but serious thrombocytopenia occurs in <10% of patients.

Anemia is most commonly anemia of chronic disease or may be due to iron deficiency caused by blood loss. Autoimmune hemolytic anemia occurs in ~15% of patients and correlates with disease activity.

ESR and CRP may be increased.

Abnormal serum proteins frequently occur.

- Biologically false-positive (BFP) test for syphilis is very common; occurs in <20% of patients. *This may be the first manifestation of SLE and may precede other features by many months; 7% of asymptomatic individuals with BFP test for syphilis ultimately develop SLE.*

MISC

♦ Polyclonal gammopathy. Serum γ-globulin is increased in 50% of patients; a continuing rise may indicate poor prognosis. α_2-globulin is increased; albumin is decreased. Immunoglobulins may be increased.

Tissue biopsy of skin, muscles, kidney, and lymph node may be useful.

Laboratory findings reflecting specific organ involvement

- Renal: Serologic changes may appear months before clinical renal involvement; urine findings are stronger indication to modify therapy. Urine findings indicate acute nephritis, nephrotic syndrome, chronic renal impairment, secondary pyelonephritis. Sediment is the same as in chronic active glomerulonephritis. >3.5 g/24 hours indicates severe progressive renal damage; increasing levels indicate increasing renal damage. Patients with azotemia and marked proteinuria usually die in 1 to 3 years. High antibody titer to native DNA associated with decreased serum complement indicates lupus nephritis. Disease activity often disappears when renal failure occurs. Recurrence in allograft is rare. Renal biopsy may not be indicated without significant proteinuria or urinary sediment abnormalities. Complement levels are especially low with renal involvement. (See Chapter 14)
- CNS: Manifestations due to vascular changes causing occlusions, uremia, electrolyte imbalance, coagulopathy, hypertension, antineuronal antibodies, infection. (*Rule out complicating TB and cryptococcosis.*) CSF findings of aseptic meningitis (increased protein and pleocytosis are found in 50% of these patients).
- Cardiovascular: Bacterial and nonbacterial endocarditis; increased prevalence of coronary arteriosclerosis and valvular lesions.
- Pulmonary (acute or chronic disease) findings may be present. Pleural effusions are exudate in type.
- Joint involvement occurs in 90% of patients.
- Anti-Ro/SSA antibodies in pregnancy indicates risk for neonatal lupus syndrome. Neonates of mothers with SLE may have discoid lupus, hematologic or serologic abnormalities due to transplacental passage of Ro antibodies. Later may develop complete heart block.
- Inflammatory manifestations become less common and thrombotic events become more common with long term disease.

Laboratory findings reflecting diseases due to autoantibodies

- Hashimoto thyroiditis
- Sjögren syndrome
- Myasthenia gravis
- Autoimmune thrombocytopenia in ≤25% of SLE patients
- Circulating lupus anticoagulants; antiphospholipid antibody syndrome in 50% of patients (see Chapter 11)

Laboratory findings due to complications

- Various bacterial and viral opportunistic infections (e.g., herpes zoster) caused by immunodeficiency (from SLE as well as from therapy).
- Osteonecrosis
- Malignancy—increased risk for lymphoma and soft tissue sarcomas.

SLE should be ruled out in asymptomatic patients (especially women of child-bearing age) with false-positive VDRL, various unexplained conditions (e.g., thrombocytopenia, leukopenia, proteinuria or abnormal urine sediment, positive Coombs test, prolonged aPTT).

Lupus syndromes due to prolonged administration of drugs. Some drugs may induce ANA without symptoms. Drug-induced ANA is histone dependent, but in idiopathic SLE, histone dependence is found in only 30% of patients and histone-dependent antibodies are never the only ANA.

- High risk
   Procainamide (15%–100% develop ANA within 1 year and 5%–30% develop SLE; does not induce antibodies to dsDNA)
   Hydralazine (24%–50% develop ANA and 8%–13% develop SLE)
- Low risk (e.g., ethosuximide, hydantoins, isoniazid, lithium, quinidine, thiouracils)
- Possible (rare) association (e.g., D-penicillamine, chlorpromazine, reserpine)

- Unlikely association (e.g., allopurinol, gold salts, griseofulvin, methysergide, oral contraceptives, penicillin, streptomycin, sulfonamides, tetracycline)

◆ *Antihistone antibodies are present in >95% of cases of drug-induced lupus*; if negative, drug-induced lupus is unlikely. Other antibodies that are frequently seen in SLE (e.g., anti-dsDNA and anti-Sm) are usually absent.

- Usually high titer ANA and absent dsDNA antibodies.
- Renal and CNS manifestations are very unusual.

LE Cell Test has been replaced by ANA tests. May be found in smears from CSF, joint, pleural, pericardial, pericardial and blister fluids.

Hematoxylin Bodies
Homogeneous round extracellular material.

May be found in SLE, RA, multiple myeloma, and cirrhosis. In SLE, they may be found without LE cells in the same sample.

Lupus Band Test (LBT)
Direct immunofluorescence to detect IgG in biopsy of skin
Use
In patients without sufficient clinical manifestations of SLE (e.g., only renal or CNS findings).
In patients whose symptoms and other laboratory tests show remission due to steroid therapy.
In differentiation of early SLE from RA.
Interpretation
Is positive in SLE patients in ≤80% with active multisystem (especially renal) disease; and ~40% with inactive disease; in discoid lupus is found only in skin lesions.
Specificity for SLE increases with the number of immunoglobulins and complement components found.
May be positive in dermatomyositis, undifferentiated collagen-vascular disease and other nonrheumatic diseases but usually only one immunoglobulin is found.

Lupus, Discoid
About 10% of patients develop SLE.
ANA and other laboratory tests are negative.
◆ Characteristic biopsy of skin lesions in classic cases shows deposition of complement and Ig.
Lupus band test on fresh tissue is positive.

Mixed Connective Tissue Disease (MCTD)
Combines clinical features of RA, polymyositis, SLE, and especially scleroderma; ~10% of SLE patients fulfill criteria for MCTD.

◆ ANA Profile: *High titer of anti-RNP in >95% of patients without anti-Sm and other antibodies is characteristic of MCTD.*
ANA positive with speckled pattern.

Polymyositis/Dermatomyositis
Syndrome may include pulmonary fibrosis, Raynaud syndrome, dry cracked skin on hands ("mechanics' hands"). Often associated with cancer.

See Chapter 10.
◆ ANA Profile: Anti-Jo-1 (PM-1; histidyl-transfer RNA synthetase antibody) in 50% of polymyositis and 10% of dermatomyositis patients; strong association with interstitial lung disease. Rarely detected in other diseases.

MISC

○ Increased serum CK and aldolase.
♦ Abnormal findings on biopsy of muscle.

Rheumatoid Arthritis (RA)

See Chapter 10.
♦ ANA Profile: RA nuclear antigen is found in 85% to 95% of patients.
♦ RF is present in ~80% of patients. Frequently present in Sjögren syndrome; less often in other connective tissue diseases; occasionally in chronic infections (e.g., SBE, gammopathies).

ANAs are absent; low titer anti-native DNA may be present.
Histones are found in 20% of patients.

Sjögren Syndrome (SS)

Primary systemic chronic autoimmune disease associated with decreased salivary and lacrimal gland secretion or may be secondary to RA, SLE, scleroderma, or vasculitis in one half to two thirds of patients. 90% of patients are female.

♦ **Diagnostic Criteria**

A. Primary SS
   1. Symptoms and objective signs of dry eyes *and*
   2. Symptoms and objective signs of mouth including biopsy of minor salivary gland *and*
   3. Laboratory evidence of systemic autoimmune disease

      a) Increased RF titer ≥1:320 (RF is present in ≤90% of primary and secondary SS).
      b) Increased ANA titer ≥1:320 *or*
      c) Presence of anti-SS-A (Ro) or SS-B (La) antibodies

B. Secondary SS
   • SLE is found in 4%–5% of patients with SS; SS is found in 50%–98% of patients with SLE.
   • RF is found in ≤75% of patients with SS; SS is found in 20%–100% of patients with RA.
   • Primary biliary cirrhosis is found in 3% of patients with SS; SS is found in 50%–100% of patients with biliary cirrhosis.
   • Polymyositis, generalized scleroderma

C. Not caused by sarcoidosis, HIV, HTLV, HBV, HCV, preexisting lymphoma, fibromyalgia, or causes of keratitis sicca or enlarged salivary glands

---

♦ Biopsy of salivary gland is a hallmark.
♦ ANAs in speckled or homogeneous pattern are present in 65% of patients, more frequently in those with primary type. Anti-SS-A (Ro) is present in ~70% of patients with primary type and <10% of those with secondary SS. Anti-SS-B (La) is present in ~60% of patients with primary SS and <5% of those with secondary SS. Anti-SS-A and anti-SS-B without other antibodies indicates probable Sjögren syndrome; with other ANA probably indicates SLE. If SS-B is present, it usually accompanies SS-A. Virtually absent in normal persons. ANA is not required for diagnosis. Anti-salivary duct antibody is rare (<30%) in primary SS and frequent (76%–83%) in secondary SS. Patients with primary SS also have higher levels of tissue antibodies (e.g., thyroglobulin [in 35%], gastric parietal, smooth muscle). Anti-dsDNA is not found.
Mild normochromic, normocytic anemia occurs in 50% of patients.
Leukopenia occurs in up to one third of patients.
ESR is usually increased.

Serum protein electrophoresis shows polyclonal hyperglobulinemia largely caused by IgG. Cryoglobulins may be present.

Laboratory findings due to concomitant diseases.

Immune complex GN may occur, but chronic tubulointerstitial nephritis is more characteristic.

Progressive Systemic Sclerosis (Scleroderma)[3]

Multisystem disease of unknown etiology characterized by specific autoantibodies, organ fibrosis, small vessel vasculopathy. Clinical course varies from mild disease to rapid progressive organ failure.

See Table 16-1.

♦ Biopsy of skin or other involved tissue may establish diagnosis.

Laboratory tests are generally not diagnostic; no antibodies may be present.

ANA are found in low titers in 40% to 90% of patients; not required for diagnosis. High titer of anti-nRNP alone may indicate risk of developing scleroderma. RNP, SS-A, SS-B at low titers

♦ Anti-Scl-70 is found in 30% to 70% of patients with diffuse cutaneous scleroderma and is highly specific but occurs late in disease when diagnosis is obvious. Suggests a worse prognosis. More prevalent in severe scleroderma than in CREST.

♦ Antinucleolar pattern is most specific for scleroderma; is highly specific when no other antibody is present. Is rarely found in early scleroderma. High titer in 40% to 50% of patients

CREST syndrome is outmoded acronym for limited form of scleroderma with **c**alcinosis, **R**aynaud phenomenon, **e**sophageal dysfunction, **s**clerodactyly, **t**elangiectasia). May be present in early stage when only Raynaud phenomenon is present. Anticentromere antibody is said to be S/S; is only antibody in 70% to 85% of CREST patients; moderate to high titers; rare in other disorders.

May be found in 20% of other rheumatic diseases in association with other antibodies.

RF present in 30% of patients.

ESR is normal in one third of patients, mildly increased in one third of patients, markedly increased in one third of patients.

Eosinophilia is described in all scleroderma syndromes.

Mild hypochromic microcytic anemia present in 10% of patients.

Serum γ-globulins are increased in 25% of patients (usually slight increase) and has no predictive value.

Abnormal serum proteins occasionally occur, as revealed by BFP test for syphilis (5% of patients), positive RA test (35% of patients), cold agglutinins, cryoglobulins, etc.

Laboratory findings reflect specific organ involvement:

• Malabsorption syndrome due to GI tract involvement (≤90% of patients)
• Abnormal urinary findings, renal function tests, and uremia due to renal involvement
• Myocarditis, pericarditis, secondary bacterial endocarditis
• Pulmonary fibrosis, secondary pneumonitis

Vitiligo

Considered to be an autoimmune response against melanocytes in skin.

May be a marker for presence of other autoimmune diseases (e.g., Addison disease, inflammatory bowel disease, hypothyroidism) and autoantibodies (e.g., thyroid microsomal and peroxidase, gastric parietal cell, ANAs).

Other Autoimmune Disorders

See related chapters: Diabetes Mellitus (type I), Goodpasture Syndrome, Grave Disease, Multiple Sclerosis, Myasthenia Gravis, Pernicious Anemia, Polyarteritis Nodosa, etc.

[3]Clements PJ, Furst DE. Systemic Sclerosis. Second Ed. Lippincott William & Wilkins. Phila. 2004.

MISC

Miscellaneous Disorders

Allergic Diseases[4]

○ Increased serum total IgE is not a sensitive test and is of limited clinical value but extreme values may be helpful:

* Very low levels (<50 μg/L) help exclude atopic disease but not IgE sensitivity to special allergens such as penicillin or hymenoptera venoms.
* If >900 μg/L, atopic disease is likely but tests for specific allergens are needed.
* Very high levels (2,000–>60,000 μg/L) are found in asthma associated with severe atopic dermatitis, allergic bronchopulmonary aspergillosis, Buckley syndrome (staphylococcal infections with hyper-IgE), systemic parasitic infestations, IgE myeloma, immune deficiency.
* Principal value in infants is to alert the clinician to the possibility of allergic disease when this is not the presumptive diagnosis.

○ • RAST (_r_adio_a_llergosorbent _t_est) in-vitro measures total serum IgE antibodies as well as specific allergens. Useful when skin testing cannot be done (e.g., children, risk of anaphylaxis) or when skin testing is unreliable (e.g., generalized dermatitis, dermographism). Less sensitive than skin and bronchial provocation tests. Largely replaced by FEIA (_f_luorescent _e_nzyme _i_mmuno_a_ssay).

○ Blood eosinophil count >450/μL in adults and >750/μL in children suggest allergic disorders. Significant number of false positive and false negative results occur.

○ Nasal cytology smears (Hansel-stained) showing >5% eosinophils, >1% basophils, and/or >50% goblet/epithelial cells suggest allergic disease of respiratory tract. Does not correlate with blood eosinophilia. Many neutrophils suggest infection. Both eosinophils and neutrophils suggest chronic allergy with superimposed infection. Significant number of false-positive and false-negative results occur.

Measurement of serum complement is not useful.

Amyloidosis[5]

Extracellular deposition of nonbranching rodlike fibril proteins in a β-pleated sheet conformation in various tissues. Classified according to protein component.

◆ Diagnosis is established by demonstration of amyloid in tissue. Congo red stain of tissue deposits is positive and shows apple-green birefringence under polarized light in one third of patients with primary amyloidosis and about two thirds of patients with secondary amyloidosis.

* Subcutaneous abdominal fat biopsy is positive in 85% of patients with AL amyloidosis.
* Gingival or rectal biopsy is positive in one half to two thirds of patients.
* Needle biopsy of kidney is useful when gingival and rectal biopsies are not helpful and there is a differential diagnosis of nephrosis.
* Bone biopsy in positive in 30% of patients; also useful to identify multiple myeloma.
* Needle biopsy of liver is often positive but beware of intractable bleeding or rupture.
* Skin biopsy is taken from sites of plaque formation.
* Tissue from carpal-tunnel decompression is positive in 90% of amyloidosis cases.
* Other areas of involvement include GI tract, spleen, and respiratory tract.
* Immunohistochemical staining shows reaction of fibrils with kappa or lambda antisera.
* Electron microscopy is the most specific diagnostic method. EM and immuno-EM of tissues have been used to characterize cases of cardiac amyloidosis.

Evans blue dye is retained in serum.

---

[4]Gendo K, Larson EB. Evidence-based diagnostic strategies for evaluating suspected allergic rhinitis. *Ann Int Med* 2004;140:278.
[5]Falk RH, Comenzo RL, Skinner M. The systemic amyloidoses. *New Eng J Med* 1997;337:898.

Table 16-3.   Classification of Amyloidosis*

	Underlying Condition	Examples of Associated Diseases	Predominant Location of Amyloid Deposits	Major Amyloid or Precursor
Reactive (Secondary)	Chronic inflammation	TB, bronchiectasis, osteomyelitis, leprosy, skin-popping of heroin	Kidney, liver, spleen, adrenals	AA
	Autoimmune disorders	RA (especially juvenile), Crohn disease		
	Neoplasms	Hodgkin's disease, renal cell carcinoma		
Light Chain (Primary)	Plasma cell dyscrasias (see Ch. 11)	Multiple myeloma, other monoclonal B cell proliferation	Kidney, heart, blood vessels, respiratory, nerves, skin, tongue	AL (κ, λ) AH (IgG, γ)
	No apparent disease			
Hemodialysis-associated	Renal failure		Nephrotic syndrome may occur	β_2-microglobulin
Hereditary	Familial Mediterranean fever	See Ch. 12	Nephropathy in ≤60% of patients. Also blood vessels, spleen, respiratory tract	AA
	Familial polyneuropathy, Types I, II, III			Transthyretin (prealbumin)
Endocrine	Medullary carcinoma of thyroid			Pro-calcitonin
	Islets of Langerhans	Type II diabetes		Islet amyloid polypeptide
	Others e.g., pheochromocytoma, stomach carcinoma			
Cerebral	Cerebral	Alzheimer disease	Brain	Aβ
Cardiac	Isolated atrial amyloid			Atrial natriuretic factor (AANF)
	Senile cardiac	Myopathy, arrhythmias		Transthyretin
Nodular deposits	Lung, larynx, skin, bladder, tongue, etc.			
Others				

*WHO-IUIS Nomenclature Subcommittee. Nomenclature of amyloid and amyloidosis. Bull WHO 1993;71:105.

MISC

(AA) Reactive (Secondary) Systemic (Amyloid A Protein)

BJ proteinuria is absent. Fifty percent die within 5 years.

Due To

Chronic inflammation (e.g., chronic infections [most common cause prior to antibiotic era (e.g., TB, bronchiectasis, osteomyelitis, leprosy, "skin-popping" of narcotics)])

Autoimmune diseases (e.g., RA, inflammatory bowel disease, heroin skin-popping, ankylosing Spondylitis)

Neoplasms (e.g., Hodgkin disease, nonlymphoid solid tumors [e.g., renal and bladder carcinoma])

Heredofamilial systemic amyloidosis:

* Familial Mediterranean fever (AA type) (see Chapter 12)
* Neuropathic types (I, II, III, IV)—serum protein electrophoresis and immunoelectrophoresis are normal.

Increased concentration of serum amyloid A protein (an acute phase protein)

♦ Immunohistochemical staining of tissue for AA protein.
♦ About 25% present with proteinuria leading to nephrotic syndrome, azotemia, ESRD.

(AL) Light Chain Amyloid (Primary) or (AH) Heavy Chain[6]

Paraprotein disorder characterized by monoclonal Ig deposits in tissues; BJ proteinuria occurs; derived from malignant clone of plasma cells in neoplastic type or small nonproliferative population of plasma cells in nontumor type.

○ One third of cases show overt myeloma; occurs in ~15% of cases of multiple myeloma. Primary when there is no evidence of associated disease (e.g. myeloma). May also be associated with Waldenstrom macroglobulinemia, heavy-chain disease, etc.

○ One organ usually shows predominant involvement.

* Cardiovascular system—involved in almost all cases; congestive failure in 25% of cases
* Proteinuria and azotemia occur in most cases; nephrotic range proteinuria (>3 g/d) occurs in 45% of cases. Amyloidosis should always be ruled out in patients > age 30 years with unexplained nephrotic syndrome.
* Liver—33% have concomitant nephrotic syndrome. Increased ALP (86%), AST (80%), total bilirubin (21%), cholesterol (80%), ESR (62%).
* Evidence of hyposplenism (e.g., Howell-Jolly bodies) (28%).
* Tongue is enlarged in 20% of cases.
* Peripheral neuropathy in 16% of cases; CNS is not involved.
* Carpal tunnel syndrome in 20%.
* GI tract (e.g., malabsorption).
* Bone marrow involved in 30%.
* Respiratory system is usually involved, but decreased pulmonary function is rare.
* Others (adrenals, thyroid, etc).

○ Serum protein electrophoresis shows hypogammaglobulinemia in 25% and an abnormal Ig (monoclonal spike) in another 45% of cases.

○ Immunoelectrophoresis/immunofixation detects a monoclonal protein in 90% of cases. About 25% of patients have a free monoclonal light chain in serum (BJ proteinemia). Lambda light chains are more common (65%) than kappa light chains (35%) in contrast to multiple myeloma. Tissue extracts for biochemical analysis may supplement and confirm this.

○ Urine contains free light chains in >75% of cases, two thirds of these are lambda-type BJ proteins; monoclonal peak is often hidden by nephrotic protein loss. Sensitivity for detection of free-light chains is increased by concentration of urine (100×–500×), and by immunoelectrophoresis and immunofixation. Low levels of urine monoclonal light chains (<200 mg/24 hrs) may indicate an immunocytic malignancy (multiple myeloma, chronic lymphocytic leukemia or non-Hodgkin lymphoma) even when serum is negative for M proteins and thus occult malignancy should be ruled out. *Monoclonal proteins are not found in secondary, senile, familial, or localized amyloidosis.*

Serum creatinine >1.3 mg/dL is associated with a shorter survival time; some renal insufficiency in ~50% of cases.

Mild anemia in 50% of cases.

---

[6]Park MA, et al. Primary [AL] hepatic amyloidosis. *Medicine* 2003;82:291.

Platelet count may be increased ($>500,000/\mu L$ in ~10% of cases); may be caused by functional hyposplenism.
WBC is frequently increased.
ESR is increased.
Bone marrow shows >5% plasma cells in 50% of cases.
Demonstration of clonal plasma cell disorder. See Multiple Myeloma
Staining tissue deposits for κ and λ Ig light chains, antisera to amyloid A (AA) and to transthyretin are a useful panel.[7]

Familial Transthyretin Associated (ATTR)

Autosomal dominant diseases; most commonly caused by mutant transthyretin.

♦ Many different types of abnormal transthyretin identified by isoelectric focusing of serum or DNA test for mutant transthyretin gene. Mass spectroscopy for transthyretins of abnormal molecular weight has been used as a screening tool.
Renal disease less common than in AL.
No tongue involvement.

Local Amyloidosis Types

BJ proteinuria is absent.

Senile cardiac amyloid (SSA) (formed from prealbumin)—found in 24% of patients >70 years old; may cause heart failure.
Familial amyloid (AF) (formed from prealbumin)—autosomal dominant with cardiac, renal, neuropathic involvement
Cerebral amyloid (CAA) (subunit protein is called A4 or β)—in cerebral vessels, plaques and neurofibrillary tangles in Alzheimer disease
Systemic amyloid (A-β_2-M) (from β_2-microglobulin) due to dialysis
Amyloid of type II diabetes (IAPP) (from islet polypeptide)
Amyloid of medullary cancer of thyroid (AE) (from calcitonin)
Laboratory findings due to associated diseases (see above)
Laboratory findings due to involvement of specific organs (e.g., liver, kidney, GI system, endocrine, skin, synovia and tendons in carpal-tunnel syndrome, lung, bladder, skin, larynx; see appropriate separate sections)
Monoclonal Ig are not found in serum or urine.

Angioedema, Hereditary

Syndrome of episodes of upper airway obstruction, cramping abdominal pain, absence of urticaria; attacks precipitated by trauma; positive family history in 75% to 85% of cases. Caused by autosomal dominant congenital deficiency of inhibitor of first component of complement (C1 INH).

○ Serum C4 is the single most reliable screening test; is decreased even when patient is asymptomatic. If borderline, repeat at height of attack since C4 falls during episode.
♦ Low (0%–30% of normal) C1 INH is necessary to confirm diagnosis. Do not use for screening.
    RIA will not detect the 15% of cases of variant form in which C1 INH antigen is present but nonfunctioning; for these cases more difficult functional assay for C1 INH is needed. (Test is performed only at reference laboratories.)
CBC and ESR are usually normal when the manifestation is peripheral or facial angioedema, but they may be abnormal when the manifestation is diarrhea and abdominal pain.

Factitious Disorders[8]

♦ Should always be suspected when there is significant discrepancy between various laboratory data, impossible laboratory results, or laboratory values discordant with clinical picture.

[7]Kaplan B, et al. Biochemical subtyping of amyloid in formalin-fixed tissue samples confirms and supplements immunohistologic data. *Am J Clin Pathol* 2004;121:794
[8]Wallach J. Laboratory diagnosis of factitious disorders. *Arch Int Med* 1994;154:1690.

Gastrointestinal[6,9]

Cause	Method of Detection
Self-induced vomiting	Hypochloremic metabolic alkalosis with increased serum bicarbonate, hyponatremia, and hypokalemia. Urine-increased potassium (>10 mEq/L) and decreased chloride.
Vomiting due to ipecac	Ipecac identified in stool as emetine by thin-layer chromatography. In stool and urine by HPLC. (Not by routine toxicology.)
Diuretic abuse	Urine assay can detect thiazides, furosemide, ethacrynic acid, carbonic anhydrase inhibitors. Increased urine potassium (>10 mEq/L). *Any urine with potassium >30 mEq/L should be tested for diuretic agents.*
Diarrhea due to laxative abuse*	Hyperchloremic metabolic acidosis with decreased serum bicarbonate and potassium. Potassium is low in urine (<10 mEq/L) and increased in fecal fluid. Detect laxative in urine (e.g., castor oil, phenolphthalein, bisacodyl, senna) and stool (e.g., phenolphthalein, mineral oil, anthraquinones, magnesium, sulfate, phosphate, bisacodyl [Dulcolax]). Alkalinization of stool causes color change caused by phenolphthalein, some anthraquinones, bisacodyl. Detect high concentration of sodium sulfate in stool when due to Glauber's salt (sodium sulfate) or high concentration of phosphate when caused by Na_2PO_4. Sodium bicarbonate abuse causes hypokalemic metabolic alkalosis.
"Diarrhea" caused by dilution of stool with water (or another dilute fluid)*	Stool osmolality is very low (<250 mOsm/kg); is lower than plasma osmolality. Is normal when defecation is supervised or colon contents are sampled endoscopically. Stool sodium, potassium, chloride, and magnesium concentrations are very low.
Vomiting and diarrhea due to salt poisoning	Very high sodium (>150 mEq/L) in serum and urine
Bleeding due to surreptitious ingestion of warfarin or brodifacoum (rodenticide) or trauma	Identify anticoagulant in plasma, prolonged PT
Abdominal pain (pancreatitis)	Saliva was added to urine and is of salivary rather than pancreatic origin

*Suspect if high daily stool volume (>500 mL/d), unexplained hypokalemia, or decreased serum bicarbonate with metabolic acidosis, melanosis coli on colonoscopy, cathartic colon on barium enema. See also Osmotic Gap.

Hematological*

Hemorrhagic diathesis	
Ingestion of warfarin	Prolonged PT which is restored to normal by administration of vitamin K. Warfarin can also be assayed in plasma. Prolonged PT due to "super warfarin" (a rodenticide-brodifacoum) may not be controlled by standard doses of vitamin K. Warfarin assay is negative; requires a separate assay
Heparin injection	Prolonged aPTT but PT is normal; repeated aPTT rapidly becomes normal while patient is under observation.

[6]Park MA, et al. Primary [AL] hepatic amyloidosis. *Medicine* 2003;82:291.
[9]Phillips S, Donaldson BS, Geisler K et al. Stool composition in Factitial Diarrhea: A 6-year experience with stool analysis. *Ann Int Med* 1995;123:97.

	Prolonged thrombin time (TT) and normal Reptilase time. TT becomes normal upon addition of protamine sulfate. Prolonged aPTT and TT are corrected after removal of heparin by an anion exchange resin or heparinase. Assay can demonstrate heparin in plasma.
Anemia due to self-blood letting	Diagnosed by ^{59}Fe-elimination rates and other erythrokinetic studies.
Thrombocytopenia due to ingestion of drugs causing antiplatelet antibodies	Demonstrate antiplatelet antibodies
Pancytopenia due to ingestion of alkylating agents	

*Blood doping may also be done to improve athletic performance. See Factitious Polycythemia, Chapter 11.

Endocrine

Hyperthyroidism (see Chapter 13)
Hypoglycemia (see Chapter 13)
Cushing syndrome (see Chapter 13)

Genitourinary

Proteinuria	Waxing and waning proteinuria. Unusual urine electrophoresis patterns Nonhuman protein is demonstrated by isoelectric focusing or immunofixation or immunodiffusion. Serum albumin remains normal.
Hematuria	RBC morphology is not of renal origin; no RBC or Hb casts.
Calculi	Analysis shows stones to be mineral (e.g., quartz, feldspar) or pepper grains.
Increased creatinine and potassium	Dilution of blood sample tube with urine.

Infections

Bacteremia	May be polymicrobial. No evident source in obstruction of GI, GU, or biliary tracts.

Respiratory

Inhalation of talc simulating asthma	Analysis of crystals in lung biopsy by electron microscopy and spectroscopy is identical to baby powder.

Diffuse Fasciitis with Eosinophilia[10]

Typically deep fibrosis of skin of extremities. May be a scleroderma variant. See Lyme disease, Chapter 15.

♦ Diagnosis is confirmed by characteristic findings in a deep biopsy of skin down to and including muscle.
○ Eosinophilia and increased total eosinophil count.
Diffuse hypergammaglobulinemia and increased ESR may be present.
Increased serum aldolase with normal CK may indicate disease activity.
ANA may occur but in low titer, not specific for scleroderma.

[10]Bolster MB, Silver RM. Other fibrosing skin disorders. In: Clements PJ, Furst DE. Systemic Sclerosis. 2nd Ed. Philadelphia: Lippincott William & Wilkins. 2004.

MISC

Multiple Organ Dysfunction Syndrome

Sequela of certain severe conditions especially in surgical ICU (e.g., ruptured aneurysm, acute pancreatitis, surgical complications, burns, trauma), septic shock; four clinical stages with 40% mortality in early stage ranging to 90% in late stage.

* Episode of physiologic shock
* Active resuscitation lasting up to 24 hours
* Stable hypermetabolism (hyperglycemia, hyperlacticemia, polyuria, urine urea nitrogen >15 g/d) lasting 7 to 10 days with appearance of acute lung injury and repeated septic episodes
* Onset of liver and kidney failure (serum bilirubin >3 mg/dL after 7–10 days with progressive rise followed by increase in serum creatinine); encephalopathy, consumption coagulopathy, GI bleeding, and recurrent infection.

Progressive increase in blood glucose, lactate, urine nitrogen excretion and fall in serum albumin, transferrin, and other liver proteins.

Increasing consumption coagulopathy and thrombocytopenia.

Failure of immune system marked by bacteremia (especially Gram-negative organisms) and positive cultures from urine, wounds, tracheal aspirate, invasive lines. *Candida* sp., viruses (especially HSV), and CMV can be cultured.

In one clinical variant, there is no clinically evident lung injury. In another clinical type (usually associated with a primary lung injury such as aspiration), liver and kidney failure does not manifest until a few days before death.

Poor prognostic findings are

* Initial mean pO_2:FiO_2 ratio <250 (normal = 400)
* Serum lactate on day 2 ≥3.4 mg/dL (normal <1.5 mg/dL)
* Liver failure by day 6 with mean serum bilirubin = 8.5 mg/dL and rising
* Kidney failure by day 12 with mean serum creatinine = 3.9 mg/dL and rising

Organ Transplantation

See Bone Marrow; Liver Transplantation; Heart Transplantation; Kidney Transplantation.

Preoperative Assessment (Recipient and Donor)

* Immunology and tissue typing
  ABO and Rh cross match
  HLA typing
  Panel reactive antibodies
* Microbiology/virology
  Hepatitis B and C
  CMV
  HIV
  HTLV I and II
  Herpes zoster and varicella
  Epstein-Barr virus
  Syphilis
  Toxoplasmosis
  Blood and urine cultures (donor)

Organ Function Panels

Liver
Kidney
Bone
Nutrition
Glucose
Electrolyte/acid-base
Hematology (coagulation, CBC)

Postoperative Monitoring of Recipient

* Monitoring of graft function
* Rejection

- Nephrotoxicity
- Wound infection
- Opportunistic infection (e.g., CMV, Pneumocystis)
- Neoplasms (e.g., posttransplantation lymphoproliferative disorders)
- Bone demineralization
- Hypertension
- Recurrence of primary disease

♦ Most difficult distinction is between infection and rejection for which organ biopsy is most diagnostic.

Sarcoidosis[11]

Multisystem granulomatous disease of unknown cause characterized by non-caseating granulomas.

♦ Diagnosis is established by tissue biopsy that shows noncaseous granulomas at several sites for which a specific cause (e.g., fungal, acid-fast bacillus infection, or berylliosis) has been excluded with a compatible clinical picture. Kveim test may be used in place of another tissue biopsy.

- Needle biopsy of liver shows granulomas in ≤75% of patients even if there is no impairment of liver function.
- Lymph node biopsy is likely to be positive if lymph node is enlarged.
- Muscle biopsy is likely to be positive if arthralgia or muscle pain is present.
- Skin and transbronchial lung biopsies have higher yield, greater specificity, and less morbidity than liver and mediastinal lymph node biopsies.
- Other sites of biopsy are synovium, eye, lung, minor salivary glands of lower lip.
- Bone marrow is involved in <40%
- Percentage of cases with organ system involvement
  Pulmonary >90%
  Peripheral lymph nodes 50% to 75%
  Liver 60% to 80%
  Skin 35%
  Heart 30%
  Bone 1% to 35%
  Eye ~25%
  Spleen 15%
  Salivary glands 5%
  CNS 5%
  Joints

Kveim reaction (skin biopsy 4–6 weeks after injection of human sarcoid tissue shows a noncaseating granulomatous reaction at that site) has reported S/S = 35% to 88%/75% to 99%.

- A positive reaction is less frequent if there is no lymph node involvement, if the disease is long standing and inactive, and during steroid therapy.
- Positive Kveim tests may occur in other diseases with enlarged lymph nodes (e.g., TB, leukemia). Kveim test material is not available commercially; a few medical centers have limited quantities with variable specificities; not approved by the FDA.

♦ Serum Angiotensin-Converting Enzyme (ACE)

Produced primarily by endothelial and epithelial cells; may also be synthesized by activated macrophages in granulomas. Values vary between laboratories even with same method. See Chapter 13.

Use
Monitor activity of disease and response to therapy.
Little diagnostic value because of poor specificity. Increased in 50% to 80% of cases.

[11]Newman LS, Rose CS, Maier LA. Sarcoidosis. *New Eng J Med* 1997;336:1224.

MISC

May be Increased In (False-positive rate = 2%–4%.)

- Active pulmonary sarcoidosis (50%–75% of patients but only 11% with inactive disease (increase is >35 units/mL by radioassay in adults and >50 units/mL if <19 years old)
- Gaucher disease (100%)
- Diabetes mellitus (>24%)
- Hyperthyroidism (81%)
- Leprosy (53%)
- Chronic renal disease
- Cirrhosis (25%)
- Silicosis (>20%)
- Berylliosis (75%)
- Amyloidosis
- TB, MAI infection

Normal In

- Lymphoma
- Lung cancer

○ Serum globulins are increased in 75% of patients, producing reduced A/G ratio and increased total protein (in 30% of patients). Is often the first clue to diagnosis.
○ Serum protein electrophoresis shows decreased albumin and increased globulin (especially γ) with characteristic "sarcoid-step" pattern.
WBC is decreased in 30% of patients. Eosinophilia (>5%) occurs in 25% of patients.
Mild normocytic, normochromic anemia occurs.
ESR is increased.
○ Serum calcium may be mildly to markedly increased in ~10% of patients; often transiently.
Increased urine calcium occurs twice as often as hypercalcemia. Increased frequency of renal calculi and of nephrocalcinosis in some patients.
Serum and urine calcium abnormalities are frequently corrected by cortisone; often within normal range in one week.
Increased sensitivity to vitamin D is often present.
Increased serum 1,25-hydroxyvitamin D which is abnormally regulated.
Serum phosphorus is normal.
Increased serum uric acid may occur even with normal renal function in ≤50% of patients.
Mumps complement-fixation test, which is positive in presence of negative mumps skin test (due to dissociation between normal circulating antibodies and defective cellular antibody response), supports the diagnosis but is not specific.
Serum lysozyme (muramidase) is increased in ~70% of cases but does not distinguish stable from progressive disease. Also increased with other chest diseases (e.g., TB, lung cancer).
Laboratory findings reflect specific organ involvement.

- Lung
    - ♦ Diagnostic method of choice is transbronchial biopsy.
    Bronchoalveolar lavage (BAL) shows 3 to 5× increase in cells; T-lymphocytes are increased to 36%; B-lymphocytes = 4%; macrophages decreased to 55%; neutrophils and eosinophils are <5%. BAL or induced sputum shows CD4/CD8 ratio >2.5.
    ^{67}Ga scan lacks specificity. Gas exchange is usually normal early in disease; later pO_2 is decreased with marked fall after exercise. BAL and ^{67}Ga scan have been used to assess disease activity.
- Kidney—renal function is decreased (because of hypercalcemia or increased uric acid with resultant nephrocalcinosis or renal calculi).
- Liver—cholestatic pattern in less than one third of patients with increased serum ALP and relatively normal transaminases.
- Spleen—hypersplenism may occur (anemia, leukopenia, thrombocytopenia).
- Bone marrow involved in <40%
- CNS—CSF may be normal or may show no characteristic changes (e.g., moderate to marked increase in protein, and pleocytosis [chiefly lymphocytes]). Sugar is

sometimes decreased. In neurosarcoidosis, ACE is increased in serum or CSF in 50% to 70%, ESR in 40%, and serum calcium 17% of cases. Oligoclonal bands may be present.
• Pituitary—diabetes insipidus, hypopituitarism or hyperprolactinemia may occur.

Scleredema[12]

May be associated with insulin resistant diabetes mellitus or with gammopathy or multiple myeloma.

WBC, ESR, and other laboratory tests are usually normal.

Nonsuppurative Panniculitis (Relapsing Febrile Nodular; Weber Christian Disease)

Group of disorders characterized by subcutaneous nodules and inflammatory cells in fat lobules without vasculitis.

♦ Biopsy of involved area of subcutaneous fat.
WBC may be increased or decreased.
Mild anemia may occur.

Biochemical Changes in Cancer

Use
Prevention of misinterpretation of various findings in patients with cancer.
Awareness of certain complications of cancers (e.g., anemia, hypercalcemia)
Decreased
Serum glucose
Serum protein and albumin (due to malnutrition, blood loss, etc.)
Anemia (due to hemorrhage, malnutrition, hemolysis, anemia of chronic disease, myelophthisis, etc.)
Increased
Serum uric acid
Serum calcium—occurs in ~20% of cancer patients, usually due to bone metastases, which sometimes cannot be detected. >14 mg/dL suggests cancer rather than hyperparathyroidism. (See Hypercalcemia of Malignancy)
Serum globulin (e.g., multiple myeloma), especially α_2-globulin
Serum lactic acid
Development of hemolytic anemia, autoantibodies (e.g., minimal change glomerular disease in Hodgkin disease, membranous GN in solid tumors)
Occult blood in stool
ESR is often normal in patients with cancer and therefore is not a good test for screening and a normal value does not exclude metastases. In patients with known cancer, ESR >100 mm/hr is usually associated with metastases.
WBC may be increased due to tumor necrosis, secondary infection, etc.
Hypercoagulable state with recurrent thromboembolism
Laboratory findings due to metastatic tumor (e.g., liver, brain, bone)
Laboratory findings due to obstruction (e.g., ureters, bile ducts, intestine)
Laboratory findings due to metastases that interfere with endocrine secretion (e.g., adrenal, pituitary)
Laboratory findings due to fluid in body cavities (pleural, abdominal, CSF)
Laboratory findings due to myelophthisis (anemia, leukopenia, thrombocytopenia)
Laboratory findings due to complications of anticancer therapy

• Blood dyscrasias including secondary leukemia
• Bladder cancer after prolonged Cytoxan therapy
• Cardiotoxicity (e.g., doxorubicin hydrochloride [Adriamycin])

MISC

[12]Clements PJ, Furst DE. Systemic Sclerosis. Second Ed. Lippincott Williams & Wilkins. Phila. 2004.

- Pulmonary fibrosis (e.g., methotrexate, bleomycin)
- Sterility
- Teratogenic effects
- Diseases that occur with particular frequency in association with neoplasms (e.g., polymyositis, dermatomyositis)

Tumor Markers[13]

Use

Not generally useful to establish a definite diagnosis or for screening

May be useful to monitor effect of therapy or recurrence of lesion, to follow the clinical course, to pinpoint the tissue of origin.

May sometimes be useful to assess the extent of tumor and to estimate prognosis.

Contents may help to distinguish cystic lesions of pancreas.

Should never rely solely on result of a single test.

Should obtain baseline level before surgery, radiation, or chemotherapy.

Beware of interferences (e.g., renal failure affecting clearance of marker).

If available, more than one marker increases S/S.

With serial testing, tests should be performed by same laboratory using same assay kit.

Interpretation

Enzymes Increased

- Serum ALP and GGT in liver metastases; increase is predictive of positive liver scan but not of positive bone scan for metastases from breast cancer. Also in bone metastases, osteogenic sarcoma, myeloid leukemia. Placental isoenzyme of ALP increased in 30% of ovarian cancer (especially serous cystadenocarcinoma), some cancers of endometrium, lung, breast and 40% of seminomas (75% in metastatic seminoma); may also be increased in smokers. Intestinal isoenzyme is associated with hepatomas and malignant tumors of GI tract.
- 5'-Nucleotidase (5'N) in metastatic carcinoma of liver but not bone
- Serum GGT in metastatic carcinoma of liver
- Serum LD in metastatic carcinoma of liver, acute leukemia, lymphomas; less useful than GGT and 5'N in evaluating space-occupying lesions of liver
- Serum LD total and LD-1 in testicular cancer; see LD isoenzymes
- Serum CK total and CK-BB in various cancers (e.g., prostate, breast, ovary, colon, small cell carcinoma of lung) in ~30% of early cases and ~45% with extensive cancer; rarely macromolecular forms of CK occur.
- Serum acid phosphatase in 80% of men with metastatic prostate cancer and 25% of those without metastases
- Neuron-specific enolase (NSE) in APUD tumors including small cell carcinoma of lung, neuroblastoma, medullary carcinoma of thyroid, islet cell carcinoma of pancreas. Thirty-two percent accompanied by increased CK-BB.
- Serum amylase in 8% to 40% of cases of carcinoma of pancreas
- Terminal deoxynucleotidyl transferase (Tdt)—large amounts in blast cells of acute lymphoblastic leukemia but little or none in nonlymphoid leukemia or nonleukemic cells; useful to differentiate acute lymphoid and acute myeloid leukemia
- β-glucuronidase has been reported to be increased in 75% of patients with metastatic leptomeningeal adenocarcinoma and 60% of patients with acute myeloblastic leukemia involving CNS (see p. 273).

Oncofetal Antigens

- Serum α-fetoprotein (AFP) in hepatocellular carcinoma, teratoblastoma, yolk sac tumor; also increased in normal pregnancy
- Serum carcinoembryonic antigen (CEA) in carcinoma of GI tract, breast, >40% of small cell carcinomas of lung
- hCG in choriocarcinoma

Specific Products of Hormone-Producing Tumor of Primary Organ or Ectopic

- Renin-producing tumor of kidney

[13]Schwartz MK. Tumor Markers. in Diagnostic Endocrinology and Metabolism. *Am Assoc Clin Chem* 1997;15:365.

- VMA, catecholamines in pheochromoblastoma, neuroblastoma by neural crest tumors, pheochromocytoma (see Chapter 13)
- Urinary 17-KS in adrenal cortical carcinoma, androgenic arrhenoblastoma
- HIAA in carcinoid
- Erythropoietin in paraneoplastic erythrocytosis
- Thyroglobulin in patients with total thyroidectomy; detectable level indicates recurrent thyroid cancer (see Chapter 13)
- Prolactin (see Chapter 13)
- ACTH in Cushing syndrome (e.g., due to adrenal tumor, due to oat cell carcinoma)
- β-hCG subunit (in blood or urine)
- C-peptide in insulinoma
- Estrogen and progesterone receptors (see Steroid Receptor Assays)
- Parathormone-related protein produced by lung, ovarian, thymoma, carcinoid, islet cell tumor of pancreas, medullary carcinoma of thyroid
- Anti-diuretic hormone produced by small cell cancer of lung, carcinoid, Hodgkin disease, bladder
- Calcitonin produced by medullary carcinoma of thyroid (see Chapter 13), breast, liver, kidney, lung carcinoid
- Gastrin in gastrinoma, gastric carcinoma; part of MEN-1 syndrome, carcinoma of pancreas, parathyroid, pituitary
- Isoenzymes of alkaline phosphatase (Regan, Nagao)

Mucins

- CA-125.
- CA 19-9.
- CA 15-3.

Other proteins

- Prostate specific antigen (see Chapter 14)
- Immunoglobulins in multiple myeloma, lymphomas, Waldenstrom macroglobulinemia.
- β_2 microglobulin is increased in multiple myeloma, Waldenstrom macroglobulinemia, B-cell lymphoma, CLL.
- Interleukin 2 Receptor may be increased in serum in adult T cell leukemia.
- Squamous cell carcinoma antigen (SCC)
- Plasma chromogranin A in pheochromocytoma (See Chapter 15.)
- Tumor-associated antigen (TA-90) in urine and sera of patients with metastatic melanoma (occult or clinical) with S/S, predictive values ~75%.[14]
- Bladder tumor associated antigen (BTA)and nuclear mitotic apparatus proteins (NMP22) (see Chapter 14.)
- Osteopontin S/S = ~80% for distinguishing early stage ovarian cancer from normal at cutoff of 252 ng/mL; also expressed in other tissues.

Philadelphia chromosome (Ph[1]) in chronic myeloid leukemia
Her-2/*neu* and estrogen receptors in breast cancer (requires tissue).
Paraneoplastic syndromes

- One third of these patients show ectopic hormone production (e.g., bronchogenic carcinoma).
- One third show evidence of connective tissue (e.g., polymyositis, dermatomyositis) and dermatologic disorders (e.g., acanthosis nigricans).
- One sixth show psychiatric and neurologic syndromes.
- Remainder show immunologic, gastrointestinal (e.g., malabsorption), renal (e.g., nephrotic syndrome), hematologic (e.g., anemia of chronic disease, DIC), paraproteinemias (e.g., multiple myeloma), or amyloidosis.

Circulating DNA of tumor cells in peripheral blood may have a poorer prognosis in some tumors.[15]

MISC

[14]Kelley MC, et al. Tumor-associated antigen TA-90 immune complex assay predicts subclinical metastasis and survival for patients with early stage melanoma. *Cancer* 1998;83:1355.
[15]Cristofanilli M, Budd GT, Ellis MJ, et al. Circulating tumor cells, disease progression, and survival in metastatic breast cancer. *N Engl J Med* 2004;351(8):781–791.

It has been suggested that combined panel of markers can distinguish high from low tumor burden.[16]

A-Fetoprotein (AFP), Serum

α-globulin found in fetal blood; originates in fetal liver, GI tract, yolk sac.

Use

Tumor marker for hepatocellular carcinoma (hepatoma)

* Screening in high prevalence areas (e.g., China, Eskimos).
* Patients with chronic active hepatitis or cirrhosis positive serology for HCV or HBV should be screened with serum AFP and ultrasound.
* Changes reflect the patient's course.

Tumor marker for germ cell tumors of ovary and testis (see Chapter 13)

* Embryonal carcinoma (increased in 27% of cases)
* Malignant teratoma (increased in 60% of cases)
* *Should be used in conjunction with hCG and LD and LD-1; more often increased with advanced disease. These are useful to monitor chemotherapy; may predict relapse before clinical or x-ray evidence.*

To distinguish neonatal hepatitis (most patients have concentrations >40 ng/mL) from neonatal biliary atresia (most patients have concentrations <40 ng/mL).
Screening for fetal defects and placental disease during pregnancy (see Chapter 12)

Interpretation

ng/mL is essentially diagnostic of AFP-producing tumor)

Primary cancer of liver (hepatocellular carcinoma; hepatoma) (see Chapter 8)

* Serum AFP may be increased for up to 18 months before symptoms; is sensitive indicator of recurrence in treated patients but a normal postoperative level does not ensure absence of metastases. Levels >500 ng/dL in adults strongly suggest hepatoma. Levels >100× URL have S/S =60%/100%. In ≤30% of hepatoma cases AFP is <4× URL and such increases are common in chronic HBC and HCV alone.
* May be markedly increased (>1,000 ng/mL in ~50/% of cases which usually indicates tumor >3 cm in size). Increased in almost 100% of cases in children and young adults.
* Ninety percent of cases of hepatoma have AFP >200 and 70% have concentrations >400 ng/mL, but in benign liver diseases, AFP >400 ng/mL is extremely rare. More likely to be increased in immature type of hepatocellular carcinoma compared to mature type.
* High initial concentrations indicate a poor prognosis.
* Failure to return to normal after surgery indicates incomplete resection or presence of metastases.
* Changes in concentrations can indicate effects of chemotherapy.
* Postoperative decreased concentration followed by an increase suggests recurrence. Short doubling time suggests occult metastases at time of surgery.

Increases associated with nonmalignant conditions are usually temporary and concentrations subsequently fall but in malignant disease, concentrations continue to rise.

Increased In[17]

Other Cancers

* Testicular teratocarcinomas (75%) (see Chapter 13)
* Pancreatic (23%)
* Gastric (18%)
* Bronchogenic (7%)
* Colon (5%)

Benign Liver Diseases

* Viral hepatitis (27%)

[16]Motiwala N, et al. High vs Low Tumor Burden in Selected Hematologic Malignancies Can Be Distinguished by Vascular Growth Factor (VRGF), IL-6, Tumor Necrosis Factor α (TNF-α), and C-Reactive Protein (CRP). *Am J Clin Pathol* 2004;122:648.
[17]Aziz DC. Clinical use of tumor markers based on outcome analysis. *Lab Med* 1996;27:817.

- Postnecrotic cirrhosis (24%)
- Laennec cirrhosis (15%)
- Primary biliary cirrhosis (5%)

Some patients with liver metastases from carcinoma of stomach or pancreas
Ataxia-telangiectasia
Hereditary tyrosinemia
Hereditary persistence of AFP

Absent In

Normal persons after first weeks of life
Various types of cirrhosis and hepatitis in adults
Seminoma of testis
Choriocarcinoma, adenocarcinoma, and dermoid cyst of ovary

CA 15-3[18]

Glycoprotein expressed on various adenocarcinomas, especially breast.

Use

FDA approval only to detect breast carcinoma recurrence before symptoms and to
monitor response to treatment. Significant change is ±25%.
Not approved for screening although increased values may occur ≤9 months before
clinical evidence of disease.

Interpretation

Reported PPV = 77% and NPV = 90% at 49 U/mL.
Increases are directly related to stage of disease; increased in ~20% of stage I or II disease and 70% to 80% of patients with metastatic or recurrent breast cancer. >30 U/L
indicates shorter survival.
Increases in 75% of patients with progressive disease and decreases in 38% of those
responding to therapy.

Increased In

Benign breast and liver diseases causing low specificity.

CA-199, Serum

Detects high molecular weight mucin.

Use

Detection, diagnosis, and prognosis of pancreatic cancer.
To determine preoperative resectability. Very high concentrations predict unresectable
cancer—only 5% of patients with concentrations >1,000 U/mL are surgically
resectable; 50% of patients with concentrations <1,000 U/mL are surgically
resectable.
Monitor response to therapy (e.g., postsurgical recurrence correlates with increased
concentrations).
May be a useful adjunct to CEA for diagnosis and to detect early recurrence of certain
cancers.
May indicate development of cholangiocarcinoma in patients with primary sclerosing
cholangitis.

Increased (>37 U/mL) In

Carcinoma of pancreas (S/S = 70%/87%) (see Chapter 8).
Pancreatitis—concentrations are usually <75 U/mL but are much higher in pancreatic
cancer.
Hepatobiliary cancer (22%–51%)
Gastric cancer (42%)
Colon cancer (20%) is associated with very poor prognosis. Not recommended for
screening, diagnosis, or monitoring.
False-negative in 7% of US population negative for Lewis[ab] blood group since CA 199 is
a Le[ab] antigen.

---

[18]Duffy MJ, et al. High Preoperative CA 15-3 Concentrations Predict Adverse Outcome in Node-
Negative and Node-Positive Breast Cancer: Study of 600 Patients with Histologically Confirmed
Breast Cancer. *Clin Chem* 2004;50:559.

MISC

CA 27-29, Serum
Tumor marker similar to CA 15-3 antigen.

Use
Recently approved by FDA in conjunction with other procedures to monitor recurrence of Stage II or III breast cancer.
Reported sensitivity = 58%; false-positive = 6%

CA-125, Serum
See Ovarian Cancer, Chapter 13.

Carcinoembryonic Antigen (CEA), Serum
High molecular weight glycoprotein.

Use
Monitoring for persistent, metastatic, or recurrent adenocarcinoma of colon after surgery; increased in >30% of patients with breast, lung, liver, pancreas adenocarcinomas.
Determination of prognosis in patients with colon cancer.
Not usually useful for diagnosis of local recurrence.
Not recommended for screening because of low S/S, especially in early stages of malignant disease because CEA reflects tumor bulk.
♦ Diagnosis of malignant pleural effusion (see Chapter 6).

Interpretation
♦ *Monitoring of Disease Course*[19]
Same methodology should be used to monitor an individual patient. A significant change in plasma concentration is +25%.
After complete removal of colon cancer, CEA should fall to normal in 6 to 12 weeks. Failure to decline to normal concentrations postoperatively suggests incomplete resection. Immunohistochemistry of resected specimen is used to identify 20% of these cancers that do not express CEA for whom monitoring is misleading. In such cases, may use serum ALP and diagnostic imaging.
Recurrence of colon cancer is indicated by progressive increase earlier than other methods but for most patients, this is not useful therapeutically although increasing concentrations may precede clinical evidence of recurrence by 2 to 6 months. Monitor for recurrence every 2 to 3 months in patients with stage II or stage III disease for 2 or more years. In ~50% of patients with advanced cancer, there may be a latent phase of 4 to 6 weeks from onset of therapy to change in CEA concentrations. Sensitivity = 97% for detecting recurrence of colon cancer in patients with preoperative elevation but only 66% in those with normal preoperative CEA. Specificity is >90% and positive predictive value is >70%. Increased concentrations indicates a poorer prognosis within a given stage; >3.0 ng/mL in ≤28% of Dukes stage A, 45% of stage B, and 70% of stage C cancers.
About 30% of patients with metastatic colon cancer do not have increased CEA.
Undifferentiated or poorly differentiated tumors do not produce CEA.
♦ *Prognosis*
Is related to serum concentration at time of diagnosis (stage of disease and likelihood of recurrence). CEA concentrations <5 ng/mL before therapy suggests localized disease and a favorable prognosis, but a concentration >10 ng/mL suggests extensive disease and a poor prognosis; >80% of colon carcinoma patients with values >20 ng/mL have recurrence within 14 months after surgery. Plasma CEA >20 ng/mL correlates with tumor volume in breast and colon cancer and are usually associated with metastatic disease or with a few types of cancer (e.g., cancer of the colon or pancreas); however, metastases may occur with concentrations <20 ng/mL. Values <2.5 ng/mL do not rule out primary, metastatic, or recurrent cancer. Increased values in node-negative colon cancer may identify poorer-risk patients who may benefit from chemotherapy.
Patterns of CEA change during chemotherapy

• Uninterrupted increase indicating failure to respond.

[19]Pfister DG, et al. Surveillance strategies after curative treatment of colorectal cancer. *N Engl J Med* 2004;350:2375.

- Decrease indicating response to therapy.
- Surge in CEA for weeks followed by a decrease indicating response.
- Immediate, sustained decrease followed by an increase indicating lack of response to therapy.
- Significant is 25% to 35% change from baseline of $\geq$ values during first 2 months of therapy. Survival is significantly longer if titer decreases below this baseline.

Increased in

Cancer. There is a wide overlap in values between benign and malignant disease. Increased concentrations are suggestive but not diagnostic of cancer.

- Seventy-five percent of patients with carcinoma of entodermal origin (colon, stomach, pancreas, lung) have CEA titers >2.5 ng/mL, and two thirds of these titers are >5 ng/mL. Increased in about one third of patients with small cell carcinoma of lung and about two thirds with non-small-cell carcinoma of lung.
- Fifty percent of patients with carcinoma of nonentodermal origin (especially cancer of the breast, head and neck, ovary) have CEA titers >2.5 ng/mL, and 50% of the titers are >5 ng/mL. Increased in >50% of breast cancer with metastases, 25% of cases without metastases, but not associated with benign lesions.
- Forty percent of patients with noncarcinomatous malignant disease have increased CEA concentrations, usually 2.5 to 5.0 ng/mL.
- Increased in 90% of all patients with solid-tissue tumors, especially with metastases to liver or lung but only 50% of patients with local disease or only intra-abdominal metastases.
- May be increased in effusion fluid due to these cancers (see Chapter 6). Active nonmalignant inflammatory diseases (especially of the GI tract [e.g., ulcerative colitis, regional enteritis, diverticulitis, peptic ulcer, chronic pancreatitis]) frequently have elevated concentrations that decline when the disease is in remission.

Liver disease (alcoholic, cirrhosis, chronic active hepatitis, obstructive jaundice) because metabolized by liver.

Others disorders

- Renal failure
- Fibrocystic disease of breast

Smoking

- Ninety-seven percent of healthy nonsmokers have plasma CEA concentrations <2.5 ng/mL.
- Nineteen percent of heavy smokers and 7% of former smokers have CEA concentrations >2.5 ng/mL.

Interferences
Heparinized patients or plasma collected in heparinized tubes may interfere with accuracy of CEA assay.
Human antimouse antibodies may cause increased values.

Human Chorionic Gonadotropin (β-hCG), Serum
Glycoprotein produced by syncytiotrophoblast cell after trophoblast differentiation.

Use
Diagnosis and monitor course and evaluate prognosis of gestational trophoblastic tumors (with AFP).
Routine pregnancy test (see Pregnancy Test); may also be used to gauge success of artificial insemination or in vitro fertilization.
Differentiation of ectopic pregnancy from other causes of acute abdominal pain. In ectopic pregnancy and in abortion, serial hCG levels will usually decrease over 48 hours (see Chapter 14).
Prenatal screening for Down syndrome (see Chapter 12).

Increased In
Gestational trophoblastic tumors, benign or malignant, (see Germ Cell Tumors of Ovary and Testicle). Is valuable marker for management as changes in concentration reflect success/failure of therapy.

- Hydatidiform mole (sometimes markedly increased; after 12 weeks of pregnancy, >500,000 IU/24 hours usually are associated with moles; >1,000,000 are almost always associated with moles).
- Choriocarcinoma (see p. 681) in virtually 100% of cases, sometimes markedly. Elevated levels are most useful for monitoring remission after treatment; failure to fall to an undetectable level or a rise after an initial fall signals residual tumor or progression of disease and need for another form of therapy. Measure weekly during therapy; every 2 weeks for 6 months after therapy; then less frequently. After uterine evacuation, average disappearance times were 99 days for hydatidiform mole, 59 days for partial mole, 51 days for hydropic degeneration; therefore, if levels show a steady fall, they may become negative by 100 days regardless of chemotherapy.
- Much poorer prognosis is indicated by failure to decline by 50% in 7 days for AFP and 3 days for β-hCG.

Nonseminomatous germ cell tumors of testicle (found in 10% of patients with pure seminoma); should be used with α-fetoprotein.

Some nontrophoblastic neoplasms (e.g., cancers of ovary, cervix, GI tract, lung, breast)
Normal pregnancy (secreted first by trophoblastic cells of conceptus and later normal pregnancy (see Chapter 3).

Interferences
False-positive results have been found in

- Postorchiectomy patients (secondary to decreased testosterone)
- Marijuana smokers

Not increased in
Endodermal sinus tumors
Nonpregnant state
Fetal death

Micrometastases, Detection
Immunocytochemistry with manual microscopy can detect as few as one tumor cell in a million normal cells.
Flow cytometry has potential sensitivity of one cell in 10^6 or 10^7.
RT-PCR has theoretical detection sensitivity of one cell in 10^7 or 10^8.
Automated cell imaging with immunocytochemistry staining may identify one cell in 10^8 normal bone marrow cells.

Neuron-Specific Enolase (NSE), Serum
Enolase isoenzyme in glycolytic pathway identified by immunoassay found mostly in neurons and neuroendocrine cells.

Use
Principal use to monitor treatment and predict relapse in small cell lung cancer.
Increased In
Neuroendocrine tumors

- Especially small cell carcinoma of lung; found in 68% of patients with limited disease and 87% with extensive disease. Other lung cancers in 17% of cases.
- Monitor patients with neuroblastoma, carcinoid, pancreatic islet cell tumor, pheochromocytoma, medullary carcinoma of thyroid.

Wilms tumor, malignant lymphoma, seminoma; 20% of cancers of breast, GI tract, prostate
Occasional patients with benign liver diseases.

Prostate-Specific Antigen (PSA) and Prostatic Acid Phosphatase (PAP), Serum
See Cancer of Prostate, Chapter 14

SCC, Serum
Antigen purified from squamous cell carcinoma of uterine cervix.

Table 16-4. Comparison of Assays for Tumor Chemosensitivity Testing

Assay	Specimen	Specimens that Can Be Evaluated (%)	Accuracy in Determining Resistance (%)	Sensitivity (%)	Reporting Time (days)
Clonogenic	Single cell	40–60	90	70	10–21
Subrenal	Tumor fragments	80–90	80	80–90	7–10
Capsule	In vivo				
Rotman fluorescent cytoprint	Tumor fragments	95–98	90	90–95	7–10

Source: Woltering EA. Tumor chemosensitivity testing: an evolving technique. *Lah Med* 1990;21(2):82.

Use
Has been reported useful to monitor and detect recurrence of squamous cell carcinoma of uterine cervix, head and neck, esophagus, lung, skin, anus. In uterine cancer, is reported increased in 29% of stage I and 89% of stage IV.
Increased in ≤50% of patients with renal failure.
Further studies are needed to define exact role.

Tumor Chemosensitivity Testing
Assays to predict sensitivity/resistance of a tumor to specific chemotherapeutic agents.

See Table 16-4.
Requires sterile preparation transported on ice in cold tissue transport medium. Avoid freezing. Setup in tissue culture media within 24 hours.
Clonogenic assay

• Minced solid tumor or fluids containing tumor (e.g., malignant effusions, urine, CSF)
• Incubated for 1 hour with test drug, then incubated on cell culture plates. Colonies are counted after 10 to 14 days and compared with control plates to determine percent decrease in tumor-colony-forming units.

Subrenal capsule assay

• Tumor fragments (not individual cells) injected into immunocompetent mouse.
• Reported as percent change in implantation weight.

Rotman in vitro chemosensitivity (fluorescent cytoprint) assay

• Measures ability of viable human tumor cells in culture to transport and hydrolyze fluorescein diacetate and retain fluorescein. Tumor is incubated with drug in media for 48 hours. Sensitivity = 100% cell death at lowest drug dose currently used.

Neoplastic Diseases

Best Diagnostic Sensitivity of Antigens for Cancers[20]
Breast = CA 15-3 (63%)
Lung = CEA (47%)
Pancreas = CA 195 (100%), CA 19-9 (66%)
Stomach = CA 50 (70%), CA 242 (70%), CA 19-9 (63%)

[20]Hall M, et al. A comparison of 11 tumor antigens for the serodiagnosis of breast, lung, and gastrointestinal cancers. *Am J Clin Pathol* 2004;122:639.

Breast Cancer[21]

♦ Diagnosis is established by microscopic examination of tumor biopsy.
♦ Serum CEA increase becomes more frequent with increasing stage and tumor burden. More frequent with bone and visceral involvement than with soft tissue involvement.

• An increasing concentration usually reflects disease progression and a decreasing concentration usually reflects remission.
• An increased or rising concentration may precede recurrence by 1 to 31 months.
• May be increased in CSF in metastases to CNS, meninges or spine but not in primary brain tumors.
• Not useful for screening or diagnosis of early breast cancer.

○ Serum CA 15-3 (see p 904).

High surviving measured by RT-PCR is said to be independent predictor of poor prognosis.[22]
Other markers (mucinlike carcinoma-associated antigen, MAM-6, mammary serum antigen) await further study of utility.
Mutations for [breast cancer susceptibility genes] *BRCA1* are present in ≤7.5% and for *BRCA2* in ≤2.7% in patients with family history of breast/ovarian cancer syndrome.[23]

♦ *Steroid Receptor Assays*

Ligand-activated transcription factors in family of nuclear hormone receptors.

Use
Prognosis and treatment of breast carcinoma. Determination of both receptors yields best information on response to hormone therapy.
Estrogen receptor (ER) is positive (>10 femtomoles/mg cytoplasmic protein) in ~50% of breast tumor specimens; levels are higher in post- than in premenopausal patients, but this is not so for progesterone receptors (PR).
When ER is negative, there is <10% chance of obtaining a favorable response to any endocrine therapy; thus chemotherapy would be the primary approach. There is a greater likelihood of visceral metastases (>50%) with ER-negative than with ER-positive patients (<6%).
When ER is positive, there is 55% to 60% chance of favorable response (i.e., tumor shrinkage and/or clinical improvement).
When ER and PR are both positive, response rate is 75% to 80%. No response to endocrine therapy in 10% to 15% of patients with ER/PR positive tumors. Predictive value of assay is increased if ER and PR levels are both high

• ER titer >100 femtomoles/mg protein (fmol/mg protein)
• PR (progesterone receptor assay) is also positive, especially >100 fmol/mg protein.

Prognostic value
    Recurrence rate is significantly greater for ER-negative tumors, both Stage I (negative axillary lymph nodes) and Stage II (positive axillary lymph nodes).
    Overall response rate to endocrine therapy is about 50%

	Response Rate to Endocrine Therapy
ERA >100 fmol/mg protein	~75%
ERA <100 fmol/mg protein	~40%
ERA <3 fmol/mg protein	~12%
ERA positive/PRA positive (60% of total group)	~80%
ERA negative/PRA negative (31% of total group)	~5%
ERA positive/PRA negative	~26%
ERA negative/PRA positve (4% of total group; this small group may be due to inaccuracy in assay procedures)	~50%

ERA, Estrogen receptor assay; PRA, progesterone receptor assay.

[21]Duffy MJ. Predictive markers in breast and other cancers: a review. *Clin Chem* 2005;51:494.
[22]Span PN, et al. Survivin is an independent prognostic marker for risk stratification of breast cancer patients. *Clin Chem* 2004;50:1986.
[23]Claus EB, et al. Prevalence of *BRCA1* and *BRCA2* mutations in women diagnosed with ductal carcinoma in situ. *JAMA* 2005;293:964.

Receptor assay should also be performed on recurrent carcinoma even when the original tumor has been previously assayed. Initial ER positives are later found negative in 19% and initial ER negatives are later positive in 13%. Initial PR negatives are later positive in 8% and initial PR positives are later reported negative in 28% to 44% of cases. These discordance rates may be up to 75% in patients receiving antiestrogen tamoxifen within 2 months.

Receptor assay may sometimes be useful in differential diagnosis of metastatic undifferentiated carcinoma in women.

Unfixed tissue specimen should be frozen immediately after removal.

HER-2/neu Oncogene[24] (human epidermal growth factor receptor-2)

Oncogene located on chromosome 17q is amplified >25%. Overexpression produces a glycoprotein product (HER-2) that can be measured by FISH, immunohistochemistry or ELISA (for its receptor protein p185).

Use

* Prognosis: Occurs in 25% to 30% of cases of metastatic breast cancer which show rapid tumor progression, metastasize at a faster rate.
* Response to therapy: May show poor response to tamoxifen therapy alone, increased sensitivity to doxorubicin therapy. Should be positive by both FISH and IHC for full response to anti-HER-2 antibody therapy, (Herceptin; trastuzumab is humanized monoclonal antibody that binds with high affinity to extracellular domain of HER-2/*neu*). Response to Herceptin is indicated by decline in HER-2.
* Earlier detection of disease progression.

DNA ploidy strongly correlates with histopathological grade—poorly differentiated tumors are more likely to be DNA aneuploid. DNA aneuploidy predicts shorter mean survival, independent of stage. Four year relapsefree rate is 72% for patients with DNA diploid tumors compared to 43% for DNA aneuploid tumors. ERA and PRA negative tumors are more likely to be DNA aneuploid.

Mast Cell Disease (Mastocytosis)[25]

Rare condition with functional secretion or abnormal proliferation of tissue mast cells.

Localized: Cutaneous (typically as urticaria pigmentosa[26]) or solitary

Systemic: Mast cell infiltration of bone marrow; may also show diffuse mast cell infiltration of multiple organs, especially skin, liver, spleen, lymph nodes, GI tract—10% to 30% of cases.

♦ Diagnosis by biopsy of tumor sites (e.g., skin [urticaria pigmentosa], lymph nodes, spleen, bone). Marrow biopsy is positive in ~90% of cases but marrow smears are less useful. Immunohistochemical stains with monoclonal antibodies against mast-cell markers (CD117 and tryptase) confirms the diagnosis.

* Serum tryptase is increased in >83% of cases and is highly specific marker for mastocytosis.
* Histamine is increased in blood, urine, and tissues. Increased levels of metabolites of histamine in random and 24-hour urine specimens; is more specific and sensitive than determination of histamine itself. Test is inadequate because histamine release is intermittent. Assay with mass spectroscopy is very accurate but not widely available. Not required for diagnosis. May also be increased in some patients with myeloproliferative disorders, carcinoid syndrome, insulinoma, medullary thyroid carcinoma, pheochromocytoma, VIPoma, glucagonoma. False increase may occur from basophil degranulation during phlebotomy or if urine bacteria change histidine to histamine.

[24]Carney WP, Neumann R, Lipton A, et al. Potential clinical utility of serum HER-2/neu oncoprotein concentrations in patients with breast cancer. *Clin Chem* 2003;49:1579–98.

[25]Sawalha A, et al. Clinical problem solving. Step by step. *N Engl J Med* 2003;349:2253.

[26]Topar G, et al. Urticaria pigmentosa: a clinical, hematopathologic, and serologic study of 30 adults. *Am J Clin Path* 1997;109:279.

MISC

During severe episodes, transient increase of aPTT (restored to normal by addition of protamine) but normal PT due to release of histamine.

Gastric acid is increased; there is a higher incidence of peptic ulcer; but hypochlorhydria and achlorhydria have been reported.

Urinary 5-HIAA is normal.

Laboratory findings due to specific organ involvement may occur

• Bone—abnormal hematologic findings in ≤70% of patients.

May include:

Progressive anemia and thrombocytopenia

WBC may be increased or decreased

Eosinophilia and occasionally basophilia may occur.

Mast cells are uncommon in peripheral blood which may contain ≤10% mast cells. Rarely progresses to mast cell leukemia or develop other leukemias, lymphoma or carcinoma.

• Liver—fibrosis, portal hypertension, hypersplenism
• Spleen—myelofibrosis
• GI tract—malabsorption, diarrhea

Tumor Lysis Syndrome, Acute

Preventable metabolic emergency due to effective induction chemotherapy of rapidly growing neoplasms (e.g., acute leukemia, malignant, lymphoma, Burkitt lymphoma), commonly 1 to 2 days after onset of chemotherapy; persists for several days; unrelated to treatment in some patients.

Associated with higher WBC count in leukemias or very large tumors, inadequate urine output, high pretreatment serum LD levels that rise further. Occurs in one third of nonazotemic and virtually all azotemic patients. Changes are greater in those with pre-existing azotemia or who develop acute renal failure.

• Abrupt onset oliguria (urine output <400 mL/24 hours)
• Hyperuricemia (often increases above elevation prior to therapy)
• Hyperkalemia begins within 12 hours.
• Hypocalcemia as low as 2.8 mg/dL.
• Severe hyperphosphatemia—occurs only after chemotherapy; peaks in 48 to 96 hours (≤65 mg/dL); is criterion for dialysis to avoid acute renal failure that may be caused.

May cause rapid decrease in serum calcium. Pretreatment with allopurinol and diuresis may prevent syndrome unless there is concomitant renal failure.

• Often acidotic and volume-depleted.
• Changes due to precipitation of urates, phosphate and calcifium, which may cause or worsen azotemia and further accentuate the above changes.

Von Hippel-Lindau Disease

Rare autosomal dominant disorder due to mutations at tumor-suppressor locus on chromosome 3p25-p26 with predisposition to develop tumors.

Renal cell cysts and carcinoma in ≤60% of cases (see Chapter 14)

Pheochromocytoma in 14% of carriers (see Chapter 13).

Islet cell carcinoma of pancreas (see Chapter 13)

Hemangioblastomas of cerebellum and retina

Cystadenomas of pancreas and epididymis

○ DNA polymorphism analysis can identify persons likely to carry this gene among asymptomatic members of disease families focusing on those who should have periodic screening.

17 Disorders Due to Physical and Chemical Agents

PHYS/CHEM

Drugs of Abuse and Addiction

See Table 17-1.
Substance Abuse and Mental Health Services Administration (SAMHSA) proposes new rules:

- Head hair, oral fluid, sweat, in addition to urine and blood; urine specimen must be collected when oral fluid is collected
- Change cutoff for cocaine from 300 ng/mL to 150 ng/mL

- Change cutoff for amphetamine from 1,000 ng/mL to 500 ng/mL
- Changed cutoff for THC from 100 ng/mL to 50 ng/mL
- Creatinine level in urine (to detect adulteration) changed from 5 mg/dL to 2 mg/dL and specific gravity cutoff <1.010 or >1.0200

Sympathomimetic Drug Intoxication

Includes amphetamines [e.g., amphetamine, methamphetamine, ephedrine, fenfluramine, etc., and their "designer" derivatives], cocaine, phencyclidine, caffeine, theophylline

Laboratory findings due to rhabdomyolysis, myocardial necrosis, metabolic acidosis, renal and liver function abnormalities, e.g.,
　Increased serum total-CK, LD, AST, myoglobin, potassium
　Increased CK-MB, cTns, leucocytosis
Increased BUN, creatinine
　Ketonuria, myoglobinuria
Heroin is a common addiction drug
Persistent absolute and relative lymphocytosis; lymphocytes are often bizarre and atypical, and may resemble Downey cells.
Eosinophilia is seen in 25% of patients.
Liver function tests commonly show increased serum AST and ALT (increased in 75% of patients). Higher frequency of positive tests is evident on routine periodic repeat of these tests. This probably represents a mild, chronic, viral hepatitis. Serum protein electrophoresis is usually normal.
HBsAg is found in 10% of patients.
Liver biopsy shows abnormal morphology in 25% of patients; foreign particles are particularly suggestive.
Laboratory findings due to preexisting glucose-6-PD deficiency may be precipitated (by quinine, which is often used to adulterate heroin).
Laboratory findings due to malaria transmitted by common syringes may occur. *(Malaria is not frequent; may be suppressed by quinine used for adulteration of heroin.)*
Laboratory findings due to active duodenal ulcer may occur.
Laboratory findings due to TB, which develops with increased frequency in narcotics addicts.
Laboratory findings due to staphylococcal pneumonia or septic pulmonary emboli secondary to skin infections or bacterial endocarditis (conditions that are more frequent in narcotics addicts) may be present.
Laboratory findings due to infective endocarditis

- Right-sided—usually *Staphylococcus aureus* affecting previously normal tricuspid valve
- Left-sided—may be due to *Candida* superimposed on previously normal valve

Laboratory findings due to syphilis and other sexually transmitted diseases, which occur with increased frequency in narcotics addicts, may occur. BFP tests for syphilis also occur with increased frequency.
Laboratory findings due to tetanus (which occurs with increased frequency in narcotics addicts because of "skin-popping") may occur. *(Tetanus causes 5%–10% of addicts' deaths in New York City.)*
Laboratory findings due to other infections (e.g. pyelonephritis, phlebitis, abscesses).
Laboratory findings due to concomitant use of sedatives, especially alcohol, barbiturates, and glutethimide (Doriden), may occur.
Oral and IV glucose tolerance curves are often flat (explanation for this finding is not known).
Urinalysis is usually normal unless renal failure due to endocarditis occurs.
Complications of drug addiction during pregnancy may also include premature rupture of membranes, abruptio placentae, stillbirth, and meconium aspiration.
♦ **Some Drug Testing Thresholds** (to report test as positive or negative)[1]

[1]Gerson B. Drug monitoring and toxicology, No. DM 91-4. ASCP Check Sample 1991:12.

PHYS/CHEM

Table 17-1. Drugs of Abuse

Drug	Street Names	Route	Usual Dose	Toxic Dose	Half-Life (hrs)	Duration of Effect (hrs)	% Not Changed in Urine
Stimulants							
Cocaine[a]	Coke, crack, snow	Nasal, smoke, IV, oral	1.5 mg/kg	>1.2 g	2–5	1–2	<10
Amphetamine[b] (Benzedrine, Dexedrine)	Bennies, dexies, uppers	Oral, IV	10 mg	30–500 mg	4–24	2–4	~30
Methamphetamine (Desoxyn, Methedrine)	Speed, meth, crystal	Oral, IV	5–10 mg	>1 g	9–24	2–4	10–20
Methylphenidate (Ritalin)		Oral, IV	5–20 mg	>2 g	2–3	2–4	<1
Phenmetrazine (Preludin)		Oral, IV	75 mg		8	12	15–20
Cannabis							
Marijuana,[c] hashish	Grass, Mary Jane, pot, THC, hash	Smoke, oral, IV		50–200 µg/kg	14–38	2–4	<1
Narcotics							
Heroin[d]	Horse, smack, white lady, scag	IV smoke, nasal	5–10 mg	100–250 mg	1–1.5	3–6	<1
Codeine[e] (e.g., with aspirin)		Oral, IV, IM	15–60 mg	500–1,000 mg	2–4	3–6	5–20
Morphine[f] (morphine sulfate, Duramorph)	M, junk, morpho, white stuff	IV, IM, oral, smoke	5–10 mg	50–100 µg/kg	2–4	3–6	<10
Methadone[g] (Dolophine, Amidone)	Methadose	Oral, IV, IM	40–100 mg	100–200 mg	15–60	12–24	5–50
Meperidine (Demerol, Mepergan, Pethidine)		IV, IM, oral	25–100 mg	500–2,000 mg	2–5	3–6	5
Propoxyphene[h] (Darvon, Darvocet, Dolene)	Yellow footballs	Oral	65–400 mg	500 mg	8–24	1–6	<1

Barbiturates[i]							
Pentobarbital (Nembutal)	Yellow jackets, yellows	Oral, IV, IM	50–200 mg	2–10 g	15–48	3–6	1
Amobarbital (Amytal, Tuinal)	Blues, bluebirds, rainbows	Oral, IV, IM	30–200 mg	1.5–10 g	12–60	3–24	<1
Secobarbital (Seconal, Tuinal)	Reds, red devils, M & Ms	Oral, IV IM	100–200 mg	2–5 g	15–40	3–6	5
Butabarbital (Butisol)		Oral	15–100 mg	>2 g	30–40	3–6	5–10
Butalbital (Fiorinal)		Oral	50–100 mg	>1 g	30–40	3–6	5
Phenobarbital (Luminal)	Downers	Oral, IV, IM	50–200 mg	6–20 g	48–120	10–20	20–35
Benzodiazepines[j]							
Alprazolam (Xanax)		Oral	0.25–1 mg		7–13	4–8	20
Chlordiazepoxide (Librium)		Oral, IM	5–100 mg	>500 µg	6–27	4–8	<1
Diazepam (Valium)		Oral, IV, IM	5–30 mg	>250 mg	20–50	4–8	<1
Flurazepam (Dalmane)		Oral	15–30 mg	>500 mg	2–3	4–12	<1
Lorazepam (Ativan)		Oral, IV, IM	0.5–2 mg	25–100 mg	9–16	4–8	<1
Antidepressants							
Tricyclics, e.g., imipramine (Tofranil, Janimine)		Oral, IM	100–500 mg	>1 g	12–30		<1
Phenothiazines, e.g., chlorpromazine (Thorazine)		Oral, IV, IM, rectal	5–800 mg	>1 g	7–120		<1
Sedatives, Depressants							
Ethanol		Oral		100 g	2–14	2–6	2–10
Methaqualone[k] (Quaalude)	'Ludes, soapers	Oral	150–500 mg	2 g	20–60	4–8	<1
Meprobamate (Equanil, Miltown, Pathibamate)		Oral	400–1,000 mg	2–5 g	6–16	4–8	5
Glutethimide (Doriden)		Oral	150–500 mg	5 g	5–22	4–8	<2
Chloral hydrate (Noctec)	Mickey Finn, joy juice	Oral, rectal	300–1,000 mg	3 g	<1	5–8	<1

(continued)

Table 17-1. *continued*

Drug	Street Names	Route	Usual Dose	Toxic Dose	Half-Life (hrs)	Duration of Effect (hrs)	% Not Changed in Urine
Hallucinogens							
Phencyclidine[l]	PCP, angel dust, killer weed	Oral, nasal, smoke, IV	0.25 mg/kg	10–20 mg	7–16	2–4 (psychosis may last wks)	30–50
LSD	Acid, white lightning, microdots	Oral	1–2 µg/kg	100–200 µg	3–4	8–12	1
Amphetamine analogs	STP, DOM	Oral, IV	2 mg		4–8		20
Ketamine (Ketalar)		IV, IM	1–4.5 mg/kg	>500 mg	3–4	0.5–2	2–5
Mescaline	Peyote, mesc, buttons	Oral		200–700 mg	6	8–12	50–60

LSD, lysergic acid diethylamide.

Detection Times in Urine with EMIT Methods

[a]Cocaine   Up to 48 hrs after a single dose.
[b]Amphetamines   Detectable within 24–48 hrs after ingestion. Cold medicines that contain ephedrine, pseudoephedrine, or phenylpropanolamine may cause positive reaction.
[c]Marijuana   ≤5 days after occasional use; 21–32 days after last dose in habitual users.
[d]Heroin   One 10-mg dose detectable for up to 24 hrs. 4–5 days in habitual users.
[e]Codeine   Excreted as morphine. 120-mg dose detectable for up to 48 hrs.
[f]Morphine   Single 10-mg dose detectable for 24–48 hrs.
[g]Methadone   ~3 days. Interference from high levels of chlorpromazine, promethazine, and dextromethorphan may occur.
[h]Propoxyphene   Up to 48 hrs.
[i]Barbiturates   Up to 9 days after one 250-mg dose of phenobarbital; other common barbiturates can be detected for 1–2 days.
[j]Benzodiazepine   Not usually positive after one dose with normal renal function. Up to 5–7 days in habitual users.
[k]Methaqualone   ≥5 days after a typical dose.
[l]Phencyclidine   1 wk after a single dose. Up to 2 wks after last dose in habitual users.

Source: *Clin Chem News Laboratory Guide to Abused Drugs.* Compiled by Wilson J for Roche Diagnostic Systems.

Table 17-2. Lower Detectability Limits for Screening Urine for Drugs of Abuse

Drug Abuse Screen (Urine)	Lower Limit of Detectability
Alcohol	300 µg/mL
Amphetamines	500 ng/mL
Barbiturates	1,000 ng/mL
Benzodiazepines	300 ng/mL
Benzoylecgonine	150 ng/mL
Cocaine	150 ng/mL
Opiates	300 ng/mL
Phencyclidine	25 ng/mL
Tetrahydrocannabinol carboxylic acid	15 ng/mL

Adapted from Leavelle DE, ed. *Mayo medical laboratories' test catalog*. Rochester, MN: Mayo Medical Laboratories, 1995.

Drug	Screen (ng/mL)	Confirm (ng/mL)
Marijuana metabolites	20–100	15
Cocaine metabolites	300	150
Opiate metabolites (Morphine, Codeine)	2,000	2,000
6-Monoacetylmorphine		25
Amphetamine, Methamphetamine	1,000	500
Phencyclidine (PCP)	25	25
Benzodiazepines	300	300
Methadone	300	300
Methaqualone	75	75

Positive screening tests should always be confirmed by GC/MS (see Table 17-2).
♦ Blood levels only detect recent ingestion, but do not predict toxicity. Have no clinical value but can be used to calculate when drug was used. Higher ratio of cocaine to benzoylecgonine (cocaine metabolite) indicates more recent use.

• Chewing of coca leaves (practiced by Peruvian Indians)—usually 300 to 400 ng/mL
• Snorting cocaine—600–800 ng/mL; snorting one line (~25 mg) produces level[2] of ~50 ng/mL
• IV cocaine—may reach 1,200 to 1,400 ng/mL
• Considerable overlap between lethal and recreational levels; death not usually dose related

Urine screen detection time (approximate)
  Alcohol: 6 to 12 hours
  Cocaine: 6 to 9 days in neonate; 2 to 4 days in adult
  Amphetamines: 2 to 4 days
    (Cocaine and amphetamines are difficult to detect >48 hours after use.)
  Opiates: 2 to 5 days
  Marijuana: <30 days
  PCP: ≤8 days
♦ Assay of hair permits estimate of cocaine use for previous several months and can indicate isolated or steady pattern (average hair growth = 1.3 cm [0.5 in] in 30 days). Thus, 8 cm length of hair can detect cocaine user over a period of ~6 months.
♦ RIA of hair for cocaine or heroin has S/S = 97% and 83% to 100% respectively.

[2]*The adulteration information booklet*. Tampa, FL: Chimera Research & Chemical, Inc.

Interferences[3,4]

Adulterants consist of either household substances (e.g., bleach, vinegar, soap, detergents, liquid drain cleaner, lemon juice, salt, eye drops) or commercial products sold for this purpose (e.g., "Klear," "Urine Luck"). There are >400 different adulterants on the market.

Positive subject identification, assurance that specimen really comes from testee, and chain of custody should be assured.

To detect adulteration,[5] check physical characteristics (e.g., color, including change in dipstick), chemical composition, other possible adulterants.

- Temperature taken promptly after specimen collection should be within 1°C or 1.8°F of body temperature.
- Appearance: dark color may be caused by goldenseal tea.
- Liquid soap may cause turbidity and foaming on shaking.
- Bleach (sodium hypochlorite) or vinegar may impart its own odor.
- pH: Should be in range of 4.6 to 8.0 for preliminary screening. Acidification of urine (e.g., vinegar, lemon juice) may speed elimination of PCP or amphetamine before test. Alkalinization of urine may slow excretion during testing period.
- Liquid drain cleaner (Drano) may mask amphetamines.
- Outside of physiologic range, e.g.,
    - Creatinine <15 mg/dL or specific gravity <1.003 may be due to external dilution of specimen, ingesting large amounts of fluids or use of diuretics.
    - Creatinine <10 mg/dL may indicate replacement by water.
    - NaCl (table salt) will cause specific gravity >1.035 or NaCl >200 mmol/L.
- Nitrite >500 μg/mL indicates adulteration. Is present in some commercial adulterants composed of KNO_3^- (e.g., "Klear," "Whizzies"). <6 μg/mL may be due to medications (e.g., nitroglycerine). <36 μg/mL may be due to bacterial urinary infection.
- Pyridinium chlorochromate (PCC) ("Urine Luck") is an effective adulterant for urine drug testing for opiates and THC. Suspect if abnormally low pH or orange tint to urine. Can be detected with spot tests using potassium iodide or hydrogen peroxide or for chromium ion in PCC. Also produces a darker purple color with nitrate dipstick. Confirm by direct GC/MS analysis for pyridine.
- Phosphates, as when testee puts motor oil on fingers and lets urine hit them while urinating.
- Commercial test strips for spot checks are available that screen for pH, specific gravity, creatinine, nitrite, glutaraldehyde, and PCC.

The clinician should be aware of which drugs are included in the screen, causes of false reactions, and detection levels for the particular methodology.

False-negative EMIT immunoassays may result from:

- Adulteration by adding various substances (e.g., acids, bases, Visine [benzalkonium], glutaraldehyde, etc.) to urine (see above)
- Brief time after drug use
- Ibuprofen may interfere with GC/MS confirmation for marijuana
- In urine testing for cannabinoids (marijuana metabolites), EMIT lower level of 100 ng/mL failed to detect 25% to 40% of cases identified by thin-layer chromatography (lower level ~25 ng/mL).
- Traces of marijuana may be present by EMIT up to 1 week after use or, in a heavy user, up to 4 weeks; 15% false positives by EMIT and 2% by HPLC.
- Screening tests not generally available for designer drugs, LSD, mescaline, psilocybin.

False-positive EMIT immunoassays may result from:

- Barbiturates and benzodiazepines: Ibuprofen ingestion
- Opiates: Dextromethorphan, poppy seeds. Eating poppy seeds may cause a false-positive EMIT for heroin confirmed by GC/MS. Poppy seed ingestion as the only source of urinary morphine and codeine can be ruled out if: urine codeine >300 ng/mL, urine morphine >5,000 ng/mL, morphine >1,000 ng/mL when no codeine is present, and morphine:codeine ratio <2.

[3]Dasgupta A. *Med Lab Obs* Feb 2003:26.
[4]Dasgupta A, et al. Rapid spot tests for detecting the presence of adulterants in urine specimens submitted for drug testing. *Am J Clin Pathol* 2002;117:325.
[5]Wu AHB, et al. Adulteration of urine by "Urine Luck." *Clin Chem* 1999;45:1051.

- Quinolone antibiotics (e.g., ciprofloxacin) may cause false positive for morphine at a threshold of 300 ng/mL by EMIT.
- Amphetamines: Ingestion of ephedrine, other sympathomimetics

Some factors that affect urine drug levels include:

- Renal function (drug excretion) and volume of fluid intake before collection
- Liver function (drug metabolism)
- Kinetics of drug distribution
- Time and size of last dose; single versus multiple doses

Laboratory Findings Due to Complications of Cocaine Abuse
(See appropriate separate sections.)
Catecholamine blood levels may reach several thousand ng/mL
Sudden death due to acute myocardial infarction—may occur in relatively young persons (i.e., <40 years old) and without evidence of coronary artery obstruction (e.g., coronary artery spasm with arrhythmias).
Acute myocarditis, acute cardiomyopathy
Bacterial endocarditis
Aortic rupture
Pneumopericardium
Acute rhabdomyolysis that may cause acute renal failure and DIC, etc.
Cerebral vasculitis with cerebral and subarachnoid hemorrhage
Hyperthyroidism
Pulmonary hemorrhage and hemoptysis, pulmonary edema, "crack lung"
Laboratory Findings Due to Phencyclidine (PCP) Abuse
Massive ingestion may cause

- Rhabdomyolysis
- Acute tubular necrosis
- Hypoglycemia

Cannabinoids (Marijuana, Hashish)
Testing (for tetrahydrocannabinol) is done to detect drug abuse rather than for therapeutic monitoring. Lower limit of detectability <15 ng/mL by definitive GC/MS. ≤25 mg/mL can be due to passive inhalation.
May be detected in plasma up to 6 days after smoking one marijuana cigarette.
In chronic marijuana users, cannabinoid metabolites have been detected in the urine ≤46 days after last use.
Urine adulterated with bleach, detergent, blood, salt, vinegar may produce negative tests with EMIT (enzyme immunoassay) methods.
Screening tests positive with one method (e.g., EMIT, RAI) should be confirmed with another method (e.g., GC/MS). Qualitative EMIT screen has occasional false positives.

Allergic Diseases/Serum Sickness

Allergic Diseases

Increased serum total IgE is not a sensitive test and is of limited clinical value; but extreme values may be helpful.

- Very low levels (<50 µg/L) help exclude atopic disease but not IgE sensitivity to special allergens such as penicillin or hymenoptera venoms.
- If >900 µg/L, atopic disease is likely but tests for specific allergens are needed.
- Very high levels (2,000 to >60,000 µg/L) are found in asthma associated with severe atopic dermatitis, allergic bronchopulmonary aspergillosis, Buckley syndrome (staphylococcal infections with hyper-IgE), systemic parasitic infestations, IgE myeloma, immune deficiency.
- Principal value in infants is to alert the clinician to the possibility of allergic disease when this is not the presumptive diagnosis.

Radioallergosorbent test (RAST; serum IgE antibodies specific for various allergens) measures IgE specific for individual allergies. Useful when skin testing cannot be done (e.g., children, risk of anaphylaxis) or when skin testing is unreliable (e.g., generalized dermatitis, severe dermographism). Less sensitive than skin and bronchial provocation tests.

PHYS/CHEM

Blood eosinophil counts >450/μLI in adults and >750/μL in children suggest allergic disorders. Significant numbers of false-positive and false-negative results occur.

Nasal cytology smears stained with Wright-Giemsa showing >5% eosinophils, >1% basophils, and/or >50% goblet/epithelial cells suggest allergic disease of respiratory tract. Does not correlate with blood eosinophilia. Large numbers of neutrophils suggest infection. Both eosinophils and neutrophils suggest chronic allergy with superimposed infection. Significant numbers of false-positive and false-negative results occur.

Measurement of serum complement is not useful.

Serum Sickness

Decreased WBC due to decreased polynuclear neutrophils; occasionally WBC is increased.

Eosinophils are usually normal.

ESR is normal.

Heterophil agglutination test is often positive and is decreased by guinea pig kidney absorption.

Accidents

Burns

Decreased plasma volume and blood volume. Greatest fall in plasma volume occurs in the first 12 hours and continues at a much slower rate for only 6 to 12 hours more. In a 40% burn, plasma volume falls to 25% below preburn levels.

Infection—burn sepsis: Gram-positive organisms predominate until the third day, when gram-negative organisms become dominant; reflects hospital flora. By fifth day, untreated infection is active. *Fatal burn-wound sepsis shows no noteworthy spread of bacteria beyond wound in half the cases. Before antibiotic therapy, this caused 75% of deaths due to burns; it now causes 10% to 15% of deaths.*

♦ Diagnosis by quantitative biopsy of eschar showing >10^5 bacteria/gm of tissue and histologic evidence of bacterial invasion in underlying unburned tissue. Surface cultures do not accurately predict incipient burn wound sepsis. Local and systemic infection due to *Candida* and *Phycomycetes*.

Laboratory findings due to pneumonia, which now causes most deaths that result from infection. Two-thirds of pneumonia cases are airborne infections. One third are hematogenous infections and are often due to septic phlebitis at sites of old cutdowns.

Laboratory findings due to inhalation injury

- ♦ Carbonaceous sputum is pathognomonic; there may be casts composed of mucin, fibrin, WBCs, cell debris.
- Hypoxemia
- Increased carboxyhemoglobin (>15%)

Cyanide toxicity should be suspected if metabolic acidosis is present with apparently sufficient oxygen delivery.

Laboratory findings due to renal failure. Reported frequency varies—1.3% of total admissions to 15% of patients with burns involving >15% of body surface.

Laboratory findings due to GI complications

- Curling ulcer occurs in 11% of burn patients. *Gastric ulcer is more frequent in general, but duodenal ulcer occurs twice as often in children as in adults. Gastric lesions are seen throughout the first month with equal frequency in all age groups, but duodenal ulcers are most frequent in adults during the first week and in children during the third and fourth weeks after the burns.*
- Others include acute pancreatitis, superior mesenteric artery syndrome, adynamic ileus.

Laboratory findings due to complications of topical antibacterial therapy

- Mafenide (Sulfamylon)—Metabolic acidosis (carbonic anhydrase inhibition)
- Silver nitrate—Methemoglobinemia due to nitrate-to-nitrite conversion by some strains of *Enterobacter cloacae*. Agyria does not occur.
- Silver sulfadiazine (Silvadene)—Hemolysis in patients with G-6-PD deficiency

Blood viscosity rises acutely; remains elevated for 4 to 5 days although Hct has returned to normal.

Fibrin split products are increased for 3 to 5 days.
Other findings that may occur in all types of trauma

- Platelet count rises slowly, lasting for 3 weeks
- Platelet adhesiveness is increased
- Fibrinogen falls during first 36 hours, then rises steeply for up to 3 months
- Factors V and VIII may be 4 to 8 times normal level for up to 3 months

Carbon Monoxide Poisoning, Acute

Binds to Hb. Displaces oxyhemoglobin dissociation curve causing tissue hypoxia. Cherry red skin color is useful clue.

♦ Gas chromatography is reference method. CO-oximeter (dedicated spectrophotometer that measures total Hb, COHb, metHb, and oxyhemoglobin) makes a rapid definitive diagnosis of increased COHb. Is diagnostic.

Symptoms are correlated with the percentage of carbon monoxide in Hb:

% COHb	Symptoms
0%–2%	Asymptomatic
2%–5%	Found in moderate cigarette smokers; usually asymptomatic but may be slight impairment of intellect
5%–10%	Found in heavy cigarette smokers; slight dyspnea with severe exertion
10%–20%	Dyspnea with moderate exertion; mild headache
20%–30%	Marked headache, irritability, disturbed judgment and memory, easy fatigability
30%–40%	Severe headache, dimness of vision, dizziness, confusion, weakness, nausea
40%–50%	Headache, confusion, fainting, ataxia, collapse, hyperventilation
50%–60%	Coma, intermittent convulsions
>60%	Respiratory failure, hypotension, and death if exposure is long continued
80%	Rapidly fatal

Blood pH is markedly decreased (metabolic acidosis due to tissue hypoxia).
Arterial pO_2 is normal, although O_2 is significantly decreased.
Arterial pCO_2 may be normal or slightly decreased.
♦ Increased CO in patient's exhaled air or in ambient air at site of exposure can help confirm diagnosis if COHb has already fallen substantially.

Drowning and Near Drowning

Hypoxemia (decreased pO_2)
Metabolic acidosis (decreased blood pH)
In severe freshwater aspiration

- Decreased serum sodium and chloride
- Increased serum potassium
- Increased plasma Hb

In severe seawater aspiration

- Hypovolemia
- Increased serum sodium and chloride
- Normal plasma Hb

These changes follow aspiration of very large amounts of water. Electrolytes return toward normal within 1 hour following survival, even without therapy.
In near drowning in fresh water, often

- Normal serum sodium and chloride
- Variable serum potassium
- Increased free plasma Hb; hemoglobinuria may occur.
- Oliguria with transient azotemia and proteinuria may develop.
- Fall in RBC, Hb, and Hct in 24 hours

In near drowning in seawater, often

- Moderate increase in serum sodium and chloride
- Normal or decreased serum potassium
- Normal Hb, Hct, and plasma Hb

Blood Hb may appear normal even when considerable hemolysis is present because usual methodology does not distinguish between Hb within RBC and free Hb in serum. Decrease in Hb and Hct may be delayed 1 to 2 days.

Electric Current Injury (Including Lightning)

Increased WBC with large immature granulocytes
Albuminuria; hemoglobinuria in presence of severe burns
CSF sometimes bloody
Myoglobinuria and increased serum AST, CK, etc., indicate severe tissue damage.

Exercise, Severe

May occur with variable severity and in variable number of persons

- Increased serum enzyme and cardiac markers concentration due to muscle injury (e.g., CK-total, CK-MB, LD, AST, cTn, aldolase, malate dehydrogenase)
- Changes due to mechanical destruction of RBCs (e.g., increased serum and urine myoglobin, increased serum indirect bilirubin)
- Increased serum uric acid

Inflammatory reaction to tissue injury (e.g., increased WBC and neutrophils)

Heat Stroke

Acute disruption of temperature-regulation mechanisms indicated by CNS depression, lack of sweating, core body temperature >41°C, severe biochemical abnormalities

Multiorgan dysfunction
Acute hepatic failure with abnormal liver function and increased muscle-enzyme values

- Uniformly increased serum AST (mean is 20× normal), ALT (mean is 10× normal), and LD (mean is 5× normal) reach peak on third day and return to normal by 2 weeks. Lethal outcome is associated with significantly higher serum values that continue to increase in next 12 to 24 hours. Consecutive normal values rule out diagnosis of heat stroke.

Hemoconcentration
Evidence of kidney damage may vary from mild proteinuria and slight abnormalities of urine sediment, azotemia, to acute oliguric renal insufficiency.
Serum sodium is often decreased but may be high, especially in exertional heatstroke.
Acute respiratory distress syndrome
Respiratory alkalosis occurs early; lactic acidosis and hyperkalemia later
Hypoglycemia may occur.
Increased WBC count is usual.
DIC is common in severe cases.
Rhabdomyolysis (with increased CK-total and CK-MM), DIC, and acute renal failure are relatively uncommon in elderly because exertional heat stroke is less common in elderly.
CSF AST, ALT, and LD are normal.

Hypothermia

Core body temperature in mild hypothermia: 34°C–36°C.; moderate to severe hypothermia: ≤33°C

Acid-base disturbances are very common.

- Initial hyperventilation causes respiratory alkalosis followed by respiratory acidosis due to CO_2 retention.
- Metabolic acidosis due to lactate accumulation. During re-warming, metabolic acidosis may become worse as lactic acid is mobilized from poorly perfused tissues.

Hemoconcentration is common.

Decreased platelets. WBC frequently falls, but differential is usually normal.

DIC may occur during rewarming.

"Cold diuresis," glycosuria, and natriuresis may occur; oliguria suggests complicating hypovolemia, acute tubular necrosis, rhabdomyolysis, or drug overdose.

Pancreatitis is a frequent complication.

Marked abnormalities in liver function tests are unusual.

Hyponatremia, hyperglycemia, hyperphosphatemia. Extreme hyperkalemia (>6.8 mEq/L) is a good indicator of death during acute hypothermia.

Infection is frequent sequela.

Bites of Insects/Spiders/Snakes

Insect and Spider Bites

Due to ticks, lice, fleas, bugs, beetles, ants, flies, bees, wasps, etc.

No specific laboratory findings if no disease transmission or wound infection.

Black Widow Spider (Latrodectus mactans)

Moderately increased WBC

Findings of acute nephritis

Brown Recluse Spider (Loxosceles reclusa)[6]

Diagnosis depends on proof of the spider bite, which is usually self-limited and self-healing.

New ELISA assay for venom may be useful.

Hemolytic anemia with hemoglobinuria and hemoglobinemia

Increased WBC

Thrombocytopenia

Proteinuria

Snake Bites[7]

Mortality <0.5% in United States; 95% of cases are due to rattlesnakes. In United States, all native snakes with elliptical pupils are poisonous.

Laboratory findings indicate severity of envenomation, which varies with snake species and size, amount and toxicity of venom, bite location, and timing of definitive treatment.

Due To

Pit vipers (e.g., rattlesnake, copperhead, water moccasin); 25% of bites do not cause envenomation

Elapidae (e.g., coral snakes, kraits, cobras)

○ Consumptive coagulopathy: fibrinogen levels are very low or absent, fibrin split products can be detected, PT and aPTT are increased considerably. As a screening test, blood drawn into a modified Lee-White clotting tube that fails to clot within a few minutes of constant agitation is a reliable indication of envenomation.

○ Platelets may be decreased to $<20,000/\mu L$.

Hemolytic manifestations may occur.

RBCs may show burrs.

Increased WBC ($20,000-30,000/\mu L$)

Albuminuria may be found.

Monitor patients with CBC, platelet count, fibrinogen, PT, aPTT, BUN, electrolytes, bilirubin, after each infusion of antivenom for at least 8 hours. May also test CK, O_2 saturation, etc., depending on symptoms. Platelet count and fibrinogen are most sensitive.

$\leq 80\%$ of patients treated with antivenom will develop serum sickness reaction.

Blood alcohol $>0.1\%$ in 40% of people bitten.

[6]Swanson DL, Vetter RS. Bites of brown recluse spiders and suspected necrotic arachnidism. *N Engl J Med* 2005;352:700.
[7]Gold BS, Dart RC, Barish RA. Bites of venomous snakes. *New Eng J Med* 2002; 347:347.

PHYS/CHEM

Table 17-3.	Stages of Acute Alcoholic Intoxication		

Ethanol Concentration
(% Weight/Volume)

Blood	Urine	Stage of Alcohol Influence	Effects
0.01–0.05	0.01–0.07	Sobriety	Little effect on most persons
0.04–0.12	0.03–0.16	Euphoria	Decreased inhibitions, decreased judgment, loss of fine control, increased reaction time ($\leq$20%)
0.09–0.20	0.07–0.30	Excitement	Uncoordination, loss of critical judgment, memory loss, increased reaction time ($\leq$100%)
0.15–0.30	0.12–0.40	Confusion	Disorientation Impaired emotional balance, slurred speech, disturbed sensation
0.25–0.40	0.20–0.50	Stupor	Paralysis, incontinence
0.30–0.50	0.25–0.60	Coma	Depressed reflexes, decreased respiration, possible death

Drugs and Poisons

Acetaminophen Poisoning

♦ Blood levels

- 200 μg/mL within 4 hours after ingestion or >50 μg/mL at 12 hours predicts severe liver damage, and treatment with acetylcysteine should begin.
- <150 μg/mL at 4 hours or <30–35 μg/mL at 12 hours indicates no liver damage will occur.
- Toxicity is dose dependent but exaggerated by starvation and drugs, *especially alcohol.*
- *Liver toxicity cannot be predicted from blood levels earlier than 4 hours.*
- *Exact time of ingestion is often difficult to ascertain.*
- *Patients taking other drugs or with concomitant cirrhosis may develop liver toxicity at different blood levels.*
- *Toxicity is less common in children <5 years old, and changes in liver function tests may be mild when serum drug levels are in toxic range.*

With hepatotoxicity (see Acute Hepatic Failure)

- During first 12 to 24 hours, increased AST and ALT are found in only ~50% of patients and serum drug levels are the chief guide to therapy; this is the only stage when treatment can prevent liver damage.
- During next 24 to 48 hours, AST, ALT, serum bilirubin, prothrombin time are increased. AST and ALT are very high (typically >4,000 U/L, often >10,000 U/L). AST/ALT ratio <2 in ~90% of cases.
- On third to fourth day, liver function abnormalities peak; hypoglycemia, secondary renal failure may occur.

Alcohol Abuse

See Tables 17-3, 17-4, and 17-5.

Ethanol

Also used for treatment of methanol or ethylene glycol poisoning, desirable blood concentration = 100 mg/dL

Criterion for driving an automobile while intoxicated = 100 mg/dL (= 0.1%; 1,000 μg/mL)

Table 17-4.   Diagnostic Efficiency of Some Markers for Alcoholism

Test	Sensitivity	Specificity	Predictive Value Positive	Predictive Value Negative
GGT (>50 U/L)	69	59	55	73
MCV	73	76	67	80
AST (>40 U/L)	69	68	55	74
ALT (>35 U/L)	58	57	49	66
AST/ALT (>1)	69	46	47	68

Source: Kwoh-Gain I, et al. Desialylated transferrin and mitochondrial aspartate aminotransferase compared as laboratory markers of excessive alcohol consumption. *Clin Chem* 1990;36:841.

For diagnosis of alcoholism

- A major criterion
    Blood concentration >150 mg/dL without gross evidence of intoxication
- Minor criteria
    Blood concentration >300 mg/dL at any time
    Blood concentration >100 mg/dL in routine examination

Toxic concentration: ≥200 mg/dL
Lower limit for detection = 100 μg/mL
Interference
False-positive values ≤690 mg/L due to elevated lactate and LD concentrations using EMIT, but not protein-free ultrafiltrates or gas chromatography
♦ Laboratory findings due to alcohol ingestion[8]

- Blood alcohol level >300 mg/dL at any time or >100 mg/dL in routine examination. (*Blood alcohol level >150 mg/dL without gross evidence of intoxication suggests alcoholic patient's increased tolerance.*) In high-dose coma, blood alcohol should be >300 mg/dL; otherwise, rule out other etiologies, especially diabetic acidosis and hypoglycemia (see Table 17-3).
- Rules of thumb to estimate blood alcohol level
    Peak is reached 1/2 hour to 3 hours after last drink.
    Each ounce of whisky, glass of wine, or 12 ounces of beer raises blood alcohol 15 to 25 mg/dL.
    Women absorb alcohol much more rapidly than do men and show a 35% to 45% higher blood alcohol level. During premenstrual period, peak occurs more rapidly and reaches a higher peak. Birth control pills cause a higher, more sustained level.
    Elderly become intoxicated more quickly than young persons.

Table 17-5.   Comparison of Poisoning by Various Alcohols

Alcohol*	Metabolic Acidosis with I AG	Osmolal Gap	Serum Acetone	Urine Ketones	Urine Oxalate Crystals
Ethanol	V	I	V	V	–
Methanol	+	+	–	–	–
Isopropanol	–	I	+	+	–
Ethylene glycol	I	I	–		One-third of cases

+, present; –, absent; AG, anion gap; I, increased; V, varies—finding on presence of lactic acidosis or alcoholic ketoacidosis.
*Measured by gas chromatography.

[8]Laposata M. Assessment of ethanol intake. Current tests and new assays on the horizon. *Am J Clin Pathol* 1999;112:443.

PHYS/CHEM

- Urine concentration is not well correlated with blood levels; cannot be used to determine level of intoxication or impairment.
- Breath test (Breathalyzer) has certain constraints and limitations.
- Alcohol content in saliva—determined by using cotton swab inserted into kit device. Method is used in drug abuse centers, hospital ER, and trauma units. Enzyme strip is colored in several minutes, which is compared with a color scale to determine level of intoxication. One kit detects concentrations >0.02%. Saliva to blood ratio = 1:1. Breath to blood ratio = .00048:1.
- Serum osmolality (reflects blood alcohol levels)—every 22.4 increment >200 mOsm/L reflects 50 mg/dL alcohol. Increased osmolar gap (difference between measured and calculated osmolality is increased >10). Absence of increased gap is evidence against elevated blood level of ethanol, methanol, or ethylene glycol.
- Laboratory findings due to other drugs of abuse may be present.
- Laboratory findings resulting from alcohol ingestion
  Hypoglycemia
  Hypochloremic alkalosis
  Low magnesium level
  Increased lactic acid (see Chapter 12)
  Metabolic acidosis with increased anion gap (see Chapter 12)
  Alcoholic ketoacidosis is preponderantly due to beta-hydroxybutyrate; therefore increased ketone levels in blood and urine are often negative or only weakly positive because nitroprusside test detects acetoacetic but not beta-hydroxybutyric acid. As the patient improves, the ketone test may become more strongly positive (although total ketone level declines) because the improved liver function slows the conversion of acetoacetate to beta-hydroxybutyrate.
- Thrombocytopenia
- Anemia most often due to folic acid deficiency; less frequently due to iron deficiency, hemorrhage, etc. (see appropriate separate sections).
- Alcohol is the most common cause of ring sideroblasts
- Three types of hemolytic syndromes may occur (spur cell anemia, acquired stomatocytosis, Zieve syndrome).

○ Increase in the following blood values with no other known cause that would arouse suspicion of alcoholism (see Table 17-4)

- MCV (e.g., >97) (26% of cases) with round macrocytosis
- Serum GGT (>50 U/L)
- Uric acid (10% of cases)
- ALT, AST (48% of cases)
- ALP (16% of cases)
- Bilirubin (13% of cases)
- Triglycerides

After 4 weeks of abstention, alcohol challenge in "moderate drinkers" causes increased AST and GGT in 24 hours with slow decline thereafter. ALT, LD, ALP show little or no change.

Decrease of GGT after 1 week of abstinence or decrease of MCV after 1 to 12 months are markers of alcoholism in cirrhosis; persistent decrease of GGT to <2.5× ULN is marker of abstinence in alcoholic liver disease.

♦ The following have been reported as biochemical markers of alcohol abuse[9]

- Carbohydrate-deficient transferrin (CDT): Ingestion of >60 g ethanol (5 beers or 5 glasses of wine, or 4 mixed drinks) for 7 to 10 consecutive days causes liver to produce CDT. Reversible by 14–21 days of abstinence. The disialotransferrin glycoform shows a relative increase over other glycoforms after >2 weeks of heavy drinking and may require >1 month to return to baseline (measured by HPLC).[10]
- Hemoglobin-associated acetaldehyde (HAA): Acetaldehyde is first degradation product of alcohol metabolism. Free (plasma and RBCs) peaks 30 minutes after last drink, returns to baseline in ~3.5 hours. Protein bound (90% is HAA) is increased for ~1 month. Whole blood (protein bound and free) acetaldehyde measured by HPLC.

[9]Bean P. Latest trends in alcohol abuse diagnosis using new biomarkers. *Am Clin Lab* Mar 2001:8.
[10]Helander A, et al. Improved HPLC method for carbohydrate-deficient transferrin in serum. *Clin Chem* 2003;49:1881.

- Early detection of alcohol consumption (EDAC) score of 12 to 36 constituents includes CBC with indices, complete chemistry and lipid profile, electrolytes, liver function tests.

Clinical Application of Some Biochemical Markers of Alcohol Abuse

	CDT	EDAC	WBAA
Screen for abuse	±	+++	++
Binge drinking	+	++	+++
Chronic/heavy drinking	+++	+++	+++
Confirm suspicion	+++	+++	+++
Monitor drinking status	+++	++	+

Source: Bean P. Latest trends in alcohol abuse diagnosis using new biomarkers. *Am Clin Lab* Mar 2001:8.)

Declining serum potassium level to hypokalemia during alcohol withdrawal is said to be a reliable predictor of delirium tremens.
Laboratory findings due to major alcohol-associated illnesses (see these appropriate separate sections)

- Fatty liver (see Chapter 8), alcoholic hepatitis (see Chapter 8), cirrhosis, esophageal varices, peptic ulcer, chronic gastritis, pancreatitis, malabsorption, vitamin deficiencies
- Head trauma, Korsakoff syndrome, delirium tremens, peripheral neuropathy, myopathy
- Cardiac myopathy
- Various pneumonias, lung abscess, TB
- Associated addictions

Isopropanol (Rubbing Alcohol)

Converted by alcohol hydrogenase to acetone

♦ Increased blood levels of isopropanol. In absence of acetone, usually indicates an artifact.

- \>400 mg/L—severe toxicity
- \>1,000 mg/L—coma

Severe metabolic acidosis with increased anion gap is not feature (as in ethanol poisoning but in contrast to methanol and ethylene glycol poisoning) unless lactic acid acidosis is present. Dialysis is seldom necessary.
○ Presence of acetone in blood and urine especially in high levels suggests isopropanol poisoning.
○ Osmolal gap increases 0.17 mOsm/L for every 1 mg of isopropanol; increase of 1 mOsm/L represents an isopropanol increase of 6 mg/dL.

Methyl Alcohol (Wood Alcohol)

Methanol is metabolized to formic acid, a metabolic dead end, and accumulates, causing metabolic acidosis with latent period of 12–72 hours. Production of formic acid can be halted by alcohol dehydrogenase inhibitor [4-methyl pyrazole; fomepizole]. Due to drinking illicit liquor [e.g., from stills, "bathtub" gin] contaminated with methyl alcohol.

See Table 17-5.
♦ Severe metabolic acidosis with increased anion gap and increased osmolar gap similar to ethanol intoxication and ethylene glycol poisoning should always arouse suspicion of alcohol poisoning. Lactic acid also contributes to metabolic acidosis. Is not excluded by low osmolar gap (<20 mOsm/kg), especially if late after ingestion.
○ Frequent concomitant acute pancreatitis
Mortality rate

- 20% if plasma bicarbonate <20 mmol/L.
- 50% if plasma bicarbonate <10 mmol/L (severe acidosis).

Treat with ethyl alcohol to achieve blood alcohol level 100 to 150 mg/dL and maintain until methyl alcohol level <10 mg/dL, formate <1.2 mg/dL, normal AG, and acidosis resolves.

Institute hemodialysis if blood methyl alcohol >50 mg/dL and severe resistant acidosis or renal failure. Lethal concentration = 80 mg/dL.

Ethylene and Diethylene Glycol (Antifreeze)

○ Severe metabolic acidosis with increased anion gap and osmolal gap
◆ Detect ethylene glycol and its metabolite glycolic acid in serum
○ Oxalate and hippurate crystals in urine
○ Characteristic oxalate crystals in renal biopsy
○ Urine may fluoresce under Wood's lamp due to fluorescence added to antifreeze.

Dialysis if glycol level >50 mg/dL, renal failure, or persistent severe acidosis.

Treat by IV ethyl alcohol to achieve level >100 mg/dL.

Aluminum Toxicity

Acceptable level = <10 μg/L; action level = 60 μg/L

Due To
Iatrogenic (e.g., dialysis, IV fluids, drugs)
Occupational (e.g., aluminum smelting)
For patients on long-term dialysis treatment

◆ • Serum aluminum should always be <200 μg/L (7.4 μmol/L); frequent monitoring and close observation for toxicity if serum >100 μg/L. Can be prevented by treatment of dialysate water (e.g., reverse osmosis) so that final aluminum concentration in dialysate is <15 μg/L.

Microcytic hypochromic anemia (non-iron-deficient type)

Osteomalacic osteodystrophy is progressive, associated with a myopathy, resists treatment with vitamin D or its metabolites; may be associated with hypercalcemia. Metastatic calcification is common. Bone biopsy (special technique) is most reliable test.

Dialysis encephalopathy

Chelation treatment with deferoxamine increases serum level with decrease in protein-bound fraction.

Anticonvulsants

e.g., electroshock, hypoglycemic therapy

Increased CSF AST and LD peak (≤3× normal) in 12 hours; return to normal by 48 hours

Apresoline (Hydralazine Hydrochloride) Reaction
Used for hypertension therapy

Anemia and pancytopenia occur infrequently.
◆ Prolonged use causes a syndrome resembling SLE (microscopic hematuria, leukopenia, increased ESR, presence of LE cells, altered serum proteins with increased gamma globulin). After cessation of drug, remission is aided by administration of ACTH.

Arsenic Poisoning
Due to insecticides, rodenticides, herbicides, industrial products, or therapeutic arsenic, [e.g., Fowler's solution].

See Table 17-6.

Chronic

◆ Increased arsenic appears in urine (usually >0.1 mg/L; in acute cases, may be >1.0 mg/L). Can be present for up to 10 days after a single exposure. With high industrial exposure, urine level may reach 1,600 μg/L. After large seafood meal, level may reach 400 μg/L in 4 hours.

Table 17-6. Reported Reference Ranges of Some Common Toxic Substances and Trace Metals

Chemical	Specimen*	Normal Range	Toxic Concentration
Arsenic	Hair or nails	<1.0 μg/gm	
	Serum	<0.07 μg/mL	
	Urine	<25 μg/specimen	>150 μg/specimen
Cadmium	Blood	<5.0 ng/mL	
	Urine	<3 μg/24 hr	
Carbon monoxide	Blood	<7%	>20%
		<15% in heavy smokers	
Chromium	Serum	0.3–0.9 μg/L	
	Urine	<8.0 μg/specimen	
Copper	Serum	0.70–1.40 μg/mL (men)	
		0.80–1.55 μg/mL (women)	
		1.20–3.00 μg/mL (pregnancy)	
		0.80–1.90 μg/mL (children 6–12 yrs old)	
		0.20–0.70 μg/mL (infants)	
	Urine	15–60 μg/specimen	
	Liver tissue	10–35 μg/g dry weight	
Ethanol	Blood		Toxic >2,000 μg/mL
Ethylene glycol	Serum		Toxic >2 mmol/L, lethal >20 mmol/L
Lead	Blood	<0.2 μg/mL	
	Serum	0.8-2.5 ng/mL	
	Urine	<80 μg/specimen; abnormal, > 400 μg/specimen; inconclusive, 80–400 μg/specimen	
	Hair or nails	<25 μg/gm	
Manganese	Serum or plasma	0.4–1.1 ng/mL	
	Whole blood	7.7–12.1 ng/mL	
	Urine	<0.3 μg/specimen	
Mercury	Blood	<0.005 μg/mL	>0.05 μg/mL
	Urine	<20 μg/specimen	>50 μg/specimen
	Hair or nails	<1.0 μg/gm	
Selenium	Serum	46–143 ng/mL	
	Whole blood	58–234 ng/mL	
	Urine	7–160 μg/L	
	Hair	0.2–1.4 μg/gm	
Silver	Serum	<0.2 μg/mL	
	Urine	<1.0 μg/specimen	
Thallium	Serum	<10 ng/mL	
	Urine	<10 μg/specimen	
Zinc	Plasma	0.70–120 μg/mL	
	Serum	5%–15% higher than plasma	
	Urine	0.15-1.0 mg/day	

*Urine concentration is reported as per 7-mL aliquot of 24-hr urine collection.
Source: Some data from Jacob RA, Milne DB. Biochemical assessment of vitamins and trace metals. *Clin Lab Med* 1993;13:371.

PHYS/CHEM

♦ Increased arsenic appears in hair (normal = 0.05 mg/100 gm of hair; chronic toxicity = 0.1–0.5 mg/100 gm of hair; acute toxicity = 1–3 mg/100 gm of hair); may take several weeks to appear.
♦ Increased arsenic appears in nails 6–9 months after exposure.
Moderate anemia is present; commonly normocytic, normochromic, basophilic stippling.
Moderate leukopenia occurs (2,000–5,000/μL), with mild eosinophilia.
Pancytopenia, aplastic anemia, and leukemia are associated with arsenic poisoning.
Liver function tests show mild abnormalities.
Abnormal renal function is frequent (oliguria, proteinuria, hematuria, casts).
Increased CSF protein (>100 mg/dL) is frequent; easily confused with Guillain-Barré syndrome.

Acute (e.g., arsine gas [hydrogen arsenide]) causes hemolysis with hemoglobinuria; may cause oliguric renal failure.

♦ Cleared from blood in 10 hours; 40% is excreted in 48 hours and 70% within 1 week of ingestion; thus toxic blood levels may be missed. Urine levels are most useful to detect current (1–3 days previously) poisoning.
Laboratory findings due to

• Vomiting
• Profuse watery or bloody diarrhea
• Circulatory collapse
• Renal damage (oliguria, proteinuria, hematuria)

Barbiturate Overdose

• Correlation between serum concentrations of barbiturates and state of intoxication in patients who have taken only a short-acting barbiturate, who are not habitual drug users, and who have no medical complications:

<6 μg/mL	Alert
6–10 μg/mL	Drowsy
11–17 μg/mL	Stuporous
16–20 μg/mL	Coma 1
20–24 μg/mL	Coma 2
24–28 μg/mL	Coma 3
28–40 μg/mL	Coma 4

If the serum drug level is less than expected for the state of intoxication, look for medical complications (e.g., aspiration pneumonia, head trauma) or presence of other drugs.

Bromism

Should always be ruled out in the presence of mental symptoms or psychosis

♦ Serum and urine bromide levels are increased.
CSF protein is increased in acute bromide psychosis.
False increase of serum "chloride" when measured by AutoAnalyzer. *If result of chloride determination with AutoAnalyzer is increased out of proportion to result with Cotlove coulimetric titrator, bromism should be ruled out.* Anion gap may be low or negative due to increased serum chloride.

Cigarette Smoking

♦ Cotinine increased in plasma or urine. Use to assess compliance in smoking cessation programs and to identify passively exposed nonsmokers. Has a longer half-life than nicotine, is more sensitive and specific than other markers to distinguish smokers from nonsmokers.

Reference ranges (HPLC)

	Plasma	Urine
Nonsmoker or passive exposure	0–8 μg/L	0.0–0.2 mg/L
Smoker	>8 μg/L	>0.2 mg/L

Increased blood carbon monoxide

Increased risk of coronary artery disease and cancers (especially of lung)

Cyanide Poisoning

Potassium cyanide is in rodenticides, insecticides, laboratory reagents, film developer, amygdalin, silver polish, and acetonitrile used to remove artificial fingernails. Hydrogen cyanide is in insecticides and fumigants and is released by the burning of plastics and synthetics. Odor of bitter almonds is useful clue. Reversibly binds to and inhibits reoxidation of cytochrome A preventing cellular respiration.

♦ CO-oximeter (dedicated spectrophotometer that measures total Hb, COHb, metHb, and oxyhemoglobin) makes a rapid definitive diagnosis of increased metHb.

pO_2 and oxygen saturation are normal except in severe cases when respiratory failure occurs.

Patient may first have respiratory alkalosis due to hyperventilation caused by tissue hypoxia.

Then severe lactic (metabolic) acidosis with increased AG gap develops.

With respiratory depression, respiratory acidosis may occur.

Increased venous oxygen with decreased arteriovenous oxygen difference due to decreased tissue extraction of oxygen

♦ Blood cyanide is increased; toxic concentration: >50 μg/dL

Treat with nitrites to form metHb level >30%; then treat with sodium thiosulfate IV to form thiocyanate. Antidote now sold commercially by Eli Lily Co.

Iron Poisoning, Acute

Occurs in children who have ingested medicinal iron preparations

Increased serum iron. Peak usually occurs 2 to 4 hours after ingestion. Levels begin to fall after 6 hours. If the first sample was taken 1 to 2 hours after ingestion, a second sample should be obtained several hours later. Serum should be obtained after absorption is complete and before peak serum level falls due to protein binding and tissue distribution.

- <350 μg/dL is rarely significant clinically; may have mild symptoms
- 350 to 500 μg/dL frequently have symptoms but risk of serious abnormality is mild; usually do not require prolonged chelation. 10% develop coma or shock.
- >500 μg/dL within 6 hours of ingestion with severe intoxication; need urgent chelation treatment in hospital. 25% develop coma or shock.
- >1000 μg/dL may be lethal; may require hemodialysis or exchange transfusion. 70% may develop coma or shock.

Increased total iron-binding capacity (TIBC) itself is unreliable and not useful. Poor prognostic sign when serum iron greatly exceeds TIBC. Spuriously increased by deferoxamine chelation therapy.

Serum glucose >150 mg/dL or WBC >15,000/cu mm and radiopaque material on flat plate of abdomen correlate with increased serum iron level.

In deferoxamine challenge (50 mg/kg up to 1 gm IM) chelates free iron in circulation (100 mg binds 9 mg of iron, chiefly ferric); later appears in urine bound to iron causing light orange to dark red-brown ("vin rose") color. Parenteral chelation should continue until serum iron <100 μg/dL or urine loses vin rose color.

Renal changes may occur (e.g., acute renal failure, nephrotic syndrome, specific tubular defects).

Metabolic acidosis, DIC, increased serum AST, ALT, bilirubin.

In chronic iron poisoning damage to various organs occurs (e.g., liver, heart, stomach).

Lead Poisoning (Plumbism)

Lead inhibits heme synthesis; see Fig. 12-7

See Tables 17-7, 17-8, and 17-9, Fig. 17-1.

PHYS/CHEM

Table 17-7.	Centers for Disease Control and Prevention (CDC) Classification of Whole Blood Lead in Children 6–72 Mos Old for Prevention and Control

Level (μg/dL)	Classification
≤9	Not considered lead poisoning
>10*	Rescreen; intervention; search for source
10–14	Need for more frequent screening of child and search for source
15–19	Rescreen; educational and nutritional intervention
20–44	Evidence of increased lead exposure; remedy environment; consider chelation
45–69	Chelation therapy; environmental intervention
>70	Emergency treatment should begin immediately

*CDC has recently lowered the intervention level from 25 to 10 μg/dL.
Source: Centers for Disease Control and Prevention. *Preventing lead poisoning in young children.* Washington, DC: U.S. Department of Health and Human Services, Public Health Service, 1994.

Due To

- In adults, usually occupational (storage batteries, lead smelters, lead solder) or environmental exposure (improperly glazed earthenware, illicitly distilled whisky, gun range)
- In children, usually due to pica
- In adolescents, may be due to gasoline sniffing
- In all groups, epidemics may be due to contamination of water supply by lead pipes, using contaminated pottery, traditional Asian remedies, etc.

♦ Measurement of zinc protoporphyrin (ZPP) (hematofluorometer) and free erythrocyte protoporphyrin (FEP) in blood using rapid micromethods are more sensitive indicators of lead poisoning than delta-ALA acid in urine. Especially useful for screening children. ZPP appears only in new RBCs and remains for life of RBC; therefore ZPP does not increase until several weeks after onset of lead exposure and remains high long after lead exposure has ended; therefore is good indicator of total body burden of lead. FEP is sensitive measure of chronic exposure; increased whole blood level is sensitive measure of acute exposure. After therapy or removal of exposure, blood lead becomes normal weeks to months before RBCs. CDC now recommends determination of whole blood lead in children because ZPP is not reliable below ~25 μg/dL. If capillary blood is used for screening, values >10 μg/dL require venous blood confirmation. Other causes of increased FEP are iron deficiency, anemia of chronic disease, sickle cell disease, erythropoietic protoporphyria. FEP ≥190 μg/dL is almost always due to

Table 17-8.	CDC Classification of Blood Lead Levels for Pediatric Screening

Blood Level (μg/dL)	Classification	Interpretation
<10	I	
10–14	II A	Rescreen with venous blood within 1 month. Educate; repeat within 3 months.
15–19	II B	Confirm within 1 month. Check exposure history. Educate; repeat within 2 months.
20–44	III	Confirm within 1 week. Check environment, history, physical examination. Possible chelation therapy.
45–69	IV	Confirm within 2 days; then environmental and medical intervention with chelation therapy.
>70	V	Confirm immediately; medical emergency. Begin chelation therapy.

Source: Centers for Disease Control and Prevention. Screening young children for lead poisoning. Guidance for state and local public health officials. Atlanta GA. US Dept of Health and Human Services, Public Health Service November 1997. http://www.cdc.gov/nceh/lead/guide/guide97.htm.

Table 17-9. Screening for Lead Poisoning in High-Risk Children

Lead (μg/dL)	FEP (μg/dL)[a]		
	≤34	35–109	110–249	≥250
≤24	Retest in 1 yr	Rule out other causes of I FEP[b]; retest in 3 mos	Rule out iron deficiency; retest in 3 mos	Rule out erythropoietic proto-porphyria; retest in 3 mos
25–49	Retest next visit	Retest in 1–3 mos, then every 3–6 mos[c]	Rule out iron deficiency; retest in 2–4 wks[c]	
50–69	Usual pattern; retest to confirm	Retest in 2 wks, then every 1–3 mos[d]	Retest stat; rule out iron deficiency[d]	Retest stat; mobilization test or treat
≥70	Unusual pattern; retest to rule out contaminated specimen	Retest stat and treat	Retest stat and treat	Hospitalize stat

FEP, free erythrocyte protoporphyrin.

[a]Other causes of increased FEP are iron deficiency, anemia of chronic disease, sickle cell disease, and erythropoietic protoporphyria.

[b]Iron deficiency and thalassemia should be ruled out even if lead level is increased because iron deficiency and lead poisoning can occur together. Use blood lead and zinc protoporphyrin (ZPP) together for possible lead poisoning; blood ZPP with serum iron and ferritin for iron deficiency.

[c]Consider mobilization test if lead is ≥35 μg/dL.

[d]Consider mobilization test if lead = 35–55 μg/dL. Treat if lead = 56–69 μg/dL.

Source: Westchester County (N.Y.) Department of Health (Rev. 8.85).

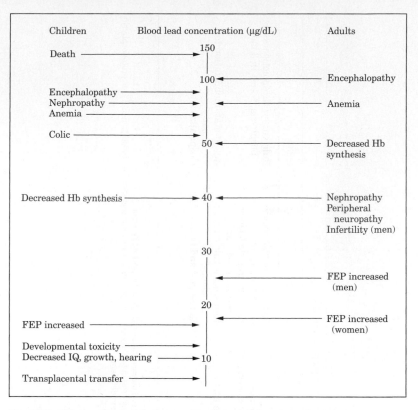

Fig. 17-1. Effects of lowest lead concentration on laboratory changes.

lead intoxication. Iron deficiency and thalassemia should be ruled out even if lead level is increased since iron deficiency and lead poisoning can occur together. Use blood lead and ZPP together for possible lead poisoning, blood ZPP with serum iron and ferritin for iron deficiency.

♦ Delta-aminolevulinic acid (delta-ALA) is increased in urine. Since it is increased in 75% of asymptomatic lead workers who have normal coproporphyrin in urine, it can be used to detect early excess lead absorption. Is not increased until blood lead >40 μg/dL.

♦ Confirm diagnosis with assay of blood lead—a single determination cannot distinguish chronic from acute exposure; reflects equilibrium between body compartments and therefore relatively recent exposure. *All blood and urine specimens for lead must be collected in special containers.*

Blood lead concentration in adults

- <10 μg/dL: In most adults without occupational exposure
- <25 μg/dL: Considered normal
- 25 μg/dL: Report to state occupational health agency; consider chelation therapy
- >60 μg/dL: Remove from occupational exposure; chelation therapy

Urine lead level

- <150 μg/L: Normal for adults
- <80 μg/L: Normal for children
- >500 μg/24 hours in children: Indicates excess mobile total body lead burden and suggests chelation therapy

Lead mobilization test—administer 500 mg/m² (up to 1,000 mg) of edetate calcium disodium followed by measurement of 8-hour urine excretion of lead. Ratio of total urine lead (μg) divided by edetate infused (mgm) >0.6 is considered positive. Difficulty in collecting urine usually makes test obsolete; begin chelation if blood lead >45 μg/dL.

◆ Increased coproporphyrin in urine is a reliable sign of intoxication and is often demonstrable before basophilic stippling (but one should rule out a false-positive reaction due to drugs such as barbiturates and salicylates). This is a useful rapid screening test.

○ Anemia is common, is usually mild (rarely <9 gm/dL). Is normochromic, normocytic, or hypochromic and microcytic. Is often the first manifestation of chronic lead poisoning; due to decreased heme synthesis (Hb production) and increased hemolysis. In acute lead poisoning, hemolytic crisis may occur. Anemia may be seen at blood lead levels of 50 to 80 μg/dL in adults and 40 to 70 μg/dL in children.

Anisocytosis and poikilocytosis may be found, and a few nucleated RBCs may be seen. Some polychromasia is usual.

Stippled RBCs occur later in ~2% of cases (due to inhibition of 5'-pyramidine nucleotidase). Basophilic stippling is not pathognomonic of lead poisoning. Amount of stippling not correlated with severity of lead toxicity.

Bone marrow shows erythroid hyperplasia, and 65% of erythroid cells show stippling, some of which are ringed sideroblasts (thus this may be considered a secondary sideroblastic anemia).

Osmotic fragility is decreased, but mechanical fragility is increased.

Hematologic changes of lead poisoning are more marked in patients with iron deficiency.

Urine urobilinogen and uroporphyrin are increased.

Porphobilinogen is normal or only slightly increased in urine (in contrast to acute intermittent porphyria).

Renal proximal tubular damage occurs, with Fanconi syndrome (hypophosphatemia, aminoaciduria, and glycosuria), usually in very severe or very chronic cases. Albuminuria, increased WBC, and transient rising BUN may occur. With chronic exposure, interstitial nephritis develops with increased serum uric acid (saturnine gout); is most frequent renal finding.

CSF protein is increased, and frequently ≤100 mononuclear cells/cu mm are present in encephalopathy, which is rare with blood lead <100 μg/dL.

In children, acute encephalopathy may be seen with blood lead ≥80 μg/dL; abdominal and GI symptoms may occur with levels of 50 μg/dL but usually indicate levels ≥70 μg/dL.

Laboratory changes due to drug therapy using dimercaprol (BAL)

- Check daily for hematuria, proteinuria, cast formation
- Check every other day for hypokalemia and hypercalcemia
- Rule out G6PD deficiency and liver disease before starting therapy

Lipid-Lowering Drugs, Side Effects

Statins (e.g., Lipitor)

- Increased ALT, AST

Nicotinic acid may cause

- Dramatic lowering (often) of blood triglyceride in hyperlipidemia, Types II and IV and probably also Types III and V
- Increased blood sugar
- Increased blood uric acid
- Abnormal liver function tests
- Jaundice (rarely)

Cholestyramine in the form of a chloride salt may cause

- Lowering of cholesterol in familial Type II hyperlipidemia
- Mild hyperchloremic acidosis

Mercury Poisoning[11]

Due To

Methyl mercury: Consumption of fish high up on food chain (e.g., salt water—sharks, swordfish, tuna; fresh water—pike, bass). EPA has reduced safe daily intake from 0.5 μg/kg body weight to 0.1 μg/kg body weight.

[11]Clarkson TW, et al. The toxicology of mercury—current exposures and clinical manifestations. *N Engl J Med* 2003;349:1731.

PHYS/CHEM

Ethyl mercury: Ingredient of preservative thimerosal used in vaccines.
Inorganic mercury: Dental amalgams causes vapor inhalation (causes urine level = 2–4 μg/L; increased by excessive chewing.). Occupational exposure or home exposure levels = 20–50 μg/L.
♦ *Concentrations*
Levels of mercury in serum, urine, and CSF are increased.
95% of asymptomatic normal people (not exposed to mercury) have a urine value <20 μg/L and blood level <3 μg/L. Urine and blood levels are nondiagnostic, in that they vary among patients with symptoms, and daily urine levels vary in the same patient. Thus in one epidemic, urine levels ≤1,000 μg/L occurred in asymptomatic patients, whereas other patients had symptoms at levels of 200 μg/L. The above values apply to mercury vapor and inorganic mercury salts.
Organic mercury (e.g., ethyl and methyl mercury) is more toxic; accumulates in RBCs and CNS. Most is slowly excreted in feces with half-life of 70 days. Only 10% is excreted in urine; urine levels may be normal even with significant exposure. Phenyl and methoxyethyl mercuries are less toxic and show higher urine levels.
Clinical correlation with organic mercury

	Whole Blood Total Mercury (μg/L or ng/mL or ppm)
Safe level	<10; urine <30 ng/mL
Probably no symptoms; recheck periodically	100–200
Symptoms occasionally present	>650
Symptoms usually present; toxic	>1000

Methemoglinemia

See Chapter 11.

Milk Sickness ("Trembles")

Poisoning from goldenrod, snakeroot, richweed, etc., or from eating poisoned animals

Acidosis
Hypoglycemia
Increased NPN (particularly guanidine)
Acetonuria

Mothballs (Camphor, Paradichlorobenzene, Naphthalene)

Produced synthetically from turpentine

Paradichlorobenzene inhalation may cause liver damage.
Naphthalene ingestion may cause hemolytic anemia in patients with RBCs deficient in glucose-6-PD.

Organophosphorus Insecticides (e.g., Parathion, Malathion, etc.)

Irreversibly binds and inhibits acetylcholinesterase and other serine hydrolases [e.g., pseudocholinesterase, RBC cholinesterase]

♦ RBC and serum acetylcholinesterase (AChE) decreased by ≥50% due to inhibition of AChE by organic phosphate pesticides (e.g., diazinon, malathion) and carbamates (e.g., carbaryl)

• Decrease in serum of 30% to 50% when first symptoms of acute ingestion appear
• Decrease in serum of 80% when neuromuscular effects occur
• Chronic low level exposure may be asymptomatic even with decreased levels

♦ RBC assay is surrogate marker and better reflects AChE activity in nerve tissue (synaptic AChE inhibition) than serum assay.
Workers experiencing industrial exposure should not return to work until these values rise to >75% of normal. RBC AChE regenerates at rate of 0.5% to 1% per day and returns to baseline in 5 to 7 weeks. Serum AChE regenerates at rate of 25% in 7 to 10 days and returns to baseline in 4 to 6 weeks.

Because of wide normal range, patient may lose 50% of their cholinesterase activity and still be within normal range. Therefore baseline levels should be determined for all workers at risk with organophosphates or carbamates. A decrease of 30% to 50% from baseline indicates toxicity even if still within normal range.

Without baseline levels, retrospective diagnosis by serial measurements that increase after exposure

Normal variation of ±20% in serum activity and ±10% in RBC activity prevents assessment of mild toxicity and recovery by only one or two assays.

Nonketotic hyperglycemia and glucosuria are common.

Serum amylase increase may reflect pancreatitis.

Serum cholinesterase may also be decreased in

- Liver diseases
    Especially hepatitis (30%–50% decrease). Lowest level corresponds to peak of disease and becomes normal with recovery.
    Cirrhosis with ascites or jaundice (50%–70% decrease). Persistent decrease may indicate a poor prognosis.
    Some patients with metastatic carcinoma (50%–70% decrease), obstructive jaundice, congestive heart failure
- Congenital inherited recessive decrease. Such patients are *particularly sensitive to administration of succinylcholine during anesthesia.*
- Some conditions that may have decreased serum albumin (e.g., malnutrition, amenia, infections, dermatomyositis, acute myocardial infarction, pregnancy, recent surgery, liver diseases—see above)
- Other drugs (e.g., prostigmine, quinine, fluoride, neostigmine, tetramethylammonium chloride, carbamate insecticides)

Oxalate Poisoning

Due to ingestion of stain remover or ink eradicator containing oxalic acid

Hypocalcemic tetany due to formation of insoluble calcium oxalate that may precipitate in various organs

Normal blood level = 1.4 to 2.4 mg/L

Normal urine excretion = 8 to 40 mg/day; >40 to 50 mg/day indicates occupational or other exposure

Toxic oral lethal dose = 15 to 30 g

Phenacetin—Chronic Excessive Ingestion

Laboratory findings due to increased incidence of peptic ulceration, especially of stomach, often with bleeding, may be present.

♦ Laboratory findings associated with increased incidence of papillary necrosis and interstitial nephritis may be present.

- Proteinuria is slight or absent.
- Hematuria is often present in active papillary necrosis.
- WBC is increased in urine in absence of infection.
- Papillae are passed in urine.
- Creatinine clearance is decreased.
- Renal failure may occur.

Anemia is common and frequently precedes azotemia.

Phenol and Lysol Poisoning

Severe acidosis often occurs.

Acute tubular necrosis may develop.

Phenytoin Sodium (Dilantin) Therapy, Complications

Megaloblastic anemia may occur. It is completely responsive to folic acid (even when Dilantin therapy is continued) but not always to vitamin B_{12}. Is the most common hematologic complication.

Rarely pancytopenia, thrombocytopenia alone, or leukopenia, including agranulocytosis may occur.

PHYS/CHEM

Laboratory findings of hepatitis may be present.
Laboratory findings resembling those of malignant lymphomas may be present.
Laboratory findings resembling those of infectious mononucleosis may occur, but heterophil agglutination is not increased.
Increased T_3 uptake, but RAIU, serum cholesterol, etc., are normal (because of competition for binding sites of thyroxin-binding globulin).
Dilantin therapy may induce a lupus-like syndrome.

Phosphorus (Yellow) Poisoning

Used in rat poisons; damage by thermal injury and general protoplasmic poisoning

No single test confirms the diagnosis.
Liver, kidney, and CNS are injured. Acute yellow atrophy of liver may occur.
Vomitus may glow in the dark and have a garlic odor.

Potassium Chloride, Enteric-Coated

Laboratory findings due to small-intestine ulceration, obstruction, or perforation

Procainamide Therapy

♦ Procainamide therapy may induce the findings of SLE. Positive serologic tests for SLE are very frequent, especially in dosage of ≥1.25 gm/day, and may precede clinical manifestations.

• LE cell tests become positive in 50% of patients.
• Anti-DNP tests become positive in 65% of patients.
• Anti-DNA tests become positive in 35% of patients.
• One of these tests becomes positive in 75% of patients.

Perform serologic tests for SLE on all patients receiving procainamide.

Salicylate Intoxication

Due to aspirin, sodium salicylate, oil of wintergreen, methylsalicylate

♦ Increased serum salicylate (correlation does not apply to chronic ingestion or enteric-coated aspirin)

• >10 mg/dL when symptoms are present
• 19 to 45 mg/dL when tinnitus is first noted
• >40 mg/dL when hyperventilation is present
• At ~50 mg/dL, severe toxicity with acid-base imbalance and ketosis
• At 45 to 70 mg/dL, death
• >100 mg/dL, hemodialysis indicated

Peak serum level is reached 2 hours after therapeutic and at least 6 hours after toxic dose. Serum levels drawn <6 hours after ingestion cannot be used to predict severity of toxic reaction using Dones nomogram although they will confirm salicylate overdose. Dones nomogram cannot be used for enteric-coated aspirin.

• 15 to 30 mg/dL for optimal anti-inflammatory effect; 5 to 27 mg/dL in patients with rheumatoid arthritis on dose of 65 mg/kg/day

When awaiting laboratory measurement, can estimate peak salicylate levels:

$$\text{mg/dL of salicylate} = \frac{(\text{mg of salicylate ingested})}{70\% \text{ of body weight (in g)}^*} \times 100$$

* = Total body water

In older children and adults, serum salicylate level corresponds well with severity; in younger children, correlation is more variable.
Gastric lavage may increase salicylate level <10 mg/dL.
Early, serum electrolytes and CO_2 are normal.
Early respiratory alkalosis followed by metabolic acidosis; 20% of patients have either one alone.

Later, progressive decrease in serum sodium and pCO_2 occurs. 80% of patients have combined primary respiratory alkalosis and primary metabolic acidosis; change in blood pH reflects the net result. (*Infants may show immediate metabolic acidosis with the usual initial respiratory alkalosis. In older children and adults, the typical picture is respiratory alkalosis.*)
Hypokalemia accompanies the respiratory alkalosis. Dehydration occurs.
○ Urine shows paradoxic acid pH despite the increased serum bicarbonate.

* Ferric chloride test is positive on boiled as well as unboiled urine (thus differentiating salicylate from ketone bodies); it may have a false-positive result because of phenacetin.
* Tests for glucose (e.g., Clinistix), reducing substances (e.g., Clinitest), or ketone bodies (e.g., Ketostix) are positive. All positive urine screening tests should be confirmed by serum sample.
* RBCs may be present.
* Number of renal tubular cells is increased because of renal irritation.

Hypoglycemia occurs, especially in infants on restricted diet and in diabetics.
Serum AST and ALT may be increased.
Hypoprothrombinemia after some days of intensive salicylate therapy is temporary and occasional; rarely causes hemorrhage.
Hydroxyproline is decreased in serum and urine.
Monitor patient by following blood glucose, potassium, pH.

Steroids, Side Effects That Cause Laboratory Changes

Endocrine effects (e.g., adrenal insufficiency after prolonged use, suppression of pituitary or thyroid function, development of diabetes mellitus)
Increased susceptibility to infections
Gastrointestinal effects (e.g., peptic ulcer, perforation of bowel, infarction of bowel, pancreatitis)
Musculoskeletal effects (e.g., osteoporosis, pathologic fractures, arthropathy, myopathy)
Decreased serum potassium, increased WBC, glycosuria, ecchymoses, etc.

Theophylline

Bronchodilator used for treatment and prevention of asthma

Therapeutic range: 10 to 20 μg/mL (adults), 5–20 μg/mL (children); <5 μg/mL is usually ineffective
Toxic concentration: >20 μg/mL is toxic in 75% of persons
Concentrations are usually measured at peak rather than trough.
Peak occurs 2 hours after oral standard form and about 5 hours after sustained release form.

Vitamins

Hypervitaminosis A

Acute intoxication after ingestion of 150 to 600 mg (500,000–2,000,000 IU)
Chronic hypervitaminosis after ingestion of 7.5 to 90 mg/day (25,000–300,000 IU) for minimum of 1 month up to 2 years
♦ Plasma vitamin A = 300 to 1,000 μg/dL
♦ Increased tissue levels of vitamin A and retinoic acid derivatives
May also show

* Increased ESR
* Increased serum ALP, GGT, bilirubin
* Decreased serum albumin
* Decreased Hb
* Slight protoinuria
* Slightly increased serum carotene
* Increased PT

Abnormal liver biopsy

Vitamin D Intoxication

See Chapter 13.

18

Therapeutic Drug Monitoring and Drug Effects

The determination of toxic and effective therapeutic concentration of drugs has become one of the most important and widely used functions of the laboratory. In the past, drugs were measured by their effects (e.g., warfarin prolonged prothrombin time, antimicrobials inhibited growth of microorganisms). Newer methodologies now permit determinations of drug concentrations in the blood that were previously impossible or not available.

The clinician must be aware of the various influences on pharmacokinetics—factors such as half-life, time to peak and to steady state, protein binding, and excretion—that are not within the province of this book but are useful for the physician in prescribing these drugs appropriately.

The route of administration and sampling time after last dose of drug must be known for proper interpretation. For some drugs (e.g., quinidine), different assay methods produce different values, and the clinician must know the normal range for the test method used for the patient.

In general, peak concentrations alone are useful when testing for toxicity, and trough concentrations alone are useful for demonstrating a satisfactory therapeutic concentration. Trough concentrations are commonly used with such drugs as lithium, theophylline, phenytoin, carbamazepine, quinidine, tricyclic antidepressants, valproic acid, and digoxin. Trough concentrations can usually be drawn at the time the next dose is administered *(this does not apply to digoxin)*. Both peak and trough concentrations are used to avoid toxicity but ensure bactericidal efficacy (e.g., gentamicin, tobramycin, vancomycin). IV and IM administration should usually be sampled 1/2 to 1 hour after administration is ended to determine peak concentration.

Concentrations are meant only as a general guide; the laboratory performing the tests should supply its own values.

Blood should be drawn at a time specified by that laboratory (e.g., 1 hour before the next dose is due to be administered). This trough concentration should ideally be greater than the minimum effective serum concentration.

If a drug is administered by IV infusion, blood should be drawn from the opposite arm. The drug should have been administered at a constant rate for at least 4 to 5 half-lives before blood samples are drawn.

Unexpected test results may be due to interference by complementary and alternative medicines (e.g., high digoxin levels may result from interference from danshen, Chan Su, or ginseng).

TDM/DRUG EF

Indications for Therapeutic Drug Monitoring

Symptoms or signs of toxicity
Therapeutic effect not obtained
Suspected noncompliance
Drug has narrow therapeutic range
To provide or confirm an optimal dosing schedule
To confirm cause of organ toxicity (e.g., abnormal liver or kidney function tests)
Other diseases or conditions exist that affect drug utilization
Drug interactions that have altered desired or previously achieved therapeutic concentration are suspected
Drug shows large variations in utilization or metabolism between individuals
Need medicolegal verification of treatment, cause of death or injury (e.g., suicide, homicide, accident investigation), detect use of forbidden drugs (e.g., steroids in athletes, narcotics)
Differential diagnosis of coma

Criteria for Therapeutic Drug Monitoring

Available methodology must be specific and reliable.
Blood concentration must correlate with therapeutic and toxic effects.
Therapeutic window is narrow with danger of toxicity on therapeutic doses.
Correlation between blood concentration and dose is poor.
Clinical effect of drug is not easily determined.

Drugs for Which Drug Monitoring May Be Useful

Antiepileptic drugs (e.g., phenobarbital, phenytoin [Dilantin])
Theophylline
Antimicrobials (aminoglycosides [gentamicin, tobramycin, amikacin], chloramphenicol, vancomycin, flucytosine [5-fluorocytosine])
Antipsychotic drugs
Antianxiety drugs
Cyclic antidepressants
Lithium
Cardiac glycosides, antiarrhythmics, antianginal, antihypertensive drugs
Antineoplastic drugs
Immunosuppressant drugs
Antiinflammatory drugs (e.g., NSAIDs, steroids)
Hematologic drugs (e.g., erythropoietin [see Chapter 11], iron, folate, B_{12})
Total parenteral nutrition
At present, four drugs (digoxin, phenytoin, phenobarbital, theophylline) account for ~50% of drug monitoring
Cannabinoids, other drugs of abuse
Athletic performance enhancement drugs (e.g., androgenic anabolic steroids, erythropoietin)

Antiarrhythmic Agents and Cardiovascular Drugs

Antihypertensive Drugs (Apresoline [Hydralazine Hydrochloride])

There is little correlation between plasma concentration and clinical effect.
Anemia and pancytopenia occur infrequently.
❍ Prolonged use causes a syndrome resembling SLE (see Chapter 16).

Digitoxin
Used to treat congestive heart failure and atrial fibrillation and flutter

Draw blood just before next dose or >6 hours after last dose.
Therapeutic range: 9 to 25 ng/mL
Toxicity is common with concentration >30 ng/mL.

Table 18-1.	Examples of Reported Reference Ranges of Some Common Drugs	
	Therapeutic Concentration	Toxic Concentration
Antimicrobial Drugs		
Amikacin		
Peak	20–25 mg/L	30 mg/L
Trough	5–10 mg/L	10 mg/L
Chloramphenicol		
Peak	15–25 mg/L	30 mg/L
Trough	5–10 mg/L	15 mg/L
Gentamicin		
Peak	4–8 mg/L	8 mg/L
Trough	1–2 mg/L	2 mg/L
Kanamycin		
Peak	20–25 mg/L	
Trough	5–10 mg/L	
Netilmicin		
Peak	4–8 mg/L	8 mg/L
Trough	1–2 mg/L	2 mg/L
Streptomycin		
Peak	5–20 mg/L	40 mg/L
Trough	<5 mg/L	40 mg/L
Tobramycin		
Peak	5–8 mg/L	8 mg/L
Trough		>2 mg/L
TMP/SMX (Trimethoprim/sulfamethoxazole)		
Peak (trimethoprim)	4–8 mg/L	8 mg/L
Peak (sulfamethoxazole)	1–2 mg/L	>2 mg/L
Vancomycin		
Peak not recommended		
Trough	5–10 mg/L	>40 mg/L
Analgesics		
Acetaminophen (e.g., Anacin, Dristan, Excedrin, Tylenol)	<50 mg/L	>120 mg/L
Salicylates	150–300 mg/L (adults)	>300 mg/L
Anticonvulsants		
Carbamazepine	8–10 mg/L	>12 mg/L
Ethosuximide	40–70 mg/L	100 mg/L
Phenobarbital	20–40 mg/L (adults)	>55 mg/L
	15–30 mg/L (children)	
Pentobarbital (for reducing intracranial pressure)	30–40 mg/L	
Phenytoin (Dilantin)	10–20 mg/L (total)	≥20 mg/L (total)
	1–2 mg/L (free)	≥2.0 mg/L (free)
Primidone (should be assayed with metabolite phenobarbital)	5–12 mg/L (adults)	≥15 mg/L
	7–10 mg/L (children <5 years old)	
Valproic acid	50–120 mg/L	500 mg/L
Bronchodilators		
Caffeine (diet)	15 mg/L	60 mg/L
Theophylline	10–20 mg/L (adults)	>20 mg/L
	5–20 mg/L (children)	
Cardiovascular Drugs		
Amiodarone	1.5–2.5 mg/L	>3.5 mg/L
Dicoumarol (warfarin)	2–5 mg/L	>10 mg/L
Digitoxin	9–25 ng/mL	>30 ng/mL
Digoxin	0.5–2.0 ng/mL	>2.5 ng/mL
Lidocaine (Xylocaine)	2–5 mg/L	≥6.0 mg/L

(continued)

TDM/DRUG EF

Table 18-1. *(continued)*		
	Therapeutic Concentration	Toxic Concentration
Procainamide should be assayed with NAPA	4–8 mg/L	12 mg/L
N-Acetyl Procainamide (NAPA)	<30 mg/L	>30 mg/L
Propranolol	50–100 ng/mL	≥1,000 ng/mL
Quinidine (P)	2–5 mg/L	>7.0 mg/L
Warfarin	7 mg/L	10 mg/L
Immunosuppressants		
Cyclosporine (WB)	0.4 mg/L	
Sirolimus (whole blood)	3.0–18.0 ng/mL (trough)	>18.0 ng/mL
Psychotropic Drugs		
Amitriptyline + Nortriptyline	75–225 ng/mL	>500 ng/mL
Nortriptyline only	50–150 ng/mL	>500 ng/mL
Chlordiazepoxide (Librium)	5–10 mg/L	≥15 mg/L
Chlorpromazine (Thorazine)	>50 ng/mL	>1,500 ng/mL
Desipramine	0.3 mg/L	
Diazepam (Valium)	0.2–0.8 mg/L	
Nordiazepam	0.2–1.0 mg/L	
Total for both	0.4–1.8 mg/L	≥5.0 mg/L
Doxepin	0.3 mg/L	1.0 mg/L
Lithium	0.8–1.2 mEq/L	≥1.5 mEq/L

Digoxin

Used to treat congestive heart failure and atrial fibrillation and flutter

Draw blood 6 to 8 hours (or 8–24 hrs) after last oral dose after steady state has been achieved in 1–2 weeks

Therapeutic range: 0.5 to 2.0 ng/mL

Toxic range: >2.5 ng/mL but 10% of patients may show toxicity at <2 ng/mL

- Pediatric toxic concentration may be higher. Therapeutic index is very low (i.e., small difference between therapeutic and toxic blood concentration). However, ~10% of patients have serum concentration 2 to 4 ng/mL without evidence of toxicity. On dose of 0.25 mg/day, mean serum concentration = 1.2 ± 0.4 ng/mL; on dose of 0.5 mg/day, mean serum concentration = 1.5 ± 0.4 ng/mL; on dose of 0.1 mg/day, mean serum concentration = 17 ± 6 ng/mL. Digitalis leaf dose of 0.1 gm/day produces same serum concentration as 0.1 mg/day of crystalline digitoxin. ECG evidence of toxicity in one third to two thirds of patients with no symptoms or signs.

Toxicity may occur at lower blood concentration in presence of hypokalemia, hypercalcemia, hypomagnesemia, hypoxia, chronic heart disease.

Some drugs that may cause increased digoxin blood concentration: quinidine, verapamil, amiodarone, indomethacin, cyclosporine A.

False low results may be due to spironolactone.

Endogenous digoxin-like substances may produce positive test results in persons who have not received the drug, especially in:

- Uremia
- Severe agonal states and postmortem—therefore, a high postmortem concentration may not have been high before death and a normal postmortem concentration suggests that the antemortem concentration was not toxic. Only high-performance liquid chromatography (HPLC) or mass spectrometry can definitively identify digoxin as a possible cause of death.

Because most methods measure both endogenous digoxin-like substances and inactive metabolites of digoxin, therapeutic monitoring should mostly be used to assess patient compliance and to confirm drug toxicity.

Amiodarone (Cordarone)/Desethylamiodarone
Used for supraventricular and some ventricular arrhythmias

Therapeutic range: 1.5 to 2.5 mg/L
Toxic concentration: ≥3.5 mg/L
Effect on other laboratory test values

- Abnormal TSH and T_4 values are common and should be monitored during therapy.
- Changes in laboratory results due to pulmonary fibrosis, which occurs in >2% of patients.

Drug interactions may increase the plasma concentration of digoxin, diltiazem, phenytoin, procainamide, quinidine.
Concentration may be increased by severe liver disease (amiodarone) or decreased renal function (desethylamiodarone).

Flecainide (Tambocor)
Used for ventricular arrhythmias

Therapeutic range: Trough plasma concentration of 0.2 to 1.0 mg/L
Toxic concentration: >1.0 mg/L

Lidocaine (Xylocaine)
Used for prevention and treatment of ventricular arrhythmias

Draw blood 12 hours after beginning therapy.
Indications for monitoring

- Repeat every 12 hours when drug clearance is altered by liver disease, heart failure, acute myocardial infarction
- Suspected toxicity
- Ventricular arrhythmias occur despite therapy

Therapeutic range: 1.4 to 6 mg/L
Toxic concentration: 6 to 8 mg/L
Concentration may be falsely low if blood is collected in some rubber-stoppered tubes

Mexiletine (Mexitil)
Used for many cardiac arrhythmias, e.g., ventricular arrhythmias

Therapeutic range: Plasma trough concentration of 0.5 to 2.0 mg/L
Toxic concentration: >2.0 mg/L
Some drugs that may cause decreased plasma mexiletine concentration: Phenobarbital, phenytoin, rifampin

Procainamide (Pronestyl)
Used for ventricular and supraventricular arrhythmias

Is measured along with its active metabolite N-acetylprocainamide (NAPA)
Therapeutic range: Procainamide, 4 to 10 mg/L; NAPA, ≤30 mg/L; both, ≤30 mg/L
Toxic concentration: Procainamide, 10 to 12 mg/L, NAPA, >30 mg/L
○ May cause drug-induced lupus with antihistone antibodies in 95% of cases, especially in dosage of ≥1.25 g/day, and may precede clinical manifestations (see Chapter 16).
Perform serologic tests for SLE on all patients receiving procainamide.

Quinidine
Used for ventricular and supraventricular arrhythmias

Therapeutic range: 2.0 to 5.0 mg/L
Toxic concentration: >6.0 mg/L

Tocainide (Tonocard)
Used for long term use of lidocaine-responsive ventricular arrhythmias

Therapeutic range: Plasma concentration of 5–12 mg/L
Toxic concentration: ≥15 mg/L (peak)

TDM/DRUG EF

Effect on other laboratory test values

- ANA antibodies or lupus syndrome is rare (in contrast to procainamide)
- Agranulocytosis is rare
- Hepatitis

Diltiazem

Calcium channel blocker used for angina pectoris and hypertension

Therapeutic range: Plasma concentration 40 to 200 ng/mL
Effect of diltiazem on other laboratory tests: Increased bleeding time due to platelet dysfunction

Nifedipine

Calcium channel blocker used for angina pectoris and hypertension

Therapeutic range: Serum concentration 25 to 100 ng/mL
Effect on other laboratory tests: Decreased glucose tolerance in normal and diabetic patients
The concentration of some drugs may be increased by nifedipine (e.g., digoxin).

Verapamil (Calan) or Norverapamil

Calcium channel blocker used for supraventricular dysrhythmias, angina pectoris, hypertension

Therapeutic range: Serum concentration 50 to 200 ng/mL (peak).
Toxic concentration: ≥400 ng/mL (peak)
Some drug concentrations that may be increased by verapamil: carbamazepine, digoxin
Rifampin may decrease verapamil serum concentration.

Anticonvulsants

Used for treatment of seizure disorders

Carbamazepine (Tegretol)

Therapeutic range: 4 to 12 mg/L
Toxic concentration: >12 mg/L

Phenobarbital (Luminal)

Also a long-acting sedative-hypnotic drug

Draw blood just before next oral dose, after steady state has occurred (11–25 days in adults; 8–15 days in children).
Therapeutic range: 10 to 40 mg/L in adults; 15 to 30 mg/L in children
Toxic concentration: >40 mg/L
Monitoring is indicated when patients are poorly controlled, have toxic symptoms, or 2 to 3 weeks after change in dose or drug (e.g., primidone and mephobarbital, which are metabolized to phenobarbital).
Valproic acid may cause increased serum concentrations.

Phenytoin (Dilantin)

Monitoring therapeutic oral maintenance in seizure disorders

Patient should be on stable dose for at least 1 week; draw blood just before next dose. Draw trough sample 1 week after beginning treatment and again in 3 to 5 weeks. After IV administration, draw blood 2 to 4 hours after loading dose.
Therapeutic drug monitoring (TDM) is indicated when

- Medication or dosage has changed (allow 1 week to reach steady state)
- Seizures are poorly controlled

- Toxic symptoms occur
- Patients are children (10–13 years old); monitor every 3 to 4 months until stable concentration occurs

Therapeutic range: Total = 10 to 20 mg/L; free = 1 to 2 mg/L

Toxic concentration: total ≥20 mg/L; free ≥2.0 mg/L

May be artifactually increased in uremia by various methods (e.g., immunoassay) compared to HPLC

Therapeutic or toxic effects may occur at a lower blood concentration in presence of decreased serum albumin, increased bilirubin, increased BUN.

Some drugs that may cause increased phenytoin blood concentration: Isoniazid, phenylbutazone, bishydroxycoumarin, diazepam, and chlorpromazine.

Some drugs that may cause decreased phenytoin blood concentration: Ethanol, valproic acid, and carbamazepine.

Effect on other laboratory tests: Decreased serum-free testosterone and increased total testosterone

Not altered by dialysis

Complications

Megaloblastic anemia may occur. It is completely responsive to folic acid (even when Dilantin therapy is continued) but not always to vitamin B_{12}. Is the most common hematologic complication.

Rarely pancytopenia, thrombocytopenia alone, or leukopenia, including agranulocytosis may occur.

Laboratory findings of hepatitis may be present.

Laboratory findings resembling those of malignant lymphomas may be present.

Laboratory findings resembling those of infectious mononucleosis may occur, but heterophil agglutination is not increased.

Increased T_3 uptake, but RAIU, serum cholesterol, etc., are normal (because of competition for binding sites of thyroxin-binding globulin).

Dilantin therapy may induce a lupuslike syndrome.

Newer anticonvulsants include topiramate, lamotrigine (Lamictal), gabapentin (Neurontin), and felbamate—used when response to other anticonvulsants is not optimal.

Antiinflammatory and Nonsteroidal Drugs (NSAIDs)

Includes

- Salicylates (aspirin, diflunisal) and acetaminophen (Tylenol) are analgesic and antipyretic. Aspirin is also used as anticoagulant.
- Acetaminophen is not a useful anti-inflammatory.
- Propionic acids (ibuprofen [Motrin], diclofenac, naproxen [Naprosyn], oxicams, piroxicam)
- Indoleacetic acids (indomethacin, sulindac)

Except for salicylates, serum concentration does not correlate with drug effects, therapeutic ranges have not been established, and routine drug monitoring is not clinically useful.

TDM of salicylates is indicated because of:

- Unreliability of clinical symptoms (e.g., tinnitus) as an indication of toxicity
- Narrow anti-inflammatory
  Therapeutic range: 150 to 300 mg/L
  Toxic concentration: >300 mg/L
- Intraindividual variation of up to 300%
- Drug interaction may significantly lower serum salicylate concentration (e.g., antacids, ACTH, prednisone)
- After 4 weeks of therapy, serum salicylate concentrations decline to 65% to 80% of 1-week concentration.

Acetaminophen Poisoning (Tylenol)

♦ Blood levels
- Therapeutic range: 10 to 30 mg/L

- Toxic concentration: >200 mg/L
- 200 mg/L within 4 hours after ingestion or >50 mg/L at 12 hours predicts severe liver damage, and treatment with acetylcysteine should begin.
- <150 mg/L at 4 hours or <30 to 35 mg/L at 12 hours indicates no liver damage will occur.
- Toxicity is dose dependent but exaggerated by starvation and drugs, *especially alcohol.*
- *Liver toxicity cannot be predicted from blood levels earlier than 4 hours.*
- *Exact time of ingestion is often difficult to ascertain.*
- *Patients taking other drugs or with concomitant cirrhosis may develop liver toxicity at different blood levels.*
- *Toxicity is less common in children <5 years old, and changes in liver function tests may be mild when serum drug levels are in toxic range.*

With hepatotoxicity (see Acute Hepatic Failure, Chapter 8)

- During first 12 to 24 hours, increased AST and ALT are found in only ~50% of patients and serum drug levels are the chief guide to therapy; this is the only stage when treatment can prevent liver damage.
- During next 24 to 48 hours, AST, ALT, serum bilirubin, and prothrombin time are increased. AST and ALT are very high (typically >4,000 U/L, often >10,000 U/L). AST/ALT ratio <2 in ~90% of cases.
- On third to fourth day, liver function abnormalities peak; hypoglycemia, secondary renal failure may occur.

Salicylate Intoxication

Aspirin is used as analgesic, antiinflammatory, antipyretic, anticoagulant; due to aspirin, sodium salicylate. Oil of wintergreen [methylsalicylate] is used for local skin application.

Therapeutic range: 150 to 300 mg/L
Toxic concentration: >300 mg/L
♦ Increased serum salicylate (correlation does not apply to chronic ingestion or enteric-coated aspirin)
- >10 mg/L when symptoms are present
- 19 to 45 mg/L when tinnitus is first noted
- >40 mg/L when hyperventilation is present
- At ~50 mg/L, severe toxicity with acid-base imbalance and ketosis
- At 45–70 mg/L, death
- >100 mg/L, hemodialysis is indicated

Peak serum level is reached 2 hours after therapeutic and at least 6 hours after toxic dose.
Serum levels drawn <6 hours after ingestion cannot be used to predict severity of toxic reaction using Dones nomogram although they will confirm salicylate overdose. Dones nomogram cannot be used for enteric-coated aspirin.

- 15 to 30 mg/L for optimal antiinflammatory effect; 5 to 27 mg/L in patients with rheumatoid arthritis on dose of 65 mg/kg/day

When awaiting laboratory measurement, can estimate peak salicylate levels as follows:

$$\text{mg/L of salicylate} = \frac{\text{(mg of salicylate ingested)}}{70\% \text{ of body weight (in g)*}} \times 100$$

* = Total body water

In older children and adults, serum salicylate level corresponds well with severity; in younger children, correlation is more variable.
Gastric lavage may increase salicylate level <10 mg/L.
In early phase, serum electrolytes and CO_2 are normal.
Early respiratory alkalosis followed by metabolic acidosis; 20% of patients have either one alone.
Later, progressive decrease in serum sodium and pCO_2 occurs. 80% of patients have combined primary respiratory alkalosis and primary metabolic acidosis; change in

blood pH reflects the net result. *(Infants may show immediate metabolic acidosis with the usual initial respiratory alkalosis. In older children and adults, the typical picture is respiratory alkalosis.)*
Hypokalemia accompanies the respiratory alkalosis. Dehydration occurs.
Urine shows paradoxic acid pH despite the increased serum bicarbonate.

- Ferric chloride test is positive on boiled as well as unboiled urine (thus differentiating salicylate from ketone bodies); it may have a false-positive result because of phenacetin.
- Tests for glucose (e.g., Clinistix), reducing substances (e.g., Clinitest), or ketone bodies (e.g., Ketostix) are positive. All positive urine screening tests should be confirmed by serum sample.
- RBCs may be present.
- Number of renal tubular cells is increased because of renal irritation.

Hypoglycemia occurs, especially in infants on restricted diet and in diabetics.
Serum AST and ALT may be increased.
Hypoprothrombinemia after some days of intensive salicylate therapy is temporary and occasional; rarely causes hemorrhage.
Hydroxyproline is decreased in serum and urine.
Monitor patient by following blood glucose, potassium, pH.

Phenacetin, Chronic Excessive Ingestion
Analgesic often used for various types of arthritis

Laboratory findings due to increased incidence of peptic ulceration, especially of stomach, often with bleeding, may be present.
○ Laboratory findings associated with increased incidence of papillary necrosis and interstitial nephritis may be present.
- Proteinuria is slight or absent.
- Hematuria is often present in active papillary necrosis.
- WBC is increased in urine in absence of infection.
- Papillae are passed in urine.
- Creatinine clearance is decreased.
- Renal failure may occur.

Anemia due to bleeding is common and frequently precedes azotemia.

Antineoplastic Drugs

Despite the large number of classes and drugs available, monitoring is clinically useful in the following instance and the clinical result is improved only with methotrexate:

Methotrexate
Folic acid antagonist antimetabolite; also used as immunosuppressant to treat psoriasis, RA, some collagen vascular diseases

Therapeutic concentration: $\leq 1.0 \times 10^{-7}$ mol/L
Toxic concentration: 1.0×10^{-5}, 1.0×10^{-6}, 1.0×10^{-7} mol/L at 24, 48 and 72 hours respectively

Immunosuppressant Drugs

Cyclosporine
Used as immunosuppressant to prevent rejection of organ [heart. kidney, liver] and marrow transplants. Possible use in graft-versus-host disease and treatment of autoimmune diseases. Acts by selective inhibition of certain T-lymphocytes; does not affect granulocytes. Often used in combination with corticosteroids.

TDM/DRUG EF

Initial oral dose 4 to 12 hours prior to transplantation surgery. Oral dose needs to be decreased (e.g., 5%) during the following weeks or months to maintain constant blood concentration. Half-life = 4 to 6 hours. Peak concentration 2 to 6 hours after oral dose. Trough concentration 12 to 18 hours after maintenance oral dose but longer after initial oral dose. Trough concentration about 12 hours after one IV dose.

Therapeutic range: 100 to 300 ng/mL (trough) in whole blood for kidney transplants. No immunosuppression with trough whole blood <100 ng/mL. For first weeks after transplantation, rejection occurs with trough values <170 ng/mL; quiescence is usually maintained at ≥200 ng/mL; requirements diminish to 50 to75 ng/mL by about 3 months and are maintained for rest of patient's life.

Monitoring: Draw blood just before next dose (trough concentration). Periodic monitoring (e.g., daily for liver transplant, three times per week for kidney transplant) should be performed, but this is not recommended as a stat procedure.

Threshold for renal toxicity: ≥400 ng/mL in whole blood. Nephrotoxicity occurs in up to half of renal transplant cases and about one thired of heart and liver transplant cases. Urine sediment unchanged.

- Nephrotoxicity includes four discrete syndromes:

    1. Delayed graft function in 10% of cases without cyclosporine and 35% of cases with cyclosporine therapy; resolves when cyclosporine is withdrawn
    2. Acute reversible functional impairment begins to occur at concentration of 200 ng/mL and is universal >400 ng/mL. Serum creatinine begins to rise 3 to 7 days after rise in cyclosporine and falls 2 to 14 days after cyclosporine is reduced. Decreased GFR, hyperkalemia, acidosis.
    3. Hemolytic-uremic syndrome
    4. Chronic nephropathy with interstitial fibrosis causes irreversible loss of renal function.

- Hepatotoxicity in 4% to 7% of cases is mild, transient, dose-related; is monitored by increased serum total bilirubin, AST, ALT, ALP, liver biopsy showing hepatocyte damage.
- Lymphoma and epithelial malignancy are uncommon (0.1%–0.4%); increase with combined immunosuppression.

Acute graft rejection occurs in 50% of patients after renal, heart, liver transplants. It may be difficult to differentiate from renal failure and renal biopsy may be indicated. Monitoring T-cell subsets is reported not useful by some while others have used rise in T4 and decline in T8 counts to reflect graft rejection. To distinguish nephrotoxicity from renal graft rejection, tests of complement-dependent cytotoxicity, antibody-dependent cell-mediated cytotoxicity and lymphocyte-mediated cytotoxicity to donor spleen cells obtained at time of donor nephrectomy. Also in bacterial or viral infection, all target cells are destroyed, but with graft rejection, only donor cells are destroyed.

RIA measures parent compound and certain metabolites; HPLC measures only parent compound. Serum concentrations are ~60% lower than whole blood.

Some drugs that may cause increased serum cyclosporine concentrations: amphotericin B, cimetidine, corticosteroids, diltiazem, erythromycin, furosemide, ketoconazole, nicardipine.

Some drugs that may cause decreased serum cyclosporine concentrations: carbamazepine, glutethimide, phenobarbital, phenytoin, rifampin with isoniazid, sulfadimidine, TMP/SMX.

Because cyclosporine contains ethanol, drug interactions may occur with: disulfiram (Antabuse), cefamandole, cefoperazone, chlorpropamide (Diabinase), metronidazole (Flagyl), moxalactam.

Sirolimus (Rapamycin; Rapamune)

Immunosuppressant used to prevent rejection of organ transplants; used synergistically with cyclosporine and corticosteroids

Therapeutic range: 3.0 to 18.0 ng/mL (trough) in whole blood
Toxic level: >18.0 ng/mL
Side effects: increased serum cholesterol, triglycerides, creatinine. Decreased GFR, WBCs, RBCs, platelets, potassium
Measured by LC/MS/MS

Flucytosine (5-Fluorocytosine)

Used as antimycotic agent [e.g., Cryptococcus neoformans, Candida] with amphotericin B

Therapeutic range: Serum concentration of 50 to 100 mg/L. Most susceptible organisms are killed at 0.5 to 12.5 mg/L concentrations. Serum and CSF fungistatic concentration of 10 to 40 mg/L. Bone marrow toxicity becomes prominent at serum concentration >125 mg/L or in presence of renal dysfunction.

In addition to drug monitoring, patients should be monitored for liver, kidney, and bone marrow toxicity.

Psychotropic Drugs

Haloperidol (Haldol)

Used for treatment of psychoses, Tourette syndrome, unresponsive hyperexcitable children

TDM is used to distinguish unresponsiveness from noncompliance or to detect high concentration in patients with abnormal liver function.

Therapeutic range: 5 to 16 ng/mL

Routine monitoring not indicated with good response to low-dose therapy.

Allow >1 week for steady state. Collect serum 12 hours after last dose.

Lithium

Used for treatment of mania, and as prophylaxis for manic and depressive episodes in bipolar disorders

Therapeutic concentration: 0.4 to 1.0 mEq/L based on serum trough concentration drawn 12 ± 1/2 hour after evening dose; significant time differences can be misleading. Blood should be drawn after steady state (3–10 days) has been achieved. About 25% of manic patients do not respond; concentration of 1.5 to 2.0 mEq/L can be tried if closely monitored. Patient compliance is a major problem in these patients.

Toxic concentration: >1.5 mEq/L; >3.0 mEq/L can be lethal

Thyroid and renal function tests should be monitored along with lithium concentration and clinical progress.

Peak concentration: 1 to 2 hours after lithium carbonate or citrate, 4 hours after slow-release preparations

Recommended blood screening tests before beginning lithium therapy: Sodium, potassium, calcium, phosphate, BUN, creatinine, TSH, T_4, CBC, urinalysis with specific gravity and osmolality

Some drugs that may cause increased serum lithium concentration: Indomethacin, hydrochlorothiazide, diclofenac

Some drugs that may cause decreased serum lithium concentration: Theophylline, aminophylline, acetazolamide, sodium bicarbonate, spironolactone, urea

Drug interactions (e.g., methyldopa, tetracycline) may cause lithium toxicity at low lithium concentration

Effect of lithium on other laboratory test values

- Increased TSH in 30% of patients (clinically euthyroid)
- Increased parathormone with resultant increased serum calcium and decreased phosphorus
- Decreased serum testosterone
- May affect TRH, growth hormone, ADH

Serum lithium values may be increased by

- Decreased glomerular filtration rate (GFR) (e.g., aging)
- Sodium deprivation and dehydration

Serum lithium values may be decreased

- By increased GFR (e.g., pregnancy, hemodialysis)
- In burn patients

TDM/DRUG EF

Tricyclic Antidepressants

TDM is usually requested because of lack of clinical response.

Utility is decreased by the lack of objective monitoring criteria, poor correlation of plasma concentration with clinical response, and the presence of active metabolites.

Some conditions that may increase tricyclic antidepressant plasma concentration: Aging, alcoholic liver disease, chloramphenicol, cimetidine, haloperidol, methylphenidate, renal failure

Some conditions that may decrease tricyclic antidepressant plasma concentration: barbiturates, chloral hydrate, smoking

Should maintain uniformity of collection (e.g., time related to last dose, serum versus plasma, type of container)

Pentobarbital

Short-acting sedative-hypnotic drug; has also been used to reduce intracranial pressure

Therapeutic range: 1 to 5 mg/L
Target for reducing intracranial pressure: 30 to 40 mg/L
Toxic concentration: ≥10 mg/L

Barbiturate Overdosage

♦ Correlation between serum concentrations of barbiturates and state of intoxication in patients who have taken only a short-acting barbiturate, who are not habitual drug users, and who have no medical complications:

<6 mg/L	Alert
6–10 mg/L	Drowsy
11–17 mg/L	Stuporous
16–20 mg/L	Coma 1
20–24 mg/L	Coma 2
24–28 mg/L	Coma 3
28–40 mg/L	Coma 4

If the serum drug level is less than expected for the state of intoxication, look for medical complications (e.g., aspiration pneumonia, head trauma) or presence of other drugs.

Other Drug Effects

Beta-Adrenergic Antagonists (Beta Blockers)

e.g., propanolol

Drug levels are not useful for determining overdosage.

Bromism

Should always be ruled out in the presence of mental symptoms or psychosis; found in "Alka-Seltzer"

Therapeutic concentration: 750 to 1,250 mg/L
Toxic concentration: >1,250 mg/L
♦ Serum and urine bromide levels are increased.
CSF protein is increased in acute bromide psychosis.
♦ False increase of serum "chloride" when measured by AutoAnalyzer. *If result of chloride determination with AutoAnalyzer is increased out of proportion to result with Cotlove coulimetric titrator, bromism should be ruled out.* Anion gap may be low or negative due to increased serum chloride.

Lipid-Lowering Drugs, Side Effects

Used to lower blood triglycerides, LDL-C, and total cholesterol

Various drugs may cause laboratory findings due to myopathy, rhabdomyolysis, abnormal liver function tests, increased blood sugar, and uric acid. The reader should consult pharmacology sources for more specific details.

Potassium Chloride, Enteric-Coated

Laboratory findings due to small intestine ulceration, obstruction, or perforation

Steroids, Side Effects That Cause Laboratory Changes

Multiple uses including immunosuppressant, antiinflammatory, hormone replacement

Endocrine effects (e.g., adrenal insufficiency, suppression of pituitary or thyroid function, development of diabetes mellitus)
Increased susceptibility to infections
Gastrointestinal effects (e.g., peptic ulcer, perforation of bowel, infarction of bowel, pancreatitis)
Musculoskeletal effects (e.g., osteoporosis, pathologic fractures, arthropathy, myopathy)
Decreased serum potassium, increased WBC, glycosuria, ecchymoses, etc.

Vitamin A Intoxication

Acute intoxication after ingestion of 150 to 600 mg (500,000–2,000,000 IU)
Chronic hypervitaminosis after ingestion of 7.5 to 90 mg/day (25,000–300,000 IU) for minimum of 1 month up to 2 years
♦ Plasma vitamin A = 300 to 1,000 mg/L
♦ Increased tissue levels of vitamin A and retinoic acid derivatives
May also show:

* Increased ESR
* Increased serum ALP, GGT, bilirubin
* Decreased serum albumin
* Decreased Hb
* Slight proteinuria
* Slightly increased serum carotene
* Increased PT

Abnormal liver biopsy

Vitamin D Intoxication

See Chapters 10 and 12.

19 Body Substances

Amniotic Fluid (AF)

See Chapter 14.
Normal values
Differentiation from urine (e.g., premature rupture of membranes)
Prenatal diagnosis of genetic disorders (see Chapter 13)
  Hypophosphatemia
  Sickle cell, thalassemia
  Coagulopathies
Hemolytic disease of newborn (see Chapter 11)
  Determine need for intrauterine transfusion
  Determine need for induced labor
Fetal/placental status
Diabetes mellitus (see Chapter 13)
Fetal lung maturity
Prenatal/neonatal infection (e.g., rubella, CMV, toxoplasmosis, syphilis, AIDS)
Amniotic fluid embolism (see Chapter 11)
Cell-free fetal messenger RNA (mRNA) can be detected in AF for gene expression changes in fetus.[1]

Ascitic Fluid

See Chapter 7.

Bile

See Chapter 8.
CEA in bile is increased in patients with cholangiocarcinoma and intrahepatic stones but not in patients with benign stricture, choledochal cysts, sclerosing cholangitis. Increases with progression of disease and declines with tumor resection. Does not correlate with serum bilirubin or ALP. Serum CEA is usually normal.
Crystals—types of calculi (see Choledocholithiasis, Chapter 8)

Breath

Tests

Helicobacter pylori (see Chapter 7)
Lactase deficiency (see Chapter 7)
Alcohol—breathalyzer (drunkometer) for DWI testing
Ratio of breath to blood alcohol = 0.00048:1
Malabsorption

Odors[2]	Possible Toxic Substance
Acetone	Acetone, isopropyl alcohol
	Metabolic acidosis (e.g., salicylates, diabetic ketoacidosis)
Airplane glue	Ethchlorvynol, toluene
Alcohol	Ethanol (no odor with vodka or ethylene glycol)
Ammonia	Ammonia (e.g., uremia)
Bitter almonds	Cyanide (half of population cannot detect this odor)
Bleach	Hypochlorite
Carrots	Cicutoxin of water hemlock
Coal gas	Illuminating gas of gas stoves, heating units
Disinfectant	Creosote, phenol
Formaldehyde	Formaldehyde, methanol
Foul odor	Bromides, lithium
	Foreign body in orifices
	Lung abscess
Garlic	Arsenic, dimethylsulfoxide, malathion, parathion, yellow phosphorus, selenium, tellurium, zinc phosphide

[1]Larrabee PB, et al. Global gene expression analysis of the living human fetus using cell-free messenger RNA in amniotic fluid. *JAMA* 2005;293:836.
[2]Viccellio P. *Handbook of medical toxicology.* Boston: Little, Brown, 1993.

Hemp	Marijuana
Mothballs	Camphor, naphthalene, paradichlorobenzene
Peanuts	Rodenticide (Vacor)
Pears	Chloral hydrate, paraldehyde
Rotten eggs	Sulfides (disulfiram, hydrogen sulfide), mercaptans, N-acetylcysteine
	Hepatic failure
Shoe polish	Nitrobenzene
Violets (urine)	Turpentine
Vinyl shower curtain	Ethchlorvynol
Wintergreen	Salicylate

Cerebrospinal Fluid

See Chapter 9.

Conjunctival Secretions

Smear (cytology)

Duodenal Contents

See Chapters 7 and 8.

Gastric Contents

See Chapter 7.
Toxicology

Hair

Hair grows 1 to 2 cm per month and integrates biochemical events at the hair follicle over its entire length.

Disorder	Finding
Kwashiorkor	Pigmentary banding ("flag" sign)
Menkes kinky-hair syndrome	Twisted hair
Argininosuccinicaciduria	Trichorrhexis nodosa
Ectodermal dysplasia	Misshapen hair
Radiation and chemotherapy	Hair loss
Thallium poisoning	Specific changes in hair roots
Genetic mosaicism	Plucked hair roots
Low-sulfur hair syndrome	Polarizing light shows alternating light and dark zones (barber pole pattern), sharp cross breaks, low sulfur content, napkin-like folds Found in various conditions (e.g., dwarfism, ichthyosis, photosensitivity, complementation-positive xeroderma pigmentosum)
Enzymatic heterozygosity	
Early deficiency of proteins or total calories	—
Cystic fibrosis	Increased sodium and chloride
	Drugs
Hair loss (2–4 months after beginning use)	Antihyperlipidemic, anticoagulants, interferons, retinol and its derivatives
Hirsutism	Testosterone, danazol, corticotropin, glucocorticoids, anabolic steroids, metyrapone
Hypertrichosis	Cyclosporinem diazoxide, minoxidil

Not useful for nutritional status of vitamins, minerals, other elements.[3]

[3]Seidel S, et al. Assessment of commercial laboratories performing hair mineral analysis. *JAMA* 2001;285:67.

Drug Testing

Use (GC/MS is method of choice)

- Drug screening (e.g., jails, workplaces, military forces)
- Drug fatalities when other samples are not available (e.g., decayed or fragmented corpses)
- Screen neonate to detect drug abuse by mother during pregnancy
- Evaluate compliance in long-term drug therapy (e.g., antihypertensive, antipsychotic) or drug withdrawal in rehabilitation centers
- Detect doping (e.g., athletes, racehorses)
- Detection of
  Heavy metals (e.g., mercury, arsenic, lead, cadmium, uranium)
  Drugs of abuse
    Opiates (e.g., morphine, codeine)
    Cocaine and metabolites, heroin
    Amphetamine/methamphetamine
    Hallucinogens (e.g., cannabis)

Hair analysis for forensic purposes should not be used without corroborative evidence because some substances (e.g., cocaine, benzoylecgonine) may also be incorporated from environmental exposure.[4]

Advantages for determination of drugs of abuse in hair include:

- Specimen easily obtained
- Easy retesting of a second sample
- Not affected by short periods of abstinence (in contrast to urinalysis) since hair grows at an average rate of 1 to 2 cm per month. Only the most recent 6 cm should be analyzed; telogen portion of hair may contain drug not used for more than 1 year.
- Iron content has been described as a possible marker to monitor therapy in iron-deficient patients.[5]
- Not useful for zinc, copper, aluminum

Interferences

Contamination due to selenium shampoo or lead-containing antigraying formulas[6]

Milk

Infection: $>10^6$ WBC/mL and $>10^3$ bacterial colonies/mL compared to noninfectious inflammation or clogged duct; usually due to *S. aureus* or *S. epidermidis* (penicillin resistant)

Develops in ~2.5% of nursing mothers, usually 2 to 5 weeks postpartum

Nails

See Table 19-1.
Heavy metal poisoning
Scrapings from under nails of victim in forensic cases

Nasal Secretions

Increased neutrophils in infection
Increased eosinophils in allergy (Hansel stain)
Increased eosinophils and neutrophils in infection superimposed on chronic allergy
Rapid antigen detection for RSV
Differentiate nasal secretions from CSF in possible skull fracture (see Head Trauma, Chapter 9)

---

[4]Kintz, P, ed. *Drug testing in hair.* New York: CRC Press, 1996.
[5]Bisse E, et al. Hair iron content: possible marker to complement monitoring therapy of iron deficiency in patients with chronic inflammatory bowel disease? *Clin Chem* 1996;42:1270.
[6]Crounse RG. The diagnostic value of microscopic examination of human hair. *Arch Pathol Lab Med* 1987;111:700.

Table 19-1.   Nail Appearance and Associated Disorders

Nail Disorder	Nail Appearance	Associated Disorders	Drugs
Blue nails	Blue lunulae	Wilson disease Hemochromatosis Ochronosis	Minocycline Silver nitrate Anti-malarials
Brown nails		Melanoma Addison disease Hemochromatosis	Gold
Yellow nail syndrome	Diffuse yellow to green color; thickened; slow growth; increased side-to-side curvature	Systemic disease (usually pulmonary effusion, bronchiectasis), cancer (e.g., lymphoma, melanoma)	
Half and half	Proximal 1/2—dull and white, obliterates lunula Distal 1/2—pink or brown	Uremia (10% of patients)	
Terry's nails	Proximal 2/3—white Distal 1/2—red	Congestive heart failure Cirrhosis with decreased serum albumin	
Muehrcke's lines	Paired horizontal narrow white and normal color bands	Nephrotic syndrome with decreased serum albumin	
Splinter hemorrhage		Multisystem disease (e.g., SBE) Trauma	
Koilonychia	Soft thin nail plates causing concave or spoon-shaped nails	Iron deficiency Raynaud syndrome Hemochromatosis Trauma May be autosomal dominant trait	
Oncholysis (Plummer disease)	Separation of nail plate from nail bed	Hyperthyroidism Psoriasis Trauma	Chemicals
Nail fold telangiectasia		Dermatomyositis, SLE	

- Transferrin by immunoelectrophoresis: CSF shows a double band; other body fluids (nasal secretions, tears, saliva, serum, lymph) show a single band
- Glucose by test tape or tablets positive in CSF but negative in nasal secretions; not reliable since may normally be positive in nasal secretions

Pancreatic Secretions
See Chapter 7; Pancreatic Pseudocyst (Chapter 8).

Pleural/pericardial Fluid
See Chapter 6.

Prostatic Fluid
WBC and Gram stain for infection/inflammation

Saliva[7-9]

Salivary glands produce almost 1 L/day of serous and mucinous saliva.

Therapeutic drug monitoring (e.g., digoxin, phenytoin, lithium, theophylline, phenobarbital, dexamethasone)

Testing for drugs of abuse (e.g., ethanol, amphetamines, barbiturates, benzodiazepines, cocaine, marijuana, heroin, codeine, PCP, nicotine [cotine]). Check winners of horse races for race fixing.

Diagnosis of infection in certain patients (e.g., HIV, hepatitis A and B, rabies)

Hormone assay, e.g., Cortisol (5–10× less than serum), 17 alpha-hydroxyprogesterone, progesterone[10]

DHEA

Estriol, unconjugated estriol

Androstenedione

Testosterone (not sensitive enough for diagnostically accurate results to assess individual patients)

Radioactive iodine in hyperthyroidism, hypothyroidism (see Chapter 13)

Sjögren syndrome (increased sodium, chloride; anti-Ro and anti-La antibodies)

Cystic fibrosis (see Chapter 8)

Secretory IgA

Interferences

Contamination with blood (due to chewing, flossing, etc.) can greatly change values.

Saliva Test for Blood Alcohol

Use

Rapid identification of blood alcohol concentration of >0.02%

Saliva to blood ratio = 1:1

Interferences

Alcohol vapors in air
Methyl and allyl alcohols
Peroxidases
Strong oxidizers
Ascorbic acid
Tannic acid
Pyrogallol
Mercaptans and tosylates
Oxalic acid
Uric acid
Bilirubin
L-dopa
L-methyldopa
Methampyrone
Internet-based non-FDA-approved tests offer kits for cholesterol, PSA, etc.

Semen

See Chapter 13.
Infertility
Adequacy of vasectomy
Rape/sexual assault (see Chapter 14)

---

[7]Malamud D, Tabak L, eds. Saliva as a diagnostic fluid. *Ann NY Acad Sci* 1993;694. ASCP Clinical Chemistry Check Sample CC 96-4.

[8]Millwe AM. Saliva: new interest in a nontraditional specimen. *Medical Lab Observer* 1993;Apr; 31–35.

[9]Xiang S, et al. Physiologic determinants of endothelin concentrations in human saliva. *Clin Chem* 2003;49:2012.

[10]Groeschl M, et al. Circadian rhythm of salivary cortisol, 17 alpha-hydroxyprogesterone, and progesterone in healthy children. *Clin Chem* 2003;49:1694.

Skin

Fluid from pustule for cytology (inclusion bodies for various viral diseases), culture for
some bacteremias (meningococcemia, Rocky Mountain spotted fever)
Fibroblasts for tissue culture for various genetic diseases

Sputum/Bronchoalveolar Lavage (BAL)

See Chapter 6.
Cytology
Infection
Allergy
Pulmonary alveolar proteinosis—BAL fluid shows increased total protein, albumin,
phospholipids, CEA

Stool

See Chapter 7.

SWEAT

Color
    Brown: Ochronosis
    Red: Rifampin overdose
    Blue: Occupational exposure to copper
    Blue-black: Idiopathic chromhidrosis (in black persons, axillary chromhidrosis may
      also be yellow, blue-green)
Electrolytes
    Cystic fibrosis (Chapter 8)
    Fucosidosis (Chapter 12)
Odor
    Maple syrup urine disease (Chapter 12)
    Organic acidemias (Chapter 12)
    Drug testing[11] (e.g., amphetamines, cannabis, cocaine, opiates)

Synovial fluid

See Chapter 10.

Tears

Decreased Volume In (Schirmer Test, Hamano Thread Test)

Sjögren syndrome
Horner syndrome
Decreased facial nerve function
Dehydration

Lysosomal Diseases that Can Be Identified by Enzyme Deficiency in Tears

See separate section for each disorder in Chapter 12.
Tay-Sachs disease
Sandhoff disease
Fabry disease
Fucosidosis
Mannosidosis
Gm_1-gangliosidosis
Type II glycogenosis
Hurler and Scheie syndrome
Metachromatic leukodystrophy

---

[11]de la Torre R, Pichini S. Usefulness of sweat testing for the detection of cannabis smoke. *Clin Chem* 2004;50:1961.

Mucosulfatidosis
Glucose sensing is described.[12]

Urine

See Chapters 4 and 14.

Vaginal Secretions

See Chapter 14.
Fibronectin
Forensic (e.g., rape/intercourse) (Chapter 14)
 Typing and DNA of rapist
Pregnancy (fern test)
Pap smear
 Hormone status
 Screening/monitoring gynecological atypias/cancers
Fibronectin (see Chapter 14)
Infection (e.g., cultures, bacterial stains, wet mounts)
 Trichomonas/Candida

Vitreous[13–15]

Postmortem glucose for diagnosis of hyperglycemia or diabetes mellitus, especially
 when ketones are also present and when blood is not available. Because glucose
 decreases after death, may not be useful to establish hypoglycemia.
Postmortem BUN for diagnosis of uremia when blood not available
Sodium, chloride, CO_2 reflect antemortem values
Increase potassium 12 mEq/L 100 hours after death. Sometimes fluid is taken from
 both eyes at different times and the rate of change is used to establish the time of
 death.
Alcohol can be measured in vitreous even if body has been embalmed.

[12]Alexeev VL, et al. Photonic crystal glucose-sensing material for noninvasive monitoring of glucose
in tear fluid. *Clin Chem* 2004;50:2353.
[13]Coe JI. Postmortem chemistries on human vitreous humor. *Am J Clin Path* 1969;51:741.
[14]Coe JI. Postmortem chemistry: practical considerations and a review of the literature. *J Forensic
Sci* 1974;19:13.
[15]Burkhard M, Hensage C. Eye changes after death. In Knight B., ed. *The estimation of the time
since death in the early postmortem period.* London: Edward Arnold,1995:106.

Appendices

APPENDIX A

Abbreviations and Acronyms

AA	amyloid A, atomic absorption
Ab	antibody
ABG	arterial blood gas
ACE	angiotensin-converting enzyme
Ach	acetylcholine
AChR	acetylcholine receptor
ACTH	adrenocorticotropic hormone
ADH	antidiuretic hormone
AF	amniotic fluid
AFB	acid fast bacillus
AFP	alpha-fetoprotein
Ag	antigen
AG	anion gap
A/G	albumin:globulin ratio
AHF	antihemophilic factor
AIDS	acquired immunodeficiency syndrome
ALA	aminolevulinic acid
ALL	acute lymphoblastic leukemia
ALP	alkaline phosphatase
ALT	alanine aminotransferase (see SGPT)
AMI	acute myocardial infarction
AML	acute myeloblastic leukemia
	acute myelocytic leukemia
	acute myelogenous leukemia
ANA	antinuclear antibody
ANCA	anti-neutrophil cytoplasmic antibody
aPTT	activated partial thromboplastic time
ARC	AIDS-related complex (see AIDS)
ARDS	acute respiratory distress syndrome
ASOT	antistreptolysin-O titer
AST	aspartate aminotransferase (see SGOT)
ATP	adenosine triphosphate
BAL	bronchoalveolar lavage
BCG	bacillus Calmette-Guerin
BJ protein	Bence-Jones protein
BT	bleeding time
BUN	blood urea nitrogen
CA-125	cancer antigen 125
CAD	coronary artery disease
CAH	congenital adrenal hyperplasia
cAMP	cyclic adenosine monophosphate
CBC	complete blood count
CDC	Centers for Disease Control and Prevention
CEA	carcinoembryonic antigen
CF	complement fixation, cystic fibrosis
CHD	congenital heart disease
ChE	cholinesterase

CHF	congestive heart failure
CIE	Counter (-current) immunoelectrophoresis
CK	creatine kinase
CK-MB	creatine kinase MB band
CK-MM	creatine kinase MM band
CLL	chronic lymphocytic leukemia
CMV	cytomegalovirus
CNS	central nervous system
COPD	chronic obstructive pulmonary disease
CRH	corticotropin-releasing hormone
CRP	C-reactive protein
CSF	cerebrospinal fluid
CT	computed tomography
CVA	cerebrovascular accident
d	day
D	decreased
DFA	direct fluorescent antibody
DHEA	dehydroepiandrosterone
DHEA-S	dehydroepiandrosterone sulfate
DIC	disseminated intravascular coagulation
DKA	diabetic ketoacidosis
dL	deciliter
DM	diabetes mellitus
DNA	deoxyribonucleic acid (also see the Glossary)
DOC	deoxycorticosterone
EBV	Epstein-Barr virus
ECG	electrocardiogram
EDTA	edetic acid
EIA	enzyme immunoassay
ELISA	enzyme-linked immunosorbent assay
EM	electron microscopy
EMIT	enzyme multiplied immunoassay technique
ENA	extractable nuclear antigen
EPA	Environmental Protection Agency
ERCP	endoscopic retrograde cholangiopancreatography
ESR	erythrocyte sedimentation rate
Fab	antigen-binding fragment of immunoglobulin
FAB	French-American-British classification for acute leukemias
FBS	fasting blood sugar
Fc	crystallizable fragment of immunoglobulin
FDA	Food and Drug Administration
FISH	fluorescence in-situ hybridization (also see the Glossary)
fL	femtoliter
FNA	fine needle aspiration
FSH	follicle-stimulating hormone
FTA	fluorescent treponemal antibody
FTA-ABS	fluorescent treponemal antibody absorption test
FTI	free thyroxine index
FT_4	free thyroxine
g	gram
GC/MS	chromatography/mass spectrometry
GFR	glomerular filtration rate
GGT	gamma-glutamyl transferase
GI	gastrointestinal
GN	glomerulonephritis
G6PD	glucose-6-phosphate dehydrogenase
GTT	glucose tolerance test
GU	genitourinary
H	hour
HA	hemagglutination
HAI	hemagglutination inhibition
Hb	hemoglobin
	(may be followed by types: HbC, HbD, HbE, HbF, HbH, HbS)

HbA$_{1c}$	glycosylated hemoglobin, hemoglobin A1c
HAA	hepatitis-associated antigen
HAV	hepatitis A virus
HBcAb	hepatitis B core antibody
HBcAg	hepatitis B core antigen
HBeAb	hepatitis B e antibody
HBeAg	hepatitis B e antigen
HBIG	hepatitis B immune globulin
HBsAb	hepatitis B surface antibody
HBsAg	hepatitis B surface antigen
HBV	hepatitis B virus
HCV	hepatitis C virus
HDV	hepatitis delta virus
Hct	hematocrit
HDL	high-density lipoprotein
HDN	hemolytic disease of the newborn
hGH	human growth hormone
hCG	human chorionic gonadotropin
H&E	hematoxylin and eosin (stain)
HI	hemagglutination inhibition
HIAA	hydroxyindole acetic acid
HIV	human immunodeficiency virus
HLA	human leukocyte antigen
HPF	high-power field
HPLC	high-pressure liquid chromatography
HPV	human papillomavirus
HSV	herpes simplex virus
HTLV	human T-cell leukemia virus
	human T-cell lymphotropic virus
HUS	hemolytic uremic syndrome
HVA	homovanillic acid
ICDH	isocitric dehydrogenase
ICU	intensive care unit
IDDM	insulin-dependent diabetes mellitus
IEP	immunoelectrophoresis
IF	immunofluorescence
IFA	indirect immunofluorescent assay
Ig	immunoglobulin
	(can be found as IgA, IgD, IgE, IgG, IgM)
IHA	indirect hemagglutination
IM	infectious mononucleosis, intramuscular
INH	isoniazid
IRMA	immunoradiometric assay
ITP	idiopathic thrombocytopenic purpura
IU	International unit
IV	intravenous
17-KGS	17-ketogenic steroids
KOH	potassium hydroxide
17-KS	17-ketosteroids
L	liter
LA	latex agglutination
LAP	leucine aminopeptidase
LD	lactate dehydrogenase
LDL	low-density lipoprotein
LE	lupus erythematosus
LH	luteinizing hormone
MAO	monoamine oxidase
MCH	mean corpuscular hemoglobin
MCHC	mean corpuscular hemoglobin concentration
MCV	mean corpuscular volume
MEN	multiple endocrine neoplasia (syndrome)
mEq	milliequivalent
MHA-TP	micro-hemagglutination test (for treponema pallidum)

μL	microliter
mg	milligram
mol	mole
mmol	millimol
mm Hg	millimeters of mercury
MoM	multiples of the median (also see the Glossary)
MRI	magnetic resonance imaging
mRNA	messenger RNA (also see the Glossary)
N	normal
NANB	non-A, non-B hepatitis (hepatitis C)
NBT	nitroblue tetrazolium
NPV	negative predictive value
NIDDM	non—insulin-dependent diabetes mellitus
NSAIDs	nonsteroidal anti-inflammatory drugs
5'-NT	5'-nucleotidase
OGTT	oral glucose tolerance test
17-OHKS	17-hydroxyketosteroids
O & P	ova and parasites
PA	pernicious anemia
PAP	prostatic acid phosphatase
Pap	Papanicolaou smear
pCO_2	partial pressure of carbon dioxide
PCV	packed cell volume
PCR	polymerase chain reaction (also see the Glossary)
PDW	platelet distribution width
pg	picogram
Ph	Philadelphia chromosome
PK	pyruvate kinase
PKU	phenylketonuria
PMN	polymorphonuclear neutrophil
PNH	paroxysmal nocturnal hemoglobinuria
PO	by mouth (Latin, *per os*)
pO_2	partial pressure of oxygen
POC	point of care
ppm	parts per million
PRA	plasma renin activity
PSA	prostate-specific antigen
PSP	phenolsulfonphthalein
PPV	positive predictive value
PT	prothrombin time
PTH	parathyroid hormone
RA	refractory anemia, rheumatoid arthritis
RAIU	thyroid uptake of radioactive iodine
RAST	radioallergosorbent test
RBC	red blood cell
RDW	red cell distribution width
RE	reticuloendothelial
RF	rheumatic fever, rheumatoid factor
Rh	rhesus factor
RIA	radioimmunoassay
RNA	ribonucleic acid
ROC	receiver-operating characteristic
RSV	respiratory syncytial virus
rT_3	reverse T_3
s	second (as time measurement)
SBE	subacute bacterial endocarditis
SD	standard deviation
SGOT	serum glutamic oxaloacetic transaminase (see aspartate aminotransferase, AST)
SGPT	serum glutamic pyruvic transaminase (see alanine aminotransferase, ALT)
SI	Système Internationale d'Unites
SIADH	syndrome of inappropriate antidiuretic hormone secretion

SLE	systemic lupus erythematosus
S/S	sensitivity/specificity
STD	sexually transmitted disease
T_3	triiodothyronine
T_4	thyroxine
TB	tuberculosis
TBG	thyroxine-binding globulin
TDM	therapeutic drug monitoring
TGT	thromboplastic generation time
THC	marijuana (delta-9-tetrahydrocannabinol)
TIBC	total iron-binding capacity
TLC	thin-layer chromatography
TMP/SMX	trimethoprim and sulfamethoxazole
TORCH	toxoplasma, others, rubella, cytomegalovirus, herpes simplex
TP	total protein
TPN	total parenteral nutrition
TRH	thyrotropin-releasing hormone
TSH	thyroid-stimulating hormone
TSI	thyroid-stimulating immunoglobulin
TT	thrombin time
TTP	thrombotic thrombocytopenic purpura
TTP/HUS	thrombotic thrombocytopenic purpura hemolytic uremic syndrome
U	unit
UIBC	unsaturated iron-binding capacity
ULN	upper limit of normal
URI	upper respiratory infection
UTI	urinary tract infection
UV	ultraviolet
V	variable
VCA	viral capsid antigen
VDRL	Venereal Disease Research Laboratory (test for syphilis)
VIP	vasoactive intestinal polypeptide
VLDL	very-low-density lipoprotein
VMA	vanillylmandelic acid
VZV	varicella-zoster virus
vWF	von Willebrand factor
WBC	white blood cell
WHO	World Health Organization
Z-E	Zollinger-Ellison (syndrome)

Glossary[1]

Chromosome	an individual portion of DNA containing some or all genes of a cell or virus. Humans have 23 pairs of chromosomes.
DNA	deoxyribonucleic acid: double-helix strands composed of nucleotides (A, C, G, T) with A on one strand paired with T and C paired with G on the other strand. The order of nucleotides determines genetic information.
FISH	fluorescent in-situ hybridization: technique for fluorescent staining of molecules (e.g., used for gene mapping and to identify chromosome abnormalities).
Gene	functional unit in genome of cells and viruses that encode RNA and proteins.
Genotype	individual's genetic makeup indicated by their DNA sequence.
Haplotype	group of adjacent alleles inherited together.
Heterozygous	two different alleles at a specific autosomal gene locus (or X chromosome in a female).
Homozygous	two identical alleles at a specific autosomal gene locus (or X chromosome in a female).

ABBREV

MoM	multiples of the median: Unit used to express marker concentrations in maternal serum that allows for variations in concentration during gestation and between laboratories (see alpha-fetoprotein).
mRNA	messenger RNA: template for protein synthesis. Sequence of a strand of mRNA is based on sequence of a complementary strand of DNA.
Mutation	permanent change in structure of DNA.
Nucleic acids	chains of nucleotides that form DNA and RNA.
Oncogene	gene with ability to convert noncancer cell to a cancer cell. Proto-oncogenes are genes able to contribute to formation of cancer due to mutations in nucleotide sequence or organization, e.g., retroviral oncogenes are derived from proto-oncogenes.
PCR	polymerase chain reaction: quick way to make unlimited number of copies of any piece of DNA.
Phenotype	clinical expression of specific genes and/or environmental factors, e.g., hair color, presence of a disease.
Retrovirus	class of viruses, including HIV and RNA tumor viruses, that replicate by copying RNA genome into DNA form by reverse transcriptase.
Reverse transcriptase	enzyme that copies RNA into DNA carried by retroviruses.
RNA	ribonucleic acid: delivers DNA messages to cytoplasm of cell where proteins are made. Similar to a single strand of DNA but uracil (U) is substituted for (T) in genetic code. Order of nucleotides is usually determined by a corresponding sequence in DNA.
Southern blot	named for Dr. Southern. Procedure used to identify and locate DNA sequences that are complementary to another piece of DNA (called a *probe*).
Tyrosine kinase	enzymes that add phosphate to tyrosine in proteins (many encoded by proto-oncogenes). Some (e.g., *ABL* and *EGF* receptor tyrosine-kinases) are inhibited by anticancer drugs (e.g., Gleevec).
WB	western blot: procedure used to identify and locate proteins using specific antibodies that bind to these proteins.

[1]Gutmacher AE, Collins FS. Genomic medicine—a primer. *N Engl J Med* 2002;347:1512.

Symbols

>	greater than
≥	equal to or greater than
<	less than
≤	equal to or less than; up to
×	times, e.g., 4× increase = fourfold increase
±	plus or minus
~	Approximately
↑ to ↑↑↑↑	increased to markedly increased
↓ to ↓↓↓↓	decreased to markedly decreased

Conversion Factors between Conventional and Système International Units

This list is included to assist the reader in converting values between conventional units and the newer SI units (Système International d'Unites) that have been mandated by some journals. Only common analytes are included.

Table B-1. Hematology

Analyte	Conventional Units	SI Units	Conversion Factors Conventional SI Units	SI to Conventional Units
WBC count (leukocytes)				
(B)	/μL	cells x 10^9/L	0.001	1,000
(CSF)	μg/L	10^6/L	1	1
(SF)	/μL	/L	10^6	10^{-6}
Platelet count	10^3/μL	10^9/L	1	1
Reticulocytes	/μL	10^9/L	0.001	1,000
RBC count (erythrocytes)				
(B)	10^6/μL	10^{12}/L	1	1
(CSF)	μg/L	10^6/L	1	1
Hct (packed cell volume [PCV])	%	Volume fraction	0.01	100
	pg	fmol	0.6206	1.611
Mean corpuscular volume (MCV; volume index)	μ^3 (cubic microns)	fL	1	1
Mean corpuscular hemoglobin (MCH; color index)	pg (or $\mu\mu$g) pg	pg fmol	0.06206 0.6206	16.11 1.611
Mean corpuscular hemoglobin concentration (MCHC; saturation index)	g/dL g/dL	g/L mmol/L	10 0.6206	0.1 1.611
Hemoglobin (Whole blood)	g/dL	mmol/L	0.155	6.45
Hemoglobin (Plasma)	mg/dL	μmol/L	0.155	6.45
Fetal hemoglobin	%	mol/mol (May omit symbol	0.01	100
Haptoglobin	mg/dL	mg/L	10	0.1
Fibrinogen	mg/dL	g/L	0.01	100

For abbreviations, see Table B-2 footnotes.

Table B-2.	Chemistry			

			Conversion Factors	
Analyte	Conventional Units	SI Units	Conventional to SI Units	SI to Conventional Units
ACTH	pg/mL	ng/L	1	1
	pg/mL	pmol/L	0.2202	4.541
Aldosterone (S)	ng/dL	nmol/L	0.0277	36.1
Aldosterone (U)	mEq/24 hr	mmol/d	1	1
	nmol/mL/min	nkat/L	16.67	
Androstenedione	ng/dL	pmol/L	34.92	
Angiotensin II	ng/dL	ng/L	10	0.1
	pg/mL	ng/L	1	1
Angiotensin-converting enzyme (ACE) (U) μg/24 hr	nmol/mL/min	U/L	1	1
	nmol/d	2.774	0.36	1
Antidiuretic hormone (ADH; vasopressin)	pg/mL	ng/L	1	1
Albumin (S)	g/dL	g/L	10	0.1
Albumin (CSF, AF)	mg/dL	mg/L	10	0.1
Alpha₁-antitrypsin	mg/dL	g/L	0.01	100
Alpha-fetoprotein (AFP) (S)	ng/mL	μg/L	1	1
	ng/dL	ng/L	10	0.1
	mg/dL	g/L	0.01	100
	mg/dL	mg/L	10	0.1
	μg/dL	μg/L	10	0.1
Ammonia (P)	μg/dL	μmol/L	0.714	1.4
	μg/dL	μmol/L	0.5872	1.703
Anion gap	mEq/L	mmol/L	1	1
Base excess	mEq/L	mmol/L	1	1
Bicarbonate	mEq/L	mmol/L	1	1
Bilirubin	mg/dL	μmol/L	17.1	0.0584
Calcitonin	pg/mL	ng/L	1	1
Catecholamines (U)				
Norepinephrine	μg/24 hr	nmol/d	5.91	0.169
	μg/mg creatinine	μmol/mol creatinine	669	0.00149
	pg/mL	pmol/L	5.91	0.169
	ng/mL	nmol/L	5.91	0.169
Epinephrine	μg/24 hr	nmol/d	5.46	0.183
	μg/mg creatinine	μmol/mol creatinine	617	0.00162
	pg/mL	pmol/L	5.46	0.183
	ng/mL	nmol/L	5.46	0.183
Normetanephrine	ng/mL	nmol/L	5.46	0.183
	mg/g creatinine	μmol/mmol creatinine		
Dopamine	μg/24 hr	nmol/d	6.53	0.153
	μg/mg creatinine	μmol/mol creatinine	738	0.00136

(continued)

Table B-2. *(continued)*

| | | | Conversion Factors | |
Analyte	Conventional Units	SI Units	Conventional to SI Units	SI to Conventional Units
	pg/mL	pmol/L	6.53	0.153
	ng/mL	nmol/L	6.53	0.153
Metanephrines	mg/24 hr	μmol/d	5.07	
	mg/g creatinine	μmol/mol creatinine	0.5736	
Catecholamines (P)				
Epinephrine	pg/mL	pmol/L	5.458	
Norepinephrine	pg/mL	nmol/L	0.0059	
Chorionic gonadotropin (hCG), beta-subunit	mU/mL U/24 hr	IU/L IU/d	1 1	1 1
Calcium (S)	mg/dL	mmol/L	0.25	4.0
	mEq/L	mmol/L	0.5	2.0
Calcium (U)	mg/24 hr	mmol/d	0.025	40
Carbon dioxide total (content CO_2 + bicarbonate)	mEq/L	mmol/L	1	1
CO_2 partial pressure, tension (pCO_2)	mm Hg	kPa	0.133	7.52
Standard bicarbonate (hydrogen carbonate)	mEq/L	mmol/L	1	1
Carotene	μg/dL	μmol/L	0.0186	
Chloride	mEq/L or mg/dL	mmol/L	1	1
CEA	ng/mL	μg/L	1	1
	μg/mL	mg/L	1	1
Ceruloplasmin	mg/dL	mg/L	10	0.1
Cholesterol	mg/dL	mmol/L	0.0259	38.61
HDL-cholesterol	mg/dL	mmol/L	0.0259	38.61
LDL-cholesterol	mg/dL	mmol/L	0.0259	38.61
Apolipoprotein, A1 or B	mg/dL	mg/L	10.00	
Copper (S)	μg/dL	μmol/L	0.157	6.37
Copper (U)	μg/24 hr	μmol/d	0.0157	63.69
Coproporphyrins (I and III) (U)	μg/dL μg/24 hr	nmol/L nmol/d	15 1.5	0.067 0.67
Coproporphyrins (F)	μg/g	nmol/g	1.5	0.67
Cortisol (S)	μg/dL	μmol/L	0.028	35.7
	ng/mL	nmol/L	2.76	0.362
17-OHKS (cortisol) (U)	mg/24 hr μg/24 hr	μmol/d nmol/d	2.759 2.759	0.3625 0.3625
Creatine (S)	mg/dL	μmol/L	76.3	0.0131
Creatinine (S, AF)	mg/dL	μmol/L	88.4	0.0113

(continued)

CONVERSIONS

> **Table B-2.** *(continued)*

Analyte	Conventional Units	SI Units	Conversion Factors Conventional to SI Units	SI to Conventional Units
Creatinine (U)	g/24 hr	mmol/d	8.84	0.1131
	mg/24 hr	mmol/d	0.00884	113.1
Creatinine (U)	mg/kg/24 hrs	μmol/kg/d	8.84	0.113
Creatinine (C)	mL/min/1.73m^2	mL/sec/m^2	0.00963	104
cAMP (cyclic adenosine monophosphate)				
cAMP (S)	μg/L	nmol/L	3.04	0.329
cAMP (B)	ng/mL	nmol/L	3.04	0.329
cAMP (U)	mg/24 hr	μmol/d	3.04	0.329
	mg/g creatinine	μmol/mol creatinine	344	0.00291
Dehydroepiandrosterone sulfate (DHEA-S)				
(DHEA-S) (S)	μg/mL	μmol/L	2.6	0.38
(DHEA-S) (AF)	ng/mL	nmol/L	2.6	0.38
17-Ketosteroids (17-KS) (as dehydroepiandros-terone) (U)	mg/24 hr mg/g creatinine	μmol/d μmol/mmol creatinine	3.467 0.3921	0.2904
17-Ketogenic steroids (17-KGS) (as dehydroepiandros-terone) (U)	mg/24 hr mg/g creatinine	μmol/d μmol/mmol creatinine	3.467 0.3921	0.2904
17-Hydroxycortico-steroids (17-OHCS) (U)	mg/g creatinine	mg/mol creatinine	113.1	0.00884
11-Deoxyortico-sterone (DOC) (S)	pg/mL	pmol/L	3.03	0.33
Glucose	mg/dL	mmol/L	0.0555	18.02
Ferritin	ng/mL	μg/L	1	1
Gastrin	pg/mL	ng/L	1	1
Growth hormone (S)	ng/mL	μg/L	1	1
Growth hormone (U)	ng/24 hr	ng/d	1	1
Homovanillic acid (HVA) (U)	mg/24 hr μg/24 hr	μmol/d μmol/d	5.49 0.00549	0.182 182
	μg/mg creatinine	mmol/mol creatinine	0.621	1.61
5-Hydroxyindole-acetic acid (5-HIAA) (U)	mg/24hr	μmol/d	5.2	0.19
Hormone receptors (T)				
Progesterone receptor assay (PRA)	fmol/mg protein	nmol/kg protein	1	1
Estrogen protein assay (ERA)	fmol/mg protein	nmol/kg protein	1	1
Iron	μg/dL	μmol/L	0.179	5.587
Iron-binding capacity	μg/dL	μmol/L	0.179	5.587

(continued)

Table B-2. *(continued)*

Analyte	Conventional Units	SI Units	Conversion Factors Conventional to SI Units	SI to Conventional Units
Iron saturation	%	fraction	0.01	100
Lactate	mg/dL	mmol/L	0.111	9.01
Lead (S)	μg/dL	μmol/L	0.0483	20.72
	mg/dL	μmol/L	48.26	
Lead (U)	μg/24 hr	μmol/d	0.00483	
Lipids (total)	mg/dL	g/L	0.01	100
Magnesium (S)	mEq/L	mmol/L	0.5	2
	mg/dL	mmol/L	0.414	2.433
Magnesium (U)	mg/24 hr	mmol/d	0.414	2.433
Osmolality	mOsmol/kg	mmol/kg	1.00	1.00
O_2 partial pressure, (p(a)O2)	mm Hg	kPa	0.133	7.5
Osteocalcin	ng/mL	μg/L	1.00	
Parathyroid hormone	pg/mL	ng/L	1	1
	μLEq/ml	mLEq/L	1	1
Phosphate (inorganic phosphorus) (S)	mg/dL	mmol/L	0.323	3.10
Phosphate (inorganic phosphorus) (U)	g/24 hr	mmol/d	32.3	0.031
pH	nEq/L	nmol/L	1	1
Porphobilinogen (PBG) (U)	mg/24 hr	μmol/d	4.42	0.226
Potassium (S)	mEq/L	mmol/L	1	1
Potassium (U)	mEq/24 hr	mmol/L	1	1
	mg/24 hr	mmol/d	0.02558	39.1
Protein, total (S)	g/dL	g/L	10	0.1
Protein, total (U)	mg/24 hr	g/d	0.001	1,000
Protein, total (CSF)	mg/dL	mg/L	10	0.1
Renin activity; (PRA) (plasma)	ng/mL/hr	μg/L/hr	1	1
Serotonin (S)	ng/mL	μmol/L	0.00568	176
Sodium (S)	mEq/L	mmol/L	1	1
Sodium (U)	mEq/24 hr	mmol/L	1	1
	mg/24 hr	mmol/d	0.0435	22.99
Testosterone (total) (S)	ng/dL	nmol/L	0.0347	28.8
Thyroid-binding globulin (TBG)	mg/dL	mg/L	10	0.1
	μg/dL	μg/L	10	0.1
Thyroglobulin	ng/mL	μg/L	1	1
TSH (thyroid stimulating hormone)	μU/mL	mIU/L	1	1
Thyrotropin releasing hormone (TRH)	pg/mL	ng/L	1	1
	pg/mL	pmol/L	2.759	

(continued)

| Table B-2. | (continued) |

Analyte	Conventional Units	SI Units	Conventional to SI Units	SI to Conventional Units
Triiodothyronine (T3) total	ng/dL	nmol/L	0.0154	65.1
Triiodothyronine (fT3) free	pg/dL	nmol/L	15.4	
Reverse T3 (rT3)	ng/dL	nmol/L	0.0154	65.1
Thyroxine (T4) total	μg/dL	nmol/L	12.9	0.0775
Thyroxine (fT4) free	ng/dL	pmol/L	12.9	
Transferrin (TIBC)	mg/dL	g/L	0.01	100
Triglycerides	mg/dL	mmol/L	0.0113	88.5
Urea nitrogen (S)	mg/dL	mmol/L	0.357	2.8
Urea nitrogen (U)	g/24 hr	mol/d	0.0357	28
Uric acid (S)	mg/dL	mmol/L	0.05948	16.9
Uric acid (U)	mg/24 hr	mmol/d	0.0059	169
Uroporphyrin	μg/24 hr	nmol/d	1.204	
	μg/g creatinine	nmol/mmol creatinine	0.1362	
Vanillylmandelic acid (VMA) (U)	mg/24 hr	μmol/d	5.05	0.198
	μg/mg creatinine	mmol/moL creatinine	0.571	1.75
Viscosity (S)	Centipoise	same		
Vitamin A	μg/dL	μmol/L	0.0349	28.65
Vitamin B6	ng/mL	nmol/L	5.982	
Folate	ng/mL	nmol/L	2.266	
Vitamin B-12 (Cyanocobalamine)	pg/mL	pmol/L	0.738	1.355
Unsaturated B-12 binding capacity (S)	pg/mL	pmol/L	0.738	1.355
Vitamin C (Ascorbic acid)	mg/dL	μmol/L	56.78	0.176
Vitamin D (calcitriol; 1,25-dihydroxy)	pg/mL	pmol/L	2.400	0.417
Vitamin D (25-hydroxy)	ng/mL	nmol/L	2.496	
Vitamin E (alpha-tocopherol)	ng/mL	nmol/L	23.22	
Xylose (U)	mg/dL	mmol/L	0.0666	15.01
	g/5 hr	mmol/5 hr	6.66	0.15

AF = amniotic fluid; C = clearance; d = day; F = feces; fmol = fentamols; g = grams; IU = international units; L = liter; mEq = milliequivalent; mg = milligrams; mL = milliliter; mL/min = milliliter/minute; mL/sec = milliliter/second; mmol = millimols; mU = milliunits; ng = nanograms; nmol = nanomols; pg = picograms; S = serum; SF = synovial fluid; T = tissue; U = units; U = urine; μ = microns; μmol = micromols
All reference is to serum unless otherwise stated

Table B-3. Therapeutic and Toxic Drugs

Analyte	Conventional Units	SI Units	Conversion Factors	
			Conventional to SI Units	SI to Conventional Units
Acetaminophen	μg/mL	μmol/L	6.62	0.151
Amikacin	μg/mL	μmol/L	1.71	0.585
Amitryptyline	ng/mL	nmol/L	3.61	0.277
Amobarbital	μg/mL	μmol/L	4.42	0.226
Amphetamine	ng/mL	nmol/L	7.4	0.135
	μg/mL	μmol/L	7.4	0.135
Bromide	μg/mL	mmol/L	0.0125	79.9
Caffeine	μg/mL	μmol/L	5.15	0.194
Carbamazepine (Tegretol, others)	μg/mL	μmol/L	4.23	0.236
Carbenicillin	μg/mL	μmol/L	2.64	0.378
Chloral hydrate	μg/mL	μmol/L	6.69	0.149
Chloramphenicol	μg/mL	μmol/L	3.09	0.323
Chlordiazepoxide (Librium, others)	ng/mL	μmol/L	0.00334	300
Chlorpromazine (Thorazine)	ng/mL	nmol/L	3.14	0.319
Chlorpropamide (Diabinese)	μg/mL	μmol/L	3.61	0.227
Cimetidine (Tagamet)	μg/mL	μmol/L	3.96	0.252
Clonazepam (Clonopin)	ng/mL	nmol/L	3.17	0.316
Clonidine (Catapres)	ng/mL	nmol/L	4.35	0.230
Cocaine	ng/mL	nmol/L	3.3	0.303
Codeine	ng/mL	nmol/L	3.34	0.299
Demerol (Meperidine)	ng/mL	nmol/L	4.04	0.247
Desipramine (Norpramin)	ng/mL	nmol/L	3.75	0.267
Diazepam (Valium)	ng/mL	μmol/L	0.0035	285
Digitoxin	ng/mL	nmol/L	1.31	0.765
Digoxin	ng/mL	nmol/L	1.28	0.781
Dilaudid	ng/mL	nmol/L	4.85	0.206
Disulfiram	μg/mL	μmol/L	12.12	0.0761
Doxepin (Sinequan)	ng/mL	nmol/L	3.58	0.279
Ethanol	mg/dL	mmol/L	0.217	4.61
Ethchlorvynol (Placidyl)	μg/mL	μmol/L	6.92	0.145
Ethosuximide (Zarontin)	μg/mL	μmol/L	7.08	0.141
Gentamicin	μg/mL	μmol/L	2.09	0.478
Glutethimide (Doriden)	μg/mL	μmol/L	4.60	0.217
Haloperidol (Haldol)	ng/mL	nmol/L	2.66	0.376
Ibuprofen	μg/mL	μmol/L	4.85	0.206
Imipramine (Tofranil)	ng/mL	nmol/L	3.57	0.28
Isoniazid	μg/mL	μmol/L	7.29	0.137

(continued)

Table B-3. *(continued)*

Analyte	Conventional Units	SI Units	Conversion Factors Conventional to SI Units	SI to Conventional Units
Kanamycin (Kantrex)	μg/mL	μmol/L	2.06	0.485
Lidocaine (Xylocaine)	μg/mL	μmol/L	4.27	0.234
Lithium	mEq/L	mmol/L	1	1
Lorazepam	ng/mL	nmol/L	3.11	0.321
LSD (Lysergic acid diethylamide)	μg/mL	μmol/L	3.09	0.323
Meprobamate	mg/L	μmol/L	4.58	0.218
Methadone	ng/mL	μmol/L	0.00323	309
Methaqualone (Quaalude)	μg/mL	μmol/L	4.0	0.250
Methotrexate	ng/mL	nmol/L	2.2	0.454
Methsuximide	μg/mL	μmol/L	5.29	0.189
Methyldopa (Aldomet)	μg/mL	μmol/L	4.73	0.211
Morphine	ng/mL	nmol/L	3.5	0.285
	ng/mL	μmol/L	0.0035	285
Nortriptyline	ng/mL	nmol/L	3.8	0.263
Oxazepam	μg/mL	μmol/L	3.49	0.287
Paraldehyde	μg/mL	μmol/L	7.57	0.132
Pentobarbital (Nembutal)	μg/mL	μmol/L	4.42	0.179
Percodan	ng/mL	nmol/L	3.17	0.315
Phenacetin	μg/mL	μmol/L	5.58	0.179
Phenobarbital (Luminal)	μg/mL	μmol/L	4.31	0.232
Phenylbutazone (Butazolidin)	μg/mL	μmol/L	3.08	0.324
Phenytoin (Dilantin)	μg/mL	μmol/L	3.96	0.253
Primidone	μg/mL	μmol/L	4.58	0.218
Procainamide (Pronestyl)	μg/mL	μmol/L	4.23	0.236
Procaine (Novocain)				
Propoxyphene (Darvon)	μg/mL	μmol/L	3.07	0.326
Propranolol	ng/mL	nmol/L	3.86	0.259
Quinidine	μg/mL	μmol/L	3.08	0.324
Quinine	μg/mL	μmol/L	3.08	0.324
Salicylic acid	μg/mL	μmol/L	7.24	0.138
Secobarbital (Seconal)	μg/mL	μmol/L	4.2	0.238
Theophylline (Aminophylline)	μg/mL	μmol.L	5.55	0.180
Tobramycin	μg/mL	μmol/L	2.14	0.467
Valproic acid	μg/mL	μmol/L	6.93	0.144
Vancomycin	μg/mL	mg/L	1	1
Warfarin (Coumadin)	μg/mL	μmol/L	3.24	0.308

Table B-4. Measurements

Factor	Fraction	Decimal	Name	Prefix	Symbol
10^{-1}	1/10	0.1	One tenth	deci	d
10^{-2}	1/100	0.01	One hundredth	centi	c
10^{-3}	1/1,000	0.001	One thousandth	milli	m
10^{-4}	1/10,000	0.000 1			
10^{-5}	1/100,000	0.000 01			
10^{-6}	1/1,000,000	0.000 001	One millionth	micro	μ
10^{-7}	1/10,000,000	0.000 000 1			
10^{-8}	1/100,000,000	0.000 000 01			
10^{-9}	1/1,000,000,000	0.000 000 001	One billionth	nano	n
10^{-10}	1/10,000,000,000	0.000 000 000 1			
10^{-12}	1/1,000,000,000,000	0.000 000 000 001	One trillionth	pico	p
10^{-15}	1/1,000,000,000,000,000	0.000 000 000 000 001	One quadrillionth	femto	f
10^{-18}	1/1,000,000,000,000,000,000	0.000 000 000 000 000 001	One quintillionth	atto	a
10^{-21}	1/1,000,000,000,000,000,000,000	0.000 000 000 000 000 000 001	One sextillionth	zepto	z
10^{-24}	1/1,000,000,000,000,000,000,000,000	0.000 000 000 000 000 000 000 001	One septillionth	yocto	y

Factor	Fraction	Name	Prefix	Symbol
10^{0}	1	standard unit	none	
10^{1}	10	ten	deka	da/dk
10^{2}	100	hundred	hecto	h
10^{3}	1,000	thousand	kilo	k
10^{4}	10,000	ten thousand	myria	my
10^{5}	100,000			
10^{6}	1,000,000	million	mega	M
10^{7}	10,000,000			
10^{8}	100,000,000			
10^{9}	1,000,000,000	billion	giga	G
10^{10}	10,000,000,000			
10^{12}	1,000,000,000,000	trillion	tera	T
10^{15}	1,000,000,000,000,000	quadrillion	peta	P
10^{18}	1,000,000,000,000,000,000	quintillion	exa	E
10^{21}	1,000,000,000,000,000,000,000	sextillion	zetta	Z
10^{24}	1,000,000,000,000,000,000,000,000	septillion	yotta	Y

Summary of Causes of and Diagnostic Tests for Spurious Laboratory Results

Effect of Artifacts on Laboratory Test Values

See Table C-1.

Spurious values are false results due to various interferences in laboratory analysis but not due to clerical error, improper performance of tests, instrument failure, or poor reagents. They are sufficiently frequent that the clinician and laboratorian should be aware of them, especially in the face of discrepant laboratory results. Particular methodologies, reagents, and instruments are all important in determining these occurrences, and opposite results may derive from different technologies. Only those spurious results of greatest clinical significance and frequency are noted here. This section does not include discussion of the effect of drugs on laboratory test values that are even more numerous, factitious disorders (Munchausen syndrome), or technician or clerical errors.

Common causes of spurious chemical values are hemolysis and lipemia.

- *Hemolysis* releases RBC analytes and enzymes into serum, characteristically increasing serum LI, potassium, acid phosphatase and prostatic acid phosphatase, cholesterol (if hemolysis is marked); AST, ALT, creatine kinase, iron, and magnesium may be affected to a lesser extent.
- *Lipemia* may cause hyponatremia, hypokalemia, hyperchloremia, and negative ion gap by means of three mechanisms:

    Turbidity due to light scattering caused by lipid particles interfering with photometry.

    Partitioning errors that cause the analyte to enter the lipid, nonpolar phase, making it inaccessible for the chemical reaction.

    Fat replacing serum water and altering the distribution and concentration of electrolytes in the total volume of the specimen. This does not become a problem until triglycerides are >1,500 mg/dL, at which time serum is milky rather than just cloudy. Serum sodium decreases 1.5 mEq/L for every 1,000-mg/dL increase in triglycerides. Serum iron may be decreased.

In addition to spurious blood cell counts, histograms are often abnormal and may vary from one instrument to another. All histograms must be carefully scrutinized when spurious blood counts are suspected.

Table C-1. Summary of Causes of and Diagnostic Tests for Spurious Laboratory Results

Spurious Manifestation	Cause	Diagnostic Clue or Confirmation
Decreased platelet count	(a) Temperature-dependent agglutinins	(a) Accurate platelet count when sample is maintained at 37°C
	(b) EDTA-dependent agglutinins	(b) Associated low WBC, high Hb or Hct. Accurate platelet count using citrate- or heparin-anticoagulated blood
		(a,b) Histograms may be abnormal. Blood smear shows normal number of platelets; may show clumping. Normal blood smear from finger stick.
	(c) Overfilling of faulty vacuum blood collection tubes	(c) Use different lot of vacuum tubes
Increased platelet count	(a) Platelet clumping due to EDTA in patient with rheumatoid arthritis. Particles counted as platelets on automated blood cell counters.	(a) Rheumatoid factor present
	(b) Bacteremia	(b) Bacteria on blood smear
	(c) Leukemic blast cell fragments	(c) Low MPV; leukemic cells present
	(d) RBC fragmentation	(d) High MPV
	(e) Small RBCs	(e) Blood smear, manual RBC count
	(f) Cryoglobulinemia due to globulin crystals being counted	(f) Normal manual platelet count or with warming; cryoglobulin deposits seen on blood smear; abnormal histogram
Increased WBC	Particles counted as WBCs on automated blood cell counters	
	(a) Clumped platelets	(a) Blood smear does not show increased WBCs; clumped platelets seen
	(b) Incomplete RBC lysis	(b) Abnormal hemoglobins or severe liver disease present
	(c) Cryoglobulinemia due to globulin crystals being counted in automated blood cell counters	(c) Normal manual WBC or with warming; cryoglobulin deposits seen on blood smear; abnormal histogram
	(d) Platelet satellitosis	(d) Satellitosis seen on blood smear of EDTA specimen but not on heparinized sample

(continued)

Table C-1. *(continued)*

Spurious Manifestation	Cause	Diagnostic Clue or Confirmation
Decreased WBC	(a) Cold-induced clumping (cold agglutinins, cryofibrinogenemia) (b) Leukocyte fragility due to immunosuppressive and antineoplastic drugs (c) Overfilled blood tubes causing inadequate mixing (d) Monoclonal gammopathies	(a) Clumped WBCs on blood smear; abnormal WBC histogram. Corrected by count at 37°C (b) Corrected by manual count (c) Associated low platelet count, high Hb and Hct (d) Protein electrophoresis
High reticulocyte count	Massive *Plasmodium* infection	*Plasmodium* seen on blood smear
Increased hemoglobin	(a) Turbidity due to high WBC (b) Markedly increased serum bilirubin	(a) Normal manual WBC and blood smear (b) Interference with Hb determination may occur at >30 mg/dL of bilirubin; MCHC and MCH may also be increased
Increased MCH and MCHC; Hb may be disproportionately high	Hyperlipidemia interferes with Hb determination, especially with triglycerides >1,000 mg/dL	Normal count after replacing patient plasma with diluent; abnormal WBC histograms
Increased RBC count, decreased WBC and platelet counts	Inadequate mixing of blood tube before testing	Compare counts on properly and improperly prepared specimens
Increased MCV	(a) Increased blood glucose (600–2,000 mg/dL) (b) Delayed testing for 24—48 hrs stored at 25°C (c) Fibrin strands	(a) Repeat CBC when glucose is normal (b) Compare with prompt testing or storage at 5°C (c) Repeat CBC using properly drawn specimen; fibrin strands may be seen on blood smear; falsely increased WBC and decreased platelet counts may be present with normal RBC count and histogram
Increased MCV with decreased MCHC	(d) Increased WBC >50,000/µL	(d) Manual WBC
Increased MCV, anisocytosis	(e) Reticulocytosis >50% Cold agglutination of RBCs	(e) Reticulocyte count Perform CBC at 37°C
Decreased automated RBC count, increased MCV, decreased Hct	Cold agglutination of RBCs	Perform CBC at 37°C
Decreased RBC, WBC, platelet counts	Collection through catheter, diluting blood	Compare with correctly collected specimen

Decreased ESR	(a) Polycythemia (b) Abnormal RBC shapes (c) Very high WBC (d) Hypofibrinogenemia
Decreased serum glucose	In vitro utilization of glucose by WBCs, platelets, or organisms
	(a) Hct, RBC count (b) Smear for sickle cells, spherocytes, acanthocytes (c) WBC (d) Evidence of DIC, massive hepatic necrosis
	Increased number of cells (e.g., leukemic WBCs, nucleated RBCs, reticulocytes) or organisms (e.g., trypanosomiasis)[d]
Decreased serum sodium	(a) Specimen drawn distal to IV infusion of hypotonic fluid (b) Hyperlipidemia interferes with flame photometry but not with ion-specific electrode methods.[a] (c) Hyperproteinemia[b] (d) Hyperglycemia[c]	(a) Measure glucose in same specimen; draw repeat specimen from another site (b) Repeat analysis with ion-specific electrode instrument
Increased serum sodium	Umbilical blood sample drawn through catheter coated with cationic benzalkonium chloride, which causes increased sodium and potassium with some ionselective electrodes	Serum potassium also increased. Draw blood from other sites or without catheter or do not use ion-selective electrode methodology
Decreased serum potassium	Gross lipemia [see "Decreased serum sodium" (a)]	
Increased serum potassium	(a) Hemolytic anemia (b) In vitro cell lysis of markedly increased platelets or WBCs	(a) Evidence of hemolytic process (b) Very high WBC or platelet count (e.g., >1 million/μL; serum level higher than simultaneously drawn plasma potassium level) (c) Compare with specimen drawn without tourniquet (d) Repeat analysis of appropriately collected specimen
	(c) Tight or prolonged tourniquet use (d) In vitro lysis of RBCs due to improper specimen collection or handling	
	(e) Umbilical blood sample drawn through catheter coated with cationic benzalkonium chloride, which causes increased sodium and potassium with some ion-selective electrodes	(e) Serum sodium also increased. Draw blood from other sites or without catheter or do not use ion-selective electrode methodology.

(continued)

Table C-1. *(continued)*

Spurious Manifestation	Cause	Diagnostic Clue or Confirmation
Increased serum chloride, negative anion gap	Hyperlipidemia causes light scattering in colorimetric assay	Hyponatremia also present; remove lipid before assay
Increased serum chloride	Bromide in serum	Test for serum bromide
Decreased serum chloride	Same as for "Decreased serum sodium"	
Increased serum phosphate	Multiple myeloma	Evidence of multiple myeloma. May have normal serum calcium and renal function; normal value if serum is first deproteinized
Increased or decreased serum calcium	Increased or decreased serum albumin[e]	Increased or decreased serum albumin or total protein
Decreased blood CO_2 and bicarbonate, increased anion gap	(a) Dilutional effect of sodium heparin solution in blood sample	(a) Different blood collection system
	(b) Loss of CO_2 by evaporation from sampling curvette may be up to 8.8 in 2 hrs	(b) Prompt analysis of simultaneously drawn samples
	(c) Underfilling of blood collection tubes	(c) Repeat with properly filled tubes
Decreased serum creatinine	Extreme hyperbilirubinemia interferes with creatinine measurement on certain instruments	Use different instrument (e.g., Astra-8 instead of Dupont ACA or Abbot-VP). BUN not affected
Increased serum creatinine	Acetoacetate as in diabetic ketoaacidosis interferes with Jaffé method	BUN not affected
Increased PO_2	Exposure of blood to air bubbles, especially with microsampling	Repeat after proper collection and transport
Hypoxemia shown by pulse oximetry	Very increased WBCs (500,000 μL) or platelets, which utilize oxygen	Higher oxygen saturation shown by pulse oximetry
Spurious O_2 and CO_2 shown by pulse oximetry	Abnormal hemoglobins (carboxyhemoglobin, methemoglobin); TV administration of methylene blue	Arterial blood gases; demonstrate abnormal hemoglobins

Increased serum TSH, CEA, hCG, or CA-125	Patient's sera contains antimouse antibodies (or those of other animal such as rabbit) used in test kit	No other evidence of causative disease (e.g., hypothyroidism). Adding mouse serum or IgG produces normal TSH results.
Increased antibody titer for infectious agents	Treatment with IV immunoglobulins	Measure titers on suspected lots of IgG and on patient's serum obtained before treatment
Positive infectious mononucleosis rapid slide test	Very high levels of horse RBC agglutinins in patient sera	Minimal absorption with test guinea pig kidney or beef RBC suspensions
Stool-positive guaiac test for blood	Toilet sanitizers present in toilet bowl	Compare with test of stool not collected from toilet bowl
Stool-negative test for blood	Blood leached from fecal surface into water	Compare with test of blood not collected from toilet bowl
Decreased urine creatinine	Cotton or rayon sponges in diapers or diaper material selectively absorb creatinine	Use alternate urine collection methods

[a] DIC, disseminated intravascular coagulation; CEA, carcinoembryonic antigen; hCG, human chorionic gonadotropin.
[b] Same mechanism as for hyperlipidemia and cationic effect of paraproteins, which displace sodium, decreasing sodium 0.7 mEq/L for each 1 g/dL of monoclonal protein.
[c] Osmotic effect of hyperglycemia decreases sodium 1.6 mEq/L for each 100-mg/dL increase in serum glucose.
[d] Even with a normal blood count, glucose decreases at a rate of 7 mg/dL hour at room temperatur if blood cells are not separated from serum.
[e] 0.8 mg of calcium is bound to 1.0 g of albumin in serum, allowing for correction of serum calcium values. Binding to globulin only affects toal calcium if globulin is >6 g/dL. Serum albumin and total protein should always be measured simultaneously with calcium determinations.

Source: Data from Yucel D, Dalv K. Effect of in vitro hemolysis on 25 common biochemical test. *Clin Chem* 1992;38;575. Kroll MH, Elin RJ. Interference with clinical laboratory analysis. *Clin Chem* 1994;40:1990.

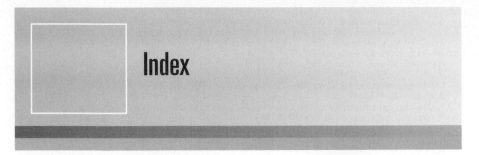

Index

Note: Page numbers followed by *b* indicate boxes; *f* indicate figures; page numbers followed by *t* indicate tables.

INDEX